Tresch and Aronow's Cardiovascular Disease in Older Adults

The seventh edition of *Tresch and Aronow's Cardiovascular Disease in Older Adults* thoroughly updates the material in the sixth edition by renowned experts in geriatric cardiology. New features include a short list of key points at the start of each chapter to help guide the reader; a new chapter on cardio-oncology in older adults, a topic of increasing importance; and new sections on geroscience, lifestyle factors in cardiovascular disease prevention, and cardiac amyloidosis added to existing chapters. These new features will enhance the value and relevance of this book as the definitive text in this growing field.

Key features:

- Provides a comprehensive and accessible overview of the epidemiology, pathophysiology, and treatment of cardiovascular disorders in older patients
- Useful for adult cardiologists, primary care providers, geriatricians, cardiac nurses, nurse practitioners, physician assistants, cardiac rehabilitation teams, physical and occupational therapists, and other practitioners working with older patients

Tresch and Aronow's Cardiovascular Disease in Older Adults

Seventh Edition

Edited by
Wilbert S. Aronow
Professor of Medicine and Director of Cardiology Research
Westchester Medical Center/New York Medical College
Jerome L. Fleg
Division of Cardiovascular Sciences, National Heart, Lung, and Blood Institute, National Institutes of Health
Michael W. Rich
Professor of Medicine
Washington University School of Medicine

CRC Press
Taylor & Francis Group
Boca Raton London New York

CRC Press is an imprint of the
Taylor & Francis Group, an **informa** business

Designed cover image: Shutterstock Image Id: 2291576643

Seventh edition published 2026
by CRC Press
2385 NW Executive Center Drive, Suite 320, Boca Raton FL 33431

and by CRC Press
4 Park Square, Milton Park, Abingdon, Oxon, OX14 4RN
CRC Press is an imprint of Taylor & Francis Group, LLC

Sixth edition published by CRC Press 2020

ISBN: 978-1-032-94095-3 (hbk)
ISBN: 978-1-032-94096-0 (pbk)
ISBN: 978-1-003-56893-3 (ebk)

DOI: 10.1201/9781003568933

Typeset in Minion Pro
by Deanta Global Publishing Services, Chennai, India

Contents

Preface

We are in the midst of a dramatic increase in the number of older adults in the United States and around the world. Since 2010, the total population of the US has increased by about 9.5%, while the number of Americans 65 years of age or older has increased by 57.1%, the number 75 years or older has increased by 64.2%, the number 85 years or older has increased by 94.7%, and the number of centenarians has doubled. This marked increase in the number of older adults over the past 15 years has set the stage for an exponential growth of the very old population in the next 25 years. Thus, current projections suggest that the total US population will increase by a modest 6.7% over the next quarter century, but the over 85 population will increase by 147% and the number of centenarians will more than triple—from 107,000 in 2025 to about 357,000 in 2050.[1] On a global scale, the number of people age 65 or older is expected to double in the next 25 years, while the number over 75 and over 85 are both expected to triple.

A critical implication of population aging for global health is that there will be a concomitant marked increase in the incidence and prevalence of cardiovascular disease (CVD) for the simple reason that age is the single strongest risk factor for heart disease, vascular disease, and stroke. And while it is widely recognized that CVD is the leading cause of death in the US and most developed countries, it is less well appreciated that more than half of all CVD deaths occur in the 8% of the population 75 years of age or older! Indeed, in the US, cancer is the leading cause of death in adults up to age 75, whereas CVD becomes the dominant cause after age 75.

But the high prevalence of CVD in older individuals also implies that practitioners—including general practitioners, internists, cardiologists, geriatricians, physician assistants, nurse practitioners, and others—have considerable experience caring for older patients with heart and vascular disease. Why, then, do we need a textbook dedicated to the diagnosis and treatment of CVD in older adults? First, and most important, CVD in older adults almost always occurs in the context of multiple other chronic conditions, both cardiac and noncardiac, as a result of which management must be individualized and nuanced. Second, geriatric syndromes, such as cognitive impairment, frailty, and polypharmacy, are also highly prevalent, and the implications of these conditions for prognosis and response to therapy must also be taken into consideration in designing a management plan. Third, there is considerable variability among older adults with respect to life expectancy, goals of care, and health care preferences, factors that must remain at the forefront of medical decision-making. Fourth, older individuals, especially those of very advanced age, those with multiple comorbidities, and nursing home residents, have been markedly underrepresented in clinical trials, so that the evidence base to guide care in these patients is fundamentally deficient. In sum, management of older adults with CVD is inevitably a complex undertaking, and there is thus a compelling need for authoritative guidance by experts in the field.

As with prior editions of this text, the primary objective of the present volume is to provide an up-to-date and in-depth, yet clinically relevant and "readable" overview of the epidemiology, pathophysiology, evaluation, and treatment of cardiovascular disorders in older adults. To the extent possible, clinical recommendations are "evidence based," but it is also acknowledged that existing data are often very limited, and that careful consideration of each patient's unique clinical and psychosocial circumstances, medical and nonmedical needs, and personal preferences is required in designing an individualized care plan. Indeed, it is perhaps in the compassionate management of these challenging patients where the "art of medicine" most clearly flourishes.

This edition appears 7 years after the sixth edition, which was published in 2019. During the intervening period, an extensive body of new research relevant to the diagnosis and treatment of cardiovascular disorders in older adults has been published. In addition to an expanding literature derived from population-based observational studies, an increasing number of clinical trials focusing on older adults have been undertaken, and practice guidelines are increasingly providing explicit commentary on the diagnosis and management of older patients. In the current edition, we have thoroughly revised and updated all chapters, while at the same time shortening the text and deleting outdated references. We have also eliminated three chapters, combined two chapters from the sixth edition (percutaneous coronary intervention and coronary bypass surgery), and added a new chapter on cancer and cardiovascular disease in older adults. Finally, we have updated the book title from *Cardiovascular Disease in the Elderly* to *Cardiovascular Disease in Older Adults*.

We would like to thank all of the contributors for their outstanding work. We also wish to express our gratitude to Shivangi Pramanik and Kanchi Shridhar at Taylor & Francis Group for their dedication and support in bringing the seventh edition to fruition. Finally, we want to thank you, the reader, for your commitment to providing the best possible care for your older patients with cardiovascular disease. We hope you will find this volume to be a valuable resource as you strive to help your older patients enjoy both longer and fuller lives. We welcome any comments you may have.

Michael W. Rich, MD, FACC, AGSF
Wilbert S. Aronow, MD, FACC, FAHA
Jerome L. Fleg, MD, FACC, FAHA

NOTE

1 US Census Bureau. 2023 National Population Projections Tables. Available at: https://www.census.gov/data/tables/2023/demo/popproj/2023-summary-tables.html (accessed July 19, 2025).

Editors

Wilbert S. Aronow, MD, is Professor of Medicine and Director of Cardiology Research at Westchester Medical Center and New York Medical College in Valhalla, NY, USA. Dr. Aronow received his MD degree from Harvard Medical School. He has edited 24 books and is an author of 1,956 papers, 225 book chapters in 118 books, 993 commentaries, 50 Letters to the Editor, and 1,230 abstracts. Dr. Aronow is a Fellow of the ACC, AHA, ACP, ACCP, ASPC, AGS, and GSA. He has been a member of 185 editorial boards of medical journals. He has received 90 awards. Dr. Aronow has been a member of 4 national guidelines committees including being an author of the 2010 AMDA guidelines for heart failure, a co-chair and first author of the 2011 ACC/AHA expert consensus document on hypertension in the elderly, an author of the 2015 AHA/ACC/ASH scientific statement on treatment of hypertension in patients with coronary artery disease, and an author of the 2017 ACC/AHA guidelines for the management of patients with hypertension. He has been a committee member of numerous professional societies and a consultant to many government agencies. Dr. Aronow has mentored more than 1,200 physicians and medical students for papers listed on PubMed. He is on the lists of best scientists in medicine in the United States and in the world.

Jerome L. Fleg, MD, FACC, FAHA, FAPS, FHFSA, is a Medical Officer in the Division of Cardiovascular Sciences at the National Heart, Lung, and Blood Institute in Bethesda, Maryland. Dr. Fleg received his MD from the University of Cincinnati and trained in internal medicine and cardiovascular disease at Washington University in St. Louis. He has published over 400 peer-reviewed journal articles, book chapters, and reviews related to cardiovascular aging and disease. He serves on multiple journal editorial boards and is an associate editor for the *Journal of Cardiopulmonary Rehabilitation and Prevention.*

Michael W. Rich, MD, FACC, AGSF, is Professor of Medicine, Washington University School of Medicine; and Director, Cardiac Rapid Evaluation Unit, Barnes-Jewish Hospital, St. Louis, Missouri. Dr. Rich received his MD from the University of Illinois College of Medicine, Chicago. He has published over 300 journal articles and more than 90 books and book chapters. Dr. Rich is an associate editor for the *American Journal of Medicine* and the *Journal of the American Geriatrics Society.*

Contributors

Nathaniel Abittan
Departments of Cardiology and Medicine
Westchester Medical Center and New York Medical College
Valhalla, New York

Hasan Ahmad
Departments of Cardiology and Medicine
Westchester Medical Center and New York Medical College
Valhalla, New York

Ali Ahmed
Veterans Affairs Medical Center
and
George Washington University
and
Georgetown University
Washington, DC

Mahmoud Samy Ahmed
Departments of Cardiology and Medicine
Westchester Medical Center and New York Medical College
Valhalla, New York

Wilbert S. Aronow
Departments of Cardiology and Medicine
Westchester Medical Center and New York Medical College
Valhalla, New York

Patrick Berchie
Department of Medicine
Piedmont Healthcare
Athens, Georgia

Jeanna D. Blitz
Wake Forest University
Winston-Salem, North Carolina

Khalifa Bshesh
Johns Hopkins School of Medicine
Baltimore, Maryland

Howard A. Cooper
Departments of Cardiology and Medicine
Westchester Medical Center and New York Medical College
Valhalla, New York

Abdulla A. Damluji
Cardiovascular Center on Aging
Department of Cardiovascular Medicine
Cleveland Clinic Foundation
Cleveland, Ohio

Subrat K. Das
Departments of Cardiology and Medicine
Westchester Medical Center and New York Medical College
Valhalla, New York

Efrat Dotan
University of Pennsylvania
Philadelphia, Pennsylvania

Samuel C. Durso
Johns Hopkins University
Baltimore, Maryland

Gregory A. Fishbein
University of California, Los Angeles
Los Angeles, California

Michael C. Fishbein
University of California, Los Angeles
Los Angeles, California

Jerome L. Fleg
Division of Cardiovascular Sciences
National Heart, Lung, and Blood Institute
Bethesda, Maryland

Daniel Forman
Department of Medicine (Cardiology and Geriatrics)
University of Pittsburgh
and
Pittsburgh Geriatrics, Research, Education and Clinical Center (GRECC)
VA Pittsburgh Healthcare System
Pittsburgh, Pennsylvania

William H. Frishman
Departments of Cardiology and Medicine
Westchester Medical Center and New York Medical College
Valhalla, New York

Parag Goyal
Program for the Care and Study of the Aging Heart
Department of Medicine
Weill Cornell Medicine
New York City, New York

Eman Hamad
Temple University
Philadelphia, Pennsylvania

Thomas Horton
HCA Memorial Health University Medical Center
Mercer University School of Medicine
Macon, Georgia

Hsinhui Hua
University of Michigan
Ann Arbor, Michigan

Dina Ioffe
Temple University
Philadelphia, Pennsylvania

Sei Iwai
Departments of Cardiology and Medicine
Westchester Medical Center and New York Medical College
Valhalla, New York

Jason T. Jacobson
Departments of Cardiology and Medicine
Westchester Medical Center and New York Medical College
Valhalla, New York

Sherrie Khadanga
Division of Cardiology
Department of Internal Medicine
University of Vermont Medical Center
Burlington, Vermont

Dae Hyun Kim
Beth Israel Deaconess Medical Center
Harvard Medical School
Boston, Massachusetts

Jennifer S. Lawton
Johns Hopkins University School of Medicine
Baltimore, Maryland

Michael Liu
Department of Cardiovascular Diseases
Mayo Clinic
Phoenix, Arizona

Emma M. Loebel
Department of Neurology
Icahn School of Medicine at Mount Sinai
New York City, New York

Aaquib H. Malik
Departments of Cardiology and Medicine
Westchester Medical Center and New York Medical College
Valhalla, New York

Seth S. Martin
Johns Hopkins School of Medicine
Baltimore, Maryland

Giulia Matteucci
Department of Geriatrics
University of Florence and Careggi University Hospital
Florence, Italy

Lona Mody
University of Michigan
Ann Arbor, Michigan

Srihari S. Naidu
Departments of Cardiology and Medicine
Westchester Medical Center and New York Medical College
Valhalla, New York

Michael G. Nanna
Yale University School of Medicine
New Haven, Connecticut

Christine Y. Nguyen
Beth Israel Deaconess Medical Center
Harvard Medical School
Boston, Massachusetts

Sade Solola Nussbaum
Departments of Cardiology and Medicine
Westchester Medical Center and New York Medical College
Valhalla, New York

Esther S. Pak
Philadelphia Corporal Michael J. Crescenz VA Medical Center
Hospital of the University of Pennsylvania
Philadelphia, Pennsylvania

Haris Patail
Departments of Cardiology and Medicine
Westchester Medical Center and New York Medical College
Valhalla, New York

Akshay Pendyal
Cardiovascular Medicine Section
Duke University School of Medicine
Durham, North Carolina

Rylie Pietrowicz
Temple University
Philadelphia, Pennsylvania

Yasser Radwan
Departments of Cardiology and Medicine
Westchester Medical Center and New York Medical College
Valhalla, New York

Martina Rafanelli
Department of Geriatrics
University of Florence and Careggi University Hospital
Florence, Italy

Michael W. Rich
Washington University School of Medicine
and
Cardiac Rapid Evaluation Unit
Barnes-Jewish Hospital
St. Louis, Missouri

Atsuko Seki
Tokyo Women's Medical University Hospital
Tokyo, Japan

Win-Kuang Shen
Department of Cardiovascular Diseases
Mayo Clinic
Phoenix, Arizona

Laura K. Stein
Department of Neurology
Icahn School of Medicine at Mount Sinai
New York City, New York

Joshua M. Stolker
Mercy Medical Group
Washington, Missouri
and
St. Louis University
St. Louis, Missouri

Kevin S. Tang
Mary and Steve Wen Cardiovascular Division
University of California, Irvine
Irvine, California

Andrea Ungar
Department of Geriatrics
University of Florence and Careggi University Hospital
Florence, Italy

Bharathi Upadhya
Cardiovascular Medicine Section
Duke University School of Medicine
Durham, North Carolina

Nathan D. Wong
Division of Cardiology
University of California, Irvine
Irvine, California

1

Cardiovascular changes with aging

JEROME L. FLEG

Key points

- Aging is accompanied by multiple cardiovascular changes, even in apparently healthy adults. Although many of these cardiovascular aging changes are considered "normative," they may lower the threshold for development of cardiovascular disease.
- Thickening and stiffening of the large arteries cause systolic blood pressure to rise with age, while diastolic blood pressure generally declines after the sixth decade.
- In the left ventricle, modest concentric wall thickening occurs due to cellular hypertrophy, but cavity size does not change.
- Although left ventricular systolic function is preserved across the age span, the early diastolic filling rate declines 30%–50% between the third and ninth decades. However, an age-associated increase in late diastolic filling preserves end-diastolic volume.
- Aerobic exercise capacity declines approximately 10% per decade in cross-sectional studies; in longitudinal studies, this decline is accelerated in the elderly. Reductions in peak heart rate and peripheral oxygen utilization, but not stroke volume, mediate the age-associated decline in aerobic capacity.
- Deficits in both cardiac β-adrenergic receptor density and in the efficiency of postsynaptic β-adrenergic signaling contribute significantly to the reduced cardiovascular performance during exercise in older adults.
- Conduction disorders, including sinus node and atrioventricular node dysfunction and bundle branch blocks, and both supraventricular and ventricular arrhythmias become more common with age. The prognostic significance of any arrhythmia or conduction disturbance depends primarily on the presence and severity of associated heart disease.

DOI: 10.1201/9781003568933-1

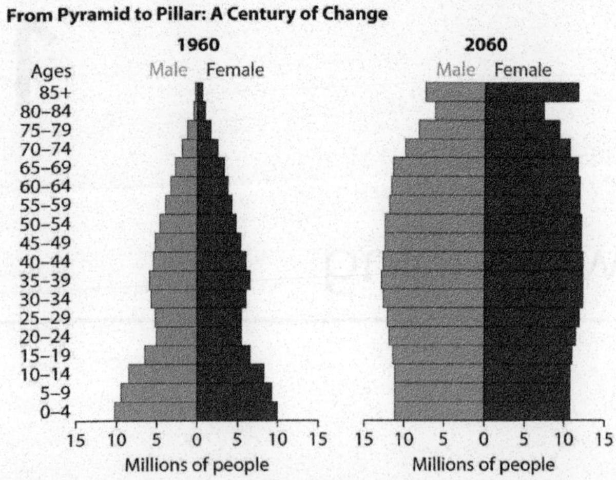

Figure 1.1 Projected growth of the US population between 1960 and 2060, stratified by age group. (From United States Bureau of the Census, www.census.gov/population/www/estimates/popest.html, March 13, 2018.)

INTRODUCTION

By 2030, one in six people, 1.4 billion, in the world will be aged 60 years or older. By 2050, the world's population of people aged 60 years and older will increase to 2.1 billion. Even more striking, the number of persons aged 80 years or older is expected to triple between 2020 and 2050 to 426 million. Although this shift in distribution of the world's population toward older ages, i.e., population aging, began in high-income countries, it is now low- and middle-income countries that are experiencing the greatest change. By 2050, an estimated two thirds of the world's population over 60 years will live in low- and middle-income countries. The fastest-growing age group, comprising those 85 years or older, has more than quadrupled since 1960 and will exceed 20 million in the United States by 2060 (Figure 1.1) (1).

Given the dramatic increase in both the prevalence and incidence of cardiovascular (CV) disease that occur with advancing age, this "graying" of the population has created a huge number of older adults requiring treatment. However, aging per se need not be accompanied by CV disease. This chapter will set the stage for those that follow by delineating the changes in the CV system that occur during the aging process in the absence of detectable CV disease. This is a challenging task, given the many factors that blur their separation. Nonetheless, it is important to define normal CV structure and function in older adults to facilitate the accurate diagnosis of CV disease in this rapidly growing segment of society.

Another important goal of this chapter will be to demonstrate how "normative" aging changes in the CV system may themselves predispose to the development of CV disease. The enhanced age-associated CV risk points to important interactions between mechanisms that underlie aging and those that underlie CV diseases. These interactions are complex and involve both mechanisms of aging plus multiple defined and undefined risk factors. However, quantitative information on age-associated alterations in CV structure and function is essential to define and target the specific characteristics of CV aging that render it such a major risk factor. Such information is also required to differentiate between the limitations of an elderly person that are within expected normal limits versus those that indicate CV disease.

METHODOLOGICAL ISSUES

Numerous methodological issues must be addressed in defining "normal" aging. Because the population sample from which norms are derived will strongly influence the results obtained, it should be representative of the general population. Thus, neither a seniors running club nor nursing home residents would provide appropriate normal values for maximal exercise capacity that could be applied to the majority of older adults. In addition, the degree of screening used to define "normal" can profoundly influence the results. In clinically healthy older adults, a resting electrocardiogram (ECG), echocardiogram, or exercise perfusion imaging study will often identify silent CV disease, especially coronary artery disease (CAD). If multiple screening tests are used, only a small proportion of the older population may qualify as normal, limiting the applicability of findings to the majority of older adults. Furthermore, the inclusion limits chosen for body fatness, blood pressure, smoking status, and other constitutional or lifestyle variables will significantly influence the normal range for CV variables. For example, if a systolic blood pressure of ≥130 mmHg is considered hypertension as per current guidelines, and if hypertension is considered a disease, then individuals with a systolic pressure between 130 and 140 mmHg, who were previously considered normotensive, are now identified as having CV disease. Many studies have shown that individuals who show even modest elevations in systolic and pulse pressures are more likely to develop overt CV disease or die from it.

Additional methodological issues can affect the definitions of normal aging. Cross-sectional studies, which study individuals across a wide age range at a single time point, may underestimate the magnitude of age-associated changes because older normal persons included in such studies represent "survival of the healthiest." True age-induced changes are better estimated by longitudinal studies, in which individuals are examined serially over time. A reality of aging research, however, is that most data are derived from cross-sectional studies because they are easier to perform. Even longitudinal studies have their limitations—changes in methodology or measurement drift over time and development of disease in previously healthy persons. Finally, secular trends such as the downward drift in serum cholesterol or increasing obesity of Americans can influence age-related longitudinal changes.

In this chapter, emphasis will be given to data obtained from community-dwelling persons screened for the absence of clinical, and in some cases subclinical, CV disease as well as major systemic disorders. A substantial portion of the data presented derives from studies over the past several decades in community-based volunteers from the Baltimore Longitudinal Study of Aging (BLSA).

ARTERIAL CHANGES: THE ROOT CAUSE OF UNSUCCESSFUL AGING

Intimal medial thickening

Changes with age in the arterial tree of apparently healthy individuals likely have relevance to the exponential increase in CV disease with aging. Cross-sectional studies in humans have found that wall thickening and dilatation are prominent structural changes that occur within large elastic arteries over time (2). Postmortem studies indicate that aortic wall thickening with aging consists mainly of intimal thickening, even in populations with a low incidence of atherosclerosis (3). Noninvasive measurements from several epidemiological studies indicate that the carotid wall intimal–medial (IM) thickness increases nearly threefold between 20 and 90 years of age, which also was seen in BLSA participants rigorously screened to exclude carotid or coronary arterial disease (Figure 1.2a).

Some researchers believe that the age-associated increase in IM thickness in humans represents an early stage of atherosclerosis (4). Indeed, excessive IM thickening at a given age predicts increased risk of silent CAD (4). Because silent CAD often progresses to clinical CAD, it is not surprising that increased IM thickness predicts future clinical CV disease. Multiple epidemiological studies of individuals not initially screened to exclude occult CV disease have shown that increased carotid artery IM thickness on ultrasound is an independent predictor of future CV events. Note in Figure 1.2b that the degree of risk varies with the degree of arterial thickening and that the risk gradation among quintiles of IM thickening is nonlinear, with the greatest risk occurring in the upper quintile (5). Thus, older adults in the upper quintile of IM thickness may be considered to have aged "unsuccessfully" or to have "subclinical" arterial disease. The potency of IM thickness as a risk factor in older individuals equals or exceeds that of most traditional risk factors.

The common finding of age-associated IM thickening in the absence of atherosclerosis, both in laboratory animals and in humans (3), suggests that such excessive IM thickening is not necessarily "early" atherosclerosis but rather "subclinical CV disease" due to arterial aging. Interpreted in this way, the increase in IM thickness with age is analogous to the intimal hyperplasia that develops in aortocoronary saphenous vein grafts, which is independent of atherosclerosis but predisposes to its later

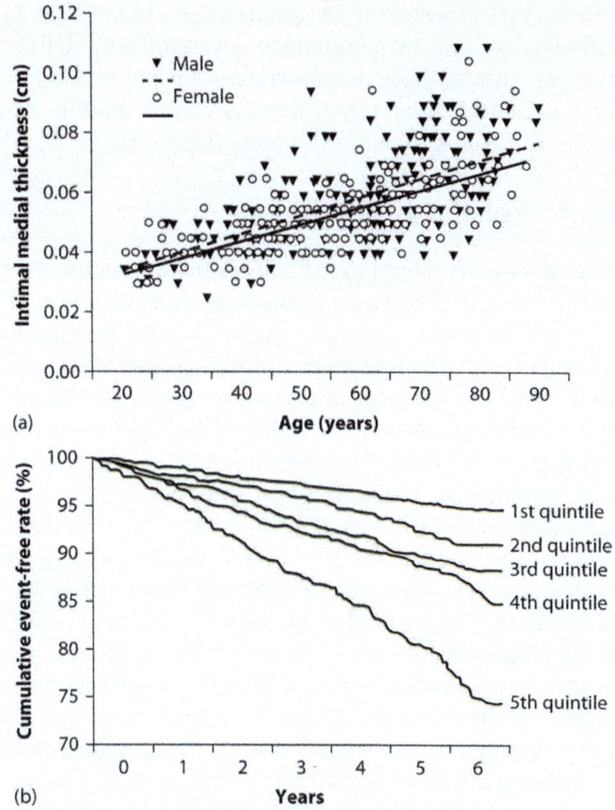

Figure 1.2 (a) The common carotid intimal–medial thickness in healthy Baltimore Longitudinal Study of Aging (BLSA) volunteers as a function of age. (b) Common carotid intimal–medial thickness predicts future cardiovascular events in the Cardiovascular Health Study. ([a] From Nagai Y et al., *Circulation*, 98, 1504–1509, 1998. [b] From O'Leary DH et al., *N Engl J Med*, 340, 14–22, 1999.)

development (6). Age-associated endothelial dysfunction, arterial stiffening, and arterial pulse pressure widening can also be interpreted similarly. Combinations of these processes occurring to varying degrees determine the overall vascular aging profile of a given individual (i.e., the degree of "unsuccessful" vascular aging). Animal data suggest that oxidative stress, inflammation, and defective cellular signaling underlie these adverse processes, initiating a vicious cycle between vascular remodeling and increasing arterial stiffness and blood pressure.

Additional risk factors (e.g., hypertension, smoking, dyslipidemia, diabetes, diet, or as-yet-unidentified genetic factors) are thought to interact with arterial aging to activate a preexisting atherosclerotic plaque. According to this view, atherosclerosis that increases with aging is not a specific disease, but an interaction between atherosclerotic plaque and intrinsic features related to vascular aging modulated by atherosclerotic risk factors. Evidence supporting this view derives from studies in which an atherogenic diet caused markedly more severe atherosclerotic lesions in older than younger rabbits and nonhuman primates despite similar elevations of serum lipids (7, 8). However, studies in populations with clinically defined vascular disease have demonstrated that pharmacological and lifestyle (diet, physical activity) interventions can retard the progression of IM thickening (9–10).

Endothelial dysfunction

The endothelial monolayer that lines the luminal surface of the vascular tree plays a pivotal role in regulating multiple arterial properties, including vessel tone, permeability, response to inflammation, and angiogenesis. Several of these functions undergo important age-associated alterations. Endothelium-derived mediators such as nitric oxide (NO) and endothelin-1 are determinants of arterial tone and compliance, suggesting that endothelial cells may modulate arterial stiffness. Brachial arterial flow-mediated dilation, mediated in large part by NO, declines with age in both sexes, even in the absence of other CV risk factors (11). A decline of ~75% in this flow-mediated vasodilation occurs in men between the ages of 40 and 70 years. This decline begins approximately a decade later in women, perhaps because of the protective effect of estrogen, but is nearly 2.5 times as steep compared with men (11). The impairment of endothelial-mediated vasodilatation with aging in humans can be partially reversed by L-arginine administration, suggesting that NO production becomes reduced with aging (12). Plasma levels of asymmetric dimethyl arginine, which reduces NO synthase (NOS) activity, also increase with age in humans (12). Age-associated changes in endothelial cell integrity, shape, and surface characteristics affect the cell's physical and chemical barrier, increasing endothelial permeability, leading to aberrant macromolecular transport (13). In contrast to endothelium-mediated vasodilation, the vasodilator response to sublingual nitroglycerin is unrelated to age (11).

Several CV risk factors and disorders are associated with endothelial dysfunction, including hypertension, hypercholesterolemia, insulin resistance, cigarette smoking, CAD, and heart failure. Furthermore, impaired endothelial vasoreactivity, in both the coronary and peripheral arterial beds, is an independent predictor of future CV events (14). Hypertensive individuals exhibit endothelial dysfunction, and the mechanisms underlying their endothelial dysfunction are similar to those that occur with normotensive aging, albeit they appear at an earlier age (15). The normotensive offspring of hypertensives also exhibit endothelial dysfunction (16), suggesting that endothelial dysfunction may precede the development of clinical hypertension. Age-associated endothelial dysfunction, arterial stiffening, and IM thickening are risk factors for arterial diseases, even after accounting for other risk factors, such as arterial pressure, plasma lipids, and smoking. The interaction between arterial wall stiffening and CV diseases may set in motion a vicious cycle. In this cycle, alterations in the mechanical properties of the vessel wall contribute to endothelial cell dysfunction and, ultimately, to arterial stiffening.

Arterial stiffness and compliance

The increase in arterial wall thickening and reduction in endothelial function with advancing age are accompanied by an increase in arterial stiffening and a reduction in compliance. Age-associated structural changes in the arterial media that increase vascular stiffness include increased collagen content, covalent cross-linking of the collagen, reduced elastin content, elastin fracture, and calcification (17). In addition, there is a substantial increase in angiotensin II levels and augmented angiotensin II signaling in aged arterial walls, which may play a pivotal role in arterial aging, given the potent pressor and mitogenic effects of angiotensin II.

Pulse wave velocity

Each systolic contraction of the ventricle generates a pressure wave that propagates centrifugally down the arterial tree, slightly preceding the luminal flow wave generated during systole. The propagation velocity of this wave is proportional to the stiffness of the arterial wall. The velocity of the pulse wave in vivo is determined not only by the intrinsic stress–strain relationship (stiffness) of the vascular wall but also by the smooth muscle tone, which is reflected by the mean arterial pressure.

Noninvasive measures of the velocity of this pulse wave allow for large-scale epidemiological studies to examine its determinants and prognostic importance. In both rigorously screened normal subjects (18) and populations with varying prevalence of CV disease (19), a significant age-associated increase in pulse wave velocity (PWV) has been observed in men and women (Figure 1.3a). In contrast to central arteries, the stiffness of muscular arteries does not increase with advancing age (20). Thus, the manifestations of arterial aging may vary among the different vascular beds, reflecting differences in the structural compositions of the arteries and, possibly, differences in the age-associated signaling cascades that modulate the arterial properties, or differences in the response to these signals across the arterial tree.

Increased PWV has traditionally been linked to structural alterations in the vascular media, such as those observed with aging. Prominent age-associated increases in PWV have been demonstrated in populations with little or no atherosclerosis, again indicating that these vascular parameters are not necessarily indicative of atherosclerosis (21). However, the data emerging from epidemiological studies indicate that increased large vessel stiffening also occurs in the context of atherosclerosis (22), metabolic syndrome (23), and diabetes (24). Thus, altered mechanical properties of the vessel wall

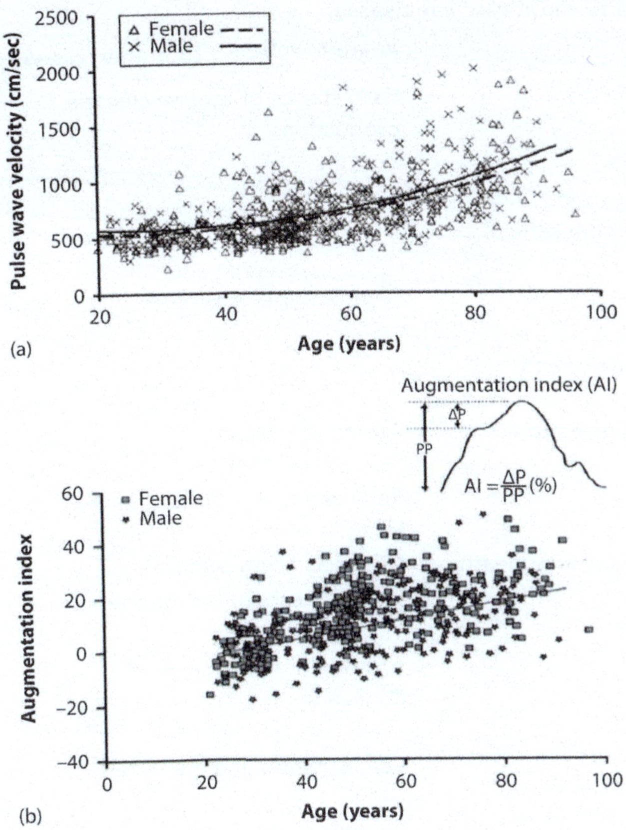

Figure 1.3 Scatter plots of aortofemoral pulse wave velocity (a), and carotid artery augmentation index (b) as a function of age in healthy non-endurance-trained Baltimore Longitudinal Study of Aging (BLSA) volunteers. A similar age-associated increase in both measures of arterial stiffness was seen in men and women. (From Vaitkevicius PV et al., *Circulation*, 88, 1456–1462, 1993.)

facilitate the development of atherosclerosis, which in turn increases arterial stiffness via endothelial cell dysfunction and other mechanisms.

Reflected pulse waves

In addition to the forward pulse wave, each cardiac cycle generates a reflected wave, originating at areas of arterial impedance mismatch, which travels back up the arterial tree toward the central aorta, altering the arterial pressure waveform. This reflected wave can be noninvasively assessed from recordings of the carotid (18) or radial (25) arterial pulse waveforms using applanation tonometry and high-fidelity micromanometer probes. Dividing the late systolic augmentation of the arterial pulse wave by the distance from the peak to the trough of the arterial waveform (corresponding to the pulse pressure) yields the augmentation index, representing the degree of late systolic pressure increase (24). The augmentation index, like the PWV, increases with age (Figure 1.3b) (17, 18).

The velocity of the reflected flow wave is proportional to the stiffness of the arterial wall. Thus, in young individuals whose vascular wall is compliant, the reflected wave does not reach the large elastic arteries until diastole. With advancing age and increasing arterial stiffening, the velocity of the reflected wave increases, and the wave reaches the central circulation earlier in the cardiac cycle, during systole. The pressure pulse augmentation provided by the early return of the reflected wave is an added load against which the aged ventricle must contract. Furthermore, the diastolic pressure augmentation seen in compliant vessels, caused by the late return of the reflected waves, is lost in the elderly, decreasing diastolic blood pressure; this decrease in diastolic pressure may reduce coronary blood flow because most coronary flow occurs during diastole.

Numerous studies (19, 26) indicate that increased arterial stiffness, over and above blood pressure, is an independent predictor of hypertension, atherosclerosis, CV events, and mortality. Kaess et al. (27) and others have demonstrated that increased arterial stiffness precedes the development of hypertension.

Thus, a “primary” increase in large artery stiffness that accompanies aging gives rise to an elevation of arterial pressure; in turn, a “secondary” increase in large artery stiffness occurs due to the increase in mean arterial pressure. Normotensive individuals who fall within the upper quartile for measures of arterial stiffness are more likely to subsequently develop hypertension. Observations such as these reinforce the concept that hypertension, at least in part, is a disease of the arterial wall. The mechanisms of age-associated changes in vascular structure and function and the putative relationship of these changes to development of CV disease are depicted in Table 1.1.

Age-associated dilation of the proximal aorta has been demonstrated in normal adults. Echocardiographic aortic root diameter increased a modest 6% in BLSA men between the fourth and eighth decades (28). In addition, the aortic arch lengthens with age due to arch widening (29). Both greater aortic diameter and arch length were independently associated with higher aortic arch PWV and left ventricular (LV) mass. Such aortic root dilation and lengthening provide an additional stimulus for LV hypertrophy (LVH) because the larger volume of blood in the proximal aorta represents a greater inertial load that must be overcome before LV ejection can begin.

Systolic, diastolic, and pulse pressure

Arterial pressure is determined by the interplay of peripheral vascular resistance and arterial stiffness; the former raises both systolic and diastolic pressure to a similar degree, whereas the latter raises systolic but lowers diastolic pressure. A rise in average systolic blood pressure across adult age has been well documented (Figure 1.4) (30). In contrast, average diastolic pressure was found to rise until about 50 years of age, level off from age 50 to 60, and decline thereafter (30). Thus, pulse pressure (systolic minus diastolic), a useful hemodynamic indicator of

Table 1.1 Relationship of cardiovascular human aging in health to cardiovascular disease

Age-associated changes	Plausible mechanisms	Possible relation to human disease
CV structural remodeling		Early stages of atherosclerosis production
↑ Vascular intimal thickness	↑ Migration of and ↑ matrix by VSMC	
	Possible derivation of intimal cells from other sources	
↑ Vascular stiffness	Elastin fragmentation	Systolic hypertension
	↑ Elastase activity	
	↑ Collagen production by VSMC stroke and	
	↑ cross-linking of collagen	
	Altered growth factor regulation/tissue repair mechanisms	Atherosclerosis
↑ LV wall thickness	↑ LV myocyte size	Retarded early diastolic cardiac filling
	↓ Myocyte number (necrotic and apoptotic death)	↑ Cardiac filling pressure
	Altered growth factor regulation	Lower threshold for dyspnea
	Focal collagen deposition	
↑ Left atrial size	↑ Left atrial pressure/volume	↑ Prevalence of lone atrial fibrillation
CV functional changes		
Altered regulation of vascular tone	↓ NO production/effects	Vascular stiffening; hypertension
	↓ β-AR responses	
↓ CV reserve	↑ Vascular load	Lower threshold for, and increased severity of, heart failure
	↓ Intrinsic myocardial contractility	
	↓ β-Adrenergic modulation of heart rate, myocardial contractility, and vascular tone	
Reduced physical activity	Learned lifestyle	Exaggerated aging changes in some aspects of CV structure and function; negative impact on atherosclerotic vascular disease, hypertension, and heart failure

Abbreviations: β-AR, β-adrenergic receptor; CV, cardiovascular; LV, left ventricular; NO, nitric oxide; VSMC, vascular smooth muscle cell.

conduit artery vascular stiffness, increases with age. These age-dependent changes in systolic, diastolic, and pulse pressures are consistent with the concept that blood pressure in younger people is determined largely by peripheral vascular resistance, whereas in older individuals it is determined more by central conduit vessel stiffness.

Because systolic pressure is higher and diastolic pressure is lower in older men and women, isolated systolic hypertension emerges as the most common form of hypertension in individuals older than 50 years (30). Isolated systolic hypertension, even when mild in severity, is associated with an appreciable increase in CV disease risk (31). On the basis of long-term follow-up of middle-aged and older subjects, however, Framingham researchers have found pulse pressure to be a better predictor of coronary disease risk than systolic or diastolic blood pressures (32). A subsequent Framingham investigation found that pulse pressure was especially informative of coronary risk in older subjects (33) because of the J- or U-shaped association between diastolic pressure and coronary risk. Thus, consideration of the systolic and diastolic pressures jointly, as reflected in pulse pressure, is preferable to consideration of either value alone.

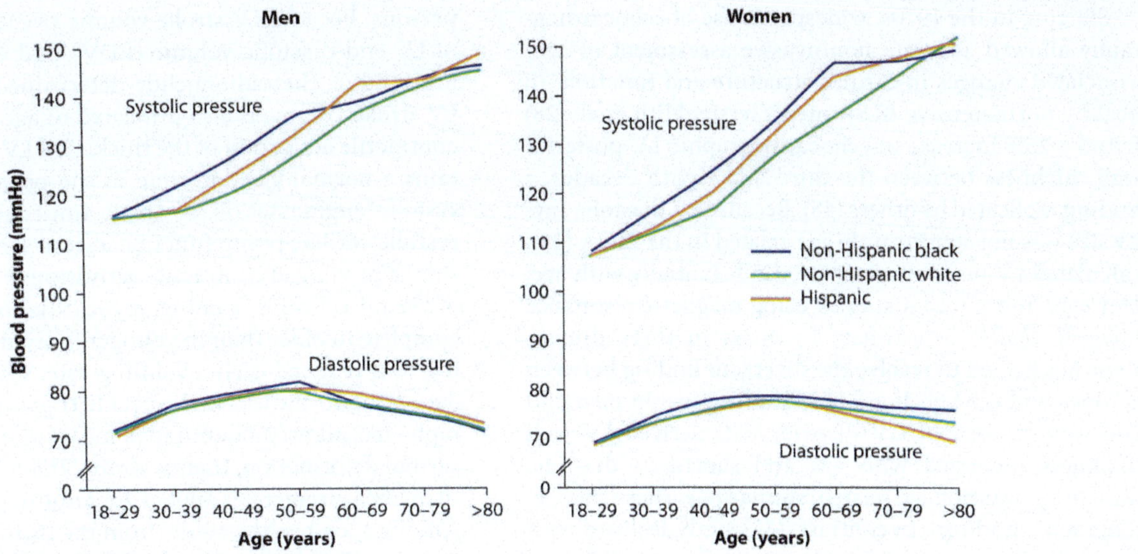

Figure 1.4 Change in blood pressure with age in healthy men and women of different ethnicities. (From Aronow WS et al., *Circulation*, 123, 2434–2506, 2011.)

INTERVENTIONS TO RETARD OR PREVENT ACCELERATED ARTERIAL AGING

Despite the deleterious effects of aging on arterial structure and function, it is noteworthy that the age increases in systolic and pulse pressures are markedly blunted in hunter-gatherer and forager-farmer societies (34). Furthermore, increasing evidence has accrued that lifestyle modifications, including aerobic exercise, and dietary modifications, including reduction in sodium intake, caloric restriction, and weight loss, can prevent or retard age-associated IM thickening (35) and arterial stiffening (36) and improve endothelial function (37). Perhaps, the most promising of these modifications is caloric restriction, which may prolong the maximal life span in laboratory animals when begun in youth or middle age. Limited studies in individuals have demonstrated decreases in CV risk factors and inflammatory markers with caloric restriction. In one study, 25 individuals aged 53 ± 12 years who had practiced voluntary caloric restriction of ~30% for an average of 6.5 years showed markedly lower blood pressure and inflammatory markers compared with controls matched for age and gender (38). In addition, the calorie-restricted group demonstrated higher transmittal early diastolic flow measures, similar to those of younger adults (38). Whether such beneficial effects can be derived by initiating caloric restriction at older ages remains unknown.

Pharmacological intervention, such as chronic angiotensin-converting enzyme inhibition or angiotensin receptor blockade, begun at an early age in animal models, markedly delays the progression of age-associated arterial remodeling. Beneficial effects include lesser IM thickening and rupture of internal elastic lamina (39), attenuated mitochondrial dysfunction, reduced reactive oxygen species, enhanced NO bioavailability, reduced fibrosis, and prolonged life (40, 41). It is thus far unproven if such treatment can prevent or retard unsuccessful aging of the vasculature in younger to middle-aged animals or humans who exhibit excessive subclinical evidence of accelerated arterial aging. Although breaking nonenzymatic collagen cross-links with a novel thiazolium agent reduces arterial stiffness in nonhuman primates (42) and humans (43), its clinical relevance is unclear.

CARDIAC STRUCTURE AND RESTING FUNCTION

Prior to the 1970s, the only method for obtaining reliable measurements of cardiac structure in normal persons was autopsy examination. However, such studies were flawed by their inherent selection bias. A large autopsy series by Linsbach et al. (44) in 7112 patients demonstrated an increase in cardiac mass of 1–1.5 g/year between ages 30 and 90 years. Given that the study included individuals with CV disease, the age-associated increase in heart weight may have derived, at least in part, from coexisting cardiac pathology. An autopsy study of 765 normal hearts from persons 20 to 99 years old who were free from both hypertension and CAD showed that heart weight indexed to body surface area was not related to age in men but increased with age in women, primarily between the fourth and seventh decades (45). In autopsies of hospitalized patients without evident CV disease, Olivetti et al. (46) observed an age-associated reduction of LV mass mediated by a decrease in estimated myocyte number, although myocyte enlargement occurred with age. These investigators subsequently found a higher prevalence of apoptotic myocytes in the hearts of older men than women, which paralleled a decline of LV mass with age in men but not in women (47).

Starting in the 1970s, widespread use of echocardiography allowed accurate noninvasive assessment of age-associated changes in cardiac structure and function. In healthy normotensive BLSA men, Gerstenblith et al. (28) found a 25% increase in echocardiographic LV posterior wall thickness between the third and eighth decades, a finding replicated by others (48). Because LV diastolic cavity size was not significantly age-related in the BLSA (28), calculated LV mass also increased substantially with age. However, more recent studies using magnetic resonance imaging (MRI) to estimate LV mass in three dimensions has helped to resolve the divergent finding between autopsy and echocardiographic studies. In 136 men and 200 women without CV disease, MRI-derived LV wall thickness increased with age and short-axis diastolic dimension was not age related, similar to earlier echocardiographic findings. In contrast, LV length declined with age in both sexes (i.e., the LV became more spherical) (49). Thus, MRI-derived LV mass was unrelated to age in women and demonstrated an age-associated decline in men (because of their lesser age-related increase in wall thickness), similar to autopsy findings (47). Three-dimensional echocardiography has confirmed this preservation of LV mass across age in women and a reduction of LV mass in older men (50). In 5004 healthy volunteers from the MESA study, cardiac MRI revealed age-related declines in both LV diastolic and systolic volumes and an increase in the LV mass/volume ratio in both sexes (51); stroke volume decreased modestly with age. Longitudinal MRI follow-up over 10 years confirmed a modest decline in LV diastolic volume and increase in LV mass/volume ratio (52). Thus, the normal LV becomes smaller, thicker, and more spherical with advancing age.

Although the mechanisms for the age-associated remodeling of the LV and increase in myocyte size are not clear, they may be adaptive responses to the arterial changes that accompany aging. Putative stimuli for cardiac cell enlargement with age are an increase in vascular load due to arterial stiffening and a stretching of cells due to dropout of neighboring apoptotic myocytes (53). Phenotypically, the age-associated increase in LV thickness resembles the LVH that develops from hypertension. This finding, coupled with the increase in systolic blood pressure that occurs over time even in healthy individuals, has led to consideration of aging as a muted form of hypertension. In older rodent hearts, which demonstrate a similar increase in LV mass and myocyte size as observed in humans, a stretching of cardiac myocytes and fibroblasts releases growth factors such as angiotensin II, a known stimulus for apoptosis. As a result, the heart becomes stiffer, that is, less compliant, with age. Increased secretion of atrial natriuretic (54) and opioid (55) peptides is also observed.

Echocardiographic LV shortening fraction (48) and radionuclide LV ejection fraction (56), the two most common measures of global LV systolic performance, are unaffected by age at rest in healthy normotensive persons. Because LV stroke volume (SV) is the difference of LV end-diastolic volume (EDV) and end-systolic volume (ESV), the radionuclide-determined supine resting LV stroke volume is also unrelated to age (56). Prolonged contractile activation of the thickened LV wall (57) maintains a normal ejection time in the presence of the late systolic augmentation of aortic impedance, preserving systolic cardiac pump function at rest. However, a downside of prolonged contractile activation is that at the time of the mitral valve opening, myocardial relaxation is less complete in older than in younger individuals, contributing to a reduced early LV filling rate. Over the last two decades, two-dimensional speckle tracking echocardiography has allowed quantitative measurement of LV myocardial deformation, that is, strain. The most widely used such measurement is global longitudinal strain (GLS). Among 1266 healthy adults from the third through ninth decades, GLS declined modestly with age, especially after 60 years (58).

In contrast to the overall preservation of resting LV systolic performance across adult age, LV diastolic performance is profoundly altered by aging. Reduced mitral valve E–F closure slope on M-mode echocardiography first documented these age changes in diastolic performance (28, 48). Pulsed Doppler (59) and radionuclide (60) techniques confirmed that the transmitral early diastolic peak filling rate declined by ~50% between the ages of 20 and 80 years (Figure 1.5). Conversely, peak A-wave velocity, which represents late LV filling facilitated by atrial contraction, increases with age (59). This greater atrial contribution to LV filling is accomplished via a modest age-associated increase in left atrial size demonstrable on echocardiography. Tissue Doppler and color M-mode techniques, both less influenced by preload and afterload

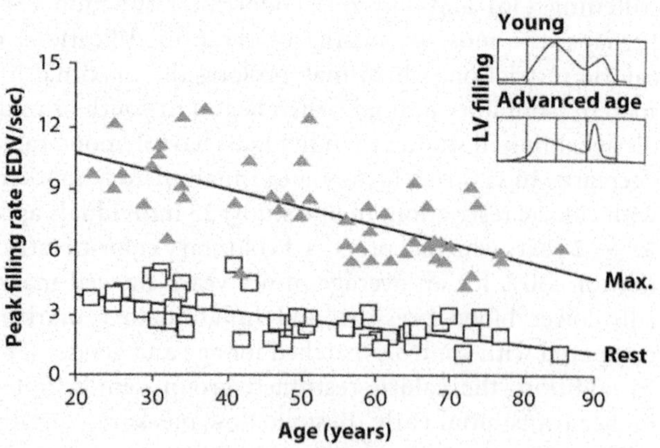

Figure 1.5 Changes with age in peak early diastolic filling rates derived from radionuclide ventriculography at rest and during maximal upright cycle ergometry. The inset shows the transmittal flow velocity profile derived from Doppler echocardiography in a young adult and older adult. Note the shift from a dominant early (E) filling wave in the young to a dominant late (A) filling wave in the elderly. (From Schulman SP et al., *Am J Physiol*, 263, H1932–H1938, 1992.)

than pulsed Doppler, have confirmed the age-associated reduction in early diastolic filling rate and increased late filling (61). Because the resting LV EDV is preserved across adult age in BLSA volunteers, the augmented atrial contribution to LV filling in older adults can be considered a successful adaptation to the reduced early diastolic filling rate in the thicker, and presumably stiffer, senescent LV. Thus, the relative importance of early and late diastolic LV filling is reversed with aging.

Reduction of early LV filling with age may derive in part from decreased LV diastolic compliance due to the increase in LV wall thickness. An age-associated reduction in ventricular compliance has been shown in animals. Studies in man have confirmed an age-associated reduction in LV compliance, which was minimally changed in older adults after a full year of endurance training (62). In both intact animal hearts and isolated cardiac muscle, studies have demonstrated prolonged isovolumic relaxation and increased myocardial diastolic stiffness. Studies in both mice and healthy volunteers have shown age-associated increases in MRI-derived extracellular volume, thought to represent myocardial fibrosis, representing another potential mechanism for reduced LV compliance with aging (63). This slower isovolumic relaxation observed in cardiac muscle from older animals may be secondary to a diminished rate of Ca^{2+} accumulation by the sarcoplasmic reticulum (64). A conceptual framework for the cardiac adaptations to age-associated arterial stiffening is shown in Figure 1.6.

Although the diminished early LV diastolic filling rate with age may not compromise resting EDV or stroke volume, an underlying reduction of LV compliance might cause a greater rise in LV diastolic pressure in older persons, especially during stress-induced tachycardia, thereby causing a lower threshold for dyspnea than in the young. It might also be anticipated that the loss of atrial contribution to LV filling that occurs during atrial fibrillation would elicit a greater deterioration of diastolic performance in older than in younger individuals. Indeed, it is attractive to speculate that the frequent occurrence of heart failure in the elderly despite preserved LV systolic function derives, at least in part, from the age-associated impairment of early diastolic filling (Table 1.1).

Information regarding aging changes in right ventricular (RV) structure and function has been limited by the difficulty in imaging the right ventricle by echocardiography. However, cardiac MRI can provide such information. In 4204 MESA participants aged 45–84 years who were free of clinical CV disease, cardiac MRI showed declines in both RV mass and volumes but a modest increase in RV ejection fraction with age (65). RVEDV, mass, and ejection fraction were positively related to systolic blood pressure and inversely related to diastolic blood pressure. The pulmonary arteries also appear to undergo age-associated remodeling, resulting in increased pulmonary artery (PA) stiffness and PA systolic pressure. In 1413 Olmsted County, Minnesota, residents ≥45 years old, PA systolic pressure estimated by Doppler echocardiography increased modestly from 26 ± 4 mmHg in persons 45–54 years old to 30 ± 6 mmHg in those 72–96 years old (66). Higher PA systolic pressure was an independent mortality predictor (hazard ratio [HR] 1.46 per 10 mmHg) (66). Healthy adults also demonstrate an exaggerated rise in

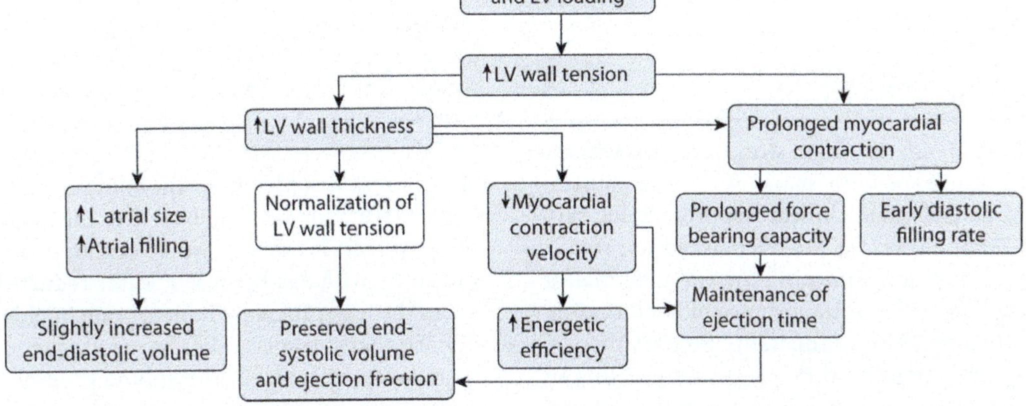

Figure 1.6 Conceptual framework for the cardiovascular adaptations to arterial stiffening that occur with aging. *Abbreviation*: LV, left ventricular.

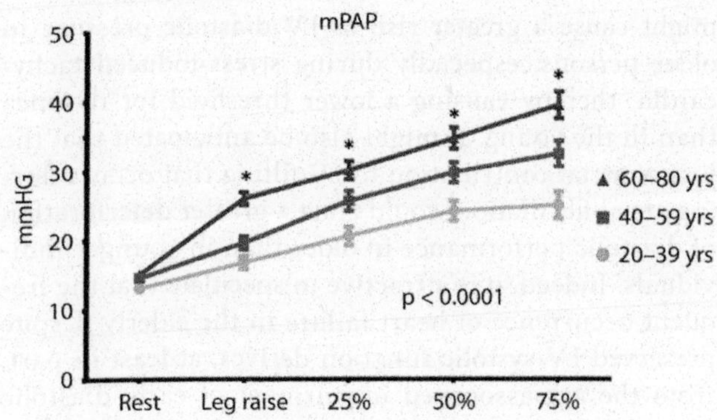

Figure 1.7 Age-associated changes in mean pulmonary artery pressure (mPAP) during leg raising and graded aerobic exercise (25%, 50%, and 75% of maximal oxygen consumption). (From Wolsk E et al., *J Am Coll Cardiol HF*, 5, 337–346, 2017.)

PA systolic and mean pressures with age during cycle ergometry (Figure 1.7) (67).

CV physical findings in older adults

During the CV examination, several age-associated alterations in CV structure and function may manifest themselves. Because of large artery stiffening, systolic blood pressure is often elevated with a normal or low diastolic blood pressure. Therefore, the carotid artery upstroke is usually brisk in older adults and may mask significant aortic valvular stenosis. The apical cardiac impulse may be difficult to palpate secondary to senile emphysema and chest wall deformities. Respiratory splitting of the second heart sound is audible in only ~30%–40% of individuals older than 60 years, presumably because of reduced compliance of the pulmonary vasculature. In contrast, an S4 gallop is commonly heard in older but not younger individuals because of the age-associated increase in late diastolic filling mediated by vigorous atrial contraction into a thicker-walled, less compliant LV. A soft basal ejection murmur occurs in 30%–60% of elders. This murmur is thought to arise from a dilated, tortuous aorta or from sclerosis of the aortic valve.

CV RESPONSE TO STRESS

The CV response of older adults to stress (e.g., to increases in arterial pressure, to postural maneuvers, or to physical exercise) is of considerable clinical importance for several reasons. First, physicians are often asked to provide advice and information concerning the CV potential of the elderly (e.g., the effect or importance of conditioning status on the maintenance of function). Second, the CV response to stress is important in assessing the ability of older individuals to respond to disease states. Third, the CV stress response is valuable in the diagnosis and management of older patients with CV disease. Despite the high prevalence of CV disease among older Americans, it is important to understand their exercise capabilities. Exercise testing is a diagnostic tool that is frequently utilized to detect and quantify the severity of CV disease. The utility of such diagnostic testing clearly depends on precise information regarding the normal limits of such stress testing procedures relative to age.

Orthostatic stress

In healthy, community-dwelling elders, arterial pressure changes little with the assumption of upright posture, and postural hypotension or acute orthostatic intolerance (i.e., dizziness or fainting when assuming an upright from a supine position or during a passive tilt) is uncommon. Orthostatic hypotension (OH), defined by a decline of systolic blood pressure by ≥20 mmHg or diastolic blood pressure by ≥10 mmHg, occurred in 16% of volunteers aged 65 and older from the Cardiovascular Health Study (CHS) (68) and in 7% of men aged 71–93 years from the Honolulu Heart Program (69); in both of these older cohorts, the prevalence of OH increased with age. In the former study, OH was associated with higher supine blood pressure, greater LV wall thickness, and smaller LV cavity size (70). In the latter study, OH was an independent predictor for mortality (relative risk [RR] = 1.64), and there was a linear relationship between the magnitude of orthostatic decline in systolic blood pressure and 4-year mortality rate (69). In contrast to healthy, community-dwelling older volunteers, OH and orthostatic intolerance are common in debilitated institutionalized elders with chronic illnesses. Within such populations, the likelihood for OH is increased among individuals who exhibit very low LV filling rates and small EDV and SV in the supine position (71). In such individuals, however, the effects of advanced age cannot be dissociated from those of profound deconditioning and multiple diseases and medications.

With advancing age, the acute heart rate increase to orthostatic stress decreases in magnitude and takes longer to achieve. The baroreceptor sensitivity (i.e., the slope of the relationship of the change in heart rate versus the change in arterial pressure) is negatively correlated with age and resting arterial pressure (72). The low-pressure baroreceptor, or cardiopulmonary reflex, also decreases with age in normotensives, but not in hypertensives.

Despite the lesser heart rate increase during orthostatic stress in older than in younger BLSA volunteers, the SV reduction tends to be less in the older group; thus, the postural change in cardiac output does not vary significantly with age because a lesser reduction in SV balances the lesser increase in heart rate in older individuals (73). Similarly, some studies have found cardiac output to be reduced with age in the supine position because of a reduced SV in older versus younger men; this age effect was abolished in the sitting position because of lesser reduction in SV in the older men on sitting.

Pressor stress

Acute increases in blood pressure represent another common CV stress. Sustained, isometric handgrip increases both arterial pressure and heart rate. The response varies in magnitude in proportion to the relative level and duration of effort. After sustained submaximal or maximal handgrip, heart rate was observed to increase more in younger than in older healthy individuals, whereas blood pressure increased more in older persons (74). In BLSA volunteers, 3 minutes of submaximal sustained handgrip elicited mild increases in echocardiographic LV diastolic and systolic dimensions and atrial filling fraction; these increases correlated positively with age (74). Thus, pressor stress accentuated the age-associated dependence on late diastolic filling.

Application of a pressor stress has also been used to assess the intrinsic myocardial reserve capacity. In healthy BLSA individuals, a 30 mmHg increase in systolic blood pressure induced by phenylephrine infusion in the presence of β-adrenergic blockade induced significant echocardiographic LV dilatation at end diastole in healthy older (60–68 years), but not in younger (18–34 years), men: the cardiac dilatation occurred in older men despite a smaller reduction in heart rate (75), analogous to the handgrip response. Thus, an apparent age-associated decrease in intrinsic myocardial contractile reserve occurs in response to an acute increase in afterload; the senescent heart dilates to preserve SV via the Frank–Starling mechanism.

Aerobic exercise capacity

The ability to perform oxygen-utilizing (i.e., aerobic) activities is a fundamental requirement of independent living and is probably the best-studied CV stressor. The accepted standard for aerobic fitness is maximum oxygen consumption rate (VO_2max), the product of cardiac output (the central component) and arteriovenous oxygen difference (the peripheral component) during exhaustive exercise. In healthy adults, VO_2max is up to 15 times greater than resting VO_2. This huge increase is accomplished by a four- to fivefold augmentation of cardiac output and up to a threefold widening of the arteriovenous oxygen difference; the latter is due to both a dramatic increase in the relative proportion of cardiac output delivered to working muscles and increased oxygen extraction by these muscles. Because the total body VO_2max is strongly influenced by muscle mass, VO_2max is typically compared across individuals by normalizing for body weight.

Multiple studies have documented that treadmill VO_2max, adjusted for body weight, declines with age. In cross-sectional studies, the decline typically approximates 50% across the adult age span (76, 77). However, the extent of the VO_2max decline with aging varies among studies, depending on age ranges, differences in body weight and composition, and differences in habitual physical activity among the individuals studied. Longitudinal studies generally report a more pronounced age-associated decline in VO_2max than do cross-sectional studies. In BLSA volunteers rigorously screened to exclude CV or lung disease, VO_2max declines by ~50% between the third and ninth decades by cross-sectional analysis (76, 77). Although such cross-sectional studies are usually interpreted to indicate that VO_2max declines linearly with age, a more detailed analysis in this same BLSA population demonstrated that the longitudinal decline in aerobic capacity is not constant across adulthood as assumed by cross-sectional studies, but accelerates markedly with successive age decades, especially in men, regardless of physical activity levels (Figure 1.8) (78). When the components of VO_2max were examined, the longitudinal decline in oxygen pulse (VO_2 per heartbeat) mirrored that of VO_2max, whereas maximal heart rate decreased only 4%–6% per decade regardless of starting age (Figure

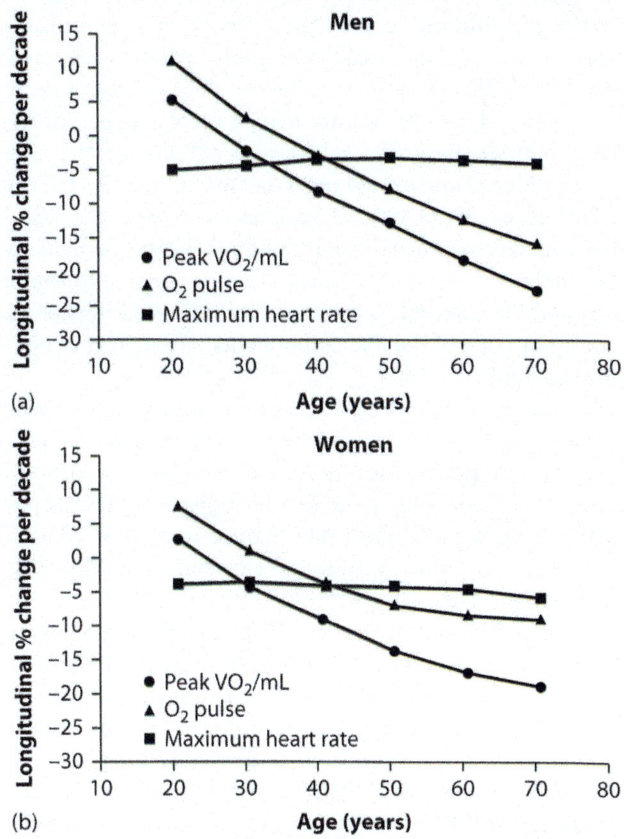

Figure 1.8 Longitudinal change in peak VO_2 and its components (maximal heart rate and O_2 pulse) in healthy Baltimore Longitudinal Study of Aging (BLSA) male (a) and female (b) volunteers. In both sexes, the decline in maximal heart rate is only ~5% per decade and is relatively constant across age. However, the decline in O_2 pulse, encompassing both stroke volume and peripheral oxygen delivery and utilization, declines more rapidly in older adults, paralleling the decline in peak VO_2. (From Fleg JL et al., *Circulation*, 112, 674–682, 2005.)

1.8). Subsequent analysis of 99 BLSA volunteers in whom both VO_2max and exercise cardiac imaging were performed during upright cycle ergometry showed that the decline in arteriovenous oxygen difference at peak effort was more strongly predictive of the longitudinal decline in peak VO_2 than the decline in cardiac output (79). Although age-associated loss of muscle mass and increase in body fat also contribute to the reduction in VO_2max with aging, the pattern of accelerated VO_2max decline with age persists even after normalizing it for fat-free mass rather than body weight (78). Despite the similar rates of decline in VO_2max with age regardless of physical activity level, it should be emphasized that at any age the more active quartiles maintain a higher VO_2max than their sedentary peers.

The accelerated decline of aerobic capacity has important implications regarding functional independence and quality of life. It should be emphasized that the data in healthy BLSA volunteers represent a best-case scenario. The superimposition of CV or pulmonary disease as well as the deconditioning and loss of muscle mass commonly seen in the elderly because of their sedentary lifestyle accentuate this decline in VO_2max. Because activities of daily living typically require a fixed aerobic expenditure, they require a significantly larger percent of VO_2max in an older than in a younger person. Once the energy required of an activity approaches or exceeds the aerobic capacity of an elderly individual, he/she will likely be unable to perform it. Thus, it is not surprising that a low aerobic capacity, represented by slow walking speed, comprises one of the five components of the "frailty phenotype" (80).

Another potential contributor to exercise intolerance with aging is a greater metabolic debt incurred during exercise that persists during recovery. For several minutes after a bout of aerobic exercise, the body continues to consume oxygen at a higher rate than at rest. This "oxygen debt" incurred during recovery can comprise 14%–20% of the total aerobic expenditure. In one study, the VO_2 consumed by healthy older persons during recovery from exercise exceeded that in the young by more than 30% (81).

The age-associated decrease in cardiac index at maximal effort during upright cycle exercise (Figure 1.9f) is due entirely to a reduction in heart rate (Figure 1.9e), as the LVSV index (LVSVI) does not decline with age in either gender (Figure 1.9d) (82). However, the manner in which SVI is achieved during maximal exercise changes importantly with aging. Although older individuals have a blunted capacity to reduce end-systolic volume index (ESVI) (Figure 1.9b) and to increase LV ejection fraction (Figure 1.9c), this deficit is offset by a larger end-diastolic volume index (EDVI) (Figure 1.9a) (82). Thus, a "stiff heart" that prohibits sufficient filling between beats during exercise does not characterize aging in healthy individuals. The larger EDVI in healthy older versus younger individuals during vigorous aerobic exercise is due in part to a longer diastolic interval (i.e., slower heart rate) and to a greater amount of blood remaining in the heart at end systole (Figure 1.9b) (82). However, an exaggerated rise in pulmonary capillary wedge pressure occurs during aerobic exercise in older adults, perhaps contributing to exercise intolerance (67).

Given the accelerated decline in VO_2max with age, an important question is whether aerobic training of sedentary older adults can improve their CV reserve capacity. It has been amply documented that physical conditioning of older persons can substantially increase their maximum aerobic work capacity. In a meta-analysis of 41 trials in 2102 individuals aged 60 and older, aerobic training elicited a 16.3% mean increase in VO_2max (83). The extent to which this conditioning effect results from enhanced central cardiac performance versus augmented peripheral mechanisms, including changes in skeletal muscle mass, likely varies with the characteristics of the population studied, the type and degree of conditioning achieved, gender, body position during study, and genetic factors.

A longitudinal study of healthy older men during upright cycle ergometry indicates that aerobic training enhances VO_2max in part by increasing the maximum cardiac output due to augmented maximum SV and in part by increasing the arteriovenous oxygen difference (84). The augmentation of maximum SV is due primarily to an augmented reduction of LVESV and, thus, a concomitant increase in LV ejection fraction; however, conditioning status had minimal effect on LVEDV during exercise in older adults. This contrasts with the effect of physical conditioning in younger persons, which substantially increases EDV and SV via the Frank–Starling mechanism, as well as via an enhanced LV ejection fraction. However, the maximal heart rate of both older and younger persons does not vary with conditioning status. Thus, physical conditioning of older persons does not appear to offset the age-associated deficiency in sympathetic modulation. Rather, increased LV ejection from aerobic training in this age group appears to derive from the reduction in vascular afterload, as reflected in a reduced PWV (85) and carotid augmentation index, with possible contribution from augmented maximum intrinsic myocardial contractility. Furthermore, aerobic training in sedentary older adults reduced their oxygen debt immediately post-exercise by nearly 30%, translating into an 18% increase in exercise efficiency; in contrast, efficiency did not change in younger persons after training (80).

MECHANISMS OF IMPAIRED LV EJECTION DURING MAXIMAL AEROBIC EXERCISE IN HEALTHY OLDER ADULTS

The ability to augment LV ejection fraction during vigorous aerobic exercise is blunted with age even after screening to exclude persons with occult CAD. The impaired ability of healthy older men and women to

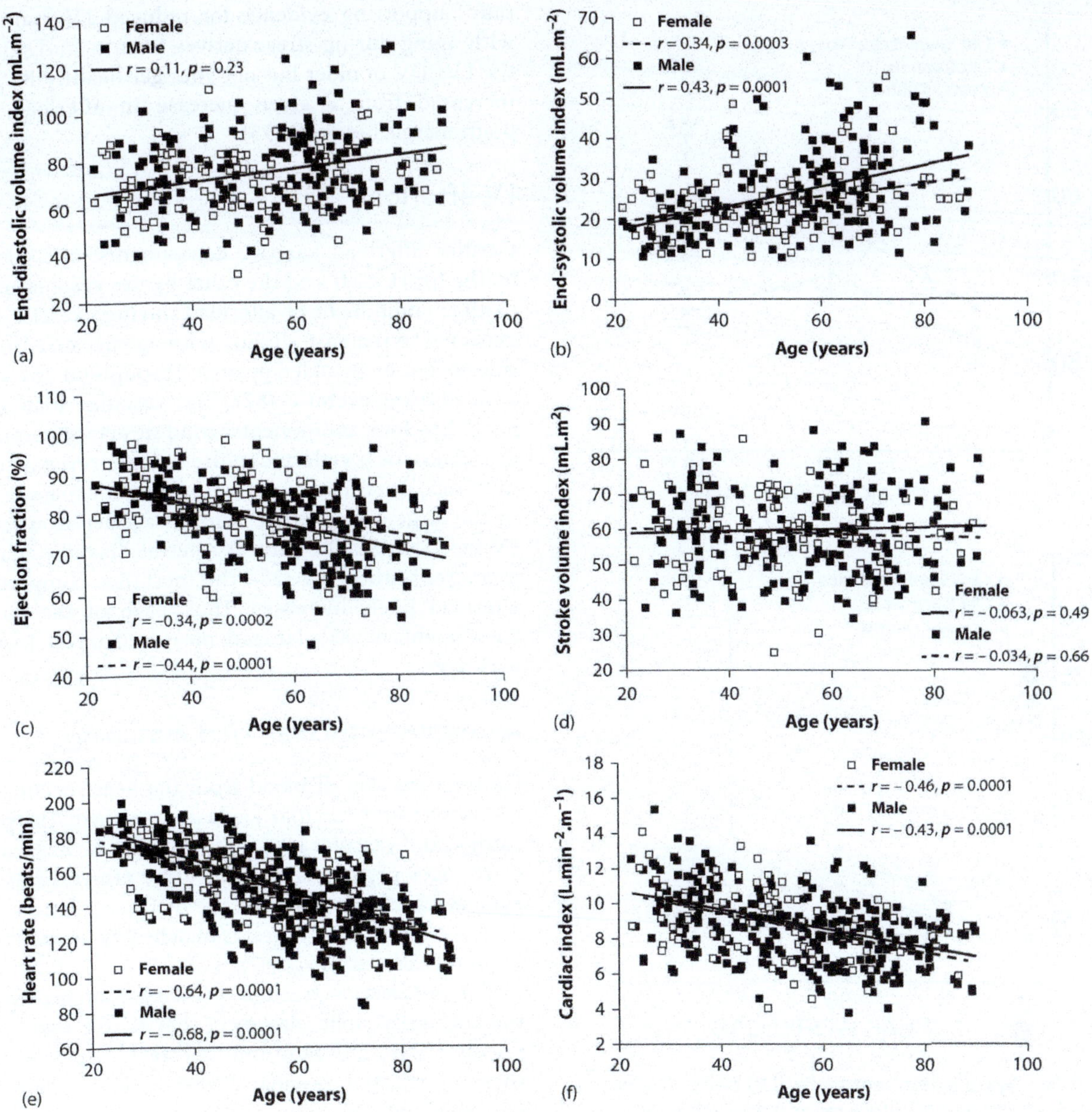

Figure 1.9 Scatter plots of left ventricular volumes (a, b), ejection fraction (c), stroke volume (d), heart rate (e), and cardiac index (f) during maximal graded upright cycle exercise in healthy Baltimore Longitudinal Study of Aging (BLSA) volunteers, carefully screened to exclude silent coronary artery disease. Note the similar age changes in men and women and the increasing heterogeneity with age in the end-systolic volume index, ejection fraction, and heart rate. (From Fleg JL et al., *J Appl Physiol*, 78, 890–900, 1995.)

reduce LVESV during vigorous exercise accounts for their smaller increase in ejection fraction from rest and their lower maximal value compared to younger individuals (Figure 1.9c) (82). A blunted LV ejection fraction response during exercise is even more prominent in older individuals with exercise-induced silent myocardial ischemia than in those without evident ischemia, due to a more pronounced inability to reduce ESVI (Figure 1.10) (86).

The underlying mechanisms for the age-associated reduction in maximum LV ejection fraction are multifactorial and include (i) a reduction in intrinsic myocardial contractility, (ii) an increase in vascular afterload, (iii) arterial–ventricular load mismatching, and (iv) a diminished effectiveness of the autonomic modulation of both LV contractility and arterial afterload. Although these age-associated changes in CV reserve per se are insufficient to produce clinical heart failure, they appear to lower the threshold for developing symptoms and signs of heart failure and adversely influence its clinical severity and prognosis for any level of disease burden (Table 1.1).

Myocardial contractility

How aging affects factors that regulate intrinsic myocardial contractility in humans is incompletely understood

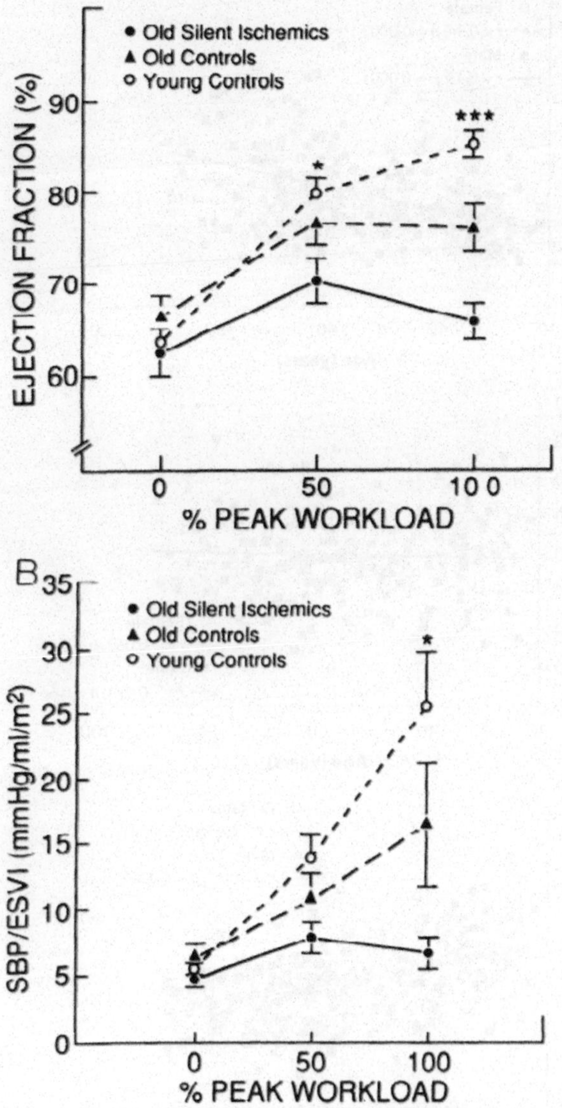

Figure 1.10 Systolic left ventricular (LV) performance as a function of age and silent myocardial ischemia during upright cycle ergometry in three groups of men from the Baltimore Longitudinal Study of Aging (BLSA) (young normal, older normal, and older age-matched men with silent ischemia). The top panel shows the LV ejection fraction response at baseline, 50% of peak workload, and maximal effort; the bottom panel shows end-systolic pressure/ESV, a more specific measure of LV contractility, at these same three time points. In both graphs, an additive negative effect of age and silent ischemia on systolic LV performance at maximal effort is evident. (From Fleg JL et al., *J Appl Physiol*, 75:499–504, 1993.)

because the effectiveness of intrinsic myocardial contractility in the intact circulation is difficult to separate from loading and autonomic modulatory influences on contractility. Given that the heart rate per se is a determinant of the myocardial contractile state, a deficit in the maximal intrinsic contractility of older persons might be expected on the basis of their reduced maximum heart rate. Supporting evidence for reduced LV contractility with aging during stress derives from a study in which the LVEDV of older but not younger healthy BLSA men increased from a given increase in afterload during β-adrenergic blockade (75).

LV afterload

Cardiac afterload has two components: one generated by the heart itself and the other by the vasculature. The cardiac component of afterload during exercise can be expected to increase slightly with age because the heart size increases in older persons throughout the cardiac cycle during exercise (82). The vascular load on the heart has four components: conduit artery compliance characteristics, reflected pulse waves, resistance, and inertance. Inertance is determined by the mass of blood in the large arteries that requires acceleration prior to LV ejection. As the central arterial diastolic diameter increases with aging (28), the inertance component of afterload likely increases. Thus, each of the pulsatile components of vascular load, measured at rest, increases with age.

Arterial/ventricular load matching

Optimal ejection of blood from the heart occurs when ventricular and vascular loads are matched. The precise cardiac and vascular load matching that is characteristic of younger persons is thought to be preserved at older ages, at least at rest, because the increased vascular stiffness in older persons at rest is matched by increased resting ventricular stiffness (87).

For the ejection fraction to increase during exercise, the LV end-systolic elastance, that is, the end-systolic pressure (ESP)/ESV ratio, must increase to a greater extent than the effective vascular elastance (EA), that is, ESP/stroke volume. With increasing age, however, end-systolic elastance fails to increase in proportion to the increase in EA; hence, the EA/ELV during exercise in older persons decreases to a lesser extent than it does in younger persons (87). This altered arterial/ventricular load matching in older versus younger persons during exercise is a mechanism for the deficit in the acute LV ejection fraction reserve that typically accompanies advancing age. Acute pharmacological reduction in both cardiac and vascular components of LV afterload by sodium nitroprusside infusions in older, healthy BLSA volunteers augments LV ejection fraction in these subjects at rest and throughout upright cycle exercise (88).

Sympathetic modulation

During acute exercise and other stresses, sympathetic modulation of the CV system increases heart rate, augments myocardial contractility and relaxation, reduces LV afterload, and redistributes blood to working muscles and skin to dissipate heat. All of the factors that have been identified to play a role in the deficient CV regulation with aging—that is, heart rate, afterload (both cardiac and vascular), myocardial contractility, and redistribution of blood flow—exhibit a deficient sympathetic modulatory component.

Sympathetic neurotransmitters

Apparent deficits in sympathetic modulation of cardiac and arterial functions with aging occur in the presence of elevated neurotransmitter levels. Plasma levels of norepinephrine and epinephrine, during any perturbation from the supine basal state, increase to a greater extent in older than in younger healthy humans (55). This increase appears to be a compensatory response to the reduced cardiac β-receptor density with advancing age (89). The age-associated increase in plasma levels of norepinephrine results from an increased cardiac spillover into the circulation and, to a lesser extent, to reduced plasma clearance. Deficient norepinephrine reuptake at nerve endings has been suggested as the primary mechanism for increased spillover. During prolonged submaximal exercise, however, diminished neurotransmitter reuptake might also be associated with reduced release and spillover in older adults, contributing to the age-associated deficit in cardioacceleration and LV systolic performance seen during such exercise (90).

Deficits in cardiac β-adrenergic receptor signaling

Numerous studies support the concept that the efficiency of postsynaptic β-adrenergic signaling declines with aging. One line of evidence derives from the observation that acute β-AR blockade changes the exercise hemodynamic profile of younger persons to resemble that of older ones. Thus, the reduction in heart rate during exhaustive aerobic exercise in the presence of acute β-adrenergic blockade is greater in younger than in older subjects, and significant β-adrenergic blockade–induced LV dilatation occurs only in the younger group (91). In addition, the age-associated deficits in early LV diastolic filling rate, both at rest and during exercise, are abolished by acute β-adrenergic blockade. However, acute β-adrenergic blockade causes SVI to increase to a greater extent in younger than in older individuals, due in part to the greater increase in LV filling time in the young, caused by greater reduction in their maximal heart rate (91).

When perspectives from intact humans to subcellular biochemistry in animal models are integrated, a diminished responsiveness to β-adrenergic modulation is among the most consistently observed CV changes that occur with advancing age. Age-associated alterations in CV function that exceed the identified limits for healthy elderly individuals most likely represent interactions of aging per se with severe physical deconditioning and/or CV disease, both of which are highly prevalent among older adults.

RELEVANT AGING CHANGES IN OTHER ORGAN SYSTEMS

Because of the close relationships between the CV system and other organs, it is important to recognize some of the more salient non-CV changes that occur with age. In the lungs, loss of elastic recoil causes reduced emptying and thus reduced vital capacity and minute ventilation during vigorous exercise. Plasma and total blood volumes decline moderately with age. Age-related loss of skeletal muscle mass, termed sarcopenia, is paralleled by reduced muscle strength, a major cause of disability and reduced quality of life in the elderly. A similar loss of bone occurs with age and is exacerbated by estrogen deficiency in postmenopausal women, leading to a marked increase in fracture risk. Additionally, age-associated nephrosclerosis results in loss of renal parenchyma and reductions in renal plasma flow, creatinine clearance, plasma rennin activity, and plasma aldosterone. These renal changes decrease the elimination of renally excreted drugs, attenuate responses to sodium restriction and volume expansion, and increase the risk for hyperkalemia. Although creatinine clearance typically declines by ~50% between the third and ninth decades, serum creatinine changes minimally because of the parallel loss of muscle mass.

ELECTROCARDIOGRAPHY AND ARRHYTHMIAS

Anatomical conduction system changes

The cardiac conduction system undergoes multiple changes with age that affect its electrical properties and, when exaggerated, cause clinical disease. A generalized increase in elastic and collagenous tissue commonly occurs. Fat accumulates around the sinoatrial node, sometimes creating partial or complete separation of the node from the atrial tissue. In extreme cases, this may contribute to the development of sick sinus syndrome. A pronounced decline in the number of pacemaker cells generally occurs after age 60; by age 75, less than 10% of the number seen in young adults remain. A variable degree of calcification of the left side of the cardiac skeleton, which includes the aortic and mitral annuli, the central fibrous body, and the summit of the interventricular system, is observed. Because of their proximity to these structures, the atrioventricular (AV) node, AV bifurcation, and proximal left and right bundle branches may be damaged or destroyed by this process, resulting in AV or intraventricular block.

Electrocardiography

Alterations in cardiac anatomy and electrophysiology with age often manifest themselves on the ECG. Because the resting ECG remains the most widely used cardiac diagnostic test, a review of these aging changes is relevant to distinguish them from those imposed by disease.

Sinus node function

Although supine resting heart rate is unrelated to age in most studies (Figure 1.11, upper panel), the phasic variation in R–R interval known as respiratory sinus arrhythmia declines with age (92, 93). Similarly, a reduced prevalence of sinus bradycardia on resting ECG is evident by the fourth decade (92). Because both sinus arrhythmia and sinus bradycardia are indices of cardiac parasympathetic activity, the age-associated reduction in parasympathetic function (93) may mediate both findings. Spectral analysis of heart rate variability has confirmed an age-related reduction of high-frequency (0.15–0.45 Hz) oscillations indicative of vagal efferent activity (Figure 1.11, lower panel) (94). Although physical conditioning status influences autonomic tone, a cross-sectional study in BLSA volunteers demonstrated that the deconditioning that usually accompanies the aging process plays only a minor role in the age-associated blunting of these high-frequency oscillations (94). Patients with organic heart disease demonstrate a reduced respiratory sinus arrhythmia compared to age-matched normal individuals. A blunting of high-frequency oscillations in apparently healthy older volunteers is predictive of future coronary events and mortality (95). Time domain indices of heart rate variability also decline substantially with age; the pattern of decline varies with the specific time domain measure. Younger men generally display higher time domain indices than younger women, but this gender difference narrows or disappears at older ages. In a Swiss population of healthy persons aged 50 years and older, CV risk factors, such as hypertension, smoking, non-high-density lipoprotein cholesterol, and C-reactive protein, were each associated with reduced heart rate variability during 24-hour ECG recordings (96).

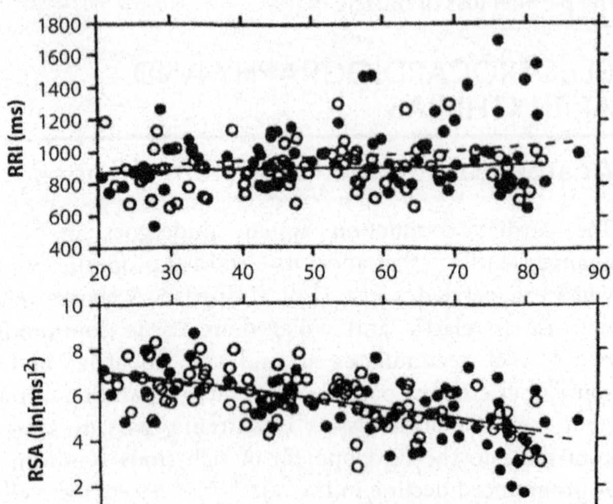

Figure 1.11 Mean RRI and RSA during 3 minutes of sitting in healthy BLSA men (closed circles and dashed line) and women (open circles and solid line). Whereas RRI (top) was unrelated to age in either sex, RSA (bottom) declined similarly with age in women ($r = 0.61$; $p < 0.001$) and men ($r = 0.59$; $p < 0.001$). *Abbreviations*: BLSA, Baltimore Longitudinal Study of Aging; RRI, RR interval; RSA, respiratory sinus arrhythmia. (From Byrne EA et al., *J Appl Physiol*, 81, 743–750, 1996.)

Sinus bradycardia below 50 bpm was found on the resting ECG in 4.1% of 1172 healthy, non-endurance-trained, unmedicated participants aged 40 years and older from the BLSA; the prevalence was similar in men (3.9%) and women (4.5%) (97). Individuals with unexplained sinus bradycardia (mean age 58 years) had a significantly greater prevalence of associated conduction system abnormalities than non-bradycardic age- and sex-matched controls, but there was no difference in the incidence of future coronary events over a 5.4-year mean follow-up period (97). Sinus bradycardia due to sick sinus syndrome is seen almost exclusively in the elderly and probably derives in part from the marked decline in the number of pacemaker cells in the sinoatrial node. In the absence of organic heart disease, such bradycardia is not associated with increased cardiac mortality (97).

P waves

The prevalence of left atrial abnormality, defined by a negative P terminal force in lead V_1 of at least 0.04 mm/s, increases with age, paralleling the echocardiographic increase in left atrial size. Among 588 institutionalized elderly, such a P terminal force was only 32% sensitive, although 94% specific, for echocardiographic left atrial enlargement (98). There is no apparent increase in ECG evidence of right atrial enlargement with age when individuals with significant chronic obstructive lung disease are excluded.

P–R interval

The P–R interval undergoes a modest but significant prolongation with advancing age (99–101). An increase in P–R interval from 159 to 175 ms in men and from 156 to 165 ms in women occurred between the ages of 30 and 72 years in BLSA volunteers (100). By high-resolution signal-averaged surface ECGs, the prolongation of AV conduction was localized proximal to the His bundle deflection, but within the P–R segment, presumably reflecting delay within the AV junction. Using the conventional upper limit of 0.20 seconds, the prevalence of first-degree AV block in healthy older men is usually 3%–4%, a prevalence severalfold greater than in young men (101). Although earlier studies found no correlation between first-degree AV block and cardiac disease or mortality (102), a 20-year follow-up of Framingham volunteers showed increased risks of atrial fibrillation, pacemaker implantation, and all-cause mortality associated with PR prolongation, even within the normal range (103).

QRS complex

Although the QRS duration shows no significant age relationship, the QRS axis shifts progressively leftward with age. In the database of 79, 743 clinically normal individuals, a shift in the mean QRS axis from 56 degrees to 8 degrees occurred between the third and ninth decades, with no gender difference (99). The corresponding lower normal limits shifted from −30 to −60 degrees. Thus, the prevalence of left-axis deviation of less than −30 degrees increases dramatically with age, reaching 20% by the tenth decade (104). This leftward QRS axis shift may be largely due to the age-related increase in LV wall thickness (28, 48). Longitudinal studies have failed to demonstrate any increase in cardiac morbidity or mortality associated with this isolated ECG finding (105).

Longitudinal (106) studies have demonstrated a decrease in R- and S-wave amplitudes with advancing age, evident by the fourth decade. At first glance, this decrease in QRS amplitude seems paradoxical, given the age-related increase in LV thickness. However, the surface ECG is influenced by extracardiac as well as cardiac factors. By increasing the distance between the heart and the chest wall, senile kyphosis and pulmonary hyperinflation in older individuals may contribute to a decrease of QRS voltage.

Despite the age-related decline in mean QRS amplitude, the prevalence of electrocardiographic LVH increases with age, probably secondary primarily to the high prevalence of hypertension, CAD, and degenerative aortic valvular disease in the elderly. Echocardiographic studies have demonstrated that the standard ECG is insensitive, although very specific, for anatomical LVH in older populations (107). In the Framingham study (107) and other older cohorts (108), ECG evidence of LVH was strongly related to the presence of hypertension and was a potent independent risk factor for future CV morbidity and mortality. Thus, the presence of ECG criteria for LVH in an older individual should generally trigger further diagnostic assessment, particularly echocardiography.

Although left and right bundle branch block (BBB) both increase in prevalence with age (109–111), these conduction defects should not be attributed to aging per se. In older populations, left BBB occurs only about half as often as right BBB. In contrast to its right-sided counterpart, left BBB is uncommon in the absence of CV disease. The prognosis of left BBB therefore reflects that of the underlying heart disease. Whereas left BBB portended a more ominous prognosis than right BBB in Framingham men, the two conduction defects had similar prognostic significance in women (109, 110). In older BLSA men with right BBB and no evident heart disease, neither exercise capacity nor CV events differed from those of age-matched controls over 8.4 years of mean follow-up (111). These findings suggest that right BBB in the absence of clinical heart disease in older men reflects a primary abnormality of the cardiac conduction system. Among 310 predominantly middle-aged individuals with BBB and no apparent heart disease, both left BBB and right BBB increased in prevalence with age, but neither was associated with increased total mortality over a 9.5-year mean follow-up (112). A nonspecific intraventricular conduction defect exceeding 120 ms occurred in only 1.9% of Framingham participants aged 70 years and older and, like left BBB, was strongly associated with clinical heart disease (113).

Q waves in two or more contiguous ECG leads are generally considered evidence of prior MI. In older, as in younger, populations, such Q waves are usually associated with clinical heart disease and increased cardiac mortality. Indeed, pathological Q waves may serve as the initial clue to the presence of CAD. Prior studies have shown that 25%–30% or more of acute infarctions are clinically silent (114–115). The incidence of such "silent" infarctions increases strikingly with age. Despite the absence of symptoms, these silent MIs portend a long-term risk of mortality similar to their symptomatic counterparts. Among the elderly, Q waves commonly occur in the absence of CAD. A QS complex in leads 3 and a VF may occasionally result from marked left-axis deviation. A pattern of poor R-wave progression in leads V_1 to V_3 is a normal age trend, because of the decrease in the initial 20 ms anterior QRS vector with age (116). Such a pattern may also result from obesity, chronic obstructive lung disease, and LVH, all of which are common in older populations.

Repolarization

Abnormalities involving the ST segment and T wave probably constitute the most prevalent age-associated findings on the ECG. In a study of 671 persons aged 70 years and older, nonspecific ST–T changes were the most common ECG abnormalities, occurring in 16% of individuals (116). In this sample and others, repolarization abnormalities were generally associated with clinical heart disease. Such an association may stem in part from the frequent use of digitalis and various antiarrhythmic drugs by elderly cardiac patients. Much of the reported increased risk attached to these nonspecific repolarization changes is likely due to the underlying heart disease that necessitated use of these cardiac medications. Even among clinically healthy older persons, however, minor ST-segment sagging or straightening is relatively common, although of questionable prognostic significance.

Reduction in the T-wave amplitude with age begins by the fourth decade (101). The spatial T-wave vector shifts leftward with age in concert with the leftward shift in QRS axis. Obesity magnifies these changes in the T waves, especially in men (101). Although isolated T wave flattening does not portend excess CV risk, definite T-wave inversion usually occurs in patients with organic heart disease and is associated with increased mortality.

In the large database of Mason et al. (99), the mean heart rate–corrected Q–T interval increased from 409 to 418 ms in women and from 391 to 407 ms in men between the third and the sixth decades. The prognostic significance of prolonged Q–T interval in apparently healthy older adults is controversial. Although no association between QTc prolongation and either sudden cardiac death or total mortality was found in the Framingham study (117), positive associations were reported in the CHS (118) and Rotterdam (119) studies. In the latter study, a QTc >456 ms in men and >470 ms in women was associated with a 2.5-fold increased risk of sudden death after adjustment for multiple CV risk factors (119). This risk was increased eightfold in persons younger than the mean age of 68 years, but only twofold in older individuals. Increased Q–T-interval dispersion, defined as the difference between the maximum and minimum QTc among the ECG leads, was also associated with a doubled risk of sudden death in this cohort (120). Table 1.2 summarizes those changes in resting ECG measurements thought to be secondary to normative aging.

Table 1.2 Normal age-associated changes in resting ECG measurements

Measurement	Change with age	Effect on mortality
R–R interval	No change	
P-wave duration	Minor increase	None
P–R interval	Increase	Possible increase
QRS duration	No change	
QRS axis	Leftward shift	None
QRS voltage	Decrease	None
Q–T interval	Minor increase	Probable increase
T-wave voltage	Decrease	None

Arrhythmias

An increase in the prevalence and complexity of both supraventricular and ventricular arrhythmias, whether detected by resting ECG, ambulatory monitoring, or exercise testing, is a hallmark of normal human aging.

Atrial arrhythmias

Isolated premature atrial ectopic beats (AEB) appear on the resting ECG in 5%–10% of individuals older than 60 years and are not generally associated with heart disease. Isolated AEB were detected in 6% of healthy BLSA volunteers older than 60 years at rest, in 39% during exercise testing, and in 88% during ambulatory 24-hour monitoring (121). Such isolated AEB on ambulatory monitoring, even if frequent, were not predictive of increased cardiac risk in this sample over a 10-year mean follow-up period (122). Among 1372 predominantly healthy persons ≥65 years old in the CHS, isolated AEB were found in 97% and were frequent in 18% of women and 28% of men (123).

Atrial fibrillation

Atrial fibrillation (AF) is found in approximately 3%–4% of subjects over age 60 (Table 1.3), a rate 10-fold higher than the general adult population (123, 124); the prevalence in octogenarians approaches 10%. Chronic AF is most commonly due to CAD and hypertensive heart disease, mitral valvular disorders, thyrotoxicosis, and sick sinus syndrome. The association between hyperthyroidism and AF is observed almost exclusively in the elderly (125); this arrhythmia may be the sole clinical manifestation of so-called apathetic hyperthyroidism in geriatric patients. In the Framingham population, AF without identifiable cause, i.e., lone AF, represented 17% of men and 6% of women with AF, with mean ages of 70.6 and 68.1 years, respectively (126). These individuals with lone AF suffered over four times as many strokes as those in sinus rhythm during long-term follow-up, although their rates of coronary events or congestive heart failure were

Table 1.3 Relationship of arrhythmias to age and mortality

Arrhythmia	Effect of age on prevalence	Effect on mortality[a]
Supraventricular ectopic beats	Increased	None
Paroxysmal supraventricular tachycardia	Increased	Probably none
Atrial fibrillation (chronic)	Increased	Increased
Ventricular ectopic beats	Increased	Possible increase if frequent
Ventricular tachycardia (short runs)	Increased	Probably none

Source: Manolio TA et al., *J Am Coll Cardiol*, 23, 916–925, 1994.
[a] *In healthy elders.*

not increased (126). Atrial flutter is a rare arrhythmia in any age group and is usually associated with organic heart disease.

Several age-associated physiological changes contribute to the high prevalence of AF among the elderly. As noted earlier, left atrial size increases modestly with age, providing an augmented late diastolic filling rate that appears to compensate for the age-related reduction in early filling. Among adults aged ≥65 years, in Olmsted County, Minnesota, who underwent clinically indicated echocardiography, both a larger left atrial volume and impaired early diastolic LV function were independent predictors of nonvalvular AF (127). In addition, both left and right atrial wavefront propagation velocities show strong inverse correlations with age, increasing the likelihood for intra-atrial reentry to occur in older individuals (128).

Paroxysmal AF also increases strikingly with age. Among CHS participants in sinus rhythm, short runs of AF were seen in ~3% of individuals during 24-hour ambulatory ECG monitoring (Table 1.3) (123). The incidence of postoperative AF, a major cause of morbidity and increased hospital costs, also rises steeply with age. Among 527 patients undergoing major elective thoracic surgery, age was the strongest predictor of postoperative AF; odds of this arrhythmia were increased 2.5-fold in persons ≥70 years old versus those <60 years (129). A study of 205 patients undergoing elective cardiac surgery demonstrated additive effects of age and left atrial volume on the 7-day incidence of postoperative AF (Figure 1.12) (130).

Paroxysmal supraventricular tachycardia

Short bursts of paroxysmal supraventricular tachycardia (PSVT) on a resting ECG are found in 1%–2% of normal individuals older than 65 years. Twenty-four-hour ambulatory monitoring studies have demonstrated short runs of PSVT (usually 3–5 beats) in 13%–50% of clinically

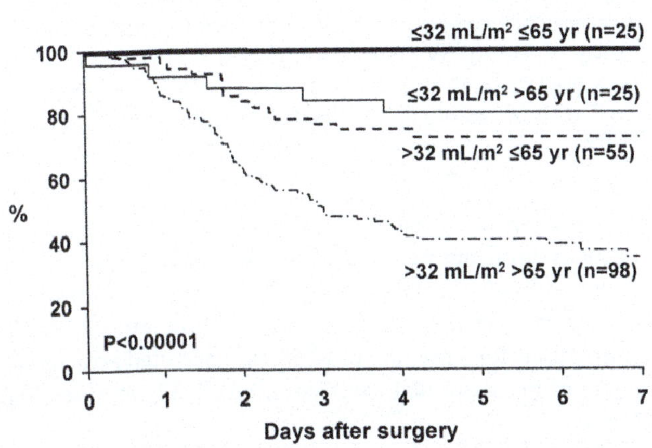

Figure 1.12 Freedom from postoperative atrial fibrillation after cardiac surgery as a function of age and left atrial volume in 205 patients. (From Osranek M et al., *J Am Coll Cardiol*, 48, 779–786, 2006.)

healthy older persons (Table 1.3) (123). Although the presence of nonsustained PSVT on ambulatory monitoring did not predict an increase in risk of future coronary events in BLSA participants, 2 of 13 individuals with PSVT later developed de novo AF, compared with only 1 of the 85 without PSVT (122). Exercise-induced PSVT has been observed in 3.5% of over 3000 maximal treadmill tests on apparently healthy BLSA volunteers (131). The arrhythmia increased sharply with age, from 0% in the 20s to approximately 10% in the 80s (Figure 1.13a); similar to PSVT on ambulatory ECG, the vast majority of these episodes were asymptomatic 3–5 beat salvos. Coronary risk factors and ECG or thallium scintigraphic evidence of ischemia occurred with similar prevalence in the 85 volunteers with exercise-induced PSVT as in age- and sex-matched controls. Of importance, the group with PSVT experienced no increase in subsequent coronary events over a 5.5-year mean follow-up period. However, 10% of the individuals with PSVT later developed a spontaneous atrial tachyarrhythmia compared with only 2% of controls (131), analogous to the results of the 24-hour ambulatory ECG.

Ventricular arrhythmias

Both in unselected populations and in those clinically free of heart disease, an exponential increase in the prevalence of ventricular ectopic beats (VEB) occurs with advancing age. Pooled data from nearly 2500 ECGs from hospitalized patients older than 70 years revealed VEB in 8% (132). Among apparently healthy BLSA volunteers with a normal ST-segment response to treadmill exercise, isolated VEB occurred at rest in 8.6% of men over age 60 years compared with only 0.5% in those 20–40 years old (121). Of note, the prevalence of resting VEB was not age related in women.

The prognostic significance of VEB detected on the resting ECG in the general elderly population is controversial. Significant increases in cardiac mortality among persons with VEB were observed in studies from Busselton (133) and Manitoba (134), with risk ratios of 3.3 and 2.4, respectively, compared with arrhythmia-free cohorts. The Framingham community, however, demonstrated no increase in the age-adjusted risk ratio for cardiac events (135). Data from the Multiple Risk Factor Intervention Trial suggest that the prognostic significance of resting VEB may vary according to age; asymptomatic White men under 50 years with frequent or complex VEB on a 2-minute resting rhythm strip suffered a 14-fold relative risk of sudden cardiac death, while in older men the risk was not significantly increased (136).

Twenty-four-hour ambulatory ECG recordings have demonstrated the presence of VEB in 69%–96% of asymptomatic elderly (122, 123). Not only the prevalence but also the density and complexity of VEB increase with age. In the CHS, VEB were found in 82% of 1372 subjects aged 65 years and older, including 7% with 3- to 5-beat runs of nonsustained ventricular tachycardia (VT). The prevalence of all VEB forms was higher in men than in women (Table 1.3) (123). Multiple studies have confirmed that the prevalence of both simple and complex VEB increases significantly with age in apparently healthy volunteers.

The prognostic importance of VEB detected on ambulatory monitoring, like those found on the resting ECG, is unclear. Over a 10-year mean follow-up period, 14 of 98 carefully screened older BLSA participants who underwent ambulatory ECG developed coronary events (122). The prevalence and complexity of VEB were virtually identical in the group that experienced an event and the group that did not. In contrast, horizontal or slowly upsloping ST-segment depression on the ambulatory ECG suggestive of silent ischemia predicted an increased risk of such events (122). However, in 456 Swedish men aged 68 years, frequent or complex VEB on 24-hour ECG were found in 35% of those without clinical CAD and predicted increased risk of myocardial infarction (MI) and CAD mortality over a 10.3-year mean follow-up (137). In 1139 older CHS volunteers with no history of heart failure and normal LV ejection fraction, those in the upper quartile of VEB frequency on 24-hour monitoring experienced a 48% higher risk of incident heart failure and 31% higher mortality over a 13.7-year median follow-up (138).

Exercise testing elicits a striking increase in the prevalence and complexity of VEB with advancing age similar to that seen on the ambulatory ECG (Figure 1.13b). In apparently healthy BLSA volunteers, isolated VEB during or after maximal treadmill exercise increased in prevalence from 11% to 57% between the third and ninth decades (121). Although LV mass index and peak exercise systolic blood pressure were higher in subjects who developed exercise-induced VEB than in those who did not, by multivariate analysis only older age independently predicted the appearance of VEB (139).

In a BLSA analysis of 1160 clinically healthy individuals who underwent an average of 2.4 maximal treadmill exercise tests per individual, 80 developed frequent VEB (≥10% of beats in any minute) or nonsustained VT on one or more tests (140). These 80 individuals were older than those free of such arrhythmias (64 vs. 50 years). Of note, the striking age-associated increase in the occurrence of these complex exercise-induced VEB was observed only in men (Figure 1.13b). The prevalence of coronary risk factors and exercise-induced ischemia by ECG and thallium scanning as well as the incidence of cardiac events (angina pectoris, nonfatal infarction, cardiac syncope, or cardiac death) were nearly identical in cases and controls matched for age and sex over a mean follow-up of 5.6 years without antiarrhythmic drug therapy (140). In contrast, over a 23-year follow-up of 6101 French men aged 42–53 years and initially free of clinical CV disease, frequent VEB during exercise predicted a 2.5-fold increased risk of CV death, independent of standard coronary risk factors (141).

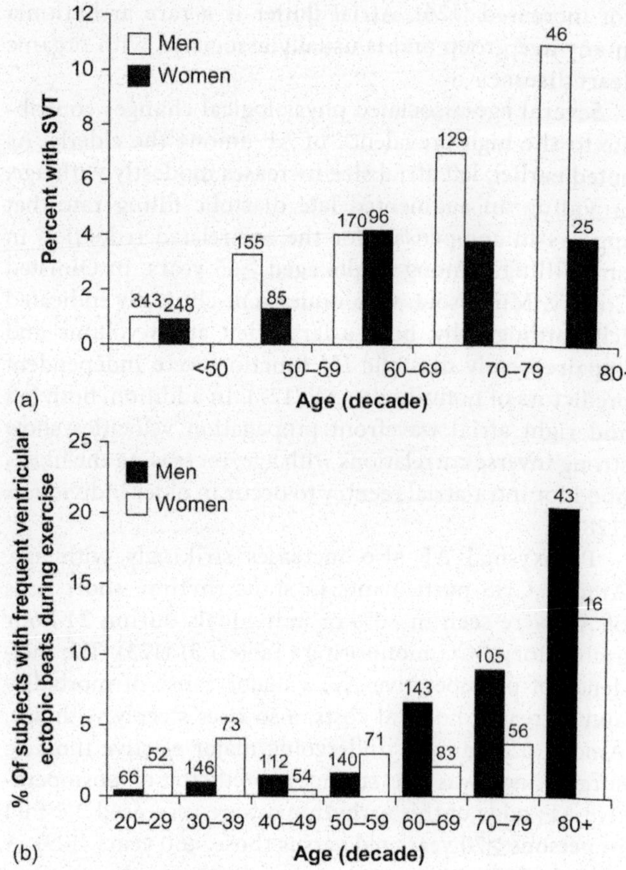

Figure 1.13 Increased prevalence of exercise-induced cardiac arrhythmias with age during the initial maximal treadmill exercise test in BLSA volunteers free from clinical cardiac disease. The numbers above each bar represent the number of persons in each age decade by gender. (a) Prevalence of exercise-induced nonsustained SVT as a function of age and sex in 1383 apparently healthy individuals. The age-associated increase in SVT prevalence was more pronounced in men ($p < 0.001$) than in women ($p = 0.09$). (b) Prevalence of frequent or repetitive ventricular ectopic beats in 1160 clinically healthy volunteers. A highly significant increase in prevalence was observed with age in men but not in women. *Abbreviations*: BLSA, Baltimore Longitudinal Study of Aging; SVT, supraventricular tachycardia. (From [a] Maurer MS et al., *Am J Cardiol*, 75, 788–792, 1995, [b] Busby MJ et al., *J Am Coll Cardiol*, 14, 1659–1665, 1989.)

Asymptomatic exercise-induced runs of VT, all <6 beats in duration, were found in 4% of apparently healthy BLSA individuals aged 65 and older, a rate 25 times that of younger persons (142). Extended follow-up of 81 such individuals for a median of 12.5 years detected no adverse effect of nonsustained exercise-induced VT on mortality (143).

Thus, the available data in older adults without apparent heart disease support a marked age-related increase in the prevalence and complexity of exercise-related VEB, at least in men; however, the prognosis conferred by frequent or repetitive VEB induced by exercise in such individuals is unclear.

A factor of major importance in determining the prognostic significance of VEB in the elderly is the milieu in which they occur. For example, among 467 patients aged 62–101 years in a long-term care facility, complex VEB occurred during 24-hour ambulatory monitoring in 21% (144). In the subset without clinical heart disease, future coronary events developed in an identical 4% of those individuals with or without complex VEB; among patients with CAD, however, such events developed in 46% with complex VEB but only 23% of patients without them. A similar doubling of risk was seen in patients with hypertension, valvular disease, or cardiomyopathy who demonstrated complex VEB. Table 1.3 summarizes the effect of age on the prevalence of various cardiac arrhythmias and their relationship to mortality in apparently healthy older adults (145).

In summary, aging is associated with multiple ECG changes in persons without evidence of CV disease. Such changes include a blunted respiratory sinus arrhythmia, a mild P–R interval prolongation, a leftward shift of the QRS axis, and increased prevalence, density, and

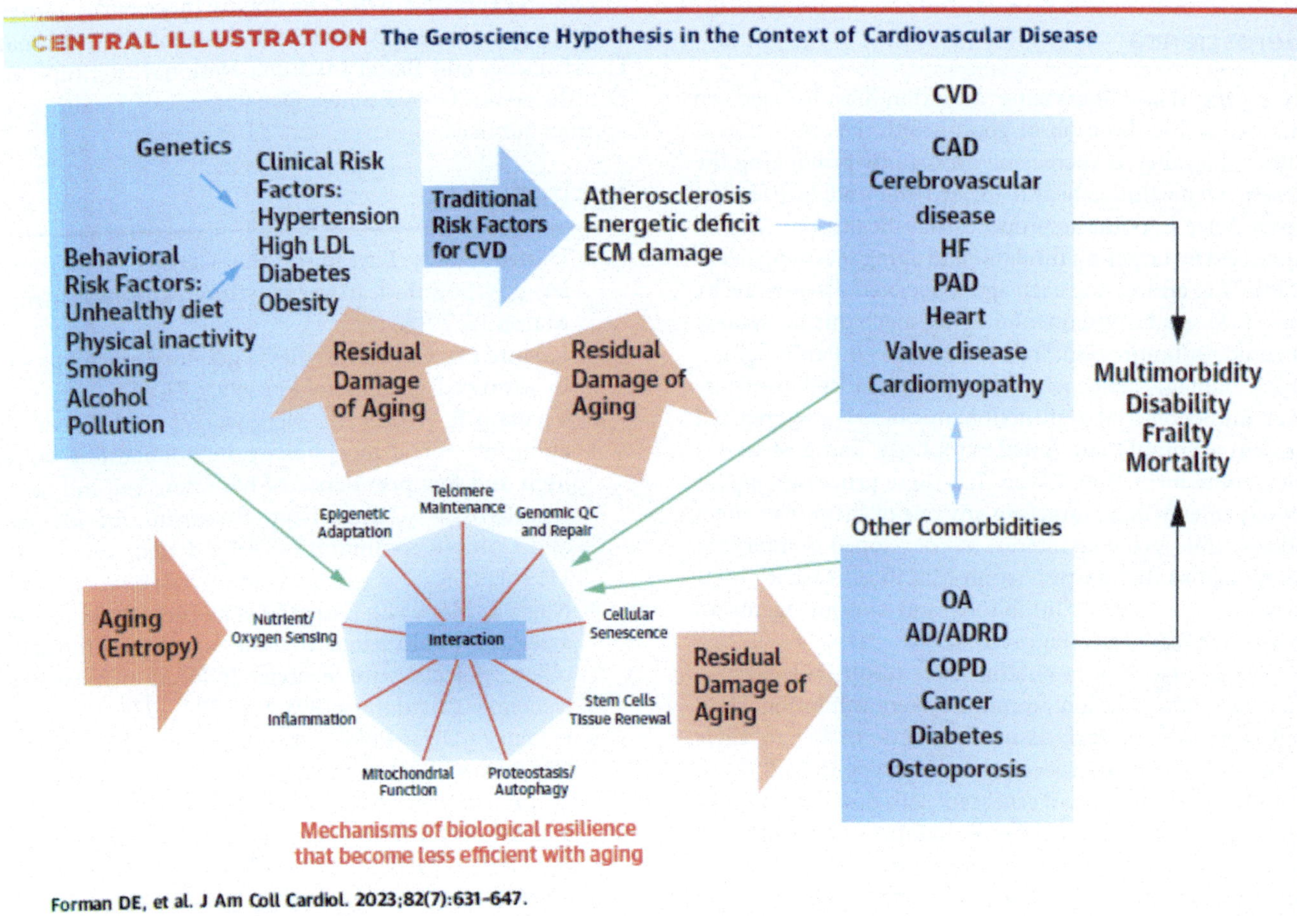

Genetic predisposition and unhealthy behaviors **(blue arrows)** contribute to major CVD risk factors and CVD in older persons. Aging itself is associated with stochastic damage to molecules and organelles **(pink arrows)** and accelerates risks of CVD, as well as multimorbidity, frailty, disability, and premature death. Whereas resilience signifies capacity to repair or replace such damaged components, resilience often diminishes over time, especially amid behavioral risk factors (eg, unhealthy diet) and chronic diseases **(green arrows)**. The geroscience hypothesis poses that enhancing resilience reduces the burden of CVD and other chronic diseases and related susceptibility to frailty and disability. AD/ADRD = Alzheimer disease and Alzheimer disease-related dementias; CAD = coronary heart disease; COPD = chronic obstructive pulmonary disease; CVD = cardiovascular disease; ECM = extracellular matrix; HF = heart failure; LDL = low-density lipoprotein; OA = osteoarthritis; PAD = peripheral arterial disease; QC = quality control.

Figure 1.14 Genetic predisposition combined with unhealthy behaviors (blue arrows) contribute to major CVD risk factors and CVD in older adults. Aging per se is associated with stochastic damage to molecules and organelles (pink arrows) and accelerates risks of CVD, multimorbidity, frailty, disability, and premature death. Although resilience indicates the capacity to repair or replace these damaged molecular and cellular components, resilience often diminishes over time, exacerbated by behavioral risk factors and chronic diseases (green arrows). The geroscience hypothesis posits that enhancing resilience reduces the burden of CVD and other chronic diseases and related susceptibility to frailty and disability.

complexity of ectopic beats, both atrial and ventricular. Although these findings generally do not affect prognosis in clinically healthy older adults, other findings that become more prevalent with age, such as increased QRS voltage, Q waves, Q–T interval prolongation, and ST–T-wave abnormalities, are generally associated with increased CV risk. Abnormalities such as left BBB or AF are strongly predictive of future cardiac morbidity and mortality among older adults, even if asymptomatic. A guiding principle for the practitioner is that the prognosis associated with a given ECG abnormality in older adults is more strongly related to the presence and severity of underlying CV disease than to the ECG finding itself.

Geroscience

In recent years, increasing attention has focused on enhancing the duration of good health, i.e., healthspan, rather than merely increasing lifespan by prolonging the period of declining health toward the end of life. The geroscience hypothesis proposes that healthspan can be increased by targeting fundamental aging mechanisms in contrast to addressing each age-associated disease one by one (146). Such fundamental aging mechanisms include chronic inflammation, often termed "inflammaging," DNA damage, epigenetic changes, stem cell dysfunction, mitochondrial dysfunction, misfolded or aggregated protein accumulation, failed autophagy, and destructive metabolite formation. Given that these processes appear closely intertwined, targeting any one of them may affect others. Thus, growing interest has developed in interventions such as dietary restriction (discussed earlier), metformin, other mTOR inhibitors, and various agents to target senescent cells (Figure 1.14).

Senescent cell accumulation can result in local and systemic inflammation, immune system inhibition, stem cell dysfunction, and tissue destruction, due to their senescence-associated secretory phenotype (SASP) (147). Between 30% and 70% of senescent cells develop this phenotype, involving release of proinflammatory, profibrotic, and proapoptotic cytokines, chemokines, tissue-destroying proteases, and other senescence-enhancing factors. A modest number of senescent cells can cause considerable dysfunction, presumably due to their SASP.

Cellular senescence contributes to multiple age-associated diseases over the lifespan. Although senescent cell burden is low in young adults, it increases with age in several tissues, including heart, lung, kidney, brain, skeletal muscle, bone, and adipose tissue, contributing to pulmonary fibrosis, cardiovascular disease, dementia, and other disorders (148, 149).

Interventions targeting fundamental aging processes have included dietary restriction, exercise training, metformin and other mTOR inhibitors, sirtuin agonists, SASP inhibitors, and senolytic agents. For example, exercise prevented senescent cell formation in mice, although it did not affect senescent cell formation in older adult cyclists (146). Bioinformatic approaches have identified over 20 agents that enhance critical senescent cell anti-apoptotic pathways that selectively eliminate senescent cells in mice and humans (148). Although clinical studies in man remain limited, several ongoing trials of senolytic drugs are addressing sequelae of Alzheimer's disease, osteoporosis, and other age-associated conditions. Figure 1.14 provides a schematic diagram focused on the geroscience hypothesis in the context of cardiovascular disease (150).

NOTE

The views expressed in this chapter are those of the author and do not necessarily represent those of the National Heart, Lung, and Blood Institute; National Institutes of Health; or the United States Department of Health and Human Services.

REFERENCES

1. United States Bureau of the Census. www.census.gov/population/www/estimates/popest.html. March 13, 2018.
2. Lakatta EG. Cardiovascular regulatory mechanisms in advanced age. *Physiol Rev* 1993; *73*: 413–467.
3. Virmani R, Avolio AP, Mergner WJ et al. Effect of aging on aortic morphology in populations with high and low prevalence of hypertension and atherosclerosis. Comparison between occidental and Chinese communities. *Am J Pathol* 1991; *139*: 1119–1129.
4. Nagai Y, Metter EJ, Earley CJ et al. Increased carotid artery intimal-medial thickness in asymptomatic older subjects with exercise-induced myocardial ischemia. *Circulation* 1998; *98*: 1504–1509.
5. O'Leary DH, Polak JF, Kronmal RA et al. Cardiovascular health study collaborative research group. Carotid artery intima and media thickness as a risk factor for myocardial infarction and stroke in older adults. *N Engl J Med* 1999; *340*: 14–22.
6. Stary HC, Blankenhorn DH, Bleakley CA et al. A definition of the intima of human arteries and its atherosclerosis-prone regions: A report from the committee on vascular lesions of the council on arteriosclerosis, American heart association. *Circulation* 1992; *85*: 391–405.
7. Spagnoli LG, Orlandi A, Mauriello A et al. Aging and atherosclerosis in the rabbit. Distribution, prevalence, and morphology of atherosclerotic lesions. *Atherosclerosis* 1991; *89*: 11–24.
8. Clarkson TB. Nonhuman primate models of atherosclerosis. *Lab Animal Sci* 1998; *48*: 569–572.
9. Heblad B, Wikstrand J, Janzon L et al. Low-dose metoprolol CR/XL and fluvastatin slow progression of carotid intima-media thickness. Main results from the b-blocker cholesterol lowering

asymptomatic plaque study (BCAPS). *Circulation* 2001; *103*: 1721–1726.

10. Lonn EM, Yusuf S, Dzavik V et al. Effects of ramipril and vitamin E on atherosclerosis. The study to evaluate carotid ultrasound changes in patients treated with ramipril and vitamin E (SECURE). For the SECURE investigators. *Circulation* 2001; *103*: 919–925.
11. Celermajer DS, Sorensen KE, Spiegelhalter DJ et al. Aging is associated with endothelial dysfunction in healthy men years before the age-related decline in women. *J Am Coll Cardiol* 1994; *24*: 471–476.
12. Bode-Boger SM, Muke J, Surdacki A et al. Oral L-arginine improves endothelial function in healthy individuals older than 70 years. *Vasc Med* 2003; *8*: 77–81.
13. Wang M, Khazan B, Lakatta EG. Central arterial aging and angiotensin II signaling. *Curr Hypertens Rev* 2010; *6*: 266–281.
14. Halcox JP, Schenke WH, Zalos G et al. Prognostic value of coronary vascular endothelial function. *Circulation* 2002; *106*: 653–658.
15. Taddei S, Virdis A, Mattei P et al. Hypertension causes premature aging of endothelial function in humans. *Hypertension* 1997; *29*: 736–743.
16. Taddei S, Virdis A, Mattei P et al. Defective L-arginine-nitric oxide pathway in offspring of essential hypertensive patients. *Circulation* 1996; *94*: 1298–1303.
17. Lakatta EG, Levy D. Arterial and cardiac aging: Major shareholders in cardiovascular disease enterprises. Part I: Aging arteries a "set up" for vascular disease. *Circulation* 2003; *107*: 139–146.
18. Vaitkevicius PV, Fleg JL, Engel JH et al. Effects of age and aerobic capacity on arterial stiffness in healthy adults. *Circulation* 1993; *88*: 1456–1462.
19. Willum-Hansen T, Staessen JA, Torp-Pedersen C et al. Prognostic value of aortic pulse wave velocity as index of arterial stiffness in the general population. *Circulation* 2006; *113*: 664–670.
20. Yin FCP. The aging vasculature and its effect on the heart. In: Weisdfeldt ML, ed. *The Aging Heart*. New York: Raven Press, 1980: pp. 137–214.
21. Avolio AP, Fa-Quan D, Wei-Qiang L et al. Effects of aging on arterial distensibility in populations with high and low prevalence of hypertension: Comparison between urban and rural communities. *Circulation* 1985; *71*: 201–210.
22. Graner M, Varpula M, Kahri J et al. Association of carotid intima-media thickness with angiographic severity and extent of coronary artery disease. *Am J Cardiol* 2006; *97*: 624–629.
23. Scuteri A, Najjar SS, Muller DC et al. Metabolic syndrome amplifies the age-associated increases in vascular thickness and stiffness. *J Am Coll Cardiol* 2004; *43*: 1388–1395.
24. Schofield I, Malik R, Izzard A et al. Vascular structural and functional changes in type 2 diabetes mellitus: Evidence for the roles of abnormal myogenic responsiveness and dyslipidemia. *Circulation* 2002; *106*: 3037–3043.
25. Chen CH, Nevo E, Fetics B et al. Estimation of central aortic pressure waveform by mathematical transformation of radial tonometry pressure. Validation of generalized transfer function. *Circulation* 1997; *95*: 1827–1836.
26. Kaess BM, Rong J, Larson MG et al. Aortic stiffness, blood pressure progression, and incident hypertension. *JAMA* 2012; *308*: 875–881.
27. Sutton-Tyrrell K, Najjar SS, Boudreau RM et al. Health ABC Study. Elevated aortic pulse wave velocity, a marker of arterial stiffness, predicts cardiovascular events in well-functioning older adults. *Circulation* 2005; *111*: 3384–3390.
28. Gerstenblith G, Frederiksen J, Yin FCP et al. Echocardiographic assessment of a normal adult aging population. *Circulation* 1977; *56*: 273–278.
29. Redheuil A, Yu W-C, Mousseaux E et al. Age-related changes in aortic arch geometry. *J Am Coll Cardiol* 2011; *58*: 1262–1270.
30. Aronow WS, Fleg JL, Pepine CJ et al. ACCF/AHA 2011 expert consensus document on hypertension in the elderly: A report of the American College of Cardiology Foundation Task Force on Clinical Expert Consensus Documents. *Circulation* 2011; *123*: 2434–2506.
31. O'Donnell CJ, Ridker PM, Glynn RJ et al. Hypertension and borderline isolated systolic hypertension increase risks of cardiovascular disease and mortality in male physicians. *Circulation* 1997; *95*: 1132–1137.
32. Franklin SS, Khan SA, Wong ND et al. Is pulse pressure useful in predicting risk for coronary heart disease? The Framingham Heart Study. *Circulation* 1999; *100*: 354–360.
33. Franklin SS, Larson MG, Khan SA et al. Does the relation of blood pressure to coronary heart disease risk change with aging? The Framingham Heart Study. *Circulation* 2001; *103*: 1245–1249.
34. Gurven M, Blackwell AD, Rodriguez SJ et al. Does blood pressure inevitably rise with age? Longitudinal evidence among forager-horticulturalists. *Hypertension* 2012; *60*: 25–33.
35. Wildman RP, Schott LL, Brockwell S et al. A dietary and exercise intervention slows menopause-associated progression of subclinical atherosclerosis as measured by intima-media thickness of the carotid arteries. *J Am Coll Cardiol* 2004; *44*: 579–585.
36. Tanaka H, Safar ME. Influence of lifestyle modification on arterial stiffness and wave reflections. *Am J Hypertens* 2005; *18*: 137–144.
37. Hamdy O, Ledbury S, Mullooly C et al. Lifestyle modification improves endothelial function in

obese subjects with the insulin resistance syndrome. *Diabetes Care* 2003; *26*: 2119–2125.
38. Meyer TE, Kovacs SJ, Ehsani AA et al. Long-term caloric restriction ameliorates the decline in diastolic function in humans. *J Am Coll Cardiol* 2006; *47*: 398–402.
39. Huang W, Alhenc Gelas F, Osborne-Pellegrin MJ. Protection of the arterial internal elastic lamina by inhibition of the renin–angiotensin system in the rat. *Circ Res* 1998; *82*: 879–890.
40. Gonzalez Bosc LV, Kurnjek ML, Muller A et al. Effect of chronic angiotensin II inhibition on the nitric oxide synthase in the normal rat during aging. *J Hypertens* 2001; *19*: 1403–1409.
41. Ferder LF, Inserra F, Basso N. Advances in our understanding of aging: Role of the renin-angiotensin system. *Curr Opin Pharmacol* 2002; *2*: 189–194.
42. Vaitkevicius PV, Lane M, Spurgeon H et al. A cross-link breaker has sustained effects on arterial and ventricular properties in older rhesus monkeys. *Proc Natl Acad Sci USA* 2001; *98*: 1171–1175.
43. Kass DA, Shapiro EP, Kawaguchi M et al. Improved arterial compliance by a novel advanced glycation end-product crosslink breaker. *Circulation* 2004; *104*: 1464–1470.
44. Linzbach AJ, Kuamoa-Boateng E. Die alternsveranderungen des menschlichen herzen. 1. Das herzgewicht im alter. *Klin Wochenschr* 1973; *51*: 156–163.
45. Kitzman DW, Scholz DG, Hagen PT et al. Age-related changes in normal human hearts during the first ten decades. Part 2 (Maturity). A quantitative anatomic study of 765 specimens from subjects 20 to 99 years old. *Mayo Clin Proc* 1988; *63*: 137–146.
46. Olivetti G, Melissari M, Capasso JM et al. Cardiomyopathy of the aging human heart: Myocyte loss and reactive cellular hypertrophy. *Circ Res* 1991; *68*: 1560–1568.
47. Olivetti G, Giordano G, Corradi D et al. Gender differences and aging: Effects in the human heart. *J Am Coll Cardiol* 1995; *26*: 1068–1079.
48. Gardin JM, Henry WL, Savage DD et al. Echocardiographic measurements in normal subjects: Evaluation of an adult population without clinically apparent heart disease. *J Clin Ultrasound* 1979; *7*: 439–447.
49. Hees PS, Fleg JL, Lakatta EG et al. Left ventricular remodeling with age in normal men versus women: Novel insights using three-dimensional magnetic resonance imaging. *Am J Cardiol* 2002; *90*: 1231–1236.
50. Khouri MG, Maurer MS, Rumberger LE et al. Assessment of age-related changes in LV structure and function by freehand three-dimensional echocardiography. *Am J Geriatr Cardiol* 2005; *14*: 118–125.
51. Cheng S, Fernandes VRS, Bluemke DA et al. Age-related left ventricular remodeling and associated risk for cardiovascular outcomes. The Multi-Ethnic Study of Atherosclerosis. *Circ Cardiovasc Imaging* 2009; *2*: 191–198.
52. Yoneyama K, Donekai S, Venkatesh BA et al. Natural history of myocardial function in an adult human population. Serial longitudinal observations from MESA. *J Am Coll Cardiol Img* 2016; *9*: 1164–1173.
53. Anversa P, Palackal T, Sonnenblick EH et al. Myocyte cell loss and myocyte cellular hyperplasia in the hypertrophied aging rat heart. *Circ Res* 1990; *67*: 871–885.
54. Esler MD, Turner AG, Kaye DM et al. Aging effects on human sympathetic neuronal function. *Am J Physiol* 1995; *268*: R278–R285.
55. Lakatta EG. Deficient neuroendocrine regulation of the cardiovascular system with advancing age in healthy humans. *Circulation* 1993; *87*: 631–636.
56. Rodeheffer RJ, Gerstenblith G, Becker LC et al. Exercise cardiac output is maintained with advancing age in healthy human subjects. *Circulation* 1984; *69*: 203–213.
57. Lakatta EG, Gerstenblith G, Angell CS et al. Prolonged contraction duration in aged myocardium. *J Clin Invest* 1975; *55*: 61–68.
58. Dalen H, Thorstensen A, Aase SA et al. Segmental and global longitudinal strain and strain rate based on echocardiography of 1266 healthy individuals: The HUNT study in Norway. *Eur J Echocardiogr* 2010; *11*: 176–183.
59. Miyatake K, Okamoto J, Kimoshita N et al. Augmentation of atrial contribution left ventricular flow with aging as assessed by intracardiac Doppler flowmetry. *Am J Cardiol* 1984; *53*: 587–589.
60. Schulman SP, Lakatta EG, Fleg JL et al. Age-related decline in left ventricular filling at rest and exercise. *Am J Physiol* 1992; *263*: H1932–H1938.
61. Hees PS, Fleg JL, Dong S-J et al. MRI and echocardiographic assessment of the diastolic dysfunction of normal aging: Altered LV pressure decline or load? *Am J Physiol Heart Circ Physiol* 2004; *286*: H782–H788.
62. Fujimoto N, Prasad A, Hastings JL et al. Cardiovascular effects of one year of progressive and vigorous exercise training in previously sedentary individuals older than 65 years of age. *Circulation* 2010; *122*: 1797–1805.
63. Neilan TG, Coelho-Filho OR, Shah RV et al. Myocardial extracellular volume fraction from T1 measurements in healthy volunteers and mice. *J Am Coll Cardiol Img* 2013; *6*: 672–683.
64. Froehlich JP, Lakatta EG, Beard E et al. Studies of sarcoplasmic reticulum function and contraction duration in young and aged rat myocardium. *J Mol Cell Cardiol* 1978; *10*: 427–438.

65. Chahal H, Johnson C, Tandri H et al. Relation of cardiovascular risk factors to right ventricular structure and function as determined by magnetic resonance imaging (results from the Multi-Ethnic Study of Atherosclerosis). *Am J Cardiol* 2010; *106*: 110–116.
66. Lam CSP, Borlaug BA, Kane GC et al. Age-associated increases in pulmonary artery systolic pressure in the general population. *Circulation* 2009; *119*: 2663–2670.
67. Wolsk E, Bakkestram R, Thomsen JH et al. The influence of age on hemodynamic parameters during rest and exercise in healthy individuals. *J Am Coll Cardiol HF* 2017; *5*: 337–346.
68. Rutan GH, Hermanson B, Bild DE et al. Orthostatic hypotension in older adults: The Cardiovascular Health Study. *Hypertension* 1992; *19*: 508–519.
69. Masaki KH, Schatz IJ, Burchfiel CM et al. Orthostatic hypotension predicts mortality in elderly men. The Honolulu Heart Program. *Circulation* 1998; *98*: 2290–2295.
70. Gottdiener JS, Yanez D, Rautaharju P et al. Orthostatic hypotension in the elderly: Contributions of impaired LV filling and altered sympathovagal balance. *Am J Geriatr Cardiol* 2000; *9*: 273–280.
71. Lipsitz LA, Jonsson PV, Marks BL et al. Reduced supine cardiac volumes and diastolic filling rates in elderly patients with chronic medical conditions: Implications for postural blood pressure homeostasis. *J Am Geriatr Soc* 1990; *38*: 103–107.
72. Gribben B, Pickering T, Sleight P et al. Effect of age and high blood pressure on baroreflex sensitivity in man. *Circ Res* 1971; *29*: 424.
73. Rodeheffer RJ, Gerstenblith G, Beard E et al. Postural changes in cardiac volumes in men in relation to adult age. *Exp Gerontol* 1986; *21*: 367–378.
74. Swinne CJ, Shapiro EP, Lima SD et al. Age-associated changes in cardiac performance during isometric exercise in normal subjects. *Am J Cardiol* 1992; *69*: 823–826.
75. Yin FC, Raizes GS, Guarnieri T et al. Age-associated decreases in ventricular response to hemodynamic stress during β-adrenergic blockade. *Br Heart J* 1978; *40*: 1349–1355.
76. Fleg JL, Lakatta EG. Role of muscle loss in the age-associated reduction in VO_2max. *J Appl Physiol* 1988; *65*: 1147–1151.
77. Talbot LA, Metter EJ, Fleg JL. Leisure-time physical activities and their relationship to cardiorespiratory fitness in healthy men and women 18–95 years old. *Med Sci Sports Exerc* 2000; *32*: 417–425.
78. Fleg JL, Morrell CH, Bos AG et al. Accelerated longitudinal decline of aerobic capacity in healthy older adults. *Circulation* 2005; *112*: 674–682.
79. AlGhatrif M, Morrell CH, Fleg JL et al. The longitudinal decline in peak VO2 with aging in a healthy population is associated with a reduction in peripheral oxygen utilization but not in cardiac output. *Am J Physiol Heart Circ Physiol* 2024; 327: H509H517.
80. Fried LP, Taugen CM, Walston J et al. CHS Collaborative Research Group. Frailty in older adults: Evidence for a phenotype. *J Gerontol* 2001; *56A*: M158–M166.
81. Woo JS, Derleth C, Stratton JR et al. The influence of age, gender, and training on exercise efficiency. *J Am Coll Cardiol* 2006; *47*: 1049–1057.
82. Fleg JL, O'Connor FC, Gerstenblith G et al. Impact of age on the cardiovascular response to dynamic upright exercise in healthy men and women. *J Appl Physiol* 1995; *78*: 890–900.
83. Huang G, Gibson CA, Tran ZV et al. Controlled endurance exercise training and VO_2max changes in older adults: A meta-analysis. *Prev Cardiol* 2005; *8*: 217–225.
84. Schulman SP, Fleg JL, Goldberg AP et al. Continuum of cardiovascular performance across a broad range of fitness levels in healthy older men. *Circulation* 1996; *94*: 359–367.
85. Tanaka H, DeSouza CA, Seals DR. Absence of age-related increase in central arterial stiffness in physically active women. *Arterioscler Thromb Vasc Biol* 1998; *18*: 127–132.
86. Fleg JL, Schulman SP, Gerstenblith G et al. Additive effects of age and silent myocardial ischemia on the left ventricular response to upright cycle exercise. *J Appl Physiol* 1993; *75*: 499–504.
87. Najjar SS, Schulman SP, Gerstenblith G et al. Age and gender affect ventricular-vascular coupling during aerobic exercise. *J Am Coll Cardiol* 2004; *44*: 611–617.
88. Nussbacher A, Gerstenblith G, O'Connor F et al. Hemodynamic effects of unloading the old heart. *Am J Physiol* 1999; *277*: H1863–H1871.
89. White M, Roden R, Minobe W et al. Age-related changes in beta-adrenergic neuroeffector systems in the human heart. *Circulation* 1994; *90*: 1225–1238.
90. Correia LCL, Lakatta EG, O'Connor FC et al. Attenuated cardiovascular reserve during prolonged submaximal exercise in healthy older subjects. *J Am Coll Cardiol* 2002; *40*: 1290–1297.
91. Fleg JL, Schulman S, O'Connor F et al. Effects of acute β-adrenergic receptor blockade on age-associated changes in cardiovascular performance during dynamic exercise. *Circulation* 1994; *90*: 2333–2341.
92. Hiss RG, Lamb LE. Electrocardiographic findings in 122,043 individuals. *Circulation* 1962; *25*: 947–961.
93. Pfeifer MA, Weinberg CR, Cook D et al. Differential changes of autonomous nervous system function with age in men. *Am J Med* 1983; *75*: 249–258.
94. Byrne EA, Fleg JL, Vaitkevicius PV et al. Role of aerobic capacity and body mass index in the age-associated decline in heart rate variability. *J Appl Physiol* 1996; *81*: 743–750.

95. Dekker JM, Crow RS, Folsom AA et al. Low heart rate variability in a 2-minute rhythm strip predicts risk of coronary heart disease and mortality from several causes. The ARIC study. *Circulation* 2000; *102*: 1239–1244.
96. Felber-Dietrich D, Schindler C, Schwartz J et al. Heart rate variability in an ageing population and its association with lifestyle and cardiovascular risk factors, results of the SAPALDI Study. *Europace* 2006; *8*: 521–529.
97. Tresch DD, Fleg JL. Unexplained sinus bradycardia: Clinical significance and long-term prognosis in apparently healthy persons older than 40 years. *Am J Cardiol* 1986; *58*: 1009–1013.
98. Aronow WS, Schwartz KS, Koenigsberg M. Prevalence of enlarged left atrial dimension by echocardiography and its correlation with atrial fibrillation and an abnormal P terminal force in lead VI of the electrocardiogram in 588 elderly persons. *Am J Cardiol* 1987; *59*: 1003–1004.
99. Mason JW, Ramseth DJ, Chanter DO et al. Electrocardiographic reference ranges derived from 79,743 ambulatory subjects. *J Electrocardiol* 2007; *40*: 228–234.
100. Fleg JL, Das DN, Wright J et al. Age-associated changes in the components of atrioventricular conduction in apparently healthy volunteers. *J Gerontol* 1990; *45*: M95–M100.
101. Simonson E. The effect of age on the electrocardiogram. *Am J Cardiol* 1972; *29*: 64–73.
102. Mymin D, Mathewson FA, Tate RB et al. The natural history of primary first-degree atrioventricular heart block. *N Engl J Med* 1986; *315*: 1183–1187.
103. Cheng S, Keyes MJ, Larson MG et al. Long-term outcomes in individuals with prolonged PR interval or first-degree atriventricular block. *JAMA* 2009; *301*: 2571–2577.
104. Golden GS, Golden LH. The "nona" electrocardiogram: Findings in 100 patients of the 90 age group. *J Am Geriatr Soc* 1974; *22*: 329–331.
105. Ostrander LD. Left axis deviation: Prevalence, associated conditions and prognosis. An epidemiologic study. *Ann Intern Med* 1971; *75*: 23–28.
106. Harlan WR Jr, Graybiel A, Mitchell RE et al. Serial electrocardiograms: Their reliability and prognostic validity during a 24-yr period. *J Chronic Dis* 1967; *20*: 853–867.
107. Levy D, Garrison RJ, Savage DD et al. Left ventricular mass and incidence of coronary heart disease in an elderly cohort. The Framingham Heart Study. *Ann Intern Med* 1989; *110*: 101–107.
108. Sunderstrom J, Lind L, Arnlov J. Echocardiographic and electrocardiographic diagnoses of left ventricular hypertrophy predict mortality independently of each other in a population of elderly men. *Circulation* 2001; *103*: 2346–2351.
109. Schneider JF, Thomas HE Jr, Kreger BE et al. Newly acquired right bundle branch block: The Framingham Study. *Ann Intern Med* 1980; *92*: 37–44.
110. Schneider JF, Thomas HE Jr, Kreger BE et al. Newly acquired left bundle branch block: The Framingham Study. *Ann Intern Med* 1979; *90*: 303–310.
111. Fleg JL, Das DN, Lakatta EG. Right bundle block: Long-term prognosis in apparently healthy men. *J Am Coll Cardiol* 1983; *1*: 887–892.
112. Fahy GJ, Pinski SL, Miller DP et al. Natural history of isolated bundle branch block. *Am J Cardiol* 1996; *77*: 1185–1190.
113. Kreger BE, Anderson KM, Kannel WB. Prevalence of intraventricular block in the general population: The Framingham Study. *Am Heart J* 1989; *117*: 903–910.
114. Kannel WB, Abbott RD. Incidence and prognosis of unrecognized myocardial infarction. An update on the Framingham Study. *N Engl J Med* 1984; *311*: 1144–1147.
115. Yano K, MacLean CJ. The incidence and prognosis of unrecognized myocardial infarction in the Honolulu Hawaii Heart Program. *Arch Intern Med* 1989; *149*: 1528–1532.
116. Mihalick MU, Fisch C. Electrocardiographic findings in the aged. *Am Heart J* 1974; *87*: 117–128.
117. Goldberg RJ, Bengston J, Chen ZY et al. Duration of the QT interval and total and cardiovascular mortality in healthy persons (the Framingham Heart Study experience). *Am J Cardiol* 1991; *67*: 55–58.
118. Robbins J, Nelson JC, Rautaharju PM et al. The association between the length of the QT interval and mortality in the Cardiovascular Health Study. *Am J Med* 2003; *115*: 689–694.
119. Strauss SM, Kors JA, DeBruyne MC et al. Prolonged QTc interval and risk of sudden cardiac death in a population of older adults. *J Am Coll Cardiol* 2006; *47*: 362–367.
120. DeBruyne MC, Hoes AW, Kors JA et al. QTc dispersion predicts cardiac mortality in the elderly: The Rotterdam Study. *Circulation* 1998; *97*: 467–472.
121. Fleg JL. Epidemiology of ventricular arrhythmias in the elderly. In: Paciaroni E, ed. *Proceedings of the 13th National Congress of Cardiology (Aging and Cardiac Arrhythmias)* I.N.R.C.A. Ancona: Istituto a Carattere Scientifico, 1991: pp. 26–30.
122. Fleg JL, Kennedy HL. Long-term prognostic significance of ambulatory electrocardiographic findings in apparently healthy subjects 60 years of age. *Am J Cardiol* 1992; *70*: 748–751.
123. Manolio TA, Furberg CD, Rautaharju PM et al. Cardiac arrhythmias on 24-hour ambulatory electrocardiography in older women and men: The Cardiovascular Health Study. *J Am Coll Cardiol* 1994; *23*: 916–925.

124. Kannel WB, Abbott RD, Savage DD et al. Epidemiologic features of chronic atrial fibrillation. *N Engl J Med* 1982; *306*: 1018–1022.
125. Staffurth JS, Gibberd MC, Fui SN. Arterial embolism in thyrotoxicosis with atrial fibrillation. *Br Med J* 1977; *2*: 688–690.
126. Brand FN, Abbott RD, Kannel WB et al. Characteristics and prognosis of lone atrial fibrillation. 30-Year follow-up in the Framingham study. *JAMA* 1985; *254*: 3449–3453.
127. Tsang TSM Gersh BJ, Appleton CP et al. Left ventricular diastolic dysfunction as a predictor of the first diagnosed nonvalvular atrial fibrillation in 840 elderly men and women. *J Am Coll Cardiol* 2002; *40*: 1636–1644.
128. Kojodjojo P, Kanagaratnam P, Markides V et al. Age-related changes in human left and right atrial conduction. *J Cardiovasc Electrophysiol* 2006; *17*: 120–127.
129. Amar D, Zhang H, Leung DH et al. Older age is the strongest predictor of postoperative atrial fibrillation. *Anesthesiology* 2002; *96*: 352–356.
130. Osranek M, Fatema K, Qaddoura F et al. Left atrial volume predicts the risk of atrial fibrillation after cardiac surgery. *J Am Coll Cardiol* 2006; *48*: 779–786.
131. Maurer MS, Shefrin EA, Fleg JL. Prevalence and prognostic significance of exercise-induced supraventricular tachycardia in apparently healthy volunteers. *Am J Cardiol* 1995; *75*: 788–792.
132. Fisch C. Electrocardiogram in the aged. An independent marker of heart disease? *Am J Med* 1981; *70*: 4–6.
133. Cullen KJ, Stenhouse NS, Wearne KL et al. Electrocardiograms and thirteen year cardiovascular mortality in Busselton Study. *Br Heart J* 1982; *47*: 209–212.
134. Rabkin SW, Mathewson FAL, Tate RB. Relationship of ventricular ectopy in men without apparent heart disease to occurrence of ischemic heart disease and sudden death. *Am Heart J* 1981; *101*: 135–142.
135. Kannel WB, Doyle JT, McNamara PM et al. Precursors of sudden death: Factors related to the incidence of sudden death. *Circulation* 1975; *57*: 606–613.
136. Abdalla ISH, Prineas RJ, Neaton JD et al. Relations between ventricular premature complexes and sudden cardiac death in apparently healthy men. *Am J Cardiol* 1987; *60*: 1036–1042.
137. Hedblad B, Janzon L, Johansson BW et al. Survival and incidence of myocardial infarction in men with ambulatory ECG-detected frequent and complex ventricular arrhythmias. *Eur Heart J* 1997; *18*: 1787–1795.
138. Dukes JW, Dewland TA, Vittinghoff E et al. Ventricular ectopy as a predictor of heart failure and death. *J Am Coll Cardiol* 2015; *66*: 101–109.
139. Mayuga R, Arrington CT, O'Connor FC et al. Why do exercise-induced ventricular arrhythmias increase with age? Role of M-mode echocardiographic aging changes. *J Gerontol Med Sci* 1996; *51A*: M23–M28.
140. Busby MJ, Shefrin EA, Fleg JL. Prevalence and long-term prognostic significance of exercise-induced frequent or repetitive ventricular ectopic beats in apparently healthy volunteers. *J Am Coll Cardiol* 1989; *14*: 1659–1665.
141. Jouven X, Zureik M, Desnos M et al. Long-term outcome in asymptomatic men with exercise-induced premature ventricular depolarizations. *N Engl J Med* 2000; *343*: 826–833.
142. Fleg JL, Lakatta EG. Prevalence and prognosis of exercise-induced nonsustained ventricular tachycardia in apparently healthy volunteers. *Am J Cardiol* 1984; *54*: 762–764.
143. Marine JE, Shetty V, Chow GV et al. Prognostic significance of exercise-induced nonsustained ventricular tachycardia in asymptomatic volunteers. *J Am Coll Cardiol* 2013; *62*: 595–600.
144. Aronow WS, Epstein S, Koenigsberg M et al. Usefulness of echocardiographic abnormal left ventricular ejection fraction, paroxysmal ventricular tachycardia, and complex ventricular arrhythmias in predicting new coronary events in patients over 62 years of age. *Am J Cardiol* 1988; *61*: 1349–1351.
145. Fleg JL. Arrhythmias and conduction disorders. In: Beers MH, Berkow R, eds. *The Merck Manual of Geriatrics*, 3rd ed. Whitehouse Station, NJ: Merck Research Laboratories, 2000: pp. 885–900.
146. Tchkonia T, Palmer AK, Kirkland JL. New horizons: Novel approaches to enhance healthspan through targeting Jour Clin cellular senescence and related aging mechanisms. *J. Clin Endocrin & Metab* 2021; 106: e1481–e1487.
147. Prata LGPL, Ovsyannikova IG, Tchkonia T, Kirkland JL. Senescent cell clearance in the immune system: Emerging therapeutic opportunities. *Semin Immunol* 2018; 40: 101275.
148. Wissler Gerdes EO, Zhu Y, Tchkonia T, Kirkland JL. Discovery, development, and future applications of senolytics: Theories and predictions. *FABSJ* 2020; 287: 2418–2427.
149. Vakka A, Warren JS, Drosatos K. Cardiovascular aging: From cellular and molecular changes to therapeutic interventions. *J Cardiovasc Aging* 2023; 3: 23. http://dx.doi.org/10.20517/jca.2023.09; PMID: 37274126.
150. Forman DE, Kuchel GA, Newman JC et al. Impact of geroscience on therapeutic strategies for older adults with cardiovascular disease. JACC Scientific Statement. *J Am Coll Cardiol* 2023; 82: 631–647.

2

Morphologic features and pathology of the aging heart

GREGORY A. FISHBEIN, ATSUKO SEKI, AND MICHAEL C. FISHBEIN

Key points

- As we age, cardiovascular structures undergo functional and structural changes that contribute to increased morbidity and mortality.
- Common age-related vascular lesions include atherosclerosis, medial calcific sclerosis (Mönckeberg's sclerosis), intimal hyperplasia, and medial hypertrophy.
- Aging-related valvular conditions include aortic stenosis, myxomatous degeneration, and mitral annular calcification.
- More than half of patients with takotsubo (stress) cardiomyopathy are over age 65.
- The most common cardiac amyloidoses involve misfolded light chains (AL) and transthyretin (ATTR), both of which are more prevalent in older individuals.

INTRODUCTION

As we age, there are numerous functional and structural changes that occur in the cardiovascular system contributing to increasing morbidity and mortality. In the United States more than a third of people over 65 report having some form of cardiovascular disease (1). This chapter reviews the major age-related changes and conditions that affect the cardiovascular system.

NONSPECIFIC CHANGES OF AGING

Some aging changes in the heart may occur in the absence of specific heart diseases. As discussed in Chapter 1, with aging there is a decrease in the functional reserve of the heart. In addition, there are major age-related structural changes, such as coronary atherosclerosis, left ventricular hypertrophy, and atrial dilatation, which predispose to conditions such as heart failure and arrhythmias (Figure 2.1) (2, 3). The number of myocytes of both ventricles decreases gradually in men and is associated with hypertrophy of the remaining myocytes; notably, no similar finding occurs in women (4).

Many consider the heart to be quite exceptional in that heart weight remains almost constant through adult life (5), while most organ weights, such as liver, kidneys, and spleen, decrease significantly with advancing age. Mean heart weight is comparable in young, middle-aged, and older adults (6). Among individuals with no apparent cardiovascular disease, some studies indicate that total heart weight, including non-myocardial components such

DOI: 10.1201/9781003568933-2

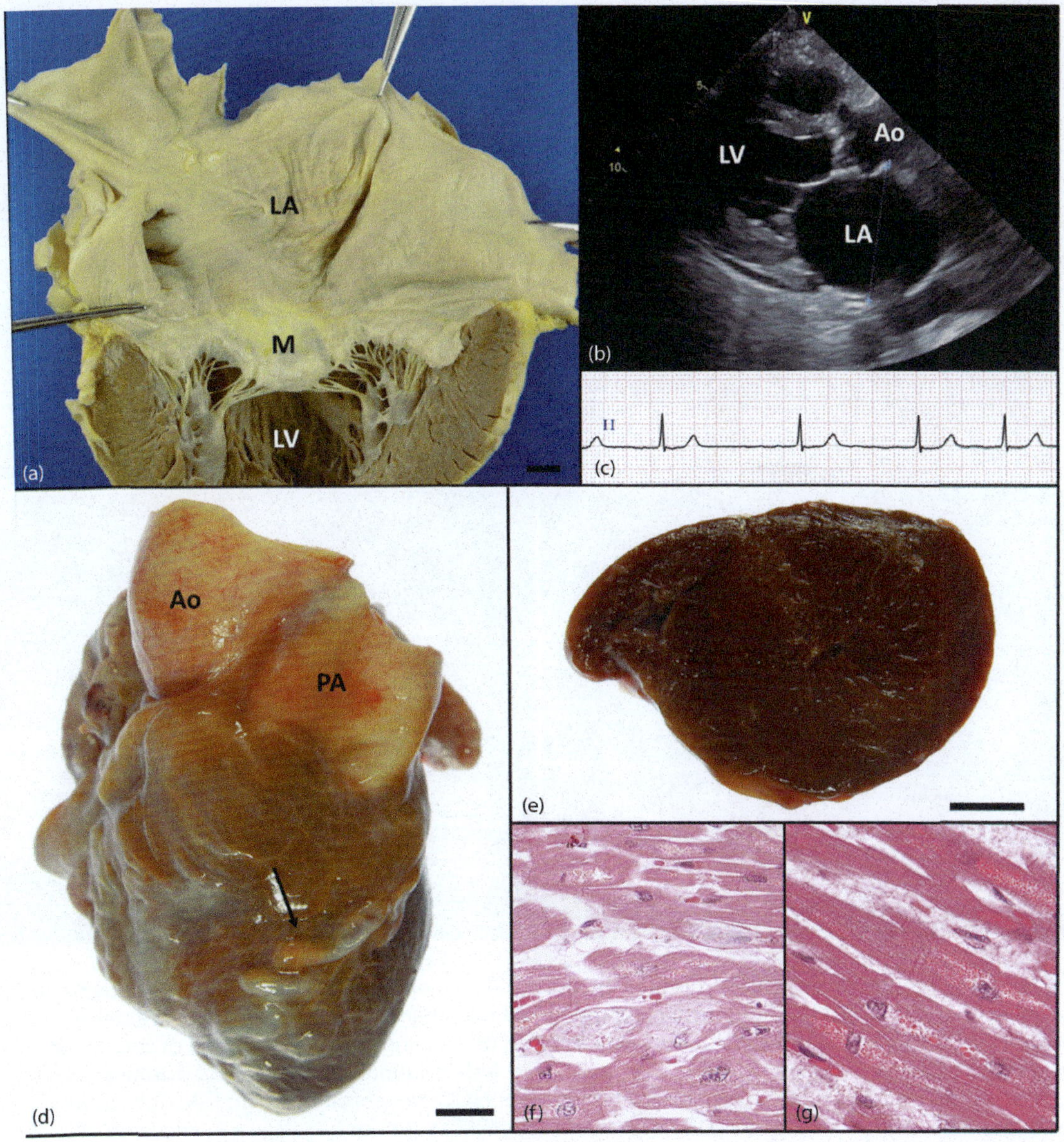

Figure 2.1 Common cardiac changes in older adults: (a) The dilated left atrium (LA) from a 93-year-old male; (b) the parasternal long axis view of a two-dimensional echocardiogram from the same patient showing dilatation of the LA (58.4 mm); and (c) this same patient also had atrial fibrillation. (d) An atrophic heart from a 100-year-old male (heart weight = 181 grams). Gelatinous changes in the epicardium (serous atrophy of fat) with tortuous coronary arteries (black arrow). Note the ascending aorta (Ao) and pulmonary artery (PA) appear disproportionately large compared to the size of the heart. (e) A transverse section of the same heart showing brown atrophy. (f) Basophilic degeneration (basophilic, finely granular materials). (g) Increased lipofuscin pigments (brown granules) of cardiomyocytes (H&E stain, ×400). *Abbreviations*: Ao, aorta; LA, left atrium; LV, left ventricle; M, mitral valve; PA, pulmonary artery. Scale bar, 1 cm. (Courtesy of Dr. Tomio Arai and Koji Chida, Tokyo Metropolitan Geriatric Hospital.)

as pericardium, coronary arteries, and valves, does not change significantly with aging (7). However, atrophy of the heart and hypertrophy of the heart do occur in older individuals. Indeed, in one study, ventricular myocardial weight gradually decreased in men, but remained constant in women at advanced age (4). There are conflicting reports of dimensional changes with aging in the heart, in part because numerous conditions that may or may not be associated with aging affect cardiac dimensions.

There are definite functional and dimensional changes that occur in the cardiovascular system with aging. Left ventricular diastolic dysfunction increases after the age of 20 years. In contrast, left ventricular systolic function is preserved in healthy older adults (3). Atrial systolic pressure increases with aging (3, 8). The "normal" aged heart, that is, the heart without any significant cardiovascular diseases, has relatively smaller ventricular cavities and larger atria than the younger adult heart (3, 7, 9, 10).

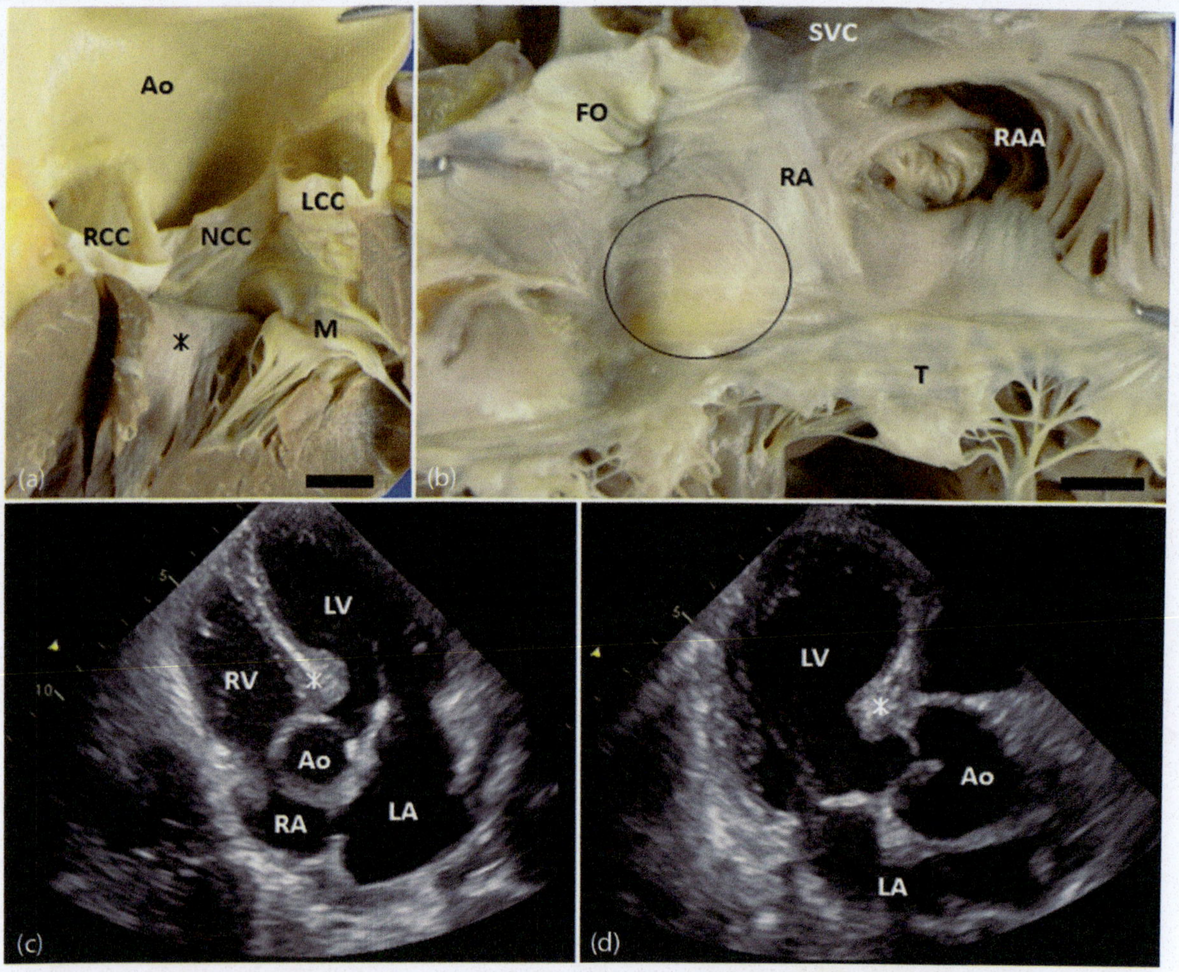

Figure 2.2 Septal bulge: (a) an angulated septum (*) from a 95-year-old female; (b) the dilated sinus of Valsalva (circled) bulges markedly toward the right atrium; (c) the apical five-chamber view from the same patient showing the apparent septal bulge (*) into the left ventricular outflow tract; (d) the angle of the long axis of the left ventricle and aorta is close to 90 degrees on the parasternal long axis view. *Abbreviations*: Ao, aorta; FO, foramen ovale; LCC, left coronary cusp; LA, left atrium; LV, left ventricle; M, mitral valve; NCC, noncoronary cusp; RA, right atrium; RAA, right atrial appendage; RCC, right coronary cusp; RV, right ventricle; SVC, superior vena cava; T, tricuspid valve Scale bar, 1 cm. (Courtesy of Dr. Koji Chida, Tokyo Metropolitan Geriatric Hospital.)

The valve rings dilate, the valve leaflets thicken, and the diameter of the aortic root increases with aging (7, 9). The shape of the left ventricular septum also changes with aging (11). "Septal bulge" refers to the base of the ventricular septum protruding prominently into the left ventricular outflow tract without left ventricular hypertrophy (Figure 2.2). Septal bulge may be associated with increased left ventricular systolic function and mitral annular calcification (12).

The prevalence of a patent foramen ovale (PFO) decreases with increasing age, from 34% during the first three decades to 20% during the ninth decade (13). Despite decreased prevalence with aging, PFO is independently associated with cryptogenic stroke in all age groups.

Undernutrition is often seen in the very elderly (5). Malnutrition is associated with the small brown heart, described as "brown atrophy." Grossly, the epicardium overlying the heart with brown atrophy has decreased adipose tissue, gelatinous degeneration of adipose tissue ("serous atrophy of fat"), and tortuous coronary arteries (Figure 2.1). As its name suggests, the myocardium in brown atrophy is brown because of increased concentration of lipofuscin pigment. Microscopically, myocytes show atrophy and increased lipofuscin granules. Lipofuscin is a perinuclear collection of yellowish-brown pigments (6, 14). The myocardium in children under 10 years of age lacks lipofuscin. Lipofuscin accumulates linearly with age in man and other mammalian species and also increases with hypertrophy of the myocardium.

VASCULAR AGING

Aging blood vessels "stiffen" via numerous processes that occur even in the absence of concomitant cardiovascular disease. Vascular remodeling, including intimal

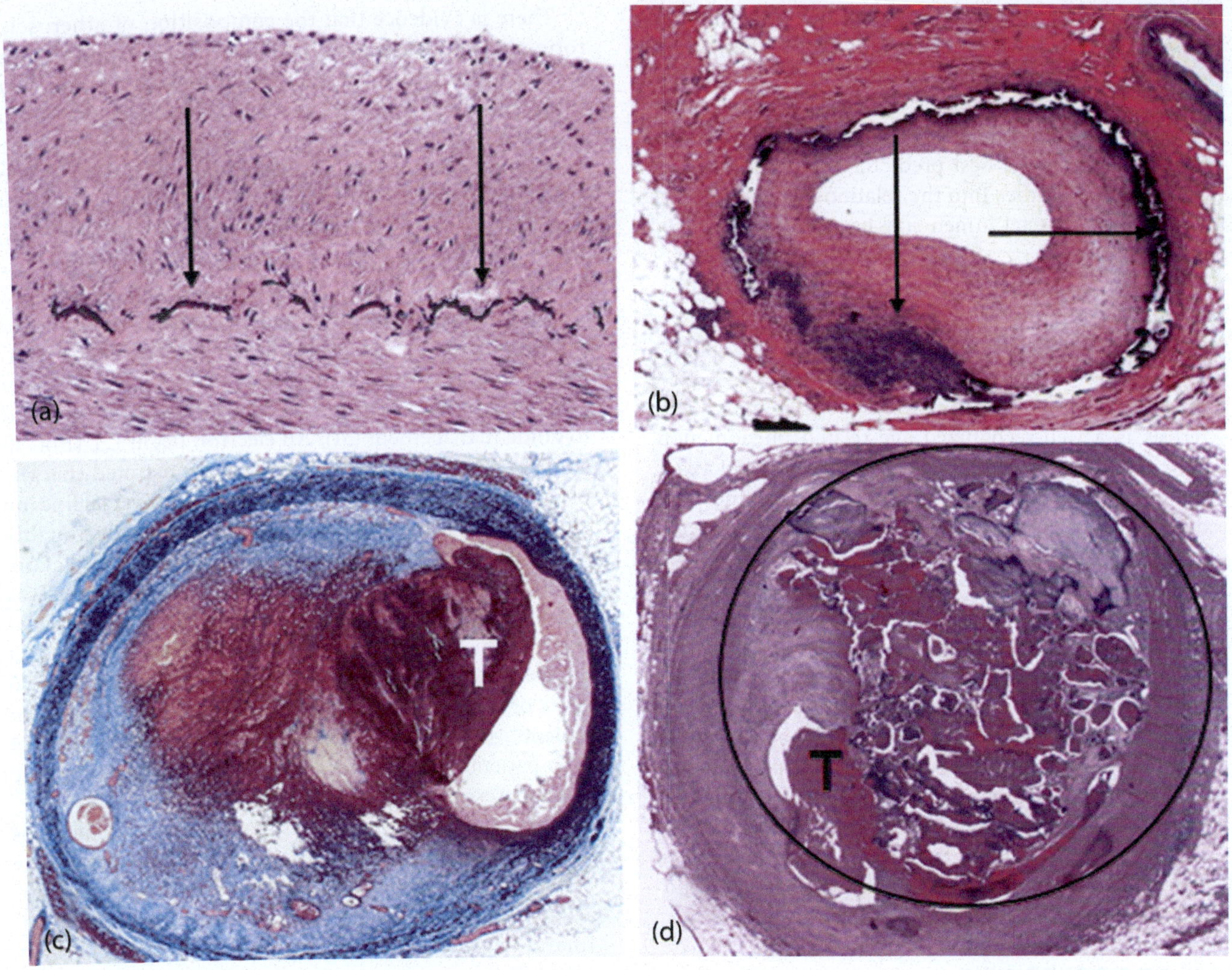

Figure 2.3 Vascular changes with aging: (a) temporal artery with intimal hyperplasia (IH) and calcification of the internal elastic lamina (arrows) (H&E stain, ×100); (b) Mönckeberg's sclerosis with calcification involving the internal elastic lamina and media of an artery (arrows) (H&E stain, ×20); (c) coronary artery with plaque rupture and luminal thrombosis (trichrome/elastic stain, ×12.5); and (d) coronary artery with heavily calcified atherosclerotic plaque (calcification in circle, H&E stain, ×12.5). There is an occlusive luminal thrombus as well. *Abbreviation*: T, thrombus.

hyperplasia and medial hypertrophy, increases the thickness of vessel walls over time, reducing compliance. Furthermore, elastic laminae become fragmented and arterial elasticity decreases. This age-related loss of elasticity has been shown to be the result of age-associated increases in glycosylated proteins, matrix metalloproteinase activity, and trophic stimuli (15). These processes are accelerated by other common conditions of aging, such as diabetes mellitus and hypertension. Increased aortic stiffening accompanies other age-associated stiffening as occurs with frailty and poor trunk flexibility (16).

Thickening of the tunica intima is seen in practically all arteries of the human body and has been described in association with aging (Figure 2.3). Originally, the intima consists of only a thin layer of endothelial cells lining the vascular lumen, with minimal subendothelial connective tissue. With aging, smooth muscle cells migrate from the tunica media and accumulate in the intima. The cells undergo a switch from a differentiated contractile to a synthetic phenotype (17). Cytoskeletal markers are reduced and cell morphology becomes more rounded, owing to an increase in rough endoplasmic reticulum and other cytoplasmic organelles. Proliferative behavior in response to growth factors increases. Slowly, over time, this proliferation results in intimal thickening. Larger arteries, such as the aorta, are most affected. Both peripherally and in the coronary vasculature, this phenomenon plays a significant role in the development of cardiovascular diseases such as hypertension and atherosclerosis.

Like the tunica intima, the tunica media also thickens with time. However, the process is not characteristically proliferative, but rather accompanies a decrease in smooth muscle cellularity with collagen accumulation (18). Space between lamellar units increases and elastin content decreases. Elastic laminae become encrusted in calcium. Medial smooth muscle cells increase in size (hypertrophy), but no increase in numbers (hyperplasia) is appreciable.

In addition to the age-associated alterations in wall composition described earlier, architectural changes are also observed, such as vessel dilatation and tortuosity. Angiographic investigation of the relationship between coronary artery morphology, heart size, and age demonstrates that age is the best predictor of coronary artery tortuosity (19). Studies into the relationship between age and coronary arterial lumen size have produced mixed results (7, 20–22).

MEDIAL CALCIFIC SCLEROSIS (MÖNCKEBERG'S SCLEROSIS)

First described in 1903 by J.G. Mönckeberg, medial calcific sclerosis is a well-recognized age-related phenomenon, rarely occurring in individuals younger than 50 years. Medial calcific sclerosis is a common incidental finding in temporal arteries, arteries of the extremities, and arteries of the breast; occasionally, coronary arteries are involved (22). The prevalence is notably increased in patients with other age-associated conditions, such as diabetes mellitus and osteoporosis. According to Mönckeberg, the sclerosis is due to a calcification process limited to the tunica media of large- and medium-sized arteries and does not result in luminal compromise (24). While the strict definition of Mönckeberg's sclerosis states the process does not affect the internal elastic lamina, calcification of the internal elastic lamina is nearly always present (Figure 2.3) (23, 25). Medial calcific sclerosis is largely considered a benign condition, usually noted as an incidental radiographic or histopathologic finding.

ATHEROSCLEROSIS

Atherosclerosis is largely considered a disease of aging. Atherosclerosis is a process that begins in adolescence but is not typically responsible for life-threatening disease until the fifth or sixth decade of life. Indeed, there is a close association between aging and the clinical manifestations of atherosclerotic disease (26). This association can partially be explained by associated age-related illnesses, such as hypertension, hypercholesterolemia, and diabetes. For example, in diabetes, the elevation of serum glucose can result in protein glycation, downregulated nitric oxide production, and increased smooth muscle cell migration, vascular inflammation, and oxidative stress that may accelerate atherogenesis (27). Over time these atherogenic risk factors intensify. In addition, there is evidence that components of vascular aging, particularly intimal thickening, are themselves atherogenic (17). While the burden of atherosclerosis progresses linearly during adulthood, this trend does not appear to continue in the very old. An autopsy study of 100 men between 30 and 89 years of age showed increasing atherosclerosis from ages 30 to 59 (28). However, there was no relationship between age and atherosclerotic burden in individuals aged 60 and older.

There is evidence that the composition of atherosclerotic plaques changes with advanced age. Van Oostrom et al. demonstrated more "atheromatous" plaques in subjects between the ages of 73 and 89 years (29). While the lipid content of atherosclerosis increased with age, the smooth muscle content decreased with age. This is an important finding, as the body of evidence suggests that plaques with increased lipid content and decreased smooth muscle are more vulnerable to plaque rupture and thrombosis (Figure 2.3) (30).

The presence of calcification in coronary arteries is used as a marker of atherosclerotic disease burden. Using computed tomography (CT), coronary artery calcium scores are calculated and used clinically for risk stratification and to guide management (31). An electron beam CT (EBCT) study of 675 men and 190 women demonstrated that the presence of calcium deposits was nearly a universal finding in older individuals (Figure 2.3) (32). After age 60, roughly 4 out of 5 men had detectable coronary artery calcium. The prevalence of coronary artery calcium in women was low until age 60, after which the prevalence approached that of men. Furthermore, the degree of calcium detected increased with age, being highest in individuals aged 70 years or older. Coronary artery calcium score data from patients ≥90 years are limited, but one autopsy study of such patients showed that coronary calcific deposits were grossly present in 95% of individuals (33).

There are numerous studies relating clinical outcomes to the location of atherosclerotic disease. Clinically, the distribution of disease may determine a patient's candidacy for percutaneous intervention after myocardial infarction (MI). The evidence suggests that coronary artery bypass graft surgery may be superior in patients with multivessel disease (34) or in some patients with left main coronary artery disease (35, 36). In an autopsy study of American octogenarians, 66% had greater than 75% atherosclerotic narrowing of at least one epicardial coronary artery (37). Three- or four-vessel coronary artery disease was present in 24%. Left main coronary artery disease was seen in 8%. Multivessel and left main coronary artery involvement was increased in individuals who died of cardiac causes. There was no statistically significant difference in atherosclerosis distribution between men and women. Autopsy studies of patients aged ≥90 years showed similar trends in atherosclerosis distribution (33).

Pulmonary arterial atherosclerosis may be seen in individuals of advanced age (38). This is likely due to the atherogenic properties of vascular aging (e.g., intimal thickening). Severe atherosclerosis of pulmonary arteries, however, is not typically encountered in the absence of pulmonary hypertension. Marked pulmonary artery atherosclerosis in conjunction with right ventricular hypertrophy is considered a reliable indicator of increased pulmonary artery pressure. Studies of pulmonary hemodynamics in the general population have demonstrated an age-associated increase in pulmonary arterial pressure and pulmonary vascular resistance (39). Nevertheless, even in nonagenarians, the age-associated increase in arterial pressure and vascular resistance is modest and does not meet the criteria for pulmonary hypertension. In concordance, some autopsy studies have demonstrated no increase in right ventricular hypertrophy associated with age (7).

MYOCARDIAL INFARCTION

Myocardial infarction (MI) is a consequence of coronary artery disease, the leading cause of death in high- and middle-income countries. The cause is often disruption of an atherosclerotic plaque in the coronary arteries. Plaque rupture is the most common coronary culprit, regardless of clinical presentation, age, sex, and continent (40). In plaque rupture, there is a luminal thrombus in continuity with the necrotic core, with a thin ruptured fibrous cap over the necrotic core. Plaque erosion is the second most common coronary culprit. The thrombus is in direct contact with the intima without plaque rupture.

The morphologic appearance of MI is dependent on the acuity of the event. Myocardial necrosis is clearly evident within 2 days of infarction (41). Histologically, findings are apparent within a few hours of coronary occlusion. Wavy fibers indicative of ischemic injury appear first. Then, necrotic fibers show increased eosinophilia, loss of cross-striation, loss of cytoplasmic granularity, and nuclear pyknosis or karyolysis. Within hours, neutrophils "marginate" in capillaries in the necrotic zone. Wavy fibers may be seen in infarcts only minutes old. By one week, fibroblastic proliferation and collagen deposition are evident, although it is not until the third week that proliferation of connective tissue is the dominant feature. The fibrotic (or healed) MI looks the same, whether it is months or years old. If reperfusion occurs related to thrombolytic therapy or angioplasty, infarcts may become hemorrhagic.

In autopsy studies by Roberts et al., morphologic evidence of MI was found in half of octogenarians and 38% of individuals ≥90 years old (33, 37). In these studies, roughly half of the individuals had systemic hypertension, while approximately 60% had significant coronary artery atherosclerosis (>75% stenosis) in at least one major coronary artery. Acute MI was present in 15% of those 90 or older. Healed MI was more prevalent, present in 27% of the ≥90 group. Similarly, Roberts's study of octogenarians showed acute MI in 24% of cases, 29% of women and 19% of men. Healed MI was present in 36% of individuals, 45% of men and 27% of women.

In octogenarians, the frequency of cardiac rupture after MI was approximately four times greater in women than in men. When cardiac rupture was found, 83% of cases involved the left ventricular free wall (Figure 2.4). The septum was involved in 29% of cases, while only 4% had rupture of a papillary muscle.

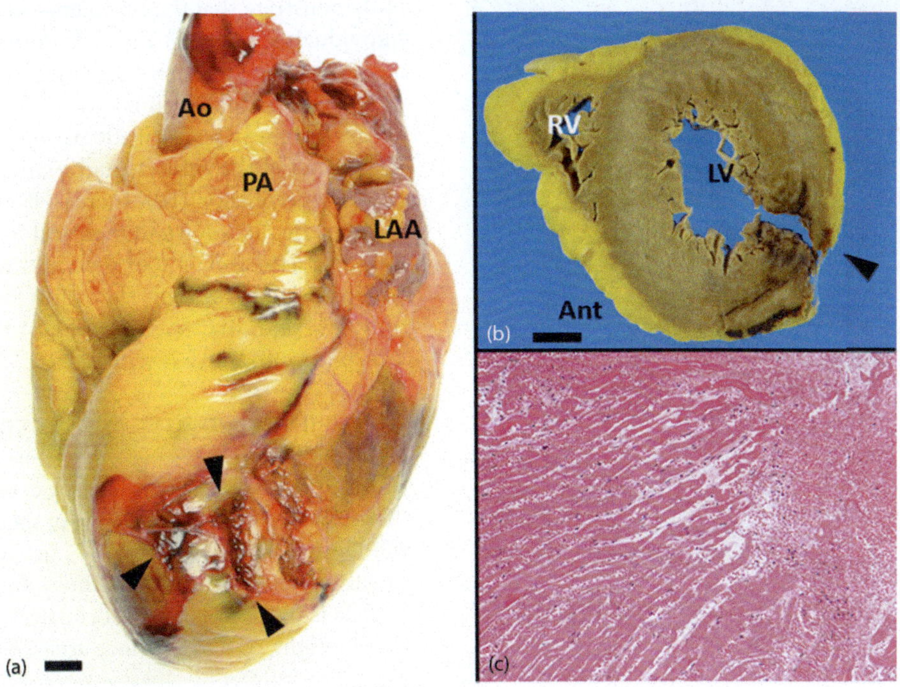

Figure 2.4 Rupture of the left ventricular free wall due to acute myocardial infarction: (a) the heart from an 80-year-old female who died suddenly due to cardiac rupture (arrowheads), who also had a long history of hypertension; (b) transverse section of the left and right ventricles from the same specimen; (c) a histologic section (H&E stain, ×200) of the rupture site. Note the necrotic myocardium (left) and hemorrhage on the rupture site (right). *Abbreviations*: Ant, anterior; Ao, aorta; LAA, left atrial appendage; LV, left ventricle; PA, pulmonary artery; RV, right ventricle. Scale bar, 1 cm.

HYPERTENSION

Hypertension is a leading cause of cardiovascular disease, affecting approximately 1.3 billion people worldwide (42). In the United States, hypertension occurs in roughly 70% of individuals over the age of 65 (43). As a result of age-related neurohumoral and vascular changes, systolic blood pressure (SBP) increases with age. In the United States, diastolic blood pressure (DBP) peaks and plateaus in late middle age, after which DBP declines modestly in both men and women. As a result of the increase in SBP and decrease in DBP, pulse pressure increases with age and is a clinical marker for vascular stiffness. The morphologic changes seen in the hypertensive heart are increased wall thickness, chamber dilatation, and a combination of the two (Figure 2.5). From middle age (about 50) to age 70, left ventricular mass index, left ventricular wall thickness, fractional shortening and left atrial diameter all increase (44). Microscopically, there is evidence of myocyte hypertrophy and interstitial fibrosis.

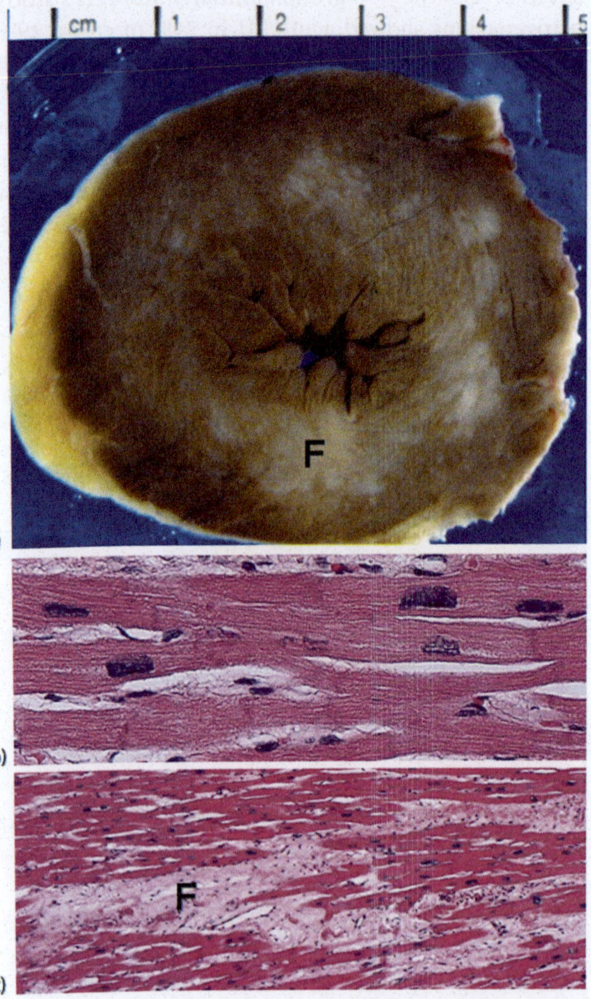

(a)
(b)
(c)

Figure 2.5 Findings in hypertrophied hypertensive hearts: (a) transverse section of left ventricle showing marked concentric hypertrophy with myocardial fibrosis (white regions); (b) hypertrophic myocytes with enlarged "boxcar" nuclei (H&E stain, ×400); and (c) interstitial fibrosis (H&E stain, ×200). *Abbreviation*: F, fibrosis.

The principal finding associated with hypertension is left ventricular hypertrophy (LVH). The classic paradigm of hypertensive heart disease teaches us that the left ventricular wall thickens in response to increased pressure (45). Through a variety of mechanisms, both mechanical and neurohumoral, cardiac myocytes increase in size, resulting in an increase in left ventricle mass and thickness. The result is concentric LVH. However, concentric hypertrophy is not the only morphologic phenotype of hypertensive heart disease. In fact, studies of hypertensive individuals demonstrate that eccentric hypertrophy is at least as common as concentric hypertrophy (46, 47). Frequently, the hypertensive heart exhibits variable degrees of both concentric and eccentric LVH.

The natural history of the hypertensive patient is variable. However, it is well established that hypertensive people who develop concentric hypertrophy may subsequently develop eccentric hypertrophy via a series of events often referred to as the "transition to failure" (47). Not surprisingly, as hypertension is a significant risk factor for other cardiovascular diseases, including coronary artery disease, the progression from concentric hypertrophy to eccentric hypertrophy often involves interval MI (46, 48). Particularly in older individuals, interval MI may go unrecognized. Data from a large study investigating age and MI susceptibility used cardiac magnetic resonance imaging (MRI) to demonstrate that the prevalence of unrecognized MI in individuals aged 67–93 is greater than previously estimated (49). In fact, the prevalence of unrecognized MI in that age group exceeds that of clinically recognized MI.

In an autopsy series of 490 patients 80–103 years of age, nearly half of the subjects had a clinical diagnosis of systemic hypertension (50). Increased heart weight, defined in this series as >400 g in men and >350 g in women, was found in 64% and 74% of men and women, respectively. Chamber dilatation, on the other hand, was present in only 33% of individuals. Both heart weight and chamber size tended to decrease with age.

VALVULAR HEART DISEASE

Valvular heart disease is a leading cause of cardiovascular disease, affecting roughly 2.5% of the adult population in the United States (51). As one ages, the mean thickness of valve leaflets increases; of note, the thickness of valve leaflets is not significantly correlated with height, weight, heart weight, or body surface area (52).

Age-related valve changes

Age-related changes are seen in all of the cardiac valves although the degree of change differs. Almost all adult aortic valves have a nodular thickening at the center of the free edges of the cusps—the so-called nodule of Arantius

(53). Lambl's excrescences, hairlike projections from the nodules, are often seen in older patients. Fenestrations of the cusps, slit-like defects between the line of closure and free edge of the cusps, are also found in aged aortic valves. None of these changes are functionally significant.

The mitral valve apparatus consists of the atrial wall, mitral valve annulus, leaflets, chordae tendineae, papillary muscles, and underlying left ventricular wall. The leaflets may display thickening with degeneration of collagen fibers, lipid accumulation, and focal calcification (52). Nodular thickening of the free edge of the anterior leaflet, referred to by some as "atheromatosis," is seen in all adults. Severity of the lipid deposition on the leaflet also correlates with age, but there are no gender differences (53). In addition, mitral annular calcification, small scars, diffuse opacity, or hooding of leaflets (myxomatous degeneration) are often seen in older hearts (52). Mitral annular calcification may be associated with mild, usually insignificant, mitral insufficiency. Age-related changes in the pulmonary valve and tricuspid valve are minor. Nodules of Arantius and fenestrations of the cusps are sometimes present in the pulmonary valve (53).

Aortic valve disease

Degenerative/calcific aortic stenosis (AS), also known as aging-related aortic stenosis, has become the most common type of valvular heart disease requiring intervention in industrialized countries, and is associated with significant morbidity and mortality (Figure 2.6) (54–56). Calcification of the aortic valve (AV) is seen in more than one fourth of individuals over 65 years and more than half of those over 85 years (56). Among octogenarians, AS was seen in 2.4%–8.1% (54, 57).

The aortic valve is chronically exposed to complex shear forces. Calcification primarily occurs on the aortic side of the cusps, along the line of coaptation (58). Calcification involves the collagenous portion of the leaflets, but calcifications can erode through the endothelial surface and even embolize to other organs (59).

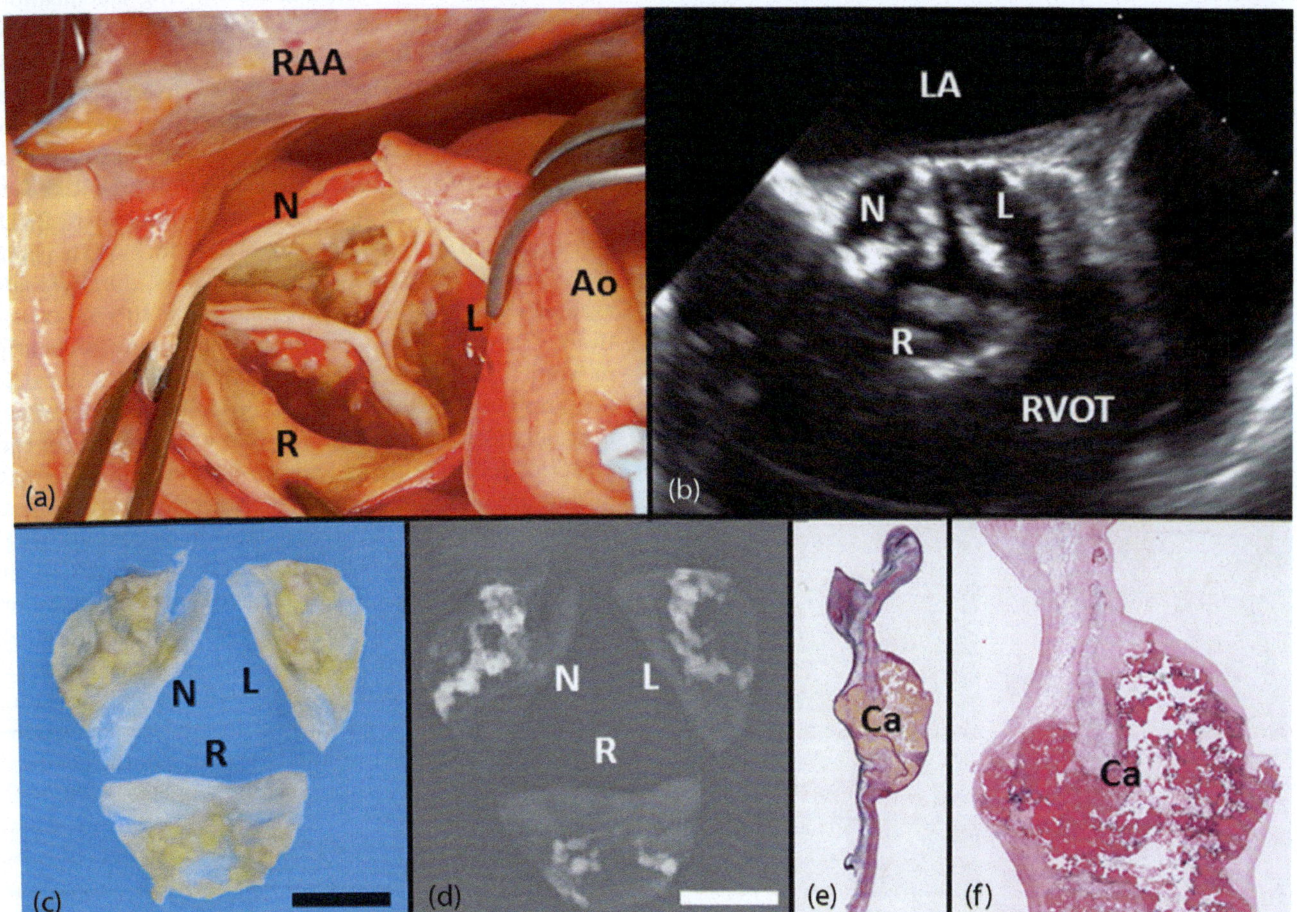

Figure 2.6 Calcific aortic stenosis in a 69-year-old female: (a) operative view of the aortic stenosis; (b) transesophageal echocardiogram of the aortic valve short axis view during systole; (c) surgically resected cusps; (d) X-ray of the same specimen, nodular calcification is found on the cusps; (e) and (f) histology of the noncoronary cusp ([e] Elastica van Gieson stain; [f] H&E stain). Calcification destroying the elastic tissue and growth on the cuspal surface. *Abbreviations*: Ao, aorta; Ca, calcification; L, left coronary cusp; LA, left atrium; N, noncoronary cusp; R, right coronary cusp; RAA, right atrial appendage; RVOT, right ventricular outflow tract. Scale bar, 1 cm. (Courtesy of Drs. Takashi Nishimura, Mitsuhiro Kawata, and Jun Tanaka, Tokyo Metropolitan Geriatric Hospital.)

The presence of calcification in the AV is associated with calcification at other sites, including the carotid arteries, coronary arteries, thoracic aorta, abdominal aorta, and iliac arteries.

Aortic regurgitation (AR) requiring surgery is less common in older adults and usually results from infective endocarditis, rheumatic fever, aortic-root dilatation or dissection, or myxoid degeneration (60, 61). Myxoid degeneration of the aortic valve is seen in 36% of cases with pure AR. There is a male predominance. Long-standing hypertension is thought to be an important underlying factor (60). In contrast to myxoid degeneration of the mitral valve (MV), myxoid degeneration of the AV is very uncommon.

Mitral valve disease

Clinically significant mitral valve disease affects 2%–3% of the adult population, resulting in about 34,000 deaths per year worldwide (62). Mitral valve regurgitation (MR), mitral stenosis (MS), mitral annular calcification (MAC), and mitral valve prolapse (MVP) are seen in older adults (Figure 2.7). Classical MS is usually post-inflammatory; most cases are due to rheumatic disease. In older patients, severe MV annular calcification with encroachment into the orifice is an uncommon cause of functional MS (63).

MR may be caused by myxomatous degeneration, infective endocarditis, collagen vascular disease, or spontaneous rupture of the chordae tendineae (64). MVP is the most common structural valvular cause of MR in older patients. The prevalence of MVP is estimated to be in the range of 3%–5% in healthy adults. Grossly, myxomatous mitral valves are characterized by floppy leaflets with elongated or ruptured chordae tendineae (Figure 2.7a). Also, the valves show an increase in leaflet thickness. The mitral valve consists of fibrosa, spongiosa, and atrialis layers. Histologically, the valve with prolapse shows collagen degeneration and disorganization, elastic fiber fragmentation, and increased thickness of the spongiosa layer (64, 65). In MVP, the leaflets contain more abundant proteoglycans, including decorin, biglycan, and versican. Ruptured mitral chordae tendineae are seen not only in myxomatous degeneration of the MV but also in chronic rheumatic valvulitis or endocarditis. Myxomatous degeneration mainly causes posterior chordae tendineae rupture, while anterior chordae tendineae rupture is more common in chronic rheumatic valvulitis (66). The cause of myxomatous degeneration remains unclear. While surgical repair is historically the treatment of choice in patients with severe MR, transcatheter edge-to-edge repair is a promising and less invasive alternative, particularly for high-risk patients (67).

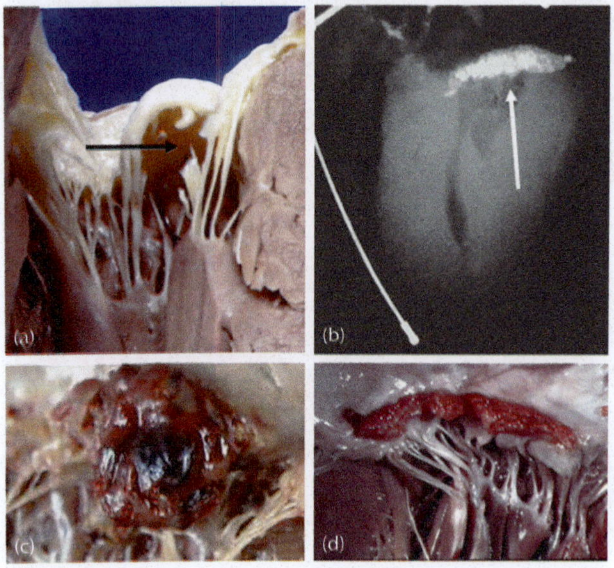

Figure 2.7 Mitral valve disease in older adults: (a) mitral valve prolapse with ruptured chorda tendinea (arrow); (b) postmortem radiograph showing mitral annular calcification (arrow); (c) fungal endocarditis with large vegetation on mitral valve; and (d) nonbacterial thrombotic endocarditis with nondestructive vegetations on valve leaflet.

The incidence of MAC, or mitral ring calcification, shows a striking increase with age. MAC is rarely found in those younger than 40 years old, except in the case of a concomitant connective tissue disorder, such as Marfan syndrome, or disorder of calcium metabolism, for example, secondary hyperparathyroidism in patients with severe chronic kidney disease (CKD) (59). Risk factors include advanced age, systemic atherosclerosis, CKD, and increased mitral stress, as occurs in hypertension, MVP, and AS (59, 68–70). The prevalences in individuals aged 66–75 and >75 years are 28.6% and 40.9%, respectively (71). Heavy calcification is seen more frequently in women (Figure 2.7b). The configuration of the calcified annulus may be J-, C-, U-, or O-shaped (72). MAC is usually located entirely in or below the annulus of the posterior mitral leaflet. Although the anterior leaflet has no true annulus, there can be anterior submitral calcification, seen much less frequently than in association with the posterior leaflet (73). Ulceration and extrusion of calcium through the cusp, extensive central necrosis, or endocarditis of the mitral valve are sometimes associated with MAC (74). Microscopically, MAC shows no evidence of previous endocarditis. Nonspecific chronic inflammatory changes are seen adjacent to calcium deposition. Rarely, MAC extends into the His bundle of the conduction system, causing atrioventricular (AV) block (70).

INFECTIVE ENDOCARDITIS

(See also Chapter 16.)

Infective endocarditis (IE) is a microbial infection of an endocardial surface of the heart. The clinical diagnosis of IE is based on culture of organisms from the blood and visualization of cardiac vegetations (Figure 2.7c). Despite current sophisticated imaging methods, IE is frequently not diagnosed until autopsy (75). Risk factors, in addition to older age, include preexisting valvular disease, artificial heart valves, intracardiac devices, and intravenous drug use (76). The prevalence of IE at autopsy has been reported to be 1.3% , and the mean age of patients is increasing (75, 76). In-hospital mortality in patients aged ≥65 is high—up to 25% (77). As in younger patients, *Staphylococcus aureus* is the most common pathogen. However, older patients have lower rates of infection by viridans streptococci group, and a higher prevalence of coagulase-negative staphylococci, enterococci, and *Streptococcus bovis* (77). Fungal endocarditis is not common, but results in larger vegetations and greater destruction of tissue.

Left-sided endocarditis is more common, but endocarditis involving right-sided structures or both right- and left-sided valves is not rare (75, 76). Right-sided endocarditis is often associated with intravenous drug use or pulmonary artery catheterization. Prosthetic valve endocarditis is a serious complication of valve replacement that often requires removal of the affected valve. Pathologically, bacterial colonies or fungal hyphae are demonstrated in untreated endocarditis. Gram stain for bacteria and Grocott–Gomori methenamine silver (GMS) stain for fungi are recommended. Infection from a native or artificial valve may spread to adjacent structures and myocardium (75). The finding of heart block indicates spread of the infection into the cardiac conduction system, and the finding of pericarditis indicates spread through the infected valve annulus—both are ominous complications. The spleen, kidneys, brain, and mesentery are common sites of embolization of infected vegetations in cases of left-sided endocarditis; the lung is a more common site in cases of right-sided endocarditis. At autopsy, gross infarction may be seen in as many as 63% of cases, but in most cases these lesions were asymptomatic.

Up to one third of patients with IE have cardiac disorders that are clinically silent, such as bicuspid aortic valve (BAV) or MVP. BAV is the most common congenital cardiac abnormality, reported to be present in 1%–2% of the population (78). Patients with endocarditis and BAV are younger, have a higher frequency of aortic perivalvular abscess, and usually require early surgery. The incidence of cardiac device-associated IE (e.g., pacemakers or implantable cardioverter-defibrillators [ICDs]) has increased over the years due to increased utilization of these technologies, especially in older adults. In one study of such patients, coexisting valve involvement was seen in 37.3%, and the most commonly infected valve was the tricuspid valve (79).

NONBACTERIAL THROMBOTIC ENDOCARDITIS

Nonbacterial thrombotic endocarditis (NBTE) is a sterile, thrombotic vegetation of the heart valves. NBTE is found in 0.3% to 9.3% of autopsy patients (80, 81). Thromboembolism may be the first manifestation; however, NBTE is usually asymptomatic, or at least not recognized clinically, in part because the patient has very severe underlying diseases, such as shock or metastatic malignancy. Accordingly, NBTE is usually first diagnosed at autopsy (80). Patients with NBTE are usually older, but NBTE is also observed in children and young adults. There is no gender predilection. NBTE is most commonly found in patients with advanced cancer, but it is also seen in patients with antiphospholipid syndrome (APS) or other autoimmune disorders characterized by hypercoagulability (80–82). NBTE may be seen in patients with disseminated intravascular coagulation (DIC) of any cause. NBTE occurs on the atrial surfaces of the mitral and tricuspid valves and the ventricular surfaces of the aortic and pulmonic valves (80). The mitral and aortic valves are most commonly involved. Histologically, NBTE shows agglutinated deposits of fibrin and platelets with no inflammatory reaction and no destruction of underlying valve tissue (80, 82). NBTE is superficial and attached to the endocardial surface along the lines of closure of the affected valves (Figure 2.7d).

CARDIOMYOPATHY

According to the 2006 American Heart Association (AHA) classification scheme, cardiomyopathy is defined as a heterogeneous group of diseases of the myocardium associated with mechanical and/or electrical dysfunction (83). Cardiomyopathies are divided into two major groups, primary and secondary. Primary cardiomyopathies are solely or predominantly confined to heart muscles and are classified as genetic, acquired, and mixed (genetic and nongenetic etiologies). There are more than a thousand disease-causing mutations (84). Morphological phenotypes and disease severity can be variable due to genetic heterogeneity and allelic variation. Genetic testing can assist diagnosis, guide clinical management, and be useful for screening of family members.

Hypertrophic cardiomyopathy

Hypertrophic cardiomyopathy (HCM) is a clinically heterogeneous hereditary heart disease characterized by unexplained hypertrophy of the left ventricle (Figure 2.8), often associated with pathogenic mutations in genes encoding sarcomeric proteins. HCM is the most common cause of sudden death in young individuals, including trained athletes, but HCM has been observed during all phases of life (85).

HCM is not rare in older adults. Maron et al. reported that the average age at diagnosis was in the fifth decade of life (86). Another study showed that approximately one quarter of HCM patients were older than 75 years (85). However, there are substantial differences in clinical manifestations across age groups. Only a minority of aged HCM patients have severe heart failure. In one study, two thirds of patients older than 75 years experienced few or no symptoms, and about 60% of those survived to age 80–96 years (87). It has also been suggested that many patients with HCM have gone undiagnosed their entire lives (86).

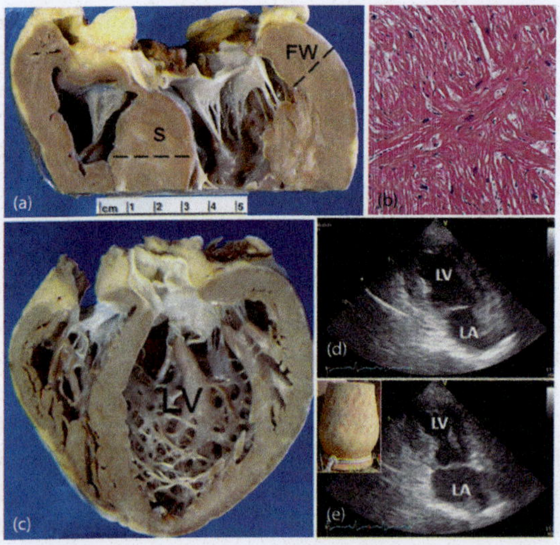

Figure 2.8 Primary cardiomyopathies and takotsubo cardiomyopathy: (a) base of heart from a patient transplanted for hypertrophic cardiomyopathy (note that the septum is thicker than the left ventricular free wall); (b) characteristic myocyte disarray seen in hypertrophic cardiomyopathy (H&E stain, ×400); and (c) heart from a patient transplanted for dilated cardiomyopathy (note dilation of left ventricle). (d, e) A 77-year-old female with the acute phase of takotsubo cardiomyopathy. Transthoracic echocardiography showing apical ballooning in end-diastole (d) and end-systole (e) that resembles the appearance of a Japanese octopus fishing pot called a *tako-tsubo* (insert). *Abbreviations*: FW, free wall; LA, left atrium; LV, left ventricle; S, septum. (Courtesy of Dr. Jun Tanaka, Tokyo Metropolitan Geriatric Hospital.)

The clinical diagnosis of HCM is usually established by echocardiography. Although characteristic pathological findings may be identified, a diagnosis of HCM should not be made by endomyocardial biopsy. Endomyocardial biopsy is useful, however, to exclude diseases that may mimic HCM, such as infiltrative or storage diseases (88). Grossly, left ventricular hypertrophy is characteristically asymmetric, with the anterior basal interventricular septum showing the greatest wall thickness (Figure 2.8a) (83, 85). Subaortic obstruction is significantly more common in older HCM patients (91). Characteristic histologic features include myocyte hypertrophy, myocyte disarray, and fibrosis. Wall thickening and luminal narrowing of intramyocardial arteries are also seen. In older patients, these morphologic features are relatively mild compared to younger patients who have died from HCM (85, 87).

Dilated cardiomyopathy

Dilated cardiomyopathy (DCM) is characterized by ventricular chamber enlargement of the left or both ventricles, and systolic dysfunction in the absence of other identifiable causes (83, 89). DCM may occur at any age, but there are onset peaks during childhood and mid-adulthood. DCM leads to progressive biventricular heart failure, ventricular and supraventricular arrhythmias, thromboembolism due to cardiac mural thrombi, and sudden cardiac death. Approximately 20%–50% of DCM cases have been reported to be familial.

DCM is a phenotype, categorized as a mixed (genetic and nongenetic) cardiomyopathy in the AHA classification (83). There are a number of potential underlying causes, including genetic mutation, toxins (such as alcohol, cocaine, and anthracyclines), viral myocarditis, Chagas disease, metabolic causes, hypersensitivity myocarditis, connective tissue disease, neuromuscular disease, and pregnancy. The etiology of DCM is not identified in approximately 50% of cases (84). In older patients, exclusion of other causes, such as ischemic heart disease and hypertensive heart disease, is essential for the diagnosis of DCM. If there is greater than 75% stenosis in the left main coronary artery, proximal left anterior descending artery, or more than two epicardial coronary arteries, ischemic cardiac disease is a more likely diagnosis (90).

Macroscopically, the heart often weighs two to three times that of a normal heart; some hearts exceed 1000 grams (so-called cor bovinum) (89). The characteristic shape of the heart is globoid and somewhat spherical with rounding of the apex due to biventricular hypertrophy and marked dilation (Figure 2.8c). Functional mitral regurgitation is very common in patients with DCM; mitral annular dilatation is a common finding. Mural thrombi may be seen in all cardiac chambers. As a consequence of diastolic dysfunction, left atrial dilation and atrial fibrillation may occur (90). Histological findings are nonspecific, including interstitial fibrosis, replacement fibrosis, irregular and hyperchromatic nuclei of myocytes, and sarcoplasmic degenerative changes. Replacement fibrosis is a consequence of myocyte injury or necrosis and is known to be a substrate for ventricular re-entrant arrhythmia. Myocardial fibrosis can predict not only the risk of sudden cardiac death but also the likelihood of LV functional recovery (91).

Takotsubo (stress) cardiomyopathy

Takotsubo cardiomyopathy is an acquired cardiomyopathy in the AHA classification (83). The name refers to the shape of the heart resembling the appearance of a Japanese octopus fishing pot called a *tako-tsubo* (octopus-pot) (Figure 2.8d and e). This cardiomyopathy is characterized by transient regional systolic dysfunction involving the left ventricular apex and/or mid-ventricle that typically recovers within a few weeks (92). Right ventricular involvement has also been reported, and has been associated with longer hospital stays and more complications (93). Diagnostic criteria from the Mayo Clinic include 1) transient akinesis or dyskinesis of the left ventricular mid-segments with or without apical involvement, 2) new ECG abnormalities (ST-segment elevation or T wave inversion), 3) no obstructive coronary disease, and 4) absence of pheochromocytoma or myocarditis (94).

Gender and age discrepancies are striking. Females comprise about 90% of reported cases, and more than half are over age 65 (95). Common symptoms include abrupt onset of angina-like chest pain and dyspnea resembling acute coronary syndrome. Symptoms are usually preceded by emotional or physical stress, such as family death, abuse, a harsh argument, exhausting work, or an earthquake (92). Sympathetic hyperactivity and increased catecholamine levels may play a role in myocardial stunning and contractile dysfunction. Plasma catecholamine levels are elevated in patients with takotsubo cardiomyopathy, and the histological findings are similar to catecholamine-induced changes, including contraction-band necrosis (92). Neurologic or psychiatric disorders are more prevalent in takotsubo cardiomyopathy (95). There is also an increased prevalence of migraine headaches and affective disorders (96). A multimodal MRI study demonstrated structural and functional alterations in regions primarily involved in cardiac control and emotional processing such as the amygdala and hippocampus (97).

There are several reports of morphological changes in takotsubo cardiomyopathy. The histology is similar to that seen in patients with ischemic electrocardiographic changes after an acute intracranial injury and cardiotoxic effects induced by catecholamines (92). Endomyocardial biopsies taken during the acute phase showed contraction bands, ultrastructural damage to contractile proteins, and vacuoles filled with cellular debris and myelin-like bodies. An autopsy case report demonstrated patchy myofibril degeneration of the myocardium with contraction band necrosis and myocyte edema at the cardiac apex (98).

AMYLOIDOSIS

Cardiac amyloidosis may be considered a secondary form of cardiomyopathy, as many forms of amyloidosis are systemic. Cardiac amyloidosis is characterized by infiltration of the myocardium by one of several misfolded proteins known as amyloid. Currently, there are more than 30 types of amyloid, 12 of which have been reported to involve the heart (99, 100). Each type has different clinicopathological features, including treatment and prognosis. In older adults, the most commonly encountered types of systemic cardiac amyloidosis are amyloid light chain (AL) and transthyretin amyloid (ATTR). Deposition of amyloid in the heart results in a thickened heart wall with a firm and rubbery consistency. Brown "waxy" deposits may be seen in the endocardium of the atria or heart valves (Figure 2.9a). Occasionally, there is a predilection

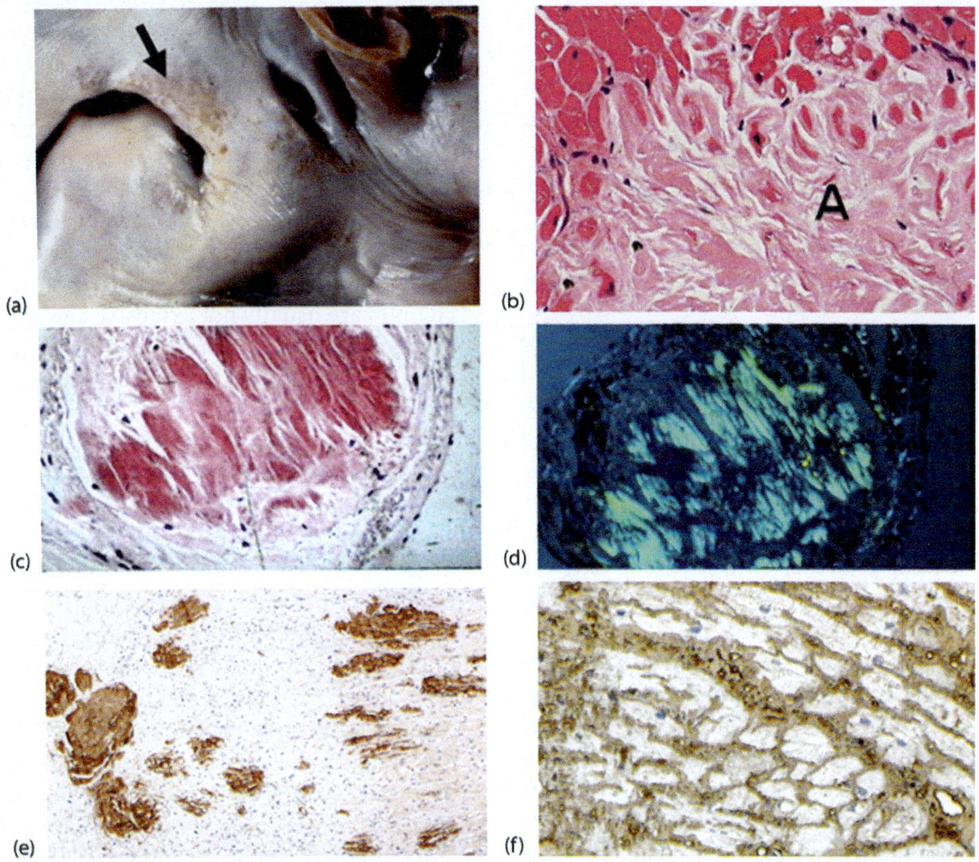

Figure 2.9 Cardiac amyloidosis: (a) gross appearance of amyloid in the left atrium (note brown "waxy" appearance (arrow); (b) H&E stain of amyloid in the myocardium; (c) Congo red stain of amyloid; (d) Congo red stain under polarized light showing characteristic green birefringence; (e) immunohistochemical staining for transthyretin from a patient with wild-type ATTR cardiac amyloidosis, ×100; and (f) immunohistochemical stain for lambda light chain from a case of AL amyloidosis in a patient with multiple myeloma. Positive immunostaining is brown (×200). *Abbreviation*: A, amyloid.

for the interventricular septum, resulting in asymmetric thickening that mimics HCM (99). The stiff heart worsens cardiac relaxation and compliance; therefore, cardiac manifestations of amyloidosis are dominated by diastolic heart failure resulting from restrictive physiology (101). As a result, the atria are often dilated. Right heart failure, conduction disturbances, and arrhythmias are common (102). When suspected clinically, the diagnosis of amyloidosis may be confirmed by biopsy. Histologically, amyloid displays an amorphous eosinophilic appearance by hematoxylin and eosin staining and shows characteristic apple-green and yellow birefringence with polarized light following Congo red staining (Figure 2.9c and d) (99). Amyloid can also be detected using fluorescent stains, such as thioflavin T or S, metachromatic dyes, such as crystal violet, and other histochemical stains, such as sulfated Alcian blue. Once confirmation of amyloid is obtained, subtyping may be attempted by immunohistochemistry and/or immunofluorescence (Figure 2.9e and f). Mass spectrometry, however, is a more reliable method that can be performed on formalin-fixed paraffin-embedded tissue (101). If transthyretin amyloid is detected, DNA mutational analysis may be performed to distinguish age-related systemic amyloidosis (wild-type transthyretin) from hereditary amyloidosis (mutated transthyretin).

AL amyloidosis is a common cause of clinically significant cardiac amyloidosis (99). A primary plasma cell dyscrasia or, less commonly, multiple myeloma are the underlying etiologies. Neoplastic plasma cells secrete monoclonal immunoglobulin light chains that form amyloid deposits in multiple organs including the heart and kidneys. Plasma cell dyscrasias are more frequent in older adults and almost exclusively affect individuals older than 40 years (103). Cardiac involvement portends a poor prognosis (104).

ATTR occurs in up to 25% of people over the age of 80 years (99, 103). Wild-type transthyretin forms amyloid deposits in various organs, although the heart is most commonly affected (103, 105, 107, 108). Both the atria and ventricles are involved. Compared to AL, ATTR is less commonly associated with cardiomegaly, heart failure, or arrhythmia (103, 105, 107, 108). Histologically, large, diffuse or multifocal, predominantly nodular amyloid deposits are present between muscle bundles. Usually the conduction system is not affected (103, 107).

Isolated atrial amyloidosis, or atrial natriuretic factor amyloidosis (AANF), is a common postmortem finding in older adults. AANF occurs in as many as 80%–90% of individuals older than 90 years (103, 108). AANF is seen in conditions associated with increased plasma concentrations of atrial natriuretic factor, such as heart failure and atrial fibrillation. Grossly, deposits of amyloid are only found in the atria, predominantly in the appendages, and beneath the endocardium (103). Histologically, amyloid deposits surround cardiac myocytes (103, 108).

Localized valvular amyloid may also be found in older patients. This amyloid deposition is associated with AV sclerosis and, less commonly, with MV dysfunction (regurgitation and stenosis) (103, 109). The exact amyloid subtype is unclear, but valvular amyloid seems to be associated with athero-inflammatory risk factors such as high shear-stress hemodynamics.

AGING CHANGES IN THE CONDUCTION SYSTEM AND ARRHYTHMIA

The prevalence rates of both conduction disturbances and arrhythmias increase with age (110). The major components of the conduction system of the heart consist of the sinoatrial (SA) node, AV node, His bundle, and bundle branches. Dysfunction of the SA node progressively increases with age regardless of gender. Even in healthy older individuals, there is an intrinsic decline in endogenous pacemaker function.

Historically, the percentage of collagen fibers within the SA node is said to increase with age (10, 111, 112); a recent quantitative study by Bois et al., however, found no such increase over time, and instead found that collagen content is highly variable across individuals (113). Mature adipose tissue is also reported to increase over time, although SA node fat content appears closely related to body mass index (BMI) (113). In contrast to prior studies asserting that nodal myocytes atrophy (114), Bois et al. also demonstrated a linear increase in nodal myocyte size after the first decade of life, and a quadratic relationship between sinoatrial nodal area with age, peaking during the sixth decade of life. Studies of the AV node in older adults show replacement by adipose tissue and an increase in elastic fibers (115, 116). However, these changes are usually not extensive enough to lead to clinical problems (115). More fibrous tissue in the His bundle and bundle branches has also been demonstrated (116).

SICK SINUS SYNDROME

Patients with sick sinus syndrome (SSS) show sinus arrest, sinoatrial exit block, or persistent sinus bradycardia. The majority of patients ultimately require implantation of a permanent pacemaker. Symptomatic SSS is mostly seen in older people and is the leading cause of pacemaker implantation. Reduction in the number of conduction cells, increased fibrosis (Figure 2.10), and infiltration of adipose tissue may contribute to SSS (115–117). In older SSS patients, there is a loss of SA node cells, resulting in decreased cellularity in the region of the SA node (116). Marked fibrosis of the SA node is found in older patients requiring permanent pacemakers for SSS (115). In cases without marked fibrosis, severe fatty infiltration is seen. Excessive fatty infiltration in the atrionodal transitional area leads to reduced atrionodal conduction with atrophy

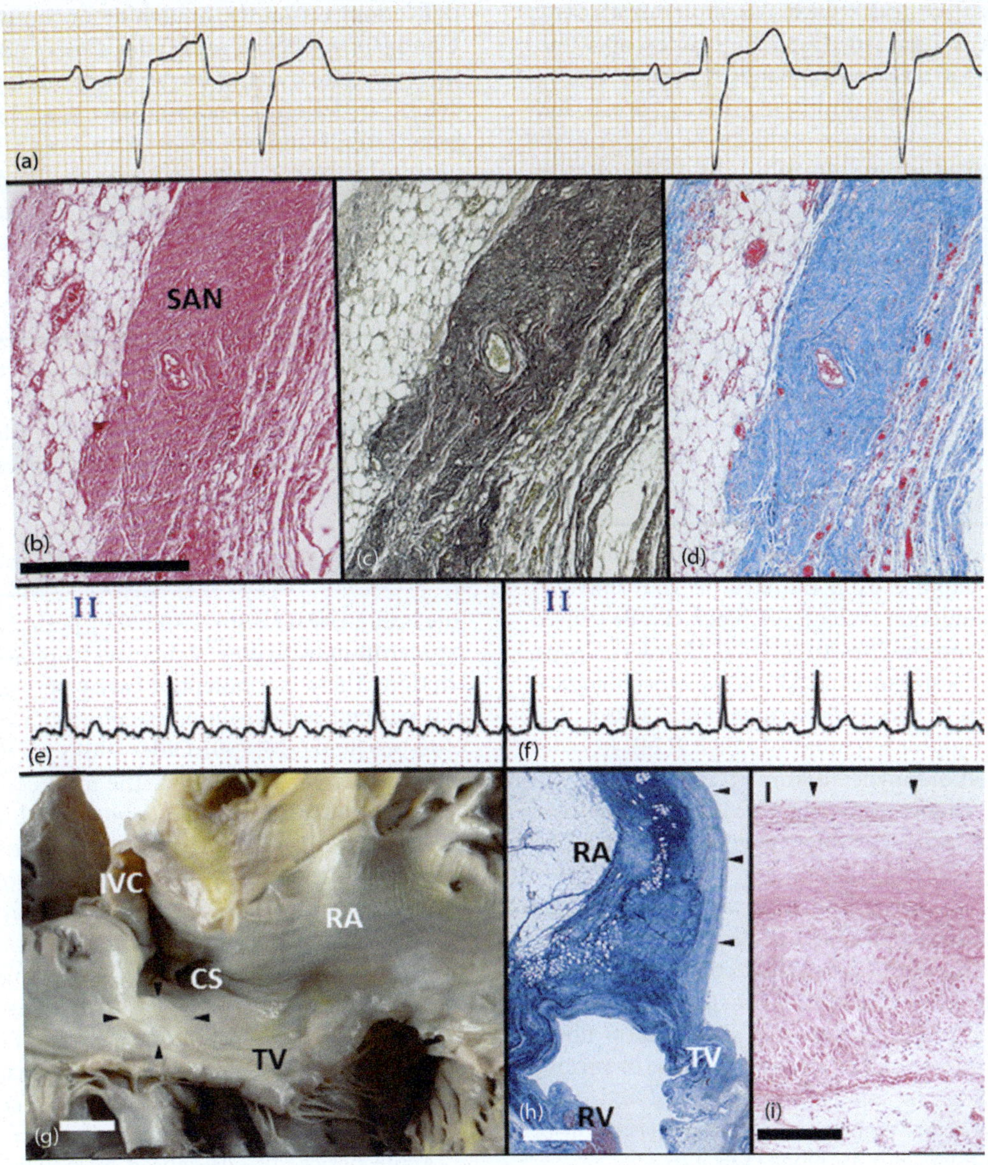

Figure 2.10 (a–d) An 80-year-old male who demonstrated sinus arrest and premature atrial contractions (a) and who underwent pacemaker implantation 8 years before death. Decreased cellularity of the sinoatrial node and increased fibrosis are present (b–d). (e–i) An 86-year-old male who demonstrated atrial flutter (e) and who underwent catheter ablation 2 years before death; (f) an electrocardiogram taken 3 months after the procedure, showing sinus rhythm; (g) macroscopic view of the right atrium 2 years after the ablation, demonstrating a white, thickened endocardium (arrowheads) between the coronary sinus and the tricuspid annulus; (h and i) histology of the ablation site showing thickened fibrotic tissue (arrowheads) without viable cardiomyocytes ([b and i], H&E stain; [c] Elastica van Gieson; [d and h] Azan). *Abbreviations*: CS, coronary sinus; IVC, inferior vena cava; RA, right atrium; RV, right ventricle; SAN, sinoatrial node; TV, tricuspid valve. White bar, 1 cm; black bar, 500 μm. (Courtesy of Dr. Koji Chida, Tokyo Metropolitan Geriatric Hospital.)

of the AV node. Fibrosis of the right atrial muscle may also be present (116).

ATRIAL FIBRILLATION

Atrial fibrillation (AF) is the most common clinically significant cardiac arrhythmia, and the prevalence of AF increases markedly with age (118). Additionally, as the population ages worldwide, its prevalence is increasing (119). There are regional and ethnic variations in the prevalence of AF; the prevalence of AF is reportedly higher in individuals of European ancestry. It is unclear, however, to what extent this increase can be attributed to better surveillance in developed countries. More than 70% of patients with AF are older than age 65 in North America and Western Europe.

Macroscopically, hearts with AF show atrial cavity dilatation (Figure 2.1a) (10, 116, 120). Microscopic findings include sinoatrial muscle cell loss or fibrosis, disruption of the internodal atrial musculature by fibrosis and/or adipose tissue, or vascular occlusion of the SA nodal artery (116, 120). Catheter ablation and the Cox maze procedure are sometimes employed for symptomatic paroxysmal or persistent AF. Macroscopically, following ablation the pulmonary vein orifices may show narrowing, and there are yellow to white lesions on the endocardium several years after the procedure (Figure 2.10g) (121, 122). Microscopic examination shows that nontransmural-to-transmural coagulative necrosis, inflammation, and fibrosis depend on the time after the procedure.

ATRIOVENTRICULAR BLOCK

AV block is defined as a delay or interruption in the transmission of an impulse from the atria to the ventricles through the conduction system. AV block can be caused by anatomical abnormalities, functional disorders, drugs, or electrolyte disturbances (123, 124). Morphological changes are seen in the AV junctional area, bifurcating His bundle, or right or left bundle branch (124). In older adults, acute and old myocardial infarction, calcific valvular disease, endocarditis, myocarditis, amyloidosis, and metastatic or primary tumors may be associated with AV block (116, 123, 124).

Lev's disease and Lenègre's disease are common causes of AV block in older people. These disorders are characterized by idiopathic progressive cardiac conduction system disease without other evidence of organic heart disease (125). According to Lev, the heart begins to show fibrosis, hyalinization, and calcification with aging in various regions, including the conduction system (126). These age-related degenerative changes lead to interruption of the conduction fibers and AV block (125, 126).

Lev reported that sclero-fibrotic changes involving the central fibrous body can cause chronic atrioventricular block (126). Fibrosis and sclero-calcification are characteristically found in the bundle of His or the proximal bundle branches (126, 127). In contrast, diffuse fibrotic degeneration of the conduction system is mainly seen in the distal parts of the bundle branches in the disease credited to Lenègre. Lenègre's disease appears to be due to a loss-of-function mutation in the gene coding for the main cardiac Na^+ channel, SCN5A (125). The disease is now thought to be hereditary. Whether Lev's disease and Lenègre's disease are the same or different entities is debatable (125–127). However, a combination of the SCN5A mutation and additional degenerative age-related changes may explain the progressive alteration of conduction velocity in both disorders.

In one autopsy study of older patients with complete AV block without any identifiable cause, the most common site of complete AV block with narrow QRS and prolonged AH interval (i.e., block proximal to the His bundle deflection) was at the branching of the His bundle (128). Complete AV block with wide QRS and prolonged HV interval (block distal to the His bundle deflection) was caused by lesions in both bundle branches. As the main penetrating bundle of His is located near the noncoronary cusp of the aortic valve and near the base of the anterior leaflet of the mitral valve, calcific deposits in either the aortic or mitral valve may cause AV block (123).

BUNDLE BRANCH BLOCK

Right bundle branch block (RBBB) and left bundle branch block (LBBB) occur at various levels of the branches of the His–Purkinje system. The prevalence of both RBBB and LBBB increases with age. RBBB and LBBB are associated with a wide range of diseases (123).

PERICARDIAL DISEASE

The human heart is surrounded by pericardial tissue. The pericardium provides structural support and reduces friction. There is a potential cavity between the visceral and parietal pericardium, usually containing 15–50 mL of serous fluid (129, 130). Older adults are not particularly prone to pericardial disease. The most common cause of acute pericarditis is thought to be viral, although the etiologic agent is usually not identified. In older patients with chest pain, the pericardium as the source of pain may not be considered in the initial differential diagnosis.

Pericardial diseases include acute and recurrent pericarditis, pericardial effusion, cardiac tamponade, pericardial constriction, and pericardial tumors. Primary malignant pericardial tumors are rare; mesothelioma is the most common type (130). In contrast, the pericardium is a common site of metastasis, especially from lung or breast primaries.

Acute pericarditis is caused by a wide range of disorders. The acute inflammatory response in pericarditis produces serous or purulent pericardial effusions or dense fibrinous exudates (131). Viral infection tends to cause serous, low-volume pericardial effusions. Neoplasms and tuberculous pericarditis cause exudative, hemorrhagic effusions. Bacterial infections cause purulent pericarditis. The cause of acute pericarditis is unclear in most patients but is often presumed to be viral (129).

Pericardial constriction (less properly referred to as constrictive pericarditis) differs in developed countries and developing countries (129, 132). Pericardial constriction is thought to be the result of chronic pericardial inflammation caused by any pericardial disease (129, 130). However, when the pericardial tissue is examined, little if any inflammation is present. In developed countries, most cases are idiopathic (often thought to be viral) or related to previous cardiac surgery or irradiation (129). Grossly, pericardial constriction is associated with thickened pericardium, fibrosis and calcification, and adhesion to the adjacent myocardium.

In contrast, in developing countries approximately 70% of large pericardial effusions and most cases of pericardial constriction are caused by tuberculosis. Mortality of tuberculous pericarditis is high, 17%–40% (132). Tuberculous pericarditis develops by retrograde lymphatic spread rather than contiguous spread from tuberculous lesions in the lungs or pleurae. The immune response to the *M. tuberculosis* bacilli penetrating the pericardium plays a fundamental role in the pathogenesis of tuberculous pericarditis. Four pathological stages of tuberculous pericarditis have been recognized: 1) fibrinous exudation with initial polymorphonuclear leukocytosis, abundant mycobacteria, and early granuloma formation; 2) serosanguineous effusion with a predominantly lymphocytic exudate with monocytes and foam cells; 3) absorption of effusion with granuloma formation, pericardial thickening, and subsequent fibrosis; and 4) constrictive scarring (132). Patients with HIV-associated tuberculous pericarditis often have associated myocarditis.

REFERENCES

1. Heart Disease Prevalence - Health, United States [Internet]. 2024 [cited 2025 Feb 26]. Available from: https://www.cdc.gov/nchs/hus/topics/heart-disease-prevalence.htm.
2. Anversa P, Rota M, Urbanek K, Hosoda T, Sonnenblick EH, Leri A, et al. Myocardial aging–a stem cell problem. *Basic Res Cardiol.* 2005 Nov;100(6):482–93.
3. Lakatta EG. Arterial and cardiac aging: major shareholders in cardiovascular disease enterprises: part II: the aging heart in health: links to heart disease. *Circulation.* 2003 Jan;107(2):346–54.
4. Olivetti G, Giordano G, Corradi D, Melissari M, Lagrasta C, Gambert SR, et al. Gender differences and aging: effects on the human heart. *J Am Coll Cardiol.* 1995 Oct;26(4):1068–79.
5. Sawabe M, Saito M, Naka M, Kasahara I, Saito Y, Arai T, et al. Standard organ weights among elderly Japanese who died in hospital, including 50 centenarians. *Pathol Int.* 2006 June;56(6):315–23.
6. Okada R. Histopathological study on the effects of aging in myocardium of hypertrophied hearts. *Jpn Circ J.* 1986;50:1018–22.
7. Chida K, Ohkawa S ichiro, Watanabe C, Shimada H, Sugiura M. A morphological study of the normally aging heart. *Cardiovasc Pathol.* 1994 Jan;3(1):1–7.
8. Juhaszova M, Rabuel C, Zorov DB, Lakatta EG, Sollott SJ. Protection in the aged heart: preventing the heart-break of old age? *Cardiovasc Res.* 2005 May;66(2):233–44.
9. Waller BF, Roberts WC. Cardiovascular disease in the very elderly: analysis of 40 necropsy patients aged 90 years or over. *Am J Cardiol.* 1983 Feb;51(3):403–21.
10. Davies MJ, Pomerance A. Quantitative study of ageing changes in the human sinoatrial node and internodal tracts. *Br Heart J.* 1972 Feb;34(2):150–2.
11. Goor D, Lillehei C, Edwards J. The "sigmoid septum." Variation in the contour of the left ventricular outt. *Am J Roentgenol Radium Ther Nucl Med.* 1969;107(2):366–76.
12. Diaz T, Pencina M, Benjamin E. Prevalence, clinical correlates, and prognosis of discrete upper septal thickening on echocardiography: the Framingham heart study. *Echocardiography.* 2009;26(3):247–53.
13. Handke M, Harloff A, Olschewski M, Hetzel A, Geibel A. Patent foramen ovale and cryptogenic stroke in older patients. *N Engl J Med.* 2007 Nov 29;357(22):2262–8.
14. Parson SJ, Russell SD, Bennett MK, Dunn JM, Gilotra NA, Rao S, et al. Increased lipofuscin on endomyocardial biopsy predicts greater cardiac improvement in adolescents and young adults. *Cardiovasc Pathol.* 2012;21(4):317–23.
15. Wang JC, Bennett M. Aging and atherosclerosis: mechanisms, functional consequences, and potential therapeutics for cellular senescence. *Circ Res.* 2012 July;111(2):245–59.
16. Gando Y, Murakami H, Yamamoto K, Kawakami R, Ohno H, Sawada SS, et al. Greater progression of age-related aortic stiffening in adults with poor trunk flexibility: a 5-year longitudinal study. *Front Physiol.* 2017;8:454.
17. Orlandi A, Bochaton-Piallat ML, Gabbiani G, Spagnoli LG. Aging, smooth muscle cells and vascular pathobiology: implications for atherosclerosis. *Atherosclerosis.* 2006 Oct;188(2):221–30.
18. Virmani R, Avolio AP, Mergner WJ, Robinowitz M, Herderick EE, Cornhill JF, et al. Effect of aging on aortic morphology in populations with high and low prevalence of hypertension and atherosclerosis communities. *Am J Pathol.* 1991;139(5):1119–29.
19. Hutchins GM, Bulkley BH, Miner MM, Boitnott JK. Correlation of age and heart weight with tortuosity and caliber of normal human coronary arteries. *Am Heart J.* 1977 Aug;94(2):196–202.
20. Johnson MR. A normal coronary artery: what size is it? *Circulation.* 1992 July;86(1):331–3.
21. Hort W, Lichti H, Kalbfleisch H, Köhler F, Frenzel H, Milzner-Schwarz U. The size of human coronary arteries depending on the physiological and pathological growth of the heart the age, the size of the supplying areas and the degree of coronary sclerosis. *Virchows Arch.* 397(1):37–59.
22. Restrepo C, Eggen DA, Guzmán MA, Tejada C. Postmortem dimensions of the coronary arteries in different geographic locations. *Lab Investig J Tech Methods Pathol.* 1973 Feb;28(2):244–51.
23. Micheletti RG, Fishbein GA, Currier JS, Fishbein MC. Mönckeberg sclerosis revisited: a clarification of the histologic definition of Mönckeberg sclerosis. *Arch Pathol Lab Med.* 2008 Jan;132(1):43–7.

24. Mönckeberg J. Über die reine Mediaverkalkung der. *Virchows Arch Für Pathol Anat Physiol Für Klin Med.* 1903;171:141.
25. Micheletti RG, Fishbein GA, Currier JS, Singer EJ, Fishbein MC. Calcification of the internal elastic lamina of coronary arteries. *Mod Pathol.* 2008;21(8):1019–28.
26. Bierman EL. Atherosclerosis and aging. *Fed Proc.* 1978 Dec;37(14):2832–6.
27. Bourantas CV, Crake T, Zhang YJ, Ozkor M, Ahmed J, Garcia-Garcia HM, et al. Intravascular imaging in cardiovascular ageing. *Exp Gerontol.* 2018 Aug;109:31–7.
28. White NK, Edwards JE, Dry TJ. The relationship of the degree of coronary atherosclerosis with age, in men. *Circulation.* 1950 Apr;1(4):645–54.
29. van Oostrom O, Velema E, Schoneveld AH, de Vries JPPM, de Bruin P, Seldenrijk C a, et al. Age-related changes in plaque composition: a study in patients suffering from carotid artery stenosis. *Cardiovasc Pathol.* 2005;14(3):126–34.
30. Virmani R, Burke AP, Farb A, Kolodgie FD. Pathology of the vulnerable plaque. *J Am Coll Cardiol.* 2006 Apr;47(8 Suppl):C13–18.
31. Raggi P, Callister TQ, Cooil B, He ZX, Lippolis NJ, Russo DJ, et al. Identification of patients at increased risk of first unheralded acute myocardial infarction by electron-beam computed tomography. *Circulation.* 2000 Feb;101(8):850–5.
32. Wong ND, Kouwabunpat D, Vo a N, Detrano RC, Eisenberg H, Goel M, et al. Coronary calcium and atherosclerosis by ultrafast computed tomography in asymptomatic men and women: relation to age and risk factors. *Am Heart J.* 1994 Feb;127(2):422–30.
33. Roberts WC. Ninety-three hearts > or = 90 years of age. *Am J Cardiol.* 1993;71(7):599–602.
34. Bangalore S, Guo Y, Samadashvili Z, Blecker S, Xu J, Hannan EL. Everolimus-eluting stents or bypass surgery for multivessel coronary disease. *N Engl J Med.* 2015 Mar 26;372(13):1213–22.
35. Stone GW, Sabik JF, Serruys PW, Simonton CA, Généreux P, Puskas J, et al. Everolimus-eluting stents or bypass surgery for left main coronary artery disease. *N Engl J Med.* 2016 Dec 8;375(23):2223–35.
36. Mäkikallio T, Holm NR, Lindsay M, Spence MS, Erglis A, Menown IBA, et al. Percutaneous coronary angioplasty versus coronary artery bypass grafting in treatment of unprotected left main stenosis (NOBLE): a prospective, randomised, open-label, non-inferiority trial. *Lancet Lond Engl.* 2016 Dec 3;388(10061):2743–52.
37. Shirani J, Yousefi J, Roberts W. Major cardiac findings at necropsy in 366 American octogenarians. *Am J Cardiol.* 1995;75(2):151–6.
38. Wagenvoort C, Heath D, Edwards J. *The Pathology of the Pulmonary Vasculature.* 1st ed. Springfield, IL: Thomas Books; 1964.
39. Lam CSP, Borlaug B a, Kane GC, Enders FT, Rodeheffer RJ, Redfield MM. Age-associated increases in pulmonary artery systolic pressure in the general population. *Circulation.* 2009 May;119(20):2663–70.
40. Falk E, Nakano M, Bentzon JF, Finn AV, Virmani R. Update on acute coronary syndromes: the pathologists' view. *Eur Heart J.* 2013 Mar 7;34(10):719–28.
41. Fishbein M, Maclean D, Maroko P. The histopathologic evolution of myocardial infarction. *Chest.* 1978 June;73(6):843–9.
42. NCD Risk Factor Collaboration (NCD-RisC). Worldwide trends in hypertension prevalence and progress in treatment and control from 1990 to 2019: a pooled analysis of 1201 population-representative studies with 104 million participants. *Lancet Lond Engl.* 2021 Sept 11;398(10304):957–80.
43. Mozaffarian D, Benjamin EJ, Go AS, Arnett DK, Blaha MJ, Cushman M, et al. Heart disease and stroke statistics--2015 update: a report from the American heart association. *Circulation.* 2015 Jan 27;131(4):e29–322.
44. Möttönen MJ, Ukkola O, Lumme J, Kesäniemi YA, Huikuri HV, Perkiömäki JS. Cardiac remodeling from middle age to senescence. *Front Physiol.* 2017;8:341.
45. Frohlich ED, Apstein C, Chobanian AV, Devereux RB. The heart in hypertension. *N Engl J Med.* 1992;327:998–1008.
46. Sehgal S, Drazner MH. Left ventricular geometry: does shape matter? *Am Heart J.* 2007 Feb;153(2):153–5.
47. Drazner MH. The progression of hypertensive heart disease. *Circulation.* 2011 Jan 25;123(3):327–34.
48. Rame JE, Ramilo M, Spencer N, Blewett C, Mehta SK, Dries DL, et al. Development of a depressed left ventricular ejection fraction in patients with left ventricular hypertrophy and a normal ejection fraction. *Am J Cardiol.* 2004 Jan;93(2):234–7.
49. Schelbert EB, Cao JJ, Sigurdsson S, Aspelund T, Kellman P, Aletras AH, et al. Prevalence and prognosis of unrecognized myocardial infarction determined by cardiac magnetic resonance in older adults. *J Am Med Assoc.* 2012 Sept;308(9):890–6.
50. Roberts WC. Morphological features of the elderly heart. In: *Cardiovascular Disease in the Elderly.* 4th ed. New York: Informa Healthcare; 2008. p. 75–98.
51. Nkomo VT, Gardin JM, Skelton TN, Gottdiener JS, Scott CG, Enriquez-Sarano M. Burden of valvular heart diseases: a population-based study. *Lancet Lond Engl.* 2006 Sept 16;368(9540):1005–11.
52. Sahasakul Y, Edwards WD, Naessens JM, Tajik AJ. Age-related changes in aortic and mitral valve thickness: implications for two-dimensional echocardiography based on an autopsy study of 200 normal human hearts. *Am J Cardiol.* 1988 Sept;62(7):424–30.

53. Pomerance A. Ageing changes in human heart valves. *Br Heart J.* 1967 Mar;29(2):222–31.
54. Shah PK. Severe aortic stenosis should not be operated on before symptom onset. *Circulation.* 2012 July 3;126(1):118–25.
55. Goldbarg SH, Elmariah S, Miller M a, Fuster V. Insights into degenerative aortic valve disease. *J Am Coll Cardiol.* 2007 Sept;50(13):1205–13.
56. O'Brien KD. Epidemiology and genetics of calcific aortic valve disease. *J Invest Med.* 2007;55(6):284–91.
57. Likosky DS, Sorensen MJ, Dacey LJ, Baribeau YR, Leavitt BJ, DiScipio AW, et al. Long-term survival of the very elderly undergoing aortic valve surgery. *Circulation.* 2009 Sept;120(11 Suppl):S127–33.
58. Fishbein GA, Fishbein MC. Pathology of the aortic valve: aortic valve stenosis/aortic regurgitation. *Curr Cardiol Rep.* 2019 July 5;21(8):81.
59. Allison MA, Cheung P, Criqui MH, Langer RD, Wright CM. Mitral and aortic annular calcification are highly associated with systemic calcified atherosclerosis. *Circulation.* 2006 Feb;113(6):861–6.
60. Allen WM, Matloff JM, Fishbein MC. Myxoid degeneration of the aortic valve and isolated severe aortic regurgitation. *Am J Cardiol.* 1985 Feb;55(4):439–44.
61. Bekeredjian R, Grayburn PA. Valvular heart disease: aortic regurgitation. *Circulation.* 2005 July 5;112(1):125–34.
62. Aluru JS, Barsouk A, Saginala K, Rawla P, Barsouk A. Valvular heart disease epidemiology. *Med Sci.* 2022 June 15;10(2):32.
63. Churchill TW, Yucel E, Deferm S, Levine RA, Hung J, Bertrand PB. Mitral valve dysfunction in patients with annular calcification: JACC review topic of the week. *J Am Coll Cardiol.* 2022 Aug 16;80(7):739–51.
64. Fishbein GA, Fishbein MC. Mitral valve pathology. *Curr Cardiol Rep.* 2019 July;21(7):61.
65. Gupta V, Barzilla JE, Mendez JS, Stephens EH, Lee EL, Collard CD, et al. Abundance and location of proteoglycans and hyaluronan within normal and myxomatous mitral valves. *Cardiovasc Pathol.* 2009;18(4):191–7.
66. Wu W, Luo X, Wang L, Sun X, Jiang Y, Huo S, et al. The accuracy of echocardiography versus surgical and pathological classification of patients with ruptured mitral chordae tendineae: a large study in a Chinese cardiovascular center. *J Cardiothorac Surg.* 2011 Jan;6(1):94.
67. Deharo P, Obadia JF, Guerin P, Cuisset T, Avierinos JF, Habib G, et al. Mitral transcatheter edge-to-edge repair vs. isolated mitral surgery for severe mitral regurgitation: a French nationwide study. *Eur Heart J.* 2024 Mar 14;45(11):940–9.
68. Fox CS, Larson MG, Vasan RS, Guo CY, Parise H, Levy D, et al. Cross-sectional association of kidney function with valvular and annular calcification: the Framingham heart study. *J Am Soc Nephrol JASN.* 2006 Feb;17(2):521–7.
69. Boon A, Cheriex E, Lodder J, Kessels F. Cardiac valve calcification: characteristics of patients with calcification of the mitral annulus or aortic valve. *Heart.* 1997 Nov 1;78(5):472–4.
70. Fulkerson PK, Beaver BM, Auseon JC, Graber HL. Calcification of the mitral annulus: etiology, clinical associations, complications and therapy. *Am J Med.* 1979 June;66(6):967–77.
71. Khalil AM, Albadarin F, Khalil ME. Prevalence and gender distribution of mitral annular calcification and associated mitral valve dysfunction across age groups: a retrospective analysis. *Eur Heart J Cardiovasc Imaging.* 2025 Jan 1;26(Supplement_1):jeae333.161.
72. Roberts C, Waller BF, Bethesda MD. Mitral valve "anular" calcium forming a complete circle or "O" configuration: clinical and necropsy observations. *Am Heart J.* 1981;101:619–21.
73. D'Cruz I, Panetta F, Cohen H, Glick G. Submitral calcification or sclerosis in elderly patients: M mode and two dimensional echocardiography in "mitral anulus calcification". *Am J Cardiol.* 1979 July;44(1):31–8.
74. Pomerance A. Pathological and clinical study of calcification of the mitral valve ring. *J Clin Pathol.* 1970 May;23(4):354–61.
75. Fernández Guerrero ML, Álvarez B, Manzarbeitia F, Renedo G. Infective endocarditis at autopsy: a review of pathologic manifestations and clinical correlates. *Medicine* (Baltimore). 2012 May;91(3):152–64.
76. Atkinson JB, Virmani R. Infective endocarditis: changing trends and general approach for examination. *Hum Pathol.* 1987 June;18(6):603–8.
77. Durante-Mangoni E, Bradley S, Selton-Suty C, Tripodi MF, Barsic B, Bouza E, et al. Current features of infective endocarditis in elderly patients: results of the international collaboration on endocarditis prospective cohort study. *Arch Intern Med.* 2008 Oct 27;168(19):2095–103.
78. Tribouilloy C, Rusinaru D, Sorel C, Thuny F, Casalta JP, Riberi A, et al. Clinical characteristics and outcome of infective endocarditis in adults with bicuspid aortic valves: a multicentre observational study. *Heart Br Card Soc.* 2010 Nov;96(21):1723–9.
79. Athan E, Chu VH, Tattevin P, Selton-Suty C, Jones P, Naber C, et al. Clinical characteristics and outcome of infective endocarditis involving implantable cardiac devices. *J Am Med Assoc.* 2012 Apr;307(16):1727–35.
80. Lopez JA, Ross RS, Fishbein MC, Siegel RJ. Nonbacterial thrombotic endocarditis: a review. *Am Heart J.* 1987 Mar;113(3):773–84.
81. Rogers LR, Cho ES, Kempin S, Posner JB. Cerebral infarction from non-bacterial thrombotic endocarditis. Clinical and pathological study including the effects of anticoagulation. *Am J Med.* 1987 Oct;83(4):746–56.

82. Silbiger JJ. The valvulopathy of non-bacterial thrombotic endocarditis. *J Heart Valve Dis*. 2009 Mar;18(2):159–66.
83. Maron BJ, Towbin JA, Thiene G, Antzelevitch C, Corrado D, Arnett D, et al. Contemporary definitions and classification of the cardiomyopathies: an American heart association scientific statement from the council on clinical cardiology, heart failure and transplantation committee; quality of care and outcomes research and Functio. *Circulation*. 2006 Apr;113(14):1807–16.
84. Burke MA, Cook SA, Seidman JG, Seidman CE. Clinical and mechanistic insights into the genetics of cardiomyopathy. *J Am Coll Cardiol*. 2016 Dec 27;68(25):2871–86.
85. Maron BJ. Hypertrophic cardiomyopathy: a systematic review. *J Am Med Assoc* [Internet]. 2002 Mar 13;287(10). [cited 2025 Feb 27] Available from: http://jama.jamanetwork.com/article.aspx?doi=10.1001/jama.287.10.1308.
86. Maron MS, Hellawell JL, Lucove JC, Farzaneh-Far R, Olivotto I. Occurrence of clinically diagnosed hypertrophic cardiomyopathy in the United States. *Am J Cardiol*. 2016 May 15;117(10):1651–4.
87. Maron BJ, Casey SA, Hauser RG, Aeppli DM. Clinical course of hypertrophiccardiomyopathy with survival to advanced age. *J Am Coll Cardiol*. 2003 Sept 3;42(5):882–8.
88. Leone O, Veinot JP, Angelini A, Baandrup UT, Basso C, Berry G, et al. 2011 Consensus statement on endomyocardial biopsy from the Association for European cardiovascular pathology and the society for cardiovascular pathology. *Cardiovasc Pathol*. 2012 July;21(4):245–74.
89. Luk a, Ahn E, Soor GS, Butany J. Dilated cardiomyopathy: a review. *J Clin Pathol*. 2009 Mar;62(3):219–25.
90. Japp AG, Gulati A, Cook SA, Cowie MR, Prasad SK. The diagnosis and evaluation of dilated cardiomyopathy. *J Am Coll Cardiol*. 2016 June 28;67(25):2996–3010.
91. Gulati A, Jabbour A, Ismail TF, Guha K, Khwaja J, Raza S, et al. Association of fibrosis with mortality and sudden cardiac death in patients with nonischemic dilated cardiomyopathy. *J Am Med Assoc*. 2013 Mar 6;309(9):896–908.
92. Akashi Y, Nef H, Lyon A. Epidemiology and pathophysiology of takotsubo syndrome. *Nat Rev Cardiol*. 2015;12(7):387–97.
93. Elesber AA, Prasad A, Bybee KA, Valeti U, Motiei A, Lerman A, et al. Transient cardiac apical ballooning syndrome: prevalence and clinical implications of right ventricular involvement. *J Am Coll Cardiol*. 2006 Mar 7;47(5):1082–3.
94. Prasad A, Lerman A, Rihal CS. Apical ballooning syndrome (Tako-Tsubo or stress cardiomyopathy): a mimic of acute myocardial infarction. *Am Heart J*. 2008 Mar;155(3):408–17.
95. Templin C, Ghadri JR, Diekmann J, Napp LC, Bataiosu DR, Jaguszewski M, et al. Clinical features and outcomes of Takotsubo (stress) cardiomyopathy. *N Engl J Med*. 2015 Sept 3;373(10):929–38.
96. Tornvall P, Collste O, Ehrenborg E. A case-control study of risk markers and mortality in takotsubo stress cardiomyopathy. *J Am Coll Cardiol*. 2016;67(16):1931–6.
97. Klein C, Hiestand T, Ghadri JR, Templin C, Jäncke L, Hänggi J. Takotsubo syndrome - predictable from brain imaging data. *Sci Rep*. 2017 July 14;7(1):5434.
98. Aoki Y, Kodera S, Watanabe T. Autopsy findings in takotsubo cardiomyopathy with special reference to the autonomic nervous system. *Int J Cardiol*. 2016;203:236–7.
99. Maleszewski JJ. Cardiac amyloidosis: pathology, nomenclature, and typing. *Cardiovasc Pathol*. 2015;24(6):343–50.
100. Eletta O, Ali M, Grieff A, Puri S, Matsuda K, Bongu A, et al. Clinically occult amyloidosis derived from leukocyte chemotactic factor 2 (ALECT 2) with cardiac involvement complicating renal transplantation: case report and literature review. *Cardiovasc Pathol*. 2021;55:107375.
101. Kapoor P, Thenappan T, Singh E, Kumar S, Greipp PR. Cardiac amyloidosis: a practical approach to diagnosis and management. *Am J Med*. 2011 Nov;124(11):1006–15.
102. Shah KB, Inoue Y MMR. Amyloidosis and the heart. *Arch Intern Med*. 2006;166:1805–13.
103. Kholová I, Niessen HWM. Amyloid in the cardiovascular system: a review. *J Clin Pathol*. 2005 Feb;58(2):125–33.
104. Falk RH. Cardiac amyloidosis. *Circulation*. 2011 Aug 30;124(9):1079–85.
105. Ueda M, Horibata Y, Shono M, Misumi Y, Oshima T, Su Y, et al. Clinicopathological features of senile systemic amyloidosis: an ante- and post-mortem study. *Mod Pathol*. 2011 Dec;24(12):1533–44.
106. Rapezzi C, Merlini G, Quarta CC, Riva L, Longhi S, Leone O, et al. Systemic cardiac amyloidoses: disease profiles and clinical courses of the 3 main types. *Circulation*. 2009 Sept;120(13):1203–12.
107. Crotty TB, Li CY, Edwards WD, Suman VJ. Amyloidosis and endomyocardial biopsy: correlation of extent and pattern of deposition with amyloid immunophenotype in 100 cases. *Cardiovasc Pathol*. 1995 Jan;4(1):39–42.
108. Cornwell GG, Johnson KH, Westermark P. The age related amyloids: a growing family of unique biochemical substances. *J Clin Pathol*. 1995 Nov;48(11):984–9.

109. Kristen AV, Schnabel P a, Winter B, Helmke BM, Longerich T, Hardt S, et al. High prevalence of amyloid in 150 surgically removed heart valves–a comparison of histological and clinical data reveals a correlation to atheroinflammatory conditions. *Cardiovasc Pathol.* 2010;19(4):228–35.
110. Chow GV, Marine JE, Fleg JL. Epidemiology of arrhythmias and conduction disorders in older adults. *Clin Geriatr Med.* 2012 Nov;28(4):539–53.
111. Lev M. Aging changes in the human sinoatrial node. *J Gerontol.* 1954 Jan 1;9(1):1–9.
112. Comunoglu C, Comunoglu N, Eren B, Tanrlöver O, Türkmen N, Gündogmuş UN, et al. Age-related histopathological changes in the cardiac conducting system in the Turkish population: an evaluation of 202 autopsy cases. *Folia Morphol.* 2012 Aug;71(3):178–82.
113. Bois MC, Wu CW, Martinez CM, Castonguay MC, Jenkins SM, Maleszewski JJ. Age-related histologic features of the sinoatrial node from normal human hearts during the first 10 decades of life: a study of 200 cases. *Cardiovasc Pathol.* 2021 May 1;52:107327.
114. Shiraishi I, Takamatsu T, Minamikawa T, Onouchi Z, Fujita S. Quantitative histological analysis of the human sinoatrial node during growth and aging. *Circulation.* 1992 June;85(6):2176–84.
115. Chida K, Imai T, Taniguchi T. Implications of marked fatty infiltration around and in the atrophic atrioventricular node in elderly patients with permanent pacemaker implantation for symptomatic sick sinus syndrome. *Jpn Circ J.* 1999;63(5):343–9.
116. Ohkawa S. Clinicopathologic correlations in various kinds of arrhythmias with special references to the histopathology of the conduction system. *J Arrhythmia.* 2000;16:312–29.
117. Bharati S, Lev M. The pathologic changes in the conduction system beyond the age of ninety. *Am Heart J.* 1992 Aug;124(2):486–96.
118. Rahman F, Kwan GF, Benjamin EJ. Global epidemiology of atrial fibrillation. *Nat Rev Cardiol.* 2014 Nov;11(11):639–54.
119. Chugh SS, Havmoeller R, Narayanan K, Singh D, Rienstra M, Benjamin EJ, et al. Worldwide epidemiology of atrial fibrillation: a global burden of disease 2010 study. *Circulation.* 2014 Feb 25;129(8):837–47.
120. Waller B, Gering L, Branyas N, Slack J. Anatomy, histology, and pathology of the cardiac conduction system: part I. *Clin Cardiol.* 1993;252:249–52.
121. Kasirajan V, Sayeed S, Filler E, Knarik A, Koneru JN, Ellenbogen KA. Histopathology of bipolar radiofrequency ablation in the human atrium. *Ann Thorac Surg.* 2016 Feb;101(2):638–43.
122. Matsuyama T aki, Asano T, Inoue S, Kobayashi Y. Pathology in the late phase after extensive and ostial pulmonary vein ablation for atrial fibrillation: findings in 2 postmortem cases. *Heart Rhythm.* 2015 Feb;12(2):425–9.
123. Waller BF, Gering LE, Branyas NA, Slack JD. Anatomy, histology, and pathology of the cardiac conduction system--Part VI. *Clin Cardiol.* 1993 Aug;16(8):623–8.
124. Waller BF, Gering LE, Branyas NA, Slack JD. Anatomy, histology, and pathology of the cardiac conduction system--Part V. *Clin Cardiol.* 1993 July;16(7):565–9.
125. Royer A, van Veen T a B, Le Bouter S, Marionneau C, Griol-Charhbili V, Léoni AL, et al. Mouse model of SCN5A-linked hereditary Lenègre's disease: age-related conduction slowing and myocardial fibrosis. *Circulation.* 2005 May;111(14):1738–46.
126. Lev M. The normal anatomy of the conduction system in man and its pathology in atrioventricular block*. *Ann N Y Acad Sci.* 1964 June;111(3):817–29.
127. Stéphan E, Aftimos G, Allam C. Familial fascicular block: histologic features of Lev's disease. *Am Heart J.* 1985 June;109(6):1399–401.
128. Ohkawa S, Sugiura M, Itoh Y, Kitano K, Hiraoka K, Ueda K, et al. Electrophysiologic and histologic correlations in chronic complete atrioventricular block. *Circulation.* 1981 Aug;64(2):215–31.
129. Khandaker MH, Espinosa RE, Nishimura R a, Sinak LJ, Hayes SN, Melduni RM, et al. Pericardial disease: diagnosis and management. *Mayo Clin Proc Mayo Clin.* 2010 June;85(6):572–93.
130. Peebles CR, Shambrook JS, Harden SP. Pericardial disease–anatomy and function. *Br J Radiol.* 2011 Dec;84 Spec No:S324–37.
131. Tingle LE, Molina D, Calvert CW. Acute pericarditis. *Am Fam Physician.* 2007 Nov;76(10):1509–14.
132. Syed FF, Mayosi BM. A modern approach to tuberculous pericarditis. *Prog Cardiovasc Dis.* 2007;50(3):218–36.

3

General principles on caring for older adults

CHRISTINE Y. NGUYEN AND DAE HYUN KIM

Key points

- The US health care system faces challenges in addressing the aging population when using a traditional focus on disease-centric care.
- Cardiovascular disease is a major contributor to mortality, disability, and health care costs among older adults.
- Cardiovascular disease management in older adults should account for age-related physiologic changes and common geriatric syndromes like frailty, multimorbidity, and cognitive impairment.
- Existing clinical trials and guidelines highlight the need for patient-centered, goal-directed care tailored to older adults.

INTRODUCTION

Population aging is a global demographic trend with important implications for managing older adults with cardiovascular disease (CVD). In the United States, the number of people 65 years and older is projected to almost double in the next 50 years, and one in four Americans will be 65 years and older in 2050.[1] Nearly 75% of people 60–79 years old and 86% of those 80 years and older have some form of CVD.[2] Despite efforts to control risk factors and advancements in therapies, CVD remains the leading cause of death, health care utilization, and functional limitations, costing over $700 billion annually.[3] In addition, economic disparities exist across subgroups of the older population, and higher proportions of older people are living alone or requiring institutional care.[1] These trends present significant challenges to clinicians in providing care for people who have complex needs due to CVD and other chronic medical and geriatric conditions, functional limitations, and limited social and economic resources. Therefore, it is crucial to consider age-related changes, geriatric conditions, and contextual factors such as financial status and social support when treating older adults with CVD to ensure collaborative, patient-centered care.

PHYSIOLOGIC CHANGES OF AGING

Aging is characterized by gradual loss and alterations in function in multiple organ systems. The rate of these changes varies and can be accelerated by an individual's lifestyle, risk factors, diseases, and environment, which culminates in the considerable heterogeneity of older populations. As these changes accumulate, an individual's physiologic capacity to withstand stressors and maintain homeostasis is diminished, a state referred to as "homeostenosis." Consequently, older individuals become more vulnerable to diseases and adverse effects of drug therapy and invasive procedures.

Age-associated changes in the anatomy and physiology of the cardiovascular system are described in Chapters 1 and 2. Decreased elasticity and increased stiffness of the arterial system lead to isolated systolic hypertension.

DOI: 10.1201/9781003568933-3

Stiffness and delayed relaxation of the left ventricle predispose to diastolic heart failure. Reduced responsiveness to beta-adrenergic stimulation and circulating catecholamines limits the maximum heart rate response and peak cardiac output, contributing to decreased exercise tolerance. Fibrosis of the cardiac skeleton and conduction system coupled with a decrease in sinus node pacemaker cells increase the risk of atrial fibrillation and other arrhythmias. Calcification of fibrous valve rings increases the prevalence of calcific aortic and mitral stenosis. Decreased sensitivity of carotid baroreceptors predisposes to orthostatic hypotension, syncope, falls, and adverse effects of cardiovascular drug therapy (e.g., diuretics, beta-blockers).

Age-associated changes in other systems interact with the manifestations and management of CVD. Aging is associated with progressive decline in glomerular surface area for filtration in the kidney (decrease of 8 mL/min/1.73 m^2 per decade after age 40) and decreased ability to maintain fluid and electrolyte balance.[4] Older adults are subsequently at increased risk for volume overload, electrolyte imbalance, and cardiorenal syndrome. Age-related renal decline also affects pharmacokinetics of drugs due to decreased drug clearance; thus, close monitoring is appropriate when these drugs (e.g., digoxin, angiotensin-converting enzyme [ACE] inhibitors, antiarrhythmic drugs, beta-blockers) are used.[5] In the respiratory system, there is increased collapsibility of the alveoli and terminal conducting airways, and increased ventilation–perfusion mismatch. The ventilatory response to hypoxic or hypercapnic stimuli is blunted, which contributes to dyspnea and reduced exercise capacity. Changes in the neurohumoral system include impaired autoregulation of cerebral perfusion, diminished reflexes and proprioception, and impaired thirst mechanisms, all of which can increase the risk of syncope, falls, and volume depletion in response to cardiovascular drug therapy. In addition, anemia is prevalent in older adults with CVD due to ineffective erythropoiesis and inflammation. Increased levels of coagulation factors, platelet activity, and fibrinolysis inhibition may predispose older individuals to arterial and venous thrombosis. The risk of bleeding with antiplatelet, anticoagulant, and fibrinolytic therapy is increased, in part due to the high prevalence of risk factors for bleeding, such as decreased renal function, higher risk of falls, and drug–drug interactions.[6] In pharmacokinetics, decreased lean body mass and increased fat in aging lead to an increased half-life in lipophilic drugs. Decreased albumin leads to a lower binding capacity for highly protein-bound drugs, increasing the free drug concentration. Drug bioavailability is variable depending on metabolism due to reduced liver size, blood flow, and metabolic capacity. As a result, the bioavailability of drugs such as propranolol, verapamil, and labetalol is increased due to reduced first-pass hepatic extraction, while prazosin is reduced. In pharmacodynamics, changes in receptor number, affinity, and signaling pathways can alter drug sensitivity. Finally, the high prevalence of vision and hearing impairment may present as a barrier to communication and implementation of treatment plans in older adults with CVD.

In summary, understanding age-associated changes to the structure and function of the cardiovascular system as well as other organ systems is fundamental to individualizing treatment decisions and to delivering effective and safe therapy for CVD.

GERIATRIC SYNDROMES IN OLDER ADULTS WITH CVD

Geriatric syndromes refer to common multifactorial conditions in older adults, such as frailty, falls, functional decline, cognitive impairment, and delirium, that do not fit into classic disease categories.[7] Although age-associated physiologic changes by themselves do not represent pathology, accumulation of such changes and diseases in multiple organ systems, including CVD and noncardiovascular conditions, predisposes to geriatric syndromes. The presence of one geriatric syndrome may increase the risk of another geriatric syndrome (e.g., hospitalization-associated delirium may lead to falls). Furthermore, geriatric syndromes are associated with poor outcomes of CVD, suggesting a bidirectional relationship.[8]

Coexistence of CVD and noncardiovascular conditions may increase the risk of geriatric syndromes and adverse clinical outcomes (disease–disease interaction). Additionally, drug therapy for CVD may worsen one or more noncardiovascular conditions or geriatric syndromes, and vice versa (drug–disease interaction). Drugs for different conditions may synergistically heighten the risk of treatment-related adverse events (drug–drug interaction). The likelihood of such interactions increases with the number of conditions and medications. Importantly, older adults with multiple chronic conditions and geriatric syndromes have limited remaining life expectancy, such that they may derive little benefit from preventive cardiovascular therapy or may not tolerate the acute stress from hospitalizations, invasive procedures, and adverse drug reactions. Therefore, clinicians should be able to identify and understand the impact of common geriatric syndromes that affect CVD management (Table 3.1).

MULTIMORBIDITY

More than two thirds of older adults have two or more chronic conditions, or multimorbidity.[9] Individuals with multimorbidity are at increased risk for death, disability, hospitalization, nursing facility stay, and health care utilization. The prevalence of multimorbidity increases with age; over 80% of people 85 years and older have at least two conditions and approximately 50% have at least four conditions. More than 50% of older individuals with heart failure, stroke, and atrial fibrillation have five or more chronic conditions.[10] Common noncardiovascular conditions in those with CVD include arthritis, anemia,

Table 3.1 Common geriatric conditions and implications for cardiovascular care

Condition	Significance	Assessment	Management

Multimorbidity	• Older patients with multimorbidity excluded from clinical trials of CVD treatments
	• Guideline-based CVD treatments may not be feasible or effective
	• CVD treatment may worsen coexisting conditions
	• Non-CVD conditions account for almost half of readmissions after CVD admissions
		• Identify coexisting non-CVD conditions requiring treatments that may compete with CVD treatments	• Adopt patient-centered care that aligns treatments with personal goals and preference
			• Consider the following aspects:
			  • Likelihood of benefits vs. harms
			  • Prognosis (life expectancy)
			  • Functional impairment and frailty
			  • Treatment feasibility

Polypharmacy	• CVD medications are responsible for 25% of preventable drug-related adverse events • ↑Risk of drug-drug interactions • ↑Risk of drug-disease interactions • ↓Treatment adherence • ↑Financial burden • ↑Caregiver stress	• Assess total treatment burden from • Nonpharmacological treatment • Pharmacological treatment (total number of medications and treatment complexity) • Assess treatment adherence	• Identify medications with high likelihood of harms and questionable benefits using an expert consensus checklist (e.g., Beers criteria) • Discontinue nonessential treatments to maximize adherence to essential treatments

Frailty	• Underdiagnosed
	• CVD is a risk factor for frailty
	• ↑Risk for hospitalization, nursing home admission, functional decline, and mortality
	• Useful for risk stratification before invasive procedure (e.g., transcatheter aortic valve replacement)
		• Use a validated frailty screening and assessment:
		  • Gait speed
		  • Clinical Frailty Scale
		  • Frailty phenotype
		  • Comprehensive geriatric assessment-based frailty index (CGA-FI)
			• No effective pharmacological interventions exist for prevention or treatment of frailty
			• Comprehensive geriatric assessment and exercise program can prevent functional decline and nursing home admission
			• Use frailty assessment to predict prognosis and guide individualized treatment decisions

Cognitive impairment	• Underdiagnosed
	• CVD is a risk factor for cognitive impairment
	• ↓Treatment adherence and disease monitoring
	• ↑Risk for hospitalization and mortality in heart failure
		• Use a validated cognitive screening tool:
		  • Mini-Mental State Examination
		  • Montreal Cognitive Assessment
		  • Mini-Cog test
			• Simplify CVD treatments for better adherence
			• Utilize support system to improve adherence and disease monitoring

Delirium	• Under-diagnosed
	• ↑Risk for hospitalization, nursing home admission, functional decline, and mortality
	• May lead to persistent cognitive impairment after cardiac surgery
		• Use a validated screening and diagnostic tool:
		  • CAM
		  • 3-D CAM
		  • Ultra-Brief CAM
			• Use nonpharmacological interventions to prevent delirium
			• No effective pharmacological interventions exist for prevention or treatment of delirium

(Continued)

Table 3.1 (Continued) Common geriatric conditions and implications for cardiovascular care

Condition	Significance	Assessment	Management

Functional decline	• Underdiagnosed
	• CVD can cause functional decline
	• ↓Treatment adherence and disease monitoring
	• ↑Risk for hospitalization, nursing home admission, and mortality
		• Use a validated instrument:
		  • Katz index of activities of daily living
		  • Lawton index of instrumental activities of daily living
		  • Nagi scale
			Utilize support system to improve adherence and disease monitoring

Falls	• Underdiagnosed
	• Symptomatic heart failure and certain CVD medications may contribute to fall risk
	• ↓Adherence to exercise intervention
		• Use a validated screening tool:
		  • Number of falls in the past year
		  • Self-reported difficulty in gait or balance
		  • Timed Up and Go test
			• Start CVD medications at low dose and gradually increase
			• Refer high-risk patients to gait and balance training program or to a fall specialist for multidisciplinary assessment and targeted interventions

Abbreviations: ACEI, angiotensin-converting enzyme inhibitor; CAM, Confusion Assessment Method; CVD, cardiovascular disease.

chronic kidney disease, cataracts, chronic obstructive pulmonary disease, dementia, and depression,[10] which add to the complexity of CVD management in older adults. These noncardiovascular conditions account for almost half of readmissions after an index admission for heart failure or myocardial infarction.[11] Moreover, older adults with multimorbidity are often excluded from clinical trials of cardiovascular therapy. Therefore, it remains unclear whether clinical trial evidence on the benefits and risks can be generalized to patients with multimorbidity.

Although multimorbidity and comorbidity are related concepts, a multimorbidity-based framework provides a useful approach to manage older adults with CVD. In the comorbidity framework, CVD is implied as the central condition, while other conditions are considered secondary entities.[12] Treatment is focused on the CVD, although coexisting conditions may affect the choice of therapy. Most CVD clinical practice guidelines were developed under this construct. In the multimorbidity framework, the patient is the central focus, and all conditions can be considered equally important as long as they impact patient-centered outcomes, such as quality of life and function.[12] Treatment is targeted at multiple conditions simultaneously with a goal to optimize these measures. To effectively achieve this goal, identifying common patterns of conditions provides a useful context to consider trade-offs between different conditions. Clinicians should prioritize interventions for CVD and other coexisting noncardiovascular conditions that have the highest impact on patient-centered outcomes.

POLYPHARMACY

Medications frequently used by older adults in the United States include cardiovascular drugs. Over 40% of older individuals take five or more medications, which is referred to as polypharmacy.[13] Polypharmacy is strongly associated with multimorbidity and prescribing practices aligned with disease-based clinical practice guidelines.[13] The consequences of polypharmacy are broad and potentially serious. In a 2011 national survey, 15% of older adults were at risk for a major drug-drug interaction; the most common interacting regimen involving prescription drugs was concurrent use of amlodipine and simvastatin.[14] In a national study of Medicare beneficiaries, 23% were taking at least one medication that could potentially worsen a coexisting condition. For example, use of nonsteroidal anti-inflammatory drugs for osteoarthritis may increase the risk of CVD and reduce the efficacy of cardiovascular therapy (e.g., ACE inhibitors, angiotensin receptor blockers, diuretics) in patients with CVD.[15] Cardiovascular drugs are responsible for 25% of preventable adverse events.[16] Other consequences of polypharmacy include lower adherence, financial burden, and caregiver stress.[17,18]

When a new cardiovascular drug is considered, clinicians should assess the incremental benefit and harm of the new drug in older patients who already have a complex regimen. A post hoc analysis of a clinical trial of anticoagulation therapy in patients with atrial fibrillation showed that the efficacy of apixaban compared with warfarin on thromboembolic events was consistent across the number of concomitant drugs used, but the protective effect of apixaban on major bleeding diminished with increasing numbers of concomitant drugs.[19] Since clinical trials often exclude patients with polypharmacy, the possibility of benefit and harm by the number of concomitant drugs remains uncertain for most cardiovascular drugs. Another important consideration is that patients with polypharmacy are more likely to have multimorbidity and frailty; such patients may not live long enough to benefit from a preventive cardiovascular therapy. In a meta-analysis evaluating the time to benefit of statins for primary prevention of cardiovascular events in older adults aged 50 to 75 years, findings suggested a benefit in statins if patients had a life expectancy of at least 2.5 years. For older adults at the end of life or with advanced illness, deprescribing statins or deferring initiation of statins can be considered.[20]

When there is a major change in the patient's general health or functional status (e.g., falls, functional or cognitive decline, delirium, hospitalization, institutionalization), clinicians should reassess the ongoing need for each medication and consider deprescribing medications with questionable benefit or high risk of harm. Standard checklists, such as the American Geriatrics Society Beers list[5] or STOPP/START criteria,[21] can be used to identify high-risk medications. A time-limited withdrawal may help clinicians determine the need for ongoing therapy when the indication for a medication is unclear. When deprescribing cardiovascular drugs, a gradual tapering off may be necessary to reduce rebound or withdrawal symptoms.

FRAILTY

Frailty is a clinical state characterized by diminished physiologic reserve and increased vulnerability to adverse health outcomes.[22] Frailty is more common with aging, as the prevalence of frailty in community-dwelling persons ranged from 11% in those age 50 to 59 years to 51% in those aged 90 years or older. Among older adults with CVD, prevalence estimates were 36% in patients with coronary artery disease,[23] 19%–52% in those with heart failure,[24] and up to 70% in patients undergoing transcatheter aortic valve replacement.[25,26] While frailty is a consequence of accumulated age-associated changes and diseases in multiple physiologic systems,[27] CVD seems to play an important role in the development of frailty. In the Cardiovascular Health Study, frailty was associated with clinical CVD as well as subclinical CVD.[28] In particular, the strongest association was found for heart failure. Individuals with frailty are more likely to develop heart failure,[29] and frailty was associated with poor outcomes in heart failure.[8] Frailty also predicts mortality and poor functional status after major cardiac surgery and transcatheter aortic valve replacement.[30,31] Given the bidirectional relationship between frailty and CVD, whether it is possible to lessen or reverse frailty by optimizing CVD management is an area of active investigation.

Frailty assessment can be useful in individualizing cardiovascular therapy, since older adults with CVD and severe frailty have a shorter life expectancy and increased risk for treatment-related harms. Several validated instruments assess frailty in older adults, each focusing on different domains.[32] The *frailty phenotype* is the most widely used assessment that is based on unintentional weight loss, weak grip strength, exhaustion, slow gait, and physical inactivity.[33] A patient is frail if they meet three or more of these components, and each component can be targeted by interventions. The deficit-accumulation *frailty index* is an alternative measure that quantifies frailty as a proportion of deficits in medical, physical, cognitive, and nutritional domains assessed during a comprehensive geriatric assessment. A frailty index can have a value between 0 and 1, with frailty defined as 0.25 and above.[34,35] Very few people have a frailty index greater than 0.7, suggesting that an individual with more than 70% of deficits has a very high mortality risk.[36] In other words, a patient whose frailty index is close to 0.7 has little reserve to withstand additional stress from adverse drug reactions, invasive procedures, or hospitalizations. Compared with frailty phenotype, the frailty index offers better prediction of adverse health outcomes.[37]

In choosing a frailty instrument for clinical use, feasibility (e.g., equipment needs, space, time, training) and specific characteristics of patients that may influence their participation in the assessment should be considered. Interactive web-based calculators for commonly used frailty assessment tools are available (eFrailty.org).[38] As an alternative to assessments of frailty phenotype or frailty index, simple instruments are available and include: Timed Up and Go test,[39] gait speed,[40] Clinical Frailty Scale,[41] and FRAIL questionnaire.[42] Since these simple instruments generally have high sensitivity and moderate specificity,[40] they can be a useful screening tool for identifying high-risk patients, and a positive test should be followed by a comprehensive geriatric assessment. For the development of individualized care plans and interventions, more comprehensive assessments are necessary.

COGNITIVE IMPAIRMENT

The prevalence of dementia, now termed major neurocognitive disorder,[43] is 14% in the older population of the United States, ranging from 5% in people 71–79 years of age to 37% in people 90 years and older.[44] More people have mild cognitive impairment (minor neurocognitive disorder), a less severe but measurable cognitive decline that may progress to dementia at an annual rate of 12%.[45] Cognitive impairment is more common in older adults with CVD, affecting 35% of patients undergoing coronary artery bypass grafting[46] and 47% of those with heart failure.[47] Cognitive decline after coronary revascularization

Three Word Recall	Clock Drawing
Give three words for person to repeat and remember. After the clock drawing, ask the person to recall the three words. Example: Banana Sunrise Chair	Instruct person to draw a clock. First put in all the numbers, then set the hands at 10 past 11. 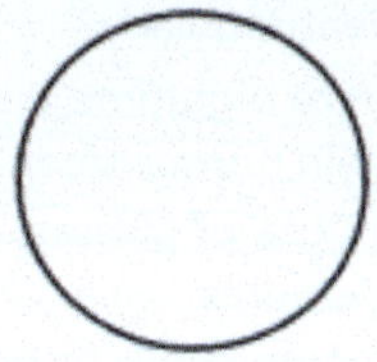
Scoring	
Word Recall: _____ (0-3 points)	1 point for each word recalled without cueing
Clock Draw: _____ (0 or 2 points)	Normal clock = 2 points Abnormal clock = 0 points
Total Score: _____ (0-5 points)	Cut point of <3 points has been validated for dementia screening

Figure 3.1 The Mini-Cog test. (From Borson S et al., *Int J Geriat Psychiatry*, 15, 1021–1027, 2000.)

does not seem different between coronary artery bypass graft surgery and percutaneous coronary intervention.[48] Risk factors for CVD, such as hypertension, diabetes, hyperlipidemia, smoking, and obesity, are associated with cerebral infarcts, microhemorrhage, hypoperfusion, inflammation, and oxidative stress.[49] These changes lead to gray matter atrophy, white matter lesions, and damage to subcortical white matter pathways.[50] Cognitive impairment associated with CVD is characterized by executive dysfunction that is critical in maintaining independence. Those with executive dysfunction have more difficulty following complex treatment regimens, contributing to low adherence, readmission, and mortality.[47,51,52] Among several validated instruments to assess cognitive function, the Mini-Cog test is a brief screening tool that consists of a three-word recall test for memory and a clock drawing test for executive function (Figure 3.1).[53] An abnormal Mini-Cog test should prompt further cognitive testing. Poor performance on the Mini-Cog test predicts readmission or mortality after heart failure hospitalization.[54]

DELIRIUM

Delirium is an acute confusional state that affects up to 35% of older patients on general medical wards, 50% of cardiac surgical patients,[55] and 75% of patients in an intensive care unit.[56] It develops as a result of a complex interaction between predisposing factors (e.g., preexisting cognitive impairment, functional limitations, multimorbidity, frailty) and precipitating factors (e.g., psychoactive drugs, surgery, anesthesia, pain, dehydration, sleep–wake cycle reversal, acute illness, inflammation).[57] Delirium is associated with prolonged hospitalization, functional and cognitive decline, institutionalization, mortality, and increased health care costs.[57] Although delirium has traditionally been considered transient, emerging literature suggests otherwise: persistent delirium is common, with 33% prevalence at 1 month and 21% at 6 months after discharge.[58] Delirium was associated with persistently lower cognitive function at 1 year after cardiac surgery[59] and increased risk of dementia over 4 years.[60] Despite these clinical and public health implications, delirium is underrecognized by clinicians, especially in the case of hypoactive ("quiet") delirium. However, hypoactive delirium is more common and associated with worse prognosis than hyperactive delirium.[55]

The Confusion Assessment Method (CAM) is the most widely used diagnostic algorithm, with a sensitivity of 94%–100% and specificity of 90%–95% against a reference standard clinical examination.[61,62] The CAM algorithm establishes the diagnosis of delirium according to the presence or absence of four features: (1) acute onset and fluctuating course, (2) inattention, (3) disorganized thinking, and (4) altered level of consciousness.[63] Brief instruments, such as the CAM for Intensive Care Unit,[64] the 3-Minute Diagnostic Assessment (3-D CAM),[65] and Ultra-Brief CAM,[66] can be adopted in clinical practice.

Currently, no pharmacological interventions are proven effective for the prevention or treatment of delirium. Therefore, prevention is the key to avoiding negative ramifications.[67] There is strong evidence to recommend nonpharmacological multifactorial interventions to address cognitive impairment, sleep deprivation, immobility, dehydration, and sensory impairment (Table

Table 3.2 Nonpharmacologic strategies for delirium prevention

Category	Intervention
Cognitive orientation	• Provide clocks and calendars • Reorient regularly
Sleep hygiene	• Minimize nighttime disruptions • Maintain normal sleep–wake cycle
Sensory deficits	• Ensure use of glasses, hearing aids, and dentures
Environment	• Encourage family to bring familiar objects • Provide adequate lighting • Minimize noise and overstimulation
Mobility and function	• Involve physical and occupational therapy • Promote early and regular mobilization
Nutrition	• Monitor fluid intake • Offer meal assistance • Assess and treat swallowing difficulties
Pain management	• Regular pain assessment • Minimize opioid analgesics as appropriate
Medication management	• Deprescribe and avoid medications that may worsen or cause delirium
Urinary and bowel habits	• Maintain regular bowel movements • Assess and treat urinary retention • Implement scheduled toileting

3.2).[67] Medications that increase the risk of delirium (e.g., drugs with anticholinergic properties, benzodiazepines, sedatives) should be avoided. Due to inconsistent efficacy and concerns for serious harms, such as cardiac arrhythmias, sedation, extrapyramidal side effects, aspiration pneumonitis, stroke, and even mortality, antipsychotics should not be routinely used for delirium prevention or treatment. In case of severe agitation that presents a substantial risk of harm to self or others, clinicians should prescribe the lowest effective dose antipsychotic for the shortest duration possible.[68] Because antipsychotics appear to have similar efficacy, the choice is often based on adverse effects.[69] Adequate management of precipitating factors, such as pain and acute medical illness, is also key in mitigating the duration and severity of delirium.

Functional decline

Patients with a higher burden of clinical and subclinical CVD experience accelerated functional decline and spend more years with disability.[70,71] Those who experience functional decline are more likely to develop CVD events.[72] In particular, the risk of functional decline is high when older adults are hospitalized with an acute illness. In addition to the negative effect of acute illness and complications like delirium, hospitalization is associated with restricted mobility, enforced dependence and limited encouragement of independence (e.g., bed alarms and bed rest), limited access to food and liquids (e.g., "nil per os" orders), and polypharmacy.[73] The effect of bed rest on sarcopenia, defined as loss in skeletal muscle mass and function, is well documented.[74,75] In healthy older adults, bed rest resulted in a loss of 630 grams of muscle mass per week compared with 100–200 grams per week in younger adults.[74] The loss in knee extensor peak torque after 10 days of bed rest was consistent with a reduction in stair-climbing power.[75] The effect of bed rest on sarcopenia is expected to be more substantial in hospitalized patients with an acute illness (e.g., acute CVD event) that is associated with a high catabolic state.[76] As a result, functional decline acquired during an acute hospitalization may require rehabilitation discharge or home health services. The period of restricted activity may persist after hospital discharge, and this can precipitate new or worsening disability in older adults.[77] Frail patients are more likely to experience functional decline than non-frail patients, even after less invasive transcatheter aortic valve replacement.[31]

Clinicians can measure functional status using a validated questionnaire, such as the Nagi scale,[78] activity of daily living scale,[79] or instrumental activity of daily living scale.[80] Considering the multifactorial nature of functional decline, prevention requires a multicomponent intervention. Evidence supports the consumption of high-quality protein (1-1.2 grams per kilogram of body weight per day),[81] with the exception of some people with advanced kidney disease not on dialysis, and exercise in close temporal proximity to protein-enriched meals as effective strategies for preventing muscle loss due to bed rest.[76] Nonpharmacological interventions to prevent delirium can reduce delirium, functional decline, and hospital falls.[67,82] In older adults who are scheduled for a cardiovascular procedure, a prehabilitation program that addresses modifiable risk factors for functional decline prior to the procedure has potential to improve postoperative outcomes and facilitate functional recovery.[83] Such programs should be individualized based on patient characteristics, available expertise, resources, and costs. As facility-based programs may not be cost-effective or feasible for many patients, a home-based program may be a suitable alternative. More research is needed to identify the best prehabilitation model for patients undergoing cardiovascular procedures.

FALLS

One in three older adults in the community falls every year. As the leading cause of injury (e.g., soft tissue injury, hip fracture, head trauma) in people 65 years and older,[84] falls have major consequences on older individuals' independence, quality of life, and medical costs. Most falls are multifactorial, with major risk factors including gait and balance impairment, muscle weakness, sensory impairment, medications, orthostatic hypotension, functional limitations, cognitive impairment, and urinary incontinence.[85] Patients with clinical CVD, in particular hypotension, heart failure, and arrhythmia, are at increased risk for falls.[86] Other cardiovascular conditions related to falls include carotid sinus hypersensitivity, vasovagal syncope, and postprandial hypotension. Symptomatic CVD can cause mobility impairment, reduced muscle strength, functional limitation, and cognitive impairment, thereby contributing to the risk of falls. Moreover, medications commonly consumed by older adults with CVD, such as antihypertensives,[87,88] loop diuretics,[89] and psychoactive drugs,[87–90] have been linked to falls. The risk may be higher after initiation of a new cardiovascular drug or dose increase compared with chronic use. On the other hand, fall history can influence CVD management. Individuals with fall history or fear of falling may exercise caution to avoid injury during physical activity. Concerns about falling are the most commonly cited reason by clinicians for not initiating anticoagulation in older adults with atrial fibrillation.[91] Since the risk of major bleeding and intracranial bleeding is higher in older adults with fall history than those without, it is important to assess fall risk before anticoagulation therapy.[92] To assess fall risk, clinicians should first ask about history of falls in the past year and difficulty with walking or balance. A mobility test, such as Timed Up and Go test, can be useful.[93] Patients at high risk for falls should receive a comprehensive evaluation followed by targeted interventions, including gait and balance training.[94]

APPROACHES TO EVALUATION AND MANAGEMENT OF OLDER ADULTS WITH CVD

The main goal of cardiovascular therapy is to improve quality of life, functional status, and survival by reducing CVD symptoms and preventing future CVD events. A frailty-guided approach to CVD management in older adults takes into account the complex interplay between frailty and cardiovascular conditions to provide patient-centered care and focuses on outcomes such as quality of life, functional status, and overall survival as opposed to CVD-free survival. Consequently, the benefit of cardiovascular therapy may be offset by exacerbation of noncardiovascular or geriatric conditions, treatment-related adverse events, and decreased adherence to complex treatment regimens. Before prescribing medications or recommending invasive procedures for CVD, clinicians should consider the severity and prognosis related to CVD as well as the impact of noncardiovascular conditions and geriatric syndromes on the overall quality of life, functional status, and prognosis.

Limitations of clinical trial evidence and clinical practice guidelines

The management of CVD is driven by evidence from clinical trials. A study comparing Medicare beneficiaries to the participants of 141 trials referenced by CVD guidelines found that trial participants were younger and more likely to be male.[95] In addition, since clinical trials primarily focus on mortality or cardiovascular events, the effect of therapeutic and preventative interventions on quality of life or functional status is not well studied. While a patient's willingness to take a medication for primary prevention may be influenced by the risk of adverse effects rather than potential benefit,[96] these patients are less likely to participate in clinical trials. Therefore, there is insufficient evidence on treatment harms from clinical trials.

Clinical practice guidelines derived from clinical trial evidence carry similar limitations. Although many guidelines include age, few guidelines discuss conflicting recommendations or the need for treatment modifications in the presence of multimorbidity.[17] Such a myopic focus on a single disease is not only impractical but potentially harmful. Therapeutic competition, which refers to the potential for standard of care treatment of one condition to introduce harm in the context of another illness, was observed in 23% of community-dwelling older adults.[15] Clinical practice guidelines that fail to address patient preferences may contribute to low adherence and suboptimal care.[17] Over time, medical literature has recognized the need for incorporating patient values and preferences,[97] including guidelines from the American Heart Association and American College of Cardiology that focus on a patient-centered, team-based approach when managing major CVD.[98]

Adopting patient-centered, goal-directed care

Fragmented care, combined with clinical practice guidelines under the comorbidity framework, often leads to conflicting recommendations. A patient-centered, goal-directed care model has been proposed as a potential remedy to the aforementioned issues. This model is centered on the achievement of patient-defined health outcome goals and care preferences.[99–101] Health outcome goals refer to specific outcomes that patients aim to accomplish through their health and health care (e.g., improvement of function, symptom relief). Care preferences are essentially what trade-offs are allowed (e.g., frequent lab monitoring, dietary changes, financial limitations), and how these trade-offs weigh into what an individual patient is willing to do. By aligning goals on patient-defined outcomes and preferences rather than individual diseases, the health care team is united in its efforts to achieve the same outcomes.

The process starts with the identification of patient goals by a member of the health care team. Here the position of the member is less important than their communication skills and ability to guide an interaction and craft meaningful goals with patients and their caregivers. Outcomes should be specific, measurable, actionable, reliable, and time-bound ("SMART").[99] Specific roles can then be established, with responsibilities delegated to the most appropriate members of the health care team and one clinician taking responsibility to coordinate care in general. Working with geriatricians and other clinicians with experience and expertise in caring for older patients is critical to the success of this model. Developing quality metrics that reflect high-value care from the patient's perspective can facilitate goal-directed care.[102]

Assessing time to benefit and prognosis

Another important consideration in treatment decisions is to assess the likelihood of a clinically meaningful treatment benefit. This involves comparing the patient's remaining life expectancy with the time to benefit from a treatment.[103] Several prognostic models exist to estimate the mortality risk at a specified time period or the remaining life expectancy.[104] The time to benefit represents the length of time needed to accrue a clinically meaningful benefit for a specific outcome.[103] For example, the time to benefit for statins to prevent a major adverse cardiac event in adults aged 50–75 years was 2.5 years.[105] If a patient's remaining life expectancy is shorter than the time to benefit from a treatment, the treatment is unlikely to provide a meaningful benefit and may be futile; if the remaining life expectancy is longer than the time to benefit, the treatment can be recommended. If the two estimates are similar, the decision should be guided by the patient's goals and preferences. While this concept is potentially useful to prioritize multiple, competing treatments in multimorbid patients, time to benefit is rarely reported in clinical trials. Although time to benefit has been explored by researchers,[106–108] these methods rely on statistical interpretation of benefit, rather than clinically meaningful benefit, or result in estimates that are often too uncertain (i.e., wide confidence intervals) to impact treatment decision-making.

Communicating evidence for treatment decision-making

Appropriate interpretation and effective communication of the evidence are essential to treatment decision-making. Evidence suggests that how evidence is presented to patients affects their treatment choice. Despite their widespread use in medical literature, statistics such as relative risk reduction, absolute risk, and number needed to treat (or harm) are not intuitive for clinicians and patients to understand or communicate.[109,110] Presenting relative risk reduction alone without absolute risk information can be misleading and tends to bias patients toward accepting treatment.[111] For instance, patients who have diabetes but low cardiovascular risk were 70% less likely to choose statin treatment after being presented with information about the small absolute risk reduction.[112] It is recommended to use natural frequencies with the denominator of 1000 people (e.g., 50 in 1000 people, instead of 5%, develop an event in 5 years) when expressing benefits and harms, avoid the number needed to treat, and present both absolute and relative risk reductions.[111,113–118] Use of visual decision aids can be helpful. Alternative measures of treatment effect, such as event-free or disability-free time gained or lost due to treatment,[119,120] may allow more intuitive interpretation of clinical trial results.

SUMMARY

CVD affects a large number of older people and remains a significant cause of mortality and morbidity. Due to an accumulation of age-associated physiologic changes, multiple diseases affecting the cardiovascular and other organ systems, and prevalent geriatric conditions, it is challenging to evaluate and manage the treatment of older adults with CVD. It is important to recognize that clinical trial evidence and recommendations from disease-specific clinical practice guidelines are inadequate for multimorbid or frail older adults because the net benefit of treatment to optimize CVD-specific outcomes may be negated by its adverse effect on other conditions that are equally important for quality of life and functioning. When such a trade-off is inevitable, clinicians should begin by asking about the patient's goals and preferences, and prioritizing and aligning treatments accordingly. Under the patient goal-directed care model, the emphasis is to maximize the chance of achieving the patient-defined goals, not to manage each disease according to the clinical practice guidelines. Additional research is needed to generate evidence on patient-centered outcomes and improve evidence communication strategies for informed decision-making.

GUIDELINE RECOMMENDATIONS

- Individualize care of older adults with CVD by considering the unique physiologic changes, multimorbidity, and geriatric conditions.
- Recognize the limitations of disease-specific clinical guidelines in frail or multimorbid older adults.
- Prioritize patient goals and preferences to guide treatment decisions and enhance quality of life and functional status rather than strictly targeting disease-specific metrics.

Further research should explore patient-centered outcomes and improve how evidence is communicated to support informed, shared decision-making.

REFERENCES

1. Fact Sheet: Aging in the United States. PRB. Accessed February 22, 2025. https://www.prb.org/resources/fact-sheet-aging-in-the-united-states/
2. Rodgers JL, Jones J, Bolleddu SI, et al. Cardiovascular risks associated with gender and aging. *J Cardiovasc Dev Dis*. 2019;6(2):19. doi:10.3390/jcdd6020019
3. Kazi DS, Elkind MSV, Deutsch A, et al. Forecasting the economic burden of cardiovascular disease and stroke in the United States through 2050: A presidential advisory from the American Heart Association. *Circulation*. 2024;150(4):e89e101. doi:10.1161/CIR.0000000000001258
4. Davies DF, Shock NW. Age changes in glomerular filtration rate, effective renal plasma flow, and tubular excretory capacity in adult males. *J Clin Invest*. 1950;29(5):496507. doi:10.1172/JCI102286
5. American Geriatrics Society 2023 updated AGS Beers Criteria® for potentially inappropriate medication use in older adults. doi:10.1111/jgs.18372
6. Schulman S, Beyth RJ, Kearon C, Levine MN. Hemorrhagic complications of anticoagulant and thrombolytic treatment: American College of Chest Physicians Evidence-Based Clinical Practice Guidelines (8th Edition). *Chest*. 2008;133(6 Suppl):257S298S. doi:10.1378/chest.08-0674
7. Inouye SK, Studenski S, Tinetti ME, Kuchel GA. Geriatric syndromes: clinical, research, and policy implications of a core geriatric concept. *J Am Geriatr Soc*. 2007;55(5):780791. doi:10.1111/j.1532-5415.2007.01156.x
8. Chaudhry SI, McAvay G, Chen S, et al. Risk factors for hospital admission among older persons with newly diagnosed heart failure: findings from the Cardiovascular Health Study. *J Am Coll Cardiol*. 2013;61(6):635642. doi:10.1016/j.jacc.2012.11.027
9. Salive ME. Multimorbidity in older adults. *Epidemiol Rev*. 2013;35:7583. doi:10.1093/epirev/mxs009
10. Arnett DK, Goodman RA, Halperin JL, Anderson JL, Parekh AK, Zoghbi WA. AHA/ACC/HHS strategies to enhance application of clinical practice guidelines in patients with cardiovascular disease and comorbid conditions: from the American Heart Association, American College of Cardiology, and U.S. Department of Health and Human Services. *J Am Coll Cardiol*. 2014;64(17):18511856. doi:10.1016/j.jacc.2014.07.012
11. Dharmarajan K, Hsieh AF, Lin Z, et al. Diagnoses and timing of 30-day readmissions after hospitalization for heart failure, acute myocardial infarction, or pneumonia. *JAMA*. 2013;309(4):355363. doi:10.1001/jama.2012.216476
12. Harrison C, Fortin M, van den Akker M, et al. Comorbidity versus multimorbidity: why it matters. *J Multimorb Comorbidity*. 2021;11:2633556521993993. doi:10.1177/2633556521993993
13. Pan S, Li S, Jiang S, et al. Trends in number and appropriateness of prescription medication utilization among community-dwelling older adults in the United States: 20112020. *J Gerontol A Biol Sci Med Sci*. 2024;79(7):glae108. doi:10.1093/gerona/glae108
14. Qato DM, Wilder J, Schumm LP, Gillet V, Alexander GC. Changes in prescription and over-the-counter medication and dietary supplement use among older adults in the United States, 2005 vs 2011. *JAMA Intern Med*. 2016;176(4):473482. doi:10.1001/jamainternmed.2015.8581
15. Lorgunpai SJ, Grammas M, Lee DSH, McAvay G, Charpentier P, Tinetti ME. Potential therapeutic competition in community-living older adults in the U.S.: use of medications that may adversely affect a coexisting condition. *PloS One*. 2014;9(2):e89447. doi:10.1371/journal.pone.0089447
16. Gurwitz JH, Field TS, Harrold LR, et al. Incidence and preventability of adverse drug events among older persons in the ambulatory setting. *JAMA*. 2003;289(9):11071116. doi:10.1001/jama.289.9.1107
17. Boyd CM, Darer J, Boult C, Fried LP, Boult L, Wu AW. Clinical practice guidelines and quality of care for older patients with multiple comorbid diseases: implications for pay for performance. *JAMA*. 2005;294(6):716724. doi:10.1001/jama.294.6.716
18. Choudhry NK, Fischer MA, Avorn J, et al. The implications of therapeutic complexity on adherence to cardiovascular medications. *Arch Intern Med*. 2011;171(9):814822. doi:10.1001/archinternmed.2010.495
19. Jaspers Focks J, Brouwer MA, Wojdyla DM, et al. Polypharmacy and effects of apixaban versus warfarin in patients with atrial fibrillation: post hoc analysis of the ARISTOTLE trial. *BMJ*. 2016;353:i2868. doi:10.1136/bmj.i2868
20. Yourman LC, Cenzer IS, Boscardin WJ, et al. Evaluation of time to benefit of statins for the primary prevention of cardiovascular events in adults aged 50 to 75 years: a meta-analysis. *JAMA Intern Med*. 2021;181(2):179185. doi:10.1001/jamainternmed.2020.6084
21. O'Mahony D, O'Sullivan D, Byrne S, O'Connor MN, Ryan C, Gallagher P. STOPP/START criteria for potentially inappropriate prescribing in older people: version 2. *Age Ageing*. 2015;44(2):213218. doi:10.1093/ageing/afu145
22. Kim DH, Rockwood K. Frailty in older adults. *N Engl J Med*. 2024;391(6):538548. doi:10.1056/NEJMra2301292
23. Li T, Shi W, Wang G, Jiang Y. Prevalence and risk factors of frailty in older patients with coronary heart disease: a systematic review and meta-analysis. *Arch Gerontol Geriatr*. 2025;130:105721. doi:10.1016/j.archger.2024.105721
24. Pandey A, Kitzman D, Reeves G. Frailty is intertwined with heart failure. *JACC Heart Fail*. 2019;7(12):10011011. doi:10.1016/j.jchf.2019.10.005

25. Sündermann S, Dademasch A, Praetorius J, et al. Comprehensive assessment of frailty for elderly high-risk patients undergoing cardiac surgery. *Eur J Cardio-Thorac Surg Off J Eur Assoc Cardio-Thorac Surg.* 2011;39(1):3337. doi:10.1016/j.ejcts.2010.04.013
26. Green P, Arnold SV, Cohen DJ, et al. Relation of frailty to outcomes after transcatheter aortic valve replacement (from the PARTNER trial). *Am J Cardiol.* 2015;116(2):264269. doi:10.1016/j.amjcard.2015.03.061
27. Clegg A, Young J, Iliffe S, Rikkert MO, Rockwood K. Frailty in elderly people. *Lancet Lond Engl.* 2013;381(9868):752762. doi:10.1016/S0140-6736(12)62167-9
28. Ab N, Js G, Ma M, et al. Associations of subclinical cardiovascular disease with frailty. *J Gerontol A Biol Sci Med Sci.* 2001;56(3). doi:10.1093/gerona/56.3.m158
29. Khan H, Kalogeropoulos AP, Georgiopoulou VV, et al. Frailty and risk for heart failure in older adults: the health, aging, and body composition study. *Am Heart J.* 2013;166(5):887894. doi:10.1016/j.ahj.2013.07.032
30. Kim DH, Kim CA, Placide S, Lipsitz LA, Marcantonio ER. Preoperative frailty assessment and outcomes at 6 months or later in older adults undergoing cardiac surgical procedures: a systematic review. *Ann Intern Med.* 2016;165(9):650660. doi:10.7326/M16-0652
31. Afilalo J, Lauck S, Kim DH, et al. Frailty in older adults undergoing aortic valve replacement: the FRAILTY-AVR Study. *J Am Coll Cardiol.* 2017;70(6):689700. doi:10.1016/j.jacc.2017.06.024
32. Sison SDM, Shi SM, Kim KM, et al. A crosswalk of commonly used frailty scales. *J Am Geriatr Soc.* 2023;71(10):31893198. doi:10.1111/jgs.18453
33. Fried LP, Tangen CM, Walston J, et al. Frailty in older adults: evidence for a phenotype. *J Gerontol A Biol Sci Med Sci.* 2001;56(3):M146156. doi:10.1093/gerona/56.3.m146
34. Rockwood K, Mitnitski A. Frailty defined by deficit accumulation and geriatric medicine defined by frailty. *Clin Geriatr Med.* 2011;27(1):1726. doi:10.1016/j.cger.2010.08.008
35. Jones DM, Song X, Rockwood K. Operationalizing a frailty index from a standardized comprehensive geriatric assessment. *J Am Geriatr Soc.* 2004;52(11):19291933. doi:10.1111/j.1532-5415.2004.52521.x
36. Mitnitski A, Song X, Skoog I, et al. Relative fitness and frailty of elderly men and women in developed countries and their relationship with mortality. *J Am Geriatr Soc.* 2005;53(12):21842189. doi:10.1111/j.1532-5415.2005.00506.x
37. Rockwood K, Andrew M, Mitnitski A. A comparison of two approaches to measuring frailty in elderly people. *J Gerontol A Biol Sci Med Sci.* 2007;62(7):738743. doi:10.1093/gerona/62.7.738
38. Kim DH, Cheslock M, Sison SM, Orkaby AR, Schwartz AW. eFrailty: making frailty assessment accessible to clinicians and researchers. *J Am Geriatr Soc.* 2025;73(1):318322. doi:10.1111/jgs.19138
39. Savva GM, Donoghue OA, Horgan F, O'Regan C, Cronin H, Kenny RA. Using timed up-and-go to identify frail members of the older population. *J Gerontol A Biol Sci Med Sci.* 2013;68(4):441446. doi:10.1093/gerona/gls190
40. Clegg A, Rogers L, Young J. Diagnostic test accuracy of simple instruments for identifying frailty in community-dwelling older people: a systematic review. *Age Ageing.* 2015;44(1):148152. doi:10.1093/ageing/afu157
41. Rockwood K, Song X, MacKnight C, et al. A global clinical measure of fitness and frailty in elderly people. *CMAJ Can Med Assoc J J Assoc Medicale Can.* 2005;173(5):489495. doi:10.1503/cmaj.050051
42. Morley JE, Malmstrom TK, Miller DK. A simple frailty questionnaire (FRAIL) predicts outcomes in middle aged African Americans. *J Nutr Health Aging.* 2012;16(7):601608. doi:10.1007/s12603-012-0084-2
43. Emmady PD, Schoo C, Tadi P. Major neurocognitive disorder (Dementia). In: *StatPearls.* StatPearls Publishing; 2025. Accessed May 14, 2025. http://www.ncbi.nlm.nih.gov/books/NBK557444/
44. Plassman BL, Langa KM, Fisher GG, et al. Prevalence of dementia in the United States: the aging, demographics, and memory study. *Neuroepidemiology.* 2007;29(12):125132. doi:10.1159/000109998
45. Plassman BL, Langa KM, Fisher GG, et al. Prevalence of cognitive impairment without dementia in the United States. *Ann Intern Med.* 2008;148(6):427434.
46. Silbert BS, Scott DA, Evered LA, Lewis MS, Maruff PT. Preexisting cognitive impairment in patients scheduled for elective coronary artery bypass graft surgery. *Anesth Analg.* 2007;104(5):10231028, tables of contents. doi:10.1213/01.ane.0000263285.03361.3a
47. Dodson JA, Truong TTN, Towle VR, Kerins G, Chaudhry SI. Cognitive impairment in older adults with heart failure: prevalence, documentation, and impact on outcomes. *Am J Med.* 2013;126(2):120126. doi:10.1016/j.amjmed.2012.05.029
48. Whitlock EL, Diaz-Ramirez LG, Smith AK, et al. Association of coronary artery bypass grafting vs percutaneous coronary intervention with memory decline in older adults undergoing coronary revascularization. *JAMA.* 2021;325(19):19551964. doi:10.1001/jama.2021.5150
49. Flicker L. Cardiovascular risk factors, cerebrovascular disease burden, and healthy brain aging. *Clin Geriatr Med.* 2010;26(1):1727. doi:10.1016/j.cger.2009.12.005
50. Leritz EC, McGlinchey RE, Kellison I, Rudolph JL, Milberg WP. Cardiovascular disease risk factors and cognition in the elderly. *Curr Cardiovasc Risk Rep.* 2011;5(5):407412. doi:10.1007/s12170-011-0189-x

51. Hawkins LA, Kilian S, Firek A, Kashner TM, Firek CJ, Silvet H. Cognitive impairment and medication adherence in outpatients with heart failure. *Heart Lung J Crit Care.* 2012;41(6):572582. doi:10.1016/j.hrtlng.2012.06.001
52. Zuccalà G, Pedone C, Cesari M, et al. The effects of cognitive impairment on mortality among hospitalized patients with heart failure. *Am J Med.* 2003;115(2):97103. doi:10.1016/s0002-9343(03)00264-x
53. Borson S, Scanlan J, Brush M, Vitaliano P, Dokmak A. The mini-cog: a cognitive 'vital signs' measure for dementia screening in multi-lingual elderly. *Int J Geriatr Psychiatry.* 2000;15(11):10211027. doi:10.1002/1099-1166(200011)15:11<1021::AID-GPS234>3.0.CO;2-6
54. Patel A, Parikh R, Howell EH, Hsich E, Landers SH, Gorodeski EZ. Mini-cog performance: novel marker of post discharge risk among patients hospitalized for heart failure. *Circ Heart Fail.* 2015;8(1):816. doi:10.1161/CIRCHEARTFAILURE.114.001438
55. Marcantonio ER. Postoperative delirium: a 76-year-old woman with delirium following surgery. *JAMA.* 2012;308(1):7381. doi:10.1001/jama.2012.6857
56. Ely EW, Shintani A, Truman B, et al. Delirium as a predictor of mortality in mechanically ventilated patients in the intensive care unit. *JAMA.* 2004;291(14):17531762. doi:10.1001/jama.291.14.1753
57. Inouye SK, Westendorp RGJ, Saczynski JS. Delirium in elderly people. *Lancet Lond Engl.* 2014;383(9920):911922. doi:10.1016/S0140-6736(13)60688-1
58. Cole MG, Ciampi A, Belzile E, Zhong L. Persistent delirium in older hospital patients: a systematic review of frequency and prognosis. *Age Ageing.* 2009;38(1):1926. doi:10.1093/ageing/afn253
59. Saczynski JS, Marcantonio ER, Quach L, et al. Cognitive trajectories after postoperative delirium. *N Engl J Med.* 2012;367(1):3039. doi:10.1056/NEJMoa1112923
60. Witlox J, Eurelings LSM, de Jonghe JFM, Kalisvaart KJ, Eikelenboom P, van Gool WA. Delirium in elderly patients and the risk of postdischarge mortality, institutionalization, and dementia: a meta-analysis. *JAMA.* 2010;304(4):443451. doi:10.1001/jama.2010.1013
61. Wong CL, Holroyd-Leduc J, Simel DL, Straus SE. Does this patient have delirium?: value of bedside instruments. *JAMA.* 2010;304(7):779786. doi:10.1001/jama.2010.1182
62. Wei LA, Fearing MA, Sternberg EJ, Inouye SK. The Confusion Assessment Method: a systematic review of current usage. *J Am Geriatr Soc.* 2008;56(5):823830. doi:10.1111/j.1532-5415.2008.01674.x
63. Inouye SK, van Dyck CH, Alessi CA, Balkin S, Siegal AP, Horwitz RI. Clarifying confusion: the confusion assessment method. A new method for detection of delirium. *Ann Intern Med.* 1990;113(12):941948. doi:10.7326/0003-4819-113-12-941
64. Ely EW, Inouye SK, Bernard GR, et al. Delirium in mechanically ventilated patients: validity and reliability of the confusion assessment method for the intensive care unit (CAM-ICU). *JAMA.* 2001;286(21):27032710. doi:10.1001/jama.286.21.2703
65. Marcantonio ER, Ngo LH, O'Connor M, et al. 3D-CAM: derivation and validation of a 3-minute diagnostic interview for CAM-defined delirium: a cross-sectional diagnostic test study. *Ann Intern Med.* 2014;161(8):554561. doi:10.7326/M14-0865
66. Steensma E, Zhou W, Ngo L, et al. Ultra-brief screeners for detecting delirium superimposed on dementia. *J Am Med Dir Assoc.* 2019;20(11):13911396.e1. doi:10.1016/j.jamda.2019.05.011
67. Hshieh TT, Yue J, Oh E, et al. Effectiveness of multicomponent nonpharmacological delirium interventions: a meta-analysis. *JAMA Intern Med.* 2015;175(4):512520. doi:10.1001/jamainternmed.2014.7779
68. Oh ES, Fong TG, Hshieh TT, Inouye SK. Delirium in older persons: advances in diagnosis and treatment. *JAMA.* 2017;318(12):11611174. doi:10.1001/jama.2017.12067
69. Marcantonio ER. Delirium in hospitalized older adults. *N Engl J Med.* 2017;377(15):14561466. doi:10.1056/NEJMcp1605501
70. Kim DH, Grodstein F, Newman AB, et al. Prognostic implications of microvascular and macrovascular abnormalities in older adults: cardiovascular health study. *J Gerontol A Biol Sci Med Sci.* 2014;69(12):14951502. doi:10.1093/gerona/glu074
71. Newman AB, Arnold AM, Naydeck BL, et al. "Successful aging": effect of subclinical cardiovascular disease. *Arch Intern Med.* 2003;163(19):23152322. doi:10.1001/archinte.163.19.2315
72. Kucharska-Newton A, Griswold M, Yao ZH, et al. Cardiovascular disease and patterns of change in functional status over 15 years: findings from the Atherosclerosis Risk in Communities (ARIC) Study. *J Am Heart Assoc.* 2017;6(3):e004144. doi:10.1161/JAHA.116.004144
73. Covinsky KE, Pierluissi E, Johnston CB. Hospitalization-associated disability: "She was probably able to ambulate, but I'm not sure." *JAMA.* 2011;306(16):17821793. doi:10.1001/jama.2011.1556
74. Kortebein P, Ferrando A, Lombeida J, Wolfe R, Evans WJ. Effect of 10 days of bed rest on skeletal muscle in healthy older adults. *JAMA.* 2007;297(16):17721774. doi:10.1001/jama.297.16.1772-b

75. Kortebein P, Symons TB, Ferrando A, et al. Functional impact of 10 days of bed rest in healthy older adults. *J Gerontol A Biol Sci Med Sci.* 2008;63(10):10761081. doi:10.1093/gerona/63.10.1076
76. English KL, Paddon-Jones D. Protecting muscle mass and function in older adults during bed rest. *Curr Opin Clin Nutr Metab Care.* 2010;13(1):3439. doi:10.1097/MCO.0b013e328333aa66
77. Gill TM, Allore HG, Gahbauer EA, Murphy TE. Change in disability after hospitalization or restricted activity in older persons. *JAMA.* 2010;304(17):19191928. doi:10.1001/jama.2010.1568
78. Nagi SZ. An epidemiology of disability among adults in the United States. *Milbank Mem Fund Q Health Soc.* 1976;54(4):439467.
79. Katz S, Downs TD, Cash HR, Grotz RC. Progress in development of the index of ADL. *The Gerontologist.* 1970;10(1):2030. doi:10.1093/geront/10.1_part_1.20
80. Lawton MP, Brody EM. Assessment of older people: self-maintaining and instrumental activities of daily living. *The Gerontologist.* 1969;9(3):179186.
81. Bauer J, Biolo G, Cederholm T, et al. Evidence-based recommendations for optimal dietary protein intake in older people: a position paper from the PROT-AGE Study Group. *J Am Med Dir Assoc.* 2013;14(8):542559. doi:10.1016/j.jamda.2013.05.021
82. Inouye SK, Bogardus ST, Baker DI, Leo-Summers L, Cooney LM. The Hospital Elder Life Program: a model of care to prevent cognitive and functional decline in older hospitalized patients. Hospital Elder Life Program. *J Am Geriatr Soc.* 2000;48(12):16971706. doi:10.1111/j.1532-5415.2000.tb03885.x
83. Wynter-Blyth V, Moorthy K. Prehabilitation: preparing patients for surgery. *BMJ.* 2017;358:j3702. doi:10.1136/bmj.j3702
84. CDC WISQARS Web-based Injury Statistics Query and Reporting System. Centers for Disease Control and Prevention. Accessed February 22, 2025. https://wisqars.cdc.gov/
85. Tinetti ME, Kumar C. The patient who falls: "It's always a trade-off." *JAMA.* 2010;303(3):258266. doi:10.1001/jama.2009.2024
86. Jansen S, Bhangu J, de Rooij S, Daams J, Kenny RA, van der Velde N. The association of cardiovascular disorders and falls: a systematic review. *J Am Med Dir Assoc.* 2016;17(3):193199. doi:10.1016/j.jamda.2015.08.022
87. Woolcott JC, Richardson KJ, Wiens MO, et al. Meta-analysis of the impact of 9 medication classes on falls in elderly persons. *Arch Intern Med.* 2009;169(21):19521960. doi:10.1001/archinternmed.2009.357
88. Tinetti ME, Han L, Lee DSH, et al. Antihypertensive medications and serious fall injuries in a nationally representative sample of older adults. *JAMA Intern Med.* 2014;174(4):588595. doi:10.1001/jamainternmed.2013.14764
89. Berry SD, Mittleman MA, Zhang Y, et al. New loop diuretic prescriptions may be an acute risk factor for falls in the nursing home. *Pharmacoepidemiol Drug Saf.* 2012;21(5):560563. doi:10.1002/pds.3256
90. Neutel CI, Perry S, Maxwell C. Medication use and risk of falls. *Pharmacoepidemiol Drug Saf.* 2002;11(2):97104. doi:10.1002/pds.686
91. Hylek EM, D'Antonio J, Evans-Molina C, Shea C, Henault LE, Regan S. Translating the results of randomized trials into clinical practice: the challenge of warfarin candidacy among hospitalized elderly patients with atrial fibrillation. *Stroke.* 2006;37(4):10751080. doi:10.1161/01.STR.0000209239.71702.ce
92. Rao MP, Vinereanu D, Wojdyla DM, et al. Clinical outcomes and history of fall in patients with atrial fibrillation treated with oral anticoagulation: insights from the ARISTOTLE trial. *Am J Med.* 2018;131(3):269275.e2. doi:10.1016/j.amjmed.2017.10.036
93. Panel on Prevention of Falls in Older Persons, American Geriatrics Society and British Geriatrics Society. Summary of the Updated American Geriatrics Society/British Geriatrics Society clinical practice guideline for prevention of falls in older persons. *J Am Geriatr Soc.* 2011;59(1):148157. doi:10.1111/j.1532-5415.2010.03234.x
94. Moyer VA, U.S. Preventive Services Task Force. Prevention of falls in community-dwelling older adults: U.S. Preventive Services Task Force recommendation statement. *Ann Intern Med.* 2012;157(3):197204. doi:10.7326/0003-4819-157-3-201208070-00462
95. Dhruva SS, Redberg RF. Variations between clinical trial participants and Medicare beneficiaries in evidence used for Medicare national coverage decisions. *Arch Intern Med.* 2008;168(2):136140. doi:10.1001/archinternmed.2007.56
96. Fried TR, Tinetti ME, Towle V, O'Leary JR, Iannone L. Effects of benefits and harms on older persons' willingness to take medication for primary cardiovascular prevention. *Arch Intern Med.* 2011;171(10):923928. doi:10.1001/archinternmed.2011.32
97. Zeng L, Helsingen LM, Bretthauer M, et al. A novel framework for incorporating patient values and preferences in making guideline recommendations: guideline panel surveys. *J Clin Epidemiol.* 2023;161:164172. doi:10.1016/j.jclinepi.2023.07.003
98. Virani SS, Newby LK, Arnold SV, et al. 2023 AHA/ACC/ACCP/ASPC/NLA/PCNA guideline for the management of patients with chronic coronary disease: a report of the American Heart Association/American College of Cardiology Joint Committee on Clinical Practice Guidelines. *Circulation.* 2023;148(9):e9e119. doi:10.1161/CIR.0000000000001168

99. Tinetti ME, Esterson J, Ferris R, Posner P, Blaum CS. Patient priority-directed decision making and care for older adults with multiple chronic conditions. *Clin Geriatr Med.* 2016;32(2):261275. doi:10.1016/j.cger.2016.01.012
100. Tinetti ME, Naik AD, Dodson JA. Moving from disease-centered to patient goals-directed care for patients with multiple chronic conditions: patient value-based care. *JAMA Cardiol.* 2016;1(1):910. doi:10.1001/jamacardio.2015.0248
101. Reuben DB, Tinetti ME. Goal-oriented patient care--an alternative health outcomes paradigm. *N Engl J Med.* 2012;366(9):777779. doi:10.1056/NEJMp1113631
102. Lynn J, McKethan A, Jha AK. Value-based payments require valuing what matters to patients. *JAMA.* 2015;314(14):14451446. doi:10.1001/jama.2015.8909
103. Guiding principles for the care of older adults with multimorbidity: an approach for clinicians: American Geriatrics Society Expert Panel on the Care of Older Adults with Multimorbidity. *J Am Geriatr Soc.* 2012;60(10):E1E25. doi:10.1111/j.1532-5415.2012.04188.x
104. Yourman LC, Lee SJ, Schonberg MA, Widera EW, Smith AK. Prognostic indices for older adults: a systematic review. *JAMA.* 2012;307(2):182192. doi:10.1001/jama.2011.1966
105. Yourman LC, Cenzer IS, Boscardin WJ, et al. Evaluation of time to benefit of statins for the primary prevention of cardiovascular events in adults aged 50 to 75 years: a meta-analysis. *JAMA Intern Med.* 2021;181(2):179185. doi:10.1001/jamainternmed.2020.6084
106. Holmes HM, Min LC, Yee M, et al. Rationalizing prescribing for older patients with multimorbidity: considering time to benefit. *Drugs Aging.* 2013;30(9):655666. doi:10.1007/s40266-013-0095-7
107. van de Glind EMM, Willems HC, Eslami S, et al. Estimating the time to benefit for preventive drugs with the statistical process control method: An example with alendronate. *Drugs Aging.* 2016;33:347353. doi:10.1007/s40266-016-0344-7
108. Lee SJ, Boscardin WJ, Stijacic-Cenzer I, Conell-Price J, O'Brien S, Walter LC. Time lag to benefit after screening for breast and colorectal cancer: meta-analysis of survival data from the United States, Sweden, United Kingdom, and Denmark. *BMJ.* 2013;346:e8441. doi:10.1136/bmj.e8441
109. Gigerenzer G, Gaissmaier W, Kurz-Milcke E, Schwartz LM, Woloshin S. Helping doctors and patients make sense of health statistics. *Psychol Sci Public Interest J Am Psychol Soc.* 2007;8(2):5396. doi:10.1111/j.1539-6053.2008.00033.x
110. Wegwarth O, Schwartz LM, Woloshin S, Gaissmaier W, Gigerenzer G. Do physicians understand cancer screening statistics? A national survey of primary care physicians in the United States. *Ann Intern Med.* 2012;156(5):340349. doi:10.7326/0003-4819-156-5-201203060-00005
111. Zipkin DA, Umscheid CA, Keating NL, et al. Evidence-based risk communication: a systematic review. *Ann Intern Med.* 2014;161(4):270280. doi:10.7326/M14-0295
112. Montori VM, Brito JP, Murad MH. The optimal practice of evidence-based medicine: incorporating patient preferences in practice guidelines. *JAMA.* 2013;310(23):25032504. doi:10.1001/jama.2013.281422
113. Stacey D, Légaré F, Lewis K, et al. Decision aids for people facing health treatment or screening decisions. *Cochrane Database Syst Rev.* 2017;4(4):CD001431. doi:10.1002/14651858.CD001431.pub5
114. Trevena LJ, Davey HM, Barratt A, Butow P, Caldwell P. A systematic review on communicating with patients about evidence. *J Eval Clin Pract.* 2006;12(1):1323. doi:10.1111/j.1365-2753.2005.00596.x
115. Visschers VHM, Meertens RM, Passchier WWF, de Vries NNK. Probability information in risk communication: a review of the research literature. *Risk Anal Off Publ Soc Risk Anal.* 2009;29(2):267287. doi:10.1111/j.1539-6924.2008.01137.x
116. Edwards AGK, Evans R, Dundon J, Haigh S, Hood K, Elwyn GJ. Personalised risk communication for informed decision making about taking screening tests. *Cochrane Database Syst Rev.* 2006;(4):CD001865. doi:10.1002/14651858.CD001865.pub2
117. Ahmed H, Naik G, Willoughby H, Edwards AGK. Communicating risk. *BMJ.* 2012;344:e3996. doi:10.1136/bmj.e3996
118. Akl EA, Oxman AD, Herrin J, et al. Using alternative statistical formats for presenting risks and risk reductions. *Cochrane Database Syst Rev.* 2011;2011(3):CD006776. doi:10.1002/14651858.CD006776.pub2
119. Uno H, Wittes J, Fu H, et al. Alternatives to hazard ratios for comparing the efficacy or safety of therapies in noninferiority studies. *Ann Intern Med.* 2015;163(2):127134. doi:10.7326/M14-1741
120. Kim DH, Uno H, Wei LJ. Restricted mean survival time as a measure to interpret clinical trial results. *JAMA Cardiol.* 2017;2(11):11791180. doi:10.1001/jamacardio.2017.2922

4

Systemic hypertension in older persons

WILBERT S. ARONOW AND WILLIAM H. FRISHMAN

Key points

- Hypertension in older adults is a systolic blood pressure of ≥130 mm Hg or a diastolic blood pressure of ≥80 mm Hg.
- Lifestyle measures plus antihypertensive drugs should be used to treat hypertension.
- Primary hypertension and hypertension associated with different comorbidities should be treated as recommended by the 2017 American College of Cardiology (ACC)/American Heart Association (AHA) hypertension guidelines.
- If a fourth antihypertensive drug is needed to control resistant hypertension treated with optimal doses of a thiazide diuretic, especially chlorthalidone, a calcium channel blocker (CCB), and an angiotensin-converting enzyme inhibitor (ACI) or angiotensin receptor blocker (ARB), an aldosterone antagonist should be added.
- If a fifth drug is needed, it should be a beta-blocker, and a sixth drug should be clonidine or methyldopa or hydralazine or minoxidil.
- The beneficial effects of thiazide diuretics are less when the glomerular filtration rate (GFR) is less than 40 cc/min. These patients should be given a loop diuretic such as furosemide every 12 hours.

INTRODUCTION

Hypertension in older persons used to be diagnosed if the systolic blood pressure (BP) was ≥140 mmHg or if the diastolic BP was ≥90 mmHg based on the mean of two or more properly measured seated BP readings on each of two or more office visits (1), but is currently diagnosed if the systolic BP is ≥130 mmHg or the diastolic BP is ≥80 mm (2). Isolated systolic hypertension (ISH) is currently diagnosed if the systolic BP is ≥130 mmHg with a diastolic BP <80 mmHg (2). Stage 1 hypertension is a systolic BP of 130–139 mmHg or a diastolic BP of 80–89 mmHg (2). Stage 2 hypertension is a systolic BP ≥140 mmHg or a diastolic BP ≥90 mmHg (2). An elevated BP is a systolic BP of 120–129 mmHg with a diastolic BP <80 mmHg (3). A normal BP is a BP <120/80 mmHg (2).

Pseudohypertension in the elderly is a falsely increased systolic BP resulting from markedly sclerotic arteries that do not collapse during inflation of the BP cuff (1–3). Suspect pseudohypertension is seen in elderly patients with refractory hypertension, no target organ damage, and/or symptoms of overmedication, and the diagnosis is confirmed by measuring intra-arterial pressure (2). White coat hypertension is diagnosed when the physician's office BP measurement is persistently high but daytime ambulatory BP readings are normal (1, 2). Ambulatory BP monitoring should be performed to confirm white coat hypertension in persons with office hypertension but no target organ damage (1, 2).

Ambulatory BP monitoring in older persons is also indicated when the response to therapy is unclear from office visits, when syncope or hypotensive disorders are suspected, and for evaluation of vertigo and dizziness (1, 2). Home recordings of BP should also be obtained to ensure adequate control of BP in the elderly, to avoid

DOI: 10.1201/9781003568933-4

excessive BP reduction in older persons, and for better prognostic accuracy versus office BP (1, 2).

A physical examination and complete history should be performed in patients with hypertension. What is the duration and severity of hypertension? What are the causes or exacerbations of hypertension? What are the current and previous treatments of hypertension? What are the adverse effects of antihypertensive drugs (1, 2)?

Patients with hypertension should be evaluated for other cardiovascular risk factors including smoking, dyslipidemia, diabetes mellitus (DM), age >55 years for men and 65 years for women, body mass index ≥25 kg/m^2, physical inactivity, unhealthy diet, microalbuminuria, an estimated glomerular filtration rate <60 mL/min/1.73 m^2, low socioeconomic/education status, family history of premature cardiovascular disease (<55 years in fathers or brothers and <65 years in mothers or sisters), obstructive sleep apnea, and psychosocial stress (2). Patients with hypertension should also be evaluated for target organ damage and clinical cardiovascular disease, including left ventricular hypertrophy (LVH), prior MI, angina pectoris, prior coronary revascularization, congestive heart failure (CHF), stroke or transient ischemic attack, peripheral arterial disease (PAD), nephropathy, and retinopathy (1, 2).

Routine laboratory tests that should be obtained in older patients with hypertension include a urinalysis to look for renal damage, especially albuminuria/microalbuminuria, serum electrolytes, especially serum potassium, serum creatinine, and estimated glomerular filtration rate, fasting serum total cholesterol, low-density lipoprotein cholesterol, high-density lipoprotein cholesterol, and triglycerides, fasting blood sugar, a hemoglobin A1C in diabetics, and a 12-lead electrocardiogram (1). In selected older patients with hypertension, a two-dimensional echocardiogram should be obtained to look for LVH and for an abnormal LV ejection fraction.

Interarm differences of ≥10 mmHg in systolic BP were present in 14% of 528 older adults (3) and appear to be an independent risk factor for cardiovascular disease (4). Interarm differences of ≥10 mmHg in diastolic BP were present in 5% of 528 older adults (3). The BP should be measured in both arms while in the sitting position, with the arm with the highest BP used for future measurements (1, 2). The BP must also be measured with the patient standing for 1–3 minutes to evaluate for postural hypotension or hypertension (1, 2).

Orthostatic hypotension is defined as a decrease in systolic BP of ≥20 mmHg or in diastolic BP of ≥10 mmHg within 3 minutes of standing and can result from blunting the carotid baroreflex due to increased stiffness of the carotid arteries (5). Orthostatic hypotension may result in falls and syncope (1, 2, 6).

PATHOPHYSIOLOGY

An increase in systolic BP in older persons is related to an age-associated increase in arterial stiffness due to structural changes within the arterial media (a change in the amount or nature of collagen, interstitial fibrosis, and calcification, and degradation of elastin fibers) (Figure 4.1) (7). The increased wall stiffness and tortuosity of the aorta and large arteries with aging are often reflected by an increased systolic BP and widened pulse pressure. Older persons with hypertension are more likely to have increased LV mass, increased peripheral resistance, reduced baroreceptor sensitivity, increased characteristic aortic impedance at rest, decreased LV early diastolic filling rate, decreased LV early diastolic filling volume, increased left atrial dimension, and decreased cardiovascular response to catecholamines (7).

Flow-mediated arterial dilation, primarily mediated by endothelium-derived nitric oxide, decreases markedly with aging (1). The neurohormonal profile of older adults is characterized by increased plasma norepinephrine, low renin, and low aldosterone levels (1). Many so-called normal aging changes in arterial structure and function are blunted or absent in populations not chronically exposed to high sodium/calorie diets, low physical activity levels, and high rates of obesity (1).

The decrease in baroreflex sensitivity with age and with hypertension leads to impaired baroreflex-mediated increase in total systemic vascular resistance and to an inability to increase heart rate in response to decreased BP (8). Therefore, older persons with hypertension have a greater impairment in baroreflex sensitivity and are more likely to develop orthostatic and postprandial hypotension on antihypertensive drug therapy (8).

Hypertension in older persons also increases the age-dependent decline in renal function. Of 143 older persons, mean age 73 years, with hypertension in an academic nursing home, 60 (42%) had moderate (33%) or severe (9%) renal insufficiency with an estimated glomerular filtration rate <60 mL/min/1.73 m^2 (5). Renal artery stenosis is also an important cause of secondary hypertension in the elderly (9).

PREVALENCE

Hypertension occurs in more than two thirds of persons >65 years. Hypertension was present in 57% of 1160 older men, mean age 80 years, and in 60% of 2464 older women, mean age 81 years, with two thirds of these older persons having ISH (10). Of 1819 older persons, mean age 80 years, living in the community and seen in an academic geriatrics practice, 58% had hypertension (37% with ISH) (11). In this study, hypertension was present in 52% of older

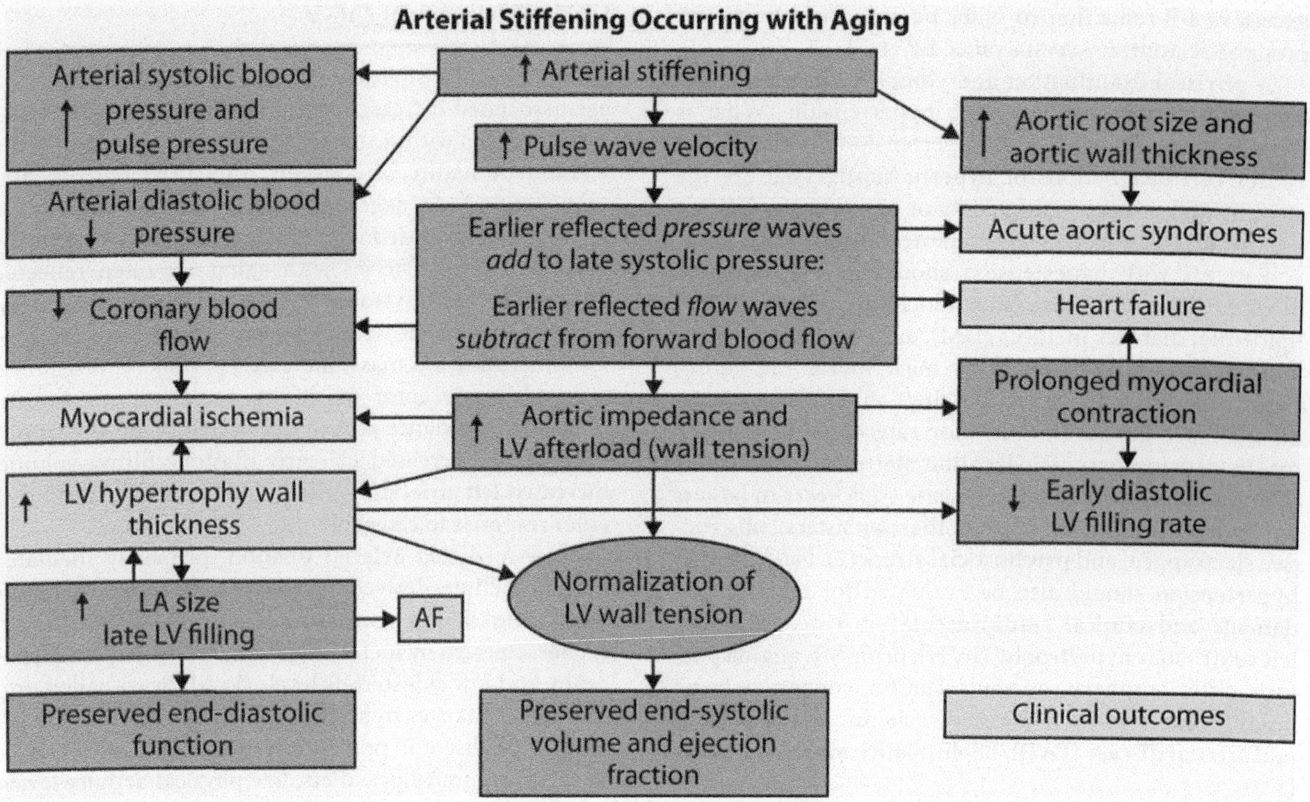

Figure 4.1 Conceptual framework for cardiovascular adaptations to arterial stiffness that occur with aging. *Abbreviations*: CBF, coronary blood flow; DBP, diastolic blood pressure; EF, ejection fraction; LA, left atrial; LV, left ventricular; SBP, systolic blood pressure; ↓ = decrease; ↑ = increased. (Modified from Fleg JL, Effects of aging on the cardiovascular system, in Lewis RP, ed., *Adult Clinical Cardiology Self-Assessment Program* (*ACCSAP 6*), American College of Cardiology Foundation, Bethesda, MD, 6–20, 2005.)

Whites, 71% of older Blacks, 61% of older Hispanics, and 64% of older Asians (12). Target organ damage, clinical cardiovascular disease, or DM was present in 70% of these older persons with hypertension (12). The prevalence of hypertension in older persons in an academic nursing home was 71% (13). The prevalence of hypertension in older persons with DM in an academic nursing home was 76% (14). Using the current guidelines for diagnosing hypertension, hypertension is present in US adults in 68% of men and 65% of women aged 55–64 years, in 75% of men and 78% of women aged 65–74 years, and in 83% of men and 86% of women aged 75-plus years (2).

HYPERTENSION AND RISK OF CARDIOVASCULAR DISEASE

The higher the systolic or diastolic BP in older persons, the higher the risk of cardiovascular morbidity and mortality. Increased systolic BP and pulse pressure are stronger risk factors for cardiovascular morbidity and mortality in older persons than is increased diastolic BP (15). An increased pulse pressure found in older persons with ISH indicates decreased vascular compliance in the large arteries and is an even better marker of risk than is systolic or diastolic BP (15). The Cardiovascular Health Study found in 5202 older men and women that a brachial systolic BP >169 mmHg increased the mortality rate 2.4 times (16).

Hypertension in older persons is a major risk factor for coronary events (1, 2, 11, 17, 18), for stroke (1, 2, 11, 18–20), for CHF (1, 2, 16, 21, 22), and for PAD (1, 2, 23–26). Hypertension is present in approximately 69% of patients with a first MI (19), in approximately 77% of patients with a first stroke (19), in approximately 74% of patients with CHF (19), and in 60% of patients with PAD (27). Hypertension is also a major risk factor for a dissecting aortic aneurysm, sudden cardiac death, angina pectoris, atrial fibrillation, DM, the metabolic syndrome, chronic kidney disease, thoracic and abdominal aortic aneurysms, LV hypertrophy, vascular dementia, Alzheimer's disease, and ophthalmologic disorders (1, 2).

At 40-month follow-up of 664 men, mean age 80 years, and at 48-month follow-up of 1488 women, mean age 82 years, hypertension increased the incidence of new coronary events in men (relative risk = 2.0, p = 0.0001) and in women (relative risk = 1.6, p = 0.0001) (17). At 42-month follow-up of 664 men, mean age 80 years, and at 48-month follow-up of 1488 women, mean age 82 years, hypertension increased the incidence of new stroke in men (relative risk = 2.2, p = 0.0001) and in women (relative risk = 2.4, p = 0.0001) (19). Hypertension was an independent risk factor for PAD in 467 men, mean age 80 years, with an odds ratio of 2.2 (p = 0.023) and in 1444 women, mean age 81 years, with an odds ratio of 2.8 (p = 0.001) (24). Hypertension was an independent risk factor for CHF in 2902 patients (926 men and 1976 women), mean age 81 years, with a risk ratio of 2.5 (p = 0.0001) (21). In 61 prospective studies of 1 million adults, coronary heart disease mortality increased with each decade from ages 40–49 to 80–89 and with each increase in systolic BP from 120–140 to 160–180 mmHg (28).

Older persons are more likely to have hypertension and ISH, to have target organ damage and clinical cardiovascular disease, and to develop new cardiovascular events. Older persons also have the lowest rates of BP control (2, 29). BP is adequately controlled in 36% of men and 28% of women aged 60–79 years and in 38% of men and 23% of women aged 80 years and older (29).

Barriers to treatment of hypertension include physicians not understanding that frail older persons should be treated according to recommended guidelines to decrease cardiovascular morbidity and mortality. Prevalent comorbidities, polypharmacy, an asymptomatic state, side effects from medications, and high cost of medications contribute to lower BP control rates in older persons (1, 2, 30). A BP <140/90 mmHg was achieved in 70% of 492 Medicaid or private insurance patients versus 38% of 122 patients who had to pay for their antihypertensive medications (p < 0.001) (30). This problem needs to be addressed if we are to reduce the great amount of cardiovascular events and mortality caused by inadequate treatment of hypertension.

EFFECT OF ANTIHYPERTENSIVE THERAPY ON LOWERING CARDIOVASCULAR EVENTS

Numerous prospective, double-blind, randomized, placebo-controlled studies have shown that antihypertensive drug therapy reduces the development of new coronary events, stroke, and CHF in older persons (1, 2, 29–37). Older persons with hypertension, if treated appropriately, will have a greater absolute reduction in cardiovascular events such as major coronary events, stroke, CHF, and renal insufficiency, and a greater reduction in dementia (28) than in younger persons.

Therapy with antihypertensive drugs reduces the incidence of all strokes: 38% in women, 34% in men, 36% in older persons, and 34% in persons >80 years (19). The overall data suggest that the decrease in stroke in older persons with hypertension is related more to a reduction in BP than to the type of antihypertensive drugs used (20).

In the Perindopril Protection Against Recurrent Stroke Study (40), perindopril plus indapamide reduced stroke-related dementia by 34% and cognitive decline by 45%. In the Systolic Hypertension in Europe trial (41), nitrendipine reduced dementia by 55% at 3.9-year follow-up. In 1900 older African Americans, antihypertensive drug treatment reduced cognitive impairment by 38% (42). In the Rotterdam Study (43), antihypertensive drugs decreased vascular dementia by 70%.

On the basis of data available at the time, Aronow (44) proposed in an editorial that unless the Hypertension in the Very Elderly Trial (HYVET) (36) found that antihypertensive drug therapy was not beneficial in patients aged 80 years and older, this group should receive antihypertensive drug treatment

In HYVET, 3845 persons aged 80 years and older (mean age 83.6 years) with a sustained systolic BP >160 mmHg were randomized to indapamide (sustained release 1.5 mg) or a matching placebo (36). Perindopril 2 mg or 4 mg, or a matching placebo, was added if needed to achieve the target BP of 150/80 mmHg. Median follow-up was 1.8 years. Antihypertensive drug treatment reduced the incidence of the primary endpoint (fatal or nonfatal stroke) by 30% (p = 0.06). Antihypertensive drug treatment reduced fatal stroke by 39% (p = 0.05), all-cause mortality by 21% (p = 0.02), death from cardiovascular causes by 23% (p = 0.06), and heart failure by 64% (p < 0.001). The significant 21% reduction in all-cause mortality by antihypertensive drug treatment was unexpected. The benefits of antihypertensive drug treatment began to be apparent during the first year of follow-up.

The prevalence of baseline cardiovascular disease was only 12% in the patients in HYVET. In a cohort of patients, mean age 80 years, with hypertension seen in a university geriatrics practice, 70% had baseline cardiovascular disease, target organ damage, or DM (12). An older population such as this one with a high prevalence of cardiovascular disease would be expected to have a greater absolute reduction in cardiovascular events resulting from antihypertensive drug therapy.

Although the results of HYVET clearly indicate that hypertensive patients aged >80 years should be treated with antihypertensive drug therapy, the study does not give us data on target BP (45). Further research is needed to answer this question (2) and was performed in the Systolic Blood Pressure Intervention Trial (SPRINT) (38, 39).

SPRINT randomized 9361 persons with a systolic BP of 130 mmHg to 180 mmHg and an increased cardiovascular risk but without diabetes mellitus, history of stroke, symptomatic heart failure within the past 6 months, a LV ejection fraction below 35%, and an estimated glomerular filtration rate below 20 mL/min/1.73 m^2 to a systolic BP goal of less than 120 mmHg or to a systolic BP goal of less than 140 mmHg (38). The participants were aged 50 years and older with a mean age of 67.9 years. Of the 9361 participants, 2636 (28.2%) were aged 75 years and older, 3332 (35.6%) were women, 5399 (57.7%) were non-Hispanic Whites, 2947 (31.5%) were Blacks, and 984 (10.6%) were Hispanics. Cardiovascular disease was present in 1877 persons (20.1%), and the Framingham 10-year cardiovascular disease risk score was 15% and higher in 5737 persons (61.3%).

At 1 year, the mean systolic BP was 121.4 mmHg in the intensive treatment group and 136.2 mmHg in the standard treatment group. The intervention was stopped after a median follow-up of 3.26 years (38).

The primary composite outcome was MI, other acute coronary syndrome, stroke, CHF, or death from cardiovascular causes and was reduced 25% ($p < 0.001$) by intensive blood pressure treatment (46). Intensive blood pressure treatment reduced all-cause mortality by 27% ($p = 0.003$), heart failure by 38% ($p = 0.002$) death from cardiovascular causes by 43% ($p = 0.005$), and the primary composite outcome or death by 22% ($p < 0.001$) (38). Intensive BP treatment nonsignificantly reduced MI by 17%, caused the same incidence of other acute coronary syndrome, and nonsignificantly reduced stroke by 11%. Intensive BP treatment significantly lowered the primary outcome by 33% in persons aged 75 years and older and significantly reduced the primary outcome by 20% in persons aged 50–74 years (38).

Serious adverse events were similar in both treatment groups (46). However, intensive BP treatment caused more hypotension (2.4% versus 1.4%, $p = 0.001$), more syncope (2.3% versus 1.7%, $p = 0.05$), more electrolyte abnormality (3.1% versus 2.3%, $p = 0.02$), and more acute kidney injury or acute renal failure (4.1% versus 2.5%, $p < 0.001$). The incidence of bradycardia, injurious falls, and orthostatic hypotension with dizziness was similar in both treatment groups (38).

Of the 2636 persons aged 75 years and older, mean age 79.9 years, in SPRINT, 33.4% of persons randomized to a systolic BP goal of less than 120 mmHg and 28.4% of persons randomized to a systolic BP goal of less than 140 mmHg were frail (47). At 3.14-year median follow-up, compared with a systolic BP goal of less than 140 mmHg, a systolic BP goal of less than 120 mmHg reduced the primary endpoint of MI, other acute coronary syndrome, stroke, CHF, or cardiovascular death by 34% ($p = 0.001$), all-cause mortality by 33% ($p = 0.009$), CHF by 38% ($p = 0.003$), and the primary outcome or death by 32% ($p < 0.001$). Absolute cardiovascular event rates were lower for the intensive treatment group within each frailty stratum. The incidence of serious adverse events was similar in both treatment groups. However, intensive BP lowering nonsignificantly increased hypotension, syncope, electrolyte abnormalities, and acute kidney injury (39).

The 2017 American College of Cardiology (ACC)/American Heart Association (AHA) guidelines contributed to by nine other professional societies recommend use of BP-lowering drugs for secondary prevention in patients with clinical cardiovascular disease and a systolic BP of 130 mmHg and higher or a diastolic BP of 80 mmHg and higher (2). These guidelines recommend use of BP-lowering drugs for primary prevention in adults with a systolic BP of 130 mmHg and higher or a diastolic BP of 80 mmHg and higher if the estimated 10-year risk of atherosclerotic cardiovascular disease is ≥10% (2). These guidelines recommend the use of BP-lowering drugs for primary prevention in adults with a systolic BP of 140 mmHg and higher or a diastolic BP of 90 mmHg and higher if the estimated 10-year risk of atherosclerotic cardiovascular disease is <10% (2). We should also be careful to monitor intensive lowering of the BP, especially in older persons with DM and coronary artery disease, as this might be poorly tolerated and might increase cardiovascular events (the J-curve phenomenon) (1, 48–52).

LIFESTYLE MEASURES

Lifestyle modification should be used in older persons to prevent mild hypertension and to decrease the dose levels of drugs needed to control hypertension. Weight reduction; consuming a diet rich in fruits, vegetables, and low-fat dairy products with a reduced amount of saturated fat and total fat; sodium reduction to not exceed 1.5 grams daily; smoking cessation; regular aerobic physical activity; avoidance of excessive alcohol intake; avoidance of excessive caffeine; and avoidance of drugs that can increase BP, including nonsteroidal anti-inflammatory drugs, glucocorticoids, and sympathomimetics, are recommended (1, 2). Implementing a national salt reduction program is likely a simple and cost-effective way of improving public health (53).

Long-term observational follow-up was performed in 744 persons in the Trials of Hypertension Prevention (TOHP) I (10 years after its end) and in 2382 persons in TOHP II (5 years after its end), in which persons with prehypertension were randomized to sodium reduction or usual diet (25%–35% greater sodium intake) (54). In these studies, sodium reduction decreased cardiovascular events by 25% ($p = 0.04$). At 31-month follow-up of 1981 Taiwanese veterans, mean age 75 years, living in a retirement home, those randomized to a potassium-enriched diet with 50% less sodium had a 41% reduction in cardiovascular mortality (95% CI, 0.37, 0.95) compared with those randomized to a regular salt diet (55).

At 14.8-year follow-up of 12,267 adults in the Third National Health and Nutrition Examination Survey, a higher sodium intake was associated with a 20% increase in all-cause mortality per 1000 mg of sodium intake per day ($p = 0.02$), whereas a higher potassium intake was associated with a 20% reduction in mortality per 1000 mg of potassium intake per day ($p = 0.01$) (56). For the sodium–potassium ratio, compared with the lowest quartile, the highest quartile increased all-cause mortality 46% ($p < 0.001$), cardiovascular mortality 46% ($p < 0.001$), and ischemic heart disease mortality 215% ($p < 0.001$) (57). Current guidelines suggest no more than 2300 mg of sodium daily in the general population and no more than 1500 mg of sodium daily in the elderly, in Blacks, and in persons with hypertension, DM, chronic kidney disease, or CHF (58).

USE OF ANTIHYPERTENSIVE DRUG THERAPY IN OLDER PERSONS

A meta-analysis of 147 randomized trials including 464,000 persons with hypertension showed that except for the extra protective effect of beta-blockers given after MI and a minor additional effect of calcium channel blockers in preventing stroke, the use of beta-blockers, angiotensin-converting enzyme (ACE) inhibitors, angiotensin receptor blockers (ARBs), diuretics, and calcium channel blockers cause a similar reduction in coronary events and stroke for a given decrease in BP (81, 82). The proportionate decrease in cardiovascular events was the same or similar regardless of pretreatment BP and the presence or absence of cardiovascular events (59, 60). Diuretics, ACE inhibitors, ARBs, calcium channel blockers, or beta-blockers may be used as initial therapy in the treatment of primary hypertension in older and younger persons. Atenolol should not be used (46, 59, 63). Beta-blockers such as carvedilol, nebivolol, and bisoprolol are preferred (2, 63).

Centrally acting agents, such as clonidine, reserpine, and guanethidine, should not be used as monotherapy in older persons because they have been associated with a high incidence of significant side effects, including sedation, depression, and constipation.

Most older persons with hypertension will need two or more antihypertensive drugs to control their BP (1, 2). If the BP is >20/10 mmHg above the goal BP, drug therapy should be initiated with two antihypertensive drugs (Table 4.1) (1, 2, 64). The initial antihypertensive drug should be given at the lowest dose and gradually increased to the maximum dose. If the antihypertensive response to the initial drug is inadequate after reaching the full dose, a second drug from another class should be given if the person is tolerating the initial drug. If there is no therapeutic response or if there are significant adverse effects, a drug from another class should be substituted. If the antihypertensive response is inadequate after reaching the full dose of two classes of drugs, a third drug from another class should be added.

Table 4.1 Rationale for combination drug therapy for hypertension

Increased antihypertensive efficacy
Additive effects
Synergistic effects
Reduced adverse events
Low-dose strategy
Drugs with offsetting actions
Enhanced convenience and compliance
Prolonged duration of action
Potential for additive target organ protection

Source: Weber MA et al., Combination drug therapy, in Frishman, WH et al., *Cardiovascular Pharmacotherapeutics*, 2nd ed., McGraw-Hill, New York, 355–368, 2003.

Before adding new antihypertensive drugs, the physician should consider possible reasons for inadequate response to antihypertensive drug therapy, including nonadherence to therapy, volume overload, drug interactions (use of nonsteroidal anti-inflammatory drugs, caffeine, antidepressants, nasal decongestants, sympathomimetics, etc.), and associated conditions such as increasing obesity, smoking, excessive ethanol intake, and insulin resistance (1, 2). Causes of secondary hypertension should be identified and treated in accordance with current guidelines (1, 2, 5).

Older persons with hypertension have a very high prevalence of associated medical conditions (1, 2). The selection of antihypertensive drug therapy in these persons depends on their associated medical conditions (1, 2).

Falls or syncope in elderly persons may be due to orthostatic or postprandial hypotension (8). Management of orthostatic and postprandial hypotension in elderly persons is discussed in detail elsewhere (8). The dose of antihypertensive drug may need to be decreased or another antihypertensive drug given. Elderly frail persons are most susceptible to orthostatic and postprandial hypotension (8). Measurements of BP in the upright position, especially after eating, are indicated in these persons.

ADVERSE EFFECTS OF ANTIHYPERTENSIVE DRUG THERAPY

All antihypertensive drugs may predispose older persons to develop symptomatic orthostatic hypotension and postprandial hypotension, and syncope or falls (8). Diuretics may cause volume depletion. Vasodilators such as ACE inhibitors, ARBs, calcium channel blockers, hydralazine, nitrates, and prazosin may cause a reduction in systemic vascular resistance and venodilation (Table 4.2) (1).

Compared with amlodipine, ramipril significantly reduced progression of renal disease in 1094 African Americans with hypertensive nephrosclerosis (65). If the older person cannot tolerate an ACE inhibitor because of cough, angioneurotic edema, rash, or altered taste sensation, an ARB should be administered (66). In the Ongoing Telmisartan Alone and in Combination with Ramipril Global Endpoint Trial (ONTARGET) (67), when compared to ramipril alone, the addition of telmisartan to ramipril in patients, mean age 67 years, with vascular disease or high-risk DM, did not decrease cardiovascular events but increased hypotensive symptoms (4.8% versus 1.7%,) syncope (0.3% versus 0.2%), and renal dysfunction (1.1% versus 0.7%) (68).

Potassium-sparing diuretics should not be given to elderly persons taking ACE inhibitors or ARBs to avoid hyperkalemia. Risk factors for renal insufficiency in older persons receiving ACE inhibitors or ARBs include renal

Table 4.2 Adverse effects of antihypertensive therapy in older persons

Drug class	Adverse effects
Thiazide and loop diuretics	Hypokalemia, hyponatremia, hypomagnesemia, volume depletion hypotension, renal impairment, hyperuricemia, gout, hyperglycemia
Potassium-sparing diuretics	Hyperkalemia, hypotension
Beta-adrenergic blockers	Sinus bradycardia, fatigue, AV nodal heart block, bronchospasm, intermittent claudication, confusion, aggravation of acute heart failure, hyperglycemia
Alpha-beta adrenergic blockers (vasodilator-beta adrenergic blockers)	Hypotension, heart block, sinus bradycardia, bronchospasm
Alpha 1-adrenergic antagonists	Orthostatic hypotension
ACE inhibitors	Cough, hyperkalemia (only with eGFR <50 mL/min), angioneurotic edema, rash, altered taste sensation, renal impairment
ARBs	Hyperkalemia, renal impairment
Central-acting drugs	Sedation, constipation, dry mouth
Calcium antagonists	
Non-dihydropyridines	Rash, exacerbation of GERD symptoms, sinus bradycardia, heart block, heart failure, constipation (verapamil), gingival hyperplasia
Dihydropyridines	Peripheral edema, heart failure, tachycardia, aggravation of angina pectoris (short-acting agents)
Direct vasodilators	Tachycardia, fluid retention, angina pectoris

Abbreviations: ACE, angiotensin converting enzyme; ARBs, angiotensin receptor blockers; AV, atrioventricular; eGFR, estimated glomerular filtration rate; GERD, gastroesophageal reflux disease.
Source: Aronow WS et al., *J. Am. Coll. Cardiol.*, 57, 2037–2114, 2011.

artery stenosis (usually bilateral); polycystic renal disease; reduced absolute or effective arterial blood volume; use of nonsteroidal anti-inflammatory drugs, cyclosporine, or tacrolimus; and sepsis (69). However, reversible renal failure may occur in older persons treated with ACE inhibitors or ARBs who are dehydrated or salt depleted. ACE inhibitors or ARBs can cause an azotemic response when there is an absolute decrease in intravascular volume due to aggressive diuresis, poor oral intake, or gastroenteritis or an effective reduction in intravascular volume in patients with severe CHF (69).

Beta-blockers depress the sinus node and the atrioventricular node and are contraindicated in patients with severe sinus bradycardia, sinoatrial disease, and marked first-degree, second-degree, and third-degree atrioventricular block (70). Beta-blockers should also not be given to patients with bronchial asthma or to patients with lung disease with severe bronchospasm (70). Beta-blockers may also cause depression or confusion in elderly persons.

Short-acting dihydropyridine calcium channel blockers have the potential to increase cardiovascular events and should be avoided (71). Verapamil and diltiazem depress the sinus node and the atrioventricular node, and are contraindicated in patients with severe sinus bradycardia, sinoatrial disease, and marked first-degree, second-degree, and third-degree atrioventricular block (71, 72).

Diltiazem and verapamil are contraindicated in treating post-infarction patients with an abnormal LV ejection fraction because they will increase coronary events and mortality as well as CHF (73, 74). Calcium channel blockers such as nifedipine, diltiazem, and verapamil exacerbate CHF in patients with CHF and abnormal LV ejection fraction (75).

In the Antihypertensive and Lipid-Lowering Treatment to Prevent Heart Attack Trial (ALLHAT), the doxazosin arm involving 9067 patients was prematurely stopped at a median of 3.3 years (76). Compared with the diuretic chlorthalidone, the alpha-blocker doxazosin significantly increased CHF 204%, stroke 19%, and combined cardiovascular disease (coronary heart disease death, nonfatal MI, stroke, angina pectoris, coronary revascularization, CHF, or PAD) 25%, angina pectoris 16%, and coronary revascularization 15%.

In an observational study of older persons, mean age 80 years, with prior MI and hypertension, those treated with alpha-blockers had a significant increase in new coronary events at 40-month mean follow-up, of 1.69 times compared with beta-blockers, of 1.50 times compared with ACE inhibitors, and of 1.35 times compared with diuretics (74). Alpha-blockers cause a high incidence of orthostatic hypotension, especially in patients receiving diuretics or other vasodilator drugs (77).

Centrally acting drugs should not be used as monotherapy in older persons because they cause a high incidence of sedation, precipitate or exacerbate depression, and cause constipation (77). Direct vasodilators may cause headache, fluid retention, and tachycardia, and may aggravate angina pectoris. Hydralazine caused a lupus-like syndrome in 6.7% of 281 patients treated with hydralazine for 3 years (78). Minoxidil may cause hirsutism and a pericardial effusion (79).

USE OF ANTIHYPERTENSIVE DRUGS IN PERSONS WITH ASSOCIATED MEDICAL CONDITIONS

Older persons with prior MI should be treated with beta-blockers and ACE inhibitors (1, 2, 57, 62, 72, 80–82). In an observational prospective study of 1212 older men and women with prior MI and hypertension treated with beta-blockers, ACE inhibitors, diuretics, calcium channel blockers, or alpha-blockers, at 40-month follow-up, the incidence of new coronary events in older persons treated with one antihypertensive drug was lowest in those treated with beta-blockers or ACE inhibitors (74). In older persons treated with two antihypertensive drugs, the incidence of new coronary events was lowest in those treated with beta-blockers plus ACE inhibitors.

Beta-blockers should be used to treat older patients with complex ventricular arrhythmias with abnormal (59) or normal (60) LV ejection fraction and with CHF with abnormal (2, 83, 84) or normal (84, 85) LV ejection fraction. Beta-blockers should also be used to treat older patients with hypertension who have angina pectoris (86), myocardial ischemia (87), supraventricular tachyarrhythmias such as atrial fibrillation with a rapid ventricular rate (88, 89), hyperthyroidism (90), preoperative hypertension (1), migraine (1), or essential tremor (1).

In addition to beta-blockers, older persons with CHF should be treated with diuretics and ACE inhibitors and with aldosterone antagonists if needed (91, 92). ACE inhibitors or ARBs should be administered to older persons with DM, chronic renal disease, or proteinuria (1, 2, 65, 66). Diuretics and ACE inhibitors are recommended to prevent recurrent stroke in older persons with hypertension (1, 2). Thiazide diuretics should be used to treat elderly persons with osteoporosis (1).

It is also very important to treat other cardiovascular risk factors in older persons with hypertension to reduce cardiovascular events and mortality (2). Smoking must be stopped (93). Dyslipidemia must be treated (48, 93–96). DM must be controlled (14, 97–99).

The Pravastatin or Atorvastatin Evaluation and Infection Therapy-Thrombolysis in Myocardial Infarction (PROVE IT-TIMI) 22 trial (100) enrolled 4162 patients with an acute coronary syndrome (acute MI with or without ST-segment elevation or high-risk unstable angina pectoris). The lowest cardiovascular event rates occurred with a systolic BP between 130 and 140 mmHg and a diastolic BP between 80 and 90 mmHg with a nadir of 136/85 mm.

An observational subgroup analysis was performed in 6400 of the 22,576 persons enrolled in the International Verapamil SR-Trandolapril Study (INVEST) (101). The study participants had DM and coronary artery disease. Persons were categorized as having tight control of their BP if they could maintain their systolic BP below 130 mmHg and their diastolic BP below 85 mmHg, usual control if they could maintain their systolic BP between 130 and 139 mmHg, and uncontrolled if their systolic BP was >140 mmHg. Using 16,893 patient-years of follow-up, a cardiovascular event rate of 12.6% occurred in patients with usual control of BP versus 19.8% in patients with uncontrolled hypertension, $p < 0.001$ (101). The incidence of cardiovascular events was 12.6% in patients with usual control of BP versus 12.7% in patients with tight control of BP (p not significant).

The Action to Control Cardiovascular Risk in Diabetes (ACCORD) BP trial (102) randomized 4733 persons with type 2 DM to intensive BP control with a target systolic BP of <120 mmHg or to standard BP control with a target systolic BP <140 mmHg. The primary composite outcome was nonfatal MI, nonfatal stroke, or death from cardiovascular causes. The mean follow-up was 4.7 years. After 1 year, the mean systolic BP was 119.3 mmHg in the intensive BP control group versus 133.5 mmHg in the standard BP control group. The annual rate of the primary outcome was 1.87% in the intensive BP control group versus 2.09% in the standard BP control group (p not significant). The annual rate of stroke, a prespecified secondary outcome, was 0.32% in the intensive BP control group versus 0.53% in the standard BP control group, $p = 0.01$ (102).

Patients with DM were excluded from SPRINT. In the ACCORD BP trial, reducing the systolic BP to <120 mmHg in 4733 persons insignificantly lowered the composite primary outcome of MI, stroke, or cardiovascular death 12%, but significantly lowered the incidence of stroke (a prespecified secondary outcome) 41% ($p = 0.01$) (102). The patients in SPRINT were older (mean age 67.9 years) than those in the ACCORD BP (mean age 62.2 years). The patients in ACCORD BP were at lower risk than the patients in SPRINT. Patients with dyslipidemia were assigned to the lipid arm and excluded from the BP arm in ACCORD BP. Patients with a serum creatinine above 1.5 mg/dL were also excluded from ACCORD BP. In addition, the use of diuretics was different in these trials. ACCORD BP often used hydrochlorothiazide, whereas SPRINT primarily used chlorthalidone (my preference).

A post hoc analysis of the results from ACCORD BP also demonstrated that the primary cardiovascular disease outcome was reduced 26% in patients randomized to intensive BP treatment and standard glycemia goals than in patients randomized to standard BP treatment and standard glycemia goals (103). In addition, targeting a systolic BP of less than 120 mmHg in ACCORD BP was associated with a 39% lower risk of electrocardiographic left ventricular hypertrophy ($p = 0.008$) (104). The ACCORD BP trial also showed that hypertensive diabetics treated to a systolic BP goal of less than 120 mmHg had a tendency for a reduced incidence of orthostatic hypotension than those randomized to a systolic BP goal of less than 140 mmHg (105, 106). The 2017 ACC/AHA hypertension guidelines recommend lowering the BP in older diabetics to <130/80 mmHg (2).

We studied the impact of baseline systolic BP on outcomes in 7785 persons with mild to moderate chronic CHF in the Digitalis Investigation Group trial (107). A baseline systolic BP ≤120 mmHg was associated during 5 years of follow-up with a 15% increase in cardiovascular mortality ($p = 0.032$), with a 30% increase in heart failure mortality ($p = 0.006$), with a 13% increase in cardiovascular hospitalization ($p = 0.008$), with a 10% increase in all-cause hospitalization ($p = 0.017$), and with a 21% increase in heart failure hospitalization ($p = 0.002$).

Randomized clinical trial data are needed to investigate the effects of a systolic BP <120 mmHg versus less than 140 mmHg on clinical outcomes in older patients with CHF and a reduced LV ejection fraction (HFrEF), in older patients with CHF and a preserved LV ejection fraction (HFpEF), and in older patients with a LV ejection fraction <35% since these patients were excluded from SPRINT. The 2017 ACC/AHA hypertension guidelines recommend treating these patients to a BP <130/80 mmHg (2).

Patients with a prior stroke and patients with an estimated glomerular filtration rate less than 20 mL/min/1.73 m^2 were also excluded from SPRINT. The 2017 ACC/AHA hypertension guidelines recommend treating these patients to a BP <130/80 mm Hg (2).

In ONTARGET, a progressive increase in the proportion of visits in which the BP was decreased to <140/90 mmHg or to <130/80 mmHg was associated with a progressive decrease in stroke, new onset of microalbuminuria or macroalbuminuria, and a return to normoalbuminuria in persons with albuminuria (108). However, the adjusted risk of cardiovascular events was reduced by increasing the frequency of BP control to <140/90 mmHg but not to <130/80 mmHg.

In ONTARGET, 9603 of 25,584 patients had DM (109). DM increased the primary outcome of cardiovascular death, nonfatal MI or stroke, or hospitalization for CHF by 48% (95% CI, 1.38–1.57). In both diabetics and nondiabetics, antihypertensive treatment reduced the primary outcome if baseline systolic BP levels ranged from 143 to 155 mmHg. Except for stroke, there was no benefit in fatal or nonfatal outcomes by lowering systolic BP below 130 mmHg.

During >12 years of median follow-up in the Cardiovascular Health Study, we found that isolated diastolic hypotension (a diastolic BP <60 mmHg with a systolic BP ≥100 mmHg) was associated with a 29% significant independent increase in incident CHF ($p = 0.003$) (110). Therefore, ISH and isolated diastolic hypotension are significant risk factors for CHF in community-dwelling older persons.

Three trials including 2272 patients with chronic kidney disease and proteinuria without DM showed that a BP target of <130/80 mmHg did not improve clinical outcomes more than a BP target of <140/90 mmHg (111).

At 2.5-year follow-up of 20,330 patients with a recent noncardioembolic stroke (112), compared with a systolic BP of 130–139 mmHg, the incidence of the primary outcome of cardiovascular death, MI, or stroke was increased 29% (95% CI, 1.07–1.56) by a systolic BP <120 mmHg, 23% (95% CI, 1.07–1.41) by a systolic BP of 140–149 mmHg, and 208% (95% CI by a systolic BP of ≥150 mmHg.

TREATMENT OF DRUG-REFRACTORY HYPERTENSION

Despite the availability of numerous effective pharmacologic agents for hypertensive patients, control of BP in the elderly is achieved in <50% of patients (1,2,29). Some data support the use of spironolactone as a fourth drug in the treatment of resistant hypertension if the serum potassium level is ≤4.5 mmol/L (113). Alternative approaches to achieving additional BP control that are under investigation in drug-refractory patients include the use of implantable carotid stimulation devices (114), devices to control the respiratory rate that can indirectly reduce BP (115), and the use of catheter-based renal sympathetic denervation (116). As of now, there are limited data available with these approaches in older persons regarding both efficacy and safety.

The Symplicity HTN-3 study randomized 535 patients with treatment-resistant hypertension to renal sympathetic denervation using a Medtronic Symplicity catheter system or to a sham-control arm (117, 118). At 6-month follow-up, the primary endpoint of the change in office systolic BP at 6 months was not significantly different between the two treated groups (117). The 1-year follow-up data from this study support no further decrease in office or ambulatory BP (118).

OTHER CLINICAL TRIALS

The Heart Outcomes Prevention Evaluation (HOPE)-3 trial randomized 12,705 persons (49% Asians, 20% Whites, 27% Hispanics, and 2% Blacks), mean age 65.7 years, without cardiovascular disease and at intermediate risk to treatment with candesartan 16 mg plus hydrochlorothiazide 12.5 mg daily or to placebo (119). The baseline mean BP was 138.1/81.9 mmHg. The reduction in BP in the drug treatment group was 6.0/3.0 mmHg. At 5.6-year median follow-up, there was no significant reduction in the composite endpoint of cardiovascular death, nonfatal MI, or nonfatal stroke. In the subgroup of patients with a systolic BP higher than 143.5 mmHg, drug therapy reduced the composite endpoint of cardiovascular death, nonfatal MI, or nonfatal stroke by 27% (95% CI, 6%–44%) (119).

Less than 40% of the persons in the HOPE-3 trial had hypertension, and the risk for cardiovascular disease was much lower in the HOPE-3 trial than in SPRINT (38, 39). The systolic BP reduction in SPRINT was 14.8 mmHg lower with intensive treatment than with standard treatment, whereas the systolic BP was reduced only 6 mmHg by drug treatment in the HOPE-3 trial (119). Chlorthalidone was used in SPRINT and has been shown to reduce cardiovascular events in clinical trials, whereas hydrochlorothiazide 12.5 mg daily used in the HOPE-3 trial has not been shown to reduce cardiovascular events (120).

A systematic review and meta-analysis were performed on 123 randomized studies of use of antihypertensive drugs, which included 613,815 participants (121). This study found that every 10 mmHg reduction in systolic BP significantly reduced major cardiovascular events by 20%, coronary heart disease by 17%, stroke by 27%, and CHF by 28%, which in the populations studied decreased all-cause mortality by 13% (121).

The REasons for Geographic and Racial Differences in Stroke (REGARDS) study is an observational study of the incidence of stroke in persons living in the stroke belt and stroke buckle regions of the United States (122). In this study, 4181 persons aged 55–64 years, 3737 persons aged 65–74 years, and 1839 patients aged 75 years and older (mean age 79.3 years) were receiving treatment with antihypertensive drugs. The median follow-up was 4.5 years for cardiovascular disease (coronary heart disease or stroke) and coronary heart disease, 5.7 years for stroke, and 6.0 years for all-cause death. We concluded from this study that in persons aged 55 years and older treated with antihypertensive drugs, a systolic BP between 120 and 139 mmHg was significantly associated with a lower risk for cardiovascular events and for all-cause death (122). The optimal diastolic BP in this study was 70–90 mmHg.

A post hoc analysis of the Secondary Prevention of Small Subcortical Strokes (SPS3) trial investigated the effects of a systolic BP goal of <130 mmHg versus 130–149 mmHg in 3020 patients, mean age 63 years, with a recent lacunar stroke (123). After 1 year, the mean systolic BP was 138 mmHg in 1519 patients and 127 mmHg in 1501 patients. Compared to a systolic BP of 138 mmHg, a systolic BP of 127 mmHg at 3.7-year follow-up nonsignificantly reduced all stroke by 19%, disabling or fatal stroke by 19%, and MI or vascular death by 16%, and significantly reduced intracerebral hemorrhage by 63% (p = 0.03) (123). These data support a systolic BP goal of less than 130 mmHg in patients with a lacunar stroke (123, 124).

Some 16.8 million US adults overall and 8.2 million US adults with treated hypertension meet the SPRINT eligibility criteria (125). The SPRINT eligibility criteria were applied to the 1999–2006 National Health and Nutrition Examination Survey and linked with the National Death Index through December 2011 (126). This study reported that intensive lowering of systolic BP of all eligible US adults could prevent 107,500 deaths per year and 46,100 cases of CHF per year but cause an increase in serious adverse events (126).

RECENT HYPERTENSION GUIDELINES

Unlike other hypertension guidelines (1, 2, 37, 70, 127–129), the 2013 Eighth Joint National Committee (JNC 8) guidelines for management of hypertension recommended lowering the BP in adults aged 60 years or older to <150/90 mmHg if they do not have DM or chronic kidney disease (130). The minority view from JNC 8 recommended lowering the BP in adults aged 60 years and older with hypertension to <140/90 mmHg (131).

The Canadian 2016 hypertension guidelines recommend that high-risk adults aged 50 years and older with a systolic BP of 130 mmHg or higher obtained by an automated office BP measurement should have a target systolic BP goal of 120 mmHg or lower (132). High-risk patients for treatment with intensive BP management include those with clinical or subclinical cardiovascular disease or chronic kidney disease or an estimated 10-year global cardiovascular risk of 15% and higher or an age of 75 years and higher (132).

The National Heart Foundation of Australia 2016 hypertension guidelines state that in selected high cardiovascular risk persons, a systolic BP goal of <120 mmHg can improve cardiovascular outcomes (133). Close monitoring should be performed in these persons to identify treatment-related adverse effects, including hypotension, syncope, electrolyte abnormalities, and acute kidney injury (133).

The American College of Physicians/American Academy of Family Physicians 2017 hypertension guidelines made three recommendations (134): (1) adults aged 60 years and older with a systolic BP of 150 mmHg and higher should have their systolic BP lowered to <150 mmHg; (2) adults aged 60 years and older with a history of stroke or transient ischemic attack should have their systolic BP lowered to <140 mmHg; and (3) adults aged 60 years and older at high cardiovascular risk should have their systolic BP reduced to <140 mmHg.

The 2017 ACC/AHA guidelines, contributed to by nine other professional societies, recommend for secondary prevention in patients with clinical cardiovascular disease a systolic BP of <130 mmHg and a diastolic BP of <80 mmHg (2). These guidelines recommend for primary prevention in adults a systolic BP of <130 mmHg and a diastolic BP of <80 mmHg if the estimated 10-year risk of atherosclerotic cardiovascular disease is ≥10%, and for primary prevention in adults a systolic BP of <140 mmHg and a diastolic BP of 90 mmHg if the estimated 10-year risk of atherosclerotic cardiovascular disease is <10% (2).

DRUG TREATMENT OF CORONARY HEART DISEASE AND OF HEART FAILURE

The 2017 ACC/AHA hypertension guidelines recommend the following drug treatment of coronary heart disease and CHF (2). Adults with stable ischemic heart disease and a BP ≥130/80 mmHg should be treated with beta-blockers plus ACE inhibitors or ARBs for compelling indications such as prior MI or stable angina pectoris as first-line therapy with the addition of other drugs such as thiazide-type diuretics, dihydropyridine calcium channel blockers, and/or mineralocorticoid receptor antagonists as needed to further control hypertension (2). In adults with stable ischemic heart disease and persistent uncontrolled hypertension, the addition of dihydropyridine calcium channel blockers to guideline-directed medical treatment (GDMT) beta-blockers is recommended. The GDMT beta-blockers include carvedilol, metoprolol tartrate, metoprolol succinate, nadolol, bisoprolol, propranolol, and timolol. In adults who have had a MI or acute coronary syndrome, it is reasonable to continue GDMT beta-blockers beyond 3 years as chronic therapy for hypertension (2).

In adults at increased risk for CHF, the optimal BP in patients with hypertension should be <130/80 mmHg (2). Adults with HFrEF should be prescribed GDMT titrated to achieve a BP <130/80 mmHg. Drugs used to treat HFrEF with hypertension include diuretics, GDMT beta-blockers (carvedilol, metoprolol succinate, or bisoprolol), ACE inhibitors or ARBs or an angiotensin receptor–neprilysin inhibitor, and mineralocorticoid receptor antagonists. Nondihydropyridine calcium channel blockers are contraindicated in patients with HFrEF (2).

In adults with CHF and HFpEF with symptoms of volume overload, diuretics should be prescribed to control hypertension (2). Adults with HFpEF and hypertension after management of volume overload should be prescribed ACE inhibitors or ARBs and beta-blockers titrated to reduce the systolic BP to <130 mmHg (2).

In 8511 older patients with hypertension, treatment to a systolic BP target of 110 to 129 mm Hg caused a lower incidence of cardiovascular events than treatment to a target systolic BP of 130 to 149 mm Hg (135). The final report of SPRINT showed that targeting a systolic BP of <120 mm Hg caused fewer major adverse cardiovascular events and lower all-cause mortality than targeting a systolic BP of <140 mm Hg both during the trial and after the trial (136). Frailty status in the SPRINT trial was a marker of high cardiovascular risk (137). Frail patients benefit similarly to other patients from intensive systolic BP control without an increased risk of serious adverse events (2). Sprint participants with higher baseline predicted cardiovascular risk had a greater absolute benefit from intensive systolic BP treatment (138). Intensive systolic BP lowering prevented malignant left ventricular hypertrophy (LVH) and reduced the composite of acute decompensated heart failure events and death in SPRINT participants with baseline malignant LVH (139). At 11.5 median follow-up of 95,545 adults with hypertension and baseline LVH, the risk for cardiovascular events was lowest with a systolic BP <139 mm Hg and a BP <80 mm Hg (140). In the Women's Health Initiative study, at a median follow-up of 19.8 years, women older than 65 years of age with low cardiovascular disease and other chronic disease risk, a systolic BP level of <130 mm Hg was associated with longevity (141).

If a fourth antihypertensive drug is needed to control resistant hypertension treated with optimal doses of a thiazide diuretic (especially chlorthalidone), a CCB, and an ACEI or ARB, an aldosterone antagonist should be added (142). If a fifth drug is needed, it should be a beta-blocker, and a sixth drug should be clonidine or methyldopa or hydralazine or minoxidil (142). The beneficial effects of thiazide diuretics are less when the glomerular filtration rate (GFR) is less than 40 cc/min. These patients should be given a loop diuretic such as furosemide every 12 hours (142). Diet and exercise can lower BP in persons with resistant hypertension (143). Resistant hypertension does not benefit from renal denervation (144). However, the US Food and Drug Administration approved renal denervation as an adjunctive treatment for patients in whom lifestyle modification and antihypertensive drugs do not adequately control BP (145). In 178,562 older patients, compared with maximizing the dose to intensify hypertension treatment, adding a new medication reduced systolic BP 1.1 mm Hg more at 1 year (146).

Sacubitril/valsartan may be used to treat older persons with hypertension (147). SGLT2 inhibitors may be second-line drugs to treat older persons with hypertension with diabetes or heart disease (148). Emerging therapies for treating resistant hypertension include selective aldosterone synthase inhibitors including baxdrostat (149) and lorundrostat (150).

REFERENCES

1. Aronow WS, Fleg JL, Pepine CJ et al. ACCF/AHA 2011 expert consensus document on hypertension in the elderly: A report of the American College of Cardiology Foundation Task Force on Clinical Expert Consensus Documents. *J Am Coll Cardiol* 2011; *57*: 2037–2114.
2. Whelton PK, Carey RM, Aronow WS et al. ACC/AHA/AAPA/ABC/ACPM/AGS/APhA/ASH/ASPC/NMA/PCNA guideline for the prevention, detection, evaluation and management of high blood pressure in adults. A report of the American College of Cardiology/American Heart Association Task Force on Clinical Practice Guidelines. *J Am Coll Cardiol* 2018; *71*: e127–e248.
3. Mendelson G, Nassimiha D, Aronow WS. Simultaneous measurements of BPs in right and left brachial arteries. *Cardiol Rev* 2004; *12*: 276–278.

4. Clark CE, Taylor RS, Shore AC et al. Association of a difference in systolic blood pressure between arms with vascular disease and mortality: A systematic review and meta-analysis. *Lancet* 2012; *379*: 905–914.
5. Joseph J, Koka M, Aronow WS. Prevalence of moderate and severe renal insufficiency in older persons with hypertension, DM, coronary artery disease, PAD, ischemic stroke, or congestive heart failure in an academic nursing home. *J Am Med Dir Assoc* 2008; *9*: 257–259.
6. Aronow WS, Lee NH, Sales FF et al. Prevalence of postural hypotension in elderly patients in a long-term health care facility. *Am J Cardiol* 1988; *62*: 336.
7. Fleg JL. Effects of aging on the cardiovascular system. In: Lewis RP, ed. *Adult Clinical Cardiology Self-Assessment Program (ACCSAP6)*. Bethesda, MD: American College of Cardiology Foundation, 2005: pp. 6–20.
8. Aronow WS. Dizziness and syncope. In: Hazzard WR, Blass JP, Ettinger WH Jr, Halter JB, Ouslander JG, eds. *Principles of Geriatric Medicine and Gerontology*, 4th ed. New York City: McGraw-Hill, 1998: 1519–1534.
9. Chiong JR, Aronow WS, Khan IA et al. Secondary hypertension: Current diagnosis and treatment. *Int J Cardiol* 2008; *124*: 6–21.
10. Aronow WS, Ahn C, Gutstein H. Prevalence and incidence of cardiovascular disease in 1160 older men and 2464 older women in a long-term health care facility. *J Gerontol: Med Sci* 2002; *57A*: M45–M46.
11. Aronow WS, Ahn C, Kronzon I et al. Congestive heart failure, coronary events and atherothrombotic brain infarction in elderly blacks and whites with systemic hypertension and with and without echocardiographic and electrocardiographic evidence of left ventricular hypertrophy. *Am J Cardiol* 1991; *67*: 295–299.
12. Mendelson G, Ness J, Aronow WS. Drug treatment of hypertension in older persons in an academic hospital-based geriatrics practice. *J Am Geriatr Soc* 1999; *47*: 597–599.
13. Koka M, Joseph J, Aronow WS. Adequacy of control of hypertension in an academic nursing home. *J Am Med Dir Assoc* 2007; *8*: 538–540.
14. Joseph J, Koka M, Aronow WS. Prevalence of a hemoglobin A1c less than 7.0%, of a BP less than 130/80 mm Hg, and of a serum low-density lipoprotein cholesterol less than 100 mg/dL in older patients with DM in an academic nursing home. *J Am Med Dir Assoc* 2008; *9*: 51–54.
15. Madhavan S, Ooi WL, Cohen H et al. Relation of pulse pressure and BP reduction to the incidence of myocardial infarction. *Hypertens* 1994; *23*: 395–401.
16. Fried LP, Kronmal RA, Newman AB et al. Risk factors for 5-year mortality in older adults. The Cardiovascular Health Study. *JAMA* 1998; *279*: 585–592.
17. Aronow WS, Ahn C. Risk factors for new coronary events in a large cohort of very elderly patients with and without coronary artery disease. *Am J Cardiol* 1996; *77*: 864–866.
18. Psaty BM, Furberg CD, Kuller LH et al. Association between BP level and the risk of myocardial infarction, stroke, and total mortality: The cardiovascular health study. *Arch Intern Med* 2001; *161*: 1183–1192.
19. Aronow WS, Ahn C, Gutstein H. Risk factors for new atherothrombotic brain infarction in 664 older men and 1,488 older women. *Am J Cardiol* 1996; *77*: 1381–1383.
20. Aronow WS, Frishman WH. Treatment of hypertension and prevention of ischemic stroke. *Curr Cardiol Rep* 2004; *6*: 124–129.
21. Aronow WS, Ahn C, Kronzon I. Comparison of incidences of congestive heart failure in older AfricanAmericans, Hispanics, and Whites. *Am J Cardiol* 1999; *84*: 611–612.
22. Levy D, Larson MG, Vasan RS et al. The progression from hypertension to congestive heart failure. *JAMA* 1996; *275*: 1557–1562.
23. Aronow WS, Sales FF, Etienne F et al. Prevalence of PAD and its correlation with risk factors for PAD in elderly patients in a long-term health care facility. *Am J Cardiol* 1988; *62*: 644–646.
24. Ness J, Aronow WS, Ahn C. Risk factors for PAD in an academic hospital-based geriatrics practice. *J Am Geriatr Soc* 2000; *48*: 312–314.
25. Ness J, Aronow WS, Newkirk E et al. Prevalence of symptomatic PAD, modifiable risk factors, and appropriate use of drugs in the treatment of PAD in older persons seen in a university general medicine clinic. *J Gerontol: Med Sci* 2005; *60A*: M255–M257.
26. Aronow WS, Ahmed MI, Ekundayo OJ et al. A propensity-matched study of the association of PAD with cardiovascular outcomes in community-dwelling older adults. *Am J Cardiol* 2009; *103*: 130–135.
27. Aronow WS, Frishman WH. Effect of antihypertensive drug treatment on cognitive function. *Clin Geriatr* 2006; *14*: 25–28.
28. Lewington S, Clarke R, Qizilbash N et al. Age-specific relevance of usual BP to vascular mortality: A meta-analysis of individual data for one million adults in 6 prospective studies. *Lancet* 2002; *360*: 1903–1913.
29. Lloyd-Jones DM, Evans JC, Levy D. Hypertension in adults across the age spectrum: Current outcomes and control in the community. *JAMA* 2005; *294*: 466–472.
30. Gandelman G, Aronow WS, Varma R. Prevalence of adequate BP control in self-pay or Medicare patients versus Medicaid or private insurance patients with

systemic hypertension followed in a university cardiology or general medicine clinic. *Am J Cardiol* 2004; *94*: 815–816.
31. SHEP Cooperative Research Group. Prevention of stroke by antihypertensive drug treatment in older persons with ISH. Final results of the Systolic Hypertension in the Elderly Program (SHEP). *JAMA* 1991; *265*: 3255–3264.
32. Kostis JB, Davis BR, Cutler J et al. Prevention of heart failure by antihypertensive drug treatment in older persons with ISH. *JAMA* 1997; *278*: 212–216.
33. Perry HM Jr, Davis BR, Price TR et al. Effect of treating ISH on the risk of developing various types and subtypes of stroke. The Systolic Hypertension in the Elderly Program (SHEP). *JAMA* 2000; *284*: 465–471.
34. Staessen JA, Fagard R, Thijs L et al. Randomised double-blind comparison of placebo and active treatment for older patients with ISH. *Lancet* 1997; *350*: 757–764.
35. Wang J-G, Staessen JA, Gong L, Liu L. Chinese trial on ISH in the elderly. *Arch Intern Med* 2000; *160*: 211–220.
36. Beckett NS, Peters R, Fletcher AE et al. Treatment of hypertension in patients 80 years of age or older. *N Eng J Med* 2008; *358*: 1887–1898.
37. Rosendorff C, Black HR, Cannon CP et al. AHA/ACC/ASH scientific statement. Treatment of hypertension in patients with coronary artery disease: A scientific statement from the American Heart Association, American College of Cardiology, and American Society of Hypertension. *J Am Coll Cardiol* 2015; *65*: 1998–2038.
38. Wright JT Jr, Williamson JD, Whelton PK et al. A randomized trial of intensive versus standard blood-pressure control. *N Engl J Med* 2015; *373*: 2103–2116.
39. Williamson JD, Supiano MA, Applegate WB et al. Intensive vs standard blood pressure control and cardiovascular disease outcomes in adults aged ≥75 years. A randomized clinical trial. *JAMA* 2016; *315*: 2673–2682.
40. Progress Collaborative Group. Randomised trial of a perindopril-based blood-pressure-lowering regimen among 6105 individuals with previous stroke or transient ischaemic attack. *Lancet* 2001; *358*: 1033–1041.
41. Forette F, Seux M-L, Staessen JA et al. The prevention of dementia with antihypertensive treatment. New evidence from the Systolic Hypertension in Europe (Syst-Eur) study. *Arch Intern Med* 2002; *162*: 2046–2052.
42. Murray MD, Lane KA, Gao S et al. Preservation of cognitive function with antihypertensive medications. A longitudinal analysis of a community-based sample of African Americans. *Arch Intern Med* 2002; *162*: 2090–2096.
43. Veld BA, Ruitenberg A, Hofman A et al. Antihypertensive drugs and incidence of dementia: The Rotterdam Study. *Neurobiol Aging* 2001; *22*: 407–412.
44. Aronow WS. What is the appropriate treatment of hypertension in elders? (editorial). *J Gerontol A Biol Sci Med Sci* 2002; *57*: M483–M486.
45. Aronow WS. Older age should not be a barrier to the treatment of hypertension. *Nat Clin Pract Cardiovasc Med* 2008; *5*: 514–515.
46. Aronow WS. Might losartan reduce sudden cardiac death in diabetic patients with hypertension? *Lancet* 2003; *362*: 591–592.
47. Frishman WH. Beta-adrenergic receptor blockers in hypertension: Alive and well. *Prog Cardiovasc Dis* 2016; *59*: 247–252.
48. Fleg JL, Aronow WS, Frishman WH. Cardiovascular drug therapy in the elderly. *Nat Rev Cardiol* 2011; *8*: 13–28.
49. Aronow WS. Hypertension guidelines. *Hypertension* 2011; *58*: 347–348.
50. Banach M, Aronow WS. Should we have any doubts about hypertension therapy in elderly patients. ACCF/AHA 2011 expert consensus document on hypertension in the elderly. *Pol Arch Med Wewn* 2011; *121*: 253–258.
51. Aronow WS, Banach M. Ten most important things to learn from the ACCF/AHA 2011 expert consensus document on hypertension in the elderly. *BP* 2012; *21*: 3–5.
52. Banach M, Aronow WS. Hypertension therapy in the elderly-do we know the answers to all the questions? The status after publication of the ACCF/AHA 2011 expert consensus document on hypertension in the elderly. *J Hum Hypertens* 2012; *26*: 641–643.
53. Webster JL, Dunford EK, Hawkes C et al. Salt reduction initiatives around the world. *J Hypertens* 2011; *29*: 1043–1050.
54. Cook NR, Cutler JA, Obarzanek E et al. Long term effects of dietary sodium reduction on cardiovascular disease outcomes: Observational follow-up of the trials of hypertension prevention (TOHP). *BMJ* 2007; *334*: 885–888.
55. Chang HY, Hu YVV, Yue CS et al. Effect of potassium-enriched salt on cardiovascular mortality and medical expenses of elderly men. *Am J Clin Nutr* 2006; *83*: 1289–1296.
56. Yang Q, Liu T, Kuklina EV et al. Sodium and potassium intake and mortality among US adults: Prospective data from the Third National Health and Nutrition Examination Survey. *Arch Intern Med* 2011; *171*: 1183–1191.
57. Aronow WS, Ahn C, Kronzon I. Effect of beta blockers alone, of angiotensin-converting enzyme inhibitors alone, and of beta blockers plus angiotensin-converting enzyme inhibitors on new coronary events and on congestive heart failure in

older persons with healed myocardial infarcts and asymptomatic left ventricular systolic dysfunction. *Am J Cardiol* 2001; *88*: 1298–1300.
58. Whelton PK. Urinary sodium and cardiovascular disease risk. Informing guidelines for sodium consumption. *JAMA* 2011; *306*: 2262–2264.
59. Kennedy HL, Brooks MM, Barker AH et al. Beta-blocker therapy in the cardiac arrhythmia suppression trial. *Am J Cardiol* 1994; *74*: 674–680.
60. Aronow WS, Ahn C, Mercando AD et al. Effect of propranolol versus no antiarrhythmic drug on sudden cardiac death, total cardiac death, and total death in patients ≥62 years of age with heart disease, complex ventricular arrhythmias, and left ventricular ejection fraction ≥40%. *Am J Cardiol* 1994; *74*: 267–270.
61. Mancia G, Laurent S, Agabiti-Rosei E et al. Reappraisal of European guidelines on hypertension management: A European Society of Hypertension Task Force document. *BP* 2009; *18*: 308–347.
62. Law MR, Morris JK, Wald NJ. Use of blood pressure lowering drugs in the prevention of cardiovascular disease: Meta-analysis of 147 randomised trials in the context of expectations from prospective epidemiological studies. *BMJ* 2009; *338*: b1665. doi:10.1136/bmj.b1665.
63. Aronow WS. Current role of beta-blockers in the treatment of hypertension. *Expert Opin Pharmaco* 2010; *11*: 2599–2607.
64. Weber MA, Neutel JM, Frishman WH. Combination drug therapy. In: Frishman WH, Sonnenblick EH, Sica DA, eds. *Cardiovascular Pharmacotherapeutics*, 2nd ed. New York: McGraw-Hill, 2003: pp. 355–368.
65. Agodoa LY, Appel L, Bakris GL et al. Effect of ramipril versus amlodipine on renal outcomes in hypertensive nephrosclerosis. A randomized controlled trial. *JAMA* 2001; *285*: 2719–2728.
66. Brenner BM, Cooper ME, de Zeeuw D et al. Effects of losartan on renal and cardiovascular outcomes in patients with type 2 diabetes and nephropathy. *N Engl J Med* 2001; *345*: 861–869.
67. The ONTARGET Investigators. Telmisartan, ramipril, or both in patients at high risk for vascular events. *N Engl J Med* 2008; *358*: 1547–1559.
68. Palmer BF. Renal dysfunction complicating the treatment of hypertension. *N Engl J Med* 2002; *347*: 1256–1261.
69. Toto RD, Mitchell HC, Lee HC et al. Reversible renal insufficiency due to angiotensin-converting enzyme inhibitors in hypertensive nephrosclerosis. *Ann Intern Med* 1991; *115*: 513–519.
70. Rosendorff C, Black HR, Cannon CP et al. Treatment of hypertension in the prevention and management of ischemic heart disease. A scientific statement from the American Heart Association Council for High BP Research and the Councils on Clinical Cardiology and Epidemiology and Prevention. *Circulation* 2007; *115*: 2761–2788.
71. Pahor M, Guralnik JM, Corti C et al. Long-term survival and use of antihypertensive medications in older persons. *J Am Geriatr Soc* 1995; *43*: 1191–1197.
72. Aronow WS. Verapamil as an antiarrhythmic agent. In: Gould LA, ed. *Drug Treatment of Cardiac Arrhythmias*. Mount Kisco, New York: Futura Publishing Company, 1983: pp. 325–341.
73. Goldstein RE, Boccuzzi SJ, Cruess D et al. Diltiazem increases late-onset congestive heart failure in postinfarction patients with early reduction in ejection fraction. *Circulation* 1991; *83*: 52–60.
74. Aronow WS, Ahn C. Incidence of new coronary events in older persons with prior myocardial infarction and systemic hypertension treated with beta blockers, angiotensin-converting enzyme inhibitors, diuretics, calcium antagonists, and alpha blockers. *Am J Cardiol* 2002; *89*: 1207–1209.
75. Elkayam U, Amin J, Mehra A et al. A prospective, randomized, double-blind, crossover study to compare the efficacy and safety of chronic nifedipine therapy with that of isosorbide dinitrate and their combination in the treatment of chronic congestive heart failure. *Circulation* 1990; *82*: 1954–1961.
76. ALLHAT Officers and Coordinators for the ALLHAT Collaborative Research Group. Major cardiovascular events in hypertensive patients randomized to doxazosin vs chlorthalidone. The Antihypertensive and Lipid-Lowering Treatment to Prevent Heart Attack Trial (ALLHAT). *JAMA* 2000; *283*: 1967–1975.
77. Frishman WH, Aronow WS, Cheng-Lai A. Cardiovascular drug therapy in the elderly. In: Aronow WS, Fleg JL, Rich MW, eds. *Cardiovascular Disease in the Elderly*, 5th ed. Boca Raton, FL, London, New York City: CRC press, 2014: pp. 67–103.
78. Cameron HA, Ramsay LE. The lupus syndrome induced by hydralazine: A common complication with low dose treatment. *Br Med J (Clin Res Ed)* 1984; *289*: 410–412.
79. Krehlik JM, Hindson DA, Crowley JJ Jr et al. Minoxidil-associated pericarditis and fatal cardiac tamponade. *West J Med* 1986; *143*: 527–529.
80. Ryan TJ, Antman EM, Brooks NH et al. Update: ACC/AHA guidelines for the management of patients with acute myocardial infarction: Executive summary and recommendations. A report of the American College of Cardiology/American Heart Association Task Force on Practice Guidelines (Committee on Management of Acute Myocardial Infarction). *Circulation* 1999; *100*: 1016–1030.

81. Aronow WS, Ahn C. Effect of beta blockers on incidence of new coronary events in older persons with prior myocardial infarction and DM. *Am J Cardiol* 2001; *87*: 780–781.
82. Aronow WS, Ahn C. Effect of beta blockers on incidence of new coronary events in older persons with prior myocardial infarction and symptomatic PAD. *Am J Cardiol* 2001; *87*: 1284–1286.
83. MERIT-HF Study Group. Effect of metoprolol CR/XL in chronic heart failure: Metoprolol CR/XL Randomised Intervention Trial in Congestive Heart Failure (MERIT-HF). *Lancet* 1999; *353*: 2001–2007.
84. Flather MD, Shibata MC, Coats AJS et al. Randomized trial to determine the effect of nebivolol on mortality and cardiovascular hospital admission in elderly patients with heart failure (SENIORS). *Eur Heart J* 2005; *26*: 215–225.
85. Aronow WS, Ahn C, Kronzon I. Effect of propranolol versus no propranolol on total mortality plus nonfatal myocardial infarction in older patients with prior myocardial infarction, congestive heart failure, and left ventricular ejection fraction ≥40% treated with diuretics plus angiotensin-converting-enzyme inhibitors. *Am J Cardiol* 1997; *80*: 207–209.
86. Aronow WS, Frishman WH. Angina in the elderly. In: Aronow WS, Fleg JL, Rich MW, eds. *Cardiovascular Disease in the Elderly*, 5th ed. Boca Raton, FL, London, New York City: CRC press, 2014: pp. 215–237.
87. Aronow WS, Ahn C, Mercando AD et al. Decrease of mortality by propranolol in patients with heart disease and complex ventricular arrhythmias is more an anti-ischemic than an antiarrhythmic effect. *Am J Cardiol* 1994; *74*: 613–615.
88. Aronow WS. Treatment of atrial fibrillation. Part 1. *Cardiol Rev* 2008; *16*: 181–188.
89. Aronow WS. Treatment of atrial fibrillation and atrial flutter Part 2. *Cardiol Rev* 2008; *16*: 230–239.
90. Aronow WS. The heart and thyroid disease. In: Gambert SR, ed. *Clinics in Geriatric Medicine, Thyroid Disease*. Philadelphia, PA: W.B. Saunders, 1995: pp. 219–229.
91. Hunt SA, Baker DW, Chin MH et al. ACC/AHA guidelines for the evaluation and management of chronic heart failure in the adult: Executive summary. A report of the American College of Cardiology/American Heart Association Task Force on Practice Guidelines (Committee to Revise the 1995 Guidelines for the Evaluation and Management of Heart Failure). Developed in collaboration with the International Society for Heart and Lung Transplantation. Endorsed by the Heart Failure Society of America. *J Am Coll Cardiol* 2001; 38: 2101–2113.
92. Yancy CW, Jessup M, Bozkurt B et al. ACCF/AHA guidelines for the management of heart failure: Executive summary. A report of the American College of Cardiology Foundation/American Heart Association Task Force on Practice Guidelines. Developed in collaboration with the American College of Chest Physicians, Heart Rhythm Society, and International Society for Heart and Lung Transplantation. Endorsed by the American Association of Cardiovascular and Pulmonary Rehabilitation. *J Am Coll Cardiol* 2013; *62*: 1495–1539.
93. Smith SC Jr, Benjamin EJ, Bonow RO et al. AHA/ACCF secondary prevention and risk reduction therapy for patients with coronary and other atherosclerotic vascular disease: 2011 update. A guideline from the American Heart Association and American College of Cardiology Foundation. *J Am Coll Cardiol* 2011; *58*: 2432–2446.
94. Grundy SM, Cleeman JI, Merz CNB et al. Implications of recent clinical trials for the national cholesterol education program adult treatment panel III guidelines. *Circulation* 2004; *110*: 227–239.
95. Stone NJ, Robinson J, Lichtenstein AH et al. ACC/AHA guideline on the treatment of blood cholesterol to reduce atherosclerotic cardiovascular risk in adults: A report of the American College of Cardiology/American Heart Association Task Force on Practice Guidelines. *J Am Coll Cardiol* 2013; *63*: 2889–2934.
96. Aronow WS. Lipid-lowering in older persons. *Arch Med Sci* 2015; *11*: 43–56.
97. American Diabetes Association. Standards of medical care in diabetes-2013. *Diabetes Care* 2013; *36* (*supplement 1*): S11–S66.
98. Ravipati G, Aronow WS, Ahn C et al. Association of hemoglobin A_{1c} level with the severity of coronary artery disease in patients with diabetes mellitus. *Am J Cardiol* 2006; *97*: 968–969.
99. Aronow WS, Ahn C, Weiss MB et al. Relation of hemoglobin A_{1c} levels to severity of peripheral arterial disease in patients with diabetes mellitus. *Am J Cardiol* 2007; *99*: 1468–1469.
100. Bangalore S, Qin J, Sloan S et al. Cannon CP, PROVE-IT -TIMI 22 trial investigators. What is the optimal BP in patients after acute coronary syndromes? Relationship of BP and cardiovascular events in the pravastatin or atorvastatin evaluation and infection therapy-thrombolysis in myocardial infarction (PROVE IT-TIMI) 22 trial. *Circulation* 2010; *122*: 2142–2151.
101. Cooper-DeHoff RM, Gong Y, Handberg EM et al. Tight BP control and cardiovascular outcomes among hypertensive patients with diabetes and coronary artery disease. *JAMA* 2010; *304*: 61–68.
102. The ACCORD Study Group. Effects of intensive blood-pressure control in type 2 DM. *N Engl J Med* 2010; *362*: 1575–1585.

103. Margolis KL, O'Connor PJ, Morgan TM et al. Outcomes of combined cardiovascular risk factor management strategies in type 3 diabetes: The ACCORD randomized trial. *Diabetes Care* 2014; *37*: 1721–1728.
104. Soliman EZ, Byington RP, Bigger JT et al. Effect of intensive blood pressure lowering on left ventricular hypertrophy in patients with diabetes mellitus: Action to control cardiovascular risk in diabetes blood pressure trial. *Hypertension* 2015; *66*: 1123–1129.
105. Fleg JL, Evans GW, Margolis KL et al. Orthostatic hypotension in the ACCORD (Action to Control Cardiovascular Risk in Diabetes) blood pressure trial. Prevalence, incidence, and prognostic significance. *Hypertension* 2016; *68*: 888–895.
106. Aronow WS. Orthostatic hypotension in diabetics in the ACCORD (Action to Control Cardiovascular Risk in Diabetes) blood pressure trial. *Hypertension* 2016; *68*: 851–852.
107. Banach M, Bhatia V, Feller MA et al. Relation of baseline systolic BP and long-term outcomes in ambulatory patients with chronic mild to moderate heart failure. *Am J Cardiol* 2011; *107*: 1208–1214.
108. Mancia G, Schumacher H, Redon J et al. BP targets recommended by guidelines and incidence of cardiovascular and renal events in the Ongoing Telmisartan Alone and in Combination with Ramipril Global Endpoint Trial (ONTARGET). *Circulation* 2011; *124*: 1727–1736.
109. Redon J, Mancia G, Sleight P et al. Safety and efficacy of low BPs among patients with diabetes. Subgroup analyses from the ONTARGET (ONgoing Telmisartan and in Combination with Ramipril Endpoint Trial). *J Am Coll Cardiol* 2012; *59*: 74–83.
110. Guichard JL, Desai RV, Ahmed MI et al. Isolated diastolic hypotension and incident heart failure in older adults. *Hypertension* 2011; *58*: 895–901.
111. Upadhyay A, Earley A, Haynes SM et al. Systematic review: BP target in chronic kidney disease and proteinuria as an effect modifier. *Ann Intern Med* 2011; *154*: 541–548.
112. Ovbiagele B, Diener HC, Yusuf S et al. Level of systolic BP within the normal range and risk of recurrent stroke. *JAMA* 2011; *306*: 2137–2144.
113. Glicklich D, Frishman WH. Drug therapy of apparent treatment-resistant hypertension: Focus on mineralocorticoid antagonist. *Drugs* 2015; *75*: 473–485.
114. Ng MM, Sica DA, Frishman WH. Rheos: An implantable carotid sinus stimulation device for the nonpharmacologic treatment of resistant hypertension. *Cardiol in Rev* 2011; *19*: 52–57.
115. Sharma M, Frishman WH, Gandhi K. RESPeRATE: Nonpharmacological treatment of hypertension. *Cardiol in Rev* 2011; *19*: 47–51.
116. Burke GM, Sica DA, Frishman WH. Renal sympathetic denervation for the treatment of systemic hypertension. *Cardiol in Rev* 2012; *20*: 274–278.
117. Bhatt DL, Kandzari DE, O'Neill WW et al. A controlled trial of renal denervation for resistant hypertension. *N Engl J Med* 2014; *370*: 1393–1401.
118. Bakris GL, Townsend RR, Flack JM et al. 12-month blood pressure results of catheter-based renal artery denervation for resistant hypertension: The SYMPLICITY HTN-3 trial. *J Am Coll Cardiol* 2015; *65*: 1314–1321.
119. Lonn EM, Bosch J, Jaramillo PL et al. Blood pressure lowering in intermediate-risk persons without cardiovascular disease. *N Engl J Med* 2016; *374*: 2009–2020.
120. Whelton PK, Reboussin DM, Fine LJ. Comparing the SPRINT and the HOPE-3 blood pressure trial. *JAMA Cardiology* 2016; *1*: 855–856.
121. Ettehad D, Emdin CA, Kiran A et al. Blood pressure lowering for prevention of cardiovascular disease and death: A systematic review and meta-analysis. *Lancet* 2016; *387*: 957–967.
122. Banach M, Bromfield S, Howard G et al. Association of systolic blood pressure levels with cardiovascular events and all-cause mortality among older adults taking antihypertensive medication. *Int J Cardiol* 2014; *176*: 219–226.
123. SPS3 Study Group, Benavente OR, Coffey CS et al. Blood-pressure targets in patients with recent lacunar stroke: The SPS3 randomised trial. *Lancet* 2013; *382*: 507–515.
124. Oparil S. SPS3 evidence supports intensive blood pressure control. *Circulation* 2016; *133*: 552–554.
125. Bress AP, Tanner RM, Hess R et al. Generalizability of SPRINT results to the U.S. adult population. *J Am Coll Cardiol* 2016; *67*: 463–472.
126. Bress AP, Kramer H, Khatib R et al. Potential deaths averted and serious adverse events incurred from adoption of the SPRINT (Systolic Blood Pressure Intervention Trial) intensive blood pressure regimen in the United States. Projections from NHANES (National Health and Nutrition Examination Survey). *Circulation* 2017; *135*: 1617–1628.
127. Mancia G, Fagard R, Narkiewicz K et al. ESH/ESC guidelines for the management of arterial hypertension: The Task Force for the Management of Arterial Hypertension of the European Society of Hypertension (ESH) and of the European Society of Cardiology (ESC). *Eur Heart J* 2013; *34*: 2159–2219.
128. Hackam DG, Quinn RR, Ravani P et al. The 2013 Canadian Hypertension Education Program recommendations for blood pressure measurement, diagnosis, assessment of risk, prevention, and treatment of hypertension. *Can J Cardiol* 2013; *29*: 528–542.

129. Weber MA, Schiffrin EL, White WB et al. Clinical practice guidelines for the management of hypertension in the community. *A Statement by the American Society of Hypertension and the International Society of Hypertension* 2014; *16*: 14–26.
130. James PA, Oparil S, Carter BL et al. Evidence-based guideline for the management of high blood pressure in adults. Report from the Panel Members Appointed to the Eighth Joint National Committee (JNC 8). *JAMA* 2014; *311*: 507–520.
131. Wright JT Jr, Fine LJ, Lackland DT et al. Evidence supporting a systolic blood pressure goal of less than 150 mm Hg in patients aged 60 years or older: The minority view. *Ann Intern Med* 2014; *160*: 499–503.
132. Padwal R, Rabi DM, Schiffrin EL. Recommendations for intensive blood pressure lowering in high-risk patients, the Canadian viewpoint. *Hypertension* 2016; *68*: 3–5.
133. Gabb GM, Mangoni A, Anderson CS et al. Guidelines for the diagnosis and management of hypertension in adults-2016. *Med J Australia* 2016; *205*: 85–89.
134. Qaseem A, Wilt TJ, Rich R et al. Pharmacologic treatment of hypertension in adults aged 60 years or older to higher versus lower blood pressure targets: A Clinical Practice Guideline from the American College of Physicians and the American Academy of Family Physicians. *Ann Intern Med* 2017; *166*: 430–437.
135. Zhang W, Zhang S, Deng Y et al. Trial of intensive blood-pressure control in older patients with hypertension. *N Engl J Med* 2021; *385*: 1268–1279.
136. The Sprint Research Group. Final report of a trial of intensive versus standard blood-pressure control. *N Engl J Med* 2021; *384*: 1921–1930.
137. Wang Z, Du X, Hua C et al. The effect of frailty on the efficacy and safety of intensive blood pressure control: A post hoc analysis of the SPRINT trial. *Circulation* 2023; *148*: 566–574.
138. Bress AP, Greene T, Derington C et al. Patient selection for intensive blood pressure management based on benefit and adverse events. *J Am Coll Cardiol* 2021; *77*: 1977–1990.
139. Ascher SB, de Lemos JA, Lee M et al. Intensive blood pressure lowering in patients with malignant left ventricular hypertrophy. *J Am Coll Cardiol* 2022; *80*: 1516–1525.
140. Lee HH, Lee H, Cho J et al. On-treatment blood pressure and cardiovascular outcomes in adults with hypertension and left ventricular hypertrophy. *J Am Coll Cardiol* 2021; *78*: 1485–1495.
141. Haring B, Andrews CA, Hovey K et al. Systolic blood pressure and survival to very old age: Results from the Women's Health Initiative. *Circulation* 2024; *149*: 1568–1577.
142. Aronow WS. Approaches for the management of resistant hypertension in 2020. *Current Hypertension Reports* 2020; *22*: 3. doi:10.1007/s11906-019-1013-0.
143. Blumenthal JA, Hinderliter AL, Smith PJ et al. Effects of lifestyle modification on patients with resistant hypertension. Results of the TRIUMPH randomized clinical trial. *Circulation* 2021; *144*: 1212–1226.
144. Ahmed M, Nudy M, Bussa R et al. A subgroup meta-analysis comparing the renal denervation sham-controlled randomized trials among those with resistant and nonresistant hypertension. *Am J Cardiol* 2023; *191*: 119–124.
145. Cluett JL, Blazek O, Brown AL et al. Renal denervation for the treatment of hypertension: A scientific statement from the American Heart Association. Hypertension 2024 Aug 5 published online ahead of print PMID 39101202.
146. Aubert CE, Sussman JB, Hofer TP et al. Adding a new medication versus maximizing dose to intensify treatment in older adults. A retrospective observational study. *Ann Intern Med* 2021; *174*: 1666–1673.
147. Malik AH, Aronow WS. Efficacy of sacubitril/valsartan in hypertension. *Am J Therap* 2022; *29*: e322–e333.
148. Gupta R, Maitz T, Egeler et al. SGLT2 inhibitors in hypertension: Role beyond diabetes and heart failure. *Trends in Cardiovasc Med* 2023; *33*: 479–486.
149. Dey S, Frishman WH, Aronow WS. Baxdrostat: An aldosterone synthase inhibitor for the treatment of systemic hypertension. *Cardiol Rev Cardiol Rev* published online ahead of print PMID 37548462
150. Feldman JM, Frishman WH, Aronow WS. Emerging therapies for treatment-resistant hypertension: A review of lorundrostat and related selective aldosterone synthase inhibitors. Published online ahead of print PMID 38358268.

5

Disorders of lipid metabolism

KHALIFA BSHESH AND SETH S. MARTIN

Key points

- Dyslipidemia remains a significant contributor to cardiovascular risk in the elderly.
- Evidence strongly supports the use of statins in high-risk older adults, demonstrating reductions in atherogenic lipid levels and atherosclerotic cardiovascular disease events.
- Additionally, studies also support the use of nonstatin lipid-lowering therapies such as ezetimibe, bempedoic acid, and PCSK9 inhibitors when additional LDL cholesterol lowering and risk reduction are needed.
- It is essential to weigh the benefits and risks of lipid-lowering therapy but not shy away from providing preventive treatment to the elderly population, who are often undertreated.
- Several clinical trials are underway that specifically aim to further explore the benefits and risks of statins in elderly individuals without established cardiovascular disease.

INTRODUCTION

Elderly persons are a rapidly growing segment of the population, and most heart attacks and strokes occur among them [1]. The most likely reason for death in an elderly person is cardiovascular disease (CVD) [1]. In the pathophysiology of the atherosclerotic process underlying these clinical outcomes, disorders of lipid metabolism play a central role. Atherosclerosis is a systemic disease that accumulates over a lifetime, therefore, the older adult population has generally had significant cumulative exposure to atherogenic lipids, and addressing disorders of lipid metabolism in the elderly is an important endeavor. Prevention remains paramount, especially given that the elderly may be prone to suffering disability following a cardiovascular event. Lack of independence with activities following a stroke and heart failure following a myocardial infarction are particularly devastating outcomes in the elderly.

An increase in age strongly increases both the global risk of CVD and the absolute benefit from risk reduction therapies. Paradoxically, the elderly are less likely to receive aggressive primary and secondary prevention therapies [2–34]. Regardless of whether an elderly person has established CVD, many will be at high risk over the next decade, and many will likely benefit from statins and other cardiovascular risk reduction therapies. Nevertheless, the increased risks of side effects and competing risks from other comorbidities can decrease the net benefits of intervention. In this regard, treatment decision-making in the elderly is different from

DOI: 10.1201/9781003568933-5

Table 5.1 Risk factors for myopathy

Medication factors	Clinical factors
Lipophilic statin	Elderly
Fibrate	Small body frame, low body mass, frailty
Nicotinic acid (rarely)	Liver, renal, or multisystem disease
Cyclosporin	Hypothyroidism
Macrolides (erythromycin, clarithromycin)	Surgery or trauma
Antifungal azole	Rheumatologic disease
HIV antiviral (protease inhibitor)	Severe illness
Amiodarone	Excessive intake of alcohol or grapefruit juice
Verapamil and diltiazem	Heavy exercise
Proton pump inhibitors	Stress or sleep deprivation

decision-making in younger patients (Table 5.1). A balanced, personalized treatment approach for each elderly individual is indicated.

More informed treatment of dyslipidemia in the elderly could help promote more successful aging in this population. The purpose of this chapter is to discuss the topic of disorders of lipid metabolism in the elderly, with a look at risk attributable to dyslipidemia, an emphasis on the preventive treatments, and special considerations for dyslipidemia management in the elderly.

DYSLIPIDEMIA AND CARDIOVASCULAR RISK IN THE ELDERLY

There is no question that dyslipidemia confers higher risk for CVD over the lifetime of an individual. However, there is some degree of disagreement among various studies in the literature about whether lipid-related measures retain their expected epidemiologic associations with CVD risk in elderly individuals. In the general population, cholesterol levels are tightly linked to coronary heart disease (CHD). Cholesterol levels are also associated with stroke; however, the relationship is less robust than with CHD [5] as some strokes are embolic and, therefore, may not be primarily driven by atherosclerosis.

Multiple studies have demonstrated the expected graded, positive relationship of atherogenic cholesterol levels with CVD in the elderly. In the Kaiser Permanente Coronary Heart Disease in the Elderly Study, 2746 White men aged 60–79 years and free of CHD at enrollment were followed for an average of 10 years [6]. CHD risk was higher in those with higher cholesterol concentrations. Moreover, the excess mortality attributable to elevated total cholesterol levels increased with age, from 2.2 deaths per 1000 person-years in those 60–64 years of age to 11.3 deaths per 1000 person-years in men aged 75–79 years.

In an elderly sample of men and women with a mean age of 72 years from the Systolic Hypertension in the Elderly Program (SHEP), baseline total cholesterol, non-high-density lipoprotein cholesterol (HDL-C), and low-density lipoprotein cholesterol (LDL-C) levels and the ratios of total cholesterol, non-HDL-C, and LDL-C to HDL-C were significantly related to CHD incidence over approximately 4 years of follow-up [7]. Furthermore, a National Heart, Lung, and Blood Institute review found that total cholesterol and LDL-C levels were significantly correlated with fatal CHD in both men and women across a broad range of age groups, including patients older than 65 years [8], at least up to 75 years of age. Even into the ninth decade of life, a cohort of both men and women with a mean age of 82 years living in a long-term healthcare facility still demonstrated an association of total cholesterol levels (over 200 mg/dL in men and over 250 mg/dL in women) with an increase in coronary events [9].

Of course, in elderly patients, competing risks from other diseases, such as cancer, are more important and can confound the association of lipids with clinical outcomes in observational studies [10]. In this context, an analysis from the Established Populations for the Epidemiologic Studies of the Elderly failed to detect an association of total cholesterol, HDL-C, or the total to HDL cholesterol ratio with cardiovascular outcomes and mortality in the elderly in 997 patients [11]. Men aged 65–74 years in the Honolulu Heart Program also did not show a relationship between lipid levels and mortality [12]. In the Framingham Heart Study, age-specific analyses suggested that as age increased, the relative risk for CHD mortality associated with a high total cholesterol level decreased [13]. The relationship with CHD mortality was significantly positive at ages 40, 50, and 60 years but was attenuated with age until the relationship was positive but not significant at age 70 years, and negative but not significant at age 80 years. Other studies have shown a differential effect in men versus women. For example, in the Bronx Aging Study, lower HDL-C levels were linked to CHD in elderly men, whereas higher LDL-C levels were linked to myocardial infarction in elderly women [14].

Perhaps differences in the populations studied, lipid-related measures examined, length of follow-up, or clinical endpoints explain part of the disagreement in the observational studies. Nevertheless, it is a key point that although the relative risk associated with dyslipidemia may decrease with age, there is an increase in absolute risk, and therefore the risk of cardiovascular events attributable to elevated cholesterol is higher. In this sense, dyslipidemia is more, not less, important to CVD risk in the elderly. Moreover, beyond epidemiologic associations, the more directly relevant clinical question is whether dyslipidemia interventions are efficacious in reducing CVD risk in the elderly, which is the topic of the next section of this chapter.

EFFICACY OF DYSLIPIDEMIA INTERVENTIONS IN THE ELDERLY

Lifestyle interventions

As in the young, a heart-healthy diet is a central component of a comprehensive approach to dyslipidemia and risk-reduction therapy. An evidence-based diet is the Dietary Approaches to Stop Hypertension (DASH) diet, which is a Mediterranean-style diet that is low in salt (<2 grams of salt/day), low in saturated and trans fats, high in fiber, and high in fruits and vegetables. When alcohol is part of one's diet, the amount of consumption should be moderate (≤2 servings a day for men, ≤1 serving a day for women; 1 serving = 12 oz of beer, 5 oz of wine, 1.5 oz liquor).

There is no strong evidence base to support any recommendations for dietary supplements, such as omega-3 fatty acid supplements, antioxidants, folic acid, flaxseed, garlic, magnesium, saw palmetto, zinc, coenzyme Q10, ginkgo biloba, or vitamins A, B, C, E [15]. When discussing dietary approaches with an elderly person, recommendations will certainly need to be individualized to the patient. Some elderly patients will be prone to malnutrition, and in this setting, a more liberalized diet is warranted.

Regular exercise is also important for the maintenance of cardiovascular health in the elderly. Moderate-intensity exercise is recommended for a minimum of 30 minutes five times per week or more. Muscle-strengthening exercises are recommended 2 days a week or more. Elderly patients may find it beneficial to wear a pedometer to monitor their walking. The Cardiovascular Health Study [16] found that greater physical activity, including walking, was inversely associated with coronary heart disease, stroke, and total CVD, even in those aged 75 years and older. Exercise interventions improve functional capacity, raise HDL-C, and lower triglyceride levels, thereby favorably altering the cardiovascular risk profile. Moreover, cardiac rehabilitation reduces the risk of recurrent CVD events, including death, following acute myocardial infarction or coronary bypass surgery, and should be recommended to such patients, as well as those with heart failure.

Overall, making changes toward a heart-healthy lifestyle is the first line of treatment for dyslipidemia and CVD risk in any patient, including the elderly. Nevertheless, in many patients, an improvement in lifestyle alone will not be an adequate intervention.

Statins

Statins (3-hydroxy-3-methylglutaryl coenzyme A reductase inhibitors) are the most robustly studied class of medications for the reduction of atherogenic lipoprotein cholesterol and CVD prevention. Guidelines from the American Heart Association/American College of Cardiology and other societies recommend statins as first-line therapy for the management of dyslipidemia in elderly patients meeting the risk threshold for therapy. The data in support of these recommendations include multiple prospective observational studies, and most importantly, randomized clinical trials, which have collected data on large numbers of older persons at high risk for CVD events, including coronary, cerebrovascular, and peripheral vascular events. Nevertheless, evidence at the extreme of old age is limited by relatively lower numbers of patients studied.

PROSPECTIVE STUDIES OF STATIN THERAPY

In a prospective study of 1410 long-term healthcare facility residents aged 60–100 years (mean age 81 years) with LDL-C ≥125 mg/dL and a history of a myocardial infarction, statin therapy was associated with a 36% reduction in the incidence of new coronary events, with consistent benefits observed across all age ranges [17]. Another prospective observational study of statin therapy in the elderly, the Cardiovascular Health Study, recorded relative risk reductions for all-cause mortality on the order of 40%–50% in patients aged 65 years and older without any history of CVD [18]. Results were consistent in participants who were 74 years of age or older at baseline.

In a secondary prevention setting, a similar relationship between statin therapy and mortality was observed in the Intermountain Heart Collaborative Study [19]. In this study, mortality was lower among statin recipients in all age groups, including those 80 years or older, in which the mortality rate was 29.5% among patients not taking a statin versus 8.5% of those taking a statin (adjusted hazard ratio [HR] 0.50, p = 0.04). Registries of patients hospitalized for myocardial infarction have shown a similar association with mortality. In an analysis of more than 40,000 Medicare beneficiaries [20] and a registry of 14,907 patients in Sweden [21], statins were associated with a mortality benefit and the benefits of statin therapy appeared to outweigh potential toxicities.

CLINICAL TRIALS OF STATIN THERAPY

Statin therapy provided a benefit to the elderly subgroup in multiple primary prevention trials. The Anglo-Scandinavian Cardiac Outcomes Trial Lipid Lowering Arm (ASCOT-LLA) of 10,305 patients aged 40–79 years with non-fasting total cholesterol concentrations of 6.5 mmol/L or less, hypertension, and other cardiovascular risk factors, randomly assigned patients to atorvastatin 10 mg or placebo. Atorvastatin reduced the risk of nonfatal myocardial infarction or fatal CHD by 36%, and the benefit was similar in patients older than 60 years (HR estimate 0.64; p = 0.003) and those 60 years and younger (0.66; p = 0.09) [22].

The Justification for the Use of statins in Prevention: An Intervention Trial Evaluating Rosuvastatin (JUPITER) was an even larger primary prevention trial that randomly assigned 17,802 apparently healthy men and women with

LDL-C levels <130 mg/dL and high-sensitivity C-reactive protein levels of ≥2.0 mg/L to rosuvastatin 20 mg daily or placebo [23]. After a median follow-up of 1.9 years (maximum 5.0), the rates of the primary composite point (myocardial infarction, stroke, arterial revascularization, hospitalization for unstable angina, or death from cardiovascular causes) were 0.77 and 1.36 per 100 person-years of follow-up in the rosuvastatin and placebo groups, respectively (HR for rosuvastatin, 0.56; 95% confidence interval [CI], 0.46–0.69; $p < 0.00001$).

There was a significant reduction in all components of the primary composite endpoint. There was also a reduction in death from any cause (HR, 0.80; 95% CI, 0.67–0.97; $p = 0.02$). Among JUPITER participants, 5695 were 70 years or older at enrollment. This group accrued 49% of confirmed primary endpoint events in the trial, and rates of the primary endpoint in this age group were 1.22 and 1.99 per 100 person-years of follow-up in the rosuvastatin and placebo groups, respectively (HR, 0.61 [95% CI, 0.46–0.82]; $p < 0.001$) [24].

Multiple clinical trials have demonstrated improved outcomes of lipid-lowering therapy in elderly patients with established CHD. The Scandinavian Simvastatin Survival Study (4S) enrolled 4444 men and women who had CHD and an age up to 70 years. In 4S, simvastatin decreased total mortality by 35% and coronary mortality by 42% in participants aged ≥60 years over 5 years [25]. Additionally, coronary procedures and cerebrovascular events were reduced in patients receiving simvastatin. Similar proportional reductions in these cardiovascular endpoints were seen in the elderly 4S participants and younger participants [26]. The absolute risk reduction for all-cause mortality and CHD mortality for statin-allocated patients was about twice as great in the elderly versus younger patients due to higher overall mortality rates in the elderly group.

Similarly, a consistent effect across age strata was shown in the Cholesterol and Recurrent Events (CARE) study [27]. CARE enrolled 4129 patients up to the age of 75 years with average cholesterol levels and a history of a prior myocardial infarction. CARE found that elderly patients benefited from a 32% reduction in major coronary events, 45% reduction in coronary death, and 40% reduction in stroke with pravastatin. Elderly patients with established CVD are at particularly high risk for future events, and therefore even the short-term number needed to treat to prevent an event can be quite low. In CARE, the number needed to treat for 5 years to prevent a major coronary event was 11. Large randomized trials of more intensive statin therapy with atorvastatin 80 mg per day, namely, Pravastatin or Atorvastatin Evaluation and Infection Therapy–Thrombolysis in Myocardial Infarction 22 (PROVE-IT) [28] and Treating to New Targets (TNT) [29], showed a benefit of the more aggressive lipid-lowering irrespective of age.

In addition to subgroup analyses from broader clinical trial populations, randomized clinical trials have specifically investigated the benefits of statin treatment in the elderly. The Prospective Study of Pravastatin in the Elderly at Risk (PROSPER) enrolled 5804 patients aged 70–82 years with established CVD or high risk for CVD [30]. After 3.2 years of follow-up, pravastatin 40 mg per day reduced LDL-C levels by 34% and triglycerides by 13%. Pravastatin treatment reduced the incidence of the composite primary endpoint of coronary death, nonfatal myocardial infarction, and fatal or nonfatal stroke by 15% and reduced CHD mortality by 24% (Figure 5.1). While an increased incidence of cancer was noted in PROSPER, this has not been confirmed in numerous other trials, and when the PROSPER investigators pooled their data with

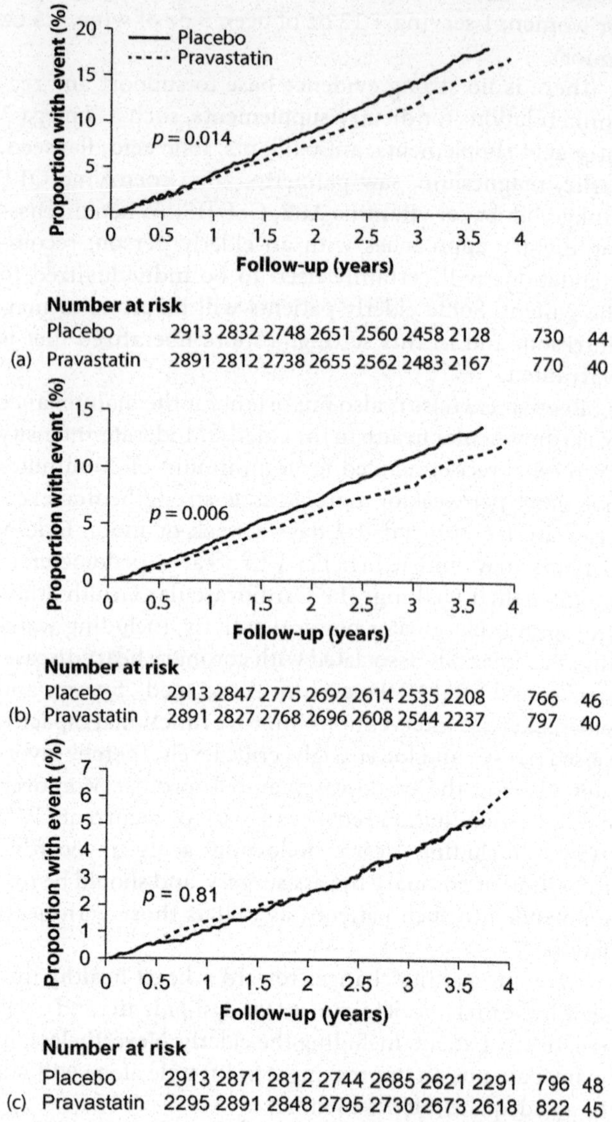

Figure 5.1 Kaplan–Meier analysis of time to primary and secondary endpoints in the PROSPER randomized clinical trial of statin therapy in the elderly: (a) coronary heart disease death, nonfatal myocardial infarction, or fatal or nonfatal stroke; (b) coronary heart disease death or nonfatal myocardial infarction; (c) fatal or nonfatal stroke. (From J. Shepherd et al., *Lancet*, 360, 1623–1630, 2002.)

Pravastatin studies	Statin	Placebo
WOSCOPS[2]	116/3302	106/3293
CARE[3]	172/2081	161/2078
LIPID[5]	379/4512	399/4502
PROSPER	245/2891	199/2913
Total	912/12786	865/12786
Other statin studies		
SSSS[1]	90/2221	96/2223
AFCAPS/TexCAPS[4]	252/3304	259/3301
HPS[6]	814/10269	803/10267
LIPS[18]	14/844	18/833
Total	1170/16638	1176/16624
All statin studies	**2082/29424**	**2041/29410**

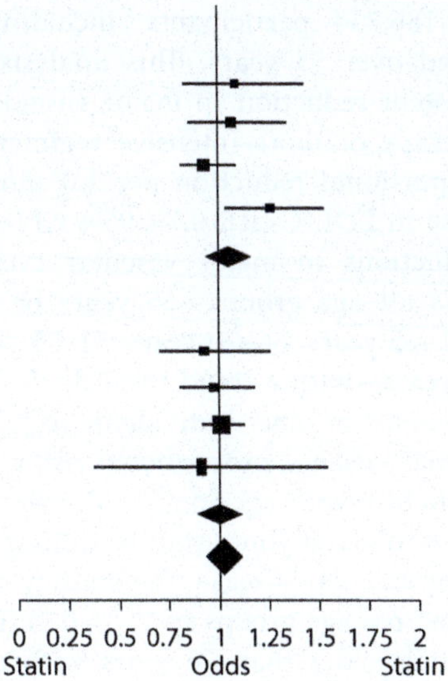

Figure 5.2 Meta-analysis of cancer incidence in major statin trials. Data are the number of individuals with cancer/number of individuals in the treatment group for each treatment group with odds ratio (95% CI) for risk of cancer in the statin-treated group relative to placebo. (From J. Shepherd et al., *Lancet*, 360, 1623–1630, 2002.)

other trials in a meta-analysis, there was no risk of cancer (Figure 5.2).

The question of whether more intensive statin therapy is beneficial in the elderly was addressed in the Study Assessing Goals in the Elderly (SAGE) [31]. In SAGE, 893 patients aged 65–85 years (mean 73 years) with CHD were randomized to atorvastatin 80 mg or pravastatin 40 mg per day and followed for 12 months. More intensive therapy with atorvastatin produced a 67% reduction in all-cause mortality ($p = 0.01$) and a nonsignificant trend (29% reduction) toward fewer major cardiovascular events ($p = 0.11$).

The totality of evidence from randomized clinical statin trials of primary and secondary prevention was summarized in a landmark Cholesterol Treatment Trialists' prospective meta-analysis of data from 170,000 participants treated over an average of 5 years in 26 randomized clinical trials [32]. In this analysis, the proportional benefit of therapy, or relative risk reduction, was relatively constant across a wide array of patient subgroups, including the elderly (Figure 5.3). Of 24,323 cardiovascular events in this meta-analysis, 8940 of them occurred in individuals aged 65–75 years, while 1872 of them occurred in those over the age of 75 years. Overall, lipid lowering with statin therapy produced proportional reductions in risk per each 1.0 mmol/L (39 mg/dL) of 22% in major cardiovascular events (RR 0.78, 95% CI 0.76–0.80; $p < 0.0001$) and 10% in all-cause mortality reduction, largely reflecting reduced coronary heart disease deaths (RR 0.80, 99% CI 0.74–0.87; $p < 0.0001$).

More recently, the Cholesterol Treatment Trialists' Collaboration provided a comprehensive assessment of the efficacy and safety of statin therapy at different ages [33]. They conducted a meta-analysis of 28 trials,

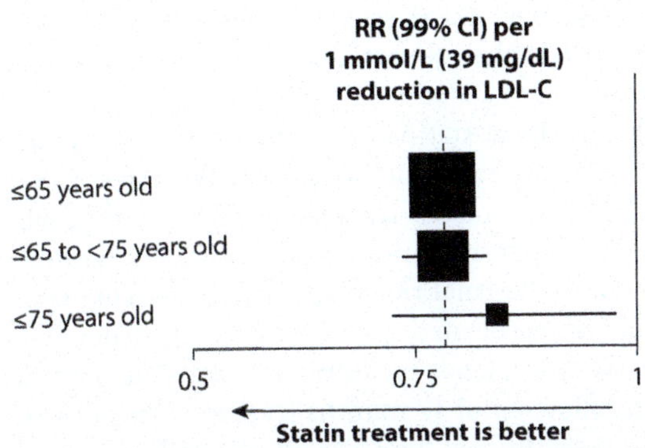

Events (% annually) Statin/more LDL-C lowering	Control/less LDL-C lowering	RR (99% CI) per 1 mmol/L (39 mg/dL) reduction in LDL-C	Heterogeneity trend test
6056 (2.9%)	7455 (3.6%)	0.78 (0.75–0.82)	
4032 (3.7%)	4908 (4.6%)	0.78 (0.74–0.83)	$\chi^2_2 = 0.70$ ($p = 0.4$)
885 (4.8%)	987 (5.4%)	0.84 (0.73–0.97)	

Figure 5.3 CTT meta-analysis showing similar relative risk reduction for major vascular events with statin therapy in the elderly compared with younger patients. Rate ratios (RRs) are plotted for each comparison of first event rates between treatment groups and are weighted per 1.0 mmol/L (39 mg/dL) LDL cholesterol (LDL-C) difference at 1 year. Missing data are not plotted. RRs are shown with horizontal lines denoting 99% CIs or with open diamonds showing 95% CIs. (Adapted from C. Baigent et al., *Lancet*, 376, 1670–1681, 2010.)

encompassing 186,854 participants, including 14,483 individuals aged over 75 years. This analysis demonstrated a consistent reduction in major vascular events with statin therapy or more intensive regimens, yielding a 21% proportional reduction per 1.0 mmol/L (39 mg/dL) decrease in LDL-C (RR 0.79, 95% CI 0.77–0.81). Significant reductions in major vascular events were observed across all age groups—55 years or younger, 56–60 years, 61–65 years, 66–70 years, 71–75 years, and older than 75 years—with a trend towards diminishing proportional benefits in older individuals (p_{trend} = 0.06). For major coronary events, proportional risk reductions also declined slightly with age (p_{trend} = 0.009), but benefits remained significant. Importantly, among patients with preexisting vascular disease, the efficacy of statins was consistent across age groups (p_{trend} = 0.2). However, among individuals older than 75 years without established vascular disease, the proportional benefits were attenuated (p_{trend} = 0.05). These findings align with prior studies demonstrating robust benefits of statin therapy in elderly patients, particularly those at high cardiovascular risk. While the analysis highlights the universal benefit of statins in reducing major vascular events, it underscores the need for further trials focusing on individuals over 75 years without preexisting vascular disease to refine treatment strategies in this subgroup.

The Statins in Reducing Events in the Elderly (STAREE) trial plans to address this critical gap in understanding the role of statins in primary prevention among individuals aged 70 years and older [34]. Unlike prior trials that primarily focused on patients with preexisting cardiovascular disease, STAREE is the first randomized, double-blind, placebo-controlled trial to investigate the effects of statin therapy in a cohort of healthy older adults. Its primary aim is to evaluate whether atorvastatin 40 mg daily can improve disability-free survival and reduce major adverse cardiovascular events, including cardiovascular death, nonfatal myocardial infarction, and stroke. Beyond cardiovascular outcomes, the trial seeks to determine the potential benefits of statins in preventing dementia, improving life expectancy, and preserving physical function, while also assessing adverse reactions and cost-effectiveness in this demographic. STAREE enrolled 9971 participants (mean age 74.7 ± 4.5 years, with 40% aged ≥75 years and 52% women) from 1583 general practices across Australia between July 2015 and March 2023. All participants were community-dwelling individuals without a history of clinical cardiovascular disease, diabetes, or dementia. At baseline, the mean LDL-C was 3.27 mmol/L (126 mg/dL), 43% of participants reported hypertension, and the mean blood pressure was 136/80 mm Hg. Cognitive and psychological measures were assessed using the Modified Mini-Mental State Examination and the Center for Epidemiologic Studies Short Depression Scale, respectively. By addressing the outcomes of disability-free survival, major cardiovascular events, and cognition, STAREE aims to provide crucial evidence for guiding statin therapy in healthy older adults, particularly as the aging population continues to grow.

Similarly, the pragmatic evaluation of events and benefits of lipid-lowering in older adults (PREVENTABLE) trial aims to assess the benefits of initiating statins for primary prevention in the elderly population [35]. The trial aims to recruit 20,000 adults >75 years living in the community who are without established dementia, CVD, or significant disability. Participants are being randomized to receive either atorvastatin 40 mg daily or a placebo. Individuals who have received statins in the past year or for greater than 5 years total and statin-intolerant individuals are excluded. The study's primary outcome is survival free of new dementia or persisting disability. Secondary outcomes include a composite of cardiovascular death and hospitalization from cardiovascular causes as well as a composite of dementia or mild cognitive impairment. As part of the trial, participants undergo baseline cognitive testing, disability screening, and a blinded lipid panel if feasible, with annual testing afterward. Overall, PREVENTABLE seeks to generate critical evidence on the role of statins in preserving cognitive and physical function in aging populations.

All-cause mortality was reduced by 10% per 1.0 mmol/L LDL-C reduction (relative risk [RR] 0.90, 95% CI 0.87–0.93; $p < 0.0001$) primarily due to protection from cardiovascular death (RR 0.80, 99% CI 0.74–0.87; $p < 0.0001$).

Another meta-analysis specifically focused on secondary prevention in the elderly [36]. The investigators included nine trials ≥6 months of follow-up with 19,569 patients ranging in age from 65 to 82 years. All-cause mortality occurred in 15.6% of elderly patients treated with statins and 18.7% given a placebo. There was a 22% relative risk reduction in all-cause mortality over 5 years (RR 0.78; 95% CI 0.65–0.89) (Figure 5.4). Statins also reduced CHD mortality by 30% (RR 0.70; 95% CI 0.53–0.83), nonfatal myocardial infarction by 26% (RR 0.74; 95% CI 0.60–0.89), need for revascularization by 30% (RR 0.70; 95% CI 0.53–0.83), and stroke by 25% (RR 0.75; 95% CI 0.56–0.94). The estimated number needed to treat to save one life was 28 (95% CI 15–56).

Like any drug, statins have side effects. Nevertheless, statins have an excellent overall safety profile and side effects that are rarely irreversible. Very low levels of LDL-C by modern standards are generally within the evolutionarily normal range and safe. A systematic overview of risks associated with statin therapy from 35 randomized clinical trials including 74,102 participants with a mean follow-up of 17 months (range 1.5–64.8 months) found no significant increase in the risk of myalgias, creatine kinase elevations, rhabdomyolysis, or discontinuation of statin therapy due to any adverse event [37]. In JUPITER, those participants attaining LDL-C levels <50 mg/dL experienced a reduction in CVD events

Study	No. Events/ Total No. of Patients: Statin	Placebo	Posterior Median Relative Risk (95% Credible Interval)
4S	67/518	96/503	0.75 (0.59, 0.89)
CARE	771640	108/643	0.76 (0.61, 0.90)
FLARE	2/179	6/187	0.74 (0.47, 0.97)
HPS	963/5366	1089/5331	0.87 (0.80, 0.93)
LIPID	287/1741	365/1773	0.80 (0.71, 0.90)
LIPS	23/324	32/299	0.75 (0.55, 0.94)
PLAC I	1 /42	2/52	0.76 (0.51, 1.00)
PROSPER	110/934	128/899	0.82 (0.69, 0.98)
REGRESS	1 /75	1/63	0.75 (0.49, 0.99)
Pooled (5 year)	**1531/9819**	**1827/9750**	**0.78 (0.65, 0.89)**

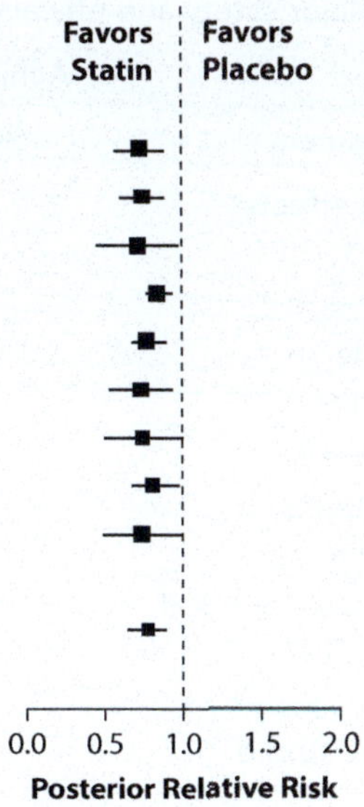

Figure 5.4 Bayesian forest plot for all-cause mortality with statin treatment in the elderly. Statin therapy reduced the incidence of all-cause mortality by 22% over 5 years as compared to placebo. The posterior median estimate of the number needed to treat was 28. (Adapted from J. Afilalo et al., *J Am Coll Cardiol*, 51, 37–45, 2008.)

and all-cause mortality without a systematic increase in reported adverse events [38].

While randomized controlled trials utilize run-in phases to select out patients who are prone to early adverse effects from statin therapy, a relatively small proportion of patients were generally excluded for side effects, and the aforementioned data indicate that statin therapy is extremely safe in those who initially tolerate therapy. What follows here is an extended general discussion of statin safety, however, the chance of side effects may increase in certain elderly patients with comorbidities (see section "Special Considerations for Dyslipidemia Management in the Elderly").

Myopathy is the most common concern with statins. In daily clinical practice, 8%–9% of statin-treated patients versus 4%–6% of untreated patients develop myopathy, of which 95% are myalgias or mild myositis [39]. Rhabdomyolysis is a rare, severe form of myopathy, with systemic myoglobin release and risk of renal failure, occurring in fewer than 1 in 10,000 patients on statin therapy [40]. Risk factors for myopathy and rhabdomyolysis on statin therapy include being elderly, as well as interacting medications and other clinical factors (Table 5.2; also see section "Special Considerations for Dyslipidemia Management in the Elderly"). Statin risk may be increased with concomitant use of P450 inhibitors, including macrolides (erythromycin, clarithromycin), antiviral drugs (protease inhibitors), systemic antifungals (itraconazole and ketoconazole), verapamil (for simvastatin), diltiazem (for lovastatin, atorvastatin), amiodarone (for simvastatin), and grapefruit juice consumption exceeding 1 quart per day can also significantly inhibit P450. The risk of myopathy may also be increased for statin use in the setting of chronic immunosuppressive therapy (cyclosporine), fibrates (gemfibrozil), niacin, or alcohol intake exceeding two drinks per day. Adverse reactions to statin treatment, including muscle toxicity, are not significantly associated with on-treatment LDL-C (Table 5.3) [41]. Reassuringly, if myopathy occurs, statin discontinuation generally leads to full recovery.

Asymptomatic transaminitis occurs with statins, but statins are not strongly tied to an increased risk of liver disease [40]. Alanine transaminase elevations exceeding three times the upper limit of normal have occurred in 0.11%–3.3% of patients on statin therapy [40]. Other systematic reviews have not found an increased risk of transaminase elevations with statin therapy [37]. In patients with mild-to-moderately elevated baseline liver tests, statins are safe and can actually lead to improvement in liver tests of many patients, perhaps explained by nonalcoholic fatty liver disease [42].

Statins are associated with a modest increase in the incidence of diabetes mellitus. There was a 9% increase (odds ratio [OD] 1.09; 95% CI 1.02–1.17) in the incidence of diabetes in a meta-analysis of 13 trials including 91,140 participants [43]. Approximately one new case of diabetes occurred per 1000 person-years of treatment; thus, the risk of diabetes mellitus is low in absolute terms and relative to the reduction in CVD events. Moreover, it is not known to what degree statin-related hyperglycemia actually confers risk in the future. Indeed, in the trials in which diabetes occurred, there was a net cardiovascular benefit with statin therapy.

An additional concern that has garnered attention is the potential for mild cognitive dysfunction with statin use. This was addressed in the 2014 NLA Task Force on Statin Safety [44]. While concerns about memory loss or confusion have been raised, most systematic reviews and

Table 5.2 Major safety and efficacy outcomes across strata of achieved LDL cholesterol (percent of subjects)

	Achieved LDL cholesterol (mg/dL)				
Safety measure	**>80–100 *n* = 256**	**>60–80 *n* = 576**	**>40–60 *n* = 631**	**<40 *n* = 193**	***p* Trend**
Muscle side effects[a]					
Myalgia	6.4	4.3	6.2	5.7	0.75
Myositis	0.4	0.6	0.6	0	0.64
CK >3 × ULN	2.3	0.7	1.9	1.0	0.18
CK >10 × ULN	0	0	0.3	0	0.45
Rhabdomyolysis	0	0	0	0	1.0
Liver side effects					
ALT >3 × ULN	3.2	3.0	3.2	2.6	0.98
Study drug discontinued because of LIT	2.0	2.6	2.4	1.6	0.83
Other					
Hemorrhagic stroke	0.4	0.2	0	0	0.12
Retinal AE	0.4	0.9	1.0	0	0.48
Suicide/trauma death	0	0	0	0	1.0
Study drug discontinued because of any AE	10.2	9.4	9.7	9.8	0.99
Major efficacy measures					
Death	1.1	1.4	1.3	0.5	0.59
CHD death	0.5	0.5	0.6	0.0	0.06
Myocardial infarction	1.0	0.7	0.5	9.6	0.009
Any stroke	0.8	0.9	0.6	1.6	0.32
Primary composite[a]	26.1	22.2	20.4	20.4	0.10

Abbreviations: AE, adverse event; ALT, alanine aminotransferase; CHD, coronary heart disease; CK, creatine kinase; LFT, liver function test; LDL, low-density lipoprotein; ULN, upper limit of normal.

Source: S.D. Wiviott et al., *J Am Coll Cardiol*, 46, 1414, 2005.

[a] Primary composite = percent of subjects with any of the following: death, myocardial infarction, stroke, unstable angina requiring rehospitalization, and revascularization. Myalgia = muscle symptoms without CK elevation; myositis = muscle symptoms with CK elevation; rhabdomyolysis = muscle symptoms with CK >10 × ULN and evidence of renal dysfunction.

Table 5.3 Statin therapy in the elderly versus younger patients

Relative risk reduction	**Similar**
Absolute risk reduction	Higher
Number needed to treat	Lower
Competing risks	Higher
Chance of adverse effects	Higher

meta-analyses indicate no conclusive evidence of a causal relationship between statin therapy and cognitive impairment. Among 14 randomized controlled trials assessed by the task force, only 2 trials reported potential adverse effects of statins on cognition consisting of a potential mild impairment in learning. Additionally, several case reports and post-marketing surveillance data continue to highlight that a subset of patients may experience reversible memory issues, which typically resolve upon discontinuation of therapy. It is hypothesized that these effects, when they occur, may be linked to individual variations in blood–brain barrier permeability, statin lipophilicity, or underlying susceptibility due to comorbid conditions. Given the overwhelming cardiovascular benefits of statins, any potential cognitive side effects should be weighed against the substantial risk reduction in cardiovascular events, and clinicians are encouraged to monitor patients closely and address concerns on a case-by-case basis.

Interestingly, a recent study in the UK investigating the symptom intensity associated with statin use found that the majority of symptoms experienced by participants were attributable to the nocebo effect [45]. In this randomized trial, 60 participants were recruited who had previously abandoned statin therapy due to side effects. They were given atorvastatin, placebo, or no treatment for a 12-month regimen. The results revealed that the symptom scores were significantly higher during statin and placebo months compared to no treatment, with no difference in symptom intensity between the statin and placebo groups. The nocebo ratio was found to be 0.90, indicating that a substantial proportion of symptoms during statin use were due to expectations or beliefs about the drug, rather than its pharmacological effects.

Overall, the potential harms of treating with statins are usually outweighed by their benefits in the majority of statin-treated patients (for circumstances where this may not be the case, see section "Special Considerations for Dyslipidemia Management in the Elderly"). Framing the well-established benefits of LDL-C lowering with statin therapy against their risks, the National Lipid Association Statin Safety Task Force stated, "For every 1 million high-risk persons treated with a statin over 100,000 heart attacks, strokes, or other major adverse cardiac event will be prevented for every 1 serious side effect. Therefore, the person should fear the heart attack not the statin" [46].

Nonstatin drugs

In combination with statin therapy, or as monotherapy in patients who are not candidates for statins, additional lipid-lowering agents are available, including bile acid sequestrants, fibrates, niacin, ezetimibe, bempedoic acid, and proprotein convertase subtilisin kexin 9 (PCSK9) inhibitors. The first three are older agents that are less used in the modern treatment era, whereas the latter three have become preferred second-line agents in the statin era as a result of favorable safety and efficacy data as add-on therapy to statins in large randomized clinical outcomes trials.

Bile acid sequestrants favorably redirect enterohepatic exchange of bile acids, increasing hepatic LDL-C receptor expression and clearance of circulating LDL-C, leading to a 5%–30% dose-dependent reduction in LDL-C levels. The Lipid Research Clinics Coronary Primary Prevention Trial (LRC-CPPT) showed significant reductions in myocardial infarction and cardiovascular death with bile acid sequestrant monotherapy [47,48]. Bile acid sequestrants remain in the gut without systemic absorption and therefore side effects are limited to gastrointestinal disturbances or impaired absorption of other drugs and can be mitigated by a once daily colesevelam suspension, which may promote the ease of patient adherence to therapy.

Fibric acid derivatives (fibrates) activate lipoprotein lipase, promote hepatic bile secretion, and reduce hepatic triglyceride production. The Helsinki Heart Study investigated gemfibrozil dosed at 600 mg twice daily in the primary prevention of heart disease in men [49]. In those with the best adherence to treatment, gemfibrozil reduced, on average, triglycerides by 45%, total cholesterol by 14%, and LDL-C by 15%, while raising HDL-C by 14%. The lipid changes seen in the gemfibrozil group were associated with a significantly lower risk of coronary events.

In the secondary prevention arena, gemfibrozil was studied in men with low levels of HDL-C in the Veterans Affairs High-Density Lipoprotein Cholesterol Intervention Trial [50]. The study included 2531 male participants who were randomized to gemfibrozil 1200 mg per day versus placebo and followed for a median of 5.1 years. Gemfibrozil therapy significantly reduced the risk of major cardiovascular events. A clinical benefit of fibrates was also seen in the Bezafibrate Infarction Prevention trial in patients with CHD [51].

Recent investigations into fibrates have continued to explore their role in cardiovascular risk reduction in patients with hypertriglyceridemia. The PROMINENT trial studied pemafibrate in patients with type 2 diabetes and mild-to-moderate hypertriglyceridemia versus placebo [52]. Among 10,497 participants, pemafibrate significantly reduced triglycerides (–26.2%), very-low-density lipoprotein cholesterol (–25.8%), and remnant cholesterol (–25.6%). However, despite these lipid changes, pemafibrate did not reduce the incidence of major cardiovascular events compared to placebo (HR 1.03; 95% CI 0.91–1.15). Additionally, pemafibrate was associated with a higher incidence of adverse renal events and venous thromboembolism, though it lowered the risk of nonalcoholic fatty liver disease. These findings highlight that while fibrates effectively modify lipid parameters, their impact on cardiovascular outcomes remains uncertain, particularly in the setting of the modern lipid-lowering treatment paradigm.

Fibrates are generally well tolerated. However, they have important interactions with other drugs that are of particular relevance in the elderly. Due to increased risk of myopathy in combination with statins, fibrates should be used in this setting with only the utmost caution and probably avoided in those with risk factors for myopathy. An interaction of warfarin with fibrates leads to an increase in warfarin levels and the international normalized ratio. Thus, warfarin is typically dosed at one third its standard dose when administered with fenofibrate and careful follow-up of the international normalized ratio is needed. Given fibric acid derivatives are excreted primarily through the kidney, if they are used in the setting of chronic kidney disease, then dose adjustment is necessary. Gastrointestinal side effects are common in patients taking fibrate therapy, including mild nausea during the first week of therapy. To reduce this potential side effect, it can be useful to start treatment with one half the normal dose for several days before increasing to a full dose.

Nicotinic acid (niacin) is a B vitamin that inhibits adenylate cyclase [53], and in daily doses of 1500–3000 mg, increases HDL-C levels by 15%–30%, reduces total cholesterol and LDL-C levels by about 10%–25%, and reduces triglyceride levels by up to 50%. In the Coronary Drug Project, niacin monotherapy provided protection from myocardial infarction and reduced long-term mortality by 11% at 15 years [54]. A series of Arterial Biology for the Investigation of the Treatment Effects of Reducing Cholesterol (ARBITER) studies have examined the effects of adding niacin on top of background statin therapy [55]. In these studies, niacin has led to slowing and even regression of atherosclerosis, as measured by carotid intima-media thickness [55,56]. Nevertheless, the absolute impact on carotid intima–media thickness was modest on average, and the clinical significance of these changes is uncertain.

From a clinical outcomes standpoint, the results for niacin as an add-on therapy to statins were disappointing from the Atherothrombosis Intervention in Metabolic Syndrome with Low HDL/High Triglycerides: Impact on Global Health Outcomes (AIM-HIGH) trial. In a secondary prevention setting, with statin and ezetimibe titrated to LDL-C levels of less than 70 mg/dL, there was no incremental clinical benefit from the addition of niacin during a 36-month follow-up period in AIM-HIGH [57]. While the study did not meet its primary endpoint for efficacy, the trial was stopped early, and there were a number of issues with the trial (e.g., change in end point during trial; low-dose niacin use in control group). In the larger Heart Protection Study 2-Treatment of HDL to Reduce the Incidence of Vascular Events (HPS2-THRIVE), in 25,673 patients with well-controlled LDL-C levels, the combination of niacin and laropiprant did not reduce a composite CVD endpoint. HPS2-THRIVE recorded a significantly increased risk of adverse events with niacin/laropiprant, with approximately 30 adverse events per 1000 treated.

Laropiprant was used in HPS2-THRIVE to inhibit the most common side effect of niacin: prostaglandin-mediated flushing. The extent of off-target effects of laropiprant is uncertain. Flushing may also be prevented or minimized by aspirin and avoidance of alcohol, monosodium glutamate, hot beverages, and spicy foods. Other side effects from high-dose niacin include a small increase in the serum glucose, a moderate increase in the serum uric acid level, and a small reduction in the serum phosphorus level.

Ezetimibe reduces LDL-C 15%–20% primarily by selectively inhibiting cholesterol absorption at the intestinal brush border. This is mechanistically attractive in combination with a statin, and safe and efficacious in the reduction of atherogenic cholesterol levels [58,59]. However, limited data are available on the use of ezetimibe in the elderly, either as a single agent or in combination with a statin. Surrogate endpoint trials, limited by the lack of a reliable correlation with clinical outcomes, have introduced doubt surrounding ezetimibe's clinical efficacy.

In the Ezetimibe and Simvastatin in Hypercholesterolemia Enhances Atherosclerosis Regression (ENHANCE) trial, involving 720 patients with heterozygous familial hypercholesterolemia, adding ezetimibe to maximal simvastatin therapy yielded greater LDL-C reduction (56% vs. 39%), but there was no difference in carotid intima–media thickness at 2 years [60]. Surprisingly, the Arterial Biology for the Investigation of the Treatment Effects of Reducing Cholesterol 6–HDL and LDL Treatment Strategies (ARBITER 6–HALTS) study observed a paradoxical increase in carotid intima–media thickness with LDL-C lowering by ezetimibe [61]. Collectively, these trials indicate that carotid intima–media thickness is a limited measure that is not a reliable surrogate endpoint.

Indeed, the Study of Heart and Renal Protection (SHARP) trial provided the first look at an ezetimibe trial powered for clinical outcomes and found that the drug added to simvastatin reduced CVD events though the comparator group was allocated a placebo, not statin monotherapy [62]. The Improved Reduction of Outcomes: Vytorin Efficacy International Trial (IMPROVE-IT) trial compared dual therapy with ezetimibe and simvastatin to simvastatin alone and found that the combination therapy group had a median LDL-C of 53.7 mg/dL compared to 69.5 mg/dL in the simvastatin-monotherapy group. IMPROVE-IT met its primary endpoint with a reduction in the composite endpoint of cardiovascular death, nonfatal myocardial infarction, unstable angina requiring rehospitalization, coronary revascularization, or nonfatal stroke. The relative risk reduction was 6%, compatible with the small magnitude of LDL-C reduction; 32.7% in the combination therapy group compared to 34.7% in the simvastatin-monotherapy group experienced events (absolute risk reduction 2%, number needed to treat 50).

Ezetimibe is generally well tolerated. In IMPROVE-IT, rates of muscle, gallbladder, and hepatic adverse effects, and cancer were no different in the ezetimibe versus control arm.

Bempedoic acid, an ATP citrate lyase inhibitor (ACL), is a newer nonstatin lipid-lowering agent with particular relevance for patients who are statin intolerant. The drug works by reducing LDL-C levels through inhibition of ACL, an enzyme upstream of HMG-CoA reductase in the cholesterol biosynthesis pathway. This inhibition leads to decreased cholesterol synthesis and increased LDL receptor activity, thereby lowering LDL-C levels in the blood [63]. This mechanism is advantageous as it minimizes the risk of muscle-related side effects, a common issue with statins, due to the liver-specific activation of the drug [64]. This occurs because ACL is not present in skeletal muscle. The most promising data to support the use of bempedoic acid comes from the CLEAR-OUTCOMES trial [65].

This randomized, placebo-controlled trial of bempedoic acid demonstrated a significant reduction in the incidence of major adverse cardiovascular events (MACE), including death from cardiovascular causes, nonfatal myocardial infarction, nonfatal stroke, and coronary revascularization, compared to placebo. At a dose of 180 mg daily, bempedoic acid reduced LDL-C levels more effectively than placebo by 21% (29.2 mg/dL). Over a median duration of follow-up of 40.6 months, the primary composite MACE endpoint was 13% lower with bempedoic acid versus placebo (819 patients [11.7%] vs. 927 [13.3%]; hazard ratio, 0.87; 95% confidence interval [CI], 0.79 to 0.96; $P = 0.004$), with significant reductions in each component, including coronary revascularization, fatal or nonfatal myocardial infarction, and a composite of cardiovascular death, nonfatal stroke, or nonfatal myocardial infarction. Although generally well tolerated, bempedoic acid was associated with an increased risk of gout and cholelithiasis (~1% absolute increases), as well as mild elevations in serum creatinine, uric acid, and hepatic enzymes. Of note, the mean age of both arms of the trial was 65.5 years, with 59.9% of the participants greater than the age of 65 in the bempedoic acid arm and 58.3% of the control group. This indicates that the results are relevant to the elderly population.

Additionally, Cordero et al. conducted an intention-to-treat meta-analysis of four clinical trials involving 17,324 patients, with 9,236 receiving bempedoic acid for a median of 46.6 months [66]. The primary outcome was the incidence of MACE, which was significantly reduced by 12% (HR 0.88; 95% CI 0.81–0.96). Specific reductions were observed in myocardial infarction (HR 0.76; 95% CI 0.66–0.89) and coronary revascularization (HR 0.82; 95% CI 0.73–0.92). No significant risk reduction was observed for stroke, cardiovascular death, or all-cause mortality. Overall, these findings suggest that bempedoic acid may offer a useful alternative for statin-intolerant patients at high cardiovascular risk, though its side effects warrant close monitoring.

INJECTABLE THERAPIES (PCSK9 INHIBITORS)

Injectable PCSK9 inhibitors have also become important lipid-lowering agents, with several well-executed clinical trials demonstrating their safety and efficacy. In the Global Assessment of Plaque Progression with a PCSK9 Antibody as measured by the Intravascular Ultrasound (GLAGOV) trial, patients randomized to evolocumab for a 76-week treatment period had a LDL-C level of 37 mg/dL compared to 93 mg/dL in the placebo group, and the percent atheroma volume decreased by 0.95% in the evolocumab group compared to no change in the placebo group. A greater reduction in atheroma volume was seen with greater reductions in LDL-C, down to levels as low as 20 mg/dL. The Further Cardiovascular Outcomes Research with PCSK9 inhibition in the Subjects with Elevated Risk (FOURIER) trial examined the safety and efficacy of evolocumab in patients on maximally tolerated statin therapy with LDL-C ≥70 mg/dL. Evolocumab significantly reduced LDL-C by 59% to 30 from 92 mg/dL, and reduced the risk of the primary endpoint, a composite of cardiovascular death, myocardial infarction, stroke, hospitalization for unstable angina, and coronary revascularization, with a 15% relative risk reduction and a number needed to treat of 67 over the short trial duration of 2 years. Importantly, there was no excess in adverse effects in FOURIER (with the exception of injection-site reactions) and no difference in cognitive function between patients allocated to evolocumab and placebo in a dedicated neurocognitive substudy, Evaluating PCSK9 Binding Antibody Influence on Cognitive Health in High Cardiovascular Risk Subjects (EBBINGHAUS).

The ODYSSEY OUTCOMES trial demonstrated that alirocumab, another PCSK9 monoclonal antibody, reduced the risk of ischemic cardiovascular events in patients who had a previous acute coronary syndrome and were treated with maximum tolerated statin [67]. The trial recruited 18,924 patients who were randomized to either alirocumab or placebo. Alirocumab significantly reduced LDL cholesterol levels and was associated with a lower incidence of major adverse cardiovascular events over a median follow-up of 2.8 years. The primary composite outcome—death from coronary heart disease, nonfatal myocardial infarction, fatal or nonfatal ischemic stroke, or hospitalization for unstable angina—occurred in 9.5% of the alirocumab group versus 11.1% of the placebo group (HR 0.85, 95% CI 0.78–0.93, $P < 0.001$). Adverse events were similar between groups, except for a higher incidence of injection-site reactions with alirocumab.

Another promising injectable treatment for hypercholesterolemia is inclisiran, a novel small interfering RNA (siRNA) therapy that targets PCSK9 production in the liver. Unlike PCSK9 monoclonal antibody therapies (evolocumab and alirocumab), which directly bind to the PCSK9 protein, inclisiran works by silencing the gene responsible for producing PCSK9, leading to long-lasting reductions in LDL-C levels. The ORION-10 and ORION-11 trials demonstrated the LDL-C lowering efficacy of inclisiran in patients with atherosclerotic cardiovascular disease or familial hypercholesterolemia [68]. In these studies, inclisiran administered every 6 months resulted in a reduction in LDL-C levels by 52.3% (95% CI 48.8–55.7) in the ORNION-10 trial and a 49.9% (CI 46.6–53.1) in the ORNION 11 trial at day 510. Notably, inclisiran was well tolerated, with injection site reactions being the most common adverse event, and no significant differences in adverse outcomes compared to placebo. In the ORION-10 trial, the mean age of participants was 66 years, with 60% of patients being 65 years or older. On subgroup analysis, there was no significant differences in efficacy between patients <65, ≥65 years, <75, or ≥75. With the potential to provide long-term cholesterol control with fewer injections, inclisiran provides a convenient option for patients needing additional LDL-C reduction. The cardiovascular outcome trials for inclisiran are ongoing.

DYSLIPIDEMIA INTERVENTION AS ONE COMPONENT OF A GLOBAL ABC APPROACH

Ultimately, dyslipidemia interventions are one component of a multifactorial, or global, approach to CVD prevention. The important lifestyle changes that help to lower cholesterol also tend to produce benefits for other components of the cardiovascular risk profile, including body mass index and blood pressure. Regarding pharmacotherapy for risk reduction, even if optimal lipid lowering is achieved in high-risk patients, the overall prognosis will remain suboptimal if other risk factors are not simultaneously addressed. In this respect, anytime dyslipidemia interventions are employed, it is imperative for clinicians to consider the other components of the global approach to risk reduction. An "ABC" or "ABCDE" approach can be practically applied in clinic, and includes (A) antiplatelet and antithrombotic agents; (B) blood pressure control; (C) cigarette smoking and cholesterol; (D) diet and diabetes control; and (E) exercise.

The benefits associated with achieving optimal global risk factor control in the primary prevention of CVD in elderly men were demonstrated in the Physicians' Health Study [69]. There were 4182 male physicians ≥65 years of age (mean age was 73 years) who enrolled in 1997. The physicians were free of CVD and diabetes at enrollment and followed for an average of 9 years. Adjusting for competing causes of mortality, a multifactorial prevention strategy was associated with considerable cardiovascular protection. Compared with control of four of four risk factors (smoking avoidance, control of non-HDL-C and blood pressure, and aspirin use) (only 6.0% of participants), control of zero of four risk factors almost quadrupled the risk of CVD (0.4% of participants; event rate 41.2%; HR 3.83, 95% CI 1.72–8.55). Control of one of four risk factors more than doubled the risk (14.2% of participants; HR 2.53, 95% CI 1.80–3.57). Most patients had partial risk factor control; with control of two of four risk factors, risk was nearly doubled (43.8% of participants; HR 1.94, 95% CI 1.41–2.69), and those with control of three of four risk factors also were at increased risk (35.6% of participants; HR 1.80, 95% CI 1.30–2.50). Depending on the number of risk factors controlled, the number needed to control to prevent one CVD event ranged from 5 to 22.

SPECIAL CONSIDERATIONS FOR DYSLIPIDEMIA MANAGEMENT IN THE ELDERLY INCREASED NEAR-TERM EFFICACY WITH INCREASED AGE

Age is a dominant factor in risk prediction models used in dyslipidemia guidelines and, therefore, a key determinant of whether a patient qualifies for treatment when using a risk score in the primary prevention setting. Moreover, given higher absolute risk with age, even small relative risk reductions can translate into large absolute benefits in the elderly [26]. Although relative risk reductions were similar in patients ≥65 years compared with those <65 years treated with pravastatin, absolute risk reductions were 1.5–2 times greater in the elderly patients [70]. The short-term benefit of statins is greatest in populations with the greatest cardiovascular risk, and even in the setting of high-risk primary prevention, the totality of evidence supports the use of statin therapy [71]. We have not yet identified an age above which, or atherogenic cholesterol level below which, patients no longer benefit from statin therapy.

Noncoronary outcomes

Multiple noncoronary outcomes are of particular interest in the elderly. As noted in this chapter, noncoronary CVD is also linked to dyslipidemia and responsive to interventions, including statin therapy. Some of the nuances of these noncoronary outcomes warrant additional discussion.

First, while many strokes are attributable to atherosclerotic vascular disease, a considerable portion is also thromboembolic, such as those related to atrial fibrillation, a disease concentrated in the elderly. There is some suggestion in the literature that statin therapy is associated with protection against atrial fibrillation in patients with coronary artery disease [72] as well as prevention of recurrence of atrial fibrillation in patients with lone atrial fibrillation after successful cardioversion [73]. In major trials of statin therapy of patients with and without known CHD, statin therapy has reduced the future incidence of stroke, which typically has been captured as a secondary outcome or component of the primary outcome.

In PROSPER, there was a trend toward reduction in transient ischemic attacks by 25% ($p = 0.05$). The Stroke Prevention by Aggressive Reduction in Cholesterol Levels (SPARCL) trial examined intensive statin therapy for protection from recurrent stroke in stroke survivors without CHD [74]. In SPARCL, statin intervention led to a 16% reduction in the risk of fatal or nonfatal stroke (HR 0.84 [0.71–0.99], $p = 0.03$). When recurrent strokes did occur, they were generally less severe in patients who were allocated statin therapy. When the data were viewed collectively, meta-analyses found a beneficial effect of statin therapy on stroke prevention [75,76], including in the elderly (Figure 5.5) [36].

Atherosclerosis affects many arterial regions throughout the body, and, therefore, beyond coronary and cerebrovascular disease, dyslipidemia may play a role in abdominal aortic aneurysm (AAA), renal artery stenosis, and peripheral arterial disease of the extremities. Accumulating evidence supports statin treatment in these settings as well. For example, in the Heart Protection Study of simvastatin, patients with peripheral arterial disease benefited from a 19% reduction in the rate of new vascular events [77].

Moreover, a frequent end-stage disease process for many patients with atherosclerosis is heart failure. Observational studies suggest a potential value of statins in patients who have heart failure with reduced systolic function [787980]. In a small single-center study, statin therapy was associated with lower mortality in patients with heart failure with preserved ejection fraction after accounting for baseline differences in hypertension,

Study	No. Events/ Total No. of Patients Statin	Placebo	Posterior Median Relative Risk (95% Credible Interval)
CARE	29/640	47/643	0.72 (0.51, 0.92)
HPS	280/5366	390/5331	0.73 (0.64, 0.84)
LIPID	104/1741	119/1773	0.80 (0.66, 1.01)
PLAC I	0/42	2/52	0.72 (0.35, 1.04)
PROSPER	45/934	53/899	0.77 (0.60, 1.02)
Pooled (5 year)	**458/8723**	**611/8698**	**0.75 (0.56, 0.94)**

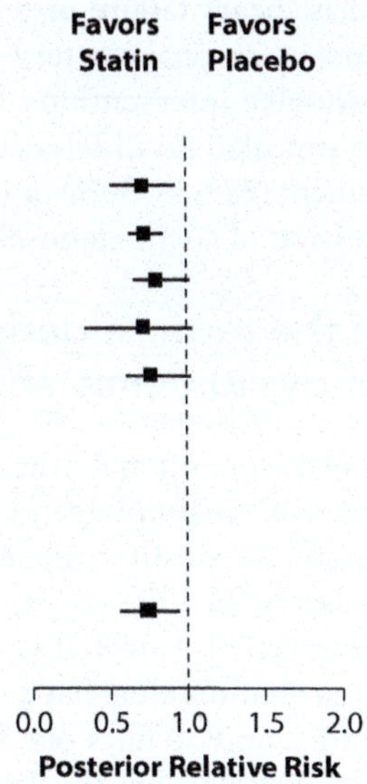

Figure 5.5 Bayesian forest plot for stroke with statin treatment in the elderly. Statin therapy reduced the incidence of stroke by 25% over 5 years as compared to placebo. The posterior median estimate of the number needed to treat was 58. (From J. Afilalo et al., *J Am Coll Cardiol*, 51, 37–45, 2008.)

diabetes, coronary artery disease, and creatinine [81]. Mechanisms beyond effects on atherosclerosis may explain how statin therapy could produce beneficial effects in heart failure patients. For example, statin therapy has been shown to reduce myocardial necrosis and preserve myocardial viability [82].

Nevertheless, randomized trials of initiating statin therapy in more advanced heart failure have been negative. In the Controlled Rosuvastatin Multinational Trial in Heart Failure (CORONA), 5011 older patients (≥60 years of age; mean age 73 years) with New York Heart Association Class II–IV ischemic, systolic heart failure (mean left ventricular ejection fraction [LVEF] 31%) were randomly assigned to receive 10 mg of rosuvastatin or placebo per day [83]. At baseline, the mean LDL-C was 137 mg/dL, and an entry requirement was that the investigator thought the patient did not need a cholesterol-lowering drug. After a median follow-up of 33 months, rosuvastatin reduced LDL-C to 76 mg/dL in the intervention group versus 138 mg/dL in the control group; however, there was not a significant reduction in the primary composite outcome of death from cardiovascular causes, nonfatal myocardial infarction, or nonfatal stroke (11.4% vs. 12.3% with placebo, HR 0.92, 95% CI 0.83–1.02), or secondary outcomes such as cardiovascular mortality (9.3% vs. 9.6%, HR 0.97), or coronary events (9.3% vs. 10.0%, HR 0.92).

Similarly, the Gruppo Italiano per lo Studio della Sopravvivenza nell'Insufficienza cardiac (GISSI-HF) trial [84] did not show a benefit of rosuvastatin 10 mg per day in 4574 patients (mean age 68 years) with ischemic or nonischemic New York Heart Association Class II–IV heart failure (mean LVEF 33%). While LDL-C was reduced from 122 to 89 mg/dL, after a median follow-up of 47 months, there was no significant difference in deaths from any cause or in the combined endpoint of death or admission to the hospital for cardiovascular causes in both ischemic and nonischemic cardiomyopathy. Thus, together the CORONA and GISSI-HF trials suggest that initiating statin therapy is not generally useful in patients with more advanced systolic heart failure who would not have otherwise met criteria for initiation of statin therapy for the purpose of primary or secondary prevention. Nevertheless, there may be more to the story—a retrospective hypothesis-generating analysis of CORONA found an interaction between high-sensitivity C-reactive protein levels and the effect of rosuvastatin on outcomes such that rosuvastatin treatment was associated with better outcomes in patients with high-sensitivity C-reactive protein levels ≥2.0 mg/L [85].

Also, of particular consideration in the elderly is calcific aortic stenosis, a disease that is associated with older age and dyslipidemia. While observational studies have suggested that statin therapy can slow the progression of aortic stenosis as measured by aortic valve area [86] or accumulation of aortic calcium [87], randomized trials have not confirmed this effect [88,89]. The prospective Simvastatin and Ezetimibe in Aortic Stenosis (SEAS) trial enrolled 1873 adults (mean age 68) with mild to moderate aortic stenosis (mean aortic jet velocity 3.1 m/s) and randomly assigned them to treatment with simvastatin plus ezetimibe or placebo [89].

After an average follow-up of 52 months, there was no difference between groups in the primary composite endpoint of cardiovascular death, aortic valve replacement, nonfatal myocardial infarction, hospitalized unstable angina pectoris, heart failure as a result of progression of aortic stenosis, coronary artery bypass grafting, percutaneous coronary interventions, and nonhemorrhagic stroke. There was also no difference in the rate of aortic valve replacement (28% vs. 30%) or in the rate of hemodynamic progression of aortic stenosis.

A note on the term "elderly" in the context of dyslipidemia and CVD risk

The medical literature often defines an elderly person as someone who is 65 years of age or older. This is a convenient cut point to stratify populations of individuals and helps to assess for differences by age at the population scale. However, of course, it is an artificial cut point when applied to an individual patient. A patient who is 64 years, 11 months, and 30 days old, becomes "elderly" on his or her 65th birthday, but this binary distinction suggests much more of a change than has occurred.

In addition, patients age differently. For clinical purposes, it is potentially useful to consider physiologic age, in addition to chronologic age. From a cardiovascular standpoint, the concept of "physiologic age" or "heart age" may be useful in understanding the absolute cardiovascular risk of a patient, and therefore the patient's potential to benefit from statins and other risk-reduction therapies. A patient who is 65 years old with cardiac risk factors may have a heart age in the 80s, and therefore, can be considered more elderly from a risk standpoint, with a larger potential role for risk-reducing therapies including statins. If the patient does not have many noncardiovascular comorbidities, the patient may be younger from the standpoint of potential statin side effects and competing risks. If so, intervention seems like a more attractive option, and in understanding that the patient's heart age is older than the chronological age, the patient may buy in more to intervention.

Conversely, a patient who is also 65 years of age with multiple noncardiovascular comorbidities, such as HIV on a protease inhibitor, alcohol abuse, and atrial fibrillation on amiodarone, is at increased risk for statin side effects, perhaps on the order of a much older, frail individual, and the attractiveness of intervention is less. Therefore, one nuance in the clinical management of dyslipidemia in the elderly is that the concept of elderly is probably best viewed more broadly than simply as chronological age.

Increased adverse effects with increased age

Common adverse events for statins and other lipid-lowering drugs were discussed earlier. It is important to consider that elderly patients are at higher risk for adverse drug effects because of the more frequent use of multiple concomitant medications, presence of multimorbidity, and impaired ability to metabolize and excrete compounds as a result of declining renal and hepatic function with age. Consequently, the safety of lipid-lowering agents, including potential drug–drug interactions, requires increased attention in this population. Indeed, age-related changes in muscle mass, total body water and fat, first-pass metabolism, and cytochrome P450 functioning can change the bioavailability of statins and other lipid-lowering drugs, altering the risk of toxicity.

Given the chance of adverse statin effects is related to the particular statin and dose, physicians may be able to reduce the likelihood of adverse drug effects in their choice of statin and dosing. The Food and Drug Administration has issued a warning on simvastatin at a dose of 80 mg per day due to a greater incidence of myopathy and serious cases of rhabdomyolysis. Therefore, this statin regimen should be avoided, especially in elderly patients. It has been suggested that the lipophilicity of statins may determine entry into muscle tissue. Hydrophilic statins, such as rosuvastatin, pravastatin, and lovastatin, may penetrate muscle tissue less than lipophilic statins, such as atorvastatin, fluvastatin, and simvastatin, and may therefore be less frequently implicated in myopathic events [90].

In elderly patients at increased risk for myopathy and other adverse drug effects, including women with low body weight, or those with hepatic or renal dysfunction, providers might consider choosing hydrophilic statins and consider initiating therapy at a lower dose than they would in younger, healthier patients. If the statin is well tolerated, the option for gradual titration remains. The highest dose of statins should be used with caution in the elderly. If severe illness, major surgery, or major trauma occurs, then it is prudent to discontinue statin use in an elderly patient until the patient has recovered.

Despite these potential issues, statin therapy is generally well tolerated in the elderly. For example, the Cholesterol Reduction in Seniors Program (CRISP) pilot study showed that lovastatin doses at 20–40 mg daily were associated with preserved health-related quality of life relative to placebo in a cohort of older adults with a mean age of 71 years [91]. A post hoc analysis from the TNT study assessed more potent treatment with atorvastatin 80 mg daily and in patients 65 years of age or older with stable CHD. High-dose atorvastatin was well tolerated and produced a 2.3% absolute reduction in major cardiovascular events and a 19% relative risk reduction compared with low-dose atorvastatin [92].

Preservation of cognitive function is a topic of particular relevance to the elderly who are at elevated risk for dementia, and there has been interest in whether statins or cholesterol lowering can impact cognitive function. Cholesterol may contribute to the pathogenesis of dementia, including both of the most common forms—Alzheimer's disease and vascular dementia. Increased midlife circulating cholesterol levels are linked with subsequent development of Alzheimer's disease [93,94]. In addition, increased non-HDL-C and decreased HDL-C are associated with an increased prevalence of vascular dementia [95].

Although cholesterol does not freely circulate between the systemic circulation and brain, patients with both Alzheimer's disease and coronary artery disease have increased cortical cholesterol levels [96]. Moreover, atherosclerosis may play a mechanistic role in the development of cognitive impairment in some patients, and cholesterol may also facilitate deposition of amyloid plaques [97]. Indeed, observational studies have found an association of statin therapy with a lower rate of dementia [98–99–100] and higher modified Mini-Mental State Examination (MMSE) scores [101].

Cancer is another topic of special importance in the elderly. With rising statin use in the 1990s, the concern arose that statin therapy could cause cancer. The Cholesterol Treatment Trialists' set out to study this issue prospectively, and the latest meta-analysis of data from clinical trials of statin therapy did not show any significant association of statin therapy with cancer. In fact, the risk estimate was exactly 1.00, indicating no effect.

In agreement, in a meta-analysis of 26 randomized controlled trials including 86,936 participants with 6662 incident cancer cases and 2407 cancer deaths, there was no association of statin therapy with the diagnosis of cancer or cancer death [102]. When the data were stratified according to cancer type, statin brand, dose, or pharmacologic characteristics, the results were consistent. These results, along with longer-term safety established in multiple clinical trials beyond 10 years, should reassure clinicians and patients.

COMPETING RISKS

Even if statins do not contribute to cancer, this does not mean that cancer, and other comorbidities that are more common in the elderly, do not impact treatment decisions. While evaluating cardiovascular risk and estimating the potential benefits of cardiovascular risk reduction therapies, providers must consider the effect of competing risks and discuss the global prognosis with patients. Of course, prognosis depends not only upon a new diagnosis of dyslipidemia and/or CVD but also on risks from other causes.

Investigators have used the declining exponential approximation for life expectancy (DEALE) to provide a framework to help clinicians gauge the effect of competing risks as a function of age [10]. In such modeling, the absolute effect of a new diagnosis on life expectancy is often relatively small, and therefore, the potential gain even from optimal therapy may also be small, at least for the endpoint of mortality. This point, combined with the added risks of therapy in old age, reduces the net benefit of intervention in the elderly and is a reason to exercise greater caution in initiating therapy or lower tolerance for side effects in elderly patients with such comorbidities.

UNDERTREATMENT IN THE ELDERLY

Despite the clear benefits of lipid lowering on cardiovascular outcomes in the elderly, undertreatment is especially prevalent in this patient population, even in those in the younger range of the elderly group. In a study published in 2006, examining male patients aged 60–75 years with acute myocardial infarction, only 29% of patients were on a lipid-lowering drug, and only 12% achieved cholesterol levels recommended by the NCEP guidelines [20]. The situation has been characterized as a treatment-risk paradox [2] in which treatment is prescribed preferentially to individuals under the age of 65 years and use is more restricted in the elderly group with higher short-term cardiovascular risk.

Low use of statins has been documented in elderly persons living in the United Kingdom [103]. Medical records were reviewed in 41,250 patients aged ≥40 years who were seen at general medical practices. In those without known CVD, use of statins and antihypertensives was assessed across age categories. Whereas antihypertensive use increased with age, as expected, statin use peaked in the 70–74 age group and then declined. Compared to a reference group aged 40–44 years, the odds ratio for taking a statin was 10.9 in the 65–69-year-old group, and similar at 10.1 for antihypertensive use. The odds ratios in the 70–74-year-old group increased to 13.6 for statins and 16.2 for antihypertensives. However, thereafter, use for statins dropped off, with an odds ratio down to 10.3 in the group aged over 80–84 years, whereas the odds ratio for antihypertensive use continued to increase up to 25.8.

Several factors might explain lower statin prescription rates in the elderly. First, the higher potential for adverse effects likely translates into a higher threshold for initiating therapy as physicians weigh the potential benefits and risks. Second, physicians may be less inclined to prescribe additional drugs to an elderly patient due to the potential for lower adherence to therapy in the setting of polypharmacy, medication costs, and cognitive decline. Third, physicians may be swayed by the potential for lower net benefits of intervention due to competing risks from multiple other comorbidities. Fourth, statins may be avoided due to shifting clinical priorities and patient preference. Fifth, clinicians may hesitate to prescribe statin therapy in very old patients (i.e., >75) for primary prevention because of the perception of too little clinical trial evidence [104] in this population and lack of clear benefit for functional status [105,106]. Ultimately, it is difficult to know for certain what portion of the lack of treatment of dyslipidemia in the elderly is due to undertreatment and what portion is due to reasonable withholding of therapy.

GUIDELINE RECOMMENDATIONS

Clinical guideline statements support treatment of high-risk elderly patients with statins and nonstatins. Recently, the European guidelines state, as a Class I recommendation, "Treatment with statins is recommended for older adults with ACSVD in the same way as for younger patients" [107]. Consistent with the aforementioned evidence, they also indicate that statin therapy for primary prevention can be appropriate in the elderly. The European guidelines state, as a Class IIb recommendation, "Initiation of statin treatment for primary prevention in older people aged >75 may be considered, if at high-risk or above." The guidelines do, however, recommend taking caution when prescribing statins for elderly people, specifically those who have renal impairment or the potential for drug interactions based on expert opinion (level of evidence C). They recommend that statins should be started at a lower dose and then titrated upward to achieve target LDL-C levels.

Similarly, the most recent ACC/AHA guidelines also recommend statin therapy for the elderly in certain clinical contexts but are a little more conservative in certain recommendations [108]. The guidelines provide a Class I recommendation to initiate high-intensity or maximal statin therapy in patients with very high risk ASCVD regardless of age. However, in those patients who have ASCVD but are not very high risk, with an age >75, the guidelines give a Class IIa recommendation to initiate moderate- or high-intensity statin, or to continue high-intensity statin therapy if the patient is on it. For patients older than 75 who have diabetes, the guidelines note that they are likely to benefit from statin therapy and offer a Class IIb recommendation for initiating therapy after clinician–patient discussion of benefits and risks, but note that benefits could be compromised by reduced longevity and increased adverse events. In the primary prevention setting, the guidelines give a Class IIb recommendation suggesting it may be reasonable to initiate moderate-intensity statin therapy for patients with an LDL-C level of 70 to 189 mg/dL, but note it may be reasonable to stop therapy when functional decline, multimorbidity, frailty, or reduced life expectancy limit benefits.

The ACC Consensus Pathway on nonstatin therapy highlights ezetimibe and PCSK9 inhibitors as key second-line agents to consider in addition to lifestyle modification and statin therapy for additional LDL-C lowering. For <25% of additional LDL-C lowering, ezetimibe was identified as the preferred agent, and for those needing greater amounts of LDL-C lowering, then a PCSK9 inhibitor was identified as the agent of choice.

CONCLUSION

With increases in life expectancy and growth of the elderly population, including the very old, the topic of dyslipidemia in the elderly is becoming increasingly important. The growth of this population also gives the opportunity for further research to incorporate these patients in even greater numbers. Ensuring informed clinicians and patients, and appropriate use of risk reduction therapies for dyslipidemia in the elderly, is vital to maintaining quality of life and avoiding preventable morbidity. A large pool of data has proven that statin treatment reduces atherogenic lipid levels and the risk of CVD as effectively in older high-risk individuals as in younger individuals. Yet, despite these benefits, many high-risk older individuals are not receiving statins and other evidence-based therapies.

Clinicians must engage patients in discussions about the benefits and risks of therapy. Physicians must use the evidence base, their knowledge of the patient, experience, and clinical judgment in deciding which patients to offer statins or other lipid-lowering treatments. Of course, the decision will also need to incorporate patient preferences for another medication and overall healthcare goals, competing risks and life expectancy, and possible side effects and quality of life. Put simply, patients should not be denied statin therapy and other dyslipidemia interventions solely on the basis of age, but therapy should reflect a careful risk–benefit analysis.

ACKNOWLEDGMENT

The authors thank Dr. Mays Ali for her prior work on this chapter.

REFERENCES

1. S. S. Martin *et al.*, "2025 heart disease and stroke statistics: A report of US and global data from the American Heart Association," *Circulation*. Jan. 2025. doi: 10.1161/CIR.0000000000001303. Epub ahead of print. PMID: 39866113.
2. D. T. Ko, M. Mamdani, and D. A. Alter, "Lipid-lowering therapy with statins in high-risk elderly patients: The treatment-risk paradox," *JAMA*, vol. 291, no. 15, pp. 1864–1870, Apr. 2004, doi: 10.1001/JAMA.291.15.1864.
3. K. P. Alexander *et al.*, "Evolution in cardiovascular care for elderly patients with non–ST-segment elevation acute coronary syndromes: Results from the CRUSADE national quality improvement initiative," *J Am Coll Cardiol*, vol. 46, no. 8, pp. 1479–1487, Oct. 2005, doi: 10.1016/J.JACC.2005.05.084.
4. S. M. Grundy, J. I. Cleeman, B. M. Rifkind, and L. H. Kuller, "Cholesterol lowering in the elderly population," *Arch Intern Med*, vol. 159, no. 15, pp. 1670–1678, Aug. 1999, doi: 10.1001/ARCHINTE.159.15.1670.
5. Eastern Stroke Coronary Heart Disease Collaborative Research, "Blood pressure, cholesterol, and stroke in eastern Asia," *Lancet*, vol. 352, no. 9143, pp. 1801–1807, Dec. 1998, doi: 10.1016/S0140-6736(98)03454-0.
6. S. M. Rubin, S. Sidney, D. M. Black, W. S. Browner, S. B. Hulley, and S. R. Cummings, "High blood cholesterol in elderly men and the excess risk for coronary heart disease," *Ann Intern Med*, vol. 113, no. 12, pp. 916–920, Dec. 1990, doi: 10.7326/0003-4819-113-12-916.

7. P. H. Frost *et al.*, "Serum lipids and incidence of coronary heart disease," *Circulation*, vol. 94, no. 10, pp. 2381–2388, Nov. 1996, doi: 10.1161/01.CIR.94.10.2381.
8. T. A. Manolio, T. A. Pearson, N. K. Wenger, E. Barrett-Connor, G. H. Payne, and W. R. Harlan, "Cholesterol and heart disease in older persons and women review of an NHLBI workshop," *Ann Epidemiol*, vol. 2, no. 1–2, pp. 161–176, Jan. 1992, doi: 10.1016/1047-2797(92)90051-Q.
9. W. S. Aronow *et al.*, "Risk factors for coronary artery disease in persons older than 62 years in a long-term health care facility," *American Journal of Cardiology*, vol. 57, no. 8, pp. 518–520, May 1986, doi: 10.1016/0002-9149(86)90827-1.
10. H. G. Welch, P. C. Albertsen, R. F. Nease, T. A. Bubolz, and J. H. Wasson, "Estimating treatment benefits for the elderly: The effect of competing risks," *Ann Intern Med*, vol. 124, no. 6, pp. 577–584, Mar. 1996, doi: 10.7326/0003-4819-124-6-199603150-00007.
11. H. M. Krumholz *et al.*, "Lack of association between cholesterol and coronary heart disease mortality and morbidity and all-cause mortality in persons older than 70 years," *JAMA*, vol. 272, no. 17, pp. 1335–1340, Nov. 1994, doi: 10.1001/JAMA.1994.03520170045034.
12. I. J. Schatz, K. Masaki, K. Yano, R. Chen, B. L. Rodriguez, and J. D. Curb, "Cholesterol and all-cause mortality in elderly people from the Honolulu Heart Program: A cohort study," *Lancet*, vol. 358, no. 9279, pp. 351–355, Aug. 2001, doi: 10.1016/S0140-6736(01)05553-2.
13. R. A. Kronmal, K. C. Cain, Z. Ye, and G. S. Omenn, "Total serum cholesterol levels and mortality risk as a function of age: A report based on the Framingham data," *Arch Intern Med*, vol. 153, no. 9, pp. 1065–1073, May 1993, doi: 10.1001/ARCHINTE.1993.00410090025004.
14. P. Zimetbaum *et al.*, "Plasma lipids and lipoproteins and the incidence of cardiovascular disease in the very elderly. The Bronx Aging Study," *Arterioscler Thromb*, vol. 12, no. 4, pp. 416–423, 1992, doi: 10.1161/01.ATV.12.4.416.
15. J. K. Grant, M. Dangl, C. E. Ndumele, E. D. Michos, and S. S. Martin, "A historical, evidence-based, and narrative review on commonly used dietary supplements in lipid-lowering," *J Lipid Res*, vol. 65, no. 2, p. 100493, Feb. 2023, doi: 10.1016/J.JLR.2023.100493.
16. L. Soares-Miranda, D. S. Siscovick, B. M. Psaty, W. T. Longstreth, and D. Mozaffarian, "Physical activity and risk of coronary heart disease and stroke in older adults: The Cardiovascular Health Study," *Circulation*, vol. 133, no. 2, pp. 147–155, Jan. 2016, doi: 10.1161/CIRCULATIONAHA.115.018323.
17. W. S. Aronow and C. Ahn, "Incidence of new coronary events in older persons with prior myocardial infarction and serum low-density lipoprotein cholesterol ≥125 mg/dl treated with statins versus no lipid-lowering drug," *American Journal of Cardiology*, vol. 89, no. 1, pp. 67–69, Jan. 2002, doi: 10.1016/S0002-9149(01)02167-1.
18. R. N. Lemaitre, B. M. Psaty, S. R. Heckbert, R. A. Kronmal, A. B. Newman, and G. L. Burke, "Therapy with hydroxymethylglutaryl coenzyme a reductase inhibitors (statins) and associated risk of incident cardiovascular events in older adults: Evidence from the Cardiovascular Health Study," *Arch Intern Med*, vol. 162, no. 12, pp. 1395–1400, Jun. 2002, doi: 10.1001/ARCHINTE.162.12.1395.
19. C. A. Allen Maycock *et al.*, "Statin therapy is associated with reduced mortality across all age groups of individuals with significant coronary disease, including very elderly patients," *J Am Coll Cardiol*, vol. 40, no. 10, pp. 1777–1785, Nov. 2002, doi: 10.1016/S0735-1097(02)02477-4.
20. J. Micale Foody *et al.*, "Hydroxymethylglutaryl-CoA reductase inhibitors in older persons with acute myocardial infarction: Evidence for an age-statin interaction," *J Am Geriatr Soc*, vol. 54, no. 3, pp. 421–430, Mar. 2006, doi: 10.1111/J.1532-5415.2005.00635.X.
21. K. Gränsbo *et al.*, "Cardiovascular and cancer mortality in very elderly post-myocardial infarction patients receiving statin treatment," *J Am Coll Cardiol*, vol. 55, no. 13, pp. 1362–1369, Mar. 2010, doi: 10.1016/J.JACC.2010.01.013.
22. P. S. Sever *et al.*, "Prevention of coronary and stroke events with atorvastatin in hypertensive patients who have average or lower-than-average cholesterol concentrations, in the Anglo-Scandinavian Cardiac Outcomes Trial - Lipid Lowering Arm (ASCOT-LLA): A multicentre randomised controlled trial," *Lancet*, vol. 361, no. 9364, pp. 1149–1158, Apr. 2003, doi: 10.1016/S0140-6736(03)12948-0.
23. P. M. Ridker *et al.*, "Rosuvastatin to prevent vascular events in men and women with elevated C-reactive protein," *N Engl J Med*, vol. 359, no. 21, pp. 2195–2207, Nov. 2008, doi: 10.1056/NEJMOA0807646.
24. R. J. Glynn, W. Koenig, B. G. Nordestgaard, J. Shepherd, and P. M. Ridker, "Rosuvastatin for primary prevention in older persons with elevated C-reactive protein and low to average low-density lipoprotein cholesterol levels: Exploratory analysis of a randomized trial," *Ann Intern Med*, vol. 152, no. 8, pp. 488–496, Apr. 2010, doi: 10.7326/0003-4819-152-8-201004200-00005.
25. Scandinavian Simvastatin Survival Study Group, "Randomised trial of cholesterol lowering in 4444 patients with coronary heart disease: The Scandinavian Simvastatin Survival Study (4S)," *The Lancet*, vol. 344, no. 8934, pp. 1383–1389, Nov. 1994, doi: 10.1016/S0140-6736(94)90566-5.
26. T. A. Miettinen *et al.*, "Cholesterol-lowering therapy in women and elderly patients with myocardial infarction or angina pectoris: Findings from

the Scandinavian Simvastatin Survival Study (4S)," *Circulation*, vol. 96, no. 12, pp. 4211–4218, 1997, doi: 10.1161/01.CIR.96.12.4211.

27. F. M. Sacks *et al.*, "The effect of pravastatin on coronary events after myocardial infarction in patients with average cholesterol levels. Cholesterol and Recurrent Events Trial investigators," *N Engl J Med*, vol. 335, no. 14, pp. 1001–1009, Oct. 1996, doi: 10.1056/NEJM199610033351401.
28. C. P. Cannon *et al.*, "Intensive versus moderate lipid lowering with statins after acute coronary syndromes," *N Engl J Med*, vol. 350, no. 15, pp. 1495–1504, Apr. 2004, doi: 10.1056/NEJMOA040583.
29. L. JC *et al.*, "Intensive lipid lowering with atorvastatin in patients with stable coronary disease," *N Engl J Med*, vol. 352, no. 14, pp. 97–99, May 2005, doi: 10.1056/NEJMOA050461.
30. J. Shepherd *et al.*, "Pravastatin in elderly individuals at risk of vascular disease (PROSPER): A randomised controlled trial," *Lancet*, vol. 360, no. 9346, pp. 1623–1630, Nov. 2002, doi: 10.1016/S0140-6736(02)11600-X.
31. P. Deedwania *et al.*, "Effects of intensive versus moderate lipid-lowering therapy on myocardial ischemia in older patients with coronary heart disease: Results of the Study Assessing Goals in the Elderly (SAGE)," *Circulation*, vol. 115, no. 6, pp. 700–707, Feb. 2007, doi: 10.1161/CIRCULATIONAHA.106.654756.
32. C. Baigent *et al.*, "Efficacy and safety of more intensive lowering of LDL cholesterol: A meta-analysis of data from 170 000 participants in 26 randomised trials," *The Lancet*, vol. 376, no. 9753, pp. 1670–1681, Nov. 2010, doi: 10.1016/S0140-6736(10)61350-5.
33. J. Armitage *et al.*, "Efficacy and safety of statin therapy in older people: A meta-analysis of individual participant data from 28 randomised controlled trials," *The Lancet*, vol. 393, no. 10170, pp. 407–415, Feb. 2019, doi: 10.1016/S0140-6736(18)31942-1.
34. S. Zoungas *et al.*, "Baseline characteristics of participants in STAREE: A randomized trial for primary prevention of cardiovascular disease events and prolongation of disability-free survival in older people," *J Am Heart Assoc*, vol. 13, no. 22, p. e036357, Nov. 2024, doi: 10.1161/JAHA.124.036357/SUPPL_FILE/JAH310335-SUP-0001-SUPINFO.PDF.
35. J. Joseph *et al.*, "Pragmatic evaluation of events and benefits of lipid lowering in older adults (PREVENTABLE): Trial design and rationale," *J Am Geriatr Soc*, vol. 71, no. 6, p. 1701, Jun. 2023, doi: 10.1111/JGS.18312.
36. J. Afilalo, G. Duque, R. Steele, J. W. Jukema, A. J. M. de Craen, and M. J. Eisenberg, "Statins for secondary prevention in elderly patients: A hierarchical Bayesian meta-analysis," *J Am Coll Cardiol*, vol. 51, no. 1, pp. 37–45, Jan. 2008, doi: 10.1016/J.JACC.2007.06.063.
37. A. Kashani *et al.*, "Risks associated with statin therapy: A systematic overview of randomized clinical trials," *Circulation*, vol. 114, no. 25, pp. 2788–2797, Dec. 2006, doi: 10.1161/CIRCULATIONAHA.106.624890.
38. J. Hsia, J. G. MacFadyen, J. Monyak, and P. M. Ridker, "Cardiovascular event reduction and adverse events among subjects attaining low-density lipoprotein cholesterol <50 mg/dl with rosuvastatin. The JUPITER trial (Justification for the Use of Statins in Prevention: An Intervention Trial Evaluating Rosuvastatin)," *J Am Coll Cardiol*, vol. 57, no. 16, pp. 1666–1675, Apr. 2011, doi: 10.1016/J.JACC.2010.09.082.
39. G. A. Nichols and C. E. Koro, "Does statin therapy initiation increase the risk for myopathy? An observational study of 32,225 diabetic and nondiabetic patients," *Clin Ther*, vol. 29, no. 8, pp. 1761–1770, Aug. 2007, doi: 10.1016/J.CLINTHERA.2007.08.022.
40. J. Armitage, "The safety of statins in clinical practice," *The Lancet*, vol. 370, no. 9601, pp. 1781–1790, Nov. 2007, doi: 10.1016/S0140-6736(07)60716-8.
41. J. H. O'Keefe, L. Cordain, W. H. Harris, R. M. Moe, and R. Vogel, "Optimal low-density lipoprotein is 50 to 70 mg/dl: Lower is better and physiologically normal," *J Am Coll Cardiol*, vol. 43, no. 11, pp. 2142–2146, Jun. 2004, doi: 10.1016/j.jacc.2004.03.046.
42. V. G. Athyros *et al.*, "Safety and efficacy of long-term statin treatment for cardiovascular events in patients with coronary heart disease and abnormal liver tests in the Greek Atorvastatin and Coronary Heart Disease Evaluation (GREACE) Study: A post-hoc analysis," *Lancet*, vol. 376, no. 9756, pp. 1916–1922, 2010, doi: 10.1016/S0140-6736(10)61272-X.
43. N. Sattar *et al.*, "Statins and risk of incident diabetes: A collaborative meta-analysis of randomised statin trials," *The Lancet*, vol. 375, no. 9716, pp. 735–742, Feb. 2010, doi: 10.1016/S0140-6736(09)61965-6.
44. T. A. Jacobson, "Executive summary NLA task force on statin safety-2014 update," 2014, doi: 10.1016/j.jacl.2014.03.003.
45. J. P. Howard *et al.*, "Side effect patterns in a crossover trial of statin, placebo, and no treatment," *J Am Coll Cardiol*, vol. 78, no. 12, pp. 1210–1222, Sep. 2021, doi: 10.1016/J.JACC.2021.07.022/SUPPL_FILE/MMC1.DOCX.
46. J. M. McKenney, M. H. Davidson, T. A. Jacobson, and J. R. Guyton, "Final conclusions and recommendations of the National Lipid Association Statin Safety Assessment Task Force," *American Journal of Cardiology*, vol. 97, no. 8 SUPPL. 1, pp. S89–S94, Apr. 2006, doi: 10.1016/j.amjcard.2006.02.030.
47. "The Lipid Research Clinics Coronary Primary Prevention Trial results: I. Reduction in incidence of coronary heart disease," *JAMA*, vol. 251, no. 3, pp. 351–364, Jan. 1984, doi: 10.1001/JAMA.1984.03340270029025.

48. "The Lipid Research Clinics Coronary Primary Prevention Trial results: II. The relationship of reduction in incidence of coronary heart disease to cholesterol lowering," *JAMA*, vol. 251, no. 3, pp. 365–374, Jan. 1984, doi: 10.1001/JAMA.1984.03340270043026.
49. M. Manttari *et al.*, "Lipoproteins and coronary heart disease in the Helsinki Heart Study," *Eur Heart J*, vol. 11, no. suppl_H, pp. 26–31, Jan. 1990, doi: 10.1093/EURHEARTJ/11.SUPPL_H.26.
50. H. B. Rubins *et al.*, "Gemfibrozil for the secondary prevention of coronary heart disease in men with low levels of high-density lipoprotein cholesterol," *New England Journal of Medicine*, vol. 341, no. 6, pp. 410–418, Aug. 1999, doi: 10.1056/NEJM199908053410604/ASSET/02830D74-5282-4321-A27F-59021B283651/ASSETS/IMAGES/LARGE/NEJM199908053410604_T5.JPG.
51. I. Goldenberg, U. Goldbourt, V. Boyko, S. Behar, and H. Reicher-Reiss, "Relation between on-treatment increments in serum high-density lipoprotein cholesterol levels and cardiac mortality in patients with coronary heart disease (from the Bezafibrate Infarction Prevention trial)," *Am J Cardiol*, vol. 97, no. 4, pp. 466–471, Feb. 2006, doi: 10.1016/J.AMJCARD.2005.09.078.
52. A. Das Pradhan *et al.*, "Triglyceride lowering with pemafibrate to reduce cardiovascular risk," *New England Journal of Medicine*, vol. 387, no. 21, pp. 1923–1934, Nov. 2022, doi: 10.1056/NEJMOA2210645/SUPPL_FILE/NEJMOA2210645_DATA-SHARING.PDF.
53. J. R. Guyton, "Niacin in cardiovascular prevention: Mechanisms, efficacy, and safety," *Curr Opin Lipidol*, vol. 18, no. 4, pp. 415–420, Aug. 2007, doi: 10.1097/MOL.0B013E3282364ADD.
54. C. PL *et al.*, "Fifteen year mortality in Coronary Drug Project patients: Long-term benefit with niacin," *J Am Coll Cardiol*, vol. 8, no. 6, pp. 1245–1255, 1986, doi: 10.1016/S0735-1097(86)80293-5.
55. A. J. Taylor, L. E. Sullenberger, H. J. Lee, J. K. Lee, and K. A. Grace, "Arterial biology for the investigation of the treatment effects of reducing cholesterol (ARBITER) 2: A double-blind, placebo-controlled study of extended-release niacin on atherosclerosis progression in secondary prevention patients treated with statins," *Circulation*, vol. 110, no. 23, pp. 3512–3517, Dec. 2004, doi: 10.1161/01.CIR.0000148955.19792.8D/ASSET/9F9C6E8A-2B60-43F1-99A6-65F74E1573CD/ASSETS/GRAPHIC/5FF3.JPEG.
56. A. J. Taylor *et al.*, "Extended-release niacin or ezetimibe and carotid intima-media thickness," *N Engl J Med*, vol. 361, no. 22, pp. 2113–2122, Nov. 2009, doi: 10.1056/NEJMOA0907569.
57. B. WE *et al.*, "Niacin in patients with low HDL cholesterol levels receiving intensive statin therapy," *N Engl J Med*, vol. 365, no. 24, pp. 2255–2267, Dec. 2011, doi: 10.1056/NEJMOA1107579.
58. A. C. Goldberg, A. Sapre, J. Liu, R. Capece, and Y. B. Mitchel, "Efficacy and safety of ezetimibe coadministered with simvastatin in patients with primary hypercholesterolemia: A randomized, double-blind, placebo-controlled trial," *Mayo Clin Proc*, vol. 79, no. 5, pp. 620–629, 2004, doi: 10.4065/79.5.620.
59. T. Feldman *et al.*, "Treatment of high-risk patients with ezetimibe plus simvastatin co-administration versus simvastatin alone to attain National Cholesterol Education Program Adult Treatment Panel III Low-Density lipoprotein cholesterol goals," *American Journal of Cardiology*, vol. 93, no. 12, pp. 1481–1486, Jun. 2004, doi: 10.1016/j.amjcard.2004.02.059.
60. J. J. P. Kastelein *et al.*, "Simvastatin with or without ezetimibe in familial hypercholesterolemia," *N Engl J Med*, vol. 358, no. 14, pp. 1431–1443, Apr. 2008, doi: 10.1056/NEJMOA0800742.
61. A. J. Taylor, T. C. Villines, and E. J. Stanek, "Paradoxical progression of atherosclerosis related to low-density lipoprotein reduction and exposure to ezetimibe," *Eur Heart J*, vol. 33, no. 23, pp. 2939–2945, Dec. 2012, doi: 10.1093/EURHEARTJ/EHS105.
62. C. Baigent *et al.*, "The effects of lowering LDL cholesterol with simvastatin plus ezetimibe in patients with chronic kidney disease (Study of Heart and Renal Protection): A randomised placebo-controlled trial," *The Lancet*, vol. 377, no. 9784, pp. 2181–2192, Jun. 2011, doi: 10.1016/S0140-6736(11)60739-3.
63. N. Ferri, E. Colombo, and A. Corsini, "Bempedoic acid, the first-in-class oral ATP citrate lyase inhibitor with hypocholesterolemic activity: Clinical pharmacology and drug–drug interactions," *Pharmaceutics*, vol. 16, no. 11, p. 1371, Oct. 2024, doi: 10.3390/PHARMACEUTICS16111371.
64. M. Ruscica, C. R. Sirtori, S. Carugo, M. Banach, and A. Corsini, "Bempedoic acid: For whom and when," *Curr Atheroscler Rep*, vol. 24, no. 10, p. 791, Oct. 2022, doi: 10.1007/S11883-022-01054-2.
65. S. E. Nissen *et al.*, "Bempedoic acid and cardiovascular outcomes in statin-intolerant patients," *New England Journal of Medicine*, vol. 388, no. 15, pp. 1353–1364, Apr. 2023, doi: 10.1056/NEJMOA2215024/SUPPL_FILE/NEJMOA2215024_DATA-SHARING.PDF.
66. A. Cordero *et al.*, "Clinical benefit of bempedoic acid in randomized clinical trials," *Am J Cardiol*, vol. 205, pp. 321–324, Oct. 2023, doi: 10.1016/J.AMJCARD.2023.07.145.
67. G. G. Schwartz *et al.*, "Alirocumab and cardiovascular outcomes after acute coronary syndrome," *New England Journal of Medicine*, vol. 379, no. 22, pp. 2097–2107, Nov. 2018, doi: 10.1056/NEJMOA180117

4/SUPPL_FILE/NEJMOA1801174_DISCLOSURES.PDF.
68. K. K. Ray *et al.*, "Two phase 3 trials of inclisiran in patients with elevated LDL cholesterol," *New England Journal of Medicine*, vol. 382, no. 16, pp. 1507–1519, Apr. 2020, doi: 10.1056/NEJMOA1912387/SUPPL_FILE/NEJMOA1912387_DATA-SHARING.PDF.
69. J. G. Robinson, C. Rahilly-Tierney, E. Lawler, and J. M. Gaziano, "Benefits associated with achieving optimal risk factor levels for the primary prevention of cardiovascular disease in older men," *J Clin Lipidol*, vol. 6, no. 1, pp. 58–65, Jan. 2012, doi: 10.1016/J.JACL.2011.10.019.
70. D. Hunt *et al.*, "Benefits of pravastatin on cardiovascular events and mortality in older patients with coronary heart disease are equal to or exceed those seen in younger patients: Results from the LIPID trial," *Ann Intern Med*, vol. 134, no. 10, pp. 931–940, May 2001, doi: 10.7326/0003-4819-134-10-200105150-00007.
71. R. Ali and K. P. Alexander, "Statins for the primary prevention of cardiovascular events in older adults: A review of the evidence," *Am J Geriatr Pharmacother*, vol. 5, no. 1, pp. 52–63, Mar. 2007, doi: 10.1016/j.amjopharm.2007.03.008.
72. Y. Young-Xu *et al.*, "Usefulness of statin drugs in protecting against atrial fibrillation in patients with coronary artery disease," *Am J Cardiol*, vol. 92, no. 12, pp. 1379–1383, Dec. 2003, doi: 10.1016/j.amjcard.2003.08.040.
73. C. W. Siu, C. P. Lau, and H. F. Tse, "Prevention of atrial fibrillation recurrence by statin therapy in patients with lone atrial fibrillation after successful cardioversion," *Am J Cardiol*, vol. 92, no. 11, pp. 1343–1345, Dec. 2003, doi: 10.1016/j.amjcard.2003.08.023.
74. A. P *et al.*, "High-dose atorvastatin after stroke or transient ischemic attack," *N Engl J Med*, vol. 355, no. 6, pp. 549–559, Aug. 2006, doi: 10.1056/NEJMOA061894.
75. M. Briel, M. Studer, T. R. Glass, and H. C. Bucher, "Effects of statins on stroke prevention in patients with and without coronary heart disease: A meta-analysis of randomized controlled trials," *Am J Med*, vol. 117, no. 8, pp. 596–606, Oct. 2004, doi: 10.1016/j.amjmed.2004.04.022.
76. M. R. Law, N. J. Wald, and A. R. Rudnicka, "Quantifying effect of statins on low density lipoprotein cholesterol, ischemic heart disease, and stroke: Systematic review and meta-analysis," *BMJ*, vol. 326, no. 7404, pp. 1423–1427, Jun. 2003, doi: 10.1136/BMJ.326.7404.1423.
77. Heart Protection Study Collaborative Group, "MRC/BHF Heart Protection Study of cholesterol lowering with simvastatin in 20 536 high-risk individuals: A randomised placebo-controlled trial," *Lancet*, vol. 360, no. 9326, pp. 7–22, Jul. 2002, doi: 10.1016/S0140-6736(02)09327-3/ASSET/E5B5008B-5BBC-4EA3-BF63-98CF918B16E7/MAIN.ASSETS/GR9.SML.
78. A. S. Go, W. Y. Lee, J. Yang, J. C. Lo, and J. H. Gurwitz, "Statin therapy and risks for death and hospitalization in chronic heart failure," *JAMA*, vol. 296, no. 17, pp. 2105–2111, Nov. 2006, doi: 10.1001/JAMA.296.17.2105.
79. J. G. Ray, Y. Gong, K. Sykora, and J. V. Tu, "Statin use and survival outcomes in elderly patients with heart failure," *Arch Intern Med*, vol. 165, no. 1, pp. 62–67, Jan. 2005, doi: 10.1001/ARCHINTE.165.1.62.
80. T. B. Horwich, W. R. MacLellan, and G. C. Fonarow, "Statin therapy is associated with improved survival in ischemic and non-ischemic heart failure," *J Am Coll Cardiol*, vol. 43, no. 4, pp. 642–648, Feb. 2004, doi: 10.1016/J.JACC.2003.07.049.
81. H. Fukuta, D. C. Sane, S. Brucks, and W. C. Little, "Statin therapy may be associated with lower mortality in patients with diastolic heart failure: A preliminary report," *Circulation*, vol. 112, no. 3, pp. 357–363, Jul. 2005, doi: 10.1161/CIRCULATIONAHA.104.519876/ASSET/A3E566F9-DCC6-4699-AC64-2E61895BD406/ASSETS/GRAPHIC/11FF3.JPEG.
82. J. Bauersachs, P. Galuppo, D. Fraccarollo, M. Christ, and G. Ertl, "Improvement of left ventricular remodeling and function by hydroxymethylglutaryl coenzyme a reductase inhibition with cerivastatin in rats with heart failure after myocardial infarction," *Circulation*, vol. 104, no. 9, pp. 982–985, Aug. 2001, doi: 10.1161/HC3401.095946.
83. J. Kjekshus *et al.*, "Rosuvastatin in older patients with systolic heart failure," *N Engl J Med*, vol. 357, no. 22, pp. 2248–2261, Nov. 2007, doi: 10.1056/NEJMOA0706201/ASSET/22D7026C-2E1A-4F35-947D-59407C18A394/ASSETS/IMAGES/LARGE/NEJMOA0706201_T4.JPG.
84. L. Tavazzi *et al.*, "Effect of rosuvastatin in patients with chronic heart failure (the GISSI-HF trial): A randomised, double-blind, placebo-controlled trial," *Lancet*, vol. 372, no. 9645, pp. 1231–1239, 2008, doi: 10.1016/S0140-6736(08)61240-4.
85. J. J. V. McMurray *et al.*, "Effects of statin therapy according to plasma high-sensitivity C-reactive protein concentration in the Controlled Rosuvastatin Multinational Trial in Heart Failure (CORONA): A retrospective analysis," *Circulation*, vol. 120, no. 22, pp. 2188–2196, Dec. 2009, doi: 10.1161/CIRCULATIONAHA.109.849117.
86. G. M. Novaro, I. Y. Tiong, G. L. Pearce, M. S. Lauer, D. L. Sprecher, and B. P. Griffin, "Effect of hydroxymethylglutaryl coenzyme a reductase inhibitors on the progression of calcific aortic stenosis," *Circulation*, vol. 104, no. 18, pp. 2205–2209, Oct. 2001, doi: 10.1161/HC4301.098249.

87. D. M. Shavelle, J. Takasu, M. J. Budoff, S. S. Mao, X. Q. Zhao, and K. D. O'Brien, "HMG CoA reductase inhibitor (statin) and aortic valve calcium," *Lancet*, vol. 359, no. 9312, pp. 1125–1126, Mar. 2002, doi: 10.1016/S0140-6736(02)08161-8.
88. S. J. Cowell *et al.*, "A randomized trial of intensive lipid-lowering therapy in calcific aortic stenosis," *N Engl J Med*, vol. 352, no. 23, pp. 2389–2397, Jun. 2005, doi: 10.1056/NEJMOA043876.
89. A. B. Rossebø *et al.*, "Intensive lipid lowering with simvastatin and ezetimibe in aortic stenosis," *N Engl J Med*, vol. 359, no. 13, pp. 1343–1356, Sep. 2008, doi: 10.1056/NEJMOA0804602.
90. D. A. Sica and T. W. B. Gehr, "Rhabdomyolysis and statin therapy: Relevance to the elderly," *Am J Geriatr Cardiol*, vol. 11, no. 1, pp. 48–55, 2002, doi: 10.1111/J.1076-7460.2002.01422.X.
91. N. C. Santanello *et al.*, "Effect of pharmacologic lipid lowering on health-related quality of life in older persons: Results from the Cholesterol Reduction in Seniors Program (CRISP) Pilot Study," *J Am Geriatr Soc*, vol. 45, no. 1, pp. 8–14, 1997, doi: 10.1111/J.1532-5415.1997.TB00971.X.
92. N. K. Wenger, S. J. Lewis, D. M. Herrington, V. Bittner, and F. K. Welty, "Outcomes of using high- or low-dose atorvastatin in patients 65 years of age or older with stable coronary heart disease," *Ann Intern Med*, vol. 147, no. 1, pp. 1–9, Jul. 2007, doi: 10.7326/0003-4819-147-1-200707030-00002.
93. I. L. Notkola *et al.*, "Serum total cholesterol, apolipoprotein E epsilon 4 allele, and Alzheimer's disease," *Neuroepidemiology*, vol. 17, no. 1, pp. 14–20, Jan. 1998, doi: 10.1159/000026149.
94. M. Kivipelto *et al.*, "Midlife vascular risk factors and late-life mild cognitive impairment: A population-based study," *Neurology*, vol. 56, no. 12, pp. 1683–1689, Jun. 2001, doi: 10.1212/WNL.56.12.1683.
95. C. Reitz, M. X. Tang, J. Luchsinger, and R. Mayeux, "Relation of plasma lipids to Alzheimer disease and vascular dementia," *Arch Neurol*, vol. 61, no. 5, pp. 705–714, May 2004, doi: 10.1001/ARCHNEUR.61.5.705.
96. D. Larry Sparks, "Coronary artery disease, hypertension, ApoE, and cholesterol: A link to Alzheimer's disease?," *Ann N Y Acad Sci*, vol. 826, pp. 128–146, 1997, doi: 10.1111/J.1749-6632.1997.TB48466.X.
97. A. Hofman *et al.*, "Atherosclerosis, apolipoprotein E, and prevalence of dementia and Alzheimer's disease in the Rotterdam Study," *Lancet*, vol. 349, no. 9046, pp. 151–154, Jan. 1997, doi: 10.1016/S0140-6736(96)09328-2.
98. B. Wolozin, W. Kellman, P. Ruosseau, G. G. Celesia, and G. Siegel, "Decreased prevalence of Alzheimer disease associated with 3-hydroxy-3-methyglutaryl coenzyme A reductase inhibitors," *Arch Neurol*, vol. 57, no. 10, pp. 1439–1443, 2000, doi: 10.1001/ARCHNEUR.57.10.1439.
99. I. Hajjar, J. Schumpert, V. Hirth, D. Wieland, and G. P. Eleazer, "The impact of the use of statins on the prevalence of dementia and the progression of cognitive impairment," *J Gerontol A Biol Sci Med Sci*, vol. 57, no. 7, 2002, doi: 10.1093/GERONA/57.7.M414.
100. K. Rockwood *et al.*, "Use of lipid-lowering agents, indication bias, and the risk of dementia in community-dwelling elderly people," *Arch Neurol*, vol. 59, no. 2, pp. 223–227, 2002, doi: 10.1001/ARCHNEUR.59.2.223.
101. K. Yaffe, E. Barrett-Connor, F. Lin, and D. Grady, "Serum lipoprotein levels, statin use, and cognitive function in older women," *Arch Neurol*, vol. 59, no. 3, pp. 378–384, 2002, doi: 10.1001/ARCHNEUR.59.3.378.
102. K. M. Dale, C. I. Coleman, N. N. Henyan, J. Kluger, and C. M. White, "Statins and cancer risk: A meta-analysis," *JAMA*, vol. 295, no. 1, pp. 74–80, Apr. 2006, doi: 10.1001/JAMA.295.1.74.
103. J. P. Sheppard, S. Singh, K. Fletcher, R. J. McManus, and J. Mant, "Impact of age and sex on primary preventive treatment for cardiovascular disease in the West Midlands, UK: Cross sectional study," *BMJ*, vol. 345, no. 7866, Jul. 2012, doi: 10.1136/BMJ.E4535.
104. D. E. Forman *et al.*, "Cardiac care for older adults. Time for a new paradigm," *J Am Coll Cardiol*, vol. 57, no. 18, pp. 1801–1810, May 2011, doi: 10.1016/J.JACC.2011.02.014.
105. A. Z. LaCroix *et al.*, "Statin use and incident frailty in women aged 65 years or older: Prospective findings from the Women's Health Initiative Observational Study," *J Gerontol A Biol Sci Med Sci*, vol. 63, no. 4, pp. 369–375, 2008, doi: 10.1093/GERONA/63.4.369.
106. S. L. Gray *et al.*, "Angiotensin-converting enzyme inhibitor and statin medication use and incident mobility limitation in community older adults. The health, aging and body composition study," *J Am Geriatr Soc*, vol. 59, no. 12, p. 2226, Dec. 2011, doi: 10.1111/J.1532-5415.2011.03721.X.
107. F. Mach *et al.*, "2019 ESC/EAS Guidelines for the management of dyslipidaemias: Lipid modification to reduce cardiovascular risk: The Task Force for the management of dyslipidaemias of the European Society of Cardiology (ESC) and European Atherosclerosis Society (EAS)," *Eur Heart J*, vol. 41, no. 1, pp. 111–188, Jan. 2020, doi: 10.1093/EURHEARTJ/EHZ455.
108. S. M. Grundy *et al.*, "2018 AHA/ACC/AACVPR/AAPA/ABC/ACPM/ADA/AGS/APhA/ASPC/NLA/PCNA Guideline on the management of blood cholesterol: A report of the American College of Cardiology/American Heart Association Task Force on Clinical Practice Guidelines," *Circulation*, vol. 139, no. 25, pp. E1082–E1143, Jun. 2019, doi: 10.1161/CIR.0000000000000625/SUPPL_FILE/WEB.

6

Diabetes mellitus and cardiovascular disease in older adults

THOMAS HORTON AND SAMUEL C. DURSO

Key points

- Diabetes is highly prevalent among older adults in the United States, affecting approximately 16.5 million individuals aged 65 years or older.
- Recent pharmacologic therapies such as glucagon-like protein-1 (GLP-1) receptor agonists and sodium-glucose cotransporter-2 (SGLT2) inhibitors have diversified treatment options and provide additional weight loss, renal, and cardioprotective benefits.
- Treatment should be tailored to the individual older adult, taking into consideration functional status, life expectancy, and what matters most.

INTRODUCTION

Diabetes mellitus is a major global health burden. In 2017 the worldwide prevalence of type 2 diabetes, the predominant form of diabetes, was estimated to be 462 million individuals, and the prevalence rate was projected to increase to 7079 individuals per 100,000 by 2030 (1). Diabetes disproportionately affects adults 65 and older, with a prevalence of over 29% or 16.5 million seniors in the United States (both diagnosed and undiagnosed) and the highest prevalence affecting non-Hispanic Black, non-Hispanic Asian, and Hispanic subgroups (2). In concert with the rising prevalence of diabetes, the cost of

DOI: 10.1201/9781003568933-6

caring for patients with diabetes is also rising. The overall cost estimate for annual diabetes-related spending in the United States in 2022 was $412.9 billion (3).

A substantial portion of this cost results from lost wages and productivity and from treating diabetes-related complications, of which cardiovascular complications are a major component (4). Diabetes confers a twofold excess risk for a wide range of macrovascular diseases, including coronary artery disease (CAD), ischemic stroke, hemorrhagic stroke, and peripheral vascular disease (5). Cardiovascular complications are associated with both increased morbidity and mortality. This is especially true for older patients, who account for more than 70% of diabetes-associated deaths (6). With the rising prevalence of diabetes mellitus in older adults, optimally preventing and treating cardiovascular complications in this patient population becomes even more critical.

CLINICAL GUIDELINES FOR MANAGEMENT OF DIABETES IN OLDER ADULTS

Care and consideration need to be taken when applying clinical guidelines for diabetes to older patients. The American Geriatrics Society (AGS) guidelines seek to recognize that older patients have marked functional and medical heterogeneity that can alter their potential treatment benefits (7).

The use of a patient-centered care plan for older adults with diabetes has been proposed to address some of the special conditions that make this population unique (8). An initial step includes considering a patient's life expectancy in the presence or absence of unusually good or poor health and function, which may help the clinician and patient assess the benefits and risks of different therapeutic choices over time. A second step includes establishing the patient's preferences and goals of care. Some older patients will prioritize independence and the ability to perform activities of daily living over longevity. Furthermore, some will view intensive insulin therapy or use of multiple medications to achieve glycemic targets as a burden that interferes with their preferred lifestyle.

Evaluating and managing comorbid geriatric syndromes are important. The AGS guidelines recommend that older patients with diabetes be screened for depression within 3 months of diagnosis and again if there is an unexplained decline in clinical status. This recognizes the increased prevalence of depression in older patients and its potential negative effect on diabetes care. Similarly, screening for cognitive impairment is recommended soon after the diagnosis of diabetes and again if a decline in health status occurs. Polypharmacy is a frequent problem for older patients with multiple medical problems and drug-drug interactions must be considered. Diabetes is associated with a higher prevalence of other common geriatric syndromes such as incontinence, falls, and persistent pain that may affect treatment outcomes and goals of care (7). Diabetes and insulin resistance are also associated with frailty, a geriatric syndrome of physiological vulnerability to stressors associated with adverse outcomes such as disability, hospitalization, and death (9–14). Evidence suggests that older individuals with severe hyperglycemia and/or insulin resistance are more likely to develop frailty up to a decade later (10, 15).

The 4Ms Framework of Age-Friendly Health Systems (What Matters, Medication, Mentation, and Mobility) is useful for gauging the intensity of therapy for glycemic control and other cardiovascular risk factors. For active, highly functioning older patients with few comorbidities and a life expectancy of greater than 10 years, motivation to achieve a hemoglobin A1C of 7%–7.5% may be appropriate. For patients with intermediate or complex health and variable life expectancy and those receiving palliative and end-of-life care, relaxed intensity that focuses on preventing therapeutic burden and harm from hypoglycemia and hyperglycemia is appropriate (16).

PATHOPHYSIOLOGY OF DIABETES MELLITUS AND INSULIN RESISTANCE

Diabetes mellitus is classified as type 1 (formerly called juvenile-onset or insulin-dependent diabetes mellitus) and type 2 (formerly called adult-onset or noninsulin-dependent diabetes mellitus).

Type 1 diabetes mellitus

Type 1 diabetes accounts for 5%–10% of all patients with diabetes. It results from a cell-mediated autoimmune destruction of the β-cells of the pancreas. The disease has a strong HLA association with linkage to the DQA and DQB genes. The immune-mediated process generally occurs in childhood and adolescence but can occur as late as the eighth decade of life. Patients with type 1 diabetes are at risk for other autoimmune diseases such as Addison's disease, Graves' disease, Hashimoto's thyroiditis, celiac sprue, vitiligo, and pernicious anemia (17).

Type 2 diabetes mellitus

Type 2 diabetes accounts for 90%–95% of all patients with diabetes. The pathogenesis of type 2 diabetes is multifactorial. Environmental factors such as diet, obesity, visceral fat, and sedentary lifestyle play a key role. There is also a strong genetic predisposition, with first-degree family members (children, siblings) having up to a six times increased risk for developing type 2 diabetes compared to those with a negative family history (18, 19). However, the genetic factors are complex and not clearly defined. Type 2 diabetes results from a combination of insulin resistance (worsened by obesity and sedentary lifestyle) and relative insulin deficiency. Unlike type 1 diabetes, there is no pancreatic β-cell destruction, and patients with type 2 diabetes do not require insulin therapy to survive (at least not initially). Over time, and with increasing insulin resistance, β-cell function worsens and can no longer compensate in many patients. This leads to relative insulin deficiency and ultimately requires exogenous insulin therapy. Ketoacidosis rarely occurs in this type of diabetes, which may go undiagnosed for many years because hyperglycemia develops gradually (17).

COMPLICATIONS OF DIABETES MELLITUS

Pathophysiologic changes

The complications of diabetes mellitus have been traditionally divided into two major categories: (i) microvascular complications including retinopathy, neuropathy, and nephropathy; and (ii) macrovascular complications including CAD, cerebrovascular disease, and peripheral vascular disease.

Microvascular complications

Diabetic microvascular complications lead to significant morbidity and cost. Diabetes mellitus is the leading cause of chronic kidney disease and can lead to the need for dialysis. Diabetic retinopathy is a leading cause of potentially reversible blindness. Further, diabetic neuropathy can lead to chronic pain, infections, and limb loss in severe cases. However, the risk of microvascular complications can be reduced with good diabetic care.

The Diabetes Control and Complications Trial (DCCT) demonstrated a delay in the onset and progression of diabetic neuropathy, retinopathy, and nephropathy by up to 70% with intensive treatment of type 1 diabetes (20). The United Kingdom Prospective Diabetes Study (UKPDS) evaluated intensive blood glucose control in patients with new-onset type 2 diabetes (21). The intensive blood glucose control group in UKPDS achieved a mean glycosylated hemoglobin of 7%, compared to the standard therapy group value of 7.9%, and showed a reduction in the risk of microvascular complications, principally through a reduction in incident photocoagulation of retinopathy and in reduction of progression to albuminuria (22, 23). An important limitation of both the DCCT and UKPDS studies is that older persons with diabetes were excluded, which some authors argue limits the generalizability of these findings to the older adult population (24).

Macrovascular complications

Diabetes mellitus is associated with atherosclerosis, which is related to the presence of chronic hyperglycemia, insulin resistance, and dyslipidemia. Both hyperglycemia and insulin resistance impair endothelium-dependent vasodilation by decreasing nitric oxide formation (25). Increased levels of endothelin-1 in patients with diabetes stimulate vasoconstriction, induce vascular smooth muscle hypertrophy, and activate the renin–angiotensin system (26). Diabetes promotes the accumulation of foam cells in the subendothelial space by increasing the production of leukocyte adhesion molecules and proinflammatory mediators (27). Plaque instability and rupture are increased in diabetes due to decreased synthesis and increased breakdown of the collagen that plays a critical role in reinforcing the fibrous cap of vulnerable plaques (28, 29).

In addition to the atherosclerotic effects of diabetes upon the arterial wall, the hematologic system is adversely affected. Diabetes promotes platelet activation by increasing platelet-surface expression of glycoprotein Ib that mediates binding to the glycoprotein IIb/IIIa (GPIIb/IIIa) receptor and to the von Willebrand factor (30). Inhibitors of platelet activity, including platelet-derived nitric oxide and endothelial prostacyclin, are decreased in diabetes. Diabetes also increases coagulation activity by stimulating production of procoagulants such as tissue factor and by reducing levels of anticoagulants such as protein C and antithrombin III (31, 32). Furthermore, decreased levels of plasminogen activator type 1 in diabetes result in impaired fibrinolysis (33).

The clinical consequences of these blood vessel changes are an increase in the incidence of atherosclerotic disease in the form of CAD, stroke, and peripheral vascular disease. Despite the risk associated with hyperglycemia, the benefit of intensive glucose control in reducing macrovascular events has not been proven. Neither DCCT nor UKPDS demonstrated a significant reduction in macrovascular events at the time of their reports. However, long-term follow-up of these cohorts has provided data on macrovascular outcomes.

The DCCT/Epidemiology of Diabetes Interventions and Complications Study (EDICS) was an observational study that followed participants from the initial DCCT (34). After a mean of 6.5 years of intensive versus standard glucose control during the DCCT, the standard glucose control group participants were offered intensive treatment, and all participants returned to their own health care providers. The difference in hemoglobin A1C dissipated in the 11 years of follow-up to 8% in the earlier intensively treated group and 8.2% in the previous standard treatment group. During follow-up, there was a significant 42% relative risk reduction of any cardiovascular disease event in the intensively treated group. The mean age of participants at follow-up was 45 years.

Similar reductions in cardiovascular complications were seen in the 10-year follow-up of the UKPDS (35). One year after the original UKPDS was completed, the hemoglobin A1C differences between the intensively treated and conventional therapy groups had dissipated. At 10-year follow-up, the intensively treated insulin/sulfonylurea arm had a significant 15% relative risk reduction for myocardial infarction (MI) compared to the conventional treatment group. A significant 33% relative risk reduction of MI was found in the intensively treated metformin arm compared to the conventional treatment group. Of note, the mean age of participants in the UKPDS follow-up study was 63 years.

GLYCEMIC CONTROL FOR MACROVASCULAR AND MICROVASCULAR RISK REDUCTION

Long-term data from the DCCT and UKPDS suggest that intensive glycemic control, for at least some period, may lower the risk of diabetic-related cardiovascular disease events. Additionally, epidemiologic data and meta-analyses showed a direct relationship between hemoglobin A1C and cardiovascular disease (36, 37). Three clinical trials (ACCORD, ADVANCE, and VADT) were undertaken to prospectively study the impact of intensive glycemic control in type 2 diabetes on reducing cardiovascular events (Table 6.1). In contrast to the older studies, these newer trials did not exclude older persons with diabetes.

The Action to Control Cardiovascular Risk in Diabetes (ACCORD) study investigated 10,252 older patients with type 2 diabetes (mean age 62 years) (38). These patients were at high risk for cardiovascular disease with 35% having a history of previous cardiovascular events, and the remaining patients having at least two cardiovascular risk factors. Study participants had a history of type 2 diabetes for a mean of 10 years and a mean baseline hemoglobin A1C of 8.2%. They were randomized to an intensive glycemic control group targeting an A1C of <6% or a standard glycemic control group targeting an A1C of 7%–7.9%. At 1 year, the intensive glycemic control group achieved a hemoglobin A1C of 6.4% compared to 7.5% in the standard glycemic control group. The study was halted at a mean of 3.5 years of follow-up due to the finding of overall increased mortality in the intensively treated group. At the time the study was stopped, the primary composite outcome (nonfatal MI, nonfatal stroke, or death from cardiovascular cause) occurred in similar numbers in both groups. However, the overall number of deaths was significantly higher in the intensively treated group compared to the standard glycemic control group (257 deaths intensive group vs. 203 deaths standard care group, hazard ratio, 1.22; 95% confidence interval [CI] 1.01–1.46; $p = 0.04$). As expected, episodes of hypoglycemia were more common in the intensively treated group. Unrecognized and untreated hypoglycemia and its sequelae have been proposed as a potential mechanism to explain the excess mortality. A follow-up to the ACCORD study reported findings of 5 years from randomization (39). After the study was halted, the intensive and standard glycemic control groups reached similar hemoglobin A1C values and had similar frequencies of hypoglycemia. However, the finding of increased overall mortality in the intensive glycemic control group persisted through this follow-up period.

Similarly, the Veterans Affairs Diabetes Trial (VADT) was designed to evaluate intensive versus standard glycemic control on cardiovascular events in type 2 diabetes (40). The study population was 1791 predominantly older men (mean age 60.4 years) with significant cardiovascular risk (40% already had a cardiovascular event). The intensive glycemic control group achieved a hemoglobin

Table 6.1 Findings from clinical trials investigating the benefits of intensive glycemic control in older adults

	ACCORD	ADVANCE	VADT
Mean age (years)	62	66	60
Duration of diabetes (years)	10	8	11.5
History of CVD	35%	32%	40%
Median baseline A1C	8.1%	7.2%	9.4%
Median duration of follow-up (years)	3.5 (terminated early)	5	5.6
Achieved median A1C intensive versus standard	6.4% vs. 7.5%	6.3% vs. 7.0%	6.9% vs. 8.5%
Definition of primary outcome	Nonfatal MI, nonfatal stroke, CVD death	Microvascular plus macrovascular (nonfatal MI, nonfatal stroke, CVD death) outcomes	Nonfatal MI, nonfatal stroke, CVD death, hospitalization for heart failure, revascularization
HR for primary outcome (95% CI)	0.90 (0.78–1.04)	0.9 (0.82–0.98); macrovascular 0.94 (0.84–1.06)	0.88 (0.74–1.05)
HR for mortality findings (95% CI)	1.22 (1.01–1.46)	0.93 (0.83–1.06)	1.07 (0.81–1.42)

Abbreviations: CVD, cardiovascular disease; A1C, hemoglobin A1C; MI, myocardial infarction; HR, hazard ratio; CI, confidence interval.
Source: Skyler JS et al., *J Am Coll Cardiol*, 53, 298–304, 2009.

A1C of 6.9% compared to 8.4% in the standard glycemic control group. After a mean of 5.6 years of follow-up, there was no difference in cardiovascular events between the groups. Unlike the ACCORD study, no difference in overall mortality was seen. There were 95 deaths in the standard glycemic control group compared to 102 in the intensive therapy group (hazard ratio, 1.07; 95% CI 0.81–1.42; $p = 0.62$).

The Action in Diabetes and Vascular Disease (ADVANCE) study looked at a similar population of 11,140 patients with type 2 diabetes (41). Study participants were older (mean age 66 years) with a mean baseline hemoglobin A1C of 7.2%. One third of the population had a history of vascular disease at baseline with the remaining two thirds having multiple risk factors. Patients were randomized to intensive glycemic control or standard glycemic control. The groups achieved mean hemoglobin A1Cs of 6.5% and 7.3%, respectively. After a mean follow-up of 5 years, there was no difference between the two groups in the rate of macrovascular events or death from cardiovascular causes. Like the VADT, there was no difference in overall mortality between the intensive and standard glycemic control groups. A total of 1031 deaths occurred, including 8.9% in the intensive control group and 9.6% in the standard control group (hazard ratio, 0.93; 95% CI 0.83–1.06; $p = 0.28$).

Given the findings of the ACCORD, VADT, and ADVANCE studies, the clinical practice of intensive glycemic control for the prevention of cardiovascular disease in type 2 diabetes has been debated. The American Diabetes Association (ADA), American College of Cardiology, and American Heart Association published a joint statement on this topic (42). Subset analyses of ACCORD, VADT, and ADVANCE suggest that patients with a shorter duration of type 2 diabetes and without a history of cardiovascular disease might gain greatest benefit in macrovascular disease risk reduction from intensive control. Alternatively, the risks of intensive glycemic control (hypoglycemia in particular) may outweigh benefits in patients with a long-standing history of diabetes, frequent hypoglycemia, advanced cardiovascular disease, or older age. Recent recommendations from the ADA recognize that the decision to achieve intensive control is not always clear (43). The guidelines recommend achieving a hemoglobin A1C <7% in adults to reduce microvascular complications and particularly in patients recently diagnosed due to the association with long-term reduction in macrovascular disease. A less stringent hemoglobin A1C goal of <8% may be appropriate for patients with a history of severe hypoglycemia, advanced microvascular or macrovascular complications, or with limited life expectancy. Findings from trials suggest that too aggressive glucose control (i.e., <6%) may not be beneficial and may be harmful.

VASCULAR CONSEQUENCES OF DIABETES MELLITUS

Coronary artery disease

The Framingham study demonstrated that diabetes is a powerful predictor of CAD (44). The older patient with diabetes is at particularly high risk for CAD; in one study 44% of octogenarians with diabetes were found to have CAD (45).

Many patients with diabetes have CAD that is not clinically apparent. This was demonstrated in a population-based autopsy series that characterized coronary atherosclerosis in 293 persons with diabetes (mean age 73 years), without clinically known CAD. Nearly 75% had high-grade coronary atherosclerosis and more than half had multivessel disease (46). In addition to clinically undiagnosed CAD, there is an increased prevalence of silent ischemia and unrecognized MI with diabetes. In a French study, the prevalence of silent ischemia was found to be approximately 30% in men with type 2 diabetes and established CAD, while the prevalence in patients without diabetes was 1%–4% (47). Specifically looking at older patients, the Framingham epidemiological study reported an increased incidence of asymptomatic MI in this population (48). A study by Aronow and Epstein demonstrated silent ischemia through Holter monitoring in about one third of older patients (49). Given the high prevalence of silent ischemia in older adults and in diabetes, older patients with diabetes present a particularly high-risk population for silent ischemia.

Currently, the ADA recommends against routine screening for CAD in asymptomatic patients. Screening has not been shown to improve outcomes in patients who are already being treated with optimized cardiovascular risk factor modifications. Furthermore, the coronary artery calcium (CAC) score measurement is not recommended for patients already on statin therapy, as statins can increase the CAC score despite reducing overall coronary atherosclerosis volume and high-risk plaque features (43, 50). However, older adults with diabetes are a heterogeneous group with respect to ASCVD risk, and a CAC score can enhance risk assessment. A minority of older diabetic patients will have a CAC score of 0 and few additional risks for ASCVD (e.g., long duration of diabetes, albuminuria, chronic kidney disease, retinopathy, neuropathy, or abnormal ankle-brachial index), leading to reclassification as lower risk, while those with elevated CAC burden may benefit from additional pharmacological therapy. In these individuals, a CAC score may increase willingness to take or intensify medication and adhere to lifestyle changes (51).

Acute coronary syndromes

MI rates are increased among people of all ages with diabetes (52). For example, in a population-based study, the 7-year incidence of first MI was 20% for type 2 diabetes but only 3.5% for people without diabetes (53). Short- and long-term outcomes following MI are worsened in patients with diabetes (54). The Framingham study determined that the overall risk of cardiac mortality, particularly post-MI, was two to three times higher in people with diabetes compared to those without diabetes.

The explanation for the worse prognosis among people with diabetes is not entirely clear. Diabetes is associated with complicated metabolic changes and alterations in coagulation parameters that may predispose to worse outcomes (55). People with diabetes tend to have fewer collateral vessels compared to those without diabetes and may have more diffuse coronary disease (56).

Stroke

The Framingham study and others have demonstrated that the risk of stroke is increased 1.5–4 times for patients with diabetes (57). Hypertension, a frequent comorbidity with diabetes, additionally increases the risk for stroke. A Finnish study prospectively followed nearly 50,000 patients without a history of stroke or CAD for incident stroke over a mean follow-up of 19 years (58). The hazard ratio for stroke was 1.98 for patients with stage II hypertension, 2.54 for patients with diabetes, and 4.50 for patients with both stage II hypertension and diabetes. Like post-MI prognosis, diabetes is also associated with a worse prognosis after stroke. In the same Finnish study, the hazard ratio for stroke mortality was 3.06 for patients with diabetes. This hazard ratio climbed to 9.27 in patients with both diabetes and stage II hypertension.

HEART FAILURE AND LEFT VENTRICULAR DYSFUNCTION

The importance of diabetes as a risk factor for heart failure (HF) was first established in the Framingham Heart Study. Among participants between the ages of 45 and 75 years, the frequency of HF was increased in both men and women with diabetes (59). Approximately 15%–25% of HF patients in large clinical trials and up to 30% of hospitalized HF patients have diabetes as a comorbid condition (60, 61). Traditional risk factors for HF, i.e., hypertension and CAD, have a high prevalence among patients with diabetes. However, even people with diabetes who lack these other traditional risk factors have a higher incidence of HF.

The term "diabetic cardiomyopathy" is defined as ventricular dysfunction occurring independently of a recognized cause such as CAD or hypertension (62). In a large cohort of American Indians, the Strong Heart Study demonstrated structural changes that a patient with diabetes may experience. Patients with diabetes had higher left ventricular mass, wall thickness, and arterial stiffness compared to patients without diabetes. These findings were independent of body mass index or blood pressure (63). Additionally, a large epidemiological study involving over 800,000 patients showed diabetes to be independently associated with the occurrence of HF after adjusting for left ventricular hypertrophy, hypertension, CAD, and atrial fibrillation (64).

Guideline-recommended therapies for HF used in patients without diabetes are appropriate for patients with diabetes. This includes angiotensin-converting enzyme (ACE) inhibitors, β-blockers, mineralocorticoid antagonists (MRA), and sodium-glucose cotransporter-2 inhibitors (SGLT2i) in appropriately selected patients (62). Additionally, glycemic control is a potential therapeutic avenue to prevent and treat HF. For each 1% elevation in hemoglobin A1C, the risk of developing HF increases by 8% (65). Early in the development of cardiomyopathy, good glycemic control can improve diastolic function and myocardial perfusion (66).

PERIPHERAL ARTERIAL DISEASE

Peripheral arterial disease (PAD) is common among patients with diabetes. The Hoorn Study found the prevalence of an ankle-brachial index <0.9 in patients with normal glucose tolerance to be 7% compared to 20.9% in patients with diabetes (67). PAD presents at an earlier age and progresses more rapidly in patients with diabetes compared to patients without diabetes. Patients with diabetes may not be offered revascularization procedures as readily as those without diabetes, and when they do undergo procedures, they tend to have a poorer prognosis and a higher risk of undergoing amputation (68). PAD may also go largely undiagnosed and untreated in diabetes until the late stages. This is due to a potential lack of claudication symptoms, which can be masked by diabetic neuropathy and decreased mobility in some older adults. One of the most important risk factors for PAD in patients with diabetes is increasing age. This has been correlated with PAD in both type 1 and type 2 diabetes (69).

Treatment and management of PAD in diabetes is similar to treatment in the non-diabetes population. Hallmarks of therapy should include lifestyle and risk factor modification. Smoking cessation, blood pressure control, and treatment of dyslipidemia have all been shown to be effective therapies. Tight glycemic control has been investigated as a potential therapeutic intervention but has not been conclusively shown to lower the risk of PAD (35). Antiplatelet therapy with aspirin or clopidogrel is usually indicated. The COMPASS trial demonstrated benefit in the use of low-dose rivaroxaban and aspirin compared to aspirin alone in patients with stable CAD and PAD. There was a reduction in major adverse cardiovascular events in the experimental group, however, with an increased incidence of bleeding (70). Regular walking to the point of calf discomfort is the primary treatment for symptomatic claudication. Cilostazol is also effective in reducing symptoms, either alone or in combination with walking. Finally, revascularization such as stenting or bypass grafting should be considered for disabling claudication or critical limb ischemia (69).

MANAGEMENT OF ACUTE CORONARY SYNDROMES IN PATIENTS WITH DIABETES MELLITUS

Few studies have specifically addressed the impact of modern medical therapies for acute coronary syndromes (ACS) in patients with diabetes. Subgroup analyses of several clinical trials, however, suggest a consistent beneficial effect of current therapies in this population. The management of ACS is similar for older patients with and without diabetes, with a few caveats, as noted later. Three key issues will be considered here: (i) optimal reperfusion therapy for ST-elevation MI (STEMI), (ii) early invasive versus early conservative management of unstable angina and non-ST-elevation MI (UA/NSTEMI), and (iii) adjunctive antiplatelet pharmacotherapy and its applicability to older patients with diabetes and ACS.

REPERFUSION THERAPY FOR STEMI

Thrombolytic therapy

Thrombolytic therapy (TT) for STEMI has been shown to be equally or more beneficial in patients with diabetes compared to those without diabetes. The Fibrinolytic Therapy Trialists (FTT) overview found a statistically greater mortality benefit in the diabetes group: 37 lives saved per 1000 treated patients with diabetes compared with 15 lives saved per 1000 treated patients without diabetes (71). Concerns about possible TT-related increased ocular hemorrhagic complications because of underlying diabetic retinopathy have not been substantiated (72). The beneficial effects of TT in patients >75 years of age are uncertain with conflicting results showing potential benefit and harm in this population (71, 73, 74). However, it is notable that the STREAM Trial, a prospective study designed to examine the safety/efficacy of pre-hospitalization fibrinolysis before percutaneous coronary intervention (PCI), found that individuals over age 75 who received a weight-adjusted reduction in dose of the fibrinolytic drug tenecteplase experienced no intracranial hemorrhage (ICH) or stroke, while achieving a high rate of pre-PCI coronary patency (75). This suggests that safety and efficacy may be achieved by protocols that utilize age-appropriate dose adjustment of fibrinolytic drugs.

Primary percutaneous coronary intervention

Acute success rates with primary PCI are comparable in the presence or absence of diabetes, although restenosis and long-term mortality rates may be higher in patients with diabetes (76, 77). An observational study comparing early and late outcomes of PCI and TT in patients with diabetes and STEMI concluded that PCI was associated with reduced early and late adverse outcomes relative to TT (78). However, mortality was similar in both groups. In this study, over one third of the patients were 65 years or older.

MANAGEMENT OF UA/NSTEMI

Beginning with the Thrombolysis in MI (TIMI) III study of early invasive versus early conservative management of UA, subgroup analyses of several randomized controlled trials have demonstrated a consistent, modest benefit of early invasive therapy in older patients (aged >65 years) and in patients with diabetes. In the Fast Revascularization During Instability in Coronary Artery Disease (FRISC) II trial, reduction in the composite endpoint of death and nonfatal MI among those assigned to the early invasive group resulted entirely from the benefit realized by the subgroup over age 65 (79). The TIMI 18 study compared outcomes of ACS patients treated with an early invasive strategy or a more conservative strategy of catheterization only if the patient demonstrated ischemia. Although no clear survival benefit was demonstrated, subgroup analysis showed that both patients over age 65 and patients with diabetes assigned to the early invasive strategy realized significant risk reductions in the composite primary endpoint of death, nonfatal MI, and rehospitalization for an ACS at 6 months (80).

Adjunctive antiplatelet therapies in ACS

The beneficial effects of aspirin in ACS have been conclusively demonstrated in many studies. Several studies have shown that patients with either type 1 or type 2 diabetes mellitus have a prothrombotic state, including enhanced platelet aggregation in response to various stimuli (81, 82), and that agents that inhibit platelet aggregation in vivo consistently reduce the incidence of thrombotic events.

Platelet aggregation is enhanced in patients with diabetes, and GPIIb/IIIa inhibitors given in addition to aspirin have been shown to improve outcomes in UA/NSTEMI. These agents have been shown to be particularly effective in patients with diabetes, likely owing to the enhanced platelet aggregation of this population. Clopidogrel was shown in the Clopidogrel in Unstable Angina to Prevent Recurrent Ischemic Events (CURE) trial to improve long-term outcomes when administered for 3–9 months to patients with UA/NSTEMI who did not undergo PCI (83).

Improved outcomes were demonstrated in patients over the age of 65 years and in patients with diabetes.

MANAGEMENT OF CHRONIC CORONARY DISEASE

Medical therapy versus revascularization

All patients with diabetes and chronic ischemia are recommended to receive maximal medical therapy. However, controversy exists regarding if and when revascularization should be performed in these patients. In high-risk patients with severe angina, early revascularization has been shown to be beneficial (84). Appropriate management of patients with less severe disease is not as clear. The Clinical Outcomes Utilizing Revascularization and Aggressive Drug Evaluation (COURAGE) trial showed that in patients with stable CAD, initial management by PCI did not improve outcomes when added to optimal medical therapy (85). These results were similar in prespecified subgroups of patients with and without diabetes. The Bypass Angioplasty Revascularization Investigation 2 Diabetes (BARI 2D) study was designed in part to help answer the question of if and when to revascularize, specifically in patients with diabetes. BARI 2D enrolled patients with type 2 diabetes who had documented coronary ischemia and at least one significant angiographic stenosis (86). Participants were evaluated prior to randomization by a local cardiologist to determine if they could be managed by initial medical therapy alone or by revascularization plus medical therapy. This led to the exclusion of patients with severe unstable angina or left main disease with left ventricular dysfunction that required immediate revascularization and for whom medical therapy alone was not an option. Once enrolled in the study and randomized, cardiologists selected the most appropriate revascularization method, either PCI or coronary artery bypass grafting (CABG), based on clinical and angiographic features for the group randomized to medical therapy plus revascularization. Comparing the medical therapy and medical therapy/revascularization groups, 5-year mortality (12% vs. 12%, $p = 0.97$) and cardiovascular event rates (23% vs. 24%, $p = 0.70$) were similar. The findings in type 2 diabetes patients were similar to the overall results from the COURAGE trial where early revascularization was not better than intensive medical management. The ISCHEMIA trial showed that in patients with stable coronary artery disease with moderate to severe reversible ischemia, early revascularization (PCI/CABG) did not provide significant benefit over medical therapy alone with respect to the primary outcome of cardiovascular death, MI, or hospitalization for cardiovascular causes (87). Results were similar in patients with or without diabetes.

Revascularization: CABG versus PCI

Revascularization may be necessary for the management of patients with diabetes and high-risk coronary anatomy or severe angina. Debate exists over which type of revascularization, CABG versus PCI, should be utilized in treating these patients.

The original BARI study provided guidance to this important clinical question. The study randomly assigned 1829 patients (most with unstable angina and multivessel disease) to CABG or PCI. In 1996, this trial reported no overall difference in the rates of death and MI when comparing the two treatment arms (88). However, in the diabetes subgroup analysis, there was a better 5.4-year survival with CABG versus PCI (76% vs. 56%; $p = 0.0011$). This was due to reduced cardiac mortality with CABG versus PCI (5.8% vs. 20.6%, $p = 0.0003$). The beneficial findings from CABG were largely confined to patients who received at least one internal mammary artery graft (89). The improved survival among patients with diabetes treated with CABG persisted at 10-year follow-up (CABG 57.8% vs. PCI 45.5%, $p = 0.025$) (90).

Two studies have reported initial 1-year outcome data comparing CABG versus PCI in diabetes.

The Coronary Artery Revascularization in Diabetes (CARDia) study randomized 510 patients with diabetes and multivessel or complex single-vessel CAD to CABG or PCI (91). At 1 year, the composite rates for death, stroke, or MI were similar in the CABG versus PCI groups (10.5% vs. 13%, $p = 0.39$). However, the PCI group experienced a higher rate of late MI (1.2% CABG vs. 5.5% PCI, $p = 0.016$) and a higher rate of revascularization at 1 year (2% CABG vs. 11.8% PCI, $p < 0.001$). The Synergy between Percutaneous Coronary Intervention with Taxus and Cardiac Surgery (SYNTAX) study compared 1-year outcomes among CABG and PCI (with paclitaxel stents) in 1800 patients (92). These patients had complex left main or three-vessel disease. There was a mix of patients with and without diabetes. In a subgroup analysis of the 452 patients with diabetes, the composite endpoint of death, stroke, and MI at 1 year was comparable between the CABG- and PCI-treated groups. Even though the groups were similar for the composite endpoint, the PCI group had a higher 1-year major adverse cardiac and cerebrovascular event rate (26% PCI vs. 14% CABG, $p = 0.003$). This was driven by an increased rate of repeat revascularization with PCI compared to CABG (20.3% PCI vs. 6.4% CABG, $p < 0.001$).

Based on current evidence, management of chronic coronary disease in diabetic patients for whom revascularization is likely to improve survival, CABG is preferred over PCI, particularly if left internal mammary artery to left anterior descending coronary anastomosis is feasible (93).

MEDICAL THERAPY FOR CARDIOVASCULAR DISEASE

Aspirin for primary prevention

Aspirin has previously been shown to have beneficial effects for the primary prevention of cardiovascular disease among the general population. The Antithrombotic Trialists' (ATT) Collaboration meta-analysis (94), which included over 95,000 patients, demonstrated a 12% reduction in risk of vascular events (relative risk 0.88, 95% CI 0.82–0.94). The ATT meta-analysis included only a modest number of patients with diabetes (~4000), but risk reduction was similar for both diabetic and nondiabetic patients. Conversely, two randomized placebo-controlled trials examined the role of aspirin for primary prevention of cardiovascular disease in patients with diabetes (95, 96), but neither trial demonstrated an overall benefit for preventing CAD or stroke.

Aspirin is no longer routinely recommended as primary prevention in older adults with or without diabetes based on findings from the ARRIVE, ASCEND, and ASPREE trials. The ARRIVE trial enrolled adults with moderate cardiovascular risk but, notably, excluded individuals with diabetes (97). Results showed that low-dose aspirin (100 mg) did not reduce major cardiovascular events but did increase bleeding compared to placebo. In the ASCEND trial, adults with diabetes without established cardiovascular disease were randomized to either aspirin versus placebo or omega-3 fatty acid supplementation versus placebo (98). In the aspirin group, there was modest reduction in vascular events (8.5% vs. 9.6%) but with increased major bleeding (4.1% vs. 3.2%). Supplementation with omega-3 fatty acids did not significantly reduce the risk of serious vascular events compared to placebo. The ASPREE trial focused on healthy older adults aged ≥70 years (≥65 years for Hispanic and Black participants) without known cardiovascular disease (99). Findings revealed no reduction in cardiovascular events or improvement in disease-free survival with aspirin, but there was a significant increase in major bleeding and all-cause mortality.

The AHA, ACC, and US Preventive Services Task Force have updated their guidelines to reflect the most recent data and do not recommend aspirin for primary prevention in the majority of adults ≥60 years of age. In addition, aspirin is listed on the updated Beers criteria as a potentially inappropriate medication.

Hypertension and diabetes mellitus

Patients with diabetes have an increased prevalence of hypertension and, conversely, hypertensive patients have an increased incidence of impaired glucose tolerance and demonstrate increased insulin release following an oral glucose load (43,100). More than 7 million people in the United States have both hypertension and diabetes, and the association between these risk factors and cardiovascular disease becomes stronger with advancing age. Epidemiological studies have demonstrated that hypertension increases the risk of atherosclerotic vascular disease in patients with diabetes more than in patients without diabetes. The Systolic Hypertension in the Elderly Program (SHEP) found almost twofold increases in the 5-year rates of major cardiovascular events, coronary events, and strokes among patients with versus without diabetes in the placebo group (101). Randomized controlled trials have shown benefit with reduction in cardiovascular events, stroke, and nephropathy with treatment of hypertension in older patients with and without diabetes (102, 103).

Because of the high prevalence, increased morbidity, and apparent benefits of treatment, patients with diabetes should be carefully screened and treated for hypertension. The ADA recommends that blood pressure be measured at every clinic visit. A goal of <130/80 is appropriate for most older diabetics if it can be achieved without side effects or undue burden (43). Lifestyle modifications such as exercise, weight loss, treatment of obstructive sleep apnea, and the Dietary Approach to Stop Hypertension (DASH) diet may be effective for patients in the elevated or stage 1 hypertension range (120–139). Most patients with blood pressures ≥140/90 require drug therapy, and the majority require multidrug therapy to achieve adequate control. Drug therapy regimens often include ACE inhibitors or angiotensin II receptor blockers (ARBs). The Heart Outcomes Prevention Evaluation (HOPE) trial investigated the effect of ramipril versus placebo in 9297 high-risk patients 55 years or older with evidence of vascular disease or diabetes plus one other cardiovascular risk factor (104). Patients with diabetes made up 38% and 39% of the treatment and placebo groups, respectively. Ramipril was found to significantly reduce the rate of MI, stroke, or death from cardiovascular causes compared to placebo. The beneficial effects of ramipril were consistently observed in patients with or without diabetes. In patients unable to tolerate ACE inhibitors due to cough, ARBs are an appropriate substitute. Like ACE inhibitors, ARBs provide protection from diabetic nephropathy. The Ongoing Telmisartan Alone and in Combination with Ramipril Trial (ONTARGET) evaluated a high-risk patient population with underlying vascular disease or diabetes with end organ damage that was similar to the HOPE trial population (105). The effects of telmisartan versus ramipril versus combination telmisartan/ramipril were compared. The impact of therapy on patients with diabetes was not a primary outcome in ONTARGET, but of the 25,620 individuals enrolled in the study, 38% (n = 9612) had diabetes. In the overall population, the primary endpoint of cardiovascular death, MI, stroke, or hospitalization for HF was reached by 1412 patients in the ramipril group (16.5%), compared with 1423 patients in the telmisartan group (16.7%; risk ratio: 1.01; 95% CI 0.94–1.09). Combination therapy of ramipril and telmisartan increased the rate of the primary endpoints. These data suggest that ARBs are a viable alternative to ACE inhibitors for providing cardiovascular protection to patients with diabetes.

Other agents are also useful for treatment of hypertension in diabetes. The Antihypertensive and Lipid Lowering Treatment to Prevent Heart Attack (ALLHAT) trial included over 33,000 patients among whom over 35% had type 2 diabetes (106). This large trial compared a thiazide diuretic (chlorthalidone), calcium channel blocker (amlodipine), and ACE inhibitor (lisinopril). In general, the drugs recommended for first-line treatment of hypertension are calcium channel blockers, ACE inhibitors or angiotensin receptor blockers, and diuretics (107).

Although treating hypertension in patients with diabetes is beneficial, the degree to which blood pressure should be lowered is not clear. To explore whether more intensive blood pressure control is associated with proportionally greater cardiovascular benefits, the ACCORD Study group followed 4733 patients with type 2 diabetes at elevated risk for cardiovascular disease (108). Participants were randomized to intensive blood pressure control (target systolic <120 mmHg) or standard blood pressure control (target systolic <140 mmHg). By 1 year the intensive therapy group had achieved a systolic pressure of 119.3 mmHg compared to 133.5 mmHg in the standard therapy arm. Over a mean follow-up of 4.7 years, no difference was seen between the two groups in the rate of fatal and nonfatal cardiovascular events, but there was a significant reduction in stroke incidence. However, the intensive therapy group experienced significantly more adverse events (hypotension, hyperkalemia, and bradycardia) compared to the standard therapy group.

Recent studies conducted in China have provided new evidence that intensive BP control may be more beneficial in diabetic older adults than previously thought. The BPROAD trial (Blood Pressure Control Target in Diabetes) enrolled individuals ≥50 years of age with type 2 diabetes and systolic blood pressure (SBP) >130 mm Hg (109). Participants were randomized to either intensive blood pressure control (target SBP <120 mmHg) or standard control (target SBP <140 mmHg) and followed for a median of 4.2 years. Intensive treatment resulted in a significantly lower incidence of major cardiovascular events compared to standard treatment (HR 0.79; 95% CI 0.69–0.90; $P < 0.001$). Serious adverse events were similar between the two groups, but symptomatic hypotension and hyperkalemia were more common in the intensive treatment group.

The ESPRIT trial also studied intensive (systolic <120 mmHg) compared to standard (systolic <140 mmHg) blood pressure targets in individuals ≥50 years of age (110). Of the participants enrolled, 39% had diabetes and 27% had a prior stroke. The results were similar to BPROAD, with the intensive group having fewer major adverse cardiac events compared with the standard target group. There was no significant difference between the two groups in the serious adverse events of electrolyte abnormality, hypotension, injurious fall, or acute kidney injury. There were, however, more syncopal events in the intensive treatment group.

When treating hypertension in older patients with diabetes, consideration should be given to their increased risk of falls and potential adverse reactions to antihypertensive medications. Autonomic dysfunction is a common complication of diabetes. Cardiovascular autonomic dysfunction may be present in up to one third of patients with type 2 diabetes (111). This can manifest clinically as abnormal heart rate fluctuations with variations in peripheral vascular tone, contributing to orthostatic hypotension. As a result, antihypertensive therapy should be titrated gradually to minimize complications (112). Screening for falls and orthostasis is important before and during antihypertensive treatment. A blood pressure goal of <130/80 is reasonable for the majority of patients, while some individuals may benefit from a target of <120/80 if this can be safely attained. A meta-analysis of blood pressure control in patients with type 2 diabetes suggests that more intensive control (<130/80) in those with stage 3 or greater CKD, CVD, or CVD risk factors is associated with reductions in stroke, progression of microalbuminuria, CVD mortality, and heart failure relative to a less intensive control target (<140/90) (113).

Lipid disorders and diabetes mellitus

Patients with diabetes commonly have two lipid disorders to consider. The first is an elevated low-density lipoprotein (LDL) cholesterol level. This leads to atherogenesis and contributes to plaque rupture and acute coronary events. The second is atherogenic dyslipidemia, which is characterized by increased triglyceride levels, depressed high-density lipoprotein (HDL) levels, and normal to mildly increased LDL levels but increased levels of small, dense (easily oxidizable) LDL particles. Both these disorders are associated with progressive atherosclerosis and increased incidence of cardiovascular events (114, 115).

Multiple clinical trials have demonstrated the beneficial effects of statin therapy on CV outcomes in patients with diabetes and history of CAD and have suggested potential benefits in primary prevention for cardiovascular disease (116). The Collaborative Atorvastatin Diabetes Study evaluated the use of atorvastatin for primary prevention of cardiovascular disease in patients with type 2 diabetes. The trial was stopped 2 years early when a prespecified early stopping rule for efficacy was met. The atorvastatin-treated patients demonstrated a 37% relative risk reduction in major cardiovascular events compared to placebo. This trial and others support the use of statin therapy in patients with diabetes to lower their LDL. The use of HDL-raising therapies (specifically niacin) is less promising. A systematic review in 2007 evaluated 31 trials looking at therapies to raise HDL and found only modest evidence to support aggressively raising HDL beyond what can be achieved with lifestyle modifications alone (117). Fibrates have also been evaluated as potential therapeutic agents to treat dyslipidemia in patients with diabetes. The Fenofibrate Intervention and Event Lowering in Diabetes (FIELD) study examined the long-term use of fenofibrate in patients with type 2 diabetes. Use of fenofibrate in this population with diabetes and no statin use at entry was not associated with a reduction in overall cardiovascular outcomes (118).

Because of the high prevalence of dyslipidemia and the proven benefits of statin therapy, the ADA recommends measuring a fasting lipid profile at least annually in patients with diabetes. Lifestyle modifications that include nutritional changes (i.e., reducing saturated fats, trans fats, and cholesterol intake) and increases in physical activity should be the initial therapy for all patients with diabetes and dyslipidemia. If no contraindications exist, a high-intensity statin should be offered to patients of all ages who have diabetes and known CAD, and to those with diabetes, age 40–75 years, including those with no other CV risk factors (119, 120).

Combination statin and other lipid-lowering therapy have not been shown to be more efficacious than statin monotherapy. The ACCORD study group investigated the effect of combination statin and fenofibrate therapy in patients with type 2 diabetes (121). All patients were treated with simvastatin and then were randomized to additional placebo or fenofibrate. Combination therapy with statin and fenofibrate did not reduce the rate of fatal cardiovascular events, nonfatal MI, or nonfatal stroke when compared to the statin and placebo group. Combination statin and extended-release niacin therapy was studied in the Atherothrombosis Intervention in Metabolic Syndrome with Low HDL/High Triglycerides (AIM-HIGH) study (122). A total of 3414 patients (1158 with diabetes) who had established cardiovascular disease were treated with statins for a goal LDL <70 mg/dL. Patients were then randomized to the addition of placebo or extended-release niacin. The study was halted early when no between-group difference was seen in the primary outcome of CV events. The REDUCE-IT trial evaluated the efficacy of icosapent ethyl in reducing cardiovascular events among patients with high triglycerides already on statin therapy. In participants with diabetes, there was a 23% relative risk reduction in the primary composite endpoint compared to placebo. These findings were similar to those in participants without diabetes and to the overall trial results (123).

Several studies have shown that the addition of ezetimibe to statin therapy is associated with significant incremental reduction in LDL. The IMPROVE-IT study randomized 18,144 patients with recent ACS to simvastatin 40 mg alone or in combination with ezetimibe 10 mg daily. Combination therapy was associated with significantly lower mean LDL (53.7 mg/dL vs. 69.5 mg/dL, $p < 0.001$) and with an absolute reduction of 2.0% in the composite outcome of CV death, nonfatal MI, nonfatal stroke, hospitalization for unstable angina, or coronary revascularization over a median follow-up of 6 years (HR 0.936, 95% CI 0.89–0.99, $p = 0.016$). In subgroup analysis, the benefits of combination therapy were greater in patients age 75 or older ($N = 2798$) than in younger patients and in patients with diabetes ($N = 4933$) compared to nondiabetics. Thus, the addition of ezetimibe is an excellent option for older patients with diabetes who fail to achieve optimal reduction in LDL on statin monotherapy (124).

For older adults with diabetes and a high risk of ASCVD who have not achieved LDL targets on maximum tolerated doses of statins and ezetimibe, proprotein convertase subtilisin/kexin type 9 (PCSK9) inhibitors are a safe and effective option. PCSK9 inhibitors, such as evolocumab and alirocumab, work by increasing the number of LDL receptors on hepatocytes, which increases uptake of circulating LDL in the liver (125). The FOURIER and ODYSSEY OUTCOMES trials demonstrated that PCSK9 inhibitors significantly reduce LDL levels by 50%–60% when added to maximally tolerated statin therapy and reduce the incidence of major cardiovascular events (126, 127).

Other studies have suggested that statins, particularly at higher doses, can lead to elevations in blood glucose; however, the potential cardiovascular benefits outweigh the minimal risk of developing diabetes (128, 129). Although niacin has been shown, in short-term trials, to exacerbate insulin resistance, the glycemic response in patients with and without diabetes is usually mild. Niacin can be used safely in patients with diabetes (130). Combination therapy of statins and fibrates can also increase the risk for adverse reactions such as transaminitis, myositis, and rhabdomyolysis (130). The risk of rhabdomyolysis is higher in patients with chronic kidney disease. Given the age-related reduction in glomerular filtration rate, special consideration should be given when using combination therapy in older patients.

LIFESTYLE MODIFICATIONS

The importance of lifestyle modifications in the management of diabetes to improve glycemic control and modify cardiovascular risk factors cannot be overstated. The Diabetes Prevention Program demonstrated that in patients with prediabetes, intensive lifestyle modification with diet, exercise, and weight loss was more effective than standard care or metformin at reducing the incidence of type 2 diabetes (131). Among patients already diagnosed with type 2 diabetes, the Look Action for Health in Diabetes (Look-AHEAD) trial provided insight into the benefits of intensive lifestyle modification. This study included 5145 patients aged 45–74 years with type 2 diabetes who were also overweight. Participants were randomized to an Intense Lifestyle Intervention (ILI) group or Diabetes Support and Education (DSE) group. The ILI group participated in group and individual meetings to achieve and maintain weight loss through decreased caloric intake and increased physical activity. At 1 year, the ILI group had lost an average of 8.6% of their initial weight versus 0.7% in the DSE group ($p < 0.001$). The mean A1C in the ILI group also dropped from 7.4% to 6.6% compared to the change in the DSE group of 7.3% to 7.2% ($p < 0.001$). Accompanying these improvements in weight and glycemic control, patients in the ILI group experienced reductions in blood pressure, dyslipidemia (i.e., increased HDL and decreased triglyceride levels), and microalbuminuria (132) that persisted after 4 years of follow-up (133).

The ADA recommends that all individuals with diabetes receive individualized nutritional therapy (134). Ideally this is done by a registered dietician familiar with diabetes nutritional therapy. Weight loss is recommended for all overweight or obese individuals with type 2 diabetes. Saturated fats should be limited to <7% of total calories, and trans-fat intake should be minimized to help with LDL and HDL control. In type 2 diabetes, moderate weight loss (5% of body weight) has been associated with decreased insulin resistance, improved glycemic and lipid control, and reduced blood pressure (135).

It is recommended that patients with diabetes perform at least 150 minutes per week of moderate-intensity aerobic exercise. This should be supplemented by resistance exercises at least two to three times per week, as resistance training has been shown to exert favorable effects on insulin resistance (43). Prior to starting an exercise regimen, clinicians should assess patients with multiple cardiovascular risk factors, but the role of stress testing and other imaging modalities (e.g., coronary artery calcium scans) to screen asymptomatic patients with diabetes for CAD remains unclear (35).

TREATMENT OF DIABETES MELLITUS

The current approach to the treatment of type 2 diabetes mellitus in older adults focuses heavily on lifestyle modifications and pharmacological management that is tailored to the patient's comorbidity, functional status, and goals of care. Overtreatment resulting in increased risk of hypoglycemia is common, particularly for older adults on complex regimens with multiple coexisting conditions and functional or cognitive impairment. Older patients with diabetes are especially vulnerable to hypoglycemia during transitions of care (e.g., hospital to post-acute care). As a general principle, pharmacologic therapy that is least burdensome, carries low risk of hypoglycemia, and has demonstrated cardiovascular and renal benefit is preferred. Guidance for simplifying and deintensifying pharmacological regimens for older adults to match patient-centered goals and comorbid and functional status is available at https://doi.org/10.2337/dc25-S009 (136).

METFORMIN

Metformin is a biguanide that remains a first-line agent for those with type 2 diabetes mellitus and may be safely used for those with an estimated GFR >30 mL/min/1.73 m^2 (137). The mechanism of action is suppression of hepatic gluconeogenesis through reduction in hepatic insulin resistance, leading primarily to reduction of fasting blood glucose. Metformin can lower hemoglobin A1C by ~1.5% when used as monotherapy or in combination (138). It does not cause weight gain and may help promote mild weight loss. Hypoglycemia is rare in the absence of high circulating blood levels such as might occur with acute renal failure.

Independent of improved glycemic control, metformin has a positive effect on arterial vasculature through lowering inflammatory cytokines and improving platelet, endothelial, and hemostatic functions, and may reduce the risks of myocardial infarction and death (35). Recent studies, such as the ongoing TAME trial, are investigating metformin's potential anti-aging effects including delayed development or progression of age-related chronic diseases.

Potential drawbacks of metformin include adverse gastrointestinal effects such as diarrhea, nausea, and abdominal cramping. These reactions can be mitigated using a slow titration beginning with 500–1000 mg daily, followed by gradual increases to a target dose of 2000 mg daily (139). An extended-release formulation of metformin generally has fewer adverse effects. Lactic acidosis due to metformin is rare in patients with normal renal function (140). Current US prescribing guidelines warn against the use of metformin in patients with eGFR <30 mL/min/1.73 m^2 and recommend against starting metformin with an eGFR between 30 and 45 mL/min/1.73 m^2.

SULFONYLUREAS

The sulfonylureas have been used for the management of diabetes longer than any other oral hypoglycemic agents. The drug class has wide variability from early ("first generation") drugs like chlorpropamide to the most recent ("third generation") agents like glimepiride. Newer third-generation drugs are associated with less fasting insulin secretory stimulation and hypoglycemia compared to first-generation sulfonylureas (141). The drugs bind to receptors on the ATP-dependent potassium channel on β-cells leading to an influx of calcium which stimulates insulin secretion (142). Reductions in hemoglobin A1C of 1%–2% can be seen when using sulfonylureas as monotherapy.

The overall effect of sulfonylureas on cardiovascular risk appears to be neutral. Available data suggest no significant effects on blood pressure, lipid profiles, or coagulant factors. Concern for potential adverse cardiovascular outcomes from sulfonylureas dates to the University Group Diabetes Program in the 1970s (143). This trial was halted early when participants treated with the first-generation sulfonylurea tolbutamide were found to have excess cardiovascular mortality compared to diet alone. This finding resulted in a black box warning for sulfonylureas, noting an increased risk of cardiovascular events. Subsequent trials have not shown similar results. Notably, the UKPDS trial was able to demonstrate a reduction in all endpoints in the intensive treatment groups (sulfonylureas or insulin) compared to conventional therapy groups. Within the intensively treated group (sulfonylureas vs. insulin) there was no difference in any of the endpoints (20).

In 2006, A Diabetes Outcome Progression Trial (ADOPT) studied 4360 patients previously untreated with oral agents. Participants were randomized to glyburide, metformin, or rosiglitazone. The study was designed to evaluate a primary outcome of time to monotherapy failure. However, there were fewer serious cardiovascular events in the glyburide group compared to the rosiglitazone group (1.8% vs. 3.4%, $p < 0.05$). There was no difference in cardiovascular events comparing glyburide- and metformin-treated patients (144).

In older patients, renal and hepatic impairment can affect the clearance of sulfonylureas and lead to hypoglycemia. Poor nutritional status, anorexia, or concurrent illnesses limiting nutritional intake can commonly occur in older patients with comorbidities, making them more vulnerable to adverse side effects. Nonetheless, sulfonylureas can be useful agents in selected patients, and newer-generation sulfonylureas may be preferable in older patients who may be susceptible to hypoglycemia. However, there is conflicting evidence regarding the effects of sulfonylureas on cardiovascular outcomes.

MEGLITINIDES

Meglitinides produce an insulin secretory effect through action on the β-cell sulfonylurea receptor at a unique site from sulfonylureas. The different activation of this ATP-dependent potassium channel causes a more rapid onset of action and shorter half-life, allowing these drugs to be taken before meals to control postprandial hyperglycemia. In general, this class of medicines modestly lowers hemoglobin A1C levels 0.5%–1.0%.

For older patients with type 2 diabetes, the meglitinides may be useful agents for glycemic control. They are helpful in reducing postprandial hyperglycemia. They also offer flexibility in dosing to match a patient's dietary intake and reduce the risk of hypoglycemia that can occur with longer-acting sulfonylureas. To date, they have not been shown to reduce cardiovascular events.

α-Glucosidase inhibitors

α-Glucosidase inhibitors competitively block the action of α-glucosidase in the gut. This enzyme is important for the enzymatic breakdown of carbohydrates. This class of agents interferes with carbohydrate digestion and absorption resulting in a blunting of postprandial glucose levels. The glucose-lowering effect of α-glucosidase inhibitors is mild with hemoglobin A1C reductions of ~0.5%. Common side effects include gastrointestinal bloating, diarrhea, and flatulence.

The cardiovascular effects of α-glucosidase inhibitors were evaluated in the Study to Prevent Noninsulin-Dependent Diabetes Mellitus (STOP-NIDDM) trial. This study randomized 1429 patients with impaired glucose tolerance to placebo or acarbose 100 mg thrice daily for prevention of type 2 diabetes. A substudy assessed the development of major cardiovascular events and hypertension. Acarbose was associated with a 49% relative risk reduction (hazard ratio 0.51; 95% CI 0.28–0.95; $p = 0.03$) and 2.5% absolute risk reduction of incident cardiovascular events (145).

Other studies have shown inconsistent findings regarding the cardiovascular effects of α-glucosidase inhibitors. A meta-analysis of seven studies with a minimum treatment time of 1 year included over 2000 patients with type 2 diabetes randomized to acarbose or placebo. This meta-analysis showed a reduced risk of MI (HR 0.36, 95% CI 0.16–0.8, $p = 0.012$) and cardiovascular events (HR 0.65, 95% CI 0.48–0.88, $p = 0.006$) (146). Conversely, a Cochrane review and meta-analysis evaluated 42 studies. Although α-glucosidase inhibitors decreased BMI by 0.17 kg/m^2 (95% CI 0.08–0.26), there was no effect on plasma lipids and no evidence of improvement in morbidity or mortality (147).

Thiazolidinediones

Thiazolidinediones (TZDs) are peripheral insulin sensitizers that work through the peroxisome proliferator-activated receptors (PPARs) to improve peripheral insulin sensitivity in skeletal muscle. The two available drugs in this class are rosiglitazone and pioglitazone, which have divergent cardiovascular effects. TZDs reduce hemoglobin A1C by ~1% to 1.5%.

This drug class does not usually cause hypoglycemia. Major adverse effects include fluid retention, weight gain, HF, and bone fractures. Pioglitazone may increase the risk of bladder cancer that appears to be related to duration and intensity of exposure. It is recommended that patients exposed for long periods or at high dose be monitored for signs of bladder cancer (148).

Pioglitazone's cardiovascular disease effects were highlighted in the PROspective pioglitAzone Clinical Trial In macroVascular Events (PROactive study) in which 5238 patients with type 2 diabetes were prospectively followed after receiving pioglitazone or placebo in addition to their regular glucose-lowering drugs (149). The primary endpoint was the composite of all-cause mortality, nonfatal MI, stroke, ACS, endovascular or surgical intervention in the coronary or leg arteries, and amputation above the ankles. The primary endpoint occurred in 19.7% of the pioglitazone group and 21.7% of the placebo group ($p = 0.095$). There was a significant reduction in the secondary composite outcome of all-cause mortality, nonfatal MI, and stroke, which occurred less frequently in the pioglitazone group than in the placebo group (HR 0.84, 95% CI 0.72–0.98, $p = 0.027$). However, there were significantly more HF events and HF admissions in the pioglitazone group, although there was no difference between groups in HF mortality.

In 2011, the FDA restricted the use of rosiglitazone due to reports of an increased risk for MI, and the drug is now only available in the United States through a special access program. A meta-analysis of 35,531 patients, including 19,509 who received rosiglitazone and 16,022 who received control therapy found that rosiglitazone significantly increased the risk for MI (OR 1.28, 95% CI 1.02–1.63, $p = 0.04$) (150). However, there was no difference between rosiglitazone and the control for all-cause or cardiovascular mortality.

In summary, rosiglitazone is associated with an increased risk for MI and has been restricted by the FDA, but pioglitazone does not seem to carry the same adverse ischemic cardiovascular risks (151). Both drugs are associated with an increased risk of HF.

INCRETIN-BASED THERAPY: GLP-1 ANALOGS AND DPP-IV INHIBITORS

Incretins are gut hormones that are released in response to oral but not intravenous glucose loads. Two known human incretins are glucagon-like peptide-1 (GLP-1) and gastric inhibitory peptide (GIP). They have glucose-dependent action, allowing their release to be augmented in the prandial period when glucose levels are rising. GLP-1 stimulates pancreatic β-cell release, inhibits hepatic gluconeogenesis, and slows gastric emptying. This combination of actions works to lower glucose levels. Because the incretins are stimulated in response to a glucose load, they are not associated with hypoglycemia.

DPP-IV is an endogenous enzyme that degrades GLP-1 and limits the time course of glucose-lowering actions of GLP-1. Inhibitors of DPP-IV have been developed. These are orally available agents that block the action of DPP-IV and allow endogenous GLP-1 to have a prolonged course of action. These agents modestly lower hemoglobin A1C levels 0.5%–1%.

The slowed gastric emptying effect of GLP-1 analogs is thought to be responsible for the common side effects of gastrointestinal symptoms such as nausea, vomiting, and diarrhea. GLP-1 analogs also frequently lead to early satiety and, as a consequence, weight loss is frequently seen. A meta-analysis evaluated the weight loss effects in patients receiving GLP-1 analogs compared to a control population treated with placebo, oral glycemic drugs, or insulin (152). The analysis included 6411 participants and demonstrated a weighted mean weight loss difference of −2.9 kg, favoring GLP-1 analogs over controls (95% CI −3.6 to −2.2). Other cardiovascular risk factor benefits from GLP-1 analogs included decreased systolic blood pressure of 3.6 mmHg (95% CI 1.7–5.5 mmHg), decreased diastolic blood pressure of 1.4 mmHg (95% CI 0.7–2.0 mmHg), and a decrease in total cholesterol of 0.1 mmol/L (95% CI 0.04–0.16 mmol/L; 3.9 mg/dL). In contrast to the GLP-1 analogs, the DPP-IV inhibitors are weight neutral and have not been shown to reduce cardiovascular risk factors.

For older patients with diabetes, the GLP-1 analogs and DPP-IV inhibitors offer favorable profiles. These drug classes do not predispose patients to hypoglycemia, and DPP-IV inhibitors can be renally dosed for use in patients with chronic kidney disease. Recent trials have reinforced the weight loss, cardiovascular, and renal protective benefits of GLP-1 receptor agonists (RAs). The ADA now recommends the use of GLP-1 RAs in individuals with type 2 diabetes and established atherosclerotic disease or multiple ASCVD risk factors to reduce the risk of major adverse cardiovascular events (MACE).

Large randomized controlled trials including LEADER, SUSTAIN-6, and REWIND have demonstrated that GLP-1 RAs, such as liraglutide, semaglutide, dulaglutide, and tirzepatide, significantly reduce cardiovascular events in this patient population. These benefits are observed irrespective of baseline metformin use, making GLP-1 RAs a valuable addition to the therapeutic regimen for patients with high cardiovascular risk. A meta-analysis of eight cardiovascular outcome trials revealed a ~14% reduction in the primary outcome of the three-component MACE (cardiovascular death, nonfatal MI, and nonfatal stroke; number-needed-to-treat 65) (153).

An emerging indication for GLP-1 analogs is heart failure with preserved ejection fraction (HFpEF). In the STEP-HF trial, treatment with semaglutide resulted in improved symptom scores, improvement in exercise function, and greater weight loss than placebo (154). Tirzepatide has also shown benefit in patients with HFpEF and obesity. When compared to placebo, treatment with tirzepatide led to a lower risk of a composite of death from cardiovascular causes or worsening heart failure (155).

Of the GLP-1 analogs, tirzepatide (a dual GLP-1/GIP receptor agonist) has shown to be most efficacious in weight loss compared to both placebo and semaglutide in a head-to-head trial. The initial tirzepatide study showed an average weight reduction of −15.0% body weight (95% CI, −15.9 to −14.2) over the 72-week study period and, when compared to semaglutide, 42.3% of the tirzepatide group (95% CI, 39.8%–44.6%) versus 18.1% of the semaglutide group (95% CI, 16.1%–20.0%) achieved 15% or greater weight loss within 365 days (156, 157).

GLP-1 analogs have shown modest renal protective effects. In the FLOW trial, semaglutide had fewer major kidney disease events in patients with CKD and type 2 DM versus placebo with a HR 0.76 (95% CI 0.66–0.88). There are ongoing studies with other GLP-1 analogs to discern further benefit. In the interim, GLP-1 RAs can be used in combination with SGLT2 inhibitors to provide complementary cardiovascular and renal benefits (158).

In summary, GLP-1 receptor agonists now play a crucial role in reducing cardiovascular events and improving overall cardiovascular health in patients with type 2 diabetes, particularly those with established CVD or multiple cardiovascular risk factors. Their multifaceted benefits now make them a cornerstone in the management of diabetes and its cardiovascular complications.

Sodium-glucose cotransporter-2 inhibitors

Sodium-glucose cotransporter-2 (SGLT2) inhibitors are a new class of glucose-lowering drugs. They lower glucose by inhibiting the reabsorption of glucose at the proximal renal tubule. Normally, virtually all filtered glucose is reabsorbed, leaving none excreted into the urine. Inhibition of renal glucose reabsorption by blocking the glucose transport protein SGLT2 results in urinary glucose excretion and reduction in hyperglycemia. These drugs work independently of insulin and can therefore be used with other classes of glucose-lowering medication. Randomized, controlled studies demonstrate that SGLT2 inhibitors result in mean reductions of hemoglobin A1C levels of −0.69% (95% CI, −0.75 to −0.62). In addition, body weight is reduced by a mean of −2.1 kg (95% CI, −2.3 to −2.0) and systolic blood pressure by a mean of −3.9 mmHg (95% CI, −4.6 to −3.3) (159).

SGLT2 inhibitors are generally well tolerated. There is an increased risk of genital mycotic and urinary tract infections. Volume contraction resulting in postural hypotension and renal failure must be considered and monitored, particularly in older adults who are susceptible. Euglycemic diabetic ketoacidosis (DKA) is another potential risk factor in older adults who are acutely ill or have decreased oral intake. These agents should be held prior to any major surgery or during hospitalization. The risk of hypoglycemia is low when used alone but increased when used with insulin or insulin secretory analogs.

The favorable benefits of SGLT2 inhibitors on the heart and kidneys in patients with diabetes have been well described in recent literature. A meta-analysis reviewing the EMPEROR-Reduced (empagliflozin) and DAPA-HF (dapagliflozin) trials demonstrated reductions in MACE outcomes, CV mortality, and heart failure hospitalizations (160). Additionally, dapagliflozin and empagliflozin have been shown to reduce worsening heart failure or cardiovascular death (HR 0.82; 95% CI 0.73–0.92) in patients with mildly reduced or preserved ejection fraction along with improvement in HF-related symptoms and 6-minute walk test distance (161–163).

The updated Kidney Disease: Improving Global Outcomes (KDIGO) guidelines recommend SGLT2 inhibitors for patients with CKD having an eGFR ≥20 ml/min per 1.73 m^2 with a urine albumin to creatinine ratio ≥200 mg/g or heart failure irrespective of albuminuria (Class 1A Recommendation) (164). The class's ability to reduce albuminuria and preserve eGFR while also reducing death from renal or cardiovascular causes has been demonstrated in various trials, most notably DAPA-CKD. Patients who were in the dapagliflozin arm compared to placebo had an HR of 0.56 (95% CI 0.4 –0.68) for the composite endpoint sustained decline in eGFR of at least 50%, ESRD, or death from renal causes. The number-needed-to-treat to prevent one primary outcome event was 19 (95% CI 15–27) (165).

Insulin

The natural history of type 2 diabetes leads to progressive β-cell dysfunction in the setting of insulin resistance. Insulin replacement therapy often becomes necessary to achieve appropriate glycemic control that cannot be accomplished with oral agents alone. Additionally, comorbidities such as liver or renal dysfunction can sometimes limit the use of oral agents necessitating the use of insulin therapy for type 2 diabetes.

Initial management with insulin typically involves a basal, long-acting insulin to provide steady levels of insulin during the day and night. This can be achieved with intermediate-acting insulins such as neutral protamine Hagedorn (NPH) or long-acting insulin analogs (glargine or detemir). These insulins are usually dosed at night and titrated to achieve a target morning glucose level. Oral agents such as metformin, sulfonylureas, pioglitazone, or DPP-IV inhibitors can be continued while basal insulin therapy is used, but dose reductions of oral agents may be necessary. β-cell dysfunction may become so severe that basal insulin alone is not sufficient to achieve desired glycemic control. Short-acting insulins given at mealtimes to assist with prandial rises in glucose may be necessary. This can be achieved with rapid-acting insulin analogs such as lispro, aspart, or glulisine (141, 142).

The advantages of insulin use include established efficacy and the ability to titrate the dosage to achieve desired glycemic control. Inherent disadvantages include weight gain and a high risk of hypoglycemia. The risk of hypoglycemia can be substantial in vulnerable older patients. Additionally, multiple daily injections of insulin require frequent self-monitoring of glucose levels for safe use. Patients must also have adequate hand–eye coordination to appropriately dose and inject insulin. This can be a potential problem in some older patients with common comorbidities, such as visual impairment or tremor. Continuous glucose monitoring (CGM) for older adults is now commonly utilized and can be useful for patients with labile blood sugars and hypoglycemia, and for those who have difficulty obtaining fingerstick readings. CGMs also provide easy access to the patient's blood sugar trends for clinicians and care partners.

CONCLUSION

The burden of diabetes mellitus continues to grow. In addition, as our population ages, older adults with type 2 diabetes mellitus will remain the fastest growing subgroup. Diabetes mellitus increases the risk of cardiovascular disease, which in turn is associated with significant morbidity and mortality. Therefore, management of older adults with diabetes mellitus should focus on cardiovascular risk reduction through control of hypertension, lipid management, antiplatelet therapy, and lifestyle modifications to include smoking cessation, weight reduction, and exercise. While tight glycemic control in non-elderly adults with type 1 and type 2 diabetes mellitus has been shown to reduce microvascular complications, a comparable benefit has not been demonstrated in older patients, and there is significant potential for harm associated with hypoglycemia. Similarly, tight glycemic control has not been shown to reduce macrovascular complications for older patients with type 1 or type 2 diabetes mellitus. Comorbidities, functional status, and life expectancy should be taken into consideration when setting glycemic goals for older patients, and therapy should be individualized to account for patient preferences and health status. For most older patients with diabetes mellitus and other significant comorbidities, a hemoglobin A1C target <8% is usually sufficient to control symptomatic hyperglycemia while avoiding hypoglycemia. In healthy older adults, tighter control with an A1C target of <7.0%–7.5% is recommended. Ongoing studies are investigating the effects of newer hypoglycemic agents on cardiovascular outcomes and the role of hyperglycemia in the development of geriatric syndromes. Additional research is needed to develop more effective strategies for the prevention and management of diabetes mellitus in older adults.

Guidelines

- Glycemic targets should be individualized based on overall health, comorbidities, cognitive and functional status, and life expectancy; for healthy older adults, the American Diabetes Association recommends an A1C goal of <7.0%–7.5%, while less stringent goals (e.g., <8.0%) are appropriate for those with complex health issues or significant comorbidities, prioritizing avoidance of hypoglycemia.
- Assess medical, psychological, functional, and social domains to help guide diabetes management, and screen for geriatric syndromes (such as cognitive impairment, depression, falls, and polypharmacy), as these can impact self-management and quality of life.
- Select anti-hyperglycemic agents with a low risk of hypoglycemia (e.g., metformin, DPP-4 inhibitors, GLP-1 receptor agonists, SGLT2 inhibitors), and avoid overtreatment; deintensify or simplify regimens, especially for those at high risk for hypoglycemia or with limited life expectancy.
- Treat hypertension and other cardiovascular risk factors to individualized targets and consider agents with proven cardiovascular and renal benefit in those with established or at high risk for atherosclerotic cardiovascular disease, heart failure, or chronic kidney disease.

REFERENCES

1. Khan MAB, Hashim, MJ, King, JK et al. Epidemiology of type 2 diabetes – Global burden of disease and forecasted trends. *J Epidemiol Glob Health* 2020 Mar; *10*(1): 107–111.
2. Statistics about diabetes. ADA: accessed February 17, 2025
3. Parker ED et al. Economic costs of diabetes in the U.S. in 2022. *Diabetes Care* 2024 Jan 1; *47*(1): 26–43.
4. Dall TM, Zhang Y, Chen YJ et al. The economic burden of diabetes. *Health Aff (Millwood)* 2010; *29*: 297–303.
5. Sarwar N, Gao P, Seshasai SR et al. Emerging Risk Factors Collaboration. Diabetes mellitus, fasting blood glucose concentration, and risk of vascular disease: A collaborative meta-analysis of 102 prospective studies. *Lancet* 2010; *375*: 2215–2222.
6. Huang ES, Basu A, O'Grady M et al. Projecting the future diabetes population size and related costs for the U.S. *Diabetes Care* 2009; *32*: 2225–2229.
7. American Geriatrics Society Expert Panel on the Care of Older Adults with Diabetes Mellitus. Guideline abstracted from the American Geriatrics Society Guidelines for improving the care of older adults with diabetes mellitus: 2013 update. *J Am Geriatr Soc* 2013; *61*: 2020–2026.
8. Durso SC. Using clinical guidelines designed for older adults with diabetes mellitus and complex health status. *JAMA* 2006; *295*: 1935–1940.
9. Bandeen-Roche K, Xue QL, Ferrucci L et al. Phenotype of frailty: Characterization in the women's health and aging studies. *J Gerontol A Biol Sci Med Sci* 2006; *61*: 262–266.
10. Barzilay JI, Blaum C, Moore T et al. Insulin resistance and inflammation as precursors of frailty: The Cardiovascular Health Study. *Arch Intern Med* 2007; *167*: 635–641.
11. Blaum CS, Xue QL, Tian J et al. Is hyperglycemia associated with frailty status in older women? *J Am Geriatr Soc* 2009; *57*: 840–847.
12. Fried LP, Tangen CM, Walston J et al. Frailty in older adults: Evidence for a phenotype. *J Gerontol A Biol Sci Med Sci* 2001; *56*: M146–M156.
13. Kalyani RR, Varadhan R, Weiss CO et al. Frailty status and altered glucose-insulin dynamics. *J Gerontol A Biol Sci Med Sci* 2011; *67(12)*: 1300–1306.

14. Walston J, McBurnie MA, Newman A et al. Frailty and activation of the inflammation and coagulation systems with and without clinical comorbidities: Results from the Cardiovascular Health Study. *Arch Intern Med* 2002; *162*: 2333–2341.
15. Kalyani RR, Tian J, Xue QL et al. Hyperglycemia and incidence of frailty and lower extremity mobility limitations in older women. *J Am Geriatr Soc* 2012; *60(9)*: 1701–1707.
16. American Diabetes Association Professional Practice Committee. 13. Older adults: Standards of care in diabetes—2025. *Diabetes Care* 2025 Jan 1; *48*: S266–S282.
17. Kaprio J, Tuomilehto J, Koskenvuo M et al. Concordance for type 1 (insulin-dependent) and type 2 (non-insulin-dependent) diabetes mellitus in a population-based cohort of twins in Finland. *Diabetologia* 1992; *35*: 1060–1067.
18. Wild S, Roglic G, Green A et al. Global prevalence of diabetes: Estimates for the year 2000 and projections for 2030. *Diabetes Care* 2004; *27*: 1047–1053.
19. Harrison TA, Hindorff LA, Kim H et al. Family history of diabetes as a potential public health tool. *Am J Prev Med* 2003; *24*: 152–159.
20. The Diabetes Control and Complications Trial Research Group. The effect of intensive treatment of diabetes on the development and progression of long-term complications in insulin-dependent diabetes mellitus. *N Engl J Med* 1993; *329*: 977–986.
21. UK Prospective Diabetes Study (UKPDS) Group. Intensive blood-glucose control with sulphonylureas or insulin compared with conventional treatment and risk of complications in patients with type 2 diabetes (UKPDS 33). *Lancet* 1998; *352*: 837–853.
22. Bilous R. Microvascular disease: What does the UKPDS tell us about diabetic nephropathy? *Diabet Med* 2008; *25*: 25–29.
23. Kohner EM. Microvascular disease: What does the UKPDS tell us about diabetic retinopathy? *Diabet Med* 2008; *25*: 20–24.
24. Finucane TE. Tight control in geriatrics: The emperor wears a thong. *J Am Geriatr Soc* 2012; *60*: 1571–1575.
25. De Vriese AS, Verbeuren TJ, Van de Voorde J et al. Endothelial dysfunction in diabetes. *Br J Pharmacol* 2000; *130*: 963–974.
26. Hopfner RL, Gopalakrishnan V. Endothelin: Emerging role in diabetic vascular complications. *Diabetologia* 1999; *42*: 1383–1394.
27. Beckman JA, Creager MA, Libby P. Diabetes and atherosclerosis: Epidemiology, pathophysiology, and management. *JAMA* 2002; *287*: 2570–2581.
28. Hussain MJ, Peakman M, Gallati H et al. Elevated serum levels of macrophage-derived cytokines precede and accompany the onset of IDDM. *Diabetologia* 1996; *39*: 60–69.
29. Uemura S, Matsushita H, Li W et al. Diabetes mellitus enhances vascular matrix metalloproteinase activity: Role of oxidative stress. *Circ Res* 2001; *88*: 1291–1298.
30. Vinik AI, Erbas T, Park TS et al. Platelet dysfunction in type 2 diabetes. *Diabetes Care* 2001; *24*: 1476–1485.
31. Ceriello A, Giacomello R, Stel G et al. Hyperglycemia-induced thrombin formation in diabetes. The possible role of oxidative stress. *Diabetes* 1995; *44*: 924–928.
32. Ceriello A, Giugliano D, Quatraro A et al. Evidence for a hyperglycaemia-dependent decrease of antithrombin III-thrombin complex formation in humans. *Diabetologia* 1990; *33*: 163–167.
33. Carr ME. Diabetes mellitus: A hypercoagulable state. *J Diabetes Complications* 2001; *15*: 44–54.
34. Nathan DM, Cleary PA, Backlund JY et al. Intensive diabetes treatment and cardiovascular disease in patients with type 1 diabetes. *N Engl J Med* 2005; *353*: 2643–2653.
35. Holman RR, Paul SK, Bethel MA et al. 10-year follow-up of intensive glucose control in type 2 diabetes. *N Engl J Med* 2008; *359*: 1577–1589.
36. Selvin E, Marinopoulos S, Berkenblit G et al. Meta-analysis: Glycosylated hemoglobin and cardiovascular disease in diabetes mellitus. *Ann Intern Med* 2004; *141*: 421–431.
37. Stettler C, Allemann S, Juni P et al. Glycemic control and macrovascular disease in types 1 and 2 diabetes mellitus: Meta-analysis of randomized trials. *Am Heart J* 2006; *152*: 27–38.
38. Gerstein HC, Miller ME, Byington RP et al. Action to control cardiovascular risk in diabetes study group. Effects of intensive glucose lowering in type 2 diabetes. *N Engl J Med* 2008; *358*: 2545–2559.
39. Gerstein HC, Miller ME, Genuth S et al. ACCORD Study Group. Long-term effects of intensive glucose lowering on cardiovascular outcomes. *N Engl J Med* 2011; *364*: 818–828.
40. Duckworth W, Abraira C, Moritz T et al. Glucose control and vascular complications in veterans with type 2 diabetes. *N Engl J Med* 2009; *360*: 129–139.
41. Patel A, MacMahon S, Chalmers J et al. Advance Collaborative Group. Intensive blood glucose control and vascular outcomes in patients with type 2 diabetes. *N Engl J Med* 2008; *358*: 2560–2572.
42. Skyler JS, Bergenstal R, Bonow RO et al. Intensive glycemic control and the prevention of cardiovascular events: Implications of the ACCORD, ADVANCE, and VA Diabetes Trials: A position statement of the American Diabetes Association and a Scientific Statement of the American College of Cardiology Foundation and the American Heart Association. *J Am Coll Cardiol* 2009; *53*: 298–304.
43. American Diabetes Association's (ADA) evidence-based practice guidelines, standards, and related

recommendations and documents for diabetes care. *Diabetes Care* 2017; *40 (Suppl. 1)*: S1–S135.
44. Kannel WB, McGee DL. Diabetes and cardiovascular risk factors: The Framingham study. *Circulation* 1979; *59*: 8–13.
45. Ness J, Nassimiha D, Feria MI et al. Diabetes mellitus in older African-Americans, Hispanics, and whites in an academic hospital-based geriatrics practice. *Coron Artery Dis* 1999; *10*: 343–346.
46. Goraya TY, Leibson CL, Palumbo PJ et al. Coronary atherosclerosis in diabetes mellitus: A population-based autopsy study. *J Am Coll Cardiol* 2002; *40*: 946–953.
47. Janand-Delenne B, Savin B, Habib G et al. Silent myocardial ischemia in patients with diabetes: Who to screen. *Diabetes Care* 1999; *22*: 1396–1400.
48. Kannel WB, Abbott RD. Incidence and prognosis of unrecognized myocardial infarction. An update on the Framingham study. *N Engl J Med* 1984; *311*: 1144–1147.
49. Aronow WS, Epstein S. Usefulness of silent myocardial ischemia detected by ambulatory electrocardiographic monitoring in predicting new coronary events in elderly patients. *Am J Cardiol* 1988; *62*: 1295–1296.
50. Arnett DK, Blumenthal RS, Albert MA et al. ACC/-AHA guideline on the primary prevention of cardiovascular disease: Executive summary: A report of the American College of Cardiology/-American Heart Association Task Force on Clinical Practice Guidelines. *J Am Coll Cardiol* 2019; *74*(10): 1376–1414.
51. Obisesan OH et al. Coronary artery calcium scores in older adults with diabetes and their association with diabetes-specific risk enhancers (from the Atherosclerosis Risk in Communities Study). *Am J Cardiol* 2023 Aug 15; *201*: 219–223.
52. Weitzman S, Wagner GS, Heiss G et al. Myocardial infarction site and mortality in diabetes. *Diabetes Care* 1982; *5*: 31–35.
53. Haffner SM, Lehto S, Ronnemaa T et al. Mortality from coronary heart disease in subjects with type 2 diabetes and in nondiabetic subjects with and without prior myocardial infarction. *N Engl J Med* 1998; *339*: 229–234.
54. Miettinen H, Lehto S, Salomaa V et al. The Finmonica Myocardial Infarction Register Study Group. Impact of diabetes on mortality after the first myocardial infarction. *Diabetes Care* 1998; *21*: 69–75.
55. Jacoby RM, Nesto RW. Acute myocardial infarction in the diabetic patient: Pathophysiology, clinical course and prognosis. *J Am Coll Cardiol* 1992; *20*: 736–744.
56. Abaci A, Oguzhan A, Kahraman S et al. Effect of diabetes mellitus on formation of coronary collateral vessels. *Circulation* 1999; *99*: 2239–2242.
57. Currie CJ, Morgan CL, Gill L et al. Epidemiology and costs of acute hospital care for cerebrovascular disease in diabetic and nondiabetic populations. *Stroke* 1997; *28*: 1142–1146.
58. Hu G, Sarti C, Jousilahti P et al. The impact of history of hypertension and type 2 diabetes at baseline on the incidence of stroke and stroke mortality. *Stroke* 2005; *36*: 2538–2543.
59. Kannel WB, Hjortland M, Castelli WP. Role of diabetes in congestive heart failure: The Framingham study. *Am J Cardiol* 1974; *34*: 29–34.
60. Croft JB, Giles WH, Pollard RA et al. National trends in the initial hospitalization for heart failure. *J Am Geriatr Soc* 1997; *45*: 270–275.
61. Polanczyk CA, Rohde LE, Dec GW et al. Ten-year trends in hospital care for congestive heart failure: Improved outcomes and increased use of resources. *Arch Intern Med* 2000; *160*: 325–332.
62. Murarka S, Movahed MR. Diabetic cardiomyopathy. *J Card Fail* 2010; *16*: 971–979.
63. Devereux RB, Roman MJ, Paranicas M et al. Impact of diabetes on cardiac structure and function: The strong heart study. *Circulation* 2000; *101*: 2271–2276.
64. Movahed MR, Hashemzadeh M, Jamal MM. Diabetes mellitus is a strong, independent risk for atrial fibrillation and flutter in addition to other cardiovascular disease. *Int J Cardiol* 2005; *105*: 315–318.
65. Iribarren C, Karter AJ, Go AS et al. Glycemic control and heart failure among adult patients with diabetes. *Circulation* 2001; *103*: 2668–2673.
66. Leung M, Wong VW, Hudson M et al. Impact of improved glycemic control on cardiac function in Type 2 diabetes mellitus. *Circ Cardiovasc Imaging* 2016; *9*(*3*): 1–9.
67. Beks PJ, Mackaay AJ, de Neeling JN et al. Peripheral arterial disease in relation to glycaemic level in an elderly Caucasian population: The Hoorn study. *Diabetologia* 1995; *38*: 86–96.
68. Jude EB, Oyibo SO, Chalmers N et al. Peripheral arterial disease in diabetic and nondiabetic patients: A comparison of severity and outcome. *Diabetes Care* 2001; *24*: 1433–1437.
69. Jude EB, Eleftheriadou I, Tentolouris N. Peripheral arterial disease in diabetes: A review. *Diabet Med* 2010; *27*: 4–14.
70. Eikelboom JW et al. Rivaroxaban with or without aspirin in stable cardiovascular disease. *N Engl J Med* 2017 Oct 5; *377*(14): 1319–1330.
71. Fibrinolytic Therapy Trialists' (FTT) Collaborative Group. Indications for fibrinolytic therapy in suspected acute myocardial infarction: Collaborative overview of early mortality and major morbidity results from all randomised trials of more than 1000 patients. *Lancet* 1994; *343*: 311–322.
72. Mahaffey KW, Granger CB, Toth CA et al. Diabetic retinopathy should not be a contraindication to thrombolytic therapy for acute myocardial

infarction: Review of ocular hemorrhage incidence and location in the GUSTO-I trial. Global Utilization of Streptokinase and t-PA for occluded coronary arteries. *J Am Coll Cardiol* 1997; *30*: 1606–1610.
73. Berger AK, Radford MJ, Wang Y et al. Thrombolytic therapy in older patients. *J Am Coll Cardiol* 2000; *36*: 366–374.
74. Thiemann DR, Coresh J, Schulman SP et al. Lack of benefit for intravenous thrombolysis in patients with myocardial infarction who are older than 75 years. *Circulation* 2000; *101*: 2239–2246.
75. Sinnaeve PR, Kannays T, Bogaerts K et al. Drug treatment of STEMI in the elderly: Focus on fibrinolytic therapy and insights from the STREAM trial. *Drugs Aging* 2016; *33*: 109–118.
76. Elezi S, Kastrati A, Pache J et al. Diabetes mellitus and the clinical and angiographic outcome after coronary stent placement. *J Am Coll Cardiol* 1998; *32*: 1866–1873.
77. Abizaid A, Kornowski R, Mintz GS et al. The influence of diabetes mellitus on acute and late clinical outcomes following coronary stent implantation. *J Am Coll Cardiol* 1998; *32*: 584–589.
78. Hsu LF, Mak KH, Lau KW et al. Clinical outcomes of patients with diabetes mellitus and acute myocardial infarction treated with primary angioplasty or fibrinolysis. *Heart* 2002; *88*: 260–265.
79. Fragmin and Fast Revascularisation during InStability in Coronary artery disease Investigators. Invasive compared with non-invasive treatment in unstable coronary-artery disease: FRISC II prospective randomised multicentre study. *Lancet* 1999; *354*: 708–715.
80. Cannon CP, Weintraub WS, Demopoulos LA et al. Comparison of early invasive and conservative strategies in patients with unstable coronary syndromes treated with the glycoprotein IIb/IIIa inhibitor tirofiban. *N Engl J Med* 2001; *344*: 1879–1887.
81. Colwell JA, Nesto RW. The platelet in diabetes: Focus on prevention of ischemic events. *Diabetes Care* 2003; *26*: 2181–2188.
82. Colwell JA. Antiplatelet agents for the prevention of cardiovascular disease in diabetes mellitus. *Am J Cardiovasc Drugs* 2004; *4*: 87–106.
83. Yusuf S, Zhao F, Mehta SR et al. Effects of clopidogrel in addition to aspirin in patients with acute coronary syndromes without ST-segment elevation. *N Engl J Med* 2001; *345*: 494–502.
84. RITA-2 trial participants. Coronary angioplasty versus medical therapy for angina: The second Randomised Intervention Treatment of Angina (RITA-2) trial. *Lancet* 1997; *350*: 461–468.
85. Boden WE, O'Rourke RA, Teo KK et al. Optimal medical therapy with or without PCI for stable coronary disease. *N Engl J Med* 2007; *356*: 1503–1516.
86. Frye RL, August P, Brooks MM et al. BARI 2D Study Group. A randomized trial of therapies for type 2 diabetes and coronary artery disease. *N Engl J Med* 2009; *360*: 2503–2515.
87. Maron DJ et al. Initial invasive or conservative strategy for stable coronary disease. *N Engl J Med* 2020 Apr 9; *382*(15): 1395–1407.
88. The Bypass Angioplasty Revascularization Investigation (BARI) Investigators. Comparison of coronary bypass surgery with angioplasty in patients with multivessel disease. *N Engl J Med* 1996; *335*: 217–225.
89. BARI Investigators. Influence of diabetes on 5-year mortality and morbidity in a randomized trial comparing CABG and PTCA in patients with multivessel disease: The Bypass Angioplasty Revascularization Investigation (BARI). *Circulation* 1997; *96*: 1761–1769.
90. BARI Investigators. The final 10-year follow-up results from the BARI randomized trial. *J Am Coll Cardiol* 2007; *49*: 1600–1606.
91. Kapur A, Hall RJ, Malik IS et al. Randomized comparison of percutaneous coronary intervention with coronary artery bypass grafting in diabetic patients. 1-year results of the CARDia (Coronary Artery Revascularization in Diabetes) trial. *J Am Coll Cardiol* 2010; *55*: 432–440.
92. Mohr FW, Morice M, Kappetein AP et al. Coronary artery bypass graft surgery versus percutaneous coronary intervention in patients with three-vessel disease and left-main disease left main coronary disease: 5-year follow-up of the SYNTAX trial. *Lancet* 2013; *3871*: 629–638.
93. Fihn SD, Blankenship JC, Alexander KP et al. ACC/AHA/AATS/PCNA/SCAI/STS focused update of the guideline for the diagnosis and management of patients with stable ischemic heart disease: A report of the American College of Cardiology/American Heart Association Task Force on Practice Guidelines, and the American Association for Thoracic Surgery, Preventive Cardiovascular Nurses Association, Society for Cardiovascular Angiography and Interventions, and Society of Thoracic Surgeons. *Am Coll Cardiol* 2014; *64(18)*: 1929–1949.
94. Baigent C, Blackwell L, Collins R et al. Antithrombotic Trialists' (ATT) collaboration, aspirin in the primary and secondary prevention of vascular disease: Collaborative meta-analysis of individual participant data from randomised trials. *Lancet* 2009; *373*: 1849–1860.
95. Ogawa H, Nakayama M, Morimoto T et al. Low-dose aspirin for primary prevention of atherosclerotic events in patients with type 2 diabetes: A randomized controlled trial. *JAMA* 2008; *300*: 2134–2141.
96. Belch J, MacCuish A, Campbell I et al. The prevention of progression of arterial disease and diabetes (POPADAD) trial: Factorial randomised placebo controlled trial of aspirin and antioxidants in

patients with diabetes and asymptomatic peripheral arterial disease. *BMJ* 2008; *337*: a1840.
97. Gaziano JM, Brotons C, Coppolecchia R et al.; ARRIVE Executive Committee. Use of aspirin to reduce risk of initial vascular events in patients at moderate risk of cardiovascular disease (ARRIVE): A randomised, double-blind, placebo-controlled trial. *Lancet* 2018 Sep 22; *392*(10152): 1036–1046.
98. Bowman L, Mafham M, Stevens W, Haynes R et al.; ASCEND Study Collaborative Group. ASCEND: A Study of Cardiovascular Events in Diabetes: Characteristics of a randomized trial of aspirin and of omega-3 fatty acid supplementation in 15,480 people with diabetes. *Am Heart J* 2018 Apr; *198*: 135–144.
99. Hawk ET, Maresso KC. The ASPREE trial: An unanticipated stimulus for greater precision in prevention? *J Natl Cancer Inst* 2021 Mar 1; *113*(3): 221–222.
100. Oldridge NB, Stump TE, Nothwehr FK et al. Prevalence and outcomes of comorbid metabolic and cardiovascular conditions in middle- and older-age adults. *J Clin Epidemiol* 2001; *54*: 928–934.
101. Curb JD, Pressel SL, Cutler JA et al. Systolic hypertension in the elderly program cooperative research group. Effect of diuretic-based antihypertensive treatment on cardiovascular disease risk in older diabetic patients with isolated systolic hypertension. *JAMA* 1996; *276*: 1886–1892.
102. Lewington S, Clarke R, Qizilbash N et al. Prospective Studies Collaboration. Age-specific relevance of usual blood pressure to vascular mortality: A meta-analysis of individual data for one million adults in 61 prospective studies. *Lancet* 2002; *360*: 1903–1913.
103. UK Prospective Diabetes Study Group. Tight blood pressure control and risk of macrovascular and microvascular complications in type 2 diabetes: UKPDS 38. *BMJ* 1998; *317*: 703–713.
104. Yusuf S, Sleight P, Pogue J et al. The Heart Outcomes Prevention Evaluation Study Investigators. Effects of an angiotensin-converting-enzyme inhibitor, ramipril, on cardiovascular events in high-risk patients. *N Engl J Med* 2000; *342*: 145–153.
105. Yusuf S, Teo KK, Pogue J et al. ONTARGET Investigators. Telmisartan, ramipril, or both in patients at high risk for vascular events. *N Engl J Med* 2008; *358*: 1547–1559.
106. ALLHAT Officers and Coordinators for the ALLHAT Collaborative Research Group. The Antihypertensive and Lipid-Lowering Treatment to Prevent Heart Attack Trial. Major outcomes in high-risk hypertensive patients randomized to angiotensin- converting enzyme inhibitor or calcium channel blocker vs diuretic: The Antihypertensive and Lipid-Lowering Treatment to Prevent Heart Attack Trial (ALLHAT). *JAMA* 2002; *288*: 2981–2997.
107. James PA, Oparil S, Carter BL et al. Evidence-based guideline for the management of high blood pressure in adults: Report from the panel members appointed to the Eighth Joint National Committee (JNC 8). *JAMA* 2014; *311*(5): 507–520.
108. Cushman WC, Evans GW, Byington RP et al. ACCORD Study Group. Effects of intensive blood-pressure control in type 2 diabetes mellitus. *N Engl J Med* 2010; *362*: 1575–1585.
109. Bi Y, Li M, Liu Y et al; BPROAD Research Group. Intensive blood-pressure control in patients with type 2 diabetes. *N Engl J Med* 2025 Mar 27; *392*(12): 1155–1167.
110. Liu J, Li Y, Ge J et al.; ESPRIT Collaborative Group. Lowering systolic blood pressure to less than 120 mm Hg versus less than 140 mm Hg in patients with high cardiovascular risk with and without diabetes or previous stroke: An open-label, blinded-outcome, randomised trial. *Lancet* 2024 Jul 20; *404*(10449): 245–255.
111. Ziegler D, Gries FA, Spuler M et al. Diabetic Cardiovascular Autonomic Neuropathy Multicenter Study Group. The epidemiology of diabetic neuropathy. *J Diabetes Complications* 1992; *6*: 49–57.
112. Aronow WS, Fleg JL, Pepine CJ et al. ACCF/AHA 2011 expert consensus document on hypertension in the elderly: A report of the American College of Cardiology Foundation Task Force on Clinical Expert Consensus Documents. *Circulation* 2011; *123*: 2434–506.
113. Bloomgarden Z. A diabetes update. *J Diabetes.* 2023 Jul; *15*(7): 542–544.
114. Laakso M. Insulin resistance and coronary heart disease. *Curr Opin Lipidol* 1996; *7*: 217–226.
115. Grundy SM. Small LDL, atherogenic dyslipidemia, and the metabolic syndrome. *Circulation* 1997; *95*: 1–4.
116. Baigent C, Keech A, Kearney PM et al. Efficacy and safety of cholesterol-lowering treatment: Prospective meta-analysis of data from 90,056 participants in 14 randomised trials of statins. *Lancet* 2005; *366*: 1267–1278.
117. Singh IM, Shishehbor MH, Ansell BJ. High-density lipoprotein as a therapeutic target: A systematic review. *JAMA* 2007; *298*: 786–798.
118. Keech A, Simes RJ, Barter P et al. Effects of long-term fenofibrate therapy on cardiovascular events in 9795 people with type 2 diabetes mellitus (the FIELD study): Randomised controlled trial. *Lancet* 2005; *366*: 1849–1861.
119. Cannon CP, Braunwald E, McCabe CH et al. Intensive versus moderate lipid lowering with statins after acute coronary syndromes. *N Engl J Med* 2004; *350*: 1495–1504.
120. Nissen SE, Tuzcu EM, Schoenhagen P et al. Effect of intensive compared with moderate lipid-lowering therapy on progression of coronary atherosclerosis: A randomized controlled trial. *JAMA* 2004; *291*: 1071–1080.

121. Ginsberg HN, Elam MB, Lovato LC et al. ACCORD Study Group. Effects of combination lipid therapy in type 2 diabetes mellitus. *N Engl J Med* 2010; *362*: 1563–1574.
122. Boden WE, Probstfield JL, Anderson T et al. AIM-HIGH Investigators. Niacin in patients with low HDL cholesterol levels receiving intensive statin therapy. *N Engl J Med* 2011; *365*: 2255–2267.
123. Bhatt DL, Steg PG, Miller M et al. REDUCE-IT Investigators. Cardiovascular risk reduction with Icosapent ethyl for hypertriglyceridemia. *N Engl J Med.* 2019 Jan 3; *380*(1): 11–22.
124. Cannon CP, Blazing MA, Giugliano RP et al.; IMPROVE-IT Investigators. Ezetimibe added to statin therapy after acute coronary syndromes. *N Engl J Med* 2015 Jun 18; *372*(25): 2387–2397.
125. Handelsman Y, Lepor NE. PCSK9 inhibitors in lipid management of patients with diabetes mellitus and high cardiovascular risk: A review. *J Am Heart Assoc* 2018 Jun 22; *7*(13): e008953.
126. Sabatine MS et al. Evolocumab and clinical outcomes in patients with cardiovascular disease. *N Engl J Med* 2017 May 4; *376*(18): 1713–1722.
127. Schwartz GG et al. Alirocumab and cardiovascular outcomes after acute coronary syndrome. *N Engl J Med* 2018 Nov 29; *379*(22): 2097–2107.
128. Preiss D, Seshasai SR, Welsh P et al. Risk of incident diabetes with intensive-dose compared with moderate-dose statin therapy: A meta-analysis. *JAMA* 2011; *305*: 2556–2564.
129. Sattar N, Preiss D, Murray HM et al. Statins and risk of incident diabetes: A collaborative meta-analysis of randomised statin trials. *Lancet* 2010; *375*: 735–742.
130. Guyton JR, Bays HE. Safety considerations with niacin therapy. *Am J Cardiol* 2007; *99*: 22C–31C.
131. Knowler WC, Barrett-Connor E, Fowler SE et al. Reduction in the incidence of type 2 diabetes with lifestyle intervention or metformin. *N Engl J Med* 2002; *346*: 393–403.
132. Pi-Sunyer X, Blackburn G, Brancati FL et al. Look AHEAD Research Group. Reduction in weight and cardiovascular disease risk factors in individuals with type 2 diabetes: One-year results of the look AHEAD trial. *Diabetes Care* 2007; *30*: 1374–1383.
133. Wing RR. Look AHEAD Research Group. Long-term effects of a lifestyle intervention on weight and cardiovascular risk factors in individuals with type 2 diabetes mellitus: Four-year results of the Look AHEAD trial. *Arch Intern Med* 2010; *170*: 1566–1575.
134. Colberg SR, Sigal RJ, Fernhall B et al. Exercise and type 2 diabetes: The American College of Sports Medicine and the American Diabetes Association: Joint position statement executive summary. *Diabetes Care* 2010; *33*: 2692–2696.
135. Klein S, Sheard NF, Pi-Sunyer X et al. Weight management through lifestyle modification for the prevention and management of type 2 diabetes: Rationale and strategies: A statement of the American Diabetes Association, the North American Association for the Study of Obesity, and the American Society for Clinical Nutrition. *Diabetes Care* 2004; *27*: 2067–2073.
136. American Diabetes Association Professional Practice Committee. 9. Pharmacologic approaches to glycemic treatment: Standards of care in diabetes-2025. *Diabetes Care.* 2025 Jan 1; *48*(Supplement_1): S181–S206.
137. Inzucchi SE et al. Metformin in patients with type 2 diabetes and kidney disease: A systematic review. *JAMA* 2014 Dec 24–31; *312*(24): 2668–2675.
138. DeFronzo RA, Goodman AM. The Multicenter Metformin Study Group. Efficacy of metformin in patients with non-insulin-dependent diabetes mellitus. *N Engl J Med* 1995; *333*: 541–549.
139. Nathan DM, Buse JB, Davidson MB et al. Medical management of hyperglycemia in type 2 diabetes: A consensus algorithm for the initiation and adjustment of therapy: A consensus statement of the American Diabetes Association and the European Association for the Study of Diabetes. *Diabetes Care* 2009; *32*: 193–203.
140. Salpeter S, Greyber E, Pasternak G et al. Risk of fatal and nonfatal lactic acidosis with metformin use in type 2 diabetes mellitus. *Cochrane Database Syst Rev* 2006: CD002967.
141. Thrasher J. Pharmacologic management of type 2 diabetes mellitus: Available therapies. *Am J Med* 2017; *130*: S8–S9.
142. Bryan J, Crane A, Vila-Carriles WH et al. Insulin secretagogues, sulfonylurea receptors and K(ATP) channels. *Curr Pharm Des* 2005; *11*: 2699–2716.
143. The University Group Diabetes Program. A study of the effects of hypoglycemic agents on vascular complications in patients with adult-onset diabetes. V. Evaluation of phenformin therapy. *Diabetes* 1975; *24*: 65–184.
144. Kahn SE, Haffner SM, Heise MA et al. Glycemic durability of rosiglitazone, metformin, or glyburide monotherapy. *N Engl J Med* 2006; *355*: 2427–2443.
145. Chiasson JL, Josse RG, Gomis R et al. Acarbose treatment and the risk of cardiovascular disease and hypertension in patients with impaired glucose tolerance: The STOP-NIDDM trial. *JAMA* 2003; *290*: 486–494.
146. Hanefeld M, Cagatay M, Petrowitsch T et al. Acarbose reduces the risk for myocardial infarction in type 2 diabetic patients: Meta-analysis of seven long-term studies. *Eur Heart J* 2004; *25*: 10–16.
147. van de Laar FA, Lucassen PL, Akkermans RP et al. Alpha-glucosidase inhibitors for patients with type 2 diabetes: Results from a Cochrane systematic

review and meta-analysis. *Diabetes Care* 2005; *28*: 154–163.

148. Tang H et al. Pioglitazone and bladder cancer risk: A systematic review and meta-analysis. *Cancer Med* 2018 Apr; *7*(4): 1070–1080.
149. Dormandy JA, Charbonnel B, Eckland DJ et al. Secondary prevention of macrovascular events in patients with type 2 diabetes in the PROactive Study (PROspective pioglitAzone Clinical Trial In macroVascular Events): A randomised controlled trial. *Lancet* 2005; *366*: 1279–1289.
150. Nissen SE, Wolski K. Rosiglitazone revisited: An updated meta-analysis of risk for myocardial infarction and cardiovascular mortality. *Arch Intern Med* 2010; *170*: 1191–1201.
151. Nagajothi N, Adigopula S, Balamuthusamy S et al. Pioglitazone and the risk of myocardial infarction and other major adverse cardiac events: A meta-analysis of randomized, controlled trials. *Am J Ther* 2008; *15*: 506–511.
152. Vilsboll T, Christensen M, Junker AE et al. Effects of glucagon-like peptide-1 receptor agonists on weight loss: Systematic review and meta-analyses of randomised controlled trials. *BMJ* 2012; *344*: d7771.
153. Sattar N et al. Cardiovascular, mortality, and kidney outcomes with GLP-1 receptor agonists in patients with type 2 diabetes: A systematic review and meta-analysis of randomized trials. *Lancet Diabetes Endocrinol* 2021; *9*: 653–662.
154. Kosiborod MN et al. Semaglutide in patients with heart failure with preserved ejection fraction and obesity. *N Engl J Med* 2023 Sep 21; *389*(12): 1069–1084.
155. Packer M, Zile MR, Kramer CM et al. Tirzepatide for heart failure with preserved ejection fraction and obesity. *N Engl J Med* 2025 Jan 30; *392*(5): 427–437.
156. Jastreboff AM et al. Tirzepatide once weekly for the treatment of obesity. *N Engl J Med* 2022 Jul 21; *387*(3): 205–216.
157. Rodriguez PJ, Goodwin Cartwright BM, Gratzl S et al. Semaglutide vs tirzepatide for weight loss in adults with overweight or obesity. *JAMA Intern Med* 2024; *184*(9): 1056–1064.
158. Perkovic V et al. Effects of semaglutide on chronic kidney disease in patients with type 2 diabetes. *N Engl J Med* 2024 Jul 11; *391*(2): 109–121.
159. Storgaard H, Gluud LL, Bennett C. et al. Benefits and harms of sodium-glucose co-transporter 2 inhibitors in patients with type 2 diabetes: A systematic review and meta-analysis. *PLoS One* 2016; *11*: e0166125.
160. Zannad F et al. SGLT2 inhibitors in patients with heart failure with reduced ejection fraction: A meta-analysis of the EMPEROR-Reduced and DAPA-HF trials. *Lancet* 2020 Sep 19; *396*(10254): 819–829.
161. Nassif ME et al. The SGLT2 inhibitor dapagliflozin in heart failure with preserved ejection fraction: A multicenter randomized trial. *Nat Med* 2021 Nov; *27*(11): 1954–1960.
162. Solomon SD et al. Dapagliflozin in heart failure with mildly reduced or preserved ejection fraction. *N Engl J Med* 2022 Sep 22; *387*(12): 1089–1098.
163. Anker SD, Butler J, Filippatos G et al. EMPEROR-Preserved Trial Investigators. Empagliflozin in heart failure with a preserved ejection fraction. *N Engl J Med* 2021 Oct 14; *385*(16): 1451–1461.
164. Stevens, Paul E. et al. KDIGO 2024 clinical practice guideline for the evaluation and management of chronic kidney disease. *Kidney Int* 2024; *105*(4): S117–S314.
165. Heerspink HJL et al. Dapagliflozin in patients with chronic kidney disease. *N Engl J Med* 2020 Oct 8; *383*(15): 1436–1446.

7

Epidemiology and prevention of coronary heart disease in older adults

NATHAN D. WONG AND KEVIN S. TANG

Key points

- Coronary heart disease (CHD) is highly prevalent in older adults, affecting 40% of men and 30% of women aged 80 years and over.
- Among persons aged 75 years and over, 79% of men and 85% of women have hypertension, with intensive blood pressure control showing similar benefit for reduction of cardiovascular outcomes as compared to younger persons; isolated systolic hypertension remains the predominant hypertensive subtype in older persons.
- Elevated LDL-C remains common in older adults, and meta-analyses of clinical trials to reduce LDL-C show similar benefit in those aged >=75 years compared to <75 years.
- The greater absolute risk of atherosclerotic cardiovascular disease (ASCVD), along with multiple other comorbidities, results in proportionately greater very high-risk ASCVD persons among older adults, where additional nonstatin treatment is recommended if the LDL-C persists >=55 mg/dL.
- About 55% of adults aged 65 years and over have advanced cardiovascular kidney metabolic (CKM) syndrome, emphasizing the need for multifactorial treatments to reduce associated risk factors, including obesity, diabetes or pre-diabetes, dyslipidemia, hypertension, and chronic kidney disease to prevent CHD.
- Adoption of healthy lifestyle habits and initiation of recommended preventive treatments early in life and in the disease course can help reduce the burden of CHD and its complications with the aging of the patient.

INTRODUCTION

With more than 70% of cardiovascular diseases (CVD) occurring among developing countries (1), where people are living to an older age due to reduced communicable diseases and improved health care, the burden of CVD, including coronary heart disease (CHD), affecting mainly those aged 65 and older is rapidly becoming a global problem. There are more than 35 million persons aged 65 and older in the United States, and this is expected to double by the year 2030, hence the need to better address primary and secondary prevention in this age group is critical (2, 3). Some 28.2% of men and 19.6% of women aged 60–79 years have CHD, and among those 80 years and over, 39.6% of men and 32.8% of women in the 2017–2020 US population have CHD (Figure 7.1) (4).

While atherosclerosis begins at an early age, its prevalence is nearly universal by the age of 65, both in men and women (5). With age being the most important risk factor for CVD, the clinical and economic implications of the demographic shift in age distribution, not only in the United States but throughout the developing world,

DOI: 10.1201/9781003568933-7

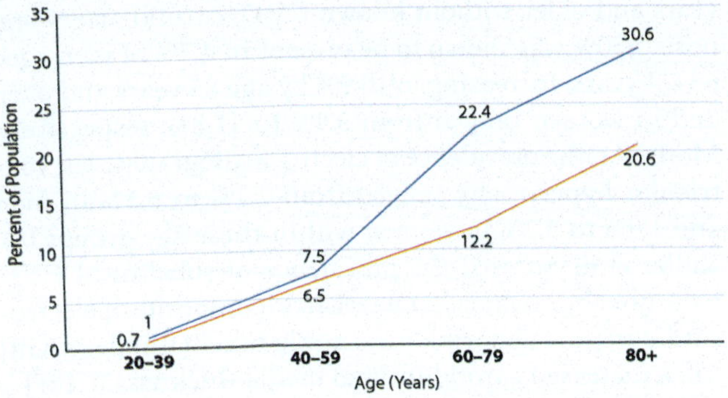

Figure 7.1 Prevalence of coronary heart disease by age and sex (NHANES 2017–2020). (Adapted from Martin SS et al., *Circulation*, 149(8), e347–e913, 2024.)

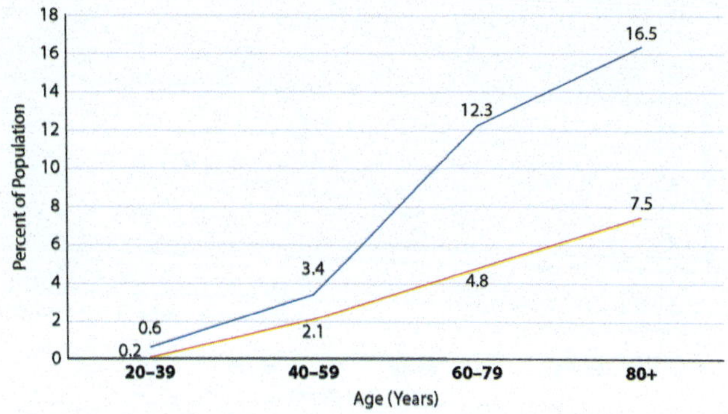

Figure 7.2 Incidence of heart attack or fatal CHD by age and sex (NHANES 2017–2020). (Adapted from Martin SS et al., *Circulation*, 149(8), e347–e913, 2024.)

are dramatic. The estimated economic costs of CHD in the United States in 2019–2020 were over $422 billion, including both direct expenditures and lost future productivity resulting from premature CHD mortality, with over half of these costs associated with those aged 65 years and older (4).

This chapter on the epidemiology of CHD in older persons will focus on the burden of CHD and its components, including the extent of subclinical atherosclerosis, as well as the key risk factors for CHD in older adults and the evidence and guidelines for managing these risk factors both in primary and in secondary prevention.

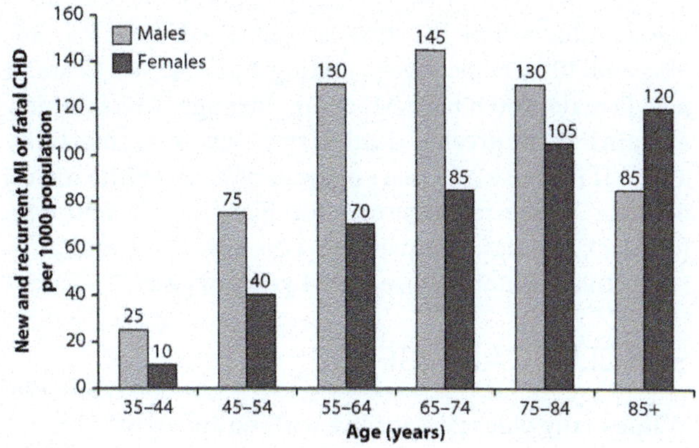

Figure 7.3 Annual number of adults per 1000 having diagnosed heart attack or fatal CHD by age and sex (ARIC surveillance 2005–2013 and CHS). (Adapted from Benjamin EJ et al., *Circulation*, 135, e146–e603, 2017.)

PRESENTATION OF CORONARY HEART DISEASE

The lifetime risk of CHD is substantial; even at age 70, the lifetime risk of a first CHD event is 34.9% in men and 24.2% in women (6). While the average age of a heart attack is 65.6 years in men, it is 72.0 years in women (4); however, early prognosis is worse for men in part because they have heart attacks at an older age. Approximately 80% of people overall who die of CHD are aged 65 and older (7). There is also variation among older individuals. In the Cardiovascular Health Study (CHS), the prevalence of any CHD ranged from 28.4% in men aged 65–74 to 35.2% in those aged 75–84, but in women ranged from 19.2% in those aged 65–74 to 36.7% in those aged 85 years and older. The large proportion of CHD was due to angina, followed by myocardial infarction (MI), coronary artery bypass, and angioplasty (8). The prognosis associated with MI in older adults is also worse than for younger persons, with recurrent MI being 1.5-fold to 3-fold greater in those aged 70 and over compared to those aged 40–69; death within 1 year is also twofold to threefold higher (9). One-year death rates from MI are 27% in White men, 29% in White women, 19% in Black men, and 31% in Black women aged 75 years and older (4). Analysis of the National Health and Nutrition Examination Survey (NHANES) 2017–2020 demonstrated rates of MI to increase approximately three- to fivefold between the ages of 40–59 and 80-plus years with substantial differences between sexes (Figure 7.2). Of interest, the rate of MI or fatal CHD peaks in men around age 65–74 years (145/1000 population) and in women age 85 years and older (120/1000 population) (Figure 7.3). In addition, the incidence of angina pectoris peaks at ages 60–79 years in men (10.3%) and 80-plus years in women (10.0%) (Figure 7.4).

The Framingham Heart Study (FHS) has previously demonstrated that among persons aged 65 and older experiencing CHD, the most common presentation for men is MI (55%), followed by angina pectoris (30%) and sudden death (15%); however, in women, angina pectoris is most common (45%), followed by MI (40%) and sudden death (12%). Of particular note is the fact that with increasing age, there is a greater proportion of MIs that are clinically unrecognized, being as high as 42% in men aged 75–84 and 46% among women aged 85 and older (10).

Prognosis following a MI is poor in older persons (4, 7). Based on pooled data from six major prospective studies between 1995 and 2012, among those ≥75 years of age, 27% of White males, 29% of White females, 19% of Black males, and 21% of Black females will die within

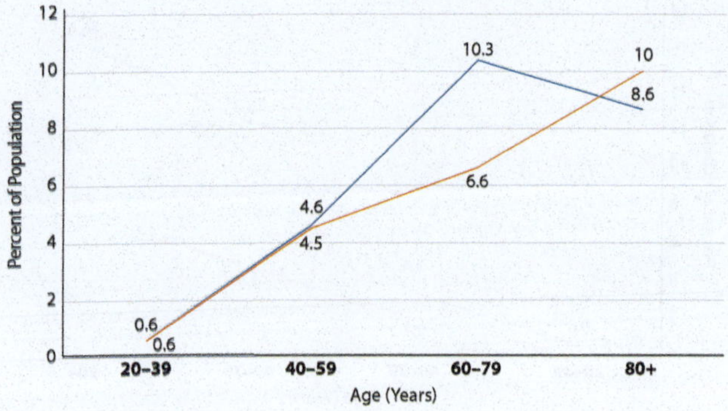

Figure 7.4 Incidence of angina pectoris by age and sex (NHANES 2017–2020). (Adapted from Martin SS et al., *Circulation*, 149(8), e347–e913, 2024.)

a year after a first MI; this is contrasted with 3%, 5%, 9%, and 10%, respectively, among those 45–64 years of age. Females often have MI at an older age, which largely explains their greater death rates. Five-year mortality after MI in those ≥75 years of age is 55% for White males, 60% for White females, 61% for Black males, and 64% for Black females, compared to 11%, 17%, 16%, and 28%, respectively, among those 45–64 years of age.

SUBCLINICAL DISEASE

While many older persons live with no apparent evidence of clinical CVD, evidence of subclinical CVD is common. In the Cardiovascular Health Study of adults aged 65 years and older without known CVD, carotid artery stenosis >50% was shown to be present in 4.3% of men aged 65–74 years, increasing to 10.9% by age 85 years and over, and in women ranged from 3.4% to 11.8%, respectively. Moreover, the prevalence of electrocardiographic left ventricular hypertrophy ranged from 2.1% to 6.3% in men and 1.9% to 5.2% in women within these age groups (8). Kuller et al. showed the prevalence of subclinical CVD measured by several characteristics (composite of electrocardiographic abnormalities, ankle brachial index [ABI] <0.9, increased carotid intimal media thickness [CIMT], echocardiographic abnormalities, angina, or claudication) to be 61%, with such persons at increased risk of future CVD events (9). Wong et al. (5), in the Multiethnic Study of Atherosclerosis (MESA), showed the prevalence of subclinical atherosclerosis defined by one of more of the following: increased CIMT >1 mm, low ABI <0.9, or the presence of coronary or abdominal aortic calcification to range from 55% in men aged 45–54 to 100% among those aged 75–84 years (and 32%–98% in women, respectively). Abdominal aortic calcification was the most common subclinical disease measure, which, unlike coronary artery calcification (CAC), occurs with nearly as high a prevalence in women as in men at most age groups (Figure 7.5). The presence and extent of abdominal aortic calcification were, in particular, strong predictors of other subclinical measures of atherosclerosis (increased CIMT, low ABI, or CAC). Importantly, a more recent report from MESA has shown over 10 years of follow-up, CAC confers increased risk of CHD events across all important

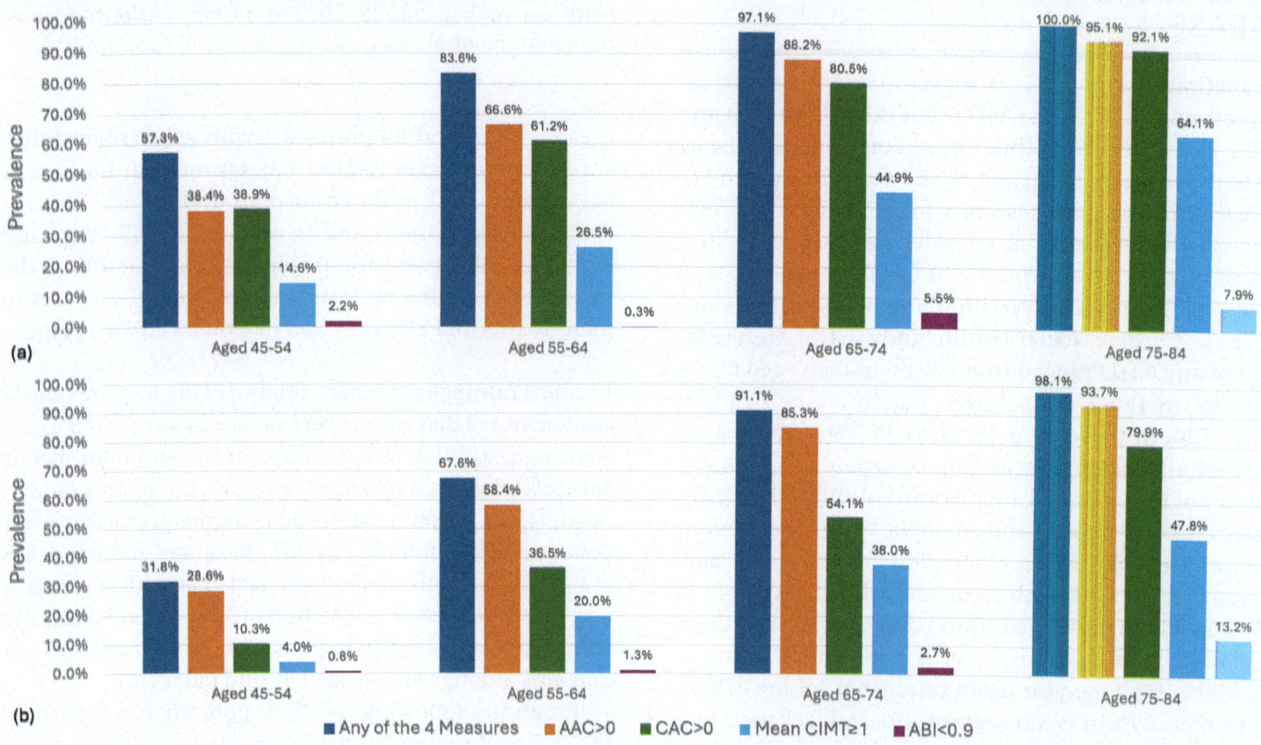

Figure 7.5 (a, b) Prevalence of AAC >0, CAC >0, CIMT ≥1 mm, ABI <0.9, or any of the four measures. Multiethnic Study of Atherosclerosis. $p < 0.001$ across age categories for men and women for each of the measures. (Adapted from Wong ND et al., *Atherosclerosis*, 214, 436–441, 2011.)

demographic subgroups; interestingly, the relative risk of CHD events conferred by increased levels of CAC (compared to a score of 0) is estimated to be slightly higher in persons aged 45–54 (hazard ratio 1.20, $p < 0.001$) compared to those aged 75–84 (hazard ratio 1.12, $p < 0.001$) (10).

RISK FACTORS

The distribution of risk for CVD rises dramatically with age, with more than half of men and nearly one third of women by the age of 70 having a ≥10% 10-year CVD risk (Figure 7.6). Data from the FHS show the risk of CHD increases more than fivefold according to the number of risk factors present (Figure 7.7). In general, as shown by the FHS, most risk factors for younger persons also hold for those in older age groups, but not consistently in both genders. While systolic blood pressure (BP) is strongly associated with CHD both in younger and older persons of both genders, diastolic BP appears to be weaker in older women; and while total cholesterol is strongly associated with CHD in younger men and women, it loses its importance in older men. Blood glucose is a powerful predictor in older and younger women and older men, but not younger men. In addition, cigarette smoking appears to be less important as a predictor in older persons of both genders than in younger persons (11).

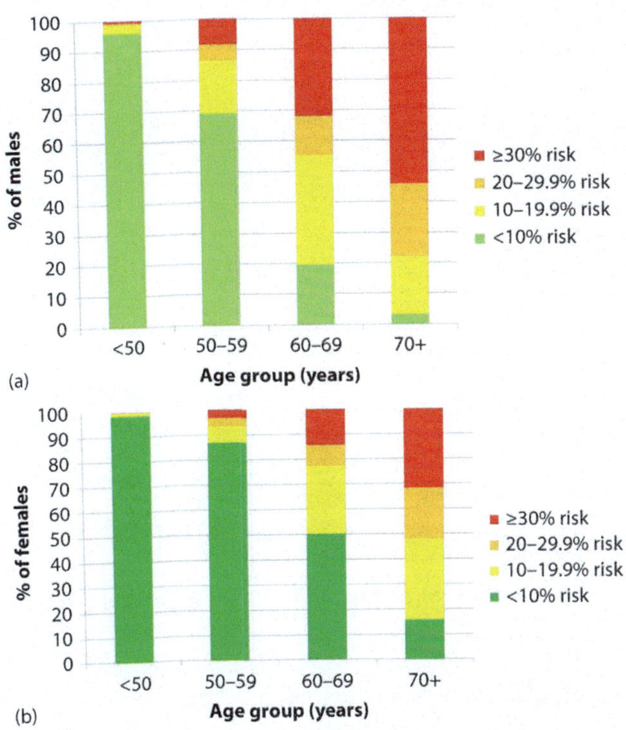

Figure 7.6 Cardiovascular risk distribution by age, Americas region: (a) men, (b) women. (Adapted from Mendis S et al., *World Health Organization*, 2011.)

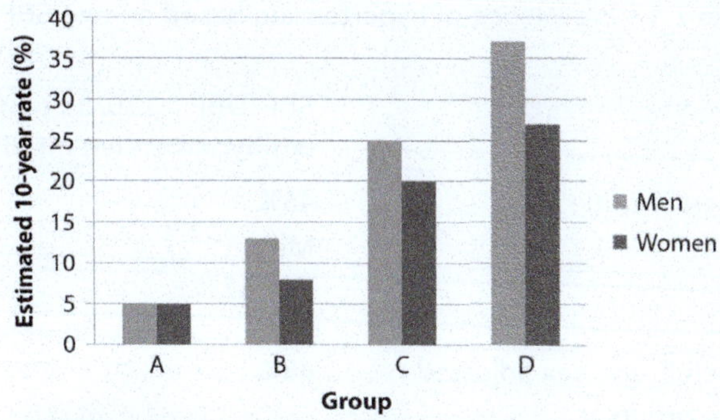

	A	B	C	D
Blood pressure	120/80	140/90	140/90	140/90
Cholesterol	200	240	240	240
HDL-C	50	50	40	40
Diabetes	No	No	Yes	Yes
Cigarettes	No	No	No	Yes

Figure 7.7 Estimated 10-year coronary heart disease risk in adults 55 years of age according to levels of various risk factors (Framingham Heart Study). (Adapted from Benjamin EJ et al., *Circulation*, 135(10), e146–e603, 2017.)

Blood pressure and hypertension

On a global basis, elevated blood pressure (BP) is responsible for more than 7 million deaths annually, more than any other risk factor (1). Hypertension among older US adults is more prevalent than any other CVD risk factor. From the most recent 2025 ACC/AHA/Multisociety Guideline for the Prevention, Detection, Evaluation and Management of High Blood Pressure in Adults (12), elevated BP, stage I hypertension, and stage II hypertension are defined as a systolic BP/diastolic BP of 120–129/<80 mmHg, 130–139/80–89 mmHg, and ≥140/90 mmHg, respectively. A goal BP of <130/80 mmHg is also specified, with encouragement in the new guideline to target the systolic BP to <120 mmHg. This has resulted in an increased overall prevalence (compared to the ≥140/90 mmHg cut-point) of hypertension from 32% to 46% and among those aged 75 and older, an increase in prevalence from 71% to 79% in men and 78% to 85% in women (Table 7.1). Among those with hypertension, we have shown that while under the age of 40 years isolated diastolic hypertension (systolic <140 mg/dL and diastolic ≥90 mmHg as defined previously) is the most common subtype, by the fifth decade of life systolic hypertension (isolated systolic and systolic diastolic combined) becomes predominant, and by the sixth decade of life, isolated systolic hypertension (ISH) becomes the most predominant subtype (13). By ages 70–79, more than 70% of individuals with hypertension have ISH (Figure 7.8), due to large artery stiffness increasing with advancing age. Moreover, in the presence of diseases that accelerate arterial stiffness, such as diabetes or chronic renal disease, ISH can develop at an earlier age (14). Furthermore, a Framingham study showed that normotensive persons reaching age 65 had a 90% lifetime risk of developing hypertension—almost

Table 7.1 Prevalence of hypertension based on two SBP/DBP thresholds

	SBP/DBP >130/80 mmHg or self-reported antihypertensive medication[a]		SBP/DBP >140/90 mmHg or self-reported antihypertensive medication[b]	
Overall, crude	46%		32%	
	Men (*n* = 4717)	Women (*n* = 4906)	Men (*n* = 4717)	Women (*n* = 4906)
Overall, age-sex adjusted	48%	43%	31%	32%
Age group, y				
20–44	30%	19%	11%	10%
45–54	50%	44%	33%	27%
55–64	70%	63%	53%	52%
65–74	77%	75%	64%	63%
75+	79%	85%	71%	78%
Race/ethnicity[c]				
Non-Hispanic White	47%	41%	31%	30%
Non-Hispanic Black	59%	56%	42%	46%
Non-Hispanic Asian	45%	36%	29%	27%
Hispanic	44%	42%	27%	32%

Abbreviations: BP, blood pressure; DBP, diastolic blood pressure; NHANES, National Health and Nutrition Examination Survey; SBP, systolic blood pressure.
Source: Adapted from Whelton PK et al., Am *Coll Cardiol*, 2017, pii: S0735-S1097(17): 41519-1.
Notes: 130/80 and 140/90 mmHg in 9623 participants (>=20 years of age) in NHANES 2011–2014. The prevalence estimates have been rounded to the nearest full percentage.
[a] BP cut-points for definition of hypertension in the present guideline.
[b] BP cut-points for definition of hypertension in JNC 7.
[c] Adjusted to the 2010 age-sex distribution of the US adult population.

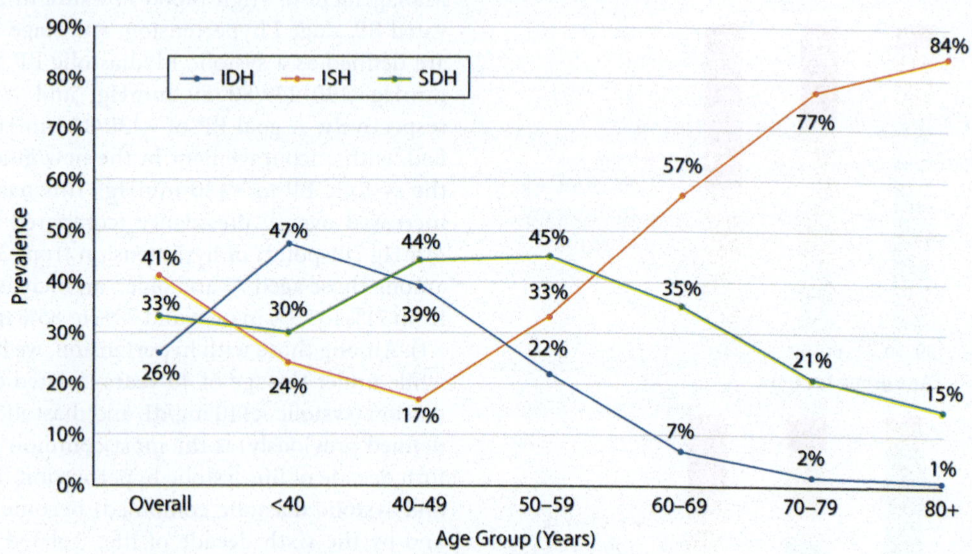

Figure 7.8 Distribution of hypertension subtype in US adults by age (NHANES). (Adapted from Tang KS et al., *Am J Hypertens*, 38(5): 303–312, 2025.)

exclusively of the ISH subtype—if they lived another 20–25 years (15). Considerable evidence, including a series of Framingham Heart Study reports, now favors the superiority of increased pulse pressure and decreased diastolic BP to that of elevated systolic BP alone in predicting cardiovascular risk in older adults. After age 50, systolic BP increases disproportionately to diastolic BP, and after 60 years of age diastolic BP falls, resulting in a further widening of pulse pressure (16). In the age range of 50–79 years, systolic BP was positively related to the incidence of CHD risk and diastolic BP was inversely related to risk, therefore supporting pulse pressure as a stronger CHD risk factor than systolic BP (17). Age is an important effect modifier in influencing BP components that predict CHD risk. Indeed, with advancing age there is a gradual shift from diastolic BP to systolic BP and eventually to pulse pressure as the strongest predictors of CHD risk (18). Furthermore, it was shown that combining systolic BP and diastolic BP was superior to systolic BP alone in predicting CVD risk (19). Systolic BP is usually superior to diastolic BP as a predictor of CVD risk from the age of 50 years onward; however, very high or very low diastolic BP adds to the systolic BP risk (19). Most recently, an analysis of over 22,000 patients in an international registry with a median 5-year follow-up found a J-shaped relationship between diastolic BP and cardiovascular events, even when controlled for pulse pressure (20) (Table 7.2).

While those aged 60–69 and 70 and older have high treatment rates for hypertension (81% and 65%), control rates are poor (54% and 33% among those treated), largely due to systolic BP being far from target. Among most persons with cardiovascular comorbidities, mean age exceeds 65 and ISH is the most predominant subtype, with systolic BP averaging 20 mmHg or more away from goal (21). Analysis of treatment failures by age revealed in the NHANES III subjects an age-related discrepancy in the successful BP control (22). Approximately 50% of younger patients who failed treatment had both systolic BP and diastolic BP that were not at target goals, representing a concordant failure in this younger population (22). In contrast, older patients who failed to achieve treatment goals had discordant failure: only 17% of patients age 50 or older were above their diastolic BP goal, but fully 82% were above their systolic BP target goal and by a significantly greater systolic BP margin (22).

While several aspects involving treatment approaches may explain the failure to optimally control ISH overall, including physician inertia and patient nonadherence, one must conclude that there is a substantial number of patients with systolic hypertension who are truly resistant to currently available medications, even when used properly. That the target systolic BP apparently becomes more difficult to achieve with aging might be explained by the presence of advanced large artery stiffness.

Table 7.2 Prediction of CVD events by SBP and DBP

SBP (mmHg)	DBP (mmHg)	HR (95% CI)
<120	<70	2.28 (1.88–2.76)
	70–79	1.54 (1.25–1.89)
	≥80	3.27 (2.00–5.33)
120–139	<70	1.48 (1.22–1.79)
	70–79	Ref (1.00)
	≥80	1.46 (1.26–1.70)
≥140	<70	1.67 (1.19–2.35)
	70–79	1.63 (1.36–1.98)
	≥80	2.36 (2.04–2.72)

Abbreviations: CI, confidence interval; CVD, cardiovascular disease; DBP, diastolic blood pressure; HR, hazard ratio; HTN, hypertension; SBP, systolic blood pressure.

Source: Vidal-Petiot E et al., *Hypertension*, 71(1), 168–176, 2018.

Numerous antihypertensive clinical trials have also shown important reductions in CVD events in older men and women. This includes the Swedish Trial in Old Patients with Hypertension among those aged 70–84 years, demonstrating a 25% reduction in fatal MI and a 67% reduction in sudden deaths and 73% reduction in fatal stroke (23), the Medical Research Council trial among those aged 65–74 showing a 25% reduction in stroke (24), the Systolic Hypertension in the Elderly study (25) among those aged 72 years on average showing a 27% reduction in nonfatal MIs and coronary death, 36% reduction in stroke, and a 49% reduction in heart failure, and in the Systolic Hypertension in Europe study (mean age 70) (26) showing a 42% reduction in stroke, but smaller nonsignificant reductions in MI and coronary mortality. Moreover, a meta-analysis of 1670 persons aged 80 years and older with hypertension showed drug therapy to reduce stroke 34%, major CVD events 22%, and heart failure 39% (27). The largest single antihypertensive clinical trial, the Antihypertensive and Lipid-Lowering Treatment to Prevent Heart Attack Trial (ALLHAT), consisting of over 40,000 patients with hypertension and a mean age of 67 years, showed after 5 years of follow-up that compared with chlorthalidone, amlodipine increased heart failure 38% and lisinopril increased combined CVD 10%, stroke 15%, and heart failure 19%, despite no statistically significant difference between the drugs in the primary endpoint of fatal CHD or nonfatal MI (relative risks of 0.98–0.99) (28). Also, in the Second Australian National Blood Pressure Study, 6083 patients with a mean age of 72 years were randomized to hydrochlorothiazide or to the ACE inhibitor enalapril, and after 4.1 years the latter resulted in a significant 11% reduction in all CVD or death from any cause (29).

Finally, with the lack of clinical trials done in those aged 80 years and older, the Hypertension in the Very Elderly Trial (HYVET) randomized over 3800 persons with a systolic BP of 160 mmHg or higher to the diuretic indapamide (sustained release, 1.5 mg) or matching placebo for 2 years and found the active treatment was associated with a 30% reduction in the rate of fatal or nonfatal stroke ($p = 0.06$), a 39% reduction in the rate of death from stroke ($p = 0.05$), and a 21% reduction in the rate of death from any cause ($p = 0.02$), with a 64% reduction in the rate of heart failure ($p < 0.001$) (Figure 7.9) (30). However, there were many questions that remained unanswered in the HYVET study, which was stopped prematurely at 18 months. The majority of recruited subjects for HYVET was healthy and robust, leading to questions about whether including a sizeable number of frail older patients would produce similar results. Second, it

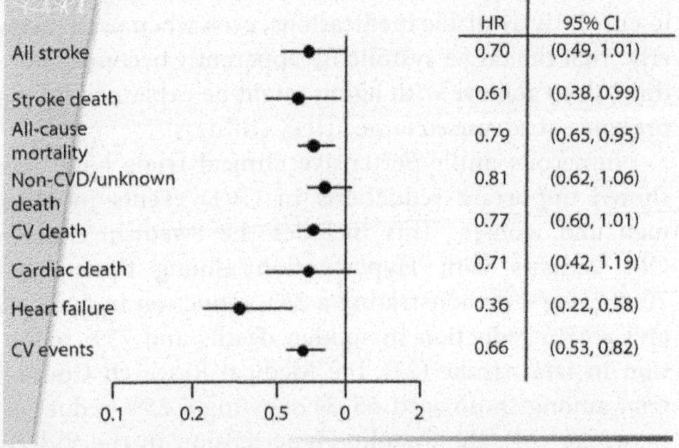

Figure 7.9 Hazard ratios for stroke and other cardiovascular endpoints in the Hypertension in the Very Elderly Trial (HYVET). (Adapted from Beckett NS et al., *N Engl J Med* 358(18), 1887–1898, 2008.)

was unclear what the optimal BP target goal for maximizing therapeutic benefit in the HYVET study was, as the authors stated that a systolic BP <150 mmHg was chosen for pragmatic reasons.

Over the past 10 years there has been a significant shift in the guideline recommendations for the treatment of BP in older adults. In 2011 expert consensus recommended BP be reduced to less than 140/90 mmHg in adults aged 60–79 years and a systolic BP to 140–145 mmHg if tolerated in adults over the age of 80 years (31). These previous guidelines were predominantly based on data from HYVET; however, the consensus recommendations for BP goals were based on expert opinion rather than on the outcome of randomized controlled trials. Furthermore, there has been no agreement on how to define "elderly," with some stating that it should be based on physiological as opposed to chronological age. Also, whether one is dealing with vigorous or frail older adults with competing illnesses has not been well considered in the past. In fact, there are no firm randomized controlled trial outcomes that provide a basis for using geriatric chronological age cut-points versus the overall general health of the patient as a guide as to how low to go with antihypertensive therapy.

In 2015, the Systolic Blood Pressure Intervention Trial (SPRINT) reported the effects of intensive (<120 mmHg) systolic BP targets compared with standard (<140 mmHg) targets in adults without diabetes (32). As compared to those with goal systolic BP <140 mmHg, those with a goal systolic BP <120 mmHg had significantly lower rates of fatal and nonfatal major CVD events (1.65% vs. 2.19% per year, hazard ration [HR] = 0.75, 95% confidence interval [CI] 0.64–0.89) and CVD death (0.25% vs. 0.43% per year, HR = 0.57, 95% CI 0.38–0.85). However, rates of serious adverse events of hypotension, syncope, electrolyte abnormalities, and acute kidney injury were higher in the intensive treatment group as compared to the standard treatment (4.7% vs. 2.5%, $p < 0.001$). Nonetheless, it was noted that the adverse events in those >75 years of age were similar to the overall cohort in the respective treatment assignment groups.

The SPRINT group conducted a similar multicenter, clinical trial in patients aged 75 years or older, randomizing them to intensive (<120 mmHg) systolic BP targets versus standard (<140 mmHg) targets (33). Among those in the intensive systolic BP group, there was a significantly lower rate of the primary outcome of nonfatal MI, acute coronary syndrome, nonfatal stroke, nonfatal acute decompensated heart failure, and death from CVD as compared to the standard systolic BP group (HR 0.66, 95% CI 0.51–0.85). Beyond the composite measure, there was a benefit in all-cause mortality in the intensive systolic BP group (HR 0.67, 95% CI 0.49–0.91). In an effort to identify if those who were more frail and older would have worse outcomes with intensive BP groups, a frailty index (34) was introduced to stratify participants into fit, less fit, and frail strata. While in the study those with worsening fitness did in fact have a greater number of events, within each frailty stratum, absolute event rates were lower for the intensive group. Serious adverse events (SAEs), including hypotension, syncope, injurious falls, electrolyte abnormalities, and bradycardia requiring hospitalization, were additionally compared between the intensive and standard blood pressure control groups. SAEs were common and essentially identical in the intensive group (48.4%) and the standard treatment group (48.3%), with no significant difference between groups in any of the SAE categories.

The SPRINT trial has largely been the driving force for the most recent 2025 guideline for BP control (12). A key advance in the 2025 guideline is the immediate consideration of pharmacologic therapy at a BP of 130/80 mmHg not only for those with known CVD or diabetes, but also if the 10-year risk of total CVD is at least 7.5% based on the new AHA Prevent Risk Score (12a) (instead of the Pooled Cohort Equation which specified a 10% ASCVD risk cutpoint in the prior 2017 guideline), which will be present in most older adults. The Prevent Risk Score incorporates similar risk factors as the Pooled Cohort Equation, but removes race and adds estimated glomerular filtration rate (eGFR) and the option to also include glycated hemoglobin, urine albumin creatinine ratio and as a social determinant of health, zip code. It predicts 10- and 30-year risk of total CVD, ASCVD, and heart failure. And even when 10-year CVD risk is below 7.5%, pharmacotherapy is still recommended if the BP remains at 130/80 mmHg or higher after a 3-6 month trial of lifestyle management alone. There is no separate distinction made for BP goals based on age. Of note, there are concerns regarding compliance, given that those in the older population often have poor vascular compliance leading to symptoms of dizziness, even with systolic BPs of 140 mmHg. In addition, adults with isolated systolic hypertension may suffer in decreasing diastolic BP at the expense at obtaining systolic BP goals. Particularly in those with CHD and diabetes, diastolic BPs below a threshold of 60 mmHg may lead to higher risks of ischemic heart disease and progressive kidney disease (35). This should be of special interest as in the SPRINT Trial for adults ≥75 years of age, mean diastolic BPs during follow-up were 62.0 mmHg in the intensive treatment group and 67.2 mmHg in the standard treatment group.

More recently, the Blood Pressure Control Target in Diabetes (BPROAD) trial examined the effect of intensive versus standard blood pressure control on a composite of nonfatal stroke, nonfatal MI, hospitalization for heart failure, or CVD mortality in patients with DM (36). In this study of over 12,000 Chinese subjects, an intensive SBP target of 120 mmHg or less resulted in a significant decrease in the primary outcome (HR 0.79, 95% CI 0.69–0.90, $p < 0.001$) compared to a conservative SBP target of 140 mmHg. Age stratification in subgroup analysis demonstrated similar effects in adults aged younger than 65 years compared to those aged 65 or older, with a non-significant trend to lower rates of the primary composite outcome in older adults (HR 0.77 vs. HR 0.81, respectively). These results further corroborated the findings of the SPRINT trial as well as the more recent Effects of Intensive Systolic Blood Pressure Lowering Treatment in Reducing Risk of Vascular Events (ESPRIT) trial, which examined over 11,000 subjects, over 75% of whom were aged 60 or older (37). The intensive BP control group with the same target of SBP 120 mmHg or less exhibited lower rates of a composite of MI, revascularization, hospitalization for heart failure, stroke, or CVD mortality compared to standard treatment to SBP 140 mmHg or less (HR 0.88, 95% CI 0.78–0.99, $p = 0.028$), regardless of the status of DM or history of stroke.

Controversy persists regarding the presence and significance of BP "J-curves" of increased cardiovascular disease risk as they relate to older people with ISH (38). A solitary diastolic BP J-curve, noted in the FHS with elevated systolic BP and pulse pressure, strongly suggests increased large artery stiffness (19); risk is defined by increased pulse pressure that results in decreased diastolic BP and increased systolic BP. In contrast, the combination of J-curves of systolic and diastolic BP, with normal-to-low pulse pressure and low mean arterial pressure (MAP), strongly suggests reverse causality (38); risk is defined by decreased diastolic and systolic BP, rather than by increased pulse pressure. Finally, in the presence of high-grade stenosis of coronary arteries, increased risk of MI with antihypertensive therapy-induced decrease in diastolic BP may well occur (39), but is by far the least common contributor to the J-curve phenomenon. Indeed, the risk of plaque disruption that leads to acute coronary syndromes depends more on plaque composition, plaque vulnerability (plaque type), and the degree of pulsatile stress than on the degree of coronary artery stenosis (plaque size) (40). Not surprisingly, therefore, the majority of MIs (>70%) occur from plaque rupture in coronary arteries that have <50% stenosis (40). Because of the many factors that result in J-curve risks, only a prospective trial with baseline and pre-event BP determinations can establish the presence and frequency of treatment-induced increased risk. On the other hand, the optimal therapeutic reduction in systolic and diastolic BP in older subjects with ISH that maximizes benefit is a separate question from the presence of a therapeutic J-curve of increased cardiovascular risk.

Importantly, the presence of white coat hypertension and masked hypertension affects the accuracy of blood pressure measurements, especially in persons of geriatric age. White coat hypertension exists if office BP is high (≥130/≥80 mmHg) but with out-of-office BP being below this point. In adults with untreated office SBP ≥130 mm Hg or DBP ≥80 mm Hg, and without office SBP ≥160 mm Hg or DBP ≥100 mm Hg, white-coat hypertension can be excluded using out-of-office BP monitoring and in those with untreated office SBP <130 mm Hg and DBP <80 mm Hg, masked hypertension can be excluded using out-of-office BP monitoring (12). In contrast, the white coat effect is the rise of BP in a medical environment regardless of daytime ABPM values in the presence or absence of antihypertensive treatment. Although the white coat effect has traditionally been viewed as independent of CVD risk (41), a recent meta-analysis found white coat hypertension to be associated with a 38% and 20% increased risk of CVD and total mortality, respectively, when compared to normotension in individuals not being treated for hypertension; however, this effect was not present in treated participants (42). In contrast, masked hypertension frequently presents as high-normal office BP, but has the CVD risk of stage 1 hypertension (43). Both masked and white coat hypertension cannot be diagnosed by office or clinic BP measurements. Furthermore, home BP monitoring does not measure daily activity or nighttime BP. Therefore, white coat and masked hypertension can best be diagnosed by ABPM.

In summary, there is overwhelming evidence that middle-aged and older adults have the highest prevalence of hypertension, predominantly of the ISH subtype, and this represents a significant burden for future CVD events. However, ISH in older adults remains more difficult to control than diastolic hypertension in younger adults. The therapeutic target goal in reducing systolic BP and diastolic BP depends in part on competing comorbidities, disabilities, and the presence of orthostatic hypotension. Future randomized controlled trials based on out-of-office BP monitoring are necessary to determine how low to go for maximum benefit of antihypertensive therapy in older adults.

Dyslipidemia

The 2024 AHA Heart Disease and Stroke Statistics reported a weighted prevalence of 34.7% and 10.0%

of total cholesterol ≥200 mg/dL and ≥240 mg/dL, respectively, in US adults per an analysis of NHANES 2017–2020, while the age-adjusted prevalences of high LDL-C (≥130 mg/dL) and low HDL-C (<40 mg/dL) were reported to be 25.5% and 16.9%, respectively, during the same time period (4). While the FHS initially showed that serum cholesterol loses its predictive value in older men (11), other cohorts have shown it remains a risk factor for new or recurrent events in both older men and women (44–47). Aronow et al. have found a 12% increase in risk for every 10 mg/dL increment in total cholesterol among 644 institutionalized elderly men and 1488 elderly women with 40–48-month follow-up (44). In a large meta-analysis of 22 US and international cohort studies, serum cholesterol appears to be a weaker predictor in both older men and women (48), although this is confounded by frailty and other comorbid conditions that, when adjusted for, appear to strengthen it as a predictor of CHD death (49). Castelli et al. also showed an important inverse relation of low HDL-C cholesterol with new coronary events (45), and Aronow et al. showed a 70% increased risk in men and 95% increased risk in women for every decrement of 10 mg/dL in HDL-C among a large institutionalized older adult cohort (44). This study did not show hypertriglyceridemia to be a risk factor in men and showed it to be a weak risk factor for CHD events in women. While total cholesterol (whose measurement alone is now obsolete) is not a consistent predictor of risk, the total cholesterol/HDL-C ratio demonstrates a nonlinear correlation with all-cause mortality (50) and may provide additional cardiovascular risk information, especially when discordant with LDL-C or non-HDL-C levels (51).

In several major clinical trials, the efficacy of LDL-C lowering with statins has been shown to be similar when comparing older to younger adults. In the Scandinavian Simvastatin Survival Study (4S), a placebo-controlled trial among high-risk persons, mostly with preexisting CHD, the statin-treated group showed a 43% reduction in CHD mortality among those aged 65 and older versus those under age 65 (52). Moreover, in the Cholesterol and Recurrent Events (CARE) study, statin therapy was actually more effective for reducing major recurrent coronary events in those aged 65 and older (32% risk reduction) compared to those under age 65 (19% risk reduction) (53). Few trials of lipid intervention have been done specifically in the older adult population. In the Prospective Study of Pravastatin in the Elderly at Risk (PROSPER) trial (54), men and women aged 70–82 years with a history of, or risk factors for, vascular disease were randomized to pravastatin (40 mg per day; $n = 2891$) or placebo ($n = 2913$). Follow-up was 3.2 years on average, with the primary endpoint a composite of coronary death, nonfatal MI, and fatal or nonfatal stroke. Pravastatin lowered LDL-C concentrations by 34% and reduced the incidence of the primary endpoint (HR 0.85, 95% CI 0.74–0.97, $p = 0.014$). CHD death and nonfatal MI risk was also reduced (0.81, 0.69–0.94, $p = 0.006$). However, new cancer diagnoses

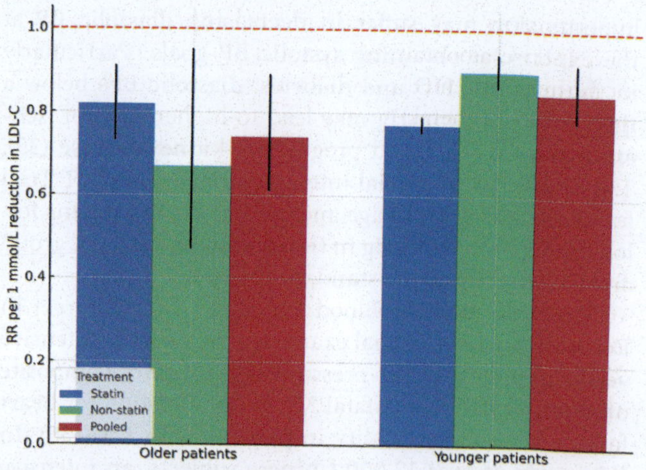

Figure 7.10 Effect of lipid-lowering therapies on risk of major vascular events in older (age ≥75) versus younger patients. (Adapted from Gencer B et al., *Lancet*, 396, 22–27, 2020.)

were more frequent on pravastatin than on placebo (1.25, 1.04–1.51, $p = 0.020$), although incorporation of this finding in a meta-analysis of all pravastatin and all statin trials showed no overall increase in risk. Importantly, the Cholesterol Treatment Trialists' collaboration (55) of over 180,000 subjects among 28 trials showed an overall benefit of lipid-lowering therapy to reduce CHD event risk by 24% per 1.0 mmol/L reduction in LDL-C, with no significant differences across age groups <65 years, 65–74 years, and 75 years and older, although the benefit appeared a bit weaker (16% risk reduction) in the latter group who do not already have ASCVD. A recent meta-analysis including over 240,000 participants pooled from 29 trials found lipid-lowering therapy to be as effective in reducing both cardiovascular events and cardiovascular death in older adults (age ≥75) compared to adults age <75 (56) (Figure 7.10). A subsequent analysis of over 60,000 individuals from the Danish national health care and administrative registries corroborated this conclusion and found the use of lipid-lowering therapies for primary prevention of ASCVD to cause similar LDL-C and major vascular event risk reductions in older adults (age ≥70) when compared to middle-aged adults (age 50–69) (57).

Metabolic syndrome, diabetes, and cardiovascular–kidney–metabolic (CKM) health

Metabolic syndrome is jointly defined by the American Heart Association, NHLBI, and IDF, among others (4), as the presence of three or more of the following factors: (1) abdominal obesity defined as a waist circumference >102 cm in men or >88 cm in women; (2) increased BP of ≥130 mmHg systolic or ≥85 mmHg diastolic or on therapy for BP; (3) impaired fasting glucose of 100 mg/dL or higher or on hyperglycemic therapy; (4) HDL-cholesterol <40 mg/

dL in men or <50 mg/dL in women or on medication for low HDL-C; and/or (5) fasting triglycerides of 150 mg/dL or higher or on medication for hypertriglyceridemia. The prevalence of metabolic syndrome in US adults increases dramatically with age, reaching 48.6% in those aged ≥60 years (4). Moreover, diabetes mellitus (DM), defined by a fasting glucose ≥126 mg/dL or on hyperglycemic therapy, also increases in prevalence with age, approaching 30% in adults age 65 and older compared to a prevalence of just 4.8% and 18.9% in those aged 18–44 and 45–64, respectively (58); the lifetime risk of DM is 25%–45% in females and 30%–55% in males (59) and varies substantially according to ethnicity and sex, being highest in non-Hispanic Asian males and Hispanic males and lowest in non-Hispanic White and Asian females (4) (Figure 7.11). Importantly, with the burden of CVD risk factors also increasing with age, estimated short-term (10-year) risk of CHD or CVD also increases with age, so that many persons with metabolic syndrome or DM who already either have CHD or CVD are at >20% 10-year risk of these conditions by the age of 65 (60, 61). In fact, 80% or more of those with diabetes over the age of 60 are at either >20% CVD risk or have preexisting CVD (61).

DM is a clear risk factor for CHD events in older men and women (44, 62) and has been associated with an approximate twofold increase in risk of new coronary events in a large study of 644 elderly men and 1488 elderly women followed for 40–48 months (44). In the FHS, increased blood glucose as well as a composite of glucose intolerance and diabetes, was a powerful risk factor for incident CHD events in 30-year follow-up (11); it is also a stronger risk factor in women, both among younger and older adults (62).

There have not been any large clinical trials examining the impact of intensive glycemic control in older persons with DM; however, several recent large trials have examined stratification of their key results according to age groups. For example, the Action in Diabetes and Vascular Disease: Preterax and Diamicron Modified Released Controlled Evaluation (ADVANCE) trial of intensive blood glucose control and vascular outcomes in 11,140 persons with type 2 DM showed intensive control to a hemoglobin (Hb) A1C to ≤6.5% showed a similar 30% reduction in combined major microvascular and macrovascular events in both those aged <65 and ≥65, although the finding did not reach statistical significance in the older subgroup; overall, this study did not show a risk reduction in major macrovascular events (63). The Action to Control Cardiovascular Risk in Diabetes (ACCORD) Study Group similarly showed no beneficial effect of intensive glucose control among 10,251 patients randomized to standard or intensive therapy to achieve an HbA1C <6.0% in either younger or older (age 65 years or greater) subgroups (64). Only recently has there been renewed excitement in the potential of hypoglycemic agents to reduce CVD risk. The Empagliflozin Cardiovascular Outcome Event Trial in Type 2 Diabetes Mellitus Patients—Removing Excess Glucose (EMPA-REG OUTCOME) trial showed that among persons with known CVD and DM, the sodium glucose cotransporter 2 (SGLT2) inhibitor empagliflozin demonstrated efficacy for reducing risk of the primary composite cardiovascular endpoint by 14%, with subgroup analyses actually showing benefit was greater for those aged ≥65 versus <65 years of age (p = 0.01 for interaction) (65). However, a more recent meta-analysis including data from EMPRA-REG OUTCOME, the Canagliflozin Cardiovascular Assessment Study (CANVAS) Program, and Dapagliflozin Effect on Cardiovascular Events—Thrombolysis in Myocardial Infarction 58 (DECLARE-TIMI 58) trial showed SGLT2 inhibitors to offer only moderate reduction in major cardiovascular events and

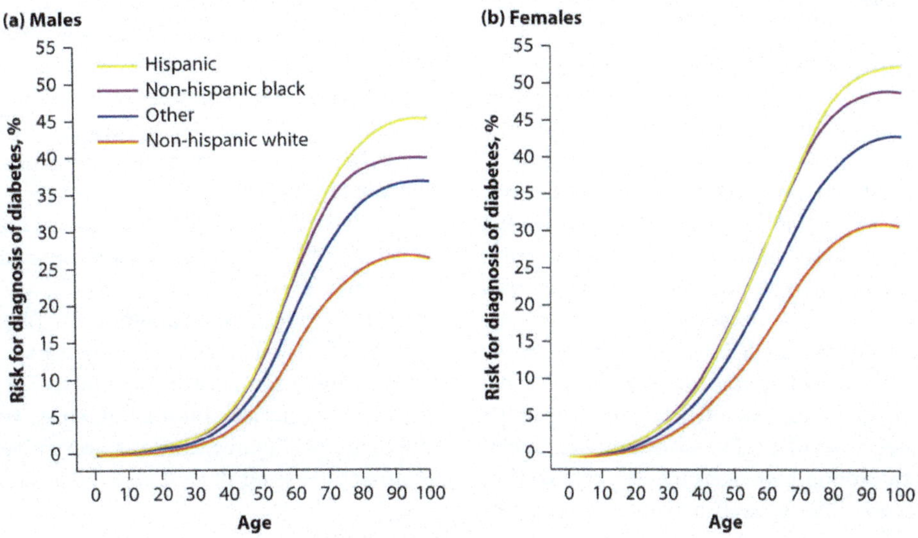

Figure 7.11 (a, b) Cumulative lifetime risk of developing diabetes by age and ethnicity. (Adapted from Ford ES et al., *Diabetes Care*, 27, 2444, 2004.)

only in patients with established atherosclerotic CVD (HR 0.89, 95% CI 0.83–0.94, $p = 0.0014$) (66), although the benefits with regard to reducing risk for hospitalization in heart failure and in slowing progression of chronic kidney disease appeared more robust. In the Liraglutide Effect and Action in Diabetes: Evaluation of Cardiovascular Outcome Results (LEADER) trial, the glucagon-like peptide-1 (GLP-1) agonist liraglutide showed in those with DM and CVD or at high risk of CVD an overall reduction in the primary cardiovascular endpoint of 14%, with similar reductions in risk in those aged ≥60 years and <60 years (10% and 22%, respectively, $p = 0.27$ for interaction) (67). Additional trials have since been published demonstrating similar efficacy of other GLP-1 agonist agents, including semaglutide (68) and dulaglutide (69), in achieving glycemic control and reducing rates of major cardiovascular events.

Most recently, the American Heart Association introduced cardiovascular–kidney–metabolic (CKM) health to reflect the connection between metabolic risk factors, chronic kidney disease, and the cardiovascular system, which has important implications for morbidity and mortality (70). This scientific advisory proposed a CKM staging construct reflecting the pathophysiology, spectrum of risk, and opportunities for prevention and care optimization within CKM syndrome: stage 0, no CKM risk factors; stage 1, excess or dysfunctional adiposity; stage 2, metabolic risk factors (hypertriglyceridemia, hypertension, diabetes, metabolic syndrome) or moderate- to high-risk chronic kidney disease; stage 3, subclinical CVD in CKM syndrome or risk equivalents (high predicted CVD risk or very high-risk CKD); and stage 4, clinical CVD in CKM syndrome. An analysis of NHANES 2011–2020 found the prevalence of advanced CKM (stages 3 and 4) to increase significantly with age, with 55.3% of adults aged 65 or older having advanced CKM compared to 10.7% and 2.1% in adults aged 45–64 and 20–44, respectively (71).

Cigarette smoking

The prevalence of cigarette smoking has seen significant decline since the first US Surgeon General's report on smoking and health in 1964, from 51% of males and 34% of females in 1965 to 15.6% and 12.0%, respectively, in 2018 (4). The latest AHA statistics report noted only 8.3% of adults aged 65 or older were current smokers, compared to 12.6% and 14.9% in adults aged 25–44 and 45–64, respectively (4). The FHS initially demonstrated that cigarette smoking was not associated with incident CHD in persons aged 65 and older; however, approximate twofold greater risks of CHD among smokers have been observed both among men aged 65–74 years in the Honolulu Heart Study (72) as well as in 40–48-month follow-up of 644 men and 1488 women with a mean age of 80 years (44). Among secondary prevention studies, the Coronary Artery Surgery Study (CASS) showed a 1.5-fold greater risk of MI or death in those aged 65–69 years of age, which increased to 2.9-fold for those age 70 and older who continued to smoke compared to those who quit smoking (73). CASS data additionally showed that the 6-year mortality rate (relative risk of 1.7) was greater among continuing smokers as compared to those who quit smoking a year prior to the study and abstained from smoking throughout the study. Importantly, there was no diminution of the beneficial effects of smoking cessation by age. These findings indicate that smoking cessation lessens the risk of MI and improves survival rates in both older and younger individuals.

Overweight and obesity

It has been well established that obesity, defined as a body mass index (BMI) ≥30 kg/m^2, is a risk factor for second coronary events in older adults with CHD. According to NHANES 2017–2020, obesity prevalence in older adults age 65 or older was 41.5%, with significant variation between sex and ethnic groups (4). While past prospective studies have shown that general and central adiposity are risk factors for CHD incidence in middle-aged men and women, fewer studies have focused on CHD in the older adult population. Data from the FHS suggests that older persons have similar risk factors for CHD as younger adults (74). While true, studies of data from both the Honolulu Heart Program and the Health Professionals Follow-Up Study (HPFS) have shown that weight gain in adults younger than 65 years of age is more strongly correlated with CHD risk than weight gain in those older than 65 (75, 76). Past cohort studies in older adults have found weak to no correlation of BMI with CHD, indicating that BMI alone may be a flawed metric for visceral and overall adiposity in this demographic (75, 76). However, these same studies did show waist circumference and fat distribution are strong predictors of CVD and CHD events (77). Using HPFS data, Rimm at al. showed that despite a weak association between BMI and risk of CHD among men ≥65 years, waist-to-hip ratio showed a relative risk of 2.76 when comparing extreme quintiles (75). This is most likely due to increased body fat in the abdominal cavity with increased age, causing the waist–hip ratio to be better than BMI as an indicator of overall fat in older persons (78).

Villareal et al. used a randomized control trial to show that lifestyle interventions of diet-induced weight loss and exercise training improved obesity-related CHD risk factors in obese older adults (79). These results indicate that CHD risk factors, including waist circumference, BP, circulating inflammatory markers, oral glucose tolerance, insulin resistance, plasma glucose, triacylglycerol and free fatty acid concentrations, were reversible, not only in younger obese adults but also older obese adults.

Physical activity

Decreased fitness and physical activity (PA) have been shown to be predictors of mortality in older adults (79).

These findings, independent of overall or abdominal adiposity, have led to recommendations for regular PA in older adults. The aerobic Physical Activity Guidelines for Americans recommends ≥150 min/week of moderate PA or ≥75 min/week of vigorous PA, or an equivalent combination of both. The 2020 NHIS found that only 24.2% of US adults met criteria for recommended PA, with the percentage decreasing progressively with increasing age regardless of sex (only 15.3% of men and 10.8% of women aged 65 and over met recommendations compared to 41.3% and 28.7% of men and women age 18–34, respectively) (4). The report also found significant variation according to ethnicity, education level, and urbanicity. PA is a significant predictor of CHD risk. Data from the Honolulu Heart Program shows a 2.2 relative risk of developing a coronary event for older men who walked less than 0.25 miles a day as compared to those who walked more than 1.5 miles a day (80). Similar results were found from the Harvard Alumni Study, in which men with a starting mean age of 66 who expended 4000 kcal/week in physical activities through recreational sports, climbing stairs, and walking found a relative risk reduction of 38% for CHD as compared to those expending less than 1000 kcal/week (81). The study found that the duration of PA did not have a different effect on relative risk as long as energy expended was the same. PA has proven beneficial for total cardiovascular health in older adults. Data from 1645 men and women older than 65 years showed that walking more than 4 hours/week was significantly associated with a reduced risk of CVD hospitalization (relative risk of 0.69) compared to those walking less than 1 hour/week after adjusting for baseline cardiovascular risk factors and general health (82). Of note, in all these studies of older cohorts, smaller proportions of individuals were older than 80 years of age. Nonetheless, data from these studies suggest that exercise by older adults has similar magnitudes of benefits of CHD risk reduction as seen in those who are younger.

Secondary prevention through PA has additionally proven effective for the reduction of mortality secondary to CHD. The British Regional Heart Study showed that of those patients diagnosed with CHD, the lowest risk for all-cause cardiovascular mortality was seen in patients with light and moderate PA (relative risks of 0.42 and 0.47, respectively) as compared to those patients who were inactive or occasionally active (83). Nonsporting activities such as heavy gardening and regular walking were seen to be more beneficial than sporting activities.

Inflammatory risk factors

Inflammatory markers increase with age, due to declining levels of sex hormones and increases in visceral adipose tissue (84). Thus, whether these inflammatory markers can be categorized as independent risk factors for CHD has become of high interest for early screening. High-sensitivity C-reactive protein (hsCRP) has been established as an acute inflammatory marker that plays a significant role in cardiovascular health. In 2002 the American Heart Association and Centers for Disease Control and Prevention suggested that hsCRP may be a useful screening mechanism for 10-year risk of CHD of between 10% and 20% (85). However, not based on data from the older adult population, these recommendations would have applied to the vast majority of American men and women over the age of 65 who have a 10-year CHD risk of at least 10% (86). Inflammatory markers have been shown to be associated with CHD risk prediction for older adults; however, their added benefit over other traditional risk factors is controversial. Most recently, the US Preventive Services Task Force found inadequate evidence to advocate for the addition of hsCRP to traditional CVS risk assessment models (87). However, there is some evidence from the LoDoCo2 Trial that low-dose colchicine can reduce the risk of major cardiovascular events in patients with chronic CHD (HR 0.69, 95% CI 0.57–0.83, $p < 0.001$ compared to placebo), accompanied by a non-significant higher incidence of non-cardiovascular death in the treatment group (HR 1.51, 95% CI 0.99–2.31) (88). The reduced risk of the primary composite endpoint was also consistent between those aged >65 versus <65 years of age.

Lipoprotein-associated phospholipase A2 (Lp-PLA2), a proatherogenic inflammatory marker, has been shown to be strongly associated with risk of incident CHD in middle-aged populations (89, 90). More recently, data using the Rancho Bernardo Study showed that Lp-PLA2 mass has demonstrated capabilities for predicting risk of CHD independent of traditional CHD risk factors in healthy older adults (91). Hazard ratios ranging from 1.89 to 1.75 were calculated for the highest Lp-PLA2 quartile when compared to the lowest quartile after adjusting for cumulative traditional CHD risk factors.

PREVENTIVE STRATEGIES

Primordial and primary prevention

Preventing CHD in older adults involves not only primary and secondary prevention approaches but also primordial prevention approaches, that is, preventing the major CHD risk factors from developing in the first place. The construct of the American Heart Association's Life's Essential 8 (92) calls for achieving normal cholesterol, BP, glucose, and body fat, reducing nicotine and tobacco exposure, following a heart-healthy diet, getting regular physical activity, and maintaining 7–9 hours of sleep each night. Recent data from the NHANES 2013–2018 showed that middle-aged and older adults on average scored significantly worse (mean score 62.2 and 62.3, respectively) on the Life's Essential 8 cardiovascular health score (possible range, 0 to 100) compared to younger adults under

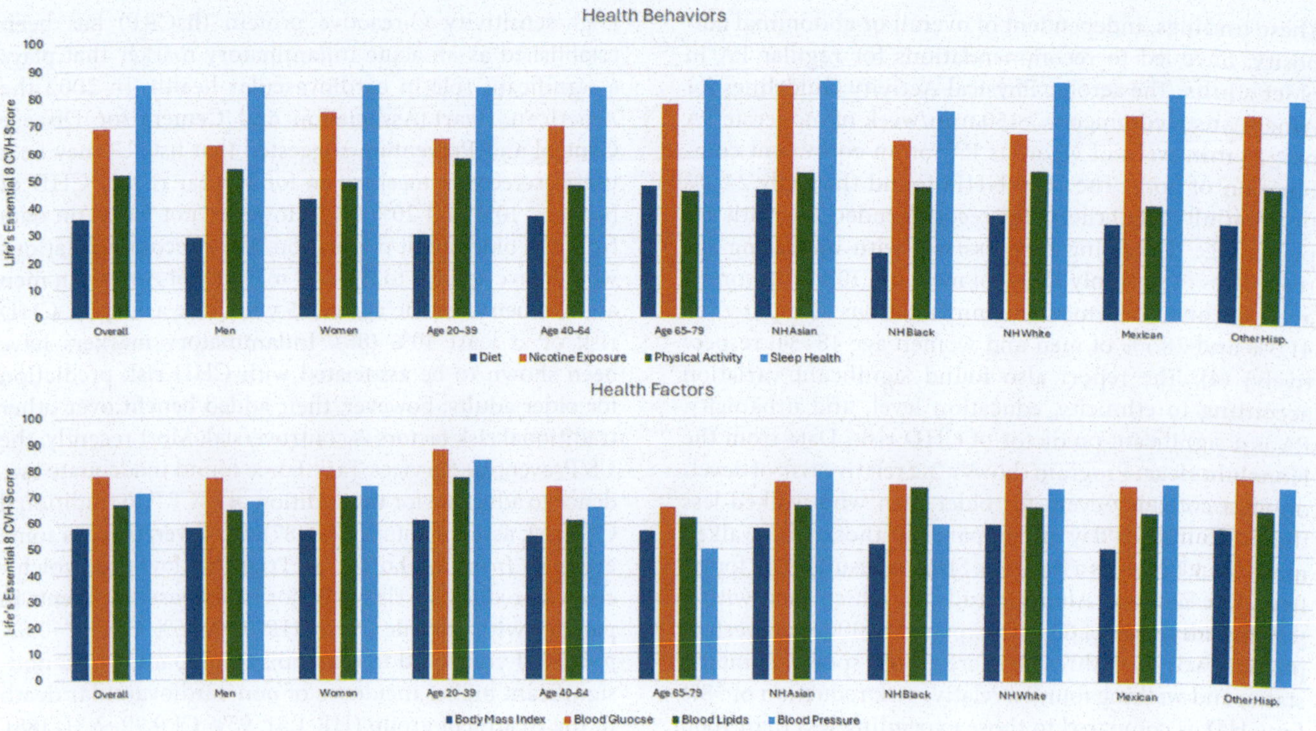

Figure 7.12 Cardiovascular health scores for (a) health behaviors and (b) health factors by age, sex, and race and ethnicity among US adults. National Health and Nutrition Examination Survey 2013–2018. (From Lloyd-Jones DM et al., *Circulation*, 146(11), 822–835, 2022.)

age 40 years (mean score 68.7) (93). Notably, those aged 65–79 years scored significantly worse on tobacco exposure, BP control, and serum glucose levels (Figure 7.12).

While the relative benefits of lowering BP and lipid intervention have been shown to be consistent across all age groups, such interventions are of particular importance in older adults, where the absolute risk for CHD events is dramatically higher than in younger persons. Thus, the absolute risk reduction resulting from risk factor interventions is dramatic and the number of preventable CHD events is substantial. For example, we have previously demonstrated among US adults with the metabolic syndrome that optimal management of dyslipidemia (LDL-C and HDL-C) and BP could potentially prevent up to 80% of CHD events, a finding that is consistent across age groups. This translates to preventing about 1.3 million CHD events in men and 530,000 CHD events in women; however, of these, approximately 600,000 of those events in men and 300,000 in women are among those aged 60 and older (94). In the same study, optimal management of BP to <120/80 mmHg would be projected to prevent up to 29% of CHD events in older men and 48% of CHD events in older women.

Cardiovascular risk assessment is the foundation for prevention of CHD. The ACC/AHA 2013 Guideline on the Assessment of Cardiovascular Risk (95) recommends the use of the Pooled Cohort Risk Calculator as the initial step in cardiovascular risk assessment, which provides an estimate of 10-year risk of ASCVD for those aged 40–79 (and lifetime risk for those aged 20–59) years. Newer risk scores such as the PREVENT risk scores may be considered in future guidelines. The guideline states that if the treatment decision is uncertain based on the risk calculator, then risk enhancing factors can be used to inform the treatment decision, such as the existence of a premature family history of ASCVD (prior ASCVD in a first-degree male relative <55 years of age or female relative <65 years of age), high sensitivity C-reactive protein >2 mg/L, ABI <0.9 (diagnostic of peripheral arterial disease), as well as certain pregnancy-related factors such as pre-eclampsia or premature menopause. Further consideration of results from coronary calcium testing can also inform the treatment decision, such as a coronary calcium score ≥100 or ≥75th percentile for age and sex.

The ACC/AHA 2019 Guideline on the Primary Prevention of Cardiovascular Disease (96) recommends consumption of a diet that emphasizes intake of vegetables, fruits, legumes, nuts, fish, and whole grains; substitutes of monounsaturated and polyunsaturated fats in place of saturated fats; and reduced intake of cholesterol, sodium, processed meats, and refined carbohydrates. Such a dietary pattern should be adapted to appropriate calorie requirements, personal and cultural food preferences, and nutrition therapy for other medical conditions (including diabetes). It is recommended that such a dietary pattern can be achieved by following plans such as the Dietary Approaches to Stop Hypertension (DASH) dietary pattern, the US Department of Agriculture (USDA) Food Pattern, or the AHA Diet. There is further evidence from an analysis of the NHANES 1999–2002 and 2019–2022 that found >2 g/day sodium consumption, >14 servings/week red meat consumption, and consumption of sugar-sweetened beverages and processed red meat were associated with a higher risk of cardiovascular death (97). As for physical activity, it is generally recommended that adults engage in aerobic physical activity to reduce LDL-C and non-HDL-C: three to four sessions a week, lasting on average 40 minutes per session, and involving moderate- to vigorous-intensity physical activity. No specific recommendations differentiate older from younger people; however, specific issues for older persons (e.g., sarcopenia, osteoporosis) must be taken into account when designing a physical activity program.

The ACC/AHA/TOC Guideline for Management of Overweight and Obesity in Adults (98) notes that even modest weight loss (3%–5% of body weight) can result in clinically meaningful benefits for triglycerides, blood glucose, glycated hemoglobin, and prevention of diabetes (type 2). It specifically suggests that overweight and obese individuals participate for ≥6 months in a comprehensive lifestyle program adhering to a lower-calorie diet, increasing physical activity, and prescribing to high-intensity (i.e., ≥14 sessions in 6 months) comprehensive weight loss interventions by a trained interventionist (dietitian, exercise physiologist). There are no age-specific recommendations for these guidelines.

As for cigarette smoking cessation, at each clinic visit, the five A's are recommended in the patient encounter, which includes asking about tobacco use, advising the patient to quit, assessing readiness to quit, assisting the patient to obtain required resources (e.g., individual or group counselling and/or pharmacologic therapy), and arranging for needed follow-up visits to provide guidance and assistance.

Given that hypertension is the single greatest cause of mortality globally (1), its prevention and control, especially among older adults who have the highest absolute risks due to CHD, is essential. Besides sodium restriction, achieving ideal body weight, moderation of alcohol consumption, and getting regular physical activity, which each can lower systolic BP 5 mmHg or more, together can have a significant impact on controlling elevated BP. The recent 2025 ACC/AHA/Multisociety high blood pressure guideline also gives consideration for potassium-based salt substitutes for prevention or treatment of elevated blood pressure and hypertension (12). Achieving better adherence to these means of lowering BP is crucial given that many older persons still have systolic BP averaging 20 mmHg or more away from goal despite being on treatment (22). With the recent 2025 ACC/AHA/Multisociety high blood pressure guideline (12) identifying more persons who should be treated for elevated BP, this will be an impetus for stronger recommendations for adherence to lifestyle management to reduce BP, before the consideration of pharmacologic therapy for those with BP>130/80 mmHg.

The 2018 ACC/AHA guidelines on the treatment of blood cholesterol to reduce ASCVD risk in adults (99) notes those eligible for statins to include (1) those with known ASCVD (described below under secondary prevention, (2) those with LDL-C ≥190 mg/dL, (3) those with diabetes aged 40–75, and (4) those without diabetes, but who are aged 40–75 years of age and have ≥20% risk of ASCVD based on the Pooled Cohort Risk Calculator, with those at borderline (5–<7.5%) or intermediate (7.5–<20%) risk indicated for further assessment of a variety of risk enhancing factors (including premature family history of ASCVD, persistently elevated LDL-C >160 mg/dL, chronic kidney disease, metabolic syndrome, conditions specific to women, inflammatory disease, high-risk ethnicity such as South Asian, and elevations in biomarkers including lipoprotein(a), hs-C-reactive protein, apolipoprotein B, and abnormal ankle brachial index) to further inform the treatment decision. Coronary calcium testing was also introduced to further inform the treatment decision if needed. The guideline noted that a clinician's discussion should guide treatment for those older than 75. There should always be a patient–clinician discussion about what the risks mean and the best ways to reduce them, including nonpharmacologic lifestyle recommendations, and the risks and benefits of any pharmacologic therapy. It has been previously noted that randomized clinical trial evidence does support the continuation of statins in those already taking and tolerating them, and that while there is a large amount of data supporting the use of moderate-intensity statins in persons over the age of 75 years, the few data supporting the initiation of high-intensity statins in this age group are unclear. In addition, data are limited supporting ASCVD risk reduction for primary prevention among those aged >75 years; thus initiation of statins in this age group requires consideration of other factors such as comorbidities, safety considerations, and priorities of care.

Tobacco use, high blood glucose, physical inactivity, overweight/obesity, and elevated cholesterol levels are the second through sixth top risk factors for death globally. Their predominance in older adults makes these important targets for primary prevention of CHD in this age group. The benefits of tobacco cessation and lipid intervention are well demonstrated in older adults, and improved weight control and greater physical activity will have benefits as well in helping to maintain healthy blood glucose levels and prevent diabetes.

Secondary prevention

Secondary prevention of CHD in older adults involves intervention on many of the same risk factors, including recommendations for lifestyle management as discussed earlier, although there are limited data that have shown the efficacy of these interventions in older persons (98). Smoking cessation can reduce overall mortality by

25%–50% in those who have suffered MI, with much of this decline in the first year (101). Smoking cessation rates in middle-aged and older persons range from 20% to 70% after 1 year (102); multiple-component programs combine strong physician advice with behavioral counseling, nicotine replacement therapy, and nurse case management for follow-up (103).

For antihypertensive therapy, meta-analyses have shown the efficacy of treatment to be particularly high in those aged 60–80 years (104), and in older persons, more strokes and heart failure are generally prevented compared to coronary events. The recent 2025 ACC/AHA/Multisociety High Blood Pressure Guideline (12) has similar targets regardless of the presence of cardiovascular disease or other comorbidities of <130/80 mmHg, despite older guidelines that suggest more lenient targets (such as a systolic BP <150 mmHg) in less complicated patients, given the lack of rigorous clinical trial evidence in the older adult population.

For lipid-lowering therapy, given the consistency of statin therapy's impact on reducing CHD events both in older and younger persons, and the greater absolute baseline CHD risk with aging, makes appropriate achievement of lipid targets an important measure in secondary prevention. It is estimated from the CARE study, where statin therapy was shown to be more effective in older patients with known CHD (32% risk reduction compared to 19% reduction in younger patients), that for every 1000 older patients treated, 225 CVD hospitalizations could be prevented compared with 121 for 1000 younger patients (105). Statin therapy in older adults has been shown to be cost-effective, with an incremental cost per quality-adjusted life year being $18,800, which will be even lower if estimated based on the cost of now widely available generic statins (106). In persons with known ASCVD, current ACC/AHA guidelines for cholesterol management recommend a high-intensity statin, or in those aged ≥75 years, a moderate-intensity statin. However, since substantial residual CVD risk exists despite statin therapy in these and other trials, recent guidance from the ACC nonstatin expert consensus decision pathway has recommended the addition of nonstatin therapies beyond maximally tolerated statin therapy when >50% LDL-C lowering or LDL-C <70 mg/dL (<100 mg/dL for non-HDL-C) is not reached in high-risk persons or LDL-C <55 mg/dL (<85 mg/dL for non-HDL-C) for those with very high risk ASCVD (two or more major ASCVD events and one major with multiple high risk conditions). These newer recommendations are particularly relevant for older persons with ASCVD, of whom many will have had multiple ASCVD events or high-risk conditions qualifying them as very high-risk ASCVD patients. This document recommended ezetimibe or a PCSK9 inhibitor as the first choice of nonstatin therapy, followed by bempedoic acid or inclisiran (107). Subgroup analyses involving the use of nonstatin therapies show the use of ezetimibe on top of simvastatin (compared to simvastatin alone) in the Improved Reduction of Outcomes: Vytorin Efficacy International Trial (IMPROVE-IT) in patients with recent acute coronary syndrome (108) among prespecified subgroup analyses showed similar benefit at 1 year in those ≥65 versus those <65 years of age (HRs of 0.89 and 0.975, respectively, $p = 0.090$ for heterogeneity) but greater benefit at 2 years in those ≥75 versus those <75 years of age (HRs 0.80 and 0.97, respectively, $p < 0.001$ for heterogeneity). The Reduction of Cardiovascular Events with Icosapent Ethyl—Intervention Trial (REDUCE-IT) involving patients with known ASCVD or DM with cardiovascular risk factors currently on statin therapy with serum triglycerides between 135–499 mg/dL found a 25% risk reduction in major cardiovascular events with the addition of icosapent ethyl (HR 0.75, 95% CI 0.68–0.83, $p < 0.001$) (109), although subgroup analysis found this effect to be attenuated for participants aged ≥65 years (HR 0.87, 95% CI 0.76–1.00 compared to HR 0.65, 95% CI 0.56-0.75 for adults <65 years, $p = 0.004$ for interaction). From use of the PCSK9 monoclonal antibody therapy evolocumab on top of statin therapy (versus statin alone) in the Further Cardiovascular Outcomes Research with PCSK9 Inhibition in Subjects with Elevated Risk (FOURIER) trial (110), there was similar efficacy in persons aged ≥65 years (HR = 0.85, 95% CI = 0.76–0.95) as compared to <65 years (HR = 0.86, 95% CI = 0.78–0.94) for the primary composite endpoint.

The control of obesity, which is an important risk factor for secondary CHD events in older persons from the FHS (111), can have important benefits on several major risk factors, including dyslipidemia, hypertension, and insulin resistance, which all impact CHD risk. It is well established that exercise training alone without a nutritional approach has only a minimal effect, thus a multidisciplinary approach combining the two, along with other behavioral interventions as needed, is critically important. There are relatively few studies specifically among older adults with CHD that have documented the effects of weight loss on outcomes. In one study of obese patients of mean age 60 who had CHD, a mean weight loss of 11 kg was associated with a 10% reduction in total and LDL-C, 24% reduction in triglycerides, and an 8% increase in HDL-C as a result of a hypocaloric diet (112).

While there is a lack of data on the efficacy of diabetes interventions in reducing CHD risk in older persons with CHD, the management of diabetes, which is often accompanied by dyslipidemia and hypertension in older adults, is crucial to preventing microvascular complications and reduces the attributable risk of CHD events, especially due to dyslipidemia and hypertension. Although an official goal of A1C <7% is generally recommended, most older persons have had long-standing diabetes and/or macrovascular disease and may have difficulty reaching this target without experiencing hypoglycemia or other adverse effects of therapy. Thus, less stringent A1C goals may be appropriate in such patients. For those with known CVD and diabetes, the most recent American Diabetes Association guidelines have recommended that early combination therapy consisting of metformin with a SGLT2 inhibitor or GLP-1 agonist be initiated based on the clinical needs for additional glycemic control or cardiorenal protection, with several of these therapies indicated for CVD risk reduction (113).

CONCLUSION

Much of the burden and costs due to hospitalizations from CHD are borne by those aged 65 and over, although with an increasing focus on biologic age, such a cut-point is quite arbitrary, and an increasing proportion of older adults can live fully functioning lives many years beyond this age. With key lifestyle recommendations and pharmacologic interventions definitively shown to prevent or reduce the development of important risk factors such as hypertension, dyslipidemia, and diabetes, and whose adverse effects have been demonstrated to be consistent in older populations, we have a significant opportunity in the next decade to keep older persons healthier and free of CHD for longer, thus exemplifying the concept of healthy aging. Updated guidelines for secondary prevention of CHD and efficacy of risk factor interventions in this group can have a significant impact on reducing the risk of recurrent events. The proliferation of new knowledge on CVD prevention offers significant opportunity for increasing CVD-free life expectancy and keeping our current young and middle-aged adult populations healthier into their senior years.

ACKNOWLEDGMENT

The authors wish to acknowledge the significant contributions Dr. Stanley S. Franklin made to understanding cardiovascular disease in older persons, especially on the role aging plays in hypertension, as well as his contributions to prior chapters in this text.

REFERENCES

1. Mendis S, Puska P, Norvving B, eds. *Global Atlas on Cardiovascular Disease Prevention and Control.* Washington, DC: World Health Organization, 2011.
2. *US Census Bureau. US Population Projects: 2010–2050.* US Department of Commerce; Washington, DC, 2008. www.census.gov/population/www/projections/summarytables.html.
3. Najjar SS, Lakatta EG, Gerstenblith G. Cardiovascular aging: The next frontier in cardiovascular prevention. In: Blumenthal RS, Foody JM, Wong ND, eds. *Preventive Cardiology: A Companion to Braunwald's Heart Disease.* New York: Elsevier, 2011.
4. Martin SS, Aday AW, Almarzooq ZI et al. American Heart Association Council on Epidemiology and Prevention Statistics Committee and Stroke Statistics Subcommittee. 2024 heart disease and stroke statistics: A report of US and global data from the American Heart Association. *Circulation* 2024; *149*(8): e347–e913.
5. Wong ND, Lopez VA, Allison M et al. Abdominal aortic calcium and multi-site atherosclerosis: The Multiethnic Study of Atherosclerosis. *Atherosclerosis* 2011; *214*: 436–441.
6. Lloyd-Jones D, Larson MG, Beiser A et al. Lifetime risk of developing coronary heart disease. *Lancet* 1999; *353*: 89–92.
7. Benjamin EJ, Blaha MJ, Chiuve SE et al. American Heart Association Statistics Committee and Stroke Statistics Subcommittee. Heart disease and stroke statistics update: A report from the American Heart Association. *Circulation* 2017; *135*(*10*): e146–e603.
8. Bild DE, Fitzpatrick A, Fried LP et al. Age-related trends in cardiovascular morbidity and physical functioning in the elderly: The Cardiovascular Health Study. *J Am Geriat Soc* 1993; *41*: 1047–1056.
9. Kuller LH, Arnold AM, Psaty BM et al. 10-year follow-up of subclinical cardiovascular disease and risk of coronary heart disease in the cardiovascular health study. *Arch Intern Med* 2006; *166*: 71–78.
10. Budoff MJ, Young R, Burke G et al. Ten-year association of coronary artery calcium with atherosclerotic cardiovascular disease (ASCVD) events: The multi-ethnic study of atherosclerosis (MESA). *Eur Heart J* 2018; *39*(*25*): 2401–2408.
11. Cupples LA, D'Agostino RB. Section 34. Some risk factors related to the annual incidence of cardiovascular disease and death using pooled repeated biennial measurements: Framingham Heart Study, 30-year follow-up. In: Kannel WB, Wolf PA, Garrison RJ, eds. *The Framingham Study: An Epidemiological Investigation of Cardiovascular Disease.* Bethesda, MD: National Heart, Lung and Blood Institute, publication No. (NIH) 87-2703, 1987.
12. Writing Committee Members; Jones DW, Ferdinand KC, Taler SJ, et al. 2025 AHA/ACC/AANP/AAPA/ABC/ACCP/ACPM/AGS/AMA/ASPC/NMA/PCNA/SGIM guideline for the prevention, detection, evaluation and management of high blood pressure in adults: A report of the American College of Cardiology/American Heart Association Joint Committee on Clinical Practice Guidelines. *Hypertension* 2025 Oct;*82*(*10*): e212–e316.

12a. Khan SS, Coresh J, Pencina MJ, et al. American heart association. novel prediction equations for absolute risk assessment of total cardiovascular disease incorporating cardiovascular-kidney-metabolic health: A scientific statement from the American Heart Association. *Circulation* 2023 Dec 12;*148*(*24*):1982–2004.

13. Tang KS, Jones JE, Fan W et al. Prevalence and mortality trends of hypertension subtypes among

US adults: An analysis of the National Health and Nutrition Examination Survey (NHANES). *Am J Hypertens* 2025; *38(5)*: 303–312.

14. Ronnback M, Fagerudd J, Forsblom C et al. Altered age-related blood pressure pattern in type 1 diabetes. *Circulation* 2004; *110*: 1076–1108.
15. Vasan RS, Beiser A, Seshadri S et al. Residual lifetime risk for developing hypertension in middle-aged women and women: The Framingham Heart Study. *JAMA* 2002; *287*: 1003–1010.
16. Franklin SS, Gustin W, Wong ND et al. Hemodynamic patterns of age-related changes in blood pressure. The Framingham Heart Study. *Circulation* 1997; *96*: 308–315.
17. Franklin SS, Khan SA, Wong ND et al. Is pulse pressure useful in predicting risk for coronary heart disease? The Framingham Heart Study. *Circulation* 1999; *100*: 354–360.
18. Franklin SS, Larson MG, Khan SA et al. Does the relation of blood pressure to coronary heart disease risk change with aging? The Framingham Heart Study. *Circulation* 2001; *103*: 1245–1249.
19. Franklin SS, Lopez VA, Wong ND et al. Single versus combined blood pressure components and risk for cardiovascular disease. The Framingham Heart Study. *Circulation* 2009; *119*: 243–250.
20. Vidal-Petiot E, Greenlaw N, Ford I et al. Relationships between components of blood pressure and cardiovascular events in patients with stable coronary artery disease and hypertension. *Hypertension* 2018; *71(1)*: 168–176.
21. Wong ND, Lopez VA, L'Italien G et al. Inadequate control of hypertension in U.S. adults with cardiovascular disease comorbidities in 2003–2004. *Arch Intern Med* 2007; *167(22)*: 2437–2442.
22. Franklin SS, Jacobs MJ, Wong ND et al. Predominance of isolated systolic hypertension among middle-aged and elderly US hypertensives. *Hypertension*. 2001; *37*: 869–874.
23. Dalhof B, Lindholm LH, Hansson L et al. Morbidity and mortality in the Swedish Trial in Old Patients with Hypertension (STOP Hypertension). *Lancet* 1991; *338*: 1281–1285.
24. MRC Working Party. Medical Research Council trial of treatment of hypertension in older adults: Principal results. *BMJ* 1992; *304*: 405–412.
25. SHEP Cooperative Research Group. Prevention of stroke by antihypertensive drug treatment in older persons with isolated systolic hypertension: Final results of the Systolic Hypertension in the Elderly Program (SHEP). *JAMA* 1991; *265*: 3255–3264.
26. Staessen JA, Fagard R, Thijs L et al. Randomised double-blind comparison of placebo and active treatment for older patients with isolated systolic hypertension. *Lancet* 1997; *350*: 757–764.
27. Gueyffier F, Bulpitt C, Boissel J-P et al. Antihypertensive drugs in very old people: A subgroup meta-analysis of randomized controlled trials. *Lancet* 1999; *353*: 793–796.
28. ALLHAT Officers and Coordinators for the ALLHAT Collaborative Research Group. Major outcomes in high-risk hypertensive patients randomized to angiotensin-converting enzyme inhibitor or calcium channel blocker vs. diuretics: The Antihypertensive and Lipid-Lowering Treatment to Prevent Heart Attack Trial (ALLHAT). *JAMA* 2002; *288*: 2981–2997.
29. Wing LMH, Reid CM, Ryan P et al. A comparison of outcomes with angiotensin-coverting enzyme inhibitors and diuretics for hypertension in the elderly. *N Engl J Med* 2003; *348*: 583–592.
30. Beckett NS, Peters R, Fletcher AE et al. HYVET Study Group. Treatment of hypertension in patients 80 years of age or older. *N Engl J Med* 2008; *358(18)*: 1887–1898.
31. Aronow WS, Fleg JL, Pepine CJ et al. ACCF/AHA 2011 expert consensus document on hypertension in the elderly: A report of the American College of Cardiology Foundation Task Force on Clinical Expert Consensus documents developed in collaboration with the American Academy of Neurology, American Geriatrics Society, American Society for Preventive Cardiology, American Society of Hypertension, American Society of Nephrology, Association of Black Cardiologists, and European Society of Hypertension. *J Am Coll Cardiol* 2011; *57*: 2037–2114.
32. SPRINT Research Group, Wright JT Jr, Williamson JD, Whelton PK et al. A randomized trial of intensive versus standard blood-pressure control. *N Engl J Med* 2015; *373(22)*: 2103–2116.
33. Williamson JD, Supiano MA, Applegate WB et al. SPRINT Research Group. Intensive vs standard blood pressure control and cardiovascular disease outcomes in adults aged ≥75 years: A randomized clinical trial. *JAMA* 2016; *315(24)*: 2673–2682.
34. Pajewski NM, Williamson JD, Applegate WB et al. Characterizing frailty status in the systolic blood pressure intervention trial. *J Gerontol A Biol Sci Med Sci* 2016; *71(5)*: 649–655.
35. Blood Pressure Lowering Treatment Trialists' Collaboration. Effects of different regimens to lower blood pressure on major cardiovascular events in older and younger adults: Meta-analysis of randomized trials. *BMJ* 2008; *336*: 1121–1123.
36. Bi YF, Li M, Liu Y et al. Intensive blood pressure control in patients with type 2 diabetes. *N Engl J Med* 2024. doi: 10.1056/NEJMoa2412006. Epub ahead of print.
37. Liu JM, Li Y, Ge JZ et al. Lowering systolic blood pressure to less than 120 mm Hg versus less than 140 mm Hg in patients with high cardiovascular risk with and without diabetes or previous stroke: An open-label, blinded-outcome, randomised trial. *Lancet* 2024; *404(10449)*: 245–255.

38. Franklin SS. Isolated systolic hypertension and the J-curve of cardiovascular disease risk. *Artery Research* 2010; *4*: 1–6.
39. Messerli FH, Mancia G, Conti CR et al. Dogma disputed: Can aggressively lowering blood pressure in hypertensive patients with coronary artery disease be dangerous? *Ann Intern Med* 2006; *144*: 884–993.
40. Falk E, Shah PK, Fuster V. Coronary plaque disruption. *Circulation* 1995; *92*: 657–661.
41. Franklin SS, Thijs L, Asayama K et al. The cardiovascular risk of white-coat hypertension. *J Am Coll Cardiol* 2016; *68*: 2033–2043.
42. Huang Y, Huang W, Mai W et al. White-coat hypertension is a risk factor for cardiovascular diseases and total mortality. *J Hypertens* 2017; *35(4)*: 677–688.
43. Franklin SS, O'Brien E, Staessen, JA. Masked hypertension: Understanding its complexity. *Eur Heart J* 2017; *38(15)*: 1112–1118.
44. Aronow WS, Ahn C. Risk factors for new coronary events in a large cohort of very elderly patients with and without coronary artery disease. *Am J Cardiol* 1996; *77*: 864–866.
45. Castelli WP, Wilson PWF, Levy D et al. Cardiovascular disease in the elderly. *Am J Cardiol* 1989; *63*: 12H–19H.
46. Wong ND, Wilson PWF, Kannel WB. Serum cholesterol as a prognostic factor after myocardial infarction: The Framingham Study. *Ann Intern Med* 1991; *115*: 697–693.
47. Belfante R, Reed D. Is elevated serum cholesterol level a factor for coronary heart disease in the elderly? *JAMA* 1990; *263*: 393–396.
48. Manolio TA, Pearson TA, Wenger NK et al. Cholesterol and heart disease in older persons and women: Review of an NHLBI workshop. *Ann Epidemiol* 1992; *2*: 161–176.
49. Corti MC, Guralnik JM, Salive ME et al. Clarifying the direct relation between total cholesterol levels and death from coronary heart disease in older persons. *Ann Intern Med* 1997; *126*: 753–760.
50. Zhou D, Liu X, Lo K et al. The effect of total cholesterol/high-density lipoprotein cholesterol ratio on mortality risk in the general population. *Front Endocrinol* 2022; *13*: 1012383.
51. Quispe R, Elshazly MB, Zhao D et al. TC/HDL-C ratio discordance with LDL-C and non-HDL-C and incidence of atherosclerotic cardiovascular disease in primary prevention: The ARIC Study. *Eur J Prev Cardiol* 2021; *27(15)*: 1597–1605.
52. Miettinen TA, Pyorala K, Olsson AG et al. Cholesterol-lowering therapy in women and elderly patients with myocardial infarction or angina pectoris: Findings from the Scandinavian Simvastatin Survival Study (4S). *Circulation* 1997; *96*: 4211–4218.
53. Lewis SJ, Moye LA, Sacks FM et al. Effect of pravastatin on cardiovascular events in older persons with myocardial infarction and cholesterol levels in the average age range: Results of the Cholesterol and Recurrent Events (CARE) trial. *Ann Intern Med* 1998; *129*: 681–689.
54. Shepherd J, Blauw GJ, Murphy MB et al. PROSPER study group. PROspective Study of Pravastatin in the Elderly at Risk. Pravastatin in elderly individuals at risk of vascular disease (PROSPER): A randomised controlled trial. *Lancet* 2002; *360*: 1623–1630.
55. Cholesterol Treatment Trialists' Collaboration. Efficacy and safety of statin therapy in older people: A meta-analysis of individual participant data from 28 randomized controlled trials. *Lancet* 2019; *393(10170)*: 407–415.
56. Gencer B, Marston NA, Im KA et al. Efficacy and safety of lowering LDL cholesterol in older patients: A systematic review and meta-analysis of randomised controlled trials. *Lancet* 2020; *396(10263)*: 21–27.
57. Andersson NW, Corn G, Dohlmann TL et al. LDL-C reduction with lipid-lowering therapy for primary prevention of major vascular events among older individuals. *J Am Coll Cardiol* 2023; *82(14)*: 1381–1391.
58. Centers for Disease Control and Prevention (CDC). (2024). National Diabetes Statistics Report. Retrieved from https://www.cdc.gov/diabetes/php/data-research/index.html.
59. Narayan KM, Boyle JP, Thompson TJ et al. Lifetime risk for diabetes mellitus in the United States. *JAMA* 2003; *290(14)*: 1884–1890.
60. Hoang K, Ghandehari H, Lopez VA et al. Global coronary heart disease risk assessment of individuals with the metabolic syndrome in the U.S. *Diabetes Care* 2008; *31*: 1405–1409.
61. Wong ND, Glovaci D, Wong K et al. Global cardiovascular disease risk assessment in United States adults with diabetes. *Diab Vas Disease Res* 2012; *9*: 146–152.
62. Aronow WS, Ahn C. Association of diabetes mellitus using old and new diagnostic criteria with incidence of new coronary events in older men and women. *Am J Cardiol* 2000; *85*: 104–105.
63. The ADVANCE Collaborative Group. Intensive blood glucose control and vascular outcomes in patients with type 2 diabetes. *N Engl J Med* 2008; *358*: 2560–2572.
64. The Action to Control Cardiovascular Risk in Diabetes Study Group. Effects of intensive glucose lowering in type 2 diabetes. *N Engl J Med* 2008; *358*: 2545–2559.
65. Zinman B, Wanner C, Lachin JM et al. EMPA-REG OUTCOME Investigators. Empagliflozin, cardiovascular outcomes, and mortality in type 2 diabetes. *N Engl J Med* 2015; *373(22)*: 2117–2128.
66. Zelniker TA, Wiviott SD, Raz I et al. SGLT2 inhibitors for primary and secondary prevention of cardiovascular and renal outcomes in type 2 diabetes: A systematic review and meta-analysis of cardiovascular outcome trials. *Lancet* 2019; *393(10166)*: 31–39.

67. Marso SP, Daniels GH, Brown-Frandsen K et al. LEADER steering committee; LEADER trial investigators. Liraglutide and cardiovascular outcomes in type 2 diabetes. *N Engl J Med* 2016; *375*(*4*): 311–322.
68. Marso SP, Bain SC, Consoli A et al. SUSTAIN-6 Investigators. Semaglutide and cardiovascular outcomes in patients with type 2 diabetes. *N Engl J Med* 2016; *375*(*19*): 1834.
69. Gerstein HC, Colhoun HM, Dagenais GR et al. REWIND Investigators. Dulaglutide and cardiovascular outcomes in type 2 diabetes (REWIND): A double-blind, randomised placebo-controlled trial. *Lancet* 2019; *394*(*10193*): 121.
70. Ndumele CE, Rangaswami J, Chow SL et al. Cardiovascular-Kidney-Metabolic health: A presidential advisory from the American Heart Association. *Circulation* 2023; *184*(*20*): 1606–1635.
71. Aggarwal R, Ostrominski JW, Vaduganathan M. Prevalence of cardiovascular-kidney-metabolic syndrome stages in US adults, 2011–2020. *JAMA* 2024; *331*(*21*): 1858–1860.
72. Belfante R, Reed D, Frank J. Does cigarette smoking have an independent effect on coronary heart disease incidence in the elderly? *Am J Pub Health* 1991; *81*: 897–899.
73. Hermanson B, Omenn GS, Kronmal RA et al. Beneficial six-year outcome of smoking cessation in older men and women with coronary artery disease: Results of the CASS registry. *N Engl J Med* 1988; *319*: 1365–1369.
74. Harris T, Cook EF, Kannel WB et al. Proportional hazards analysis of risk factors for coronary heart disease in individuals aged 65 or older. The Framingham Heart Study. *J Am Geriatr Soc* 1988; *36*(*11*): 1023–1028.
75. Rimm EB, Stampfer MJ, Giovannucci E et al. Body size and fat distribution as predictors of coronary heart disease among middle-aged and older US men. *Am J Epidemiol* 1995; *141*(*12*): 1117–1127.
76. Galanis DJ, Harris T, Sharp DS et al. Relative weight, weight change, and risk of coronary heart disease in the Honolulu Heart Program. *Am J Epidemiol* 1998; *147*(*4*): 379–386.
77. Dey DK, Lissner L. Obesity in 70-year-old subjects as a risk factor for 15-year coronary heart disease incidence. *Obes Res* 2003; *11*(*7*): 817–827.
78. Seidell JC, Visscher TL. Body weight and weight change and their health implications for the elderly. *Eur J Clin Nutr* 2000; *54*(*Suppl 3*): S33–S39.
79. Sui X, LaMonte MJ, Laditka JN et al. Cardiorespiratory fitness and adiposity as mortality predictors in older adults. *JAMA* 2007; *298*(*21*): 2507–2516.
80. Hakim AA, Curb JD, Petrovitch H et al. Effects of walking on coronary heart disease in elderly men: The Honolulu Heart Program. *Circulation* 1999; *100*(*1*): 9–13.
81. Lee IM, Sesso HD, Paffenbarger RS, Jr. Physical activity and coronary heart disease risk in men: Does the duration of exercise episodes predict risk? *Circulation* 2000; *102*(*9*): 981–986.
82. LaCroix AZ, Leveille SG, Hecht JA et al. Does walking decrease the risk of cardiovascular disease hospitalizations and death in older adults? *J Am Geriatr Soc* 1996; *44*(*2*): 113–120.
83. Wannamethee SG, Shaper AG, Walker M. Physical activity and mortality in older men with diagnosed coronary heart disease. *Circulation* 2000; *102*(*12*): 1358–1363.
84. Singh T, Newman AB. Inflammatory markers in population studies of aging. *Ageing Res Rev* 2011; *10*(*3*): 319–329.
85. Pearson TA, Mensah GA, Alexander RW et al. Markers of inflammation and cardiovascular disease: Application to clinical and public health practice: A statement for healthcare professionals from the Centers for Disease Control and Prevention and the American Heart Association. *Circulation* 2003; *107*(*3*): 499–511.
86. Kritchevsky SB, Cesari M, Pahor M. Inflammatory markers and cardiovascular health in older adults. *Cardiovasc Res* 2005; *66*(*2*): 265–275.
87. US Preventive Services Task Force, Curry SJ, Krist AH, Owens DK et al. Risk assessment for cardiovascular disease with nontraditional risk factors: US Preventive Services Task Force recommendation statement. *JAMA* 2018; *320*(*3*): 272–280.
88. Nidorf SM, Fiolet ATL, Mosterd A et al. Colchicine in patients with chronic coronary disease. *N Engl J Med* 2020; *383*(*19*): 1838.
89. Packard CJ, O'Reilly DS, Caslake MJ et al. Lipoprotein-associated phospholipase A2 as an independent predictor of coronary heart disease. West of Scotland Coronary Prevention Study Group. *N Engl J Med* 2000; *343*(*16*): 1148–1155.
90. Koenig W, Khuseyinova N, Lowel H et al. Lipoprotein-associated phospholipase A2 adds to risk prediction of incident coronary events by C-reactive protein in apparently healthy middle-aged men from the general population: Results from the 14-year follow-up of a large cohort from southern Germany. *Circulation* 2004; *110*(*14*): 1903–1908.
91. Daniels LB, Laughlin GA, Sarno MJ et al. Lipoprotein-associated phospholipase A2 is an independent predictor of incident coronary heart disease in an apparently healthy older population: The Rancho Bernardo Study. *J Am Coll Cardiol* 2008; *51*(*9*): 913–919.
92. Lloyd-Jones DM, Allen NB, Anderson CA et al. Life's essential 8: Updating and enhancing the American Heart Association's construct of cardiovascular health: A presidential advisory from the American Heart Association. *Circulation* 2022; *146*(*5*): e18–e43.

93. Lloyd-Jones DM, Ning H, Labarthe D et al. Status of cardiovascular health in US adults and children using the American Heart Association's new "Life's Essential 8" metrics: Prevalence estimates from the National Health and Nutrition Examination Survey (NHANES), 2013 through 2018. *Circulation* 2022; *146(11)*: 822–835.
94. Wong ND, Pio J, Franklin SS et al. Preventing coronary events by optimal control of blood pressure and lipids in patients with the metabolic syndrome. *Am J Cardiol* 2003; *91*: 1421–1426.
95. Goff DC Jr, Lloyd-Jones DM, Bennett G et al. American College of Cardiology/American Heart Association Task Force on Practice Guidelines. 2013 ACC/AHA guideline on the assessment of cardiovascular risk: A report of the American College of Cardiology/American Heart Association Task Force on Practice Guidelines. *J Am Coll Cardiol* 2014; *63(25 Pt B)*: 2935–2959.
96. Arnett DK, Blumenthal RS, Albert MA et al. 2019 ACC/AHA guidelines on the primary prevention of cardiovascular disease: A report of the American College of Cardiology/American Heart Association Task Force on Clinical Practice Guidelines. *Circulation* 2019; *140(11)*: e596–646.
97. Micha R, Penalvo JL, Cudhea F. Association between dietary factors and mortality from heart disease, stroke, and type 2 diabetes in the United States. *JAMA* 2017; *317(9)*: 912–924.
98. Jensen MD, Ryan DH, Apovian CM et al. American College of Cardiology/American Heart Association Task Force on Practice Guidelines; Obesity Society. 2013 AHA/ACC/TOS guideline for the management of overweight and obesity in adults: A report of the American College of Cardiology/American Heart Association Task Force on Practice Guidelines and The Obesity Society. *J Am Coll Cardiol* 2014; *63(25 Pt B)*: 2985–3023.
99. Grundy SM, Stone NJ, Bailey AL et al. 2018 AHA/ACC/AACVPR/AAPA/ABC/ACPM/ADA/AGS/APhA/ASPC/NLA/PCNA guideline on the management of blood cholesterol: A report of the American College of Cardiology/American Heart Association Task Force on Clinical Practice Guidelines. *Circulation* 2019; *139(25)*: e1082–e1143.
100. Williams MA, Fleg JL, Ades PA et al. Secondary prevention of coronary heart disease in the elderly (with emphasis of patients >=75 years of age). *Circulation* 2002; *105*: 1735–1743.
101. Sparrow D, Dawber T, Colton T. The influence of cigarette smoking on prognosis after first myocardial infarction. *J Chronic Dis* 1978; *31*: 415–422.
102. Taylor CB, Houston-Miller NH, Killen JD et al. Smoking cessation after myocardial infarction: Effects of a nurse-managed intervention. *Ann Internal Med* 1990; *113*: 118–123.
103. DeBusk RF, Houston Miller N, Superko HR et al. A case management system for coronary risk factor modification after acute myocardial infarction. *Ann Intern Med* 1994; *120*: 721–729.
104. MacMahon S, Rodgers A. The effects of blood pressure reduction in older patients: An overview of five randomized controlled trials in elderly hypertensives. *Clin Exp Hypertens* 1993; *15(6)*: 967–978.
105. Lewis SJ, Moye LA, Sacks FM et al. Effect of pravastatin on cardiovascular events in older patients with myocardial infarction and cholesterol levels in the average range. Results of the Cholesterol and Recurrent Events (CARE) trial. *Ann Intern Med* 1998; *129(9)*: 681–689.
106. Ganz DA, Kuntz KM, Jacobson GA et al. Cost-effectiveness of 3-hydroxy-3-methylglutaryl coenzyme A reductase inhibitor therapy in older patients with myocardial infarction. *Ann Intern Med* 2000; *132*: 780–787.
107. Lloyd-Jones DM, Morris PB, Ballantyne CM et al. 2022 ACC expert consensus decision pathway on the role of nonstatin therapies for LDL-cholesterol lowering in the management of atherosclerotic cardiovascular disease risk: A report of the American College of Cardiology Solution Set Oversight Committee. *J Am Coll Cardiol* 2022; *80(14)*: 1366–1418.
108. Cannon CP, Blazing MA, Giugliano RP et al. Ezetimibe added to statin therapy after acute coronary syndromes. *N Engl J Med* 2015; *372*: 2387–2397.
109. Bhatt DL, Steg PG, Miller M et al. Cardiovascular risk reduction with icosapent ethyl for hypertriglyceridemia. *N Engl J Med* 2019; *380*: 11–22.
110. Sabatine MS, Giugliano RP, Keech AC et al. Evolocumab and clinical outcomes in patients with cardiovascular disease. *N Engl J Med* 2017; *376*: 1713–1722.
111. Vokonas PS, Kannel WB. Epidemiology of coronary heart disease in the elderly. In: Tresch DD, Aronow WS, eds. *Cardiovascular Disease in the Elderly Patient*. New York: Marcel Dekker, 1994: pp. 91–123.
112. Katzel LI, Coon PJ, Dengel J et al. Effects of an American Heart Association step I diet and weight loss on lipoprotein levels in obese men with silent myocardial ischemia and reduce HDL-C. *Metabolism* 1995; *44*: 307–314.
113. Davies MJ, Aroda VR, Collins BS et al. Management of hyperglycemia in type 2 diabetes, 2022. A consensus report by the American Diabetes Association (ADA) and the European Association for the Study of Diabetes (EASD). *Diabetes Care* 2022; *45(11)*: 2753–2786.

8

Diagnosis of coronary heart disease in older adults

JEROME L. FLEG AND WILBERT S. ARONOW

Key points

- The prevalence and incidence of coronary heart disease (CHD) increase dramatically with age in both men and women.
- Myocardial ischemia in older adults is often manifest as dyspnea with or without chest pain.
- Older adults with acute myocardial infarction may demonstrate a wide variety of symptoms, including chest pain, dyspnea, neurologic symptoms, and gastrointestinal symptoms, and are less likely to show diagnostic Q waves or ST-segment elevation than younger patients. A sizeable percentage may have unrecognized infarction.
- Multiple diagnostic techniques are useful in detecting CHD in older adults, including resting and ambulatory ECG, exercise testing, and cardiac imaging.
- Stress testing using dipyridamole, adenosine, and dobutamine in combination with nuclear or echocardiographic imaging is especially useful for CHD diagnosis in older individuals unable to perform meaningful exercise.
- Both coronary computed tomographic angiography and cardiac magnetic resonance imaging are useful for diagnosis of CHD without requiring exercise.
- Invasive coronary angiography can be performed with relatively low complication rates in clinically stable older adults.

INTRODUCTION

Atherosclerosis of the coronary arterial tree is highly prevalent in Western societies. Autopsy studies from Minnesota noted coronary atherosclerosis in 70% or more of individuals ≥70 years old (1). In contrast, only ~30% of adults aged ≥75 years have clinical manifestations of coronary heart disease (CHD), with a slightly higher prevalence in men than women. For example, the prevalence of clinical CHD in the 1999–2002 National Health and Nutrition Examination Survey in community-dwelling adults increased progressively with age, reaching 18.6% in men and 16.1% in women ≥75 years (2). In a long-term care facility, clinical CHD was present in 502 of 1160 men (43%) of mean age 80 years, and in 1019 of 2464 women (41%), of mean age 81 years (3). The marked discrepancy between the clinical and autopsy prevalence of CHD in older persons in the community indicates that CHD is often silent in this age group. Studies employing exercise testing and myocardial perfusion imaging in asymptomatic volunteers have demonstrated a striking age-related increase in silent myocardial ischemia, helping to reconcile differences in CHD prevalence between clinical and autopsy studies (4).

Although CHD is so prevalent in older persons, the disease is often undiagnosed or misdiagnosed in this age group. Failure to correctly diagnose the disease in older persons may be due in part to a difference in clinical manifestations in this age group compared with those of

DOI: 10.1201/9781003568933-8

younger patients. Such differences may reflect a difference in the disease process between older and younger patients or may be related to the superimposition of normal aging changes on those of concomitant diseases that may mask the usual clinical manifestations.

Not only the prevalence, but also the extent of CHD increases with age. In the Coronary Artery Surgery Study, the prevalence of three-vessel CHD was 61% in patients aged 65 years and older versus 46% in those younger than 65 years; left main coronary artery stenosis was seen in 13% versus 9%, respectively (5). In a database of 21,573 patients undergoing cardiac catheterization between 1995 and 1998, left main coronary artery disease (CAD) increased in prevalence from 6.3% below age 70 to 13.9% in those 80 years and older (6). Multiple studies of patients undergoing percutaneous coronary interventions have also found a higher prevalence of multivessel and left main coronary disease in older adults.

Coronary artery calcium deposition is also more common in older than in younger individuals. In the community-based Rotterdam Study, 1795 volunteers (mean age 71 years) with no history of CHD underwent electron beam computed tomography to detect coronary artery calcium (7). Calcium scores >100 were observed in 49% and scores greater than 400 in 25%, both markedly higher than in younger populations. In this study, scores of 401–1000 were associated with a fourfold risk of hard CHD events compared with persons with scores ≤100, even after adjustment for standard CHD risk factors; scores exceeding 1000 increased CHD risk more than eightfold (Figure 8.1) (7). Thus, coronary artery calcium is highly prevalent in older volunteers free of clinical CHD and has similar adverse prognostic significance as in younger populations. In 532 asymptomatic participants aged 80 years and older in the Cardiovascular Health Study, 36% had a coronary artery calcium score >400 (8). The coronary artery calcium score and number of coronary calcifications in this study were directly related to age-adjusted total mortality and CHD (8). In 3382 asymptomatic participants, mean age 66.4 years, in the Multi-Ethnic Study of Atherosclerosis (MESA) with baseline coronary artery calcium scores greater than 0, at 7.6-year median follow-up, progression of coronary artery calcium was associated with an increased risk of total cardiovascular events and with an increased risk of myocardial infarction and fatal CHD (9). Participants with an annual progression of ≥300 units had adjusted hazard ratios of 3.8 for total cardiovascular events and 6.3 for myocardial infarction and fatal CHD (8). In patients, mean age 69 years, higher coronary artery calcium scores were associated with moderate or severe myocardial ischemia in the left anterior descending and left circumflex coronary artery territories on myocardial perfusion imaging (10).

MYOCARDIAL ISCHEMIA

Exertional angina pectoris caused by myocardial ischemia is commonly the first manifestation of CHD in young and middle-aged persons. It is usually easily recognized because of its typical features; however, in older persons, this may not be the case. Because of limited physical activity, many older persons with CHD will not experience exertional angina pectoris. Even when angina pectoris does occur, the patient and physician may often attribute it to a cause other than CHD. For example, myocardial ischemia, appearing as shoulder or back pain, may be misdiagnosed as degenerative joint disease, or, if the pain is located in the epigastric area, it may be ascribed to peptic ulcer disease. Nocturnal or postprandial epigastric discomfort of a burning quality is often attributed to hiatus hernia or esophageal reflux instead of CHD. Postprandial angina pectoris tends to occur among elderly and hypertensive patients with severe CHD. Furthermore, the presence of comorbid conditions, so frequent in the older patient, adds to the confusion and may lead to misdiagnosis of the patient's symptoms, which are actually due to myocardial ischemia.

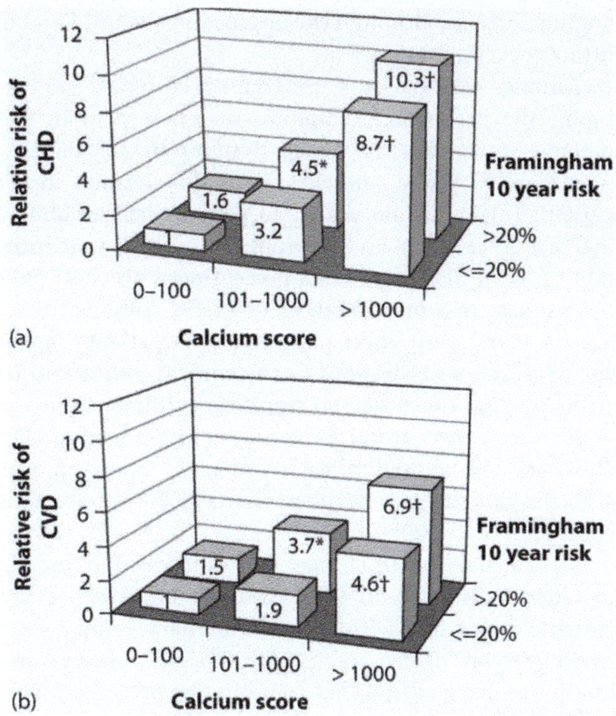

Figure 8.1 Relative risks of coronary heart disease (CHD) events (a) and cardiovascular disease (CVD) events (b) in older volunteers by coronary artery calcium score and Framingham risk categories. (From Vliegenthart R et al., *Circulation*, 112, 572–577, 2005.)

Myocardial ischemia in older patients is often manifested as dyspnea, which is considered an "angina equivalent." The dyspnea is usually exertional and is thought to be related to a transient rise in left ventricular (LV) end-diastolic pressure caused by ischemia superimposed on reduced ventricular compliance. Reduction in LV compliance may reflect normal aging changes or, more likely, is caused by coexisting hypertension and LV hypertrophy, disorders commonly present in older patients. Not infrequently, the dyspnea will occur in combination with angina pectoris, although the angina may be mild and of little concern to the patient.

Among 1053 patients undergoing coronary angiography, the presenting symptom was chest pain in 654 patients (mean age 63 years), dyspnea in 229 patients (mean age 67 years), and chest pain plus dyspnea in 117 patients (mean age 64 years); 53 patients had an abnormal stress test with no symptoms (11). The 2-year mortality was similar in patients presenting with chest pain or dyspnea. In a meta-analysis of 24,491 patients (mean age 63 years) with chest pain and 5753 patients (mean age 67 years) with dyspnea as the clinical indication for stress testing, there was no significant difference in the incidence of myocardial ischemia on stress testing (11). However, the annual mortality during follow-up was 4.9% for patients with dyspnea versus 2.3% in those with chest pain ($p < 0.001$) (12).

Myocardial ischemia may be manifested clinically in older individuals as frank heart failure, with some patients presenting with acute pulmonary edema. In a small group of older patients with CHD who had recurrent pulmonary edema that could not be prevented with medical therapy, coronary angiography demonstrated three-vessel coronary disease with preserved LV systolic function (13). Only after undergoing coronary bypass surgery was the recurrent pulmonary edema prevented in these patients. Graham and Vetrovec (14) compared patients with CHD hospitalized with acute pulmonary edema with patients hospitalized with angina pectoris without heart failure. The patients with acute pulmonary edema were older and most had preexisting hypertension. Three-vessel CHD was common in both groups, although angina pectoris was infrequent in patients with pulmonary edema. LV ejection fraction was lower in patients with pulmonary edema (42%) than in the angina pectoris group (59%).

Some older patients with CHD who present with acute pulmonary edema will demonstrate mitral valvular regurgitation that may be secondary to papillary muscle ischemia. In 40 patients (mean age 76 years) with CHD who presented with acute pulmonary edema, Stone and associates (15) found that 67% demonstrated moderate to severe mitral regurgitation on Doppler echocardiographic examination. In 74% of these patients, a murmur of mitral regurgitation was not detected despite examination by multiple observers. The authors concluded that mitral valve regurgitation is not uncommon in elderly patients with CHD who present with acute LV failure and may contribute to the genesis of pulmonary edema.

In addition to having more severe CHD than younger patients, older patients who undergo coronary arteriography demonstrate greater comorbidities, clinical instability, and CHD complications. In 21,573 patients, unstable angina pectoris was the indication for coronary arteriography in 38% of persons aged ≥70 years versus 28% in those <70 years (6). A history of heart failure was present, respectively, in 31% versus 11% of patients. Comorbidities such as cerebrovascular and peripheral vascular disease and chronic obstructive lung disease were two to three times more common in older persons (6).

In a single-center study of older patients (mean age 71 years) undergoing coronary angiography, the initial symptom in the majority was unstable ischemic chest pain; 34% of the patients presented with an acute myocardial infarction (16). In 8% of these patients, the initial manifestation was acute heart failure unassociated with an acute myocardial infarction. On cardiac catheterization, multivessel disease was common, although LV systolic function was often normal. Only 9% of the patients had an LV ejection fraction <35%. In contrast, patients <65 years more commonly sustained an acute myocardial infarction as the initial manifestation of CHD were less likely to present with heart failure and had less multivessel CHD (16).

Among 12,792 persons (55% women, median age 74 years), a polygenic risk score for CHD added to conventional risk factors was associated with a 24% incidence of CHD at 5 years (17). In community-dwelling 70-year-olds, increased visceral adipose tissue was associated with an increased incidence of myocardial infarction at 3.6-year follow-up in men but not in women (18). In patients aged >65 years and older hospitalized for myocardial infarction, Black patients were more likely than Whites to be women (65% versus 43%) (19).

Cardiac arrhythmias, particularly complex ventricular arrhythmias, may be a manifestation of myocardial ischemia in older patients with CHD. Sudden death may be the initial manifestation of CHD in older adults; in Framingham volunteers, 65–94 years old, CHD was manifest as sudden death in 15% of men and 12% of women (20).

Silent or asymptomatic myocardial ischemia is commonly seen in older patients with CHD. In a study of 185 nursing home patients with CHD, mean age 83 years, silent myocardial ischemia (SI) was detected by 24-hour ambulatory electrocardiography (AECG) in 34% (21). SI was detected by 24-hour AECG in 51 of 117 (44%) similar patients with CHD or hypertension and an abnormal LV ejection fraction (22). The reason for the frequent absence of chest pain in elderly patients with CHD is unclear. Various speculations have included (1) mental deterioration with inability to verbalize a sensation of pain, (2) better myocardial collateral circulation related to gradual progressive coronary artery narrowing, and (3) a decreased sensitivity to pain because of aging changes.

MYOCARDIAL INFARCTION

Similar to myocardial ischemia, some patients with acute myocardial infarction may be completely asymptomatic, or the symptoms may be so vague that they are unrecognized by the patient or physician as an acute infarction. In Framingham Heart Study volunteers, approximately 25% of myocardial infarctions diagnosed by pathological Q

Table 8.1 Prevalence of silent or unrecognized Q-wave myocardial infarction in older patients

Study (reference)	Unrecognized myocardial infarction		
	Age (years)	Number	Percentage age
Aronow (*n* = 110) (24)	mean, 82	23	21
Kannel et al. (*n* = 199 men) (23)	65–94	66	33
Kannel et al. (*n* = 162 women) (23)	65–94	58	36
Muller et al. (*n* = 46 men) (25)	65–95	14	30
Muller et al. (*n* = 67 women) (25)	65–95	34	51
Nadelmann et al. (*n* = 115) (26)	75–85	50	43
Sigurdsson et al. (*n* = 237) (27)	58–62	83	35
Sheifer et al. (*n* = 901) (28)	mean, 72	201	22

waves on ECG were clinically unrecognized and, of these, 48% were truly silent (23). The incidence increased with age, with 42% of infarctions clinically silent in men aged 75–84 years. In women, the proportion of unrecognized myocardial infarctions was greater than in men, but the incidence was unaffected by increasing age. Other studies (24–29) have also reported a high prevalence of silent or unrecognized myocardial infarction in older patients, with rates from 21% to 68% (Table 8.1). These studies also demonstrated that the incidence of new coronary events, including recurrent myocardial infarction, ventricular fibrillation, and sudden death, in patients with unrecognized myocardial infarction is similar to that in patients with recognized myocardial infarction (25–29). In the Rotterdam Study of 2672 men, mean age 68 years, and 3862 women, mean age 69 years, unrecognized myocardial infarction was present in 165 of 472 myocardial infarctions (35%) in men and in 205 of 335 myocardial infarctions (61%) in women (30). At 15.6-year follow-up, the hazard ratios for mortality were 1.57 for men versus 1.89 for women with recognized myocardial infarction and 1.72 for men versus 1.36 for women with unrecognized myocardial infarction (30).

When present in older patients with an acute myocardial infarction, symptoms may be extremely vague and, as with myocardial ischemia, the diagnosis may be easily missed. Numerous studies (24, 31–34) have demonstrated the atypical features and wide variability of symptoms in older patients with acute myocardial infarction (Table 8.2). Pathy (31) demonstrated in 387 older patients with acute myocardial infarction that 19% had chest pain; 56% had dyspnea, neurological, or gastrointestinal symptoms; 8% had sudden death; and 17% had other symptoms (Table 8.2). In 110 older patients with acute myocardial infarction, Aronow (24) showed that 21% had no symptoms, 22% had chest pain, 35% had dyspnea, 18% had neurological symptoms, and 4% had gastrointestinal symptoms (Tables 8.1 and 8.2).

Other studies have also shown a high prevalence of dyspnea and neurological symptoms in elderly patients with acute myocardial infarction (Table 8.2, [32–35]). In 777 older patients with acute myocardial infarction, Bayer and associates (33) reported that, with increasing age, the prevalence of chest pain decreased, whereas the prevalence of dyspnea increased. In the Multicenter Chest Pain Study, the lower prevalence in older patients of some typical features of acute myocardial infarction present in younger patients, such as pressure-like chest pain, the initial symptoms and signs led to a lower predictive value for diagnosing acute myocardial infarction in the older group (35).

Other features that differ between older and younger patients with acute myocardial infarction, and which may modify the therapy, should be emphasized. An important difference is that older patients delay longer in seeking medical assistance after the onset of chest pain (36, 37). In a study of out-of-hospital chest pain, Tresch and associates (36) reported that patients ≥80 years delayed >6.5 hours in calling paramedics, compared with a 3.9-hour delay in patients <70 years. Interestingly, this prolonged delay occurred even though over 50% of the older patients had a past history of either a myocardial infarction or coronary

Table 8.2 Prevalence of dyspnea, chest pain, neurological symptoms, and gastrointestinal symptoms associated with acute myocardial infarction in older patients

Study (reference)	Age (years)	Dyspnea	Chest pain	Neurological symptoms	Gastrointestinal symptoms
Pathy (*n* = 387) (31)	>65	77 (20%)	75 (19%)	126 (33%)	10 (3%)
Tinker (*n* = 87) (32)	mean, 74	19 (22%)	51 (59%)	14 (16%)	0 (0%)
Bayer et al. (*n* = 777) (33)	65–100	329 (42%)	515 (66%)	232 (30%)	145 (19%)
Aronow (*n* = 110) (24)	mean, 82	38 (35%)	24 (22%)	20 (18%)	5 (4%)
Wroblewski (*n* = 96) (34)	mean, 84	57 (59%)	19 (20%)	33 (34%)	24 (25%)

bypass surgery. Such delay may be one of the reasons why older patients with acute myocardial infarction are less likely to receive thrombolytic therapy or primary coronary angioplasty compared with younger patients. Sheifer et al. (37) showed in the Cooperative Cardiovascular Project that among 102,339 patients >65 years with confirmed acute myocardial infarction, 29.4% arrived at the hospital 6 hours or later after onset of symptoms.

The National Registry of Myocardial Infarction included 743,177 men and women, mean age 78 years (38). The prevalence of myocardial infarction patients who presented without chest pain was 42% for women versus 31% for men ($p < 0.001$). In patients aged 65–74 years, the in-hospital mortality was 6.9% for men versus 8.6% for women with chest pain and 18.9% for men versus 19.3% for women without chest pain ($p < 0.001$). In patients aged ≥75 years, the in-hospital mortality was 13.7% for men versus 15.2% for women with chest pain and 23.6% for men versus 21.8% for women without chest pain ($p < 0.001$) (38). The Korea Acute Myocardial Infarction Registry study included 7,288 patients, mean age 62 years, with ST-segment acute myocardial infarction undergoing percutaneous coronary intervention (39). Patients with painless myocardial infarction were older (65.2 vs. 61.4 years) and were more likely to be women (30% vs. 25%). In-hospital mortality was higher in painless myocardial infarction (5.9%) than in painful myocardial infarction (3.6%) ($p = 0.023$). The incidence of 1-year major adverse cardiac events was also higher in painless myocardial infarction (26%) than in painful myocardial infarction (19 %) ($p = 0.002$) (39).

Another important age difference found in multiple studies is the greater incidence of non-Q-wave myocardial infarctions in older persons. For example, in one study 40% of older patients with acute myocardial infarction demonstrated non-Q-wave infarction compared with only 20% of the younger patients with infarction (36). In another study, of 91 consecutive patients aged ≥70 years with acute myocardial infarction, 61 (75%) had non-Q-wave myocardial infarction (40).

In younger patients, non-Q-wave myocardial infarctions are usually associated with a more benign acute hospital course than Q-wave myocardial infarctions, although this does not necessarily pertain to older patients. Chung and associates (41) reported a 10% hospital mortality and 36% 1-year mortality in a group of older patients sustaining acute non-Q-wave myocardial infarction. In contrast, the acute hospital and 1-year mortality in younger patients were 3% and 16%, respectively. Moreover, 23% of the older patients with non-Q-wave myocardial infarction developed atrial fibrillation, and 53% had congestive heart failure. Regardless of the type of myocardial infarction, older patients with acute myocardial infarction usually demonstrate more LV dysfunction than younger patients upon hospital admission and have a more complicated hospital course. Common complications in older patients include heart failure, ventricular rupture, shock, and death (42). Not infrequently, the older patient's initial complaints will reflect these complications instead of chest pain.

Fedullo and Swinburne (43) compared complications from acute myocardial infarction in 104 patients aged 70 years and older with 157 patients 70 years or younger. Mortality was 22% in the older group versus 5% in the younger group. Cardiogenic shock occurred in 7% of the older group versus 1% of the younger group. Pulmonary edema occurred in 18% of the older group versus 4% of the younger group. Heart failure occurred in 29% of the older group versus 14% of the younger group. A rhythm disturbance requiring pacemaker implantation occurred in 5% of the older group versus 2% of the younger group (43). The increased mortality and complication rates in older patients with acute myocardial infarction suggest that an aggressive diagnostic and therapeutic approach may be beneficial in these patients. More aggressive therapy, including use of aspirin, β-blockers, angiotensin-converting enzyme inhibitors, statins, thrombolytic therapy, and coronary revascularization by percutaneous coronary angioplasty or by coronary bypass surgery, should be considered.

In patients aged ≥70 years presenting to an emergency department with suspected myocardial infarction, chest pain with radiation to both arms, exertional chest pain in the last week, and chest pain during activity had the strongest predictive value for acute myocardial infarction (44). In 1320 patients aged 70 years and older (37% women) with myocardial infarction who survived 1-month follow-up, frailty was independently associated with a 57% increased risk of major adverse cardiovascular events at 1-year follow-up (45). In 80,176 patients aged ≥70 years (43% women) with myocardial infarction, the multimorbidity burden increased 1-year hospital readmission by 42% (46). In 40,654 patients aged ≥70 years (505 women) with myocardial infarction, adjusted all-cause mortality was lower in women than men at 30 days (16% versus 19%) and at 1 year (27.7% versus 32.4%) (47). In 1388 patients (32% women) with myocardial infarction, at 998 days follow-up, poor physical performance increased mortality, and women with preserved physical performance had a better outcome than men (48). At 10-year follow-up of 31,578 patients aged ≥70 years (51% men) with myocardial infarction, men had a 17% increased risk of major adverse cardiovascular events than women with similar baseline features and evidence-based medications (49).

DIAGNOSTIC TECHNIQUES

The remaining sections of the chapter will briefly review the techniques commonly used to diagnose CHD in older individuals, ranging from the simple 12-lead ECG to various forms of stress testing, and sophisticated imaging techniques such as magnetic resonance imaging (MRI), computed tomographic angiography (CCTA), and invasive coronary arteriography.

Resting ECG

In addition to diagnosing recent or previous myocardial infarction, the resting ECG may show ischemic ST-segment depression, arrhythmias, conduction defects, and LV hypertrophy, all of which may increase the likelihood of subsequent coronary events. At 37-month mean follow-up, older institutionalized patients with ischemic ST-segment depression ≥1 mm on the resting ECG were 3.1 times more likely to develop new coronary events (myocardial infarction, primary ventricular fibrillation, or sudden cardiac death) than were those with no significant ST-segment depression (50). In this population, patients with ischemic ST-segment depression 0.5–0.9 mm on the resting ECG were 1.9 times more likely to develop new coronary events during the 37-month follow-up than were those with no significant ST-segment depression. At 45-month mean follow-up, pacemaker rhythm, atrial fibrillation, premature ventricular complexes, left bundle branch block, intraventricular conduction defect, and type II second-degree atrioventricular (AV) block were all associated with a higher incidence of new coronary events in such elderly patients (50).

Numerous studies have documented that older adults with ECG LV hypertrophy have an increased incidence of new cardiovascular events (51–55). Men and women 65–94 years of age participating in the Framingham Heart Study who had ECG LV hypertrophy had an increased incidence of new coronary events, atherothrombotic brain infarction, chronic heart failure (CHF), and peripheral arterial disease compared with persons without ECG LV hypertrophy (52). Aronow and associates (53, 54) also found that elderly patients with hypertension or CHD and ECG LV hypertrophy had an increased incidence of new coronary events, atherothrombotic brain infarction, and heart failure.

The Copenhagen Heart Study obtained ECGs in 6991 asymptomatic participants without cardiovascular disease at age 65 years and older (55). At 9.8-year follow-up, patients with an ECG abnormality increased fatal cardiovascular events by 33% ($p < 0.001$) and fatal or nonfatal cardiovascular events by 21% ($p < 0.001$) (55). In 4224 participants ≥65 years in the Cardiovascular Health Study, 8.6% developed an incident silent MI, 10.0% an incident overt MI, and 8.9% an incident ischemic stroke during a median follow-up of 9.8 years. After adjustment for demographics and comorbidities, both silent MI and overt MI were independently associated with subsequent ischemic stroke. The association between silent MI and stroke was limited to nonlacunar ischemic stroke (HR, 2.40) (56).

Ambulatory electrocardiography

Prior studies have demonstrated that complex ventricular arrhythmias in older adults without underlying cardiovascular disease are not associated with an increased incidence of new coronary events (Table 8.3) (57–59). In contrast, complex ventricular arrhythmias in elderly

Table 8.3 Association of complex ventricular arrhythmias and ventricular tachycardia on ambulatory ECG with new coronary events in older patients

Study (reference)	Mean age (years)	Cardiac status	Follow-up (months)	Incidence of new coronary events
Fleg et al. (*n* = 98) (57)	69	No heart disease	120	No association
Aronow et al. (*n* = 843) (58)	82	Heart disease	39	Increased 1.7 times by complex VA
Aronow et al. (*n* = 395 men) (759)	80	CAD	45	Increased 2.4 times by complex VA and 1.7 times by VT
Aronow et al. (*n* = 385 men) (759)	80	HT, VD, or CMP	45	Increased 1.9 times by complex VA and 1.9 times by VT
Aronow et al. (*n* = 135 men) (759)	80	No heart disease	45	No association
Aronow et al. (*n* = 771 women) (59)	81	CAD	47	Increased 2.5 times by complex VA and 1.7 times by VT
Aronow et al. (*n* = 806 women) (59)	81	HT, VD, or CMP	47	Increased 2.2 times by complex VA and 2.0 times by VT
Aronow et al. (*n* = 297 women) (59)	81	No heart disease	47	No association

Abbreviations: CAD, coronary artery disease; CMP, cardiomyopathy; HT, hypertension; LVEF, left ventricular ejection fraction; LVH, left ventricular hypertrophy; SCD, sudden coronary death; VA, ventricular arrhythmias; VD, valvular heart disease; VF, primary ventricular fibrillation; VT, ventricular tachycardia.

persons with underlying cardiovascular disease are associated with an increased incidence of new coronary events, including sudden cardiac death (58–61). The incidence of new coronary events is especially increased in elderly patients with complex ventricular arrhythmias and abnormal LV ejection fraction (60) or LV hypertrophy (61).

Complex ventricular arrhythmias detected by 24-hour AECG in elderly nursing home patients with heart disease predicted a 2.5 times greater incidence of new coronary events at a 2-year follow-up in persons with normal LV ejection fraction and 7.6 times greater incidence in those with abnormal LV ejection fraction (60). Those with heart disease, normal LV mass, and complex ventricular arrhythmias detected by 24-hour AECG experienced a 2.4-fold greater incidence of primary ventricular fibrillation or sudden cardiac death at a 27-month follow-up than those without such arrhythmias. This risk was 7.3 times higher in persons with both complex ventricular arrhythmias and echocardiographic LV hypertrophy (61).

AECG performed for 24 hours is also useful in detecting myocardial ischemia in elderly persons with suspected CHD who cannot perform treadmill or bicycle exercise stress testing because of advanced age, intermittent claudication, musculoskeletal disorders, heart failure, or pulmonary disease. Ischemic ST-segment changes demonstrated on the 24-hour AECG correlate with transient abnormalities in myocardial perfusion and LV systolic dysfunction. The changes may be associated with symptoms, or symptoms may be completely absent, which is referred to as SI. SI is predictive of future coronary events, including cardiovascular mortality in older persons with CHD (21, 22, 62–66) and in those with no clinical heart disease (21, 57).

The incidence of new coronary events is especially increased in older individuals with SI plus complex ventricular arrhythmias (65), abnormal LV ejection fraction (22), or echocardiographic LV hypertrophy (66). In a population of institutionalized elders with CHD or hypertension, at a 40-month follow-up, SI predicted a doubled incidence of new coronary events in persons with normal LV ejection fraction and a 3.2-fold increase in those with abnormal LV ejection fraction (22). The combination of complex ventricular arrhythmias plus SI was associated with a fourfold higher incidence of new coronary events; echocardiographic LV hypertrophy plus SI predicted a 3.4-fold greater incidence of new coronary events at a 31-month follow-up (66). SI was associated with an approximately doubled incidence of new coronary events over nearly 4 years of follow-up in both elderly men and women with CHD, hypertension, valvular heart disease, or cardiomyopathy. Among those without clinical heart disease, SI predicted an incidence of new coronary events 6.3-fold higher in men and 4.4-fold higher in women (65). Fleg and associates (57) showed at a 10-year follow-up of older persons without heart disease that SI on AECG was associated with a 3.8-fold increased incidence of new coronary events; two of the three persons who died suddenly had evidence of SI plus ventricular tachycardia detected by 24-hour AECG.

SI detected by 24-hour AECG has been used in the assessment of patients undergoing no cardiac surgery. Such use of 24-hour AECG may be especially beneficial in elders, who are frequently at high surgical risk and may not be able to undergo preoperative exercise stress testing because of concomitant illness. No study, however, has shown SI detected by 24-hour AECG to be more accurate than pharmacological stress testing in stratifying preoperative older patients into high- and low-risk groups.

Raby and associates (67) studied 176 patients who underwent 24-hour AECG before noncardiac surgery. Eighteen percent had signs of myocardial ischemia on their preoperative 24-hour AECG, with the ischemia silent in the majority. Preoperative myocardial ischemia was highly predictive of postoperative cardiac events. The sensitivity of preoperative myocardial ischemia for postoperative cardiac events in this study was 92%, the specificity 88%, the positive predictive value 38%, and the negative predictive value 99% (67). By multivariate analysis, preoperative myocardial ischemia was the variable correlating most strongly with postoperative cardiac events. The authors concluded that the absence of preoperative myocardial ischemia on the 24-hour AECG indicates a very low risk for postoperative cardiac events. In 38% of patients older than 69 years, preoperative myocardial ischemia was more prevalent compared with younger patients. In a study of older patients (mean age 67 years) undergoing peripheral vascular surgery, Raby and associates (68) again found preoperative SI to be the most important predictor of postoperative cardiac events. Preoperative myocardial ischemia also strongly correlated with intraoperative and postoperative ischemia, and perioperative myocardial ischemia commonly preceded clinical cardiac events.

Echocardiography

Echocardiography is useful in evaluating LV function, cardiac chamber size, and wall thickness in older adults with known or suspected CHD. Echocardiographic LV ejection fraction can help to predict new coronary events in elders with CHD (22, 60). In older adults with CHD and heart failure, cardiovascular mortality is higher among individuals with abnormal than in those with normal LV ejection fraction (69). Multivariate analysis showed that LV ejection fraction was the most important prognostic variable for mortality in such individuals with CHF associated with CHD; those with abnormal LV ejection fraction had approximately twice the mortality of persons with normal LV ejection fraction.

Numerous studies have demonstrated that older patients with echocardiographic LV hypertrophy have an increased incidence of new cardiovascular events (53, 54, 61, 66, 70). At 4-year follow-up, older adults in the

Framingham study with echocardiographic LV hypertrophy had a relative risk for new coronary events of 1.67 for men and of 1.60 for women per 50 g/m increase in LV mass/height (70). In these volunteers, echocardiographic LV hypertrophy was 15.3 times more sensitive than ECG LV hypertrophy in predicting new coronary events in men and 4.3 times more sensitive than ECG LV hypertrophy in predicting new coronary events in women.

Over 27 months of follow-up, institutionalized older adults with echocardiographic LV hypertrophy developed a 2.7-fold higher incidence of new coronary events, 3.7-fold higher rate of new atherothrombotic brain infarction (ABI), and 3.3-fold greater rate of primary ventricular fibrillation or cardiac death (61). At a 37-month follow-up of such persons with CHD or hypertension, echocardiographic LV hypertrophy predicted a doubled incidence of new coronary events and a 2.8-fold greater rate of new ABI (53). Echocardiographic LV hypertrophy was approximately four times more sensitive than ECG LV hypertrophy in predicting new coronary events or new ABI in this population. Multiple logistic regression analysis showed that echocardiographic LV hypertrophy was a strong independent risk factor in such a population for new coronary events (odds ratio of 3.2), new ABI (odds ratio of 4.2), and new CHF (odds ratio of 2.6) (53); increased risk was similar in African Americans and Whites (54).

Exercise and pharmacological stress testing

Although age per se significantly influences the cardiovascular response to aerobic exercise, treadmill or cycle ergometer exercise testing remains a useful diagnostic and prognostic tool for evaluating older patients with suspected or documented CHD. Exercise ECG is also a useful prognostic indicator of subsequent coronary events in patients with documented CHD, with or without previous myocardial infarction. Exercise testing in elderly patients should evaluate symptoms that develop during exercise (especially angina pectoris or dyspnea, which may be an anginal equivalent); the maximal workload achieved; the heart rate and blood pressure response; the presence, magnitude, and onset time of ischemic ST-segment depression or elevation; and the presence of exercise-induced arrhythmias. These variables must be interpreted in light of normative age-associated changes including a decline of maximal aerobic capacity averaging 8%–10% per decade (71, 72), a reduced maximal heart rate of approximately 1 beat/min/year, and an exaggerated rise in systolic blood pressure (73, 74). Maximal LV systolic emptying is impaired in older adults, resulting in a higher end-systolic volume and lower LV ejection fraction compared with younger individuals (73–75); stroke volume is preserved, however, by a greater reliance on the Frank–Starling mechanism to augment LV end-diastolic volume (74, 75). Exercise-induced supraventricular (76) and ventricular arrhythmias (77) both increase exponentially with age in clinically healthy volunteers but do not increase the risk for future CHD events in such a population.

In light of the lower exercise capacity of older adults, exercise-testing protocols should employ low starting work rates and smaller work increments than in younger patients. Thus, protocols such as the Naughton or Balke, in which the treadmill speed is held constant and only the elevation is increased, are ideal for the elderly. Individuals with gait disturbances can often be tested on a cycle ergometer, although their aerobic capacity and peak heart rate are usually lower than those achieved with treadmill exercise.

Diagnostic sensitivity of the exercise ECG for CHD appears to increase with age at the expense of a modest reduction in specificity. Hlatky et al. (78) found the exercise ECG to have a sensitivity of 84% and a specificity of 70% for the diagnosis of CHD in patients 60 years or older. In contrast, sensitivity was only 56% in patients younger than 40 years, although specificity was 84%. In patients aged ≥65 years, Newman and Phillips (79) found a sensitivity of 85%, a specificity of 56%, and a positive predictive value of 86% for the exercise ECG in diagnosing CHD. The increased sensitivity and higher positive predictive value of the exercise ECG with increasing age found in these two treadmill exercise studies were probably due to the greater prevalence and severity of CHD in older individuals (80). Reduced specificity is largely explained by their higher prevalence of ST-T-wave abnormalities on the pre-exercise ECG.

Prognostic utility of the exercise ECG

Multiple studies in patients with known or suspected CHD have shown that the standard treadmill exercise test provides valuable prognostic information. In 2632 patients 65 years or older undergoing clinically indicated exercise testing, a lower peak treadmill workload was a strong independent predictor of cardiac death over the subsequent 2.9-year mean follow-up period (81). Of note, neither ischemic ST changes nor angina were predictive. In a similar population, however, Glover et al. demonstrated that an ischemic ST-segment response to exercise predicted an eightfold cardiovascular mortality (17% vs. 2%) over a 2-year follow-up (82). The Duke treadmill score, which incorporates exercise duration, magnitude of ischemic ST-segment depression, and presence of exercise-induced angina, has demonstrated prognostic utility in younger populations (83) but appears to be less useful in patients aged ≥75 years (84).

Exercise testing after myocardial infarction has prognostic value in older patients, as it does in younger ones. Identification of jeopardized myocardium in such post-myocardial infarction patients may be useful because recurrent infarction and sudden cardiac death are the most common causes of 1-year mortality posthospital discharge (85). In 188 patients aged 70 years or older who underwent exercise testing a mean of 14 days post-infarction, Ciaroni et al. (86) found that a rise in systolic blood pressure of less than 30 mmHg, a maximal cycle work rate less than 60 W, and an exercise duration less than 5 minutes predicted cardiovascular death; whereas ST-segment depression and ventricular arrhythmias predicted reinfarction and the need for coronary revascularization. Similar to the general post-infarction population, older patients excluded from exercise testing after myocardial infarction have the highest cardiovascular risk. For example, Deckers et al. (87) found a mortality of 4% for patients 65 years or older who were able to perform a cycle exercise test post-infarction versus a mortality of 37% for those excluded.

Although the diagnostic and prognostic utility of exercise testing in the general population is modest, such testing may have greater value in asymptomatic older persons with multiple CHD risk factors. Older subjects embarking on a vigorous training program or those entrusted with the safety of others, such as school bus drivers, are appropriate candidates for testing.

At 27-year follow-up of 898 Rancho Bernardo Study asymptomatic participants, mean age 55 years at baseline, an integrated scoring model of submaximal treadmill stress tests using the variables ST change, inability to achieve target heart rate, abnormal heart rate recovery, and chronotropic incompetence was an independent predictor of myocardial infarction and of unrecognized myocardial infarction (88). Participants with one or two abnormalities had an increased risk of myocardial infarction (hazard ratios 1.8 or 2.3, respectively) and an increased risk of unrecognized myocardial infarction (hazard ratios 1.8 or 2.6, respectively). Participants with three or four abnormalities had an increased risk of myocardial infarction (hazard ratio 8.0) and an increased risk of unrecognized myocardial infarction (hazard ratio 3.2) (88).

Exercise cardiac imaging

Exercise stress testing incorporating thallium perfusion scintigraphy or echocardiography provides additional value in the diagnosis and prognosis of CHD compared with the exercise ECG alone. In 120 patients 70 years or older with known or suspected CHD who underwent exercise thallium-201 scintigraphy, Hilton et al. (89) showed that the combination of low peak exercise capacity and any thallium-201 perfusion defect was the most powerful predictor of new cardiac events (relative risk, 5.3 at 1 year). Individuals with an ischemic ST-segment depression of more than 2 mm and a thallium defect who failed to complete stage 1 of a Bruce protocol suffered a 47% event rate. Exercise single-photon emission computed tomography (SPECT) performed in 247 patients aged ≥75 years classified 49% as low risk and 35% of the patients as high risk by a summed stress score (90). At 6.4-year follow-up, patients classified as low risk had an annual cardiac mortality rate of 0.8%, and those classified as high risk had an annual cardiac mortality rate of 5.8%. In this study, the Duke treadmill score was not significantly associated with cardiac death. Among 247 octogenarians undergoing exercise thallium imaging, Katsikis et al. (91) found that the summed stress score during exercise and the difference score from rest were the only variables that significantly predicted all-cause and cardiac death, nonfatal myocardial infarction, and late coronary revascularization over 7.3 years mean follow-up.

Older patients with diabetes mellitus (mean age 63 years) had a significantly higher prevalence of unrecognized myocardial infarction (18% of 287 patients) detected by a treadmill exercise sestamibi myocardial perfusion stress test than age-matched and gender-matched patients without diabetes mellitus (7% of 292 patients) ($p < 0.001$) (92). Patients with diabetes mellitus also had a higher prevalence of SI without a history of angina pectoris (33%) than patients without diabetes mellitus (18%) ($p < 0.001$).

Fleg et al. (4) performed maximal treadmill exercise ECGs and thallium scintigraphy in 407 asymptomatic volunteers between 40 and 96 years old from the Baltimore Longitudinal Study on Aging. At 4.6 years follow-up, new cardiac events developed in 7% of patients who had negative results on both tests, 8% of patients with a single positive result, and 48% of patients with both results positive. Persons with both a positive exercise ECG and a thallium perfusion defect averaged 69 years of age and had 3.6 times the relative risk for new coronary events as those with negative results, independent of standard coronary risk factors (4).

Echocardiography during, or more commonly, immediately after treadmill or cycle exercise has also proven useful in the detection and prognostication of CHD. Overall sensitivity of exercise-induced wall motion abnormalities for CHD using this technique is 74%–97% with specificity of 64%–88%, similar to values using exercise thallium scintigraphy (93). As with other diagnostic modalities, the sensitivity of exercise echocardiography increases with the extent of CHD, which should result in a high sensitivity in the elderly. Although a lower technical success of echocardiographic imaging in older versus younger patients is probably responsible for a lesser utilization of exercise echocardiography in this population, recent advances in echocardiographic equipment have largely overcome this deficiency. In 2632 patients, aged 65 years or older, referred for clinically indicated exercise echocardiography, the exercise-induced changes in LV end-systolic volume and the exercise LV ejection fraction or wall motion score were predictors of cardiac events and cardiac death, independent of clinical status, resting echocardiography, and exercise duration (81) (Figure 8.2).

At 2.8-year follow-up of 1268 patients of mean age 60 years, nonfatal myocardial infarction or cardiac death occurred in 1.1% patients per year with a normal stress

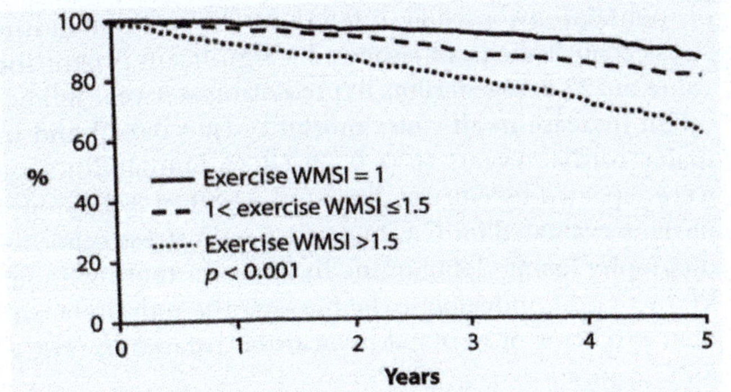

No. at risk						
<1	1094	1008	749	460	274	150
1–1.5	898	795	613	407	237	135
>1.5	640	503	363	221	133	72

Figure 8.2 Exercise echocardiographic wall motion score as a predictor of survival free of cardiac events in 2632 patients aged 65 years or older referred for exercise testing. A higher wall motion score index (WMSI) denotes worse LV function. (From Arruda AM et al., *J Am Coll Cardiol*, 37(4), 1036–1041, 2001.)

echocardiogram and in 3.6% patients per year with a normal stress ECG ($p < 0.001$) (94). Peak wall motion score index (hazard ratio = 2.55) and LV ejection fraction (hazard ratio = 0.99) were independent and incremental prognostic markers for stress echocardiography. In 2159 patients aged ≥70 years with known or suspected CHD undergoing stress echocardiography, 844 patients (38.6%) developed ischemia during exercise (95). The cumulative 5-year mortality was 29.3% in those with ischemia versus 16.8% in those without ischemia ($p < 0.001$).

PHARMACOLOGICAL STRESS TESTING

The greatest advancement in stress testing over the past few decades has been the widespread application of pharmacological stress testing on populations unable to perform diagnostically adequate exercise tests. Older adults are clearly the greatest beneficiaries of pharmacological stress testing because of their high prevalence of exercise-limiting conditions, such as obstructive lung disease, peripheral arterial insufficiency, arthritis, and neuromuscular disorders. The agents most commonly used for this purpose are the vasodilators dipyridamole and adenosine, and the synthetic catecholamine dobutamine in conjunction with either radionuclide or echocardiographic imaging.

Dipyridamole is a phosphodiesterase inhibitor that blocks the degradation of adenosine, thereby increasing plasma adenosine, which is a potent arteriolar dilator. Both dipyridamole and adenosine dilate normal coronary arteries more than stenotic vessels, creating a coronary steal that causes a myocardial perfusion defect or wall motion abnormality. With either drug, serious side effects, including bronchospasm, hypotension, and arrhythmias, occur in 2%–3% of patients but do not appear to be age-related (96, 97). In 101 subjects older than 70 years, the sensitivity and specificity of dipyridamole thallium imaging for CHD were 86% and 75%, respectively, compared with corresponding values of 83% and 70% in younger patients (96). In 92 patients aged 65 years and older who had undergone prior coronary artery bypass grafting, the dipyridamole sestamibi nuclear stress test had a sensitivity of 95%, a specificity of 50%, a positive predictive value of 96%, and a negative predictive value of 43% for graft occlusion or 50% or more new native CAD; these values were similar to those in younger patients (98).

The prognostic utility of dipyridamole in combination with echocardiography was shown in 190 patients aged ≥65 years evaluated at a mean of 10 days after uncomplicated myocardial infarction. Patients with a positive test experienced a 3-fold risk of future cardiac events and 4.4-fold risk of death compared with those with normal results (99). An abnormal dipyridamole thallium scan was the best predictor of subsequent events in 348 patients aged 70 years and older with known or suspected CHD, conferring a relative risk of 7.2 on multivariate analysis (100).

Adenosine echocardiography has also demonstrated both diagnostic and prognostic utility in older patients with known or suspected CHD. In 120 such patients 70 years or older, sensitivity for CHD was 66%, specificity 90%, and diagnostic accuracy 73% (97). Sensitivity increased from 42% in patients with single-vessel CHD to 73% in those with multivessel disease. An abnormal adenosine echocardiogram predicted a threefold risk of future cardiac events, independent of clinical CHD risk factors. The only serious effect was transient AV block, which occurred in 6% of patients, but was asymptomatic and self-limited in all (97). In another study, the risk of such transient AV block after adenosine infusion was 18% in patients 75 years or older versus 8% in younger patients (101). Combining adenosine infusion with symptom-limited treadmill exercise reduced the incidence of premature infusion termination from 15% to 5%. A study of 370 octogenarians who underwent adenosine nuclear myocardial perfusion imaging (49% with known CHD) found that 86% of patients were able to tolerate a 6-minute infusion (102). After 9.3 years, there were 124 all-cause deaths (ACDs), 62 cardiac deaths (CDs), 16 myocardial infarctions, and 35 revascularizations. Differences between survival curves of summed stress score (SSS)-based risk groups were significant for all endpoints. The inability to increase HR by >10 bpm and decrease systolic blood pressure by >10 mmHg during adenosine were also independent predictors of ACDs and CDs (102).

A potential advantage of adenosine, and probably dipyridamole, stress testing over exercise is the ability to continue β-blockers without compromising on diagnostic yield. In a study of 158 consecutive patients (mean age 66 years) who had adenosine nuclear myocardial perfusion imaging, β-blocker therapy was continued through the test in 82 patients and stopped 48 hours prior to the test in 76 patients (103). β-blocker therapy did not affect the extent, severity, and reversibility of perfusion defects on adenosine myocardial perfusion imaging. However, patients who stopped β-blockers for 48 hours had a higher incidence of angina pectoris (10%) than those who continued β-blocker therapy through the test (2%) (103).

Dobutamine is a synthetic catecholamine that is frequently used as a pharmacological stressor in older patients, in combination with echocardiography or thallium imaging. Dobutamine produces dose-related increases in heart rate and inotropy that augment coronary artery blood flow, thereby inducing ischemia by a mechanism similar to exercise in patients with CHD (104). Atropine is frequently combined with dobutamine to help ensure an adequate chronotropic response. The classic ischemic response induced by dobutamine is characterized by improved wall motion at low doses but worsening wall motion at high doses. Dobutamine is particularly useful in older patients with obstructive lung disease in whom both dipyridamole and adenosine are contraindicated. In 120 patients aged 70 years or older with known or suspected CHD, dobutamine echocardiography had a sensitivity of 87%, a specificity of 84%, and an accuracy of 86%, all higher than corresponding figures for adenosine in the same patients (Table 8.4) (105). Patients with a positive dobutamine stress test had a 7.3-fold risk for a future cardiac event compared with those with a normal test. Dobutamine nuclear perfusion scintigraphy demonstrated sensitivity of 86% and specificity of 90% in 144 patients aged 65 ± 10 years (105), numbers very similar to the echocardiographic data with this drug. Although dobutamine is generally well tolerated in all age groups, higher rates of asymptomatic hypotension and both supraventricular and ventricular arrhythmias, but a lower rate of chest pain, were reported in patients older than 70 years versus younger than 70 years (105, 106).

Large series have confirmed the prognostic value of dobutamine stress testing. At 6.5-year follow-up of 1434 patients older than 65 years who had dobutamine stress echocardiography, resting wall abnormalities (hazard ratio = 1.13) and inducible ischemia (hazard ratio = 2.1) were significant independent predictors of cardiac death or nonfatal myocardial infarction (107). Dobutamine stress echocardiography showed a significant prognostic value in 227 octogenarians in predicting at 3-year follow-up an increase in all-cause mortality ($p = 0.002$) and in major cardiac events ($p = 0.02$) (108). Similar findings were reported by Gurunathan et al. (109) in 374 octogenarians evaluated for CAD presence with stress echocardiography (using dobutamine in 92%). In those without known CAD, inducible ischemia was the only independent predictor of nonfatal myocardial infarction (HR = 8.7).

Coronary artery calcium scanning

Several studies have shown the ability of coronary artery calcium (CAC) scans without contrast injection to risk stratify older adults without known CHD. In 1795 asymptomatic patients, mean age 71 years, followed for a mean follow-up of 3.3 years, the risk of cardiovascular events was very low in patients with CAC of 0 to 100 but increased 8.2-fold in patients with CAC of 1000 (110). In a study of 559 patients (336 women) ages 70 to 99 years followed for 5 years, both CAC and carotid intima–media thickness were predictors of cardiovascular events and death. The top quartile for each measurement was associated with a more than twofold increased risk of events (111). Finally, Raggi et al. (112) followed 3560 patients >70 years (50% women) and noted a more than threefold increased mortality among those with CAC scores >400 compared to those with a score <10. The cost to identify these high-risk patients averaged only $409 for those aged 70–79 years and $248 for those ≥80 years.

MULTISLICE CORONARY COMPUTED TOMOGRAPHIC ANGIOGRAPHY AND MAGNETIC RESONANCE IMAGING

Over the past two decades, multislice coronary computed tomographic angiography (CCTA) and MRI have been increasingly used to detect CHD. Both techniques allow direct visualization of the coronary arteries rather than relying on their functional consequences. Since

Table 8.4 Comparison of dobutamine and adenosine echocardiography in detection of CAD in patients aged 70 years or older

	Dobutamine (%)	Adenosine (%)	*p* Value
Sensitivity			
Overall	87	66	<0.001
One-vessel CHD	74	42	NS
Two-vessel CHD	88	76	NS
Three-vessel CHD	91	71	0.02
Specificity	84	90	NS
Accuracy	86	73	0.01

Abbreviations: CHD, coronary heart disease; NS, not significant.
Source: Anthopoulos LP et al., *J Am Coll Cardiol*, 28(1), 52–59, 1996.

their introduction for coronary artery imaging in 2000, CT scanners have increased from 4 to 16 detectors and more recently to 64 or more detectors. Thus, new generation scanners acquire more imaging slices per rotation, allowing faster image acquisition and improved temporal and spatial resolution. As a result, these scanners require a shorter period of breath holding by the patient, allow a wider range of acceptable heart rates, and the ability to image very obese patients and those with moderate coronary artery calcium, using lower contrast volumes. All of these advances in CT imaging facilitate the imaging of older patients with suspected CHD.

In a pooled analysis, CCTA detected occluded coronary artery bypass grafts with a sensitivity of 84% and a specificity of 95% (113). Among 145 patients, mean age 67 years, 64 slice-CCTA had 98% sensitivity, 74% specificity, 90% positive predictive value, and 94% negative predictive value in diagnosing obstructive CAD (114). In 2538 patients undergoing CCTA, at 78-month follow-up, CCTA provided independent and incremental value in predicting all-cause mortality in symptomatic patients independent of age, gender, conventional risk factors, and coronary artery calcium score (115). Significant drawbacks of CCTA are the contrast dye load and the radiation exposure, both similar to those from conventional coronary angiography, and the artifacts induced by metal surgical clips from prior bypass grafts.

At 2.3-year follow-up of 24,775 patients without known CHD who had CCTA, all-cause mortality was increased 1.62 times in patients with nonobstructive CHD, 2.0 times in patients with one-vessel obstructive CHD, 2.92 times in patients with two-vessel obstructive CHD, and 3.7 times in patients with three-vessel or left main obstructive CHD (116). In patients aged 65 years and older, all-cause mortality was increased 1.63 times in patients with nonobstructive CHD, 1.96 times in patients with one-vessel obstructive CHD, 2.46 times in patients with two-vessel obstructive CHD, and 3.1 times in patients with obstructive three-vessel or left main CHD. All-cause mortality was higher in women than in men with three-vessel or left main obstructive CHD (4.21 times vs. 3.27 times) (116). In 454 asymptomatic and 742 symptomatic persons aged ≥70 years, the prevalence of significant CHD and the extent of atherosclerotic plaques on CCTA did not differ between the two groups (117). However, patients with asymptomatic CHD were less likely to be treated and had a higher 2-year mortality than patients with symptomatic CHD. Data from CCTA performed in 21,132 persons aged 40–79 years (46% women) were used to develop age- and sex-specific nomograms of global plaque burden in predicting major cardiac events (118).

The Prospective Multicenter Imaging Study for Evaluation of chest pain (PROMISE) randomized 10,003 symptomatic patients, mean age 61 years (53% women), to a strategy of initial anatomical testing with CCTA or to functional testing with either exercise ECG, nuclear stress testing, or stress echocardiography (119). Chest pain or dyspnea on exertion was present in 88% of the patients. At 25-month median follow-up, the primary endpoint of death, myocardial infarction, hospitalization for unstable angina pectoris, or major procedural complications occurred in 3.3% of CCTA patients versus 3.0% of functional testing patients (p not significant) (119). At 26.1-month median follow-up of 9102 of these patients, CCTA provided better prognostic information than functional testing in patients with stable chest pain with a low burden of obstructive CHD, myocardial ischemia, and cardiovascular events (120).

Cardiac MRI has also become another attractive method for noninvasive coronary artery imaging in recent years. This technique avoids the use of ionizing radiation and iodinated intravenous contrast material as well as the need for breath holding. Faster MRI techniques and more powerful magnets have improved the quality of coronary arterial images. A meta-analysis of 28 studies using MRI coronary angiography found a per-artery sensitivity of 72% and a specificity of 87%; 86% of the coronary arterial segments were assessable (121). However, the mean age of the patients in this analysis was 63 years, with only one very small study having a mean patient age over 65 years. As with CCTA, therefore, age-specific diagnostic accuracy is not available.

At 3.6-year median follow-up of 845 patients who underwent cardiac MRI, patients with the primary endpoint of cardiac death, nonfatal myocardial infarction, and stroke showed a larger extent of myocardial ischemia (10.7% vs. 3.7%, $p < 0.0001$) and late gadolinium enhancement (21% vs. 17.7%, $p < 0.001$) (122). A risk prediction model containing these variables was superior in comparison to all other models in predicting adverse outcomes. At 81-month median follow-up of 628 patients, mean age 60.4 years, who received either cardiac MRI or SPECT for suspected CHD, cardiac MRI was a stronger predictor of major adverse cardiovascular events (cardiovascular death, acute coronary syndrome, and unscheduled revascularization or hospitalization for a cardiovascular cause) (hazard ratio 2.77) than SPECT (hazard ratio 1.62, $p = 0.014$) (123). Six hundred patients, mean age 68 years, with chest pain and previous revascularization had a stress cardiac MRI (300 patients) or CCTA (300 patients) (124). At 762-days mean follow-up, major adverse cardiac events were lower with stress cardiac MRI (5%) than with CCTA (10%, $p < 0.010$), subsequent use of noninvasive tests (17% vs. 28%), invasive coronary angiography (20% vs. 31%), and revascularization procedures (16% vs. 24%), respectively, were significantly lower with stress cardiac MRI than with CCTA (124).

Dewey et al. (113) performed a direct comparison of CCTA with MRI for noninvasive coronary arteriography in 129 patients (mean age 64 years) with suspected CHD. Sensitivity for coronary stenoses greater than 50% of luminal diameter was 82% for CCTA versus 54% for MRI;

the respective specificities were 90% and 87%. Negative predictive value was slightly higher for CT (95% vs. 90%). In this study, 74% of patients preferred CCTA to MRI. The greater diagnostic accuracy of CCTA over MRI in this study is consistent with the meta-analytic findings of Schuijf et al. (121) from 51 studies. Thus, CCTA currently has a higher accuracy than MRI to detect or exclude significant CHD, although data specific to the elderly are lacking. As both techniques may miss significant coronary artery stenoses, they are best used in patients with a pretest probability of CHD less than 50%. In such patients, a normal coronary arteriogram by CCTA or MRI would reduce the post-test probability of CHD to less than 10%, avoiding the need for invasive coronary arteriography (125). Both techniques are thus attractive for use in emergency room settings in determining which low- to intermediate-risk patients presenting with acute chest pain should be admitted.

Coronary arteriography

Despite the recent advances in noninvasive cardiac imaging discussed earlier, invasive coronary arteriography remains the accepted standard for detection and quantitation of CHD, although it may underestimate the extent of coronary atherosclerosis compared with intravascular ultrasound. Major complications of coronary arteriography include myocardial infarction, stroke, and death. In the Coronary Artery Surgery Study (CASS) registry, each of these endpoints was approximately three times as common in patients aged 65 and older than in younger individuals (5). A single-center study between 1980 and 1990 of 242 patients 80–92 years old reported a mortality of 0.8% and nonfatal complication rate of 5%, compared with respective rates of 0.15% and 1.5% in patients younger than 80 years (126). Among 1085 consecutive patients ≥80 years (82.6 ± 2.6 years; 526 males, 544 females), who underwent 1384 cardiac catheterizations in a tertiary specialist university hospital, procedure-related complications, including vascular injuries, occurred in 2.1% after catheterization and 11.6% after PCI, suggesting an acceptable complication rate in such patients (127). The increased risk in the elderly is largely explained by their generally greater severity of underlying cardiac and noncardiac disease. Although major complication rates from cardiac catheterization and coronary arteriography have continued to decline through the years (126, 127), the elderly should still be considered at higher risk, especially those aged 80 years and older.

REFERENCES

1. Elveback L, Lie JT. Continued high prevalence of coronary artery disease at autopsy in Olmstead County, Minnesota 1950–1970. *Circulation* 1984; *70*; 345–349.
2. Tsao CW, Aday AW, Almarzook ZI et al. Heart disease and stroke statistics 2023 update: A report from the American Heart Association. *Circulation* 2023; *147*: e93–621.
3. Aronow WS, Ahn C, Gutstein H. Prevalence and incidence of cardiovascular disease in 1160 older men and 2464 older women in a long-term health care facility. *J Gerontol Med Sci* 2002; *57A*: M45–M46.
4. Fleg JL, Gerstenblith G, Zonderman AB et al. Prevalence and prognostic significance of exercise-induced silent myocardial ischemia detected by thallium scintigraphy and electro-cardiography in asymptomatic volunteers. *Circulation* 1990; *81(2)*: 428–436.
5. Gersh BJ, Kronmal RA, Frye RL et al. Coronary arteriography and coronary artery bypass surgery: Morbidity and mortality in patients ages 65 years or older. A report from the Coronary Artery Surgery Study. *Circulation* 1983; *67*: 483–491.
6. Graham MM, Ghali WA, Faris PD et al. Survival after coronary revascularization in the elderly. *Circulation* 2002; *105*: 2378–2384.
7. Vliegenthart R, Oudkerk M, Hofman A et al. Coronary calcification improves cardiovascular risk prediction in the elderly. *Circulation* 2005; *112*: 572–577.
8. Kuller LH, Lopez OL, Mackey RH et al. Subclinical cardiovascular disease and death, dementia, and coronary heart disease in patients 80+ years. *J Am Coll Cardiol* 2016; *67*: 1013–1022.
9. Budoff MJ, Young R, Lopez VA et al. Progression of coronary calcium and incident coronary heart disease events. MESA (Multi-Ethnic Study of Atherosclerosis). *J Am Coll Cardiol* 2013; *61*: 1231–1239.
10. Lai HM, Holtzman D, Aronow WS et al. Association of coronary artery calcium with severity of myocardial ischemia in left anterior descending, left circumflex, and right coronary artery territories. *Clin Cardiol* 2012; *35*: 61–63.
11. Paudel R, Beridze N, Aronow WS et al. Association of chest pain versus dyspnea as presenting symptom for coronary angiography with demographics, coronary anatomy, and 2-year mortality. *Arch Med Sci* 2016; *12*: 742–746.
12. Argulian E, Agarwal V, Bangalore S et al. Meta-analysis of prognostic implications of dyspnea versus chest pain in patients referred for stress testing. *Am J Cardiol* 2014; *113*: 559–564.
13. Kunis R, Greenberg H, Yeoh CG et al. Coronary revascularization of recurrent pulmonary edema in elderly patients with ischemic heart disease and preserved ventricular function. *N Engl J Med* 1985; *313*: 1207–1210.
14. Graham SP, Vetrovec GW. Comparison of angiographic findings and demographic variables in

patients with coronary artery disease presenting with acute pulmonary edema versus those presenting with chest pain. *Am J Cardiol* 1991; *68*: 1614–1618.
15. Stone GW, Griffin B, Shah PK et al. Prevalence of unsuspected mitral regurgitation and left ventricular diastolic dysfunction in patients with coronary artery disease and acute pulmonary edema associated with normal or depressed left ventricular systolic function. *Am J Cardiol* 1991; *67*: 37–41.
16. Tresch DD, Saeian K, Hoffman R. Elderly patients with late onset of coronary artery disease: Clinical and angiographic findings. *Am J Geriatr Cardiol* 1992; *1*: 14–25.
17. Neumann JT, Riaz M, Bakshi A et al. Prognostic value of a polygenic risk score for coronary heart disease in individual aged 70 years and older. *Circ Genom Precis Med* 2022; *15*: e003429.
18. Ballin M, Nordstrom P, Niklasson J et al. Associations of visceral adipose tissue and skeletal muscle density with incident stroke, myocardial infarction, and all-cause mortality in community-dwelling 70-year-old individuals: A prospective cohort study. *J Am Heart Assoc* 2021; *10*: e020065.
19. Demkowicz PC, Hajduk AM, Dodson JA et al. Racial disparities among older adults with acute myocardial infarction: The SILVER-AMI study. *J Am Geriatr Soc* 2023; *71*: 474–483.
20. Cupples LA, D'Agostino RB. Some risk factors related to the annual incidence of cardiovascular disease and death using pooled repeated biennial measurements: Framingham Heart Study, 30-year follow-up. In: Kannel WB, Wolf PA, Garrison RJ, eds. *The Framingham Heart Study: An Epidemiological Investigation of Cardiovascular Disease*. Bethesda, MD: National Heart, Lung, and Blood Institute, Publication No. (NIH), 1987: pp. 87–2703.
21. Aronow WS, Epstein S. Usefulness of silent myocardial ischemia detected by ambulatory electrocardiographic monitoring in predicting new coronary events in elderly patients. *Am J Cardiol* 1988; *62*: 1295–1296.
22. Aronow WS, Epstein S, Koenigsberg M. Usefulness of echocardiographic left ventricular ejection fraction and silent myocardial ischemia in predicting new coronary events in elderly patients with coronary artery disease or systemic hypertension. *Am J Cardiol* 1990; *65*: 811–812.
23. Kannel WB, Abbott RD. Incidence and prognosis of unrecognized myocardial infarction: An update on the Framingham Study. *N Engl J Med* 1984; *311*: 1144–1147.
24. Aronow WS. Prevalence of presenting symptoms of recognized acute myocardial infarction and of unrecognized healed myocardial infarction in elderly patients. *Am J Cardiol* 1987; *60*: 1182.
25. Muller RT, Gould LA, Betzu R et al. Painless myocardial infarction in the elderly. *Am Heart J* 1990; *119*: 202–204.
26. Nadelmann J, Frishman WH, Ooi WL et al. Prevalence, incidence, and prognosis of recognized and unrecognized myocardial infarction in persons aged 75 years or older: The Bronx aging study. *Am J Cardiol* 1990; *66*: 533–537.
27. Sigurdsson E, Thorgeirsson G, Sigvaldason H et al. Unrecognized myocardial infarction: Epidemiology, clinical characteristics, and the prognostic role of angina pectoris: The Reykjavik study. *Ann Intern Med* 1995; *122*: 96–102.
28. Sheifer SE, Gersh BJ, Yanez ND et al. Prevalence, predisposing factors, and prognosis of clinically unrecognized myocardial infarction in the elderly. *J Am Coll Cardiol* 2000; *35*: 119–126.
29. Aronow WS. New coronary events at four-year follow-up in elderly patients with recognized or unrecognized myocardial infarction. *Am J Cardiol* 1989; *63*: 621–622.
30. Dehghan A, Leening MJG, Solouki AM et al. Comparison of prognosis in unrecognized versus recognized myocardial infarction in men versus women >55 years of age (from the Rotterdam Study). *Am J Cardiol* 2014; *113*: 1–6.
31. Pathy MS. Clinical presentation of myocardial infarction in the elderly. *Br Heart J* 1967; *29*: 190–199.
32. Tinker GM. Clinical presentation of myocardial infarction in the elderly. *Age Aging* 1981; *10*: 237–240.
33. Bayer AJ, Chadha JS, Farag RR et al. Changing presentation of myocardial infarction with increasing old age. *J Am Geriatr Soc* 1986; *23*: 263–266.
34. Wroblewski M, Mikulowski P, Steen B. Symptoms of myocardial infarction in old age: Clinical case, retrospective and prospective studies. *Age Aging* 1986; *15*: 99–104.
35. Solomon CG, Lee TH, Cook EF et al. Comparison of clinical presentation of acute myocardial infarction in patients older than 65 years of age to younger patients: The Multicenter Pain Study experience. *Am J Cardiol* 1989; *63*: 772–776.
36. Tresch DD, Brady WF, Aufderheide TP et al. Comparison of elderly and younger patients with out-of-hospital chest pain. *Arch Intern Med* 1996; *156*: 1089–1093.
37. Sheifer SE, Rathore SS, Gersh BJ et al. Time to presentation with acute myocardial infarction in the elderly. Associations with race, sex, and socioeconomic characteristics. *Circulation* 2000; *102*: 1651–1656.
38. Canto JG, Rogers WJ, Goldberg RJ et al. Association of age and sex with myocardial infarction symptom presentation and in-hospital mortality. *JAMA* 2012; *307*: 813–822.

39. Cho JY, Jeong MH, Ahn YK et al. Comparison of outcomes of patients with painless versus painful ST-elevation myocardial infarction undergoing percutaneous coronary intervention. *Am J Cardiol* 2012; *109*: 337–343.
40. Woodworth S, Nayak D, Aronow WS et al. Comparison of acute coronary syndromes in men versus women ≥70 years of age. *Am J Cardiol* 2002; *90*: 1145–1147.
41. Chung MK, Bosner MS, McKenzie JP et al. Prognosis of patients ≥70 years of age with non-Q-wave acute myocardial infarction compared with younger patients with similar infarcts and with patients ≥70 years of age with Q-wave acute myocardial infarction. *Am J Cardiol* 1995; *75*: 18–22.
42. Rich MW, Bosner MS, Chung MK et al. Is age an independent predictor of early and late mortality in patients with acute myocardial infarction? *Am J Med* 1992; *92*: 7–13.
43. Fedullo AJ, Swinburne AJ. Intensive care for elderly patients with myocardial infarction: Age-related comparison of clinical features and outcome. *J Intens Care Med* 1988; *3*: 265–271.
44. Steiro O-T, Aakre KM, Tjora HL et al. Association between symptoms and risk of non-ST segment elevation myocardial infarction according to age and sex in patients admitted to the emergency department with suspected acute coronary syndrome: A single-centre retrospective cohort study. *BMJ Open* 2022; *12*: e054185.
45. Broek WWA van den, Gimbel ME, Hermanides RS et al. The impact of patient-reported frailty on cardiovascular outcomes in elderly patients after non-ST-acute coronary syndrome. *Int J Cardiol* 2024; *405*: 131940.
46. Gudnadottir GS, Gudnason T, Wilhelmson K et al. Multimorbidity and readmissions in older people with acute coronary syndrome. *Cardiology* 2022; *147*: 121–132.
47. Kyto V, Nuotio M, Rautava P. Sex difference in the case fatality of older myocardial infarction patients. *J Gerontol Biol Med Sci* 2022; *77*: 614–620.
48. Tonet E, Ariza-Sole A, Serenelli M et al. The impact of sex and physical performance on long-term mortality in older patients with myocardial infarction. *BMC Med* 2022; *20*: 15.
49. Kerola AM, Palomarki A, Rautava P et al. Sex differences in cardiovascular outcomes of older adults after myocardial infarction. *J Am Heart Assoc* 2021; *10*: e022883.
50. Aronow WS. Correlation of ischemic ST-segment depression on the resting electrocardiogram with new cardiac event in 1,106 patients over 62 years of age. *Am J Cardiol* 1989; *64*: 232–233.
51. Aronow WS. Correlation of arrhythmias and conduction defects on the resting electrocardiogram with new cardiac events in 1,153 elderly patients. *Am J Noninvas Cardiol* 1991; *5*: 88–90.
52. Kannel WB, Dannenberg AL, Levy D. Population implications of electrocardiographic left ventricular hypertrophy. *Am J Cardiol* 1987; *60*: 851–931.
53. Aronow WS, Koenigsberg M, Schwartz KS. Usefulness of echocardiographic and electrocardiographic left ventricular hypertrophy in predicting new cardiac events in atherothrombotic brain infarction in elderly patients with systemic hypertension or coronary artery disease. *Am J Noninvas Cardiol* 1989; *3*: 367–370.
54. Aronow WS, Ahn C, Kronzon I et al. Congestive heart failure, coronary events, and atherothrombotic brain infarction in elderly blacks and whites with systemic hypertension and with and without echocardiographic and electrocardiographic evidence of left ventricular hypertrophy. *Am J Cardiol* 1991; *67*: 295–299.
55. Jorgensen PG, Jensen JS, Marott JL et al. Electrocardiographic changes improve risk prediction in asymptomatic persons age 65 years or above without cardiovascular disease. *J Am Coll Cardiol* 2014; *64*: 898–906.
56. Merkler AF, Bartz TM, Kamel H et al. Silent myocardial infarction and subsequent risk of ischemic stroke in the Cardiovascular Health Study. *Neurology* 2021; *97*: e436–e443.
57. Fleg JL, Kennedy HL. Long-term prognostic significance of ambulatory electrocardiographic findings in apparently healthy subjects ≥60 years of age. *Am J Cardiol* 1992; *90*: 748–751.
58. Aronow WS, Epstein S, Mercando AD. Usefulness of complex ventricular arrhythmias detected by 24-hour ambulatory electrocardiogram and by electrocardiograms with one-minute rhythm strips in predicting new coronary events in elderly patients with and without heart disease. *J Cardiovasc Technol* 1991; *10*: 21–25.
59. Aronow WS, Ahn C, Mercando A et al. Prevalence and association of ventricular tachycardia and complex ventricular arrhythmias with new coronary events in older men and women with and without cardiovascular disease. *J Gerontol Med Sci* 2002; *57A*: M178–M180.
60. Aronow WS, Epstein S, Koenigsberg M et al. Usefulness of echocardiographic abnormal left ventricular ejection fraction, paroxysmal ventricular tachycardia, and complex ventricular arrhythmias in predicting new coronary events in patients over 62 years of age. *Am J Cardiol* 1988; *61*: 1349–1351.
61. Aronow WS, Epstein S, Koenigsberg M et al. Usefulness of echocardiographic left ventricular hypertrophy, ventricular tachycardia and complex ventricular arrhythmias in predicting ventricular fibrillation or sudden cardiac death in elderly patients. *Am J Cardiol* 1988; *62*: 1124–1125.

62. Dicker RC, Han LF, Mancone JJ. *Quality of Care Surveillance Using Administrative Data, 1996.* Health Care Financing Administration, 1998.
63. Gottlieb SO, Weisfeldt ML, Ouyang P et al. Silent ischemia as a marker for early unfavorable outcomes in patients with unstable angina. *N Engl J Med* 1986; *314*: 1214–1219.
64. Gottlieb SO, Gottlieb SH, Achuff SC et al. Silent ischemia on Holter monitoring predicts mortality in high-risk postinfarction patients. *JAMA* 1988; *259*: 1030–1035.
65. Aronow WS, Ahn C, Mercando AD et al. Prevalence and association of silent myocardial ischemia with new coronary events in older men and women with and without cardiovascular disease. *J Am Geriatr Soc* 2002; *50*: 1075–1078.
66. Aronow WS, Epstein S, Koenigsberg M. Usefulness of echocardiographic left ventricular hypertrophy and silent ischemia in predicting new cardiac events in elderly patients with systemic hypertension or coronary artery disease. *Angiology* 1990; *41*: 189–193.
67. Raby KE, Goldman L, Creager MA et al. Correlation between preoperative ischemia and major cardiac events after peripheral vascular surgery. *N Engl J Med* 1989; *321*: 1296–1300.
68. Raby KE, Barry J, Creager MA et al. Detection and significance of intraoperative and postoperative myocardial ischemia in peripheral vascular surgery. *JAMA* 1992; *268*: 222–227.
69. Aronow WS, Ahn C, Kronzon I. Prognosis of congestive heart failure after prior myocardial infarction in older men and women with abnormal versus normal left ventricular ejection fraction. *Am J Cardiol* 2000; *85*: 1382–1384.
70. Levy D, Garrison RJ, Savage DD et al. Left ventricular mass and incidence of coronary heart disease in an elderly cohort: The Framingham Heart Study. *Ann Intern Med* 1989; *110*: 101–107.
71. Buskirk ER, Hodgson JL. Age and aerobic power. The rate of change in men and women. *Fed Proc* 1987; *46*: 1824–1829.
72. Talbot LA, Metter EJ, Fleg JL. Leisure-time physical activities and their relationship to cardiorespiratory fitness in healthy men and women 18–95 years old. *Med Sci Sports Exerc* 2000; *32*: 417–425.
73. Stratton JR, Levy WC, Cerqueira MD et al. Cardiovascular responses to exercise. Effects of aging and exercise training in healthy men. *Circulation* 1994; *89(4)*: 1648–1655.
74. Fleg JL, O'Connor F, Gerstenblith G et al. Impact of age on the cardiovascular response to dynamic upright exercise in healthy men and women. *J Appl Physiol* 1995; *78(3)*: 890–900.
75. Fleg JL, Schulman S, O'Connor F et al. Effects of acute beta-adrenergic receptor blockade on age-associated changes in cardiovascular performance during dynamic exercise. *Circulation* 1994; *90(5)*: 2333–2341.
76. Maurer MS, Shefrin EA, Fleg JL. Prevalence and prognostic significance of exercise-induced supraventricular tachycardia in apparently healthy volunteers. *Am J Cardiol* 1995; *75*: 788–792.
77. Marine JE, Shetty V, Chow GV et al. Prevalence and prognostic significance of exercise-induced nonsustained ventricular tachycardia in asymptomatic volunteers: The Baltimore Longitudinal Study of Aging. *J Am Coll Cardiol* 2013; *62*: 595–600.
78. Hlatky MA, Pryor DB, Harrell FE et al. Factors affecting sensitivity and specificity of exercise electrocardiography: Multivariable analysis. *Am J Med* 1984; *77(1)*: 64–71.
79. Newman KP, Phillips JH. Gradual exercise testing for diagnosis of coronary artery disease in elderly patients. *South Med J* 1988; *81*: 430–432.
80. Chaitman BR, Bourassa MG, Davis K et al. Angiographic prevalence of high-risk coronary artery disease in patient subsets (CASS). *Circulation* 1981; *64*: 360–367.
81. Arruda AM, Das MK, Roger VL et al. prognostic value of exercise echocardiography in 2,632 patients ≥65 years of age. *J Am Coll Cardiol* 2001; *37(4)*: 1036–1041.
82. Glover DR, Robinson CS, Murray RG. Diagnostic exercise testing in 104 patients over 65 years of age. *Eur Heart J* 1984; *5(suppl E)*: 59–61.
83. Mark DB, Shaw L, Harrell FE et al. Prognostic value of a treadmill exercise score in outpatients with suspected coronary artery disease. *N Engl J Med* 1991; *325(12)*: 849–853.
84. Kwok JM, Miller TD, Hodge DO et al. Prognostic value of the Duke treadmill score in the elderly. *J Am Coll Cardiol* 2002; *39*: 1475–1481.
85. Smith SC Jr., Gilpin E, Ahnve S et al. Outlook after acute myocardial infarction in the very elderly compared with that in patients aged 65–75 years. *J Am Coll Cardiol* 1990; *16(4)*: 784–792.
86. Ciaroni S, Delonca J, Righetti A. Early exercise testing after acute myocardial infarction in the elderly: Clinical evaluation and prognostic significance. *Am Heart J* 1993; *126*: 304–311.
87. Deckers JW, Fioretti P, Brower RW et al. Ineligibility for predischarge exercise testing after myocardial infarction in the elderly: Implications for prognosis. *Eur Heart J* 1984; *5(suppl E)*: 97–100.
88. Park JI, Shin SY, Park SK et al. Usefulness of the integrated scoring model of treadmill tests to predict myocardial ischemia and silent myocardial ischemia in community-dwelling adults (from the Rancho Bernardo study). *Am J Cardiol* 2015; *115*: 1049–1055.
89. Hilton TC, Shaw LJ, Chaitman BR et al. Prognostic significance of exercise thallium-201 testing in patients

aged ≥70 years with known or suspected coronary artery disease. *Am J Cardiol* 1992; *69(1)*: 45–50.
90. Valeti US, Miller TD, Hodge DO et al. Exercise single-photon emission computed tomography provides effective risk stratification of elderly men and elderly women. *Circulation* 2005; *111*: 1771–1776.
91. Katsikis A, Theodorako A, Papalonnou S et al. Long-term prognostic value of myocardial perfusion imaging in octogenarians able to undergo treadmill testing. *J Nucl Cardiol* 2014; *21*: 1213–1222.
92. DeLuca AJ, Kaplan S, Aronow WS et al. Comparison of prevalence of unrecognized myocardial infarction and of silent myocardial ischemia detected by a treadmill exercise sestamibi stress test in patients with versus without diabetes mellitus. *Am J Cardiol* 2006; *98*: 1045–1046.
93. Quinones MA, Verani MS, Haichin RM et al. Exercise echocardiography versus 102 Tl single-photon emission computed tomography in evaluation of coronary artery disease. Analysis of 292 patients. *Circulation* 1992; *85(3)*: 1026–1031.
94. Mahenthiran J, Bangalore S, Yao SS et al. Comparison of prognostic value of stress echocardiography versus stress electrocardiography in patients with suspected coronary artery disease. *Am J Cardiol* 2005; *96*: 628–634.
95. Bouzas-Mosquera A, Peteiro J, Broullon FJ et al. Value of exercise echocardiography for predicting mortality in elderly patients. *Eur J Clin Invest* 2010; *40*: 1122–1130.
96. Lam JY, Chaitman BR, Glaenzer M et al. Safety and diagnostic accuracy of dipyridamole-thallium imaging in the elderly. *J Am Coll Cardiol* 1988; *ll(3)*: 585–589.
97. Anthopoulos LP, Bonou MS, Kardaras FG et al. Stress echocardiography in elderly patients with coronary artery disease: Applicability, safety and prognostic value of dobutamine and adenosine echocardiography in elderly patients. *J Am Coll Cardiol* 1996; *28(l)*: 52–59.
98. DeLuca AJ, Cusack E, Aronow WS et al. Sensitivity, specificity, positive predictive value, and negative predictive value of the dipyridamole sestamibi stress test in predicting draft occlusion or ≥50% new native coronary artery disease in men versus women and in patients aged ≥65 years versus <65 years who had prior coronary artery bypass grafting. *Am J Cardiol* 2004; *94*: 625–626.
99. Camerieri A, Picano E, Landi P et al. Prognostic value of dipyridamole echocardiography early after myocardial infarction in elderly patients. Echo Persantine Italian Cooperative (EPIC) Study Group. *J Am Coll Cardiol* 1993; *22(7)*: 1809–1815.
100. Shaw L, Chaitman BR, Hilton TC et al. Prognostic value of dipyridamole thallium-201 imaging in elderly patients. *J Am Coll Cardiol* 1992; *19(7)*: 1390–1398.
101. Hashimoto A, Palmer EL, Scott JA. Complications of exercise and pharmacologic stress tests: Differences in younger and elderly patients. *J Nucl Cardiol* 1999; *6*: 612–619.
102. Katsikis A, Theodorakos A, Papaioannou S et al. Long-term prognostic value of myocardial perfusion imaging in octogenarians able to undergo treadmill exercise stress testing. *J Nucl Cardiol* 2019; *26*: 250–262.
103. Lakkireddy D, Aronow WS, Bateman T et al. Does beta blocker therapy affect the diagnostic accuracy of adenosine single photon emission computed tomographic myocardial perfusion imaging? *Am J Therap* 2008; *15*: 19–23.
104. Hays JT, Mahmarian JJ, Cochran AJ et al. Dobutamine thallium-201 tomography for evaluating patients with suspected coronary artery disease unable to undergo exercise or vasodilator pharmacologic stress testing. *J Am Coll Cardiol* 1993; *21(7)*: 1583–1590.
105. Elhendy A, van Domburg RT, Bax JJ et al. Safety, hemodynamic profile, and feasibility of dobutamine stress technetium myocardial perfusion single-photon emission CT imaging for evaluation of coronary artery disease in the elderly. *Chest* 2000; *117(3)*: 649–656.
106. Hiro J, Hiro T, Reid CL et al. Safety and results of dobutamine stress echocardiography in women versus men and in patients older and younger than 75 years of age. *Am J Cardiol* 1997; *80(8)*: 1014–1020.
107. Sicari R, Pasanisi E, Venneri L et al. Stress echo results predict mortality: A large-scale multicenter prospective international study. *J Am Coll Cardiol* 2003; *41*: 589–595.
108. Innocenti F, Totti A, Baroncini C et al. Prognostic value of dobutamine stress echocardiography in octogenarians. *Int J Cardiovasc Imaging* 2011; *27*: 65–74.
109. Gurunathan S, Ahmed A, Pabla J et al. The clinical efficacy and long-term prognostic value of stress echocardiography in octogenarians. *Heart* 2017; *103*: 530–536.
110. Vliegenthart R, Oudkerk M, Hofman A et al. Coronary calcification improves cardiovascular risk prediction in the elderly. *Circulation* 2005; *112*: 572–577.
111. Newman AB, Naydeck BL, Ives DG et al. Coronary artery calcium, carotid artery wall thickness, and cardiovascular disease outcomes in adults 70 to 99 years old. *Am J Cardiol* 2008; *101*: 186–192.
112. Raggi P, Gongora MC, Gopal A et al. Coronary artery calcium to predict all-cause mortality in elderly men and women. *J Am Coll Cardiol* 2008; *52*: 17–23.

113. Dewey M, Teige F, Schnapauff D et al. Noninvasive detection of coronary artery stenosis with multislice computer tomography or magnetic resonance imaging. *Ann Intern Med* 2006; *145*: 407–415.
114. Ravipati G, Aronow WS, Lai H et al. Comparison of sensitivity, specificity, positive predictive value, and negative predictive value of stress testing versus 64-multislice coronary computed tomography angiography in predicting obstructive coronary artery disease diagnosed by coronary angiography. *Am J Cardiol* 2008; *101*: 774–775.
115. Ostrom MP, Gopal A, Ahmadi N et al. Mortality incidence and the severity of coronary atherosclerosis assessed by computed tomography angiography. *J Am Coll Cardiol* 2008; *52*: 1335–1343.
116. Min JK, Dunning A, Lin FY et al. Age-and sex-related differences in all-cause mortality risk based on coronary computed tomography angiography findings. *J Am Coll Cardiol* 2011; *58*: 849–860.
117. Lee HJ, Kim YJ, Hur J et al. Prevalence and extent of atherosclerotic coronary artery disease and related outcome based on coronary computed tomographic angiography in asymptomatic elderly patients: Retrospective cohort study. *Int J Cardiovasc Imaging* 2014; *30*: 669–676.
118. Naoum C, Berman DS, Ahmadi A et al. Predictive value of age-and sex-specific nomograms of global plaque burden on coronary computed tomography angiography for major cardiac events. *Circ Cardiovasc Imaging* 2017; *10*(*3*): e004896.
119. Douglas PS, Hoffmann U, Patel MR et al. Outcomes of anatomical versus functional testing for coronary artery disease. *N Engl J Med* 2015; *372*: 1291–1300.
120. Hoffmann U, Ferencik M, Udelson JE et al. Prognostic value of noninvasive cardiovascular testing in patients with stable chest pain: Insights from the PROMISE trial (Prospective Multicenter Imaging Study for Evaluation of Chest Pain). *Circulation* 2017; *135*: 2320–2332.
121. Buckert D, Cieslik M, Tibi R et al. Cardiac magnetic resonance imaging derived quantification of myocardial ischemia and scar improves risk stratification and patient management in stable coronary artery disease. *Cardiol J* 2017; *24*: 293–304.
122. Greenwood JP, Herzog BA, Brown JM et al. Prognostic value of cardiovascular magnetic resonance and single-photon emission computed tomography in suspected coronary heart disease: Long-term follow-up of a prospective, diagnostic accuracy cohort study. *Ann Intern Med* 2016; *165*: 1–9.
123. Pontone G, Andreini D, Guaricci AL et al. The STRATEGY study (stress cardiac magnetic resonance versus computed tomography coronary angiography for the management of symptomatic revascularized Patients): Resources and outcomes impact. *Circ Cardiovasc Imaging* 2016; *9*(*10*): e005171.
124. Schuijf JD, Bax JJ, Shaw LJ et al. Meta-analysis of comparative diagnostic performance of magnetic resonance imaging and multislice computed tomography for noninvasive coronary angiography. *Am Heart J* 2006; *151*: 404–411.
125. Greenland P. Who is a candidate for noninvasive coronary angiography? *Ann Intern Med* 2006; *145*: 466–467.
126. West R, Ellis G, Brooks N. Complications of diagnostic cardiac catheterisation: Results from a confidential inquiry into cardiac catheter complications. *Heart* 2006; *92*: 810–814.
127. Niebauer J, Sixt S, Zhang F et al. Contemporary outcomes of cardiac catheterizations in 1085 consecutive octogenarians. *Int J Cardiol* 2004; *93*: 225–230.

9

Angina pectoris in older persons

WILBERT S. ARONOW AND WILLIAM H. FRISHMAN

Key points

- Antianginal therapy with a beta-blocker, a calcium channel blocker (CCB), or long-acting nitrates is recommended for angina relief in patients with chronic coronary disease (CCD).
- In patients with CCD who remain symptomatic despite treatment with a beta-blocker, CCB, and long-acting nitrates, ranolazine is recommended.
- In patients with CCD, sublingual nitroglycerin or nitroglycerin spray is recommended for immediate short-term relief of angina.
- In patients with lifestyle-limiting angina despite guideline-directed medical treatment (GDMT) with significant coronary stenoses amenable to revascularization, revascularization is recommended to improve symptoms.
- In patients with CCD who have significant left main disease or multivessel disease with a left ventricular ejection fraction of ≤35%, coronary artery bypass grafting (CABG) in addition to medical therapy is recommended over medical therapy alone to improve survival.

Coronary artery disease (CAD) is the number one cause of death in older persons and also the major cause of hospitalization and rehospitalizations in this age group. Clinically, CAD manifests as both acute and chronic ischemic syndromes. Although the pathophysiology of myocardial ischemia and the treatment options are similar in older and younger patients, there are significant differences in presentation and response to treatment between the age groups. Older CAD patients with myocardial ischemia often present with "atypical" symptoms, and have more comorbid illnesses, a greater number of vessels involved, and worse left ventricular (LV) function (1–6). The pharmacokinetics of medications are altered in older patients, and there is often a greater sensitivity to medication and a greater potential for side effects and drug–drug interactions. Since older patients often present with more advanced CAD and their prognosis is often worse, there is a greater potential for gain from aggressive interventions, such as percutaneous coronary intervention (PCI) and coronary artery bypass graft (CABG) surgery, although the risks are greater compared to younger patients. Finally, older patients and their families may place different values on risk, quality of life, and the importance of prognosis, all of which must be considered by the practicing physician.

EVALUATION AND MANAGEMENT

The most common symptom of myocardial ischemia in older patients, as well as in younger patients, is exertional chest pain (angina); however, in many older patients, instead of chest pain, exertional dyspnea may be the initial manifestation of ischemia. Other common symptoms experienced by elderly patients with myocardial ischemia

DOI: 10.1201/9781003568933-9

are dizziness, mental confusion, or easy fatiguability. In some older patients with myocardial ischemia, the presentation will be the sudden onset of heart failure ("flash" pulmonary edema) (7–9) or arrhythmias, including sudden death (10). Silent ischemia is particularly common in older patients with CAD, occurring in up to one third of older patients, as documented by ambulatory electrocardiogram (ECG) monitoring (11, 12).

In a study of 1053 patients who had coronary angiography to investigate the association of chest pain versus dyspnea with demographics, coronary angiographic findings, and outcomes, 654 (62%) had chest pain, 229 (22%) had dyspnea, and 117 (11%) had chest pain and dyspnea as the presenting symptom (13). Patients presenting with dyspnea were older (67 years) than patients presenting with chest pain (63 years) but had a similar 2-year mortality (13).

The initial evaluation of the elderly patient with possible myocardial ischemia should begin with a thorough history and complete physical examination, and determination of coronary risk factors and comorbid illnesses. The assessment should determine if the patient is stable or unstable and the risk stratification of the patient. In addition to advanced age, morbidity and mortality in elderly patients with acute myocardial ischemia are directly related to LV function, the extent of CAD, and the presence of comorbidity.

Angina pectoris is a clinical syndrome reflecting inadequate oxygen supply for myocardial metabolic demands with resultant ischemia. Depending on the underlying pathophysiology, the patient will present with stable or unstable angina. The goals of therapy in older patients with angina (ischemic syndromes) are to (1) relieve the acute symptoms and stabilize the acute pathophysiological process; (2) minimize the frequency and severity of recurrent anginal attacks; and (3) prevent progression, plus cause regression of the underlying pathophysiological process. Therapeutic measures are directed at modifying the underlying pathophysiology with therapeutic agents and reducing myocardial ischemia by (1) reducing myocardial oxygen demand and (2) increasing coronary blood flow.

The main underlying pathological process in patients with angina is coronary atherosclerosis with plaque formation and narrowing of the vessel luminal diameter, plus intermittent rupture of the atherosclerotic plaque. Because thrombus formation is an important factor in the progression of atherosclerotic lesions and in the conversion of clinical to acute events after plaque rupture, antiplatelet and anticoagulant therapy are important in the management of elderly CAD patients. In addition, stabilization and regression of the atherosclerotic lesions are possible by vigorous control of the patient's serum lipids, particularly with hydroxymethylglutaryl coenzyme A (HMG CoA)-reductase inhibitors (statins), and treatment of other risk factors, such as systemic hypertension, smoking, and diabetes mellitus.

The main determinants of myocardial oxygen demand are heart rate, myocardial contractility, and intramyocardial tension, which is a function of systemic pressure and ventricular volume. Reduction of the myocardial oxygen demand includes correction of potentially reversible factors, such as heart failure, hyperthyroidism, valvular heart disorders (particularly aortic stenosis), obesity, emotional stress, hypertension, and arrhythmias, such as atrial fibrillation. Drug therapy to reduce myocardial oxygen demand is directed at reducing myocardial contractility, slowing the heart rate, and limiting myocardial tension by reducing systemic pressure (afterload) and preload.

Coronary blood flow is dependent on the duration of cardiac diastole, coronary arterial resistance, aortic diastolic pressure, and the availability of coronary collateral vessels. Improvement in coronary blood flow can be accomplished by those drugs that increase the duration of diastole, that decrease coronary artery resistance by vasodilatation by reducing intramyocardial tension, and that stimulate the development of and flow through collateral vessels.

SPECIFIC DRUG THERAPIES

The principles of drug therapy for treating angina in older patients are the same as those for younger patients (14–19). The physician treating elderly patients, however, must be aware that the pharmacokinetics of drugs may be different in this age group. Gastrointestinal disorders can potentially interfere with drug absorption, although drug bioavailability is usually unaffected by the aging process (20). The decrease in lean body mass and increase in adipose tissue associated with aging affect the volume of drug distribution. Hepatic blood flow and hepatic oxidation (phase I reactions) decrease with aging, whereas hepatic conjugation is unchanged. Not only is renal dysfunction common in elderly patients, but aging is associated with a decline in glomerular filtration rate of 30% between the fifth and ninth decades in normal patients (20). The elderly often demonstrate increased sensitivity to drugs at any given dosage and may tolerate side effects less well. The presence of comorbid conditions increases the potential for adverse drug reactions. The axiom to remember when prescribing drugs in elderly patients is to start low and titrate up slowly.

Given the pharmacological considerations of drug therapy in older patients, the specific antianginal drugs can be very effective in controlling symptoms and modifying the underlying pathophysiological process in older patients with angina. The classes of drugs commonly used include (1) nitrates, (2) beta-blockers, (3) calcium channel blockers, and (4) antiplatelet and/or anticoagulant agents.

Nitrates

Nitrates are safe, effective, and usually the first choice for treatment of angina. Denitration of the organic nitrate with the subsequent liberation of nitric oxide (NO) is necessary for the drug to have therapeutic effects. Nitric oxide stimulates guanylyl cyclase, which leads to the conversion of guanosine triphosphate to cyclic guanosine monophosphate, which causes relaxation of vascular smooth muscle with vasodilatation (20, 21). The exact mechanism by which the organic nitrates undergo denitration and thus liberate NO remains controversial (22, 23).

The active metabolite, NO, is also known as the endothelium-derived relaxing factor (EDRF) (24) and, in addition to relaxing vascular smooth muscle, reduces platelet adhesion and aggregation (25). In vessels with atherosclerosis, it has been shown that the endothelium is dysfunctional with attenuation of EDRF activity (26). Such attenuation of EDRF has been found in patients with hypercholesterolemia without overt coronary atherosclerosis (27). Due to this attenuated activity of EDRF, vascular vasoconstriction is predominant in patients with CAD. Therefore, nitrates as exogenous donors of NO would appear to be the ideal drug to use in older patients with angina (myocardial ischemia).

The mechanisms by which nitrates relieve and prevent myocardial ischemia include both a reduction in myocardial oxygen demand and an increase in myocardial oxygen supply due to the drug's potent vasodilator properties (Table 9.1). Dilatation of capacitance veins reduces ventricular volume and preload, thus lowering myocardial oxygen requirement and improving subendocardial blood flow. Dilatation of systemic conductive arteries decreases afterload, another determinant of oxygen consumption. Nitrates dilate epicardial coronary arteries with an increase in coronary flow and an improvement in subendocardial perfusion. Nitrates also dilate collateral vessels, which can improve blood flow to the areas of ischemia (28). In the doses used clinically, nitrates do not affect coronary resistance vessels (29). Thus, the risk of myocardial ischemia due to coronary steal is minimal, which has been shown to occur with drugs such as dipyridamole and short-acting calcium channel blockers that cause arteriolar dilatation (30).

Table 9.1 Cardiovascular effects of nitrates and mechanisms to relieve angina (ischemia)

Decreased myocardial O_2 demand
Venodilation → ↓ preload → ↓ wall tension
Arteriolar dilatation → ↓ afterload → ↓ wall tension
Increase myocardial blood flow (O_2)
Coronary dilatation → ↑ coronary flow → ↑ regional myocardial perfusion (subendocardial)
Increase collateral flow → ↑ myocardial perfusion (subendocardial)
Decrease coronary resistance → ↑ coronary flow

NITRATE PREPARATIONS

Short-acting nitrates

Nitroglycerin is the drug most frequently used for relief of the acute anginal attack. It is given either as a sublingual tablet or as a sublingual spray, and is absorbed rapidly, with hemodynamic effects occurring within 2 minutes after drug administration. The advantage of the spray is that sublingual tablets deteriorate when exposed to light and will need to be renewed every 4 to 6 months to ensure complete bioavailability. The other advantage of nitroglycerin spray is that it may be easier to administer in elderly patients who have difficulty with the fine motor skills necessary to administer sublingual tablets. An inhalational form of nitroglycerin has just been approved for the management of acute anginal attacks. Orally, nitrates are also available to abort acute anginal attacks that are not relieved with sublingual tablets or spray, and to prevent recurrent anginal attacks. Table 9.2 lists the different nitrate preparations and dosages (31).

Long-acting nitrates

Nitrates have been proven not only effective in relieving acute anginal pain but also beneficial in preventing recurrent anginal attacks. Long-acting nitrates also improve exercise time until the onset of angina and reduce exercise-induced ischemic ST-segment depression (32, 33). The oral preparation is usually the nitrate of choice in the prevention of angina. Standard-formulation isosorbide dinitrate is rapidly absorbed and is typically administered three times a day with a 14-hour nitrate-free interval. Sustained-release isosorbide dinitrate has a slower rate of absorption and results in a therapeutic plasma concentration for 12 h. The usual dosage schedule is twice daily in doses of 20 to 80 mg.

An isosorbide mononitrate is also available for the prevention of angina. The major advantage of the mononitrate preparation is that it is completely bioavailable because it does not undergo first-pass hepatic metabolism. To avoid drug tolerance, it is recommended that the 20–40 mg tablets be given twice daily with 7 hours between doses. A sustained-release formulation of isosorbide mononitrate is also available that provides therapeutic plasma drug concentrations for up to 12 hours each day and low concentrations during the latter part of the 24-hour period. The drug dose range is 30–240 mg given once daily.

Transdermal nitroglycerin is a topical nitroglycerin preparation that is effective in preventing angina and may be particularly beneficial in elderly patients who are taking numerous pills and have difficulty remembering drug schedules. Moreover, transdermal nitrate preparations will be more effective than oral preparations in elderly patients who have problems with gastrointestinal malabsorption. Transdermal nitroglycerin is available as an ointment or patch preparation. Both preparations are

Table 9.2 Different nitrate preparations and dosages

Medication	Usual dose (mg)	Onset of action (min)	Duration of action
Short-acting			
Sublingual nitroglycerin powder	400–800 mcg	2–5	10–30 min
Sublingual nitroglycerin	0.3–0.6	2–5	10–30 min
Aerosol nitroglycerin	0.4	2–5	10–30 min
Sublingual and chewable isosorbide dinitrate	2.5–10	3–15	1–2 h
Intravenous	5 μg/min to 30–80 μg/min	1	Sustained during infusion
Long-acting			
Oral isosorbide dinitrate	5–40	15–30	3–6 h
Oral isosorbide dinitrate (sustained release)	40	30–60	6–10 h
Oral erythrityl tetranitrate	10	30	Variable
Oral isosorbide mononitrate	5–60	30	6–8 h
Transdermal nitroglycerin	5–15	30–60	8–14 h

Source: Nifedipine/Metoprolol Trial (HINT) Research Group, *Br Heart J*, 56, 400–413, 1986.

effective, although the patch obviates some of the inherent messiness of the ointment. As with the oral preparation, a 12- to 14-hour nitrate-free interval is necessary to avoid tolerance when using nitroglycerin ointment or patches.

Sublingual nitroglycerin powder has been approved by the US Food and Drug Administration (FDA) based on its efficacy for prevention or acute relief of an attack of angina pectoris from an unpublished clinical trial in 51 patients with exertional angina pectoris (34). One or two packets (400 mcg of nitroglycerin per packet) should be placed under the tongue at the onset of an anginal attack. An additional packet may be given if needed every 5 minutes. No more than three packets should be given within a 15-minute period.

ADVERSE EFFECTS

Older patients in general tolerate nitrates without significant adverse effects, although the two major side effects, hypotension and headaches, can be extremely bothersome in certain patients. Hypotension may occur within minutes after sublingual administration of a nitrate or 1–2 hours after oral ingestion and is caused by the reduction in preload and afterload caused by the vasodilator effect of the drug. Symptoms may range from lightheadedness to syncope and are commonly positional, precipitated by standing. The hypotension related to nitrates more commonly occurs following the initial use of the drug, when hypovolemia is present, or with concomitant vasodilator therapy use, such as calcium channel blockers or other antihypertensive drugs. The hypotension episode may also be potentiated by alcohol. The episodes can be alleviated by reduction of the dose of nitrate, by correction of hypovolemia, and by avoiding an upright position after sublingual use of the drug. In certain elderly patients, the hypotension will be associated with bradycardia, similar to a typical vasovagal reaction. The hypotension associated with nitrate use can usually be alleviated by the patient lying down; in certain patients with a severe hypotensive reaction, elevation of the legs plus administration of fluid will be necessary.

The headache associated with nitrates can be a significant problem in certain elderly patients. It may be a mild, transient frontal headache, although in other patients the headache will be diffuse and throbbing, with persistent head and neck pain associated with nausea or vomiting. Such severe headaches are more common with the use of intravenous or transdermal nitrates. Nitrates may also aggravate vascular headaches and even initiate episodes of "cluster headaches." As in the management of hypotension related to nitrates, the best approach to alleviate or prevent headaches is to use the lowest doses of nitrates possible and titrate slowly upward if necessary. The use of an analgesic such as aspirin or acetaminophen in conjunction with the nitrate administration may prevent the associated headache. Commonly, due to vascular adaptation, within 7 to 10 days after initiation of nitrate use, the headache will diminish and subside. However, while waiting for adaptation to occur, elderly patients will require much reassurance to continue using the drug; and in certain elderly patients, a different antianginal drug will have to be substituted for the nitrate because the patient will not be able to tolerate the recurrent headaches.

Nitrate tolerance, defined as the loss of hemodynamic and antianginal effects during sustained therapy (35), is another consideration when treating elderly CAD patients. Tolerance has been shown to occur, regardless of the nitrate preparation, if the patient is continuously exposed to nitrates throughout a 24-hour period. The clinical impact of nitrate tolerance, however, is unknown, and the mechanism of nitrate tolerance remains unclear (35, 36). Various possible hypotheses include (1) increased intravascular blood volume; (2) depletion of sulfhydryl groups, which are needed for conversion of nitrates to NO; (3) activation of vasoconstriction hormones; and (4) an increased free-radical production by the endothelium during nitrate therapy (37–39). To prevent tolerance, it is recommended that a 12- to 14-hour nitrate-free interval be established when using long-acting nitrate preparations. During the nitrate-free interval, the use of another antianginal drug will be necessary. In elderly patients with unstable angina who are receiving continuous intravenous nitrates, tolerance is not a consideration; if tolerance develops in this setting, the dose of the nitrate should be increased.

Studies have demonstrated that abrupt withdrawal of nitrate exposure may produce nonatherosclerotic ischemic cardiac events, including myocardial infarction (MI) (40, 41). Such events are presumably due to coronary artery spasm. Therefore, caution should be exercised when high-dose nitrate therapy is discontinued in elderly patients; if possible, the nitrate dose should be slowly tapered downward before discontinuation. Phosphodiesterase inhibitors, such as sildenafil, vardenafil, and tadalafil, used in the treatment of erectile dysfunction, can be safely prescribed to men with CAD, but should not be used in men receiving long-acting nitrates (42).

Beta-adrenergic blockers

Beta-adrenergic blocking agents are effective in preventing angina and are considered by many authorities to be the drug of choice to prevent ischemic events. Beta-blockers also improve exercise time until the onset of angina and reduce exercise-induced ischemic ST-segment depression (43). Beta-blockers prevent angina mainly by causing a reduction in myocardial oxygen demand related to slowing of the heart rate, by depressing myocardial contractility, and by reducing blood pressure (Table 9.3). These effects are particularly impressive in the setting of increased emotional and physical stress, such as during exercise and high anxiety states. In addition to the reduction of myocardial oxygen demand, beta-blockers will increase myocardial oxygen supply by slowing the heart rate and extending the period of diastole.

Table 9.3 Cardiovascular effects of beta-blockers and mechanisms to relieve angina (ischemia)

Decrease myocardial O_2 demand
Decrease contractility → ↓ blood pressure and ↓ CO
Decrease heart rate → ↓ blood pressure and ↓ CO
Increase myocardial blood flow (O_2)
Decrease heart rate → ↑ diastolic perfusion time

Abbreviation: CO, cardiac output.

Beta-adrenergic blocking agents can be classified according to (1) beta-1 selectivity; (2) intrinsic sympathomimetic activity; and (3) lipophilic activity (Table 9.4). Consideration of these specific properties is important when using the drug in elderly CAD patients. Beta-1 selectivity is determined by the extent the agent is capable of blocking β_1-receptors and not β_2-receptors (44). Certain agents, such as metoprolol and atenolol, are relatively more beta-1 selective than propranolol, which makes these drugs less prone to inducing bronchospasm or peripheral arterial vasoconstriction, as compared to the nonselective agents. At higher doses, however, beta-1 selective beta-blockers react like nonselective agents with full potential for bronchospasm and peripheral arterial constriction.

Some beta-blockers, such as pindolol and acebutolol, in addition to blocking beta-adrenergic receptors, possess partial agonist properties and, therefore, are capable of producing intrinsic sympathomimetic activity (ISA) stimulation (45). The degree to which sympathomimetic activity is clinically apparent depends on the underlying sympathetic activity of the patient receiving the drugs. Beta-blockers with ISA may prevent slowing of the heart rate, depression of atrioventricular conduction, and a decrease in myocardial contractility in the setting of a low sympathetic state, such as when the patient is resting. When the sympathetic state is high, however, the effect of beta-blockers with ISA is similar to that of the usual beta-blockers, with a slowing of heart rate and a decrease in blood pressure and ventricular contractility. It should be emphasized that beta-blockers with ISA do not prevent sudden death in post-MI patients, which has been demonstrated with the use of the usual beta-blockers; therefore, these agents are not recommended in elderly patients who have had a MI (46).

The various beta-blockers differ with regard to their lipophilic properties. Some beta-blockers, such as propranolol and metoprolol, are highly lipophilic, which facilitates transfer of the drug across the blood–brain barrier and, therefore, the lipophilic agents are more likely to produce central nervous system side effects, including mood changes, depression, and sleeping disturbances (47). In contrast, the hydrophilic beta-blockers, such as atenolol and nadolol, are less likely to produce central nervous system side effects.

In general, beta-blockers are well tolerated in elderly patients, and some studies have not shown any difference in prevalence of drug side effects between older and younger patients (48). However, significant drug side effects may occur in elderly patients and may be life-threatening. Bradycardia, secondary to the drug effects on the sinus node and atrioventricular conduction may occur, and, due to attenuation of bronchodilatation, asthmatic attacks may be precipitated by the drugs. Therefore, beta-blockers are contraindicated in patients with

Table 9.4 Pharmacology of beta-blockers and dosage

Generic drug (brand)	Cardioselectivity (relative B_1 sensitivity)	ISA	Lipophilic properties	Usual maintenance dose
Propranolol (Inderal)	0	0	High	10–40 mg, q.i.d.
Propranolol LA (Inderal LA)	0	0	High	40–240 mg, q.d.
Atenolol (Tenormin)	+	0	Low	25–100 mg, q.d.
Metoprolol (Lopressor)	+	0	Moderate	25–100 mg, b.i.d.
Metoprolol ER (Toprol XL)	+	0	Moderate	50–200 mg, q.d.
Timolol (Blocadren)	0	0	Low	10–20 mg, b.i.d.
Carvedilol	0	0	Low	25 mg, b.i.d.
Acebutolol (Sectral)	+	+	Low	200–600 mg, b.i.d.
Pindolol (Visken)	0	+	Moderate	5–2 mg, t.i.d.
Labetalol (Normadyne)	0	0	Low	100–600 mg, b.i.d.
Nadolol (Corgard)	0	0	Low	40–80 mg, q.d.
Esmolol (Brevibloc injection)	+	0	Low	0.10–0.15 µg/kg/min

Abbreviations: ER, extended release; ISA, intrinsic sympathomimetic activity; LA, long-acting.

significant bradycardia, unless a pacemaker is inserted, and in persons with a history of bronchospasm. The drugs should also be avoided, or used with caution, in persons with hypotension, hypoglycemic reactions, severe peripheral vascular disease with gangrene, mental depression, and severe heart failure secondary to severe LV systolic dysfunction. The possibility of a withdrawal rebound phenomenon with activation of acute ischemic events should be considered when discontinuing beta-blockers in elderly patients. Accordingly, if possible, the dose of beta-blockers should slowly be tapered downward before discontinuation while another antianginal drug should be started; in addition, the patient should be advised to avoid strenuous activities during the tapering period.

Beta-blockers do have effects on serum lipids, which need to be considered when managing elderly CAD patients. Some studies have shown beta-blockers to increase triglycerides and to decrease HDL cholesterol, although no significant change was noted in total cholesterol or LDL cholesterol (49). Other studies have not demonstrated a significant effect of long-term propranolol use in serum lipids in elderly persons (50). Patients with angina pectoris should be treated with beta-blockers (51, 52). The beta-blockers carvedilol, metoprolol CR/XL, and bisoprolol are recommended to improve outcomes in patients with heart failure and a reduced LV ejection fraction (53, 54). The 2017 American College of Cardiology (ACC)/American Heart Association (AHA) hypertension guidelines recommend lowering the blood pressure to less than 130/80 mmHg in patients with angina pectoris (54). Angina pectoris does not predict all-cause mortality in medically treated patients with heart failure and reduced LV ejection fraction, and is improved to a greater extent by coronary artery bypass grafting than by medical therapy alone (55).

Calcium channel blockers

Calcium channel blockers are usually not considered as first-line drugs in elderly patients with acute coronary artery syndromes. Unlike beta-blockers, their effects are less predictable, and they have not been shown to reduce mortality, sudden death, or reinfarction in post-MI patients (56). The studies that have shown an increase in morbidity and mortality with the use of these drugs in treating hypertension or CAD are also disturbing (57, 58). In turn, calcium blockers have cardiovascular effects that can be beneficial in preventing and controlling angina. In general, the calcium blockers exert their effect by inhibiting the influx of calcium ions through calcium channels of cardiac and vascular smooth muscle cells. Due to this inhibition of calcium influx, myocardial contractility is decreased, dilatation of the peripheral and coronary vasculature occurs, and sinus node and atrioventricular conduction function are suppressed. Therefore, myocardial oxygen demand is reduced by the decrease in preload and afterload and the decrease in myocardial contractility. Slowing of heart rate, which occurs with the use of nondihydropyridine calcium blockers, such as verapamil and diltiazem, is also effective in decreasing myocardial oxygen demand. In addition to reducing myocardial oxygen demand, calcium blockers can improve myocardial oxygen supply by relaxing the tone of coronary arteries and by promoting the development of coronary collaterals (Table 9.5). This property of relaxing coronary vasculature tone is particularly beneficial when Prinzmetal's angina (vasospasm) is present.

Calcium channel blockers are usually divided into the dihydropyridine and non-dihydropyridine groups (Table 9.6). Nifedipine was the first dihydropyridine made available for the treatment of angina, but newer generations

Table 9.5 Cardiovascular effects of calcium blockers and mechanisms to relieve angina

Decreased myocardial O_2 demand
Arteriolar vasodilatation → ↓ afterload → ↓ wall tension
D Decrease contractility
D Decrease heart rate
I Increase myocardial blood flow (O_2)
D Decrease heart rate → ↑ diastolic perfusion time
C Coronary vasodilatation → ↑ flow

of dihydropyridine agents are now available, including nicardipine, nisoldipine, nimodipine, felodipine, amlodipine, and isradipine. Nifedipine is a potent coronary and peripheral artery vasodilator with negative inotropic properties. Significant afterload reduction occurs due to the vasodilation. At therapeutic doses, nifedipine has only a minor effect on the sinus and atrioventricular nodes; thus, due to the decrease in afterload, sympathetic reflex increases in heart rate commonly occur when the drug is administered. The increased heart rate may ameliorate the negative inotropic effect, and clinically hemodynamic indices of contractility generally are unaffected. Due to intense vasodilation of the peripheral coronary circulation, however, the possibility of a coronary steal phenomenon has to be considered when using the drug (59). Such a phenomenon is more common when using a short-acting drug preparation and in patients with severe three-vessel CAD. Therefore, a beta-blocker should be added if nifedipine is used to treat elderly patients with acute ischemic syndromes. A sustained-release preparation of nifedipine is available, which results in less sympathetic activity and is considered to be a safer agent than the shorter-acting preparations. Nevertheless, the addition of a beta-blocker with nifedipine, regardless of the type of preparation, is considered the best approach when managing elderly patients with acute ischemic syndromes. The second-generation dihydropyridines, amlodipine and felodipine, have greater vascular selectivity and less negative inotropy and have no clinical effect on the sinus or atrioventricular nodes. Therefore, coronary artery steal does not appear to be a major concern with these drugs, and the drugs can be used in elderly patients with LV systolic dysfunction.

Verapamil and diltiazem, two nondihydropyridine agents, are both potent inhibitors of sinus node activity and atrioventricular node conduction, in addition to being peripheral vasodilators (Table 9.6). Both drugs have significant negative inotropic effects. Due to these effects, the drugs are effective antianginal agents; however, caution is necessary when using the drugs in elderly patients with bradycardia and depressed LV systolic function. These drugs are contraindicated in patients with LV systolic dysfunction with or without clinical heart failure, in patients with disorders of the sinus node, and in patients with heart block. The Multicenter Diltiazem Post-Infarction study reported an increased mortality in post-infarction patients with heart failure or abnormal LV ejection fraction who were randomized to diltiazem therapy (60). Therefore, if a calcium channel blocker is necessary to control angina in elderly post-infarction patients with depressed LV systolic function, second-generation dihydropyridines, such as amlodipine and felodipine, should be used instead of diltiazem or verapamil.

Extreme caution is required when using diltiazem or verapamil in combination with a beta-blocker, particularly in elderly patients who demonstrate sinus node or atrioventricular conduction dysfunction, or in elderly patients who have depressed LV systolic function. Some authorities recommend ECG monitoring when initiating these drugs, particularly verapamil, in combination with beta-blockers.

It should be emphasized that the ACC/AHA guidelines state that there are no class I indications for using calcium channel blockers during or after MI (61). However, if angina pectoris persists despite the use of beta-blockers and nitrates, long-acting calcium channel blockers such as diltiazem or verapamil should be used as antianginal agents in elderly patients with CAD and normal LV

Table 9.6 Calcium channel blocker preparations and dosage

Generic drug (brand)	Potential for SA node and AV node depression	Potential for depression of myocardial contractility	Usual adult oral dosage (mg)
Nifedipine (Procardia) (Adalat)	0	0 to +	10–30, t.i.d.
Nifedipine GITS (Procardia XL)	0	0 to +	30–90, q.d.
Nicardipine (Cardene)	0	0 to +	20–30, t.i.d.
Amlodipine (Norvasc)	0	0	2.5–10, q.d.
Felodipine (Plendil)	0	0	2.5–20, q.d.
Diltiazem (Cardizem)	+ +	+	30–90, t.i.d.
Diltiazem CD (Cardizem CD)	+ +	+	120–300, q.d.
Verapamil (Isoptin) (Calan) (Verelan)	+ +	+ +	40–120, t.i.d.
Verapamil SR (Isoptin SR) (Calan SR)	+ +	+ +	120–240, q.d.

Abbreviations: CD, extended release; GITS, gastrointestinal therapeutic system; SR, sustained release.
Source: Nifedipine/Metoprolol Trial (HINT) Research Group, *Br Heart J*, 56, 400–413, 1986.

systolic function, and amlodipine or felodipine in patients with CAD and abnormal LV systolic function.

Aspirin

Recent knowledge of the importance of thrombus formation in acute coronary syndromes and the results of studies demonstrate a decreased incidence of MI in patients taking daily aspirin compared to patients receiving a placebo (62). The updated ACC/AHA guidelines for the management of patients with stable angina pectoris (17) and the American College of Physicians (ACP) clinical practice guidelines (16) recommend treating all patients with CAD with aspirin in a dose of 75–162 mg daily unless there are contraindications to the use of this drug. The use of enteric low-dose aspirin may be associated with aspirin resistance (a lack of an antiplatelet effect), and a 162 mg aspirin dose may need to be prescribed.

In an observational prospective study of 1410 patients, mean age 81 years, with prior MI and hypercholesterolemia, 59% of patients were treated with aspirin, and at 36-month follow-up the use of aspirin was associated with a 52% reduction in new coronary events (63).

Clopidogrel

Not all patients can tolerate aspirin, and recently an aspirin-resistance phenomenon has been described in patients where there is little to no antiplatelet effect from the drug. Clopidogrel is a useful alternative to aspirin when the drug is not tolerated, although it has its own associated toxicities (64). This may, however, be dose related in most situations.

Clopidogrel in a dose of 75 mg daily is recommended in patients who cannot tolerate aspirin (51, 52, 62, 65). Dipyridamole should not be used in patients with angina pectoris since it can cause a coronary steal syndrome and increase exercise-induced myocardial ischemia (66).

Other adjunctive treatments

ANGIOTENSIN-CONVERTING ENZYME INHIBITORS AND ANGIOTENSIN RECEPTOR BLOCKERS

Based on the results of various clinical trials, there is now strong evidence that angiotensin converting enzyme (ACE) inhibitors can reduce the frequency of new cardiovascular events in both normotensive and hypertensive patients with known vascular disease and in patients with diabetes mellitus. If tolerated, ACE inhibitors should be part of a medical regimen to treat chronic ischemic heart disease (67). Angiotensin II receptor blockers are now being studied in patients with known ischemic heart disease who have no history of a previous MI or LV systolic dysfunction.

STATINS

Numerous studies have demonstrated that statins reduce cardiovascular morbidity and mortality in elderly patients with CAD, including those with stable angina pectoris (68–76). The low-density lipoprotein cholesterol should be reduced to less than 70 mg/dL in patients with stable angina pectoris (73, 74). The updated ACC/AHA guidelines for management of patients with chronic stable angina pectoris (15), the ACP clinical practice guidelines (16), and the ACC/AHA 2013 lipid guidelines (76) recommend treating patients with chronic stable angina pectoris with high-dose statins (atorvastatin 40–80 mg daily or rosuvastatin 20–40 mg daily).

STABLE CORONARY ARTERY DISEASE

In the Clinical Outcomes Utilizing Revascularization and Aggressive druG Evaluation (COURAGE) trial, 904 of the 2085 patients aged 65 years and older (mean age 72 years) with stable CAD were randomized to optimal medical therapy or optimal medical therapy plus PCI (77). The addition of PCI to optimal medical therapy in these older patients did not improve or worsen clinical outcomes during a median follow-up of 4.6 years (77). Treatment of stable angina pectoris is not benefited (class III indication) by estrogen therapy, vitamin C, vitamin E, and beta-carotene supplementation; treatment of increased homocysteine with folate or vitamins B6 and B12; chelation therapy; garlic; coenzyme Q10; selenium; or chromium (15, 17). All patients with angina pectoris should receive an annual influenza vaccination and avoid active and passive smoking (15).

AN APPROACH TO MANAGEMENT: SPECIFIC PRACTICE CONSIDERATIONS

Unstable angina

Unstable angina is a transitory syndrome that results from disruption of a coronary atherosclerotic plaque with the subsequent cascade of pathological processes, including thrombosis formation that critically decreases coronary blood flow resulting in new onset or exacerbation of angina (ischemia) (78). Transient episodes of vessel occlusion or near occlusion by thrombus at the site of plaque injury may occur and lead to angina at rest. The thrombus may be labile and result in temporary obstruction to flow. Release of vasoconstrictive substances by platelets and vasoconstriction secondary to endothelial vasodilator dysfunction can contribute to further reduction in blood flow (79), and in some patients myocardial necrosis (non-Q-wave infarction) is documented. Table 9.7 lists the various clinical presentations that are classified as unstable angina.

In contrast to older patients with stable angina who do not require hospitalization, elderly patients with unstable

Table 9.7 Unstable angina presentations

Rest angina within 1 week of presentation
New-onset angina of Canadian Cardiovascular Society Classification (CCSC) class III or IV within 2 months of presentation
Angina increasing in CCSC class to at least CCSC III or IV
Variant angina
Non-Q-wave myocardial infarction
Postmyocardial infarction angina (>24 h)

angina are usually hospitalized and, depending on their risk stratification, may require monitoring in an intensive care unit. Severe classification schemes of risk stratification have been developed. Table 9.8 lists a classification that subdivides patients into high-, intermediate-, and low-risk groups (80). As noted by this classification, clinical characteristics are readily identifiable on the initial patient evaluation that stratify the patient into low-, intermediate-, or high-risk subgroups for hospital complications. For example, acute resting ischemic ECG abnormalities markedly worsen the prognosis. Other characteristics that identify the high-risk patient include prolonged ongoing rest pain longer than 20 minutes and signs of LV dysfunction (S_3, rales, new murmur, or mitral regurgitation). Within each subgroup of unstable angina, it is important to recognize that certain elderly patients have specific characteristics that will influence therapy. Recurrent angina after percutaneous transluminal coronary angioplasty (PTCA) is a common clinical event related to partial artery restenosis and occurs in as many as 40% of patients within the first 3–6 months post-PCI, regardless of the patient's age. The prognosis is favorable, and the elderly patient can usually be stabilized medically prior to a scheduled repeat angiogram and a possible repeat PCI. Angina after intracoronary stent placement occurs less frequently than after an isolated angioplasty and is often the result of subacute closure due to thrombus formation. These patients are at higher risk for MI and are usually managed as higher-risk patients (81). Patients with angina following CABG are another subgroup of elderly patients who require specific considerations. Since the risk of reoperation is higher than that of the initial surgery, surgeons are often reluctant to reoperate in elderly patients, especially on those elderly patients who have undergone internal mammary grafting. Medical therapy is usually the first approach to this subgroup of elderly patients with unstable angina. Other clinical subgroups of elderly patients with unstable angina who require special considerations are the patient with a non-Q-wave infarct, variant angina, and cocaine intoxication.

Table 9.9 lists the ACC/AHA stratification of patients with unstable angina into high-risk, intermediate-risk, and low-risk groups for short-term risk of death or nonfatal MI (82). Following risk stratification of the elderly patient with unstable angina, therapy should be initiated. The initial goals of therapy should be to alleviate symptoms by decreasing myocardial oxygen demand and increasing myocardial blood flow, and to stabilize the atherosclerotic plaque. Furthermore, a plan to promote regression of the atherosclerotic lesion should be initiated during the patient's hospitalization.

Therapy, including drug therapy, should be started in the emergency department; it should not be delayed until hospital admission. Reversible factors causing angina should be identified and corrected, including anemia, which may require packed red cell transfusion. ECG monitoring is important since arrhythmias can occur, and ST-T changes are a marker for an increased risk of complications. The aggressiveness of the drug dosage will depend on the severity of symptoms and will need modification during the elderly patient's hospitalization. Oxygen should be given to patients with cyanosis, respiratory distress, heart failure, or high-risk factors. Oxygen therapy should be guided by arterial saturation; its use when the baseline saturation is more than 94% is questionable. Morphine sulfate should be administered intravenously when symptoms are not immediately relieved with nitroglycerin or when acute pulmonary congestion and/or severe agitation is present.

Aspirin should be given to all patients with unstable angina unless contraindicated and continued indefinitely. Clopidogrel should be administered to patients who are unable to tolerate aspirin because of hypersensitivity or major gastrointestinal intolerance. Data from the Clopidogrel in Unstable Angina to Prevent Recurrent Events (CURE) trial favors the use of aspirin plus the use of clopidogrel for 9 months in patients with unstable angina (83). The ACC/AHA guidelines for unstable

Table 9.8 Risk stratification scheme of unstable angina based on presenting clinical characteristics

Risk class[a]	Clinical characteristics
IA	Acceleration of previous exertional angina without ECG changes
IB	Acceleration of previous exertional angina with ECG changes
II	New onset of exertional angina
III	New onset of rest angina
IV	Coronary insufficiency syndrome; protracted chest pain >20 min with persistent ECG changes

Source: Chesebro JH, Fuster V, *N Engl J Med*, 327, 192–194, 1992.

[a] IA = lowest risk for in-hospital complications; IV = highest risk for in-hospital complications.

Table 9.9 Risk stratification of patients with unstable angina for short-term risk of death or nonfatal myocardial infarction

High risk (at least 1 of following factors)	Intermediate risk (no high-risk feature but 1 of following features)	Low risk (no high- or intermediate-risk feature)
Accelerating tempo of ischemic symptoms in prior 48 h	Prior MI or CABG; peripheral or cerebrovascular disease; prior aspirin use	—
Prolonged ongoing (>20 min) rest pain	Prolonged (>20 min) rest angina, now resolved, with moderate or high likelihood of CAD; rest angina (<20 min or relieved with rest or sublingual NTG)	New-onset CCS class III or IV angina in past 2 weeks with moderate or high likelihood of CAD
Pulmonary edema; new or worsening MR murmur; S_3 or new/ worsening rales; hypotension, tachycardia, bradycardia; age >75 years	Age >70 years	—
Angina at rest with transient ST-segment changes >0.05 mV; bundle branch block, new or presumed new; sustained ventricular tachycardia	T-wave inversions >0.2 mV; pathological Q waves	Normal or unchanged ECG during episode of chest discomfort
Markedly elevated troponin T or I (>0.1 ng/mL)	Slightly elevated troponin T or I (>0.01 but <0.1 ng/mL)	Normal

Abbreviations: CABG, coronary artery bypass graft surgery; CAD, coronary artery disease; CCS, Canadian Cardiovascular Society; MI, myocardial infarction; MR, mitral regurgitation; NTG, nitroglycerin.

Source: Mark K et al., *J Am Coll Cardiol*, 27, 494–503, 1996.

angina support the use of aspirin plus clopidogrel in high-risk and intermediate-risk patients with unstable angina, with clopidogrel withheld for 5–7 days if CABG is planned (84).

Prasugrel is a thienopyridine that requires conversion to an active metabolite before binding to the platelet P2Y12 receptor. Compared to clopidogrel, it is metabolized more efficiently, has greater bioavailability, and produces a greater antiplatelet effect. In the Trial to Assess Improvement in Therapeutic Outcomes by Optimizing Platelet Inhibition with Prasugrel–Thrombolysis in Myocardial Infarction (TRITON–TIMI) 38 (85), prasugrel significantly lowered the rates of ischemic events in the prasugrel group, with a 2.3% absolute reduction and a 24% relative reduction of MI. There was also a 52% relative reduction for stent thrombosis. These benefits were seen irrespective of the type of stent used. However, patients with a prior history of stroke or transient ischemic attack (TIA) had poor clinical outcomes with a net harm from prasugrel (hazard ratio 1.54), and there was a 32% increase in relative TIMI major hemorrhage with prasugrel. Therefore, prasugrel is contraindicated in patients with history of prior stroke or TIA, while for patients weighing <60 kg and those >75 years of age, a reduced dose of the drug is suggested (85). The 2011 ACCF/AHA guidelines support the use of prasugrel or clopidogrel as an addition to aspirin in patients with acute coronary syndromes (84).

Ticagrelor is a non-thienopyridine with a plasma half-life of 12 hours. It is a reversible and direct-acting oral antagonist of the ADP receptor P2Y12. In the Study of Platelet Inhibition and Patient Outcomes (PLATO) trial (86), when compared with clopidogrel, ticagrelor significantly lowered at 1 year the rate of death from vascular causes, MI, or stroke from 11.7% to 9.8% ($p < 0.001$) in patients with acute coronary syndromes. However, the drug seemed to work better at preventing clinical events when accompanied by low-dose as opposed to high-dose aspirin based on the findings that the outcomes were superior with the new drug across the entire international trial but not in North America, where the aspirin doses were generally higher. It was approved by the FDA, provided a low dose of aspirin ≤100 mg was coadministered.

Parenteral anticoagulation with intravenous infractionated heparin or preferably with subcutaneous low-molecular-weight heparin (87–90) should be added to antiplatelet therapy in patients with high-risk or intermediate-risk unstable angina. The revised ACC/AHA guidelines for unstable angina also recommend adding a platelet glycoprotein IIb/IIIa inhibitor in addition to aspirin, clopidogrel or prasugrel, and low-molecular-weight heparin in patients with continuing ischemia or with other high-risk features, and to patients in whom PCI is planned. Eptifibatide and tirofiban are approved for this use (83). Abciximab can also be used for 12–24 hours in patients with unstable angina in whom PCI is planned within the next 24 hours (84).

As with the use of aspirin, nitrates should be instituted quickly in the emergency department. Patients whose symptoms are not fully relieved with three sublingual nitroglycerin tablets should receive continuous intravenous nitroglycerin. The initial dose is 5–10 mg/min, and the dose should be titrated every 3–5 minutes to relieve symptoms or associated hypertension. If angina is relieved, then an oral or transdermal preparation can be started after 24 hours of intravenous therapy. Beta-blockers (in addition to aspirin, heparin, and nitrates) should also be started in the emergency room unless there are contraindications. Intravenous loading (e.g., metoprolol 5 mg for 5 min, repeated every 15 min for a total of 15 mg) or propranolol followed by oral therapy is recommended. A continuous beta-blocker intravenous infusion may be used (esmolol, starting maintenance dose of 0.1 g/kg/min intravenously with titration upward in increments of 0.5 g/kg/min every 10 to 15 minutes as tolerated by blood pressure until the desired response has been obtained, limiting symptoms develop, or a dose of 0.20 mg/min is reached). An oral ACE inhibitor and a statin should also be administered unless there are contraindications.

Patients with unstable angina pectoris do not benefit from treatment with the oral selective inhibitor of the Lp-PLA$_2$ enzyme darapladib (91). Patients with unstable angina pectoris also do not benefit from treatment with the oral sPLA$_2$ inhibitor varespladib (92).

INTERVENTIONAL THERAPY

The majority of older patients with stable and unstable angina can be stabilized with medical management. Patients who continue to have unstable angina 30 minutes after initiation of therapy or who have recurrent unstable angina during the hospitalization are at increased risk for MI or cardiac death. In addition, patients who demonstrate major ischemic complications, such as pulmonary edema, ventricular arrhythmias, or cardiogenic shock associated with unstable angina, also have a poor prognosis. In these patients, emergency cardiac catheterization should be performed with the consideration of interventional therapy (CABG or PCI). Insertion of an intra-aortic balloon pump may be necessary in some of these elderly patients.

For the majority of older patients whose angina is stabilized, two alternate strategies for definitive treatment of angina need to be considered: early invasive and early conservative (18, 93). The early invasive strategy approach is to perform cardiac catheterization in all patients after 48 hours of presentation unless interventional therapy is contraindicated due to extensive comorbidities. In contrast, the early conservative strategy is to perform cardiac catheterization only in patients who have one or more of the following high-risk indicators: prior revascularization, associated congestive heart failure or depressed LV ejection fraction (<50%) by noninvasive study, malignant ventricular arrhythmia, persistent or recurrent pain/ischemia, and/or a functional study (stress test) indicating high risk. On the basis of data from the TACTICS–Thrombolysis in Myocardial Infarction 18 study, an early invasive strategy is superior to a conservative strategy in high-risk unstable angina patients (94). The revised ACC/AHA guidelines recommend an early invasive strategy for all high-risk patients with unstable angina.

A stress test can be performed 48–72 hours after the patient has stabilized. The choice of the type of stress testing (exercise, exercise with imaging, or pharmacological) will depend on the resting ECG findings and the patient's ability to exercise.

Myocardial revascularization is indicated in patients who at catheterization are found to have significant left main CAD (≥50%) or significant (≥70%) three-vessel disease with depressed LV function (LV ejection fraction <50%); patients with two-vessel disease with proximal severe subtotal stenosis (≥95%) of the left anterior descending coronary artery and depressed LV ejection fraction; and patients with significant CAD if they fail to stabilize with medical treatment, have recurrent angina/ischemia at rest or with low-level activities, and/or if ischemia is accompanied by congestive heart failure symptoms, an S_3 gallop, new or worsening mitral regurgitation, or definite ECG changes (18, 93).

The ACC/AHA guidelines recommend CABG for patients with unstable angina with significant left main CAD, three-vessel CAD, and for two-vessel CAD with significant proximal left anterior descending CAD and either abnormal LV function (ejection fraction <50%) or demonstrable ischemia on noninvasive testing (18, 84). PCI or CABG is recommended for patients with one-vessel or two-vessel CAD without significant proximal left anterior descending CAD, but with a large area of viable myocardium and high-risk criteria on noninvasive testing. PTCA is recommended for patients with multivessel CAD with a suitable coronary anatomy with normal LV function and without diabetes mellitus (18, 84).

For some patients without these high-risk features, revascularization may still be an option, depending on recurrent symptoms, test results, and patient preferences. The health care team should educate the patient and his or her family or advocate about the expected risks and benefits of revascularization and determine individual patient preferences and fears that may affect the selection of therapy. CABG with or without cardiopulmonary bypass causes a high incidence of cognitive decline (95).

Interventional therapy with PTCA, atherectomy, and/or some combination of PCI and coronary artery stenting has increased in usage in patients with CAD, diminishing the frequency of CABG. Studies comparing PCI and CABG have been performed, and generally the results of PCI and CABG are similar in terms of mortality. However, an increased incidence of recurrent angina and need for revascularization procedure occurs with PCI (96–98). On the other hand, the incidence of cognitive decline is high in older persons undergoing CABG with no difference seen when comparing the incidence of cognitive dysfunction in on-pump and off-pump bypass procedures (95).

Older, stable angina patients who are at low risk (preserved LV function and no left main CAD) can be treated as effectively with medical therapy as with interventional therapy. In patients with stable angina, the atherosclerotic lesions are predominantly advanced fibrolipoid plaques or fibrotic lesions (99). Usually no plaque ulceration or thrombosis is present, and the main cause of angina is the reduction of luminal diameter of the coronary vessel due to chronic atherosclerosis. Therefore, therapy is directed at decreasing myocardial oxygen demand and increasing coronary blood flow. In addition, prevention of plaque instability and initiation of therapy to cause regression of the atherosclerotic lesion are necessary.

Studies have not demonstrated any significant benefit of a specific class of antianginal drugs compared to other classes in the treatment of stable angina. Therefore, the choice of a single antianginal drug will depend on the clinical situation, contraindications, and the physician's preference. Surely a beta-blocker should be the first choice in elderly patients who have a history of MI or demonstrate electrocardiographic evidence of silent infarction or silent myocardial ischemia (100).

Combination drug therapy, in which a beta-blocker and a vasodilator are used, is highly advantageous in treating elderly patients with angina. Studies have shown that combination therapy with a nitrate and beta-blocker decreases the number of anginal attacks and increases the duration of time of treadmill stress testing as compared to either nitrates or beta-blockers alone (101). The combination of a beta-blocker and a calcium channel blocker has also been shown to be more effective in reducing angina and extending exercise time than monotherapy (101). Such a combination can be very beneficial when attempting to control both hypertension and angina in elderly patients. In turn, caution is necessary when using beta-blockers in combination with diltiazem or verapamil due to the potential risk of provoking serious bradycardia or precipitating heart failure. This is particularly a concern when verapamil and a beta-blocker are used in combination, and when underlying sinus or atrioventricular nodal disease or LV systolic dysfunction is present. In elderly patients whose angina is refractory to double-drug therapy, triple-drug therapy may be necessary. Such therapy would include a beta-blocker, a long-acting nitrate, and a calcium channel blocker. Such therapy may be beneficial in preventing anginal attacks. However, elderly patients taking these multiple drugs will need to be monitored closely for side effects, and the drugs should be started at low doses. Patients aged 75 years or older with angina despite standard drug therapy benefit more from coronary revascularization (102, 103).

A preventive program in elderly patients with angina is mandatory, including abstinence from smoking, treatment of hypertension, use of aspirin and ACE inhibitors, an exercise program, and control of lipids and weight (104). Treatment of associated heart failure and anemia can also prevent or relieve symptoms of angina. The recent studies that have demonstrated the efficacy of statin therapy in lowering serum lipids and in preventing future coronary events in elderly patients with CAD (68–76) compel physicians to screen elderly anginal patients for elevated serum lipids and to be aggressive in their treatment of lipid abnormalities. In the Heart Protection Study, 20,536 adults up to age 80 years with CAD, other occlusive arterial disease, or diabetes mellitus were randomized to simvastatin 40 mg daily or double-blind placebo and followed for a mean of 5 years (72). All-cause mortality, coronary events, stroke, and coronary and noncoronary revascularization were significantly reduced by simvastatin, regardless of age and initial serum lipids (72).

In addition, elderly patients will require counseling in reference to lifestyle, with avoidance of activities that trigger ischemic attacks (105). The physician will need to be aware of the potential for the development of mental depression in elderly CAD patients. The symptoms of depression may be subtle in elderly patients and will progress unless the disease is treated. Depression has also been shown to be a risk factor for future coronary events in patients with CAD (106).

The role of exercise should be emphasized when managing elderly patients with angina. Exercise programs that progressively increase physical endurance and reduce the heart rate and cardiac work at any given level of activity lead to improvement in cardiac performance and prolong exercise time before the onset of angina (107). In addition, some studies have shown stress-induced myocardial ischemia (as assessed by thallium 201 scintigraphy) to be significantly decreased after a 1-year program of supervised exercise and low cholesterol diet in patients with stable angina (108). Caution is necessary, however, when initiating an exercise program in elderly CAD patients. Elderly patients should be screened for high-risk characteristics, including results of a stress test, before starting an exercise program since exercise can provoke serious arrhythmias in high-risk patients, especially in poorly conditioned patients. Other exercise programs can be advised according to the patient's needs and preferences, such as swimming or stationary cycling.

New approaches for the management of angina

Over the years, the management of patients with angina has changed, and new approaches have developed. Some of these changes are due to increased knowledge of the underlying pathophysiology of myocardial ischemia with the development of new drugs. Other changes are related to the development of innovative mechanical devices and techniques that theoretically should relieve angina.

RANOLAZINE

Ranolazine is a piperazine derivative and a partial fatty acid oxidation inhibitor that reduces calcium overload in the ischemic myocyte by inhibition of the late sodium current (109, 110). This action decreases the magnitude of ischemia-induced sodium and calcium overload, improving myocardial function as well as myocardial perfusion. Four randomized, double-blind trials have demonstrated that ranolazine reduces the frequency of angina episodes and nitroglycerin consumption and improves exercise duration and time to anginal attacks without clinically significant effects on heart rate or blood pressure (111–114). Ranolazine's anti-ischemic mechanism is most likely due to an improvement in regional coronary blood flow in areas of myocardial ischemia (115).

Ranolazine was approved by the FDA for the treatment of patients with chronic stable angina pectoris in January 2006. Ranolazine was approved for use as combination therapy when angina is not adequately controlled with other antianginal drugs. The recommended dose of sustained-release ranolazine is 750 or 1000 mg twice daily. Ranolazine may be effective in patients with microvascular angina and endothelial dysfunction (116).

OTHER PHARMACOLOGIC APPROACHES

Other drugs under investigation to be considered for FDA approval include nicorandil, ivabradine, and trimetazidine (117). Nicorandil is a coronary vasodilator with a unique dual mechanism of action that involves a nitrate-like effect and a potassium ion channel opening action (109, 118–120). The Impact of Nicorandil in Angina (IONA) study showed at 1.6-year follow-up in patients with stable angina pectoris that 2565 patients randomized to nicorandil 20 mg twice daily had a 17% significant reduction in CAD death, nonfatal MI, or unplanned hospital admission for cardiac chest pain compared with 2561 patients randomized to placebo (120). Another study of 402 patients with stable angina pectoris showed that nicorandil added to standard antianginal therapy reduced the number of ischemic attacks by 50% (119).

Ivabradine is a heart rate–lowering drug that acts specifically on the sinoatrial node (121). Ivabradine caused dose-dependent improvements in exercise tolerance and time to development of ischemia during exercise (122). In a subgroup of patients with a heart rate of 70 beats/min or higher, ivabradine did not affect the primary endpoint of cardiovascular death or hospital admission for fatal and nonfatal MI (123). However, ivabradine did reduce the secondary endpoint of hospital admission for fatal and nonfatal MI by 36% ($p = 0.001$) and coronary revascularization by 30% ($p = 0.016$) (123). In the Systolic Heart Failure Treatment with the IF inhibitor Ivabradine Trial (SHIFT), ivabradine showed a reduction of cardiovascular outcomes in patients with heart failure and angina pectoris (124). A meta-analysis of three randomized controlled trials in 36,577 patients with stable angina pectoris showed that ivabradine was not effective in reducing cardiovascular mortality, all-cause mortality, coronary revascularization, and hospital admission for worsening of heart failure but increased adverse events (125). In a study of 2403 patients with stable angina pectoris, 636 patients were treated with a combination of ivabradine plus metoprolol (126). This study showed that ivabradine combined with metoprolol reduced angina symptoms and use of nitroglycerin and improved quality of life with a 14.7-point increase in the EQ-5D questionnaire (126). Combining ivabradine with low-dose bisoprolol in patients with stable angina pectoris caused additional antianginal and anti-ischemic benefits and improved chronotropic reserve (127). Ivabradine should be considered for use in patients with stable angina pectoris and heart failure being treated with beta-blockers in whom coronary revascularization is incomplete or unsuitable (128).

Trimetazidine is an antianginal drug that improves myocardial glucose utilization through inhibition of fatty acid metabolism. A meta-analysis of 13 randomized clinical trials showed that trimetazidine was efficacious in the treatment of patients with stable angina pectoris and reduced the number of weekly anginal episodes, reduced the weekly nitroglycerin use, caused a longer time to 1 mm of ischemic ST-segment depression, increased total work, and caused a longer exercise duration at peak exercise (129).

CELL THERAPY

Innovative approaches for the management of drug-resistant angina pectoris include the use of vascular growth factors to induce myocardial angiogenesis (130, 131). Granulocyte-macrophage colony-stimulating factor has been used to mobilize bone marrow stem cells to induce angiogenesis. In addition, stem cells are being used by direct injection to affect new vascular growth (130).

OTHER MECHANICAL APPROACHES

Recent mechanical techniques for the treatment of angina include transmyocardial laser revascularization (TMLR), enhanced external counterpulsation (EECP), and spinal cord stimulation. These approaches have been used in patients with severe angina who are not candidates for PTCA or CABG, usually due to diffuse CAD or extreme comorbidities. Such approaches would appear to be suitable for many elderly CAD patients who may have inoperable CAD and multiple comorbidities plus angina that is difficult to control with medical therapy.

TMLR employs a high-energy laser beam to create channels in the myocardium from the epicardial to the endocardial surface (132). The channels allow oxygenated LV blood to perfuse ischemic myocardial zones (133). The human myocardium contains an extensive network of sinusoids, and TMLR theoretically delivers oxygenated blood to these sinusoids with improved myocardial oxygen delivery to the ischemic region. Data on the efficacy of TMLR in improving anginal symptoms and exercise capacity are controversial (134–137).

EECP is a noninvasive outpatient treatment designed to increase coronary flow in the treatment of angina

(138–140). This treatment involves wrapping the calves, thighs, and buttocks with pneumatic cuffs. Synchronized pulsatory pressure is applied sequentially from calves to thighs during diastole, returning arterial blood to the heart to increase diastolic pressure in the coronary vessels. Pressure is relieved during systole, reducing afterload and cardiac work, thus decreasing myocardial oxygen demand. The typical course of treatment is 35 1-hour sessions over a period of 7 weeks. EECP has been shown to improve ischemia in patients who have thallium reperfusion evidence of ischemia. In one study of patients who received EECP, 75% of subjects had resolution of ischemia, demonstrated by improved thallium scintigraphy with normal thallium stress tests, except for areas scarred by previous MIs (141). In addition, the subjects showed exercise improvement. A controlled study of 139 patients showed a reduction in anginal episodes, an increase in the time to 1 mm ischemic ST-segment depression, and a trend toward reduced nitroglycerin use in the EECP group but a similar increase in exercise duration in both groups (142). In a prospective study of 47 patients with chronic refractory angina pectoris, EECP improved anginal symptoms, dyspnea on exertion, quality of life, and 6-minute walking distance at 1 year ($p < 0.001$) (143).

Spinal cord stimulation (SCS) has been demonstrated to cause clinical improvement in patients with refractory angina pectoris in the number of anginal episodes, in nitroglycerin consumption, in maximal exercise time, in exercise time until angina, in the number of episodes of myocardial ischemia, in the duration of episodes of myocardial ischemia, and in ischemic ST-segment depression at a comparable workload (144, 145). Double-blind, randomized, placebo-controlled studies have not been performed with SCS. The clinical improvement from SCS occurred despite no evidence of improvement in regional myocardial blood flow during exercise or in myocardial oxygen consumption as assessed by the heart rate times systolic pressure product at maximal exercise. The mechanisms of clinical improvement by SCS are unclear. SCS must be considered experimental at this time and is a therapeutic option for the treatment of refractory angina pectoris in patients unable to have coronary revascularization or at very high risk for coronary revascularization.

A coronary sinus reducer stent has also been found to clinically improve patients with refractory angina pectoris (146, 147). However, randomized, placebo-controlled data are necessary to evaluate this form of therapy in treating patients with refractory angina pectoris who are not candidates for coronary revascularization.

2023 AHA/ACC GUIDELINE FOR MANAGEMENT OF PATIENTS WITH CCD

These guidelines (148) recommend:

1. Antianginal therapy with a beta-blocker, a calcium channel blocker (CCB), or long-acting nitrates is recommended for angina relief in patients with chronic coronary disease (CCD).
2. In patients with CCD who remain symptomatic despite treatment with a beta-blocker, CCB, and long-acting nitrates, ranolazine is recommended.
3. In patients with CCD, sublingual nitroglycerin or nitroglycerin spray is recommended for immediate short-term relief of angina.
4. In patients with lifestyle-limiting angina despite guideline-directed medical treatment with significant coronary stenoses amenable to revascularization, revascularization is recommended to improve symptoms.
5. In patients with CCD who have significant left main disease or multivessel disease with a left ventricular ejection fraction of ≤35%, CABG in addition to medical therapy is recommended over medical therapy alone to improve survival.

Beta-blockers and CCBs have the strongest evidence in improving symptoms in patients with microvascular angina (149). The ISCHEMIA trial showed that older patients with CCD had consistent improvement in angina frequency but less improvement in angina-related health status with invasive management compared with younger patients (150). Invasive management in this study was not associated with improved clinical outcomes in older or younger patients.

REFERENCES

1. Toffler G, Muller FE, Stone PH, MILIS Study Group. Factors leading to shorter survival after acute myocardial infarction in patients ages 65 to 75 years compared with younger patients. *Am J Cardiol* 1988; *62*: 860–867.
2. Tresch D, Aronow W. Clinical manifestations and diagnosis of coronary artery disease. *Clin Geriatr Med* 1996; *12*: 89–100.
3. Wei J. Heart disease in the elderly. *Cardiol Med* 1984; *9*: 971–982.
4. Ten berg J, Bal E, Gin T et al. Initial and long-term results of percutaneous transluminal coronary angioplasty in patients 75 years of age and older. *Cathet Cardiovasc Diag* 1992; *26*: 165–170.
5. Kelsey SF, Miller DP, Holubkov R et al. Results of percutaneous transluminal coronary angioplasty in patients 65 years of age (from the 1985 to 1986 National Heart, Lung, and Blood Institute's Coronary Angioplasty Registry). *Am J Cardiol* 1990; *66*: 1033–1038.
6. Thompson RC, Holmes DR Jr, Gersh BJ et al. Percutaneous transluminal coronary angioplasty in the elderly: Early and long-term results. *Circulation* 1992; *88*: 1579–1587.
7. Siegel R, Clemens T, Wingo M et al. Acute heart failure: Another manifestation of unstable angina [abstr]. *J Am Coll Cardiol* 1991; *17*: 149.

8. Clark LT, Garfein OB, Dwyer EM. Acute pulmonary edema due to ischemic heart disease without accompanying myocardial infarction. *Am J Med* 1983; *75*: 332–336.
9. Kunis R, Greenberg H, Yeoh CB et al. Coronary revascularization of recurrent pulmonary edema in elderly patients with ischemic heart disease and preserved ventricular function. *N Engl J Med* 1985; *313*: 1207–1210.
10. Tresch D, Saeian K, Hoffman R. Elderly patients with late onset of coronary artery disease: Clinical and angiographic findings. *Am J Geriatr Cardiol* 1992; *1*: 14–25.
11. Aronow WS, Epstein S. Usefulness of silent myocardial ischemia detected by ambulatory electrocardiographic monitoring in predicting new coronary events in elderly patients. *Am J Cardiol* 1988; *62*: 1295–1296.
12. Hedblad B, Juul-Moller S, Svensson K et al. Increased mortality in men with ST segment depression during 14 h ambulatory long-term ECG recording. Results from prospective population study "Men born in 1914," from Malmo, Sweden. *Eur Heart J* 1989; *10*: 149–158.
13. Paudel R, Beridze N, Aronow WS et al. Association of chest pain versus dyspnea as presenting symptom for coronary angiography with demographics, coronary anatomy, and 2-year mortality. *Arch Med Sci* 2016; *12*: 742–746.
14. Aronow WS, Frishman WH. Angina pectoris in the elderly. In: Aronow WS, Fleg JF, Rich MW, eds. *Cardiovascular Disease in the Elderly*, 5th ed. New York: Boca Raton, London, New York, CRC Press, 2013: pp. 215–237.
15. Fihn SD, Gardin JM, Abrams J et al. 2012 ACCF/AHA/ACP/AATS/PCNA/SCAI/STS guideline for the diagnosis and management of patients with stable ischemic heart disease. A Report of the American College of Cardiology Foundation/American Heart Association Task Force on Practice Guidelines, and the American College of Physicians, American Association for Thoracic Surgery, Preventive Cardiovascular Nurses Association, Society for Cardiovascular Angiography and Interventions, and Society of Thoracic Surgeons. *J Am Coll Cardiol* 2012; *60*: e44–e164.
16. Qaseem A, Fihn SD, Dallas P et al. Management of stable ischemic heart disease: Summary of a clinical practice guideline from the American College of Physicians/American College of Cardiology Foundation/American Heart Association/American Association for Thoracic Surgery/Preventive Cardiovascular Nurses Association/Society of Thoracic Surgeons. *Ann Intern Med* 2012; *167*: 735–743.
17. Fihn SD, Blankenship JC, Alexander KP et al. 2014 ACC/AHA/AATS/PCNA/SCAI/STS focused update of the guideline for diagnosis and management of patients with stable ischemic heart disease. A report of the American College of Cardiology Foundation/American Heart Association Task Force on Practice Guidelines, and the American Association for Thoracic Surgery, Preventive Cardiovascular Nurses Association, Society for Cardiovascular Angiography and Interventions, and Society of Thoracic Surgeons. *J Am Coll Cardiol* 2014; *64*: 1929–1949.
18. Amsterdam EA, Wenger NK, Brindis RG et al. 2014 AHA/ACC guideline for the management of patients with non-ST-elevation acute coronary syndromes: Executive summary. A report of the American College of Cardiology/American Heart Association Task Force on Practice Guidelines. Developed in collaboration with the Society for Cardiovascular Angiography and Interventions, and Society of Thoracic Surgeons. Endorsed by the American Association for Clinical chemistry. *J Am Coll Cardiol* 2014; *64*: 2645–2687.
19. Ohman EM. Chronic stable angina. *N Engl J Med* 2016; *374*: 1167–1176.
20. Everitt D, Avorn J. Drug prescribing for the elderly. *Arch Intern Med* 1986; *146*: 2393–2396.
21. Katsuki S, Murad F. Regulation of adenosine cycli 3′,5′-monophosphate and guanosine cyclic 3′5′-monophosphate levels and contractility in bovine tracheal smooth muscle. *Mol Pharmacol* 1977; *13*: 330–341.
22. Axelsson KL, Wikberg JES, Andersson RGG. Relationship between nitroglycerin, cyclic GMP and relaxation of vascular smooth muscle. *Life Sci* 1979; *24*: 1779–1786.
23. Fung HL, Chung SJ, Bauer JA et al. Biochemical mechanism of organic nitrate action. *Am J Cardiol* 1992; *70*: 4B–10B.
24. Abrams J, Frishman WH. The organic nitrates and nitroprusside. In: Frishman WH, Sica DA, eds. *Cardiovascular Pharmacotherapeutics*, 3rd ed. Minneapolis, MN: Cardiotext, 2011: pp. 205–215.
25. Moncada S, Higgs A. The L-arginine-nitric oxide pathway. *N Engl J Med* 1993; *329*: 2002–2012.
26. Diodati J, Cannon RO. Effect of nitroglycerin on platelet activation in patients with stable coronary disease. *Circulation* 1991; 84(*suppl 2*): 731.
27. Hansson GK. Immune and inflammatory mechanisms of monocyte recruitment and accumulation. *Br Heart J* 1993; *69*: 9S–29S.
28. Flavahan NA. Atherosclerosis or lipoprotein induced endothelial dysfunction. Potential mechanism underlying reduction in EDRF/nitric oxide activity. *Circulation* 1985; *85*: 1927–1938.
29. Goldstein RE, Stinison EB, Scherer JL et al. Intraoperative coronary collateral function in patients with coronary occlusive disease:

Nitroglycerin responsiveness and angiographic correlations. *Circulation* 1974; *49*: 298–308.
30. Harrison DG, Bates JN. The nitrovasodilators: New ideas about old drugs. *Circulation* 1993; *87*: 1461–1467.
31. Nifedipine/Metoprolol Trial (HINT) Research Group. Early treatment of unstable angina in the coronary care unit: A randomized, double blind, placebo controlled comparison of recurrent ischaemia in patients treated with nifedipine or metoprolol or both: Report of the Holland Interuniversity Nifedipine/Metoprolol Trial (HINT). *Br Heart J* 1986; *56*: 400–413.
32. Olson HG, Aronow WS. Medical management of stable angina and unstable angina in the elderly with coronary artery disease. In: Aronow WS, Tresch DD, eds. *Clinics in Geriatric Medicine: Coronary Artery Disease in the Elderly*. Philadelphia, PA: WB Saunders, 1996: pp. 121–140.
33. Danahy DT, Burwell DT, Aronow WS et al. Sustained hemodynamic and antianginal effect of high-dose oral isosorbide dinitrate. *Circulation* 1977; *55*: 381–387.
34. Danahy DT, Aronow WS. Hemodynamics and antianginal effects of high dose oral isosorbide dinitrate after chronic use. *Circulation* 1977; *56*: 205–212.
35. No authors listed. Sublingual nitroglycerin powder (GoNitro). *Med Lett Drugs The* 2016; *58*: 156–157.
36. Parker JD, Parker JO. Nitrate therapy for stable angina pectoris. *N Engl J Med* 1998; *337*: 520–531.
37. Elkayam U. Tolerance to organic nitrates: Evidence, mechanisms, clinical relevance and strategies for prevention. *Ann Intern Med* 1991; *114*: 667–677.
38. Needleman P, Johnson EM. Mechanism of tolerance development of organic nitrates. *J Pharmacol Exp Ther* 1973; *84*: 709–715.
39. Munzel T, Giaid A, Kurz S et al. Evidence for enhanced vascular superoxide anion production in nitrate tolerance: A novel mechanism underlying tolerance and cross-tolerance. *J Clin Invest* 1995; *95*: 187–194.
40. Munzel T, Giaid A, Kurz S et al. Evidence for a role of endothelin 1 and protein kinase C in nitroglycerin tolerance. *Proc Natl Acad Sci USA* 1995; *92*: 5244–5248.
41. Lange RL, Reid MS, Tresch DD et al. Nonatheromatous ischemic heart disease following withdrawal from chronic industrial nitroglycerin exposure. *Circulation* 1972: *466*: 666–678.
42. Klock JC. Nonocclusive coronary disease after chronic exposure to nitrate. Evidence for physiologic nitrate dependence. *Am Heart J* 1975; *89*: 510–513.
43. Ravipati G, McClung JA, Aronow WS et al. Type 5 phosphodiesterase inhibitors and cardiovascular disease. *Cardiol in Rev* 2007; *15*: 76–86.
44. Aronow WS, Turbow M, Van Camp S et al. The effect of timolol vs. placebo an angina pectoris. *Circulation* 1980; *61*: 66–69.
45. Frishman WH. Alpha- and beta-adrenergic blocking drugs. In: Frishman WH, Sica DA, eds. *Cardiovascular Pharmacotherapeutics*, 3rd ed. Minneapolis, MN: Cardiotext, 2011: pp. 57–85.
46. Cocco G, Burkart F, Chu D et al. Intrinsic sympathomimetic activity of beta-adreno-receptor blocking agents. *Eur J Clin Pharmacol* 1978; *13*: 1–4.
47. Yusuf S, Peto R, Lewis J et al. Beta blockade during and after myocardial infarction: An overview of the randomized trials. *Prog Cardiovasc Dis* 1985; *27*: 335–371.
48. Westerlund A. Central nervous system side effects with hydrophilic and lipophilic beta blockers. *Eur J Clin Pharmacol* 1985; *28(suppl)*: 73–76.
49. Hjalmarson A, Herlitz J, Waagstein F. Treatment of myocardial infarction with beta blockers in elderly patients. In: Lang E, Sorgel F, Blaha L, eds. *Beta-Blockers in the Elderly*. New York: Springer-Verlag, 1982: pp. 47–55.
50. Lehtonen A. Effect of beta blockers on blood lipid profile. *Am Heart J* 1985; *109*: 1192–1196.
51. Aronow WS, Ahn C, Mercando AD et al. Effect of propranolol versus no antiarrhythmic drug on serum lipids in patients with heart disease and complex ventricular arrhythmias. *Curr Ther Res* 1994; *55*: 1442–1445.
52. Fraker TD Jr, Fihn SD, Gibbons RJ et al. 2007 chronic angina focused update of the ACC/AHA 2002 guidelines for the management of patients with chronic stable angina. A report of the American College of Cardiology/American Heart Association Task Force on Practice Guidelines Writing Group to Develop the Focused Update of the 2002 Guidelines for the Management of Patients With Chronic Stable Angina. *Circulation* 2007; *116*: 2762–2772.
53. Snow V, Barry P, Fihn SD et al. Primary care management of chronic stable angina and asymptomatic suspected or known coronary artery disease: A clinical practice guideline from the American College of Physicians. *Ann Intern Med* 2004; *141*: 562–567.
54. Rosendorff C, Lackland DT, Allison M et al. AHA/ACC/ASH scientific statement. Treatment of hypertension in patients with coronary artery disease: A scientific statement from the American Heart Association, American College of Cardiology, and American Society of Hypertension. *J Am Coll Cardiol* 2015; *65*: 1998–2038.
55. Whelton PK, Carey RM, Aronow WS et al. 2017 ACC/AHA/AAPA/ABC/ACPM/ AGS/APhA/ASH/ ASPC/NMA/ PCNA guideline for the prevention, detection, evaluation and management of high blood pressure in adults. A report of the American College of Cardiology/American Heart Association

Task Force on Clinical Practice Guidelines. *J Am Coll Cardiol* 2018; *71*: e127–e248.
56. Jolicoeur EM, Dunning A, Castelvecchio S et al. Importance of angina in patients with coronary disease, heart failure, and left ventricular systolic dysfunction. Insights from STICH. *J Am Coll Cardiol* 2015; *66*: 2092–2100.
57. Frishman WH, Sica DA. Calcium channel blockers. In: Frishman WH, Sica DA, eds. *Cardiovascular Pharmacotherapeutics*, 3rd ed. Minneapolis, MN: Cardiotext, 2011; pp. 99–120.
58. Psaty MD, Heckbert SR, Koepsell MD et al. The risk of myocardial infarction associated with antihypertensive drug therapies. *JAMA* 1995; *274*: 620–625.
59. Furberg CD, Psaty BM, Meyer JV. Nifedipine: Dose-related increase in mortality in patients with coronary heart disease. *Circulation* 1995; *92*: 1326–1331.
60. Boden WE, Korr KS, Bough KW. Nifedipine-induced hypotension and myocardial ischemia in refractory angina pectoris. *JAMA* 1985; *253*: 1131–1135.
61. The Multicenter Diltiazem Post Infarction Trial Research Group. The effect of diltiazem on mortality and reinfarction after myocardial infarction. *N Engl J Med* 1988; *319*: 385–392.
62. Ryan TJ, Antman EM, Brooks NH et al. 1999 update: ACC/AHA guidelines for the management of patients with acute myocardial infarction: Executive summary and recommendations, a report of the American College of Cardiology/American Heart Association Task Force on Practice Guidelines (Committee on Management of Acute Myocardial Infarction). *Circulation* 1999; *100*: 1016–1030.
63. Antithrombotic Trialists' Collaboration. Collaborative meta-analysis of randomised trials of antiplatelet therapy for prevention of death, myocardial infarction, and stroke in high risk patients. *Br Med J* 2002; *324*: 71–86.
64. Aronow WS, Ahn C. Reduction of coronary events with aspirin in older patients with prior myocardial infarction treated with and without statins. *Heart Dis* 2002; *4*: 159–161.
65. Lerner RG, Frishman WH, Mohan KT. Clopidogrel: A new antiplatelet drug. *Heart Dis* 2000; *2*: 168–173.
66. CAPRIE Steering Committee. A randomised, blinded, trial of clopidogrel versus aspirin in patients at risk of ischaemic events (CAPRIE). *Lancet* 1996; *348*: 1329–1339.
67. Tsuya T, Okada M, Horie H et al. Effect of dipyridamole at the usual oral dose on exercise-induced myocardial ischemia in stable angina pectoris. *Am J Cardiol* 1990; *66*: 275–278.
68. The Heart Outcomes Prevention Evaluation Study Investigators. Effects of an angiotensin converting enzyme inhibitor, ramipril, on cardiovascular events and stroke in high-risk patients. *N Engl J Med* 2000; *342*: 145–153.
69. Miettinen TA, Pyorala K, Olsson AG et al. Cholesterol-lowering therapy in women and elderly patients with myocardial infarction or angina pectoris. Findings from the Scandinavian Simvastatin Survival Study (4S). *Circulation* 1997; *96*: 4211–4218.
70. Lewis SJ, Moye LA, Sacks FM et al. Effect of pravastatin on cardiovascular events in older patients with myocardial infarction and cholesterol levels in the average range. Results of the Cholesterol and Recurrent Events (CARE) Trial. *Ann Intern Med* 1998; *129*: 681–689.
71. The Long-Term Intervention with Pravastatin in Ischaemic Disease (LIPID) Study Group. Prevention of cardiovascular events and death with pravastatin in patients with coronary heart disease and a broad range of initial cholesterol levels. *N Engl J Med* 1998; *339*: 1349–1357.
72. Aronow WS, Ahn C. Incidence of new coronary events in older persons with prior myocardial infarction and serum low-density lipoprotein cholesterol 125 mg/dL treated with statins versus no lipid-lowering drug. *Am J Cardiol* 2002; *89*: 67–69.
73. Heart Protection Study Collaborative Group. MRC/BHF Heart Protection Study of cholesterol lowering with Simvastatin in 20,536 high-risk individuals: A randomised placebo-controlled trial. *Lancet* 2002; *360*: 7–22.
74. LaRosa JC, Grundy SM, Waters DD et al. Intensive lipid lowering with atorvastatin in patients with stable coronary disease. *N Engl J Med* 2005; *352*: 1425–1435.
75. Grundy SM, Cleeman JI, Merz CNB et al. Implications of recent clinical trials for the National Cholesterol Education Program Adult Treatment Panel III guidelines. *Circulation* 2004; *110*: 227–239.
76. Deedwania P, Stone PH, Merz CNB et al. Effects of intensive versus moderate lipid-lowering therapy on myocardial ischemia in older patients with coronary heart disease. Results of the Study Assessing Goals in the Elderly (SAGE). *Circulation* 2007; *115*: 700–707.
77. Stone NJ, Robinson J, Lichtenstein AH et al. 2013 ACC/AHA guideline on the treatment of blood cholesterol to reduce atherosclerotic cardiovascular risk in adults: A report on the American College of Cardiology/American Heart Association Task Force on Practice Guidelines. *J Am Coll Cardiol* 2014; *63*: 2889–2934.
78. Teo KK, Sedlis SP, Boden WE et al. Optimal medical therapy with or without percutaneous coronary intervention in older patients with stable coronary disease: A pre-specified subset analysis of the COURAGE (Clinical Outcomes Utilizing Revascularization and Aggressive druG Evaluation) trial. *J Am Coll Cardiol* 2009; *54*: 1303–1308.

79. Theroux P, Lidon R. Unstable angina: Pathogenesis, diagnosis, and treatment. *Curr Prob Cardiol* 1993; *3*: 162–231.
80. Chesebro JH, Fuster V. Thrombosis in unstable angina. *N Engl J Med* 1992; *327*: 192–194.
81. Rizik D, Healy S, Margulis A et al. A new clinical classification for hospital prognosis of unstable angina pectoris. *Am J Cardiol* 1995; *75*: 993–997.
82. Mark K, Belli G, Ellis S et al. Subacute stent thrombosis: Evolving issues and current concepts. *J Am Coll Cardiol* 1996; *27*: 494–503.
83. Braunwald E, Antman EM, Beasle JW et al. ACC/AHA guidelines for the management of patients with unstable angina and non-ST-segment elevation myocardial infarction: Executive summary and recommendations. A report of the American College of Cardiology/American Heart Association Task Force on Practice Guidelines (Committee on the Management of Patients with Unstable Angina). *J Am Coll Cardiol* 2000; *36*: 970–1056.
84. The Clopidogrel in Unstable Angina to Prevent Recurrent Events Trial Investigators. Effects of clopidogrel in addition to aspirin in patients with acute coronary syndromes without ST-segment elevation. *N Engl J Med* 2001; *345*: 494–502.
85. Wright RS, Anderson JL, Adams CD et al. 2011 ACCF/AHA focused update of the guidelines for the management of patients with unstable angina/non-ST-elevation myocardial infarction (updating the 2007 guideline). A report of the American College of Cardiology Foundation/American Heart Association Task Force on Practice Guidelines. *J Am Coll Cardiol* 2011; *57*: 1920–1959.
86. Wiviott SD, Braunwald E, McCabe CH et al. Prasugrel versus clopidogrel in patients with acute coronary syndromes. *N Engl J Med* 2007; *357*: 2001–2015.
87. Wallentin L, Becker RC, Budaj A et al. Ticagrelor versus clopidogrel in patients with acute coronary syndromes. *N Engl J Med* 2009; *361*: 1045–1057.
88. Antman EM, McCabe CH, Garfinkel EP et al. Enoxaparin prevents death and cardiac ischemic events in unstable angina/non-Q-wave myocardial infarction. Results of the Thrombolysis in Myocardial Infarction (TIMI) 11B Trial. *Circulation* 1999; *100*: 1593–1601.
89. Antman EM, Cohen M, Radley D et al. Assessment of the treatment effect of enoxaparin for unstable angina/non-Q-wave myocardial infarction TIMI IIB-ESSENCE meta-analysis. *Circulation* 1999; *100*: 1602–1608.
90. Goodman SG, Cohen M, Bigonzi F et al. Randomized trial of low molecular weight heparin (enoxaparin) versus unfractionated heparin for unstable coronary artery disease. One-year results of the ESSENCE study. *J Am Coll Cardiol* 2000; *36*: 693–698.
91. Goodman SG, Barr A, Sobtchouk A et al. Low molecular weight heparin decreases rebound ischemia in unstable angina or non-Q-wave myocardial infarction: The Canadian ESSENCE ST Segment Monitoring Substudy. *J Am Coll Cardiol* 2000; *36*: 1507–1513.
92. O'Donoghue ML, Braunwald E, White HD et al. Effect of darapladib on major coronary events after an acute coronary syndrome. The SOLID-TIMI 52 randomized clinical trial. *JAMA* 2014; *312*: 1006–1015.
93. Nicholls SJ, Kastelein JJP, Schwartz GG et al. Varespladib and cardiovascular events in patients with an acute coronary syndrome. The VISTA-16 randomized clinical trial. *JAMA* 2014; *311*: 252–262.
94. Braunwald E, Jones RH, Mark DB et al. Diagnosing and managing unstable angina. *Circulation* 1994; *90*: 613–622.
95. Cannon CP, Weintraub WS, Demopoulo LA et al. Comparison of early invasive and conservative strategies in patients with unstable coronary syndromes treated with the glycoprotein IIb/IIIa inhibitor tirofiban. *N Engl J Med* 2001; *344*: 1879–1887.
96. van Dijk D, Spoor M, Hijman R et al. Cognitive and cardiac outcomes 5 years after off-pump vs on-pump coronary artery bypass graft surgery. *JAMA* 2007; *297*: 701–708.
97. CABRI Trial Participants. First-year results of CABRI (Coronary Angioplasty versus Bypass Revascularization Investigation). *Lancet* 1995; *346*: 1179–1184.
98. King SB III, Lembo NJ, Weintraub WS et al. A randomized trial comparing coronary angioplasty with coronary bypass surgery. *N Engl J Med* 1994; *331*: 1044–1050.
99. Hamm CW, Reimers J, Ischinger T et al. A randomized study of coronary angioplasty compared with bypass surgery in patients with symptomatic multivessel coronary disease. *N Engl J Med* 1994; *331*: 1037–1043.
100. Gallo R, Badiman JJ, Fuster V. Pathobiology of coronary ischemic events: Clinical implications. *Adv Intern Med* 1998; *43*: 203–232.
101. Aronow WS, Ahn C, Mercando AD et al. Decrease in mortality by propranolol in patients with heart disease and complex ventricular arrhythmias is more an anti-ischemic than an antiarrhythmic effect. *Am J Cardiol* 1994; *74*: 613–615.
102. Aronow WS. Medical management of stable angina pectoris. *Compr Ther* 1987; *13*: 54–60.
103. The TIME Investigators. Trial of invasive versus medical therapy in elderly patients with chronic symptomatic coronary-artery disease (TIME): A randomised trial. *Lancet* 2001; *358*: 951–957.
104. Aronow WS. Approach to symptomatic coronary disease in the elderly: TIME to change? *Lancet* 2001; *358*: 945–946.

105. Smith SC Jr, Benjamin EJ, Bonow RO et al. AHA/ACCF secondary prevention and risk reduction therapy for patients with coronary and other atherosclerotic vascular disease: 2011 update. A guideline from the American Heart Association and American College of Cardiology Foundation. Endorsed by the World Heart Federation and the Preventive Cardiovascular Nurses Association. *J Am Coll Cardiol* 2011; *58*: 2432–2446.
106. Willich SN, Lewis M, Lowel H et al. Physical exertion as a trigger of acute myocardial infarction. *N Engl J Med* 1993; *329*: 1684–1690.
107. Frasure-Smith N, Lesperance F, Talajic M. Depression following myocardial infarction. Impact on six-month survival. *JAMA* 1993; *270*: 1819–1825.
108. Aronow WS. Exercise therapy for older persons with cardiovascular disease. *Am J Geriatr Cardiol* 2001; *10*: 245–252.
109. Schuler G, Schlierf G, Wirth A et al. Low-fat diet and regular supervised physical exercise in patients with symptomatic coronary artery disease: Reduction of stress-induced myocardial ischemia. *Circulation* 1988; *77*: 172–181.
110. Frishman WH, Nawarskas JJ, Anderson JR. Ranolazine: A piperazine derivative. In: Frishman WH, Sica DA, eds. *Cardiovascular Pharmacotherapeutics*, 3rd ed. Minneapolis, MN: Cardiotext, 2011: pp. 217–222.
111. Belardinelli L, Antzelevitch C, Fraser H. Inhibition of late (sustained/persistent) sodium current: A potential drug target to reduce intracellular sodium dependent calcium overload and its detrimental effects on cardiomyocyte function. *Eur Heart J* 1994; *9(suppl 1)*: 13–17.
112. Chaitman BR, Skettino SL, Parker JO et al. Anti-ischemic effects and long-term survival during ranolazine monotherapy in patients with chronic severe angina. *J Am Coll Cardiol* 2004; *43*: 1375–1382.
113. Chaitman BR, Pepine CJ, Parker JO et al. Effects of ranolazine with atenolol, amlodipine, or diltiazem on exercise tolerance and angina frequency in patients with severe chronic angina: A randomized controlled trial. *JAMA* 2004; *291*: 309–316.
114. Rousseau MF, Pouleur H, Cocco G et al. Comparative efficacy of ranolazine for chronic angina pectoris. *Am J Cardiol* 2005; *95*: 311–316.
115. Stone PH, Gratsiansky NA, Blokhin A et al. Antianginal efficacy of ranolazine when added to treatment with amlodipine: The ERICA (Efficacy of Ranolazine in Chronic Angina) trial. *J Am Coll Cardiol* 2006; *48*: 566–575.
116. Stone PH, Chaitman BR, Stocke K et al. The anti-ischemic mechanism of action of ranolazine in stable ischemic heart disease. *J Am Coll Cardiol* 2010; *56*: 934–942.
117. Padala SK, Lavelle MP, Sidhu MS et al. Antianginal therapy for stable ischemic heart disease. *J Cardiovasc Pharmacol Ther* 2017; *22(6)*: 499–510.
118. Kloner RA, Chaitman B. Angina and its management. *J Cardiovasc Pharmacol Ther* 2017; *22*: 199–209.
119. Taira N. Nicorandil as a hybrid between nitrates and potassium channel activators. *J Cardiol* 1989; *63*: 18J–24J.
120. Jiang J, Li Y, Zhou Y et al. Oral nicorandil reduces ischemic attacks in patients with stable angina: A prospective, multicenter, open-label, randomized controlled study. *Int J Cardiol* 2016; *224*: 183–187.
121. The IONA Study Group. Effect of nicorandil on coronary events in patients with stable angina: The Impact of Nicorandil in Angina (IONA) randomised trial. *Lancet* 2002; *359*: 1269–1275.
122. DiFrancesco CD, Camm JA. Heart rate lowering by specific and selective I_f current inhibition with ivabradine. A new therapeutic perspective in cardiovascular disease. *Drugs* 2004; *64*: 1757–1765.
123. Borer JS, Fox K, Jaillon P et al. Antianginal and anti-ischemic effects of ivabradine, an I_f inhibitor, in stable angina. A randomized, double-blind, multicentered, placebo-controlled trial. *Circulation* 2003; *107*: 817–823.
124. Fox K, Ford I, Steg G et al. Ivabradine for patients with stable coronary artery disease and left ventricular systolic dysfunction (BEAUTIFUL): A randomised, double-blind, placebo-controlled trial. *Lancet* 2008; *372*: 807–816.
125. Borer JS, Swedberg K, Komjda M et al. Efficacy profile of ivabradine in patients with heart failure plus angina pectoris. *Cardiology* 2017; *136*: 138–144.
126. Mengesha HG, Weldearegawi B, Petrucka P et al. Effect of ivabradine on cardiovascular outcomes in patients with stable angina: Meta-analysis of randomized clinical trials. *BMC Cardiovasc Disord* 2017; *17*: 105.
127. Zarifis J, Kallistratos M, Katsivas A et al. Antianginal efficacy of ivabradine/metoprolol combination in patients with stable angina. *Clin Cardiol* 2016; *39*: 697–702.
128. Amosova E, Andrejev E, Zaderey I et al. Efficacy of ivabradine in combination with beta-blocker versus uptitration of beta-blocker in patients with stable angina. *Cardiovasc Drugs Ther* 2011; *25*: 531–537.
129. Godino C, Colombo A, Margonato A. Ivabradine in patients with coronary artery disease: A rationale for use in addition to and beyond percutaneous coronary intervention. *Clin Drug Investig* 2017; *37*: 105–120.
130. Peng S, Zhao M, Wan J et al. The efficacy of trimetazidine on stable angina pectoris: A meta-analysis of randomized clinical trials. *Int J Cardiol* 2014; *177*: 780–785.
131. Takano H, Komuro I. Cytokines and heart remodeling. In: Leri A, Anversa P, Frishman WH, eds.

Cardiovascular Regeneration and Stem Cell Therapy. Malden, MA: Blackwell Futura, 2007: pp. 139–147.
132. Deedwania PC, Chatterjere K. Current therapeutic options and evolving therapies for chronic stable angina/chronic coronary syndrome. *Johns Hopkins Adv Stud Med* 2006; *6 (9A)*: S827–S836.
133. Frazier OH, Cooley DA, Kadipasaoglu KA et al. Myocardial revascularization with laser: Preliminary findings. *Circulation* 1995; 92(suppl II): II-58–II-65.
134. Donovan CL, Landolfo KP, Lowe JE et al. Improvement in inducible ischemia during dobutamine stress echocardiography after transmyocardial laser revascularization in patients with refractory angina pectoris. *J Am Coll Cardiol* 1997; *30*: 607–612.
135. Lauer B, Junghans U, Stahl F et al. Catheter-based percutaneous myocardial laser revascularization in patients with end-stage coronary artery disease. *J Am Coll Cardiol* 1999; *34*: 1663–1670.
136. Schofield PM, Sharpies LD, Caine N et al. Transmyocardial laser revascularization in patients with refractory angina: A randomised controlled trial. *Lancet* 1999; *353*: 519–524.
137. Oesterle SN, Sanborn TA, Ali N et al. Percutaneous transmyocardial laser revascularisation for severe angina: The PACIFIC randomised trial. *Lancet* 2000; *356*: 1705–1710.
138. Soroff HS, Hui J, Giron F. Current status of external counterpulsation. *Crit Care Clin* 1986; *2*: 277–295.
139. Kumar A, Aronow WS. Use of enhanced counterpulsation in the treatment of refractory angina pectoris and congestive heart failure. *Compr Ther* 2009; *35*: 133–138.
140. Raza A, Steinberg K, Tartaglia J et al. Enhanced external counterpulsation therapy: Past, present, and future. *Cardiol Rev* 2017; *25*: 59–67.
141. Lawson WE, Hui JCK, Soroff HS et al. Efficacy of enhanced external counterpulsation in the treatment of angina pectoris. *Am J Cardiol* 1992; *70*: 859–862.
142. Arora R, Chou T, Jain D et al. External Counter Pulsation (MUST-EECP): Effect of EECP on exercise-induced myocardial ischemia and anginal episodes. *J Am Coll Cardiol* 1999; *33*: 1833–1840.
143. Kumar A, Aronow WS, Vadnerkar A et al. Effect of enhanced external counterpulsation on clinical symptoms, quality of life, 6-minute walking distance, and echocardiographic measurements of left ventricular systolic and diastolic function after 35 days of treatment and at 1-year follow-up in 47 patients with chronic refractory angina pectoris. *Am J Ther* 2009; *16*: 116–118.
144. Aronow WS, Frishman WH. Spinal cord stimulation for the treatment of angina pectoris. *Curr Treat Options in Cardiovasc Med* 2004; *6*: 79–83.
145. Aronow WS, Frishman WH. Spinal cord stimulation for the treatment of angina pectoris. In Frishman WH, Weintraub WI, Micozzi MS, eds. *Complementary and Integrative Therapies for Cardiovascular Disease.* Philadelphia, PA: Elsevier, 2005: pp. 390–395.
146. Banai S, Muvhar SB, Parikh KH et al. Coronary sinus reducer stent for the treatment of chronic refractory angina pectoris. A prospective, open-label, multicenter, feasibility first-in-man study. *J Am Coll Cardiol* 2007; *49*: 1783–1789.
147. Foley MJ, Rajkumar CA, Ahmed-Jushuf F et al. Coronary sinus reducer for the treatment of referactory angina (ORBITA-COSMIC): A randomized, placebo-controlled trial. *Lancet* 2024; *403*: 1543–1553.
148. Virani SS, Newby LK, Arnold SV et al. 2023 AHA/ACC/ACCP/ASPC/NLA/PCNA guideline for the management of patients with chronic coronary artery disease. A Report of the American Heart Association/American College of Cardiology Joint Committee on Clinical Practice Guidelines. *J Am Coll Cardiol* 2023; *82*: 833–955.
149. Soleymani M, Masoudkabir F, Shabani M et al. Updates on pharmacologic management of microvascular angina. *Cardiovasc Ther* 2022; *2022*: 6080258.
150. Nguyen DD, Spertos JA, Alexander KP et al. Health status and clinical outcomes in older adults with chronic coronary disease: The ISCHEMIA trial. *J Am Coll Cardiol* 2023; *81*: 1697–1709.

10

Therapy for acute myocardial infarction

JOSHUA M. STOLKER AND MICHAEL W. RICH

Key points

- Older patients comprise a large, high-risk subgroup of the acute myocardial infarction (MI) population who may derive substantial benefits from appropriately selected therapeutic interventions.
- Older patients are also at increased risk for adverse treatment effects, so therapy must be individualized, balancing the potential benefits and risks, while also considering patient preferences and goals of care.
- Older patients with acute MI tend to have more comorbidities and geriatric syndromes than younger patients, and these coexisting conditions frequently impact clinical presentation, hospital course, selection of and response to therapy, and prognosis.
- As in younger patients, reperfusion therapy, most commonly with percutaneous coronary intervention (PCI), is the mainstay of treatment for ST-elevation MI, but the utility of early angiography and PCI for non-ST-elevation MI is less certain.
- Preventive strategies, including control of risk factors and behavioral interventions, such as regular exercise and healthy diet, hold the key to reducing the burden of acute MI in older adults in the coming decades.

DOI: 10.1201/9781003568933-10

INTRODUCTION

According to the American Heart Association's 2024 statistics on cardiovascular disease, over 800,000 Americans experience an acute myocardial infarction (MI) each year, with an average age 65 years for men and 72 years

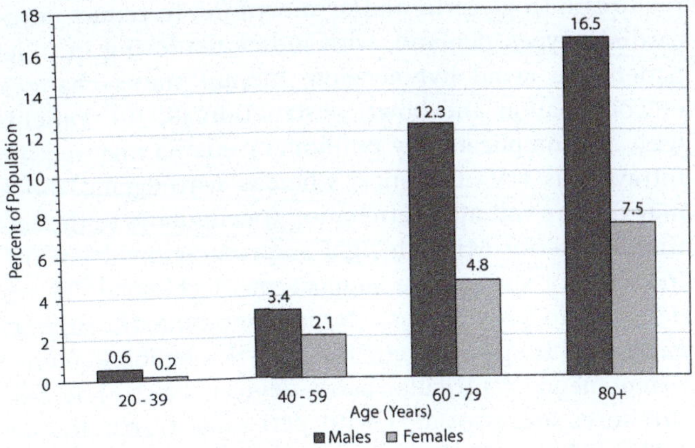

Figure 10.1 Prevalence of myocardial infarction by age and sex, United States. From the National Health and Nutrition Examination Survey (NHANES), 2017–2020. (Adapted from Martin SS et al., 2024 heart disease and stroke statistics: a report of US and global data from the American Heart Association, *Circulation*, 2024.)

for women (1). Much of this burden is disproportionally shouldered by older patients, as epidemiologic studies continue to demonstrate increasing prevalence of MI with increasing age (Figure 10.1). Although mortality rates from acute MI have been declining over the past several decades, heart disease and stroke still claim more lives annually in the US than all forms of cancer and lower respiratory diseases combined. In addition, more than one third of all cardiovascular (CV) deaths occur among patients age 85 and older, despite this subgroup comprising <5% of the overall population. Coronary disease is the primary etiology behind these deaths; in 2021, approximately 40% of CV deaths were a consequence of coronary-related events, while each of the next most common etiologies accounted for <18% of CV deaths (1). Thus, increasing age remains a potent risk factor for MI and fatal coronary events.

Outcomes after MI are consistently worse among older patients, partly due to atypical symptoms and late presentations that shorten the window for optimal intervention. For example, in the National Registry of Myocardial Infarction, chest pain was the presenting symptom in only half of MI patients age 75 and older (2), with higher rates of pulmonary edema at presentation and in-hospital mortality (2, 3). The National Cardiovascular Data Registry (NCDR) database showed that in patients with ST-elevation MI (STEMI), the in-hospital mortality was 4% in patients younger than 75 years, 12% in patients age 75–84 years, and 19% in patients age 85 years and older (4). Thus, acute MI is substantially more common in older adults, and the complication and case fatality rates are disproportionately high. This chapter reviews the treatment of older patients with acute MI, including the management of selected complications.

GUIDING PRINCIPLES

Numerous studies have demonstrated that older patients with acute MI are at increased risk for cardiovascular complications, including atrial fibrillation, heart failure (HF), myocardial rupture, cardiogenic shock, and death (5–7). Noncardiovascular events occur at higher rates in hospitalized older individuals as well, including renal dysfunction, pneumonia, venous thromboembolism, vascular access complications, bleeding events, and rapid debilitation with more prolonged hospital stays and protracted periods of recuperation. The risk of each cardiac complication is two- to fourfold higher in patients over age 65 than in younger patients. Older age thus defines a high-risk subgroup of MI patients who could potentially derive substantial benefit from aggressive therapeutic interventions. On the other hand, older patients are at increased risk for serious adverse consequences arising from fibrinolytic therapy, percutaneous coronary intervention (PCI), and cardiac surgery. In addition, the risk-benefit ratio may be modulated by the presence of comorbid conditions (e.g., diabetes, renal insufficiency, dementia), and choosing specific therapies may be further affected by social considerations and patient preferences. Thus, some older individuals prefer to focus on limiting morbidity and improving *quality* of life, even if it means foregoing more intensive therapies designed to increase *quantity* of life. In one large survey of cardiovascular patients, older individuals tended to be more concerned about the risk of experiencing stroke or MI rather than avoiding death, whereas younger subjects were more concerned about mortality risk (8). Therefore, the potential benefits and risks of each intervention must be carefully considered on an individualized basis.

While older MI patients clearly represent a high-risk subgroup, it is important to recognize that they also comprise an extremely heterogeneous subgroup, and this heterogeneity has important therapeutic implications. For example, an 85-year-old patient presenting with a large anterior MI complicated by HF and hypotension has an expected mortality of over 50%. As a result, the potential benefit to be derived from maximally aggressive therapy (e.g., immediate catheterization and PCI, with possible need for inotropic or mechanical support to stabilize cardiogenic shock) would be large, thereby justifying a moderate increase in procedural risk. In contrast, an 85-year-old individual presenting with a small inferior MI of more than 12 hours' duration who is hemodynamically stable and free of chest pain has a relatively favorable prognosis with contemporary medical therapies, and the risks associated with thrombolysis or PCI may not be justified. Accordingly, in considering the interventions described in this chapter, the clinician should keep in mind that the "sickest" patients often have the most to gain from aggressive treatment, while those with a more favorable prognosis often respond satisfactorily to conservative management—particularly when the risks of the more aggressive approach are elevated.

GENERAL APPROACH AT HOSPITAL PRESENTATION

As in younger patients, the early management of older patients with acute MI should include measures designed to relieve the patient's discomfort and to evaluate and treat any hemodynamic disturbances such as HF or hypotension (Table 10.1). Empiric administration of supplemental oxygen is appropriate if the baseline arterial saturation is less than 92%. Symptom relief often requires nitroglycerin and/or morphine to reduce myocardial oxygen demand, with judicious dosing in older patients to avoid hypotension, mental status changes, or constipation and bowel obstruction (9, 10). Patients with MI complicated by pulmonary edema may require intravenous (IV) diuretics, whereas cardiogenic shock may require volume resuscitation (particularly in the setting of inferior MI with right ventricular involvement), inotropic or vasopressor support, or mechanical devices designed to provide short-term hemodynamic support (transvenous pacemaker, intra-aortic balloon pump, percutaneous ventricular assist device). Electrolyte disturbances are associated with peri-infarct arrhythmias and should be corrected immediately. Secondary causes

Table 10.1 Early management of older patients with acute myocardial infarction

Symptom or sign	Agent	Dose	Comment
Chest pain or anginal equivalent	Oxygen	2–5 L/min	Not helpful if O_2 saturation ≥92%
	Morphine	2–4 mg IV, q 5–15 min	Watch for respiratory depression or hypotension
	Nitroglycerin	0.4 mg sublingually; 0.5–2" transdermally; 10–200 µg/min IV infusion	Watch for hypotension, especially in inferior myocardial infarction
	Metoprolol or atenolol	12.5–25 mg PO initially, only consider 2.5–5 mg IV in select patients with adequate hemodynamics	Watch for bradycardia, hypotension, heart block, bronchospasm, worsening HF
HF complicating acute MI	Oxygen	As needed to maintain arterial saturation ≥92%	
	Furosemide	20–80 mg IV	Watch for hypotension
	Bumetanide	0.5–2 mg IV	Watch for hypotension
	Nitroglycerin	0.5–2 inches transdermally; 10–200 µg/min IV	Avoid hypotension
	Echocardiography	N/A	For refractory or unexplained pulmonary edema or hypotension out of proportion to the MI
Hypotension	IV fluids	As needed to maintain adequate perfusion	Watch for worsening HF
	Dobutamine	2.5–10 µg/kg/min	Watch for arrhythmias or worsening hypotension; may aggravate ischemia
	Dopamine	2–40 µg/kg/min	May worsen ischemia
	Norepinephrine	0.5–30 mg/min	May worsen ischemia
	Transvenous pacemaker	N/A	For profound bradycardia
	Intra-aortic balloon pump or percutaneous ventricular assist device	Usually placed in cardiac cath lab	As adjunct to emergent coronary revascularization for patients with cardiogenic shock

Abbreviations: HF, heart failure; IV, intravenous; MI, myocardial infarction; PO, per os (oral administration).

of acute MI should be identified and treated, including severe hypertension, arrhythmias, thyroid dysfunction, or other medical sources of hyperadrenergic tone and increased myocardial oxygen demand (e.g., infections, severe anemia, drug or medication effects). In patients with persistent or unexplained pulmonary edema or hypotension, urgent echocardiography is warranted to assess biventricular function and evaluate for mechanical complications of acute MI.

Aside from initial symptom relief and clinical stabilization, and in the absence of an apparent secondary cause of MI, patients with acute MI are generally treated with medications directed at minimizing coronary thrombosis and obstruction to blood flow (i.e., antiplatelet, antithrombotic, and/or fibrinolytic therapies, as discussed later). Disease-modifying agents should be added as well, with careful attention to side effect profiles and potential adverse events. For example, ß-blockers are indicated to reduce left ventricular wall stress and overall ischemic and arrhythmic burden, with several studies demonstrating benefit during management of MI (9, 10). However, starting with lower doses and using oral (instead of IV) dosing helps reduce the risk of adverse effects, including worsening bradycardia, heart block, hypotension, or heart failure. Similarly, angiotensin-converting enzyme inhibitors (ACEIs) and angiotensin II receptor blockers (ARBs) should not be administered until blood pressure and renal function have stabilized. Patients with STEMI or cardiogenic shock generally require urgent triage for coronary revascularization (i.e., fibrinolytic therapy or primary PCI). However, the majority of older MI patients present with non-ST-elevation MI (NSTEMI). While most younger patients with NSTEMI undergo early invasive management including cardiac catheterization and revascularization as indicated, the benefits and risks of an early invasive strategy must be evaluated on an individual basis in older patients with NSTEMI. Elicitation of patient preferences is critical to clinical decision-making for frail older individuals, particularly those with substantial medical comorbidities or anticipated difficulty recovering from invasive procedures.

ANTIPLATELET AGENTS

Aspirin

Aspirin is of proven benefit in patients with either unstable angina or acute MI, and should be considered standard therapy in all patients presenting with acute coronary syndromes (ACS) in the absence of life-threatening allergy or severe bleeding. After several smaller studies showed benefit, definitive evidence supporting the use of aspirin for acute MI came from the second International Study of Infarct Survival (ISIS-2) (11). In this study, 17,187 patients with suspected MI were randomized to receive either aspirin 162.5 mg or placebo, and either streptokinase 1.5 million units or placebo. Overall, patients receiving aspirin experienced a 23% reduction in the risk of vascular death within 35 days of hospitalization, and this effect was independent of whether or not the patient received streptokinase. In 3411 patients over 70 years of age, aspirin was associated with a 21% reduction in vascular deaths (17.6% vs. 22.3%; $p < 0.01$), which was similar to the benefit seen in the overall trial population. Of note, the benefit of aspirin increased with increasing age, from 1% absolute reduction in vascular death for patients under age 60 years to 4.7% absolute reduction for patients age 70 and older.

With respect to aspirin dosage, the minimum loading dose in patients with acute MI is 160 mg, and doses in excess of 325 mg provide no additional benefit. Importantly, the initial dose of aspirin should be administered as soon as possible after presentation, and the non-enteric-coated form should be used to ensure rapid absorption. When possible, the first dose should be chewed rather than swallowed. Following MI, aspirin has traditionally been considered a long-term medication to be continued indefinitely at a dose of 75 to 325 mg daily or every other day (12, 13). However, newer studies have questioned the need for continued aspirin beyond the first month in ACS patients receiving PCI and ticagrelor, as ischemic benefits were similar but bleeding risks were reduced with earlier aspirin termination (14). This is also reflected in contemporary guidelines that focus on minimizing bleeding when possible (15).

Platelet $P2Y_{12}$ inhibitors

Although shorter durations of therapy have been studied among patients undergoing PCI for stable coronary artery disease, most patients with acute MI should be treated for at least 12 months with an inhibitor of the platelet $P2Y_{12}$ receptor—a critical component of platelet activation. This 12-month recommendation is based on findings from several large randomized clinical trials evaluating clopidogrel, prasugrel, and ticagrelor in patients with ACS, with some studies suggesting even longer therapy for patients at low risk of bleeding.

Thienopyridines

Clopidogrel and prasugrel are thienopyridine derivatives that inhibit platelet aggregation more effectively than aspirin by irreversibly binding the adenosine diphosphate (ADP) binding site on the platelet $P2Y_{12}$ receptor. Both thienopyridines require an oral loading dose at the time of ACS diagnosis, but prasugrel should only be considered for carefully selected MI patients undergoing PCI. In the landmark Clopidogrel in Unstable Angina to Prevent Recurrent Events (CURE) trial, the combination of clopidogrel plus aspirin reduced the risk of cardiovascular death, MI, or stroke by about 20% compared with aspirin alone during the 12-month period following hospitalization for unstable angina or MI (16). This benefit was driven by reductions in MI and recurrent angina, and absolute benefits were similar for patients younger or older than age 65.

The combination of aspirin and clopidogrel remained the standard of care after MI for many years, but in 2007 the combination of aspirin plus prasugrel was shown to be superior to aspirin plus clopidogrel among MI patients undergoing PCI in the TRial to assess Improvement in Therapeutic Outcomes by optimizing platelet inhibitioN (TRITON) (17). In this trial of 13,608 patients, median age was 61 years, and prasugrel reduced the primary composite endpoint of cardiovascular death, MI, or stroke more effectively than clopidogrel during 1-year follow-up (9.9% vs. 12.1%). However, life-threatening bleeding was significantly increased from 0.9% with clopidogrel to 1.4% with prasugrel, and among patients with a history of stroke or transient ischemic attack, intracranial hemorrhage increased from 0% on clopidogrel to 2.3% on prasugrel. Furthermore, the subgroup of patients age 75 years and older had similar rates of the primary composite endpoint with prasugrel (16.1%) or clopidogrel (16.0%), with higher rates of bleeding on prasugrel, and similar trends were noted in the subgroup of patients with body weight less than 60 kg (17). Indeed, among the subgroup of MI patients requiring coronary artery bypass graft (CABG) surgery, bleeding was 8.2 times higher with prasugrel ($p = 0.003$). Of note, prasugrel has not shown benefit over clopidogrel in ACS patients treated medically (i.e., without PCI) (18).

Based on these findings, the US Food and Drug Administration (FDA) approved prasugrel for treating patients with acute MI undergoing PCI, but with a boxed warning that prasugrel should not be used in patients with a prior stroke or transient ischemic attack, in patients with active pathological bleeding, or in patients with an urgent need for surgery, including CABG. Guidelines from the American College of Cardiology and American Heart Association also recommend against the use of prasugrel in patients age 75 years and older, in patients weighing less than 60 kg, and in patients at high risk for bleeding or requiring systemic anticoagulation therapy for other clinical indications (19). In addition, thienopyridines are associated with a substantially increased risk for perioperative bleeding. Therefore, in the absence of an emergency indication for surgery, clopidogrel should be discontinued 5 days prior to CABG or other surgery, while prasugrel should be discontinued 7 days before surgery (15, 19).

Ticagrelor

Shortly after prasugrel became available, a new drug class was introduced to the field of ACS management. Ticagrelor is a cyclopentyltriazolopyrimidine (CPTP) that reversibly binds at a different location on the platelet's $P2Y_{12}$ receptor from the ADP binding site, thus avoiding the irreversible platelet inactivation observed with the thienopyridines and potentially reducing some of the bleeding concerns with prasugrel. In the PLATelet inhibition and patient Outcomes (PLATO) trial, 18,624 patients with ACS were randomized to aspirin plus either ticagrelor or clopidogrel for 12 months, irrespective of the treatment approach (medical management, PCI, or CABG) (20). Like clopidogrel and prasugrel, ticagrelor was studied with an initial loading dose (180 mg), resulting in nearly twice the inhibition of platelet aggregation as clopidogrel in mechanistic studies of patients with stable coronary disease (21). In PLATO, the primary composite endpoint of cardiovascular death, MI, or stroke was significantly lower with ticagrelor than with clopidogrel (9.8% vs. 11.7%), a relative risk reduction of 16% and an absolute risk decrease of 1.9% (20). Unlike prasugrel, which only reduced recurrent MI in TRITON, ticagrelor reduced both MI and cardiovascular death in PLATO, with no significant difference in major bleeding between groups. About half of the benefit occurred in the first 30 days, with continued accrual of benefit during the subsequent 11 months after the acute coronary event. Findings were similar among patients treated medically versus PCI versus CABG, although the benefit was more pronounced in subgroups of patients with STEMI and NSTEMI (vs. the 15% of PLATO patients with unstable angina), and the benefit was somewhat attenuated among the 15% of trial participants over age 75 years (22). Of note, subgroup analysis of patients treated medically or with PCI (i.e., excluding the CABG subgroup) had higher rates of major bleeding on ticagrelor (4.5%) than on clopidogrel (3.8%) ($p = 0.03$), but there was no signal for increased bleeding among the subgroups previously noted to be at high risk with prasugrel (prior stroke or transient ischemic attack, age >75 years, weight <60 kg). Higher rates of dyspnea were noted with ticagrelor (14% vs. 8%), thought to be related to an adenosine-mediated effect of the drug, and nearly all of the benefit was noted in patients treated with lower-dose aspirin (≤100 mg). With its shorter duration of effect on platelets, ticagrelor only needs to be held for 3 days prior to elective CABG or other major surgery (15, 19).

A few years after the publication of PLATO, the Prevention of Cardiovascular Events in Patients with Prior Heart Attack Using Ticagrelor Compared to Placebo on a Background of Aspirin (PEGASUS-TIMI 54) clinical trial evaluated the use of ticagrelor during longer-term follow-up after MI (23). In this trial, 21,162 patients age 50 and older with prior MI (1–3 years earlier) and at least one additional risk factor for thrombotic cardiovascular events (including age ≥65 years) were randomized to aspirin plus either ticagrelor or placebo. At approximately 3-year median follow-up, the composite primary endpoint of cardiovascular death, MI, or stroke was reduced from 9.0% to 7.8%, a relative risk reduction of 16%, driven by reductions in all three components of the composite endpoint. Findings were similar among subgroups of patients age 50–64 years, 65–75 years, and >75 years, and outcomes were nearly identical between the 60 mg and 90 mg doses of twice-daily ticagrelor. However, since the comparator arm was placebo (whereas clopidogrel was the comparator in PLATO), there was a substantial increase in major bleeding with ticagrelor (0.8% with placebo vs. 1.7% with ticagrelor), and combined rates of major plus minor bleeding were increased from 1.0% to 2.4%. As reported in PLATO, higher rates of dyspnea were noted with ticagrelor in the PEGASUS trial.

Based on these findings, plus results from smaller studies and subgroup analyses evaluating longer-term antiplatelet therapy (24, 25), current guidelines recommend dual antiplatelet therapy (aspirin plus thienopyridine or ticagrelor) for the first 1 to 3 months after MI, with a preference for ticagrelor in eligible patients (15, 19). Then, in the absence of stent thrombosis or other high-risk conditions for recurrent thrombosis, aspirin may be held in favor of single-agent $P2Y_{12}$ therapy for the remainder of the 12-month period after MI. After 1 year, patients at lower risk of bleeding may be considered for longer-term clopidogrel or reduced-dose (60 mg) ticagrelor for several more years after MI, while older patients at higher risk of bleeding could be switched back to low-dose aspirin alone.

Parenteral antiplatelet agents

One concern with any of the oral antiplatelet agents is reduced gastrointestinal absorption during ACS and the potential for higher rates of stent thrombosis or other thrombotic complications, particularly among patients receiving opioids for treatment of pain (26). In addition, patients loaded with oral antiplatelet therapy experience higher rates of perioperative bleeding if urgent CABG is needed after cardiac catheterization, so many physicians avoid loading oral antiplatelet therapy until after coronary angiography has been performed. Cangrelor is an intravenous $P2Y_{12}$ inhibitor that reduced periprocedural complications during PCI (particularly stent thrombosis) when compared with clopidogrel in a clinical trial (27), with similar benefits in patients <75 and >75 years of age. This drug has not been compared to the newer, more potent oral antiplatelet agents (prasugrel, ticagrelor), and its higher cost has likely contributed to its relatively restricted use in the United States.

Older IV options for platelet inhibition include the glycoprotein (GP) IIb/IIIa inhibitors, which block the final common pathway leading to platelet aggregation. Although all three of these medications—abciximab, eptifibatide, and tirofiban—have been shown to improve outcomes in patients with ACS, most of the studies primarily evaluated NSTEMI (28) and were performed in the era before early loading of oral $P2Y_{12}$ inhibitor therapy. Furthermore, the benefits of these drugs are attenuated in patients older than 75–80 years of age (29, 30). Most notably, GP IIb/IIIa inhibitors are associated with an increased risk for major bleeding (30), with particularly high risk for those over age 75 years (31). As a result, GP IIb/IIIa inhibitors should be limited to very select older individuals with high thrombosis risk and low bleeding risk, generally as an adjunct to PCI in the catheterization laboratory, as reflected in contemporary guidelines (3, 7, 9, 10, 15, 19).

ANTITHROMBOTIC AGENTS

Antithrombotic therapy has been considered the standard of care during ACS for many decades. However, the original studies of unfractionated heparin from the 1970s and 1980s were performed with different medical and procedural techniques, and with less statistical rigor, when compared with contemporary clinical trials. Nonetheless, heparin and its successor agents have remained critical adjunctive therapies for the early management of patients with acute MI.

Unfractionated heparin

When acute MI is diagnosed, the recommended dose of heparin is 60 units/kg bolus (maximum 4000 units), followed by an infusion of 12 units/kg/hr (maximum 1000 units/hr), adjusted for an activated partial thromboplastin time (aPTT) between 60 and 80 seconds (15). Prior to the coronary reperfusion era, heparin was continued for at least 48 hours after MI diagnosis, and this approach continues to be recommended for patients treated conservatively (i.e., without thrombolysis, PCI, or CABG). Patients with large anterior MIs, atrial fibrillation, or severe left ventricular dysfunction are at increased risk for mural thrombus formation and embolization, so these subgroups of MI patients may benefit from IV heparin even after coronary revascularization (9, 10, 19). Patients who experience recurrent ischemia during the first few days after MI are at increased risk for infarct extension, and IV heparin is recommended for these individuals as well. Routine heparin therapy in MI patients without these high-risk features remains unproven. As discussed elsewhere, patients with atrial fibrillation or flutter, or those with deep venous thrombosis or pulmonary embolism, should be transitioned from heparin or a related parenteral agent (e.g., enoxaparin) to warfarin or a direct oral anticoagulant (dabigatran, rivaroxaban, apixaban, edoxaban), as indicated for longer-term therapy. As with patients hospitalized for other acute illnesses, older patients are at high risk for venous thromboembolism during MI hospitalization, and lower-dose subcutaneous heparin is also used to reduce the risk of thromboembolic complications in MI patients.

Low-molecular-weight heparin

Compared with unfractionated heparin, low-molecular-weight heparins (LMWHs) offer several advantages: once or twice daily subcutaneous dosing, no need to monitor aPTTs, and fewer side effects (especially thrombocytopenia, which is common during prolonged IV heparin infusion). Enoxaparin and dalteparin are the most commonly used LMWH products in the United States. In a meta-analysis of 14 trials involving 25,280 patients with STEMI receiving fibrinolytic therapy and aspirin, LMWH reduced the risk of reinfarction by 28% and death by 10%, but increased the risk of major bleeding and intracranial bleeding, when compared with placebo (32). When compared with unfractionated heparin, LMWH reduced the risk of reinfarction by 45%, increased the risk of minor bleeding, and had no effect on mortality or major bleeding. Subgroup analyses by age were not reported in this study, and since all patients in these trials were treated with a fibrinolytic agent, the findings may not be applicable to patients receiving primary PCI, CABG, or no reperfusion therapy. Furthermore, careful attention to dosing of LMWH is required in older patients with decreased renal function, since these drugs require renal clearance, and excess dosing increases major bleeding (33). In general, unfractionated heparin is recommended in preference to LMWH in patients with STEMI undergoing reperfusion therapy with a fibrinolytic agent (16). In other ACS patients for whom antithrombotic therapy is warranted, either unfractionated heparin or LMWH may be used.

Bivalirudin

Bivalirudin is an intravenous direct thrombin inhibitor with a rapid onset and short half-life that has demonstrated clinical benefits in patients with ACS undergoing PCI. For example, in the Harmonizing Outcomes with Revascularization and Stents in Acute Myocardial Infarction (HORIZONS-AMI) trial of 3602 patients undergoing primary PCI for STEMI (mean age 60 years), bivalirudin reduced the rate of net adverse clinical events by 17% at 1-year follow-up (absolute event rates 15.6% vs. 18.3%, $p = 0.022$) (34). However, the comparator arm involved patients treated with heparin plus a GP IIb/IIIa inhibitor, and the benefit was almost exclusively driven by a lower rate of major bleeding in the bivalirudin group (5.8% vs. 9.2%, $p < 0.0001$), while the rate of major adverse cardiovascular events was identical (11.9% in both groups). Subsequent trials of NSTEMI and other patient populations have reported similar risk for ischemic events and generally less bleeding with bivalirudin when compared with unfractionated heparin (11). Like the LMWHs, bivalirudin is renally cleared, so dosing must be carefully adjusted in patients with advanced age, low body weight, or lower creatinine clearance. Furthermore, more contemporary data among patients receiving potent oral antiplatelet agents, minimal GP IIb/IIa inhibitor use, and greater use of radial artery access for cardiac catheterization have not shown benefit for bivalirudin over unfractionated heparin (35). Current guidelines consider bivalirudin a reasonable alternative to unfractionated heparin during PCI, particularly among patients with adequate renal function who are at high risk for bleeding, or those with thrombocytopenia or other relative contraindications to unfractionated heparin (9, 10, 19).

Warfarin

Long-term anticoagulation with warfarin reduces the risk of reinfarction and cardiac death in post-MI patients, including older adults, and warfarin therapy (with or without aspirin) is superior to aspirin alone (36, 37). However, these studies were performed prior to the contemporary revascularization era and prior to the routine use of oral antiplatelet therapy. Most importantly, the addition of warfarin to aspirin substantially increases the risk of bleeding, and this risk is greatest in older patients. Current guidelines recommend warfarin in the post-MI setting for patients with other noncoronary indications for chronic systemic anticoagulation therapy, including atrial fibrillation, mechanical prosthetic heart valves, or active thromboembolic disease (9, 10). Warfarin anticoagulation for 3 months is also recommended for patients with a large anterior MI, apical akinesis, or a left ventricular mural thrombus following acute MI, although the incidence of systemic thromboembolic events in patients with MI has declined significantly over time (38).

Direct oral anticoagulants

Several studies have examined the utility of the direct oral anticoagulants (DOACs) in patients with acute or chronic coronary artery disease. The Anti-Xa Therapy to Lower Cardiovascular Events in Addition to Standard Therapy in Subjects with Acute Coronary Syndrome (ATLAS ACS 2–TIMI 51) trial randomized 15,526 patients with recent ACS to low-dose rivaroxaban (2.5 or 5 mg twice daily) or placebo in addition to standard therapy (39). Despite finding a 16% relative reduction in risk of the composite endpoint of cardiovascular death, MI, or stroke, bleeding was substantially more frequent with either dose of rivaroxaban, including both major bleeding and intracranial bleeding. Subsequently, a trial of 27,395 patients with stable vascular disease showed a beneficial effect on the primary composite outcome but increased major bleeding when adding rivaroxaban 2.5 mg twice daily to aspirin compared to aspirin alone (40). Another study evaluating apixaban 5 mg twice daily among patients with recent ACS was prematurely terminated due to increased bleeding without evidence of a reduction in ischemic events (41). Based on available evidence, oral anticoagulation among geriatric patients with recent MI should only be considered for those at high risk of ischemic events, low bleeding risk, a clear indication for systemic anticoagulation, and with consideration of early reduction of antiplatelet therapies (see section "General Bleeding Considerations").

Fondaparinux

To mitigate some of the bleeding seen with LMWH and unfractionated heparin in the acute phase of MI management, fondaparinux—a subcutaneous factor Xa inhibitor administered daily—has been compared to LMWH in patients with ACS (42). Ischemic events were similar between the two drugs, but bleeding was reduced with fondaparinux; findings were similar among patients ≥65 years versus those <65 years of age. However, catheter thrombosis was more common during PCI in patients treated with fondaparinux, and this was also noted in another trial of patients with STEMI (43). As a result, guidelines have recommended fondaparinux as a reasonable antithrombotic agent in patients managed medically for STEMI or NSTEMI, but this drug should not be used as the sole anticoagulant for those proceeding to PCI (9, 10, 15).

GENERAL BLEEDING CONSIDERATIONS

During hospitalization for MI, choosing and carefully dosing anticoagulation therapy is critical in older patients, particularly given the potential need for multiple antithrombotic therapies (aspirin, oral $P2Y_{12}$ inhibitor, possible intravenous platelet inhibitors, possible fibrinolytic agent for STEMI, anticoagulants as indicated). Although there is no precise method to quantify the risk of bleeding and accurately assess the risk-benefit ratio of using multiple drugs in an individual patient, it is worth noting that bleeding risk consistently increases with age—both from measurable sources (decreasing creatinine clearance, lower body weight, polypharmacy for multiple medical comorbidities) and from sources that are often difficult to reliably quantify (delayed clinical presentation, alterations in hemostatic and other physiologic processes, frailty, etc.). In one study evaluating the effects of LMWH and a GP IIb/IIIa inhibitor in patients receiving fibrinolytic therapy for acute MI, the GP IIb/IIIa inhibitor was associated with worse clinical outcomes among patients >75 years old, largely due to the marked increase in bleeding complications in this age group (44). In addition, advanced age has been associated with increased risk for excessive dosing and major bleeding complications in ACS patients treated with heparin, LMWH, or GP IIb/IIIa inhibitors (45). Thus, the benefits of aggressive antithrombotic therapy in reducing recurrent ischemic events must be carefully balanced against the risk of serious bleeding complications, particularly in very old patients.

Despite concerns about potential pharmacologic interactions between clopidogrel and proton pump inhibitors (PPIs), especially omeprazole, PPIs are commonly used to mitigate the risk of gastrointestinal bleeding (GIB) among patients at higher risk of gastric ulcers and upper GIB (9). In a randomized trial, patients receiving omeprazole in combination with dual antiplatelet therapy had similar rates of cardiovascular outcomes as those without PPI therapy, but with significantly lower rates of GIB and other gastrointestinal symptoms such as dyspepsia (46, 47). Findings were similar regardless of whether patients were receiving higher- or lower-dose aspirin therapy (48).

Another bleeding concern involves the growing number of patients with coronary disease who have chronic indications for systemic anticoagulation therapy. As discussed in other chapters of this book, life expectancy in the developed world has increased over time, resulting in an epidemic of older patients with atrial fibrillation, venous thromboembolism, or other conditions requiring chronic systemic anticoagulation therapy. When these individuals also require antiplatelet therapy after MI or PCI, the dilemma of "triple therapy" (aspirin plus $P2Y_{12}$ inhibitor plus anticoagulation) and associated increased bleeding risk is a clinical challenge, particularly in older patients.

In one observational study, nearly 5000 older patients with atrial fibrillation and acute MI experienced higher rates of major bleeding with triple therapy compared to dual therapy (i.e., removing the aspirin), with no difference in ischemic events between the groups (49). Randomized trial data have shown similar findings, with no difference in ischemic events but fewer bleeding events during the first year after PCI among patients receiving systemic anticoagulation and clopidogrel without aspirin, compared to those who received triple therapy (50). In some cases, bare metal stents may be used during PCI among individuals at higher risk of bleeding (51, 52) to shorten exposure to triple therapy, despite the higher risk of restenosis with bare metal stents. Overall, this important subgroup of patients with acute MI requiring anticoagulation remains challenging for clinicians, and ultimately the treatment plan must be individualized according to the thrombosis and bleeding risks of each patient.

β-BLOCKADE

Most of the major trials evaluating β-blockers for the treatment of acute MI were conducted prior to the reperfusion era. However, since some older patients with acute MI do not receive reperfusion therapy, the results of these earlier trials remain relevant to these patients. Of note, in pooled analyses of atenolol and metoprolol studies from the 1980s and 1990s, early IV β-blockade in patients with suspected MI reduced mortality by 23% in older patients ($p = 0.005$), but by only 5% in younger patients (not statistically significant) (53). These data clearly indicate that older patients, who are at higher risk for adverse outcomes, derive proportionately greater benefit from early β-blocker therapy than younger patients. As a result, β-blockers should not be withheld on the basis of age alone.

The value of IV β-blockade in combination with fibrinolytic therapy was assessed in the Thrombolysis In Myocardial Infarction (TIMI)-II trial (54, 55). In this study, 1434 patients with acute MI were treated with alteplase and then randomized to receive IV metoprolol or placebo. Although there was no difference in hospital or 6-week mortality, patients receiving metoprolol experienced significantly fewer nonfatal ischemic events during follow-up. Subsequently, the impact of early β-blocker therapy was examined in 17,809 patients with STEMI enrolled in a large German registry (56), with much greater utilization of PCI than in the previous β-blocker trials. Despite more contemporary therapies and extensive multivariable adjustment for baseline characteristics, early β-blocker treatment was associated with 30% lower hospital mortality, with the greatest benefit in high-risk patients, including those over age 65. In another large multicenter registry, 55% of 306 patients with sustained ventricular tachycardia or ventricular fibrillation and HF were treated with intravenous or oral β-blockers in the first 24 hours (57), and the use of β-blockers was associated with markedly reduced in-hospital mortality (72% relative risk reduction, $p = 0.013$) without worsening HF.

Tempering these favorable results, findings from the Clopidogrel and Metoprolol in Myocardial Infarction Trial (COMMIT) have raised questions about the value of routine IV β-blockers for acute MI during the reperfusion era (58). In 45,852 patients with acute MI in China (93% of whom had ST-elevation or left bundle branch block), IV metoprolol did not reduce the risk of death, reinfarction, or cardiac arrest, but the risk of cardiogenic shock was increased by 30% in patients randomized to metoprolol. Among 11,934 patients age 70 years or older enrolled in the trial, hospital mortality was 13.6% with metoprolol compared with 13.3% in the placebo group.

Given the higher risk of hypotension, bradycardia, and shock among MI patients with increasing age, plus baseline abnormalities of the electrical conducting system among older patients, careful dosing and titration of these drugs to minimize adverse events is imperative during the initial stages of acute MI. Current guidelines recommend prompt administration of an oral β-blocker to all patients with acute MI in the absence of contraindications (9, 15). Intravenous β-blocker therapy may be considered in stable patients with tachycardia and hypertension who have no contraindication to its use.

In contrast, the long-term use of oral β-blockers for secondary prevention following MI has been extensively investigated, again demonstrating reductions in mortality and reinfarction during long-term therapy, and again with similar or greater benefit in older patients (53). Similar findings were noted with carvedilol among patients with left ventricular ejection fraction ≤40% following acute MI, including a 23% reduction in mortality relative to placebo (59). In addition, observational studies indicate that the survival benefits of β-blockers following MI extend to patients over 75 years of age (60–62). In one study, 2-year mortality rates in patients prescribed β-blockers were 50% lower among patients 65–74 years of age, 44% lower in patients ages 75–84, and 28% lower in patients over age 85, even after multivariable adjustment for baseline patient characteristics (63).

Based on these findings, oral β-blockers are recommended for all patients following acute MI in the absence of contraindications (9, 15), with careful titration for patients with cardiac electrical system disease or borderline hemodynamics (lower blood pressure or heart rate). The benefits of these drugs appear to extend for at least 3 years after the index MI event. In very old patients, it is often advisable to reduce dosages or delay upward titration until tolerance of the lower doses has been verified. Propranolol, metoprolol, timolol, and carvedilol have all been approved for long-term use following MI. Older patients may require lower doses to avoid adverse effects, and there are data suggesting that lower doses may be as effective as higher ones for reducing mortality in older patients (63). Contraindications to β-blockers include significant bradycardia, borderline blood pressure, marked first-degree or higher levels of atrioventricular block, decompensated HF, active wheezing, or severe bronchospastic pulmonary disease. Compensated HF and chronic lung disease without bronchospasm are not contraindications to β-blocker therapy.

BLOCKADE OF THE RENIN–ANGIOTENSIN–ALDOSTERONE SYSTEM

Angiotensin-converting enzyme inhibitors

Early administration of an ACEI to acute MI patients has been evaluated in several large trials. Although worse outcomes were seen with IV enalapril (64), the third Gruppo Italiano per lo Studio della Sopravvivenza nell'Infarto Miocardico (GISSI-3) and ISIS-4 trials reported small but statistically significant reductions in mortality in patients receiving oral captopril or lisinopril within 24 hours of MI onset (65, 66). In addition, patients 70 years or older treated with lisinopril in GISSI-3 experienced a 14% reduction in the combined endpoint of death or severe left ventricular dysfunction at 6-month follow-up ($p = 0.01$) (67). The Survival of Myocardial Infarction Long-term Evaluation (SMILE) investigators randomized 1556 patients with anterior MI who were not candidates for fibrinolytic therapy to either zofenopril or placebo within the first 24 hours after symptom onset (68). The incidence of death or severe HF at 6-week follow-up was reduced 34% by zofenopril, and this benefit was maintained for 1 year. Moreover, the absolute benefit was threefold greater in individuals over 65 years of age compared with younger patients.

However, the applicability of the above findings to the general MI population is unclear, since the small benefit seen in the largest trials (absolute mortality reduction

<1%) (66, 67) may reflect a larger benefit in some patients (e.g., those with anterior MI or significant left ventricular dysfunction), but no benefit or even harm in other subgroups. At the present time, early administration of an oral ACEI is optional in the overall MI population, whereas the drugs are indicated for hemodynamically stable patients with anterior MIs, HF, or a left ventricular ejection fraction <40% in the absence of hypotension or other contraindications (15).

In contrast to early MI therapy, the value of longer-term ACEIs in post-MI patients with left ventricular dysfunction (ejection fraction <40%) or clinical HF has been well established by the Salvage and Ventricular Enlargement (SAVE) (69) and Acute Infarction Ramipril Efficacy (AIRE) trials (70, 71). In SAVE, captopril reduced mortality and other cardiac events during an average follow-up of 42 months in asymptomatic or minimally symptomatic patients with left ventricular dysfunction after MI. Similar findings were noted with ramipril in AIRE, which included post-MI patients with symptomatic HF. In both studies, therapy was initiated several days after MI, and doses were titrated upward over time. Importantly, the beneficial effects of therapy were most pronounced in older patients. For example, among 783 patients over 65 years of age enrolled in SAVE, mortality was reduced by 23% with captopril (27.9% vs. 36.1%; $p = 0.017$), whereas patients under age 65 experienced a statistically insignificant 9% mortality reduction (16.6% vs. 18.3%) (69). Similarly, ramipril significantly decreased mortality in patients over age 65 enrolled in AIRE, but not in younger patients (70). Applying these clinical trial findings to real-world practice, a retrospective observational analysis of 14,129 patients age 65 years of age or older hospitalized with acute MI confirmed that patients discharged on an ACEI had an adjusted 1-year mortality rate 15% lower than patients not receiving an ACEI, including a 27% lower mortality in patients over the age of 80 (72).

In summary, ACEIs are indicated for all patients following acute MI, including older adults, in the absence of contraindications (15). However, the clearest benefits have been seen in patients with HF or left ventricular dysfunction, and among patients initiated on ACEI several days after acute MI. Guidelines recommend ACEI therapy for hemodynamically stable patients with adequate renal function, but they may be deferred in other cases. Doses should be titrated to those proven to be effective in clinical trials while monitoring blood pressure, renal function, and serum potassium levels at regular intervals.

Angiotensin receptor blockers

Angiotensin receptor blockers (ARBs) are associated with less cough than ACEIs, but the rates of hyperkalemia and the potential for worsening renal function are similar with both drug classes. Two large trials evaluated ARBs against ACEIs in the post-MI setting. In the Optimal Trial in Myocardial Infarction with Angiotensin II Antagonist Losartan (OPTIMAAL), patients 50 years of age or older with acute MI accompanied by HF, anterior Q waves on ECG, or a left ventricular ejection fraction <35% were randomized to losartan or captopril and followed for an average of 2.7 years (73). Mortality was nonsignificantly higher in the losartan group (18.2% vs. 16.4%, $p = 0.069$), with similar outcomes in older and younger subjects. In the Valsartan in Acute Myocardial Infarction Trial (VALIANT), 14,703 patients with acute MI were randomly assigned to receive captopril, valsartan, or both drugs and followed for a median of 25 months (74). Mortality was similar in all three arms, but side effects and withdrawals were more common in patients randomized to combination therapy. More than half of the patients in VALIANT were 65 years of age or older, 3160 patients were age 75 years or older, and outcomes with respect to the three treatment groups were similar across age categories, including patients over age 85 (75).

On the basis of currently available evidence, ACEIs remain the preferred agents in patients with recent acute MI, including older individuals (15). ARBs are considered reasonable alternatives to ACEIs for patients intolerant to ACEIs. Combination therapy with an ACEI and an ARB is not recommended.

Aldosterone antagonists

In the Eplerenone Post-acute myocardial infarction Heart Failure Efficacy and Survival Study (EPHESUS), the selective mineralocorticoid receptor antagonist (MRA) eplerenone reduced mortality by 17% in patients with left ventricular dysfunction (ejection fraction <40%) and HF or diabetes after acute MI (76). However, the benefit of eplerenone was attenuated in patients 65 years of age or older, and there was no apparent benefit in patients age 75 years or older. In addition, similar to the MRA spironolactone, the risk of hyperkalemia was substantially higher in older subjects. Therefore, the value of eplerenone in older patients following acute MI remains unclear, but it would be reasonable to prescribe eplerenone to older patients with preserved renal function and left ventricular (LV) dysfunction or clinical heart failure (3), particularly if good clinical follow-up has been verified for outpatient reevaluation of renal function and serum potassium levels.

LIPID MEDICATIONS

Although statins remain controversial for primary prevention in older patients, they have consistently been shown to reduce long-term mortality and morbidity in patients up to 85 years of age with established atherosclerotic disease (77, 78). In addition, early administration of high-dose statin therapy within the first 96 hours of acute MI reduces the risk of recurrent ischemic events during the 4-month period following hospital discharge, with similar effects in older and younger patients (79). In the Pravastatin or Atorvastatin Evaluation and Infection Therapy (PROVE-IT) trial, high-dose atorvastatin was more effective than standard-dose pravastatin in reducing the composite endpoint of death, MI, hospitalization for unstable angina, coronary revascularization, or stroke among patients treated for acute MI (80). The benefit of high-dose atorvastatin appeared to be limited, however, to patients less than 65 years of age. In another study of 12,853 patients with acute MI (mean age 64 years), statin therapy reduced major adverse cardiac events at 1-year follow-up, including among patients with impaired renal function (81). Based on the totality of evidence, statin therapy is recommended for all patients with acute MI regardless of age or baseline lipid profile, and statins should be continued indefinitely for secondary prevention in the absence of contraindications (3, 15).

Although statins remain the cornerstone of lipid-lowering therapy, several alternative agents are available as adjuncts to statins to achieve lipid goals or as replacement therapy in patients with statin intolerance. Among 18,144 patients with recent ACS enrolled in the Improved Reduction of Outcomes: Vytorin Efficacy International Trial (IMPROVE-IT), the addition of ezetimibe 10 mg daily to statin therapy modestly reduced cardiovascular events over a median follow-up of 6 years when compared with a statin alone (hazard ratio 0.936, $p = 0.016$) (82). There was a trend for greater benefit in patients over age 65 ($p = 0.098$) and significantly greater benefit in those over age 75 ($p = 0.005$). Ezetimibe is inexpensive and generally well tolerated, so it represents an excellent adjunct to statins in older adults who fail to achieve low-density lipoprotein (LDL) cholesterol goals on statin monotherapy.

Since many patients are intolerant to statins or are unable to achieve lipid goals with statins (with or without the addition of ezetimibe), several newer lipid therapies have been developed to further reduce the risk of recurrent cardiovascular events after MI. Two monoclonal antibodies that inhibit the enzyme paraprotein convertase subtilisin/kexin type 9 (PCSK9) have been shown to dramatically reduce LDL cholesterol and improve outcomes in selected patients. In a trial of 18,924 patients with ACS in the previous year and low-density cholesterol ≥70 mg/dL (most of whom were already taking statin drugs), alirocumab reduced the composite endpoint of cardiovascular death, MI, stroke, or unstable angina by 15% over a median of 2.8 years of follow-up (83). Patients under age 65 derived similar benefits as older patients. In another study of 27,564 patients with chronic atherosclerotic disease, more than 80% of whom had a prior MI, evolocumab also reduced the composite primary endpoint by 15% (absolute rates of 11.3% vs. 9.8%) over a median follow-up of 2.2 years (84). Again, younger and older patient subgroups had similar benefit, although this study excluded patients over age 85. Side effects with the PCSK9 inhibitors are minimal, though they do have limitations related to subcutaneous administration and higher cost.

Another alternative is bempedoic acid, with or without ezetimibe in a combination tablet, which reduced cardiovascular events in 13,970 patients, approximately 60% of whom were age 65 years and older (and 70% with secondary prevention indications for lipid therapy) (85). After 40-month median follow-up, bempedoic acid reduced the composite primary endpoint (cardiovascular death, stroke, MI, or coronary revascularization), largely due to reductions in MI and revascularization, with similar findings in older and younger patients. In a trial of icosapent ethyl (a purified omega-3 fatty acid formulation) evaluating patients with moderate elevations of triglycerides (again, 70% with secondary prevention indications, and approximately 45% age 65 and older), all ischemic events plus cardiovascular death were reduced over 4.9 years of follow-up, at the cost of higher rates of hospitalization for atrial fibrillation (3.1% vs 2.1%, $p = 0.004$) (86). Again, findings were similar for those above or below age 65.

Taken together, these studies suggest that early and intensive lipid lowering is beneficial for patients with prior MI, and contemporary guidelines have reflected these findings, including nonstatin alternatives when indicated to achieve appropriate cholesterol targets (15, 87). Specifically, patients with prior MI should have intensification of lipid therapies to achieve a target LDL cholesterol <70 mg/dL, including older patients. Those with consistently elevated triglycerides may be considered for icosapent ethyl therapy as well. Furthermore, among patients considered "very high risk" (multiple ischemic events, multiple atherosclerotic risk factors, extensive vascular disease, etc.), a target LDL <55 mg/dL is recommended. Many patients will require combination therapies to achieve these goals, with careful attention to potential side effects (especially with higher-dose statins) in older patients.

DIABETES THERAPIES

In 7020 patients with type 2 diabetes and established vascular disease (nearly half of whom had a history of MI), the sodium-glucose cotransporter-2 (SGLT2) inhibitor empagliflozin reduced cardiovascular events when added to existing diabetes and secondary prevention therapies (88). The 13% relative reduction in the composite endpoint was primarily driven by a 38% relative reduction (2.2% absolute reduction) in cardiovascular death at a median 3.1 years of follow-up, and the magnitude of benefit was larger in patients with prior coronary events (when compared with stroke or peripheral arterial disease), as well as among the 45% of patients over age 65 in the trial. The most common adverse events were urinary tract infections and genital mycotic infections, likely related to empagliflozin's action in blocking glucose reabsorption in the renal collecting system. Another SGLT2 inhibitor, canagliflozin, also demonstrated a reduction in the composite endpoint of cardiovascular death, MI, and stroke among similar patients with type 2 diabetes and vascular disease—again with a greater magnitude of benefit in the subset of patients over age 65 years—but with increased risks for fractures and lower extremity amputations (89). In a study of dapagliflozin in diabetic patients but fewer than one third with established CAD, the same composite endpoint was again reduced, though reduction in HF endpoints was more prominent than the reduction in ischemic endpoints (90). Nonetheless, findings were similar for patients older or younger than 65 years of age. These agents may be reasonable therapies for the large proportion of older MI patients who also have type 2 diabetes, provided renal function is adequate and with careful planning to adjust other diabetes therapies or diuretics to reduce the risk of adverse effects such as hypoglycemia, dehydration, or genital yeast infections.

The glucagon-like peptide-1 (GLP-1) receptor agonists, another newer class of diabetes therapies, initially demonstrated more variable outcomes in randomized trials, with several of the older drugs demonstrating cardiovascular safety but not superiority to existing diabetes or cardiac therapies. However, the daily injectable medication liraglutide reduced the primary composite endpoint of cardiovascular death, MI, or stroke by 13% (1.9% absolute reduction) among 9340 patients with type 2 diabetes and prevalent cardiovascular disease—approximately 30% of whom had prior MI (91). Patients with prior coronary events appeared to gain the most benefit during the median 3.8 years of follow-up, but unlike the SGLT2 inhibitor trials, older patients experienced less benefit in subgroup analyses. With weekly injections of the more potent drug semaglutide, on the other hand, this same composite endpoint was reduced by 26% after only 2 years of follow-up in patients with type 2 diabetes, largely driven by a reduction in stroke (92). Again, only about one third of the patients enrolled had prior MI, but this subgroup of patients had nearly identical benefits as the rest of the trial cohort, as did the subgroups of patients above or below age 65 years. In addition, semaglutide was studied in patients with obesity and established atherosclerotic disease, but without diabetes, and 76% of these patients had prior MI (93). This study confirmed a 20% reduction in the composite cardiovascular endpoint over a median 3.5 years of follow-up, including benefit in the subgroup of patients age 65–74 years, but lesser benefit in the smaller subgroup age 75 years and older. In contrast, the weekly injectable GLP-1 agonist dulaglutide reduced cardiovascular events in the setting of diabetes and established cardiovascular disease, but without an apparent trend toward benefit in the subgroup of patients age 65 years and older (94). Gastrointestinal distress is the primary adverse event with these medications, and weight loss related to early satiety and appetite suppression is sometimes problematic in older patients (particularly given the higher prevalence of gastric or intestinal dysmotility in this population). Thus, GLP-1 agonists are a reasonable option in select older patients with prior MI, with careful surveillance for adverse drug effects.

ADDITIONAL THERAPIES FOR SYMPTOM MANAGEMENT

Nitrates are widely used in the treatment of acute MI, but two large studies (GISSI-3 and ISIS-4) failed to confirm a reduction in major adverse events when nitrates were initiated within 24 hours of MI onset (65, 66). However, among 5234 patients aged 70 years or older enrolled in GISSI-3, the combined endpoint of death or severe left ventricular dysfunction at 6-month follow-up was reduced by nitroglycerin (odds ratio 0.88; $p = 0.04$). This finding, coupled with the fact that both trials demonstrated that nitrates can be administered safely to the majority of older patients, suggests that the continued use of nitrates for treating ischemic pain and peri-infarct HF is reasonable. Routine use of nitrates in older patients without pain or pulmonary congestion is of unproven value. Nitrates are contraindicated in patients with right ventricular infarction or systolic blood pressure less than 90 mmHg in the setting of acute MI, and among patients with phosphodiesterase-5 inhibitor use within the past 72 hours (sildenafil, tadalafil, vardenafil) (9, 10).

Like nitrates, morphine has failed to reduce major cardiovascular events in patients with acute MI (9, 10). Nonetheless, morphine is commonly prescribed for persistent chest pain and appears to be relatively safe (15). Older patients receiving morphine should be monitored for respiratory depression, mental status changes, constipation or bowel obstruction, and reduced gastrointestinal absorption of other drugs.

Calcium channel blockers are another class of medications widely studied in both the acute MI and post-MI settings, but without evidence of benefit and with potential for harm when using short-acting calcium antagonists and in patients with LV systolic dysfunction (9, 10, 15). Thus, these medications are not recommended for routine use in acute MI patients, but they may be considered in select patients with continued ischemia or hypertension who have preserved ventricular function and no HF (particularly among patients who are not candidates for or experience inadequate response to β-blockers) (9).

Ranolazine, a late sodium-channel inhibitor in cardiac myocytes, has been shown to improve symptoms and exercise tolerance in chronic stable angina in both younger and older patients (95). However, side effects are more common in patients over age 65. In patients with ACS, ranolazine was shown to be safe but did not improve clinical outcomes, with similar findings in patients under or over 75 years of age (96).

ANTIARRHYTHMIC THERAPIES

Prior to the reperfusion era, ventricular arrhythmias and sudden cardiac death were common causes of early mortality after MI, and the administration of prophylactic lidocaine to patients with acute MI was once a common practice. However, multiple studies suggested that lidocaine does not improve survival and may increase the incidence of asystolic cardiac arrest, as confirmed in a meta-analysis of these data (97). Similarly, other antiarrhythmic agents such as amiodarone have not reduced mortality (with some studies showing higher mortality risk), so prophylactic use of antiarrhythmic drugs is not recommended in the absence of sustained or refractory arrhythmias complicating MI (9, 10).

An implantable cardioverter-defibrillator (ICD) is indicated for secondary prevention of sudden cardiac death in patients who develop ventricular fibrillation or hemodynamically significant sustained ventricular tachycardia more than 48 hours after acute MI (9). The value of prophylactic ICD insertion in other post-MI patients is less clear, but primary prevention of sudden cardiac death with an ICD appears to be reasonable when left ventricular ejection fraction remains ≤35% after optimization of HF medical therapies (see Chapter 19). Multiple studies have evaluated ICDs in patients with reduced ejection fraction (98–101), and the majority of the benefit in reducing sudden death occurs beyond 18 months after ICD implantation (99). Thus, routine implantation of an ICD for primary prevention following acute MI may be considered for patients with persistent left ventricular ejection fraction ≤35% more than 40 days after MI, despite optimal medical therapy and an estimated life expectancy with satisfactory functional status of at least 1 year. Of note, very few patients over age 80 years were enrolled in clinical trials of ICD therapy, and the mortality benefit from ICDs declines with age due to competing causes of death (102). Since ICDs may prolong life without improving quality of life (99, 102, 103)—an effect not necessarily considered desirable for many older patients with poor quality of life at baseline—selection of older patients for ICD placement must include a realistic appraisal of benefits versus risks, with inclusion of the patient and family in the decision-making process. There should also be a discussion of clinical scenarios in which the patient might want to consider disabling the ICD function, for example, terminal illness or unacceptably poor quality of life (104).

An additional therapy commonly prescribed for patients with MI and reduced ejection fraction is the wearable cardioverter-defibrillator (WCD), designed to treat sudden cardiac death from ventricular tachyarrhythmias while awaiting recovery of left ventricular function or eligibility for a future ICD. However, this practice was called into question with publication of the Vest Prevention of Early Sudden Death (VEST) trial in 2018, in which the WCD did not show a significant reduction in arrhythmic death in 2302 patients with reduced ejection fraction after MI (105). Perhaps the most notable finding from the trial, aside from modestly poor compliance rates with wearing the device, was the low rate of arrhythmic death after MI (<5%), perhaps related to more widespread use of early reperfusion and more intensive medical therapies in line with contemporary MI management. Thus, the role of the WCD remains unclear in older patients, but may be considered for select patients with very poor left ventricular function or high risk of ventricular arrhythmias after MI.

CORONARY REPERFUSION THERAPY

Prompt reperfusion of the infarct-related artery has been shown to reduce infarct size and peri-infarct complications, including death, in a broad range of patients with acute MI associated with ST-segment elevations or new left bundle branch block (LBBB). Although early studies of reperfusion therapy focused on administration of fibrinolytic agents, primary PCI has become the preferred reperfusion strategy for STEMI if the procedure can be performed expeditiously, usually defined as within 90 minutes of the patient's arrival to the hospital (and ideally within 90 minutes of the patient's first medical contact) (9). As discussed in more detail later, several studies have examined the role of reperfusion therapy in older patients. In a large registry study, eligibility for STEMI reperfusion was present in 87% of patients younger than 75 years, 75% of patients aged 75–84 years, and 58% of patients aged 85 years and older (4). Most of the reasons for non-eligibility were related to patient and family preferences, with only about 10% of older patients having absolute contraindications to therapy. Although patients who received reperfusion had lower in-hospital mortality than eligible patients who did not receive reperfusion for STEMI, this was only significant for patients younger than 75 years (odds ratio = 0.58; 95% confidence interval [CI], 0.40 to 0.84), with loss of mortality benefit over age 75 (4). In another study of 73 patients aged 85 to 94 years hospitalized for STEMI, primary PCI was the only independent predictor of survival at a median follow-up of 429 days (hazard ratio = 0.3, $p = 0.02$) (106). More recently, a clinical trial of 1445 patients age 75 and older with acute MI and multivessel coronary disease were randomized to culprit-lesion PCI only versus complete revascularization of all significant coronary stenoses (107). Median age was 80 years, and the multivessel PCI group experienced a 27% relative risk reduction in the primary composite endpoint at 1 year, including a 36% reduction in cardiovascular death or MI, with no difference in the safety outcome (acute kidney injury, stroke, or bleeding). Similar findings were noted above or below the age of 80. In an individual patient data meta-analysis of seven randomized trials of older patients (median age 79 years) with STEMI, multivessel PCI reduced cardiovascular death or MI at 4 years follow-up (108). Thus, complete coronary revascularization appears to benefit even very old patients with ACS, at least among those enrolled in clinical trials.

Fibrinolytic therapy

In the 1980s, a series of randomized clinical trials demonstrated that IV administration of a fibrinolytic agent within 6 to 12 hours of symptom onset in patients with STEMI or new LBBB led to a significant reduction in short-term and long-term mortality. These studies ushered in the reperfusion era and revolutionized the approach to treatment of patients with ACS. However, the value of this treatment in patients over age 75 remains controversial. In the Fibrinolytic Therapy Trialists' (FTT) meta-analysis of these trials (109), the greatest absolute benefit was seen in patients 65–74 years of age (26 fewer deaths per 1000 treated patients), with more modest benefit after age 75 years (10 fewer deaths per 1000 treated patients). Reanalysis of the FTT data, when limited to patients presenting within 12 hours of symptom onset with ST-segment elevation or LBBB, showed that among patients age 75 years or older, mortality was reduced from 29.4% to 26.0% (34 fewer deaths per 1000 treated patients, $p = 0.03$) (110). Moreover, the absolute benefit was similar to that seen in other age groups and greater than in patients younger than age 55.

In contrast to the FTT analysis, several observational studies have suggested that fibrinolytic therapy in patients over 75 years of age may be associated with higher mortality (111, 112). Other studies found lower adjusted relative risks of death or nonfatal cerebral bleeding, albeit with lower absolute benefit, and neutral effects among patients aged 85 years or older (113). In comparative-effectiveness trials involving different fibrinolytic agents, similar patterns have emerged (114–117). In the Global Utilization of Streptokinase and tPA for Occluded Arteries (GUSTO) trial, which randomized over 40,000 acute MI patients to one of four fibrinolytic regimens, alteplase was associated with lower 30-day mortality than streptokinase in patients up to the age of 85 (117). However, the absolute benefit was small in patients over 75 years of age, and alteplase was associated with a significantly higher risk of intracranial hemorrhage (ICH) compared with streptokinase in this age group (2.1% vs. 1.2%; $p < 0.05$) (118). Subsequent studies with reteplase and tenecteplase failed to demonstrate a survival advantage with these agents compared with alteplase (119, 120), and in the GUSTO-III trial, reteplase was associated with a higher rate of ICH than alteplase among patients over 75 years of age (2.5% vs. 1.7%) (119). Thus, currently available data suggest that the more fibrin-specific fibrinolytic agents (i.e., alteplase, reteplase, tenecteplase) are associated with increased risk of ICH compared with streptokinase in patients over age 75, and the merits of these agents with respect to other clinical outcomes, including mortality, have not been convincingly established in this age group.

In summary, data from randomized trials demonstrate that fibrinolytic therapy is beneficial in appropriately selected older patients, including those over 75 years of age. However, real-world population studies indicate that caution is advised in the very old and suggest that strict adherence to established criteria for use of fibrinolytic drugs is essential in patients over age 75 in order to maximize benefit and minimize risk (3). Caution is also warranted when using fibrinolytic agents in older patients at increased risk for bleeding or stroke (e.g., those with prior cerebrovascular disease or severe uncontrolled hypertension) (121–123).

Primary PCI for STEMI

PCI has several potential applications in the acute MI setting: as a primary reperfusion strategy, as an adjunct to thrombolysis, as a "rescue" procedure for failed thrombolysis, and in the management of recurrent ischemia (9, 124, 125). However, with progressive technological improvements, advances in adjunctive anticoagulant therapies, and enhanced processes of care designed to improve rapid PCI availability, primary PCI has become the dominant strategy for reperfusion during STEMI.

In several studies of older patients with STEMI, PCI was shown to be more effective than fibrinolytic therapy in recanalizing the infarct-related coronary artery (125). DeBoer et al. randomized 87 patients over 75 years of age with STEMI to streptokinase or PCI. At 30-day follow-up, patients allocated to PCI had a reduced risk of death, reinfarction, or stroke ($p = 0.01$), and this benefit persisted for at least 1 year (126). In another study involving 130 patients with STEMI 70 years of age or older receiving alteplase or PCI, treatment with PCI was an independent predictor of lower mortality, reinfarction, or revascularization for recurrent ischemia at 6-month follow-up (127). In 481 patients aged 70 years or older presenting within 12 hours of STEMI onset randomized to fibrinolytic therapy or PCI (128), PCI was associated with a 55% reduction in death, stroke, or reinfarction relative to fibrinolysis ($p = 0.05$). Of note, the benefit of PCI was limited to patients 70–79 years of age; among 131 patients aged 80 years or older, outcomes did not differ between reperfusion strategies.

The findings of these randomized trials are also supported by subgroup analysis from a systematic overview of 22 randomized trials comparing PCI with fibrinolytic therapy in 6763 patients with acute MI (124). Overall, PCI was associated with a significant 37% reduction in 30-day mortality, and the absolute benefit was greater in patients over age 65 than in younger patients. Moreover, the absolute benefit of PCI increased progressively with age, from 1.0% in patients <65 years to 4.2%, 5.1%, and 6.9% in patients ages 65–74, 75–84, and 85 or older, respectively (3).

Aside from ischemic benefits, PCI offers an advantage over fibrinolysis in terms of reducing overall bleeding risk, and ICH in particular. Nonetheless, older patients suffer higher rates of bleeding with all types of procedures (including PCI). Much of this bleeding risk may be mitigated around the time of PCI by careful attention to

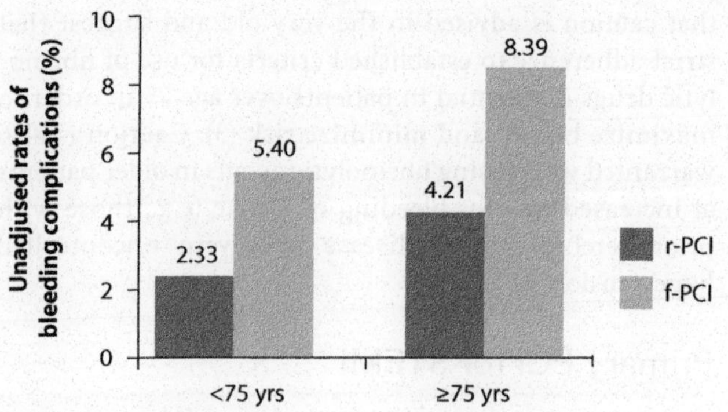

Figure 10.2 Bleeding complications within 72 hours after PCI according to age and access approach. Data obtained from the National Cardiovascular Data Registry between 2008 and 2012 involving 2.8 million PCI procedures at >1300 participating US hospitals. F-PCI indicates patients undergoing PCI via the femoral artery approach; R-PCI indicates the radial artery approach.

dosing of anticoagulant drugs, minimizing GP IIb/IIIa inhibitor use, using smaller catheters, and choosing radial access for PCI when feasible (Figure 10.2) (129, 130).

In summary, current data suggest that PCI can be performed safely in older patients with STEMI with fewer hemorrhagic strokes and more favorable clinical outcomes compared to fibrinolysis (3). In particular, very high-risk older patients, such as those with large anterior MIs or severe hemodynamic disturbances, may be most likely to benefit from this approach (131).

Of note, patients who experience recurrent ischemic pain, hemodynamic instability, or other signs of ischemia after MI are at high risk for adverse events following hospital discharge, and additional evaluation followed by revascularization with either PCI or CABG, if feasible, is indicated (9, 132). Patients with persistent ischemic pain following administration of a fibrinolytic agent, particularly when accompanied by hemodynamic instability (e.g., hypotension or HF), are at high risk for adverse outcomes, and "rescue" PCI improves prognosis in this subgroup (124, 125, 133). In a meta-analysis of eight trials including 1177 patients, rescue PCI was associated with improved clinical outcomes for patients with STEMI after failed fibrinolytic therapy (134). Thus, although cardiac catheterization and revascularization are reasonable but not mandatory for older patients initially treated medically for acute STEMI, these procedures should be strongly considered in patients with hemodynamic instability or residual ischemia in the early post-STEMI period (3, 9).

PCI for NSTEMI

In contrast to the emergent, time-dependent nature of revascularization for STEMI, patients with NSTEMI or unstable angina (NSTE-ACS, or non-ST-elevation acute coronary syndromes) should be evaluated for early invasive versus early conservative approaches to coronary care. Older age is a significant risk factor for adverse ACS outcomes, as noted previously, and as a result there are many pressures for the clinician to recommend more aggressive approaches (i.e., catheterization and coronary revascularization) to reduce ACS-related complications. Patients with high-risk features during NSTEMI (ventricular arrhythmias, recurrent angina despite medical therapy, significant left ventricular dysfunction, etc.) generally have better outcomes with revascularization than with medical management (7, 10). However, procedural complications from PCI are higher in older patients as well, both from cardiovascular issues (e.g., access site problems, complex vascular anatomy, coronary calcification precluding adequate stent delivery) and from other medical comorbidities (renal dysfunction, cognitive impairment or agitation with sedation, bleeding risks in frail patients).

Despite these concerns, most studies of older patients treated with an early invasive approach to NSTE-ACS have demonstrated reductions in death or recurrent MI (135, 136). In an unblinded trial of 457 patients ≥80 years of age with NSTE-ACS, early coronary angiography and revascularization were associated with a significant reduction in urgent revascularization or recurrent MI over a median follow-up of 1.5 years when compared with initial medical therapy alone (137). Of note, the benefit of invasive management declined with age and was no longer evident among patients ≥90 years of age. As such, the decision to pursue an invasive approach among patients with advanced age must be individualized, with consideration of anticipated benefits, potential risks, and patient preferences. Among older patients with lower-risk ACS characteristics, intensification of medical management alone is often a reasonable option.

Coronary artery bypass graft surgery

Traditional indications for CABG, whether in the setting of stable or unstable coronary disease, include left main or triple-vessel disease, multivessel disease with left ventricular dysfunction, multivessel disease with diabetes, or the need for other concomitant cardiac surgery (such as severe valvular heart disease). As with any other type of surgery, the increased risk of complications and greater likelihood of prolonged or difficult recovery in older patients must be weighed against the potential benefits of surgery. Complications of CABG are more common among patients ≥80 years of age (138), including postoperative arrhythmias such as atrial fibrillation, as well as delirium and cognitive impairment during recovery (139).

Despite these concerns, postoperative mortality rates have continued to decline over the past 2 decades in both younger and older patients despite substantial increases in comorbidity (140). Revascularization is associated with excellent long-term clinical outcomes among appropriately selected patients of advanced age (i.e., octogenarians and nonagenarians), including fewer symptoms and improved quality of life compared with medical therapy alone in the setting of stable coronary disease (141, 142). Studies evaluating PCI versus CABG for stable patients with left main or multivessel CAD have consistently demonstrated higher rates of repeat revascularization after PCI, but with similar rates of death or MI between the two approaches (143, 144). Stroke may occur at higher rates postoperatively after CABG, when compared with PCI, but rates in contemporary registry studies remain low, even among elderly patients.

These findings have been extrapolated to ACS patients, as many older individuals choose multivessel PCI over CABG, thus trading the higher perioperative risk and longer recovery time after CABG for the greater likelihood of needing repeat PCI during short-term follow-up. Coupled with additional improvements in PCI over time (greater use of radial artery access, newer stents with lower restenosis and thrombosis rates, smaller catheters, lower contrast volumes), these trends likely contribute to the continued decrease in CABG rates in the United States since 1997, while PCI rates in the geriatric population have remained relatively constant (1).

MANAGEMENT OF MI COMPLICATIONS

Older patients are at increased risk for several major complications of acute MI, including HF, hypotension, supraventricular and ventricular arrhythmias, conduction disturbances, myocardial rupture, and cardiogenic shock. In general, the management of these complications is similar in older and younger patients. In the following sections, the treatment of each of these complications is briefly reviewed, with special attention to older adults.

Heart failure

With improvements in short-term survival during the reperfusion era, many older patients are faced with residual left ventricular dysfunction and HF after recovering from acute MI (145). Several factors predispose these individuals to developing HF, including age-related changes in cardiovascular structure and function, increased prevalence of prior MI, higher prevalence of multivessel disease, more advanced grades of diastolic dysfunction, reduced contractile reserve, and increased prevalence of comorbid illnesses, both cardiac (e.g., aortic stenosis) and noncardiac (e.g., renal insufficiency) (146). As a result, HF occurs in approximately 50% of older patients with acute MI (7), and HF is often the presenting manifestation of MI in older individuals (147).

The initial treatment of acute HF includes supplemental oxygen (if the arterial oxygen saturation is less than 92%), diuretics, and nitrates. In more severe cases, morphine may be given to help relieve dyspnea. Once therapy has been initiated, it is essential to determine whether multiple etiologies of HF are present (beyond the acute MI alone), such as persistent or recurrent ischemia, significant aortic or mitral valve disease, arrhythmias (especially atrial fibrillation or runs of ventricular tachycardia), uncontrolled hypertension, diastolic dysfunction (often due to left ventricular hypertrophy or cardiac amyloidosis), inappropriate bradycardia, mechanical complications (e.g., papillary muscle rupture or ventricular septal perforation), severe renal insufficiency, or medication effects (e.g., myocardial depression from β-blockers, calcium channel antagonists, or antiarrhythmic agents). In most cases, an echocardiogram with Doppler, in conjunction with a careful review of the patient's medications and laboratory data, will be sufficient for determining the pathogenesis of HF after acute MI (9). Infrequently, supplemental studies such as pulmonary artery catheterization or transesophageal echocardiography may be necessary.

Once the etiology has been established, an effort should be made to correct treatable disorders and to reduce the dose or discontinue offending medications. If HF persists despite aggressive diuresis, placement of a pulmonary artery catheter should be considered as an aid to diagnosis and therapy. When indicated, treatment with an inotropic agent for hypotension or an IV vasodilator for persistently elevated left ventricular afterload should be considered. Dobutamine is the most frequently used IV inotrope for treating severe left ventricular dysfunction, but dobutamine may be less effective in the older patients due to an age-related decline in β-adrenergic responsiveness (148, 149). Phosphodiesterase inhibitors such as milrinone have theoretical advantages over sympathomimetic agents in coronary patients because they augment cardiac output without increasing myocardial oxygen demand (150).

Nitroglycerin and nitroprusside are the most commonly used IV vasodilators, but nitroglycerin is the only one recommended for treatment of HF in the setting of acute MI (9). Intravenous nitroglycerin has a very short half-life, which allows rapid dose titration, and it is well established for symptomatic relief of ongoing ischemia in MI patients. Hypotension is the most common serious adverse effect, so blood pressure should be monitored closely.

MI patients who fail to respond to the above measures have refractory HF, and the prognosis is grave unless a correctable problem can be identified. Additional interventions that may help stabilize patients with refractory HF include endotracheal intubation with mechanical ventilation or mechanical circulatory support devices (see later). Such therapies are usually appropriate only in patients with potentially reversible pathophysiology and otherwise favorable prognosis.

Hypotension

Hypotension in the setting of acute MI usually reflects a low cardiac output state arising from extensive myocardial damage, intravascular volume depletion, right ventricular ischemia, valvular dysfunction (especially mitral regurgitation), pericardial effusion, or electrical system disease (either tachycardia or bradycardia). Other factors that may contribute to hypotension in older patients include preexisting cardiac conditions such as aortic stenosis or cardiomyopathy, or cardiac or medical complications related to the acute MI, such as ventricular septal perforation, sepsis, bleeding (e.g., from fibrinolytic therapy or catheterization), and medications. The cause of hypotension is frequently multifactorial, and it is incumbent upon the physician to consider all potential etiologies and to perform appropriate diagnostic investigations as indicated (e.g., echocardiography, chest CT, cardiac catheterization). In the absence of HF, intravascular volume expansion is the appropriate initial treatment for hypotension. Subsequent therapy will depend on the response to fluid administration and the underlying etiology. Patients who fail to respond to IV fluids or who have coexistent HF may require pulmonary artery catheterization (9). On the basis of the hemodynamic findings and the severity of hypotension, treatment with sympathomimetic agents such as dobutamine, dopamine, phenylephrine, or norepinephrine may be necessary to maintain organ perfusion. Other supportive measures designed to reduce left ventricular workload while recovering from the acute insult include intra-aortic balloon counterpulsation or mechanical circulatory support (e.g., Impella device) (9). It is important to emphasize that all of these interventions are palliative, and unless the underlying etiology of hypotension can be corrected, the prognosis is grave for older patients with persistent hypotension after acute MI.

Arrhythmias and conduction disturbances

Older patients with acute MI are at increased risk for supraventricular arrhythmias, particularly atrial fibrillation, and for conduction disturbances such as bundle branch block and high-degree atrioventricular block. The incidence of ventricular tachycardia is similar in older and younger patients, but primary ventricular fibrillation occurs less frequently in older patients (151), possibly reflecting reduced β-adrenergic responsiveness in this age group.

New-onset atrial fibrillation following acute MI usually results from atrial distension due to an increase in ventricular diastolic pressure. Contributing factors may include preexisting atrial fibrosis, mitral or tricuspid regurgitation, atrial ischemia or infarction, pericarditis, electrolyte abnormalities (particularly hypokalemia), and medications (e.g., inotropic agents, bronchodilators). Because older patients frequently have preexisting diastolic dysfunction and an increased reliance on atrial contraction to augment ventricular filling (the "atrial kick") (146), atrial fibrillation often precipitates HF or a low cardiac output state.

Treatment of atrial fibrillation includes correcting any reversible abnormalities (e.g., hypokalemia), controlling the ventricular rate, and restoring sinus rhythm in patients with hemodynamic compromise. In patients who are hemodynamically stable, rate control with β-blockers or rate-lowering calcium channel blockers (i.e., diltiazem or verapamil) is appropriate, with careful surveillance for hypotension arising from the myocardial depressant properties of these medications. In most cases, IV heparin to maintain the aPTT in the range of 50–70 seconds is also indicated. Although effective rate control often results in spontaneous conversion to sinus rhythm, if new-onset atrial fibrillation persists longer than 24 hours, pharmacological or electrical cardioversion should be considered. Amiodarone is the most commonly used antiarrhythmic agent for the cardioversion of recent-onset atrial fibrillation. However, IV amiodarone is negatively inotropic and should be used with caution in the presence of significant left ventricular dysfunction. In patients who exhibit hypotension, severe HF, or organ hypoperfusion attributable to atrial fibrillation, immediate electrical cardioversion is the treatment of choice (9). Patients with persistent or chronic atrial fibrillation should receive long-term antithrombotic therapy with warfarin or a direct oral anticoagulant (dabigatran, rivaroxaban, apixaban, edoxaban) (152).

The treatment of peri-MI ventricular tachyarrhythmias is similar in older and younger patients and generally follows the Advanced Cardiac Life Support (ACLS) guidelines (153, 154), with subsequent therapy individualized on the basis of symptoms, severity of arrhythmia, and other factors, such as left ventricular function. Similarly, the treatment of bradyarrhythmias and conduction disturbances does not differ in younger and older patients. In general, antiarrhythmic medications, synchronized cardioversion, or defibrillation are needed for sustained ventricular tachyarrhythmias. In patients with symptomatic or hemodynamically compromising bradyarrhythmias unresponsive to atropine, temporary pacing (transthoracic or transvenous) should be considered. The ACLS guidelines should be followed for treating all life-threatening arrhythmias, regardless of age, as long as the wishes of the patient and family are honored.

Right ventricular ischemia

Right ventricular ischemia occurs in up to 50% of patients with inferior MI, with somewhat higher frequency in older than in younger patients (155). The reduction in preload to the left heart often results in hypotension requiring aggressive IV hydration and sometimes additional vasopressor support. Right ventricular function often recovers over a period of several days, at which point diuresis may be necessary to manage residual volume overload related to vigorous volume expansion. Of note, electrocardiographic evidence of right ventricular ischemia, as indicated by ST-segment elevation in the right precordial leads, is associated with a marked increase in hospital mortality in both younger and older patients (155, 156).

Myocardial rupture

Myocardial rupture is an infrequent complication of acute MI, occurring in less than 1% of patients in the era of rapid primary PCI for STEMI (157). However, when rupture does occur, the course is frequently catastrophic, with death ensuing in over 50% to almost 100% of cases, depending on the location of the rupture. There are three principal types of rupture: ventricular free wall rupture, papillary muscle rupture (PMR), and ventricular septal defect (VSD) from acute septal perforation. PMR almost always occurs following an inferoposterior or posterolateral MI, whereas septal rupture occurs somewhat more frequently following an anterior infarct. Free wall rupture can complicate an infarct of any location.

Although precise figures are not known, all forms of rupture appear to occur more frequently in patients over 65 years of age (158, 159). Other risk factors for myocardial rupture include female gender and persistent peri-MI hypertension (159). Fibrinolytic therapy may also increase the risk of myocardial rupture within the first 24 to 48 hours after treatment, particularly in older patients undergoing delayed fibrinolysis (i.e., more than 6 hours after symptom onset) (159, 160).

Impending myocardial rupture is occasionally heralded by persistent vague chest discomfort or unexplained hypotension, but sudden hemodynamic deterioration, new or worsening HF, or asystolic cardiac arrest may be the first indication of the rupture (161). The presence of a new systolic murmur, particularly in association with hemodynamic deterioration, strongly suggests the possibility of papillary muscle dysfunction or ventricular septal perforation, and prompt Doppler echocardiography should be performed (9). Pulmonary artery catheterization can provide definitive confirmation of a septal perforation by demonstrating an oxygen saturation step-up of greater than 10% at the level of the shunt (usually the right ventricle), or an elevated V-wave in the pulmonary capillary wedge pressure waveform suggesting acute mitral regurgitation.

Once a diagnosis of acute VSD or PMR has been confirmed, supportive measures should be rapidly instituted, and urgent consultation with interventional/structural cardiology and cardiac surgery should be obtained (9). Diuretics and afterload reduction with IV nitroglycerin or intra-aortic balloon counterpulsation may help stabilize the patient, along with mechanical ventilation for respiratory compromise, but urgent transcatheter or surgical repair is recommended in almost all cases of acute VSD or PMR, since medical therapy is associated with mortality rates of more than 75% (160, 161). Periprocedural mortality rates range from 10% to 70%, with global left ventricular function and the presence of cardiogenic shock being the most important factors influencing survival (162). The long-term prognosis following successful repair of acute VSD or PMR is favorable among suitable candidates.

Rupture of the left ventricular free wall usually progresses rapidly to pericardial tamponade, asystole, and death. Occasionally, however, the rupture will be locally contained as a result of pericardial adhesions or other factors, resulting in the formation of a pseudoaneurysm. Differentiation of a pseudoaneurysm from a true left ventricular aneurysm can be difficult, but echocardiography, magnetic resonance imaging, and computed tomographic angiography are all useful in making this distinction. The hemodynamic effects of a pseudoaneurysm are variable, depending on its size and location, but there is a tendency for pseudoaneurysms to undergo further rupture, resulting in pericardial tamponade (9). Although conservative management may be associated with a favorable outcome in some cases (163), surgical repair is usually recommended once an acute pseudoaneurysm has been identified (9, 164).

Cardiogenic shock

Cardiogenic shock is defined as the combination of markedly reduced cardiac output (cardiac index <1.8 L/min/m^2), increased left ventricular diastolic pressure or pulmonary wedge pressure (≥22 mmHg), hypotension (systolic blood pressure <80 mmHg), and tissue hypoperfusion (e.g., prerenal azotemia, impaired sensorium) (165). This syndrome occurs twice as frequently in older patients with acute MI as in younger subjects, and it accounts for most of the excess mortality associated with acute MI in older adults (166). Moreover, despite major advances in the treatment of acute MI over the last 30 years, the case fatality rate from cardiogenic shock remains high (166–168).

The causes of cardiogenic shock complicating acute MI are similar to the causes of HF and hypotension. Since mortality from cardiogenic shock is high in the absence of a treatable etiology, immediate evaluation for a potentially correctable problem is critical. Emergent echocardiography should be performed to assess overall left ventricular function and to rule out valvular lesions, pericardial disease, and septal or ventricular free wall perforation (9). Pulmonary artery catheterization is often indicated to facilitate diagnosis and for guiding therapy. Cardiac catheterization may be necessary in some cases if the diagnosis remains in doubt, as a prelude to PCI or corrective surgery, or to assess for stent thrombosis or occlusion of a recent PCI or bypass graft.

Although emergent catheterization and coronary revascularization have been shown to improve outcomes in patients up to age 75 with cardiogenic shock complicating acute MI, patients over age 75 may not benefit from these interventions. Specifically, in the Should We Emergently Revascularize Occluded Coronaries for Cardiogenic Shock (SHOCK) randomized trial, the subgroup of patients over age 75 did not demonstrate the same mortality benefit as seen in younger patients (169). Nonetheless, selected patients over age 75 years in the SHOCK trial registry did appear to benefit from revascularization (170). In a more recent trial of 706 patients with cardiogenic shock complicating acute MI, culprit lesion PCI was more effective than multivessel PCI for reducing mortality or severe renal failure at 30 days (171). Although this study had several important limitations (open-label design, >21% of those randomized to culprit lesion PCI crossed over to receive additional PCI procedures, exclusion of patients over age 90), the main findings were consistent across multiple subgroups, including age. Based on the preponderance of evidence, emergent revascularization is appropriate for patients under age 75 with acute MI complicated by cardiogenic shock, but careful selection is warranted for very old patients. Conversely, age alone should not be viewed as a contraindication to intervening in these critically ill patients.

In patients with a potentially reversible cause of shock, maximally aggressive therapy is indicated to stabilize the patient. In most cases, this will include IV vasoactive therapy and/or mechanical support with an intra-aortic balloon pump (172) or percutaneous ventricular assist device (Impella) (173). However, when shock is due to irreversible myocardial damage or other untreatable disorder, invasive interventions are unlikely to influence survival. For example, in a study of 598 patients with cardiogenic shock complicating acute MI (mean age 70 years) who were randomized to intra-aortic balloon support or to a control group, use of intra-aortic balloon counterpulsation did not reduce 30-day mortality (174).

Similarly, circulatory support with Impella has facilitated the performance of high-risk PCI or CABG, but mortality benefit was not demonstrated in several of the early clinical trials (175, 176), including a substudy of 355 patients with STEMI-related cardiogenic shock in which outcomes with Impella were worse for patients age 77 years and older (177). However, a more recent trial evaluating Impella specifically for STEMI-related cardiogenic shock demonstrated lower 6-month mortality, at a cost of higher rates of bleeding, limb ischemia, infection, and renal failure (178). As in previous trials of more invasive therapies for MI, the mortality benefit was attenuated among patients above the median age in the study (i.e., 67 years of age or older). Other methods of providing mechanical support (Tandem Heart, extracorporeal membrane oxygenation [ECMO], surgical ventricular assist devices) may be considered for acute stabilization of MI-related shock, but mortality benefit has not been consistently demonstrated in clinical trials, including among older patients.

Managing hyperglycemia

Multiple studies have demonstrated higher rates of adverse outcomes among patients with hyperglycemia during acute MI, particularly among patients without known diabetes prior to hospital presentation (179–182). One exploratory study suggested lower mortality with intensive therapy, including insulin during the MI hospitalization and aggressive care after discharge (183), but it was difficult to determine whether the insulin or the intensive diabetes management program was responsible for the improved outcomes. A larger follow-up study failed to demonstrate improved outcomes with more intensive insulin-based hyperglycemia management (184). Current guidelines recommend serum glucose surveillance, with therapy to keep levels below 180 mg/dL when possible (9, 10), but more intensive inpatient glucose control does not seem imperative based on available trial data. In addition, it is important to avoid hypoglycemia, especially in older patients. Nonetheless, initiating appropriate cardioprotective diabetes therapies at hospital discharge is indicated (see earlier section "Diabetes Therapies" concerning SGLT2 inhibitors and GLP-1 agonists).

Anemia, erythropoietin, and blood transfusion

Despite multiple studies demonstrating worse outcomes with lower hemoglobin levels during acute cardiac illnesses, including MI, administration of intravenous erythropoietin in patients with STEMI has been associated with an increased rate of adverse cardiovascular events, as well as concern about the potential for an increase in infarct size among older patients (185). Routine blood transfusion has not been shown to improve outcomes during acute MI, and several observational studies have suggested worse outcomes among patients receiving transfusion during an MI hospitalization (10). For patients with anemia, one small trial suggested that a liberal blood transfusion strategy provided no benefit during the first several months after MI, but potential benefit at 1 year after MI hospitalization (186). A subsequent larger randomized trial of 3504 patients with MI and anemia found that a liberal transfusion strategy (i.e., for hemoglobin <10 g/dL) failed to reduce 30-day mortality or recurrent MI compared to a more restrictive transfusion cutoff (hemoglobin <7 or 8 g/dL) (187). While this field is evolving, at present, only select patients with significant anemia should be considered for blood transfusion during MI, with careful attention to potential volume overload or other adverse reactions to transfusion.

SPECIFIC CONSIDERATIONS FOR NSTEMI

Non-ST-elevation acute coronary syndromes, including both NSTEMI and unstable angina, increase in frequency with advancing age, and NSTEMI accounts for well over 50% of all MIs in patients over the age of 70 (7). The National Registry of Myocardial Infarction showed that among 1,950,561 patients hospitalized for acute MI from 1990 to 2006, the proportion of NSTEMIs increased from 14.2% to 59.1% over that period ($p < 0.0001$) (188). In addition, the mean age of all patients increased from 64.1 to 66.4 years ($p < 0.0001$), and the proportion of women increased from 32.4% to 37.0% ($p < 0.0001$). Hospital mortality decreased in patients with STEMI from 11.5% to 8.0% ($p < 0.0001$) and in patients with NSTEMI from 7.1% to 5.2% ($p < 0.0001$). While STEMIs are usually caused by thrombosis of the infarct-related vessel (Type 1 MI) (189), the pathogenesis of NSTEMI is more variable, and thus the prognosis and treatment strategies are more variable. In older patients, NSTEMI is commonly precipitated by a sustained imbalance between myocardial oxygen supply and demand (Type 2 MI) resulting from many etiologies, including severe hypertension, hypoxemia, heart failure, atrial fibrillation, hypotension, infection, or other causes. Multivessel coronary disease is often present, but acute thrombotic occlusion of the infarct artery as the etiology for NSTEMI is less frequent than in younger populations (189).

Historically, the short-term prognosis following NSTEMI has been more favorable than for STEMI, since NSTEMIs are usually smaller and associated with greater preservation of ventricular function (190). However, patients with NSTEMI are at increased risk for recurrent ischemia and reinfarction, and long-term survival is similar to STEMI (10, 190). In one series, over 60% of all deaths within the first year after hospitalization for acute MI occurred in patients over the age of 70 presenting with NSTEMI (191).

As the clinical course following NSTEMI is distinct from that following STEMI, numerous studies have focused specifically on the management of this disorder. In general, acute pharmacotherapy should follow the same recommendations as those discussed earlier in this chapter, including aspirin, antithrombotic therapy such as LMWH or unfractionated heparin, statin, β-blocker, and ACEI or ARB when clinically stable (particularly if left ventricular function is abnormal) (7, 10). Antiplatelet therapy should be initiated in most cases, although some physicians prefer to withhold oral $P2Y_{12}$ medications until after coronary angiography has been performed (to avoid the waiting period for CABG if significant multivessel disease is found at angiography). Although cangrelor may be considered for higher-risk patients with NSTEMI while awaiting findings from the diagnostic coronary angiogram, this approach is associated with greater risks of bleeding in older patients. Nitrates or morphine should be administered for persistent or recurrent chest pain, while persistent hypertension, arrhythmias, and HF should be treated appropriately. In the absence of ST-elevation or LBBB, fibrinolytic therapy has not been shown to be efficacious and is contraindicated for NSTEMI (109).

Several studies have compared early cardiac catheterization and revascularization with conventional medical therapy in patients with NSTE-ACS (135, 136, 192–197). Although the results of earlier trials were somewhat inconsistent, with more recent trials generally showing better outcomes, overall the data suggest that early revascularization is beneficial in high-risk patients, including older individuals (7). Based on these studies, current guidelines recommend that patients with NSTEMI or unstable angina who have refractory ischemia or hemodynamic or electrical instability should undergo cardiac catheterization with the intent to revascularize ischemic myocardium in the absence of serious comorbidities or contraindications to such procedures (10). It should be noted, however, that data from quality improvement initiatives and other observational sources do not consistently demonstrate reductions in hospital mortality with an early invasive management strategy in patients 75 years of age or older with NSTE-ACS (7, 198). Therefore, selection of very old patients with NSTEMI for early catheterization and revascularization should be undertaken with due consideration for their overall health status, prognosis, personal preferences, and goals of care.

RISK STRATIFICATION AND INDIVIDUALIZED TREATMENT PLANS

The assessment of risk during and after MI has evolved from simple prediction scores to well-studied, validated approaches to selecting high-risk patients most likely to benefit from further diagnostic and therapeutic measures, and conversely, those with a favorable prognosis who may benefit from a more conservative approach (7, 15). Factors associated with an increased risk for adverse outcomes include older age, anterior MI location, spontaneous recurrent ischemia, residual ischemia on stress testing among patients who have not undergone coronary revascularization, reduced left ventricular systolic function (especially ejection fraction <40%), frequent premature ventricular contractions or higher grades of ventricular ectopy, reduced heart rate variability, higher peak cardiac biomarkers, and elevation of other biomarkers such as fibrinogen or C-reactive protein (199–201).

The prototypical risk algorithm for NSTE-ACS is the TIMI risk score (202), in which seven bedside variables obtained at hospital admission are used to predict adverse 14-day outcomes. Notably, patients with higher risk characteristics based on the TIMI risk score have been shown to benefit from more intensive therapies (early coronary angiography, higher intensity antithrombotic therapy) (203–205). Although none of the major risk stratification studies have specifically targeted older patients, key factors identified in younger individuals, particularly left ventricular dysfunction and residual myocardial ischemia, almost certainly retain their prognostic significance in older adults. In older patients who are suitable candidates for invasive treatment, further risk stratification is often appropriate and may include an echocardiogram and/or an exercise or pharmacological stress test to determine the extent of residual ischemia (if coronary angiography has not been performed) (206–208). Based on these investigations, additional interventions may be appropriate, such as more intensive anti-ischemic or HF therapies, adjustments to the timing and intensity of cardiac rehabilitation, or consideration for future ICD therapy. Although further study is needed to define the optimal approach to managing high-risk older patients, those with higher-risk markers after MI should be scheduled for early and more frequent outpatient follow-up visits after hospital discharge to allow careful adjustment of therapies designed to maximize recovery after MI and minimize the risk for recurrent events.

An important consideration in patients with ACS is the competing goal to provide evidence-based therapy for improving clinical outcomes versus a realistic appraisal of recovery in those with advanced age or frailty. In one large database of more than 565,000 patients with ACS in England between 2010 and 2015, more than 1 in 6 patients met criteria for moderate or severe frailty, and these individuals were treated with substantially lower rates of angiography and coronary revascularization (209). Although the more frail patients had higher rates of all cardiovascular events (MI, stroke, rehospitalization, bleeding events, cardiovascular death, all-cause death), revascularization in this population was associated with significantly lower rates of both 1-year and 5-year mortality. Thus, revascularization in ACS should not be withheld on the basis or age or frailty alone, as long as the patient, family, and treating physicians agree that revascularization is a suitable option following a realistic assessment of potential risks and benefits.

Noncardiac issues

As with other acute medical problems, hospitalization in older patients with acute MI often identifies other medical, functional, and psychosocial issues that require attention before hospital discharge. Some older patients are found to have concerns about self-care at home, and medication adherence and polypharmacy may challenge efforts to reduce the risk of recurrent cardiovascular events in older patients after MI. Cognitive impairment may lead to missed doses of medications, inability to recall instructions, or confusion about the multiple therapies prescribed. Substantial effort has been devoted to these issues in contemporary guidelines (7, 9, 210). Instructions must be discussed clearly with both patients and caregivers, and close attention to drug-drug interactions and medication side effects is needed. These concerns are particularly relevant for antiplatelet therapies after MI, as premature discontinuation of these agents is the primary cause of short-term stent thrombosis, reinfarction, and cardiovascular death (211).

Other supportive measures during and after MI are important as well. For example, hospitalized patients with acute MI commonly receive narcotics and are relatively bedbound (especially in the intensive care unit), so implementation of a bowel regimen is important for these individuals—many of whom already have impaired bowel function (210). Cardiac rehabilitation remains underutilized in the geriatric population despite proven reductions in mortality and improvements in quality of life (212), although referral rates have increased in recent years (213). Older patients unable to attend formal cardiac rehabilitation for logistical or transportation reasons should be referred for inpatient cardiac rehabilitation or a home-based rehabilitation program, if available.

Ethical issues

Cardiovascular guidelines and quality metrics refer to "class I indications" as those that are generally applicable to every patient with the condition, and to "class III indications" as those interventions considered contraindicated for all (or almost all) patients. However, there is substantial variability in mental status, functional status, and frailty within the geriatric population. Some 85-year-old patients live independently and play tennis regularly, while other 85-year-old patients have advanced dementia or severe orthopedic limitations and live in a nursing home. The recommendations in this chapter acknowledge that not all patients should receive every intervention, and that multiple factors must be taken into consideration during the decision-making process. Among these are the wishes of the patient, as expressed either directly or through a prior communication such as a living will; the anticipated impact of the intervention on quality of life and long-term prognosis; the potential for the intervention itself to add to versus subtract from the patient's suffering; and the concerns of the patient's family and friends. Moreover, therapies designed to reduce mortality may not always be appropriate for debilitated older patients with poor baseline quality of life; conversely, those therapies designed to provide comfort and improve health status are often not emphasized in contemporary clinical trials and guidelines (8, 214).

The clinician's role in guiding these decisions is critically important, and a high level of compassion, honesty, and respect for the patient's autonomy is required. Thus, the clinician must provide a balanced view of the available therapeutic options, including a realistic appraisal of the likelihood of various outcomes and adverse events. The clinician should avoid creating an overly grim picture, but must also avoid fostering unrealistic hopes. When the patient's condition is such that death seems inevitable, the clinician must be able to provide appropriate counsel to forego or withdraw interventions that

Table 10.2 Efficacy of selected treatments for acute myocardial infarction in older patients

Effective	Probably effective	Uncertain efficacy	Ineffective or less effective due to safety concerns
Acute phase			
Aspirin	β-Blockers[a]	Nitrates, morphine	Calcium channel blockers
IV heparin, LMWH[a]	ACE inhibitors[a]	Eplerenone[a]	Empiric magnesium
Fibrinolysis[a]	Statins	Warfarin, rivaroxaban[a]	Antiarrhythmic agents
Primary PCI[a]	Keep glucose <180 mg/dL	GP IIb/IIIa inhibitors[a]	Erythropoietin
Early revascularization[b]		Cangrelor	Prasugrel
Clopidogrel, ticagrelor		Bivalirudin[a]	
Chronic phase			
Aspirin	SGLT-2 inhibitors[c]	Warfarin, rivaroxaban[a]	Antiarrhythmic agents
β-Blockers	GLP-1 agonists[c]	Eplerenone, spironolactone[a]	Prasugrel
ACE inhibitors	Later coronary revascularization[a]		
Statins			
Clopidogrel, ticagrelor	ICD[a]		

Abbreviations: ACE, angiotensin-converting enzyme; GLP-1, glucagon-like peptide type 1; GP, glycoprotein; ICD, implantable cardioverter-defibrillator; IV, intravenous; LMWH, low-molecular-weight heparin; PCI, percutaneous coronary intervention; SGLT2, sodium-glucose cotransporter type 2.

[a] Selected subgroups; see text.

[b] For non-ST-elevation acute coronary syndromes.

are unlikely to be helpful and which will only serve to prolong the dying process. In addition, the clinician must provide comfort and emotional support for the patient and family. In this regard, the importance of the nursing staff, members of the clergy, and other health professionals (e.g., palliative care) in helping the patient and family deal with emotional issues and other concerns cannot be overemphasized.

CONCLUSION

In summary, acute MI occurs at increasing frequency with advancing age, and older patients with acute MI are at increased risk for major complications, including HF, arrhythmias and conduction disturbances, cardiogenic shock, and death. Older patients thus comprise a large high-risk subgroup of the MI population who may derive substantial benefits from appropriately selected therapeutic interventions. At the same time, many interventions are associated with increased risk in older adults, so that individualization of treatment is essential. Optimal therapy is thus based on a careful risk-benefit assessment of the available treatment options in conjunction with appropriate consideration of patient preferences and other relevant factors.

When an older individual with acute MI is considered a suitable candidate for medical and/or procedural therapies, efficacy and safety are generally extrapolated from subgroup analyses of large clinical trials, or from observational studies or smaller clinical trials focused specifically on the management of older patients. Table 10.2 summarizes the overall efficacy of selected treatments for acute MI in the geriatric population.

As the age of the population continues to increase, the number of older patients at risk for acute MI will rise commensurately. Although progressively more sophisticated interventions may result in sizable reductions in post-MI morbidity and mortality, given the high risk of adverse outcomes in the older population, prevention remains the best treatment to minimize the risk of acute cardiac events. Thus, the greatest potential for the future, as well as the greatest challenge, will be to develop more effective strategies for reducing the onset and progression of atherosclerosis and conquer the epidemic of coronary heart disease in our aging population.

GUIDELINE RECOMMENDATIONS

- The 2025 ACC/AHA guideline for the management of patients with acute coronary syndromes (ACS) offers no specific recommendations for the management of older adults or frail patients with ACS.
- The 2023 European Guidelines for the management of ACS acknowledge the paucity of data on the management of adults over 80 years of age with ACS as well as patients with frailty, but make several recommendations based on available evidence (215).
- Management should be individualized based on patient characteristics (life expectancy, comorbidities, cognitive function, functional status, frailty), patient values and preferences, and an assessment of the benefits and risks of specific interventions.

- Primary PCI should be considered in almost all patients with STEMI, regardless of age, if it can be performed in a timely manner.
- Routine assessment of frailty (e.g., Rockwood Frailty Score) and comorbidity burden (e.g., Charlson index) are recommended in older patients as an aid to clinical decision-making.

REFERENCES

1. Martin SS, et al. 2024 heart disease and stroke statistics: a report of US and global data from the American Heart Association. *Circulation* (2024). Published online January 24, 2024. doi 10.1161/CIR.0000000000001209
2. Canto JG, et al. Association of age and sex with myocardial infarction symptom presentation and in-hospital mortality. *JAMA* (2012). doi: 10.1001/jama.2012.199
3. Alexander KP, et al. Acute coronary care in the elderly, part II: ST-segment-elevation myocardial infarction. *Circulation* (2007). doi: 10.1161/CIRCULATIONAHA.107.182616
4. Forman DE, et al. Comparison of outcomes in patients aged <75, 75 to 84, and ≥85 years with ST-elevation myocardial infarction (from the ACTION Registry-GWTG). *Am J Cardiol* (2010). doi: 10.1016/j.amjcard.2010.07.008
5. Mehta RH, et al. Acute myocardial infarction in the elderly: differences by age. *J Am Coll Cardiol* (2001). doi: 10.1016/s0735-1097(01)01432-2
6. Alexander KP, et al. Evolution in cardiovascular care for elderly patients with non-ST-segment elevation acute coronary syndromes: results from CRUSADE Quality Improvement Initiative. *J Am Coll Cardiol* (2005). doi: 10.1016/j.jacc.2005.05.084
7. Alexander KP, et al. Acute coronary care in the elderly, part I: non-ST-segment-elevation acute coronary syndromes. *Circulation* (2007). doi: 10.1161/CIRCULATIONAHA.107.182615
8. Stolker JM, et al. Rethinking composite endpoints in clinical trials: insights from patients and trialists. *Circulation* (2014). doi: 10.1161/CIRCULATIONAHA.113.006588
9. O'Gara PT, et al. 2013 ACCF/AHA guideline for the management of ST-elevation myocardial infarction. *J Am Coll Cardiol* (2013). doi: 10.1007/s12350-013-9808-x
10. Amsterdam EA, et al. 2014 AHA/ACC guideline for the management of patients with non–ST-elevation acute coronary syndromes. *J Am Coll Cardiol* (2014). doi: 10.1016/j.jacc.2014.09.017
11. ISIS-2 (Second International Study of Infarct Survival) Collaborative Group. Randomised trial of intravenous streptokinase, oral aspirin, both, or neither among 17187 cases of suspected acute myocardial infarction: ISIS-2. *Lancet* (1988). PMID: 2899772
12. Antiplatelet Trialists' Collaboration. Collaborative overview of randomised trials of anti-platelet therapy. *Br Med J* (1994). PMID: 8298418
13. Antithrombotic Trialists' Collaboration. Collaborative meta-analysis of randomised trials of antiplatelet therapy for prevention of death, myocardial infarction, and stroke in high risk patients. *BMJ* (2002). doi: 10.1136/bmj.324.7329.71
14. Wiebe J, et al. Early aspirin discontinuation after coronary stenting: a systematic review and meta-analysis. *JAHA* (2021). doi: 10.1161/JAHA.120.018304
15. Rao SV, et al. 2025 ACC/AHA/ACEP/NAEMSP/SCAI guideline for the management of patients with acute coronary syndromes. *J Am Coll Cardiol* (2025). doi: 10.1016/j.jacc.2024.11.009
16. The Clopidogrel in Unstable Angina to Prevent Recurrent Events (CURE) Trial Investigators. Effects of clopidogrel in addition to aspirin in patients with acute coronary syndromes without ST-segment elevation. *N Engl J Med* (2001). doi: 10.1056/NEJMoa010746
17. Wiviott SD, et al. Prasugrel versus clopidogrel in patients with acute coronary syndromes. *N Engl J Med* (2007). doi: 10.1056/NEJMoa0706482
18. Roe MT, et al. for the TRILOGY-ACS Investigators. Prasugrel versus clopidogrel for acute coronary syndromes without revascularization. *N Engl J Med* (2012). doi: 10.1056/NEJMoa1205512
19. Lawton JS, et al. 2021 ACC/AHA/SCAI guideline for coronary artery revascularization. *J Am Coll Cardiol* (2022). doi: 10.1016/j.jacc.2021.09.006
20. Wallentin L, et al. Ticagrelor versus clopidogrel in patients with acute coronary syndromes. *N Engl J Med* (2009). doi: 10.1056/NEJMoa0904327
21. Gurbel PA, et al. Randomized double-blind assessment of the ONSET and OFFSET of the antiplatelet effects of ticagrelor versus clopidogrel in patients with stable coronary artery disease: the ONSET/OFFSET study. *Circulation* (2009). doi: 10.1161/CIRCULATIONAHA.109.912550
22. Husted S, et al. Ticagrelor versus clopidogrel in elderly patients with acute coronary syndromes: a substudy from the prospective randomized PLATelet inhibition and patient Outcomes (PLATO) trial. *Circ Cardiovasc Qual Outcomes* (2012). doi: 10.1161/CIRCOUTCOMES.111.964395
23. Bonaca MP, et al. Long-term use of ticagrelor in patients with prior myocardial infarction. *N Engl J Med* (2015). doi: 10.1056/NEJMc1508692
24. Udell JA, et al. Long-term dual antiplatelet therapy for secondary prevention of cardiovascular events in the subgroup of patients with previous myocardial infarction: a collaborative meta-analysis of randomized trials. *Eur Heart J* (2016). doi: 10.1093/eurheartj/ehv443
25. Mauri L, et al. Twelve or 30 months of dual antiplatelet therapy after drug-eluting stents. *N Engl J Med* (2014). doi: 10.1056/NEJMoa1409312
26. Kubica J, et al. Impact of morphine on antiplatelet effects of oral P2Y12 receptor inhibitors. *Int J Cardiol* (2016). doi: 10.1016/j.ijcard.2016.04.077

27. Bhatt DL, et al. Effect of platelet inhibition with cangrelor during PCI on ischemic events. *N Engl J Med* (2013). doi: 10.1056/NEJMoa1300815
28. Schneider DJ. Anti-platelet therapy: glycoprotein IIb-IIIa antagonists. *Br J Clin Pharmacol* (2011). doi: 10.1111/j.1365-2125.2010.03879.x
29. Ndrepepa G, et al. Age-dependent effect of abciximab in patients with acute coronary syndromes treated with percutaneous coronary interventions. *Circulation* (2006). doi: 10.1161/CIRCULATIONAHA.106.642306
30. De Luca G, et al. Meta-analysis of randomized trials of glycoprotein IIb/IIIa inhibitors in high-risk acute coronary syndromes patients undergoing invasive strategy. *Am J Cardiol* (2011). doi: 10.1016/j.amjcard.2010.08.063
31. Iakovou I, et al. Comparison of effect of glycoprotein IIb/IIIa inhibitors during percutaneous coronary interventions on risk of hemorrhagic stroke in patients >or=75 years of age versus those <75 years of age. *Am J Cardiol* (2003). doi: 10.1016/j.amjcard.2003.07.007
32. Eikelboom JW, et al. Unfractionated and low-molecular-weight heparin as adjuncts to thrombolysis in aspirin-treated patients with ST-elevation acute myocardial infarction: a meta-analysis of the randomized trials. *Circulation* (2005). doi: 10.1161/CIRCULATIONAHA.105.573550
33. Alexander KP, et al. Excess dosing of antiplatelet and antithrombin agents in the treatment of non-ST-segment elevation acute coronary syndromes. *JAMA* (2005). doi: 10.1001/jama.294.24.3108
34. Mehran R, et al. Bivalirudin in patients undergoing primary angioplasty for acute myocardial infarction (HORIZONS-AMI): 1-year results of a randomised controlled trial. *Lancet* (2009). doi: 10.1016/S0140-6736(09)61484-7
35. Erlinge D, et al. Bivalirudin versus heparin monotherapy in myocardial infarction. *N Engl J Med* (2017). doi: 10.1056/NEJMoa1706443
36. Hurlen M, et al. Warfarin, aspirin, or both after myocardial infarction. *N Engl J Med* (2002). doi: 10.1056/NEJMoa020496
37. van Es RF, et al. Aspirin and coumadin after acute coronary syndromes (the ASPECT-2 study): a randomised controlled trial. *Lancet* (2002). doi: 10.1016/S0140-6736(02)09409-6
38. Turpie AGG, et al. Venous thromboembolism: pathophysiology, clinical features, and prevention. *BMJ* (2002). doi: 10.1136/bmj.325.7369.887
39. Mega JL, et al. Rivaroxaban in patients with a recent acute coronary syndrome. *N Engl J Med* (2012). doi: 10.1056/NEJMoa1112277
40. Eikelboom JW, et al. Rivaroxaban with or without aspirin in stable cardiovascular disease. *N Engl J Med* (2017). doi: 10.1056/NEJMoa1709118
41. Alexander JH, et al. Apixaban with antiplatelet therapy after acute coronary syndrome. *N Engl J Med* (2011). doi: 10.1056/NEJMoa1105819
42. OASIS-V Investigators. Comparison of fondaparinux and enoxaparin in acute coronary syndromes. *N Engl J Med* (2006). doi: 10.1056/NEJMoa055443
43. Yusuf S, et al. Effects of fondaparinux on mortality and reinfarction in patients with acute ST-segment elevation myocardial infarction: the OASIS-6 randomized trial. *JAMA* (2006). doi: 10.1001/jama.295.13.joc60038
44. ASSENT-3 Investigators. Efficacy and safety of tenecteplase in combination with enoxaparin, abciximab, or unfractionated heparin: ASSENT-3. *Lancet* (2001). doi: 10.1016/S0140-6736(01)05775-0
45. Krumholz HM, et al. Use and effectiveness of intravenous heparin therapy for treatment of acute myocardial infarction in the elderly. *J Am Coll Cardiol* (1998). doi: 10.1016/s0735-1097(98)00022-9
46. Bhatt DL, et al. Clopidogrel with or without omeprazole in coronary artery disease. *N Engl J Med* (2010). doi: 10.1056/NEJMoa1007964
47. Vardi M, et al. The effects of proton pump inhibition on patient-reported severity of dyspepsia when receiving dual anti-platelet therapy with clopidogrel and low-dose aspirin: analysis from the clopidogrel and the optimization of gastrointestinal events trial. *Aliment Pharmacol Ther* (2015). doi: 10.1111/apt.13260
48. Vaduganathan M, et al. Proton-pump inhibitors reduce gastrointestinal events regardless of aspirin dose in patients requiring dual antiplatelet therapy. *J Am Coll Cardiol* (2016). doi: 10.1016/j.jacc.2015.12.068
49. Hess CN, et al. Use and outcomes of triple therapy among older patients with acute myocardial infarction and atrial fibrillation. *J Am Coll Cardiol* (2015). doi: 10.1016/j.jacc.2015.05.062
50. Dewilde WJM, et al. Use of clopidogrel with or without aspirin in patients taking oral anticoagulant therapy and undergoing percutaneous coronary intervention: an open-label, randomised, controlled trial. *Lancet* (2013). doi: 10.1016/S0140-6736(12)62177-1
51. Becker RC, et al. The primary and secondary prevention of coronary artery disease: American College of Chest Physicians evidence-based clinical practice guidelines (8th edition). *Chest* (2008). doi: 10.1378/chest.08-0685
52. Sourgounis A, et al. Coronary stents and chronic anticoagulation. *Circulation* (2009). doi: 10.1161/CIRCULATIONAHA.108.834861
53. Stolker JM, et al. Chapter 13: Diagnosis and management of heart disease in older adults. In: *Reichel's Care of the Elderly: Clinical Aspects of Aging*, eighth edition. New York, NY: Cambridge University Press (2022).
54. Roberts R, et al. Immediate vs. deferred β-blockade following thrombolytic therapy in patients with acute myocardial infarction: TIMI II-B study. *Circulation* (1991). doi: 10.1161/01.cir.83.2.422
55. The TIMI Study Group. Comparison of invasive and conservative strategies after treatment with intravenous tissue plasminogen activator in acute myocardial infarction. TIMI Phase II Trial. *N Engl J Med* (1989). doi: 10.1056/NEJM198903093201002

56. Wienbergen H, et al. Prognostic impact of acute beta-blocker therapy on top of aspirin and angiotensin-converting enzyme inhibitor therapy in consecutive patients with ST-elevation acute myocardial infarction. *Am J Cardiol* (2007). doi: 10.1016/j.amjcard.2006.12.036
57. Piccini JP, et al. Relation of mortality to failure to prescribe beta blockers acutely in patients with sustained ventricular tachycardia and ventricular fibrillation following acute myocardial infarction (from the VALIANT registry). *Am J Cardiol* (2008). doi: 10.1016/j.amjcard.2008.07.033
58. COMMIT (Clopidogrel and Metoprolol in Myocardial Infarction Trial) Collaborative Group. Early intravenous then oral metoprolol in 45,852 patients with acute myocardial infarction: randomised placebo-controlled trial. *Lancet* (2005). doi: 10.1016/S0140-6736(05)67661-1
59. The CAPRICORN Investigators. Effect of carvedilol on outcome after myocardial infarction in patients with left-ventricular dysfunction: the CAPRICORN randomised trial. *Lancet* (2001). doi: 10.1016/s0140-6736(00)04560-8
60. Soumerai SB, et al. Adverse outcomes of under use of β-blocker in elderly survivors of acute myocardial infarction. *JAMA* (1997). PMID: 8990335
61. Krumholz HM, et al. National use and effectiveness of β-blockers for the treatment of elderly patients after acute myocardial infarction. *JAMA* (1998). doi: 10.1001/jama.280.7.623
62. Krumholz HM, et al. Early β-blocker therapy for acute myocardial infarction in elderly patients. *Ann Intern Med* (1999). doi: 10.7326/0003-4819-131-9-199911020-00003
63. Rochon PA, et al. Rate of heart failure and 1-year survival for older people receiving low-dose beta-blocker therapy after myocardial infarction. *Lancet* (2000). doi: 10.1016/S0140-6736(00)02606-4
64. Swedberg K, et al. Effects of early administration of enalapril on mortality in patients with acute myocardial infarction. results of CONSENSUS II. *N Engl J Med* (1992). doi: 10.1056/NEJM199209033271002
65. Gruppo Italiano per lo Studio della Sopravvivenza nell'Infarto Miocardico. GISSI-3: effects of lisinopril and transdermal glyceryl trinitrate singly and together on 6-week mortality and ventricular function after acute myocardial infarction. *Lancet* (1994). PMID: 7910229
66. ISIS-4 Collaborative Group. ISIS-4: a randomised factorial trial assessing early oral captopril, oral mononitrate and intravenous magnesium sulphate in 58,050 patients with suspected acute myocardial infarction. *Lancet* (1995). PMID: 7661937
67. Gruppo Italiano per lo Studio della Sopravvivenza nell'Infarto Miocardico. Six-month effects of early treatment with lisinopril and transdermal glyceryl trinitrate singly and together withdrawn six weeks after myocardial infarction: the GISSI-3 Trial. *J Am Coll Cardiol* (1996). PMID: 8557903
68. Ambrosioni E, et al., for the SMILE Study Investigators. The effect of the angiotensin-converting-enzyme inhibitor zofenopril on mortality and morbidity after anterior myocardial infarction. *N Engl J Med* (1995). doi: 10.1056/NEJM199501123320203
69. Pfeffer MA, et al. Effect of captopril on mortality and morbidity in patients with left ventricular dysfunction after myocardial infarction: results of the SAVE trial. *N Engl J Med* (1992). doi: 10.1056/NEJM199209033271001
70. The AIRE Study Investigators. Effect of ramipril on mortality and morbidity of survivors of acute myocardial infarction with clinical evidence of heart failure. *Lancet* (1993). PMID: 8104270
71. Hall AS, on behalf of the AIREX Study Investigators. Follow-up study of patients randomly allocated ramipril or placebo for heart failure after acute myocardial infarction: AIRE Extension (AIREX) Study. *Lancet* (1997). doi: 10.1016/s0140-6736(97)04442-5
72. Krumholz HM, et al. Aspirin and angiotensin-converting enzyme inhibitors among elderly survivors of hospitalization for an acute myocardial infarction. *Arch Intern Med* (2001). doi: 10.1001/archinte.161.4.538
73. Dickstein K, et al. Effects of losartan and captopril on mortality and morbidity in high-risk patients after acute myocardial infarction: the OPTIMAAL randomised trial. *Lancet* (2002). doi: 10.1016/s0140-6736(02)09895-1
74. Pfeffer MA, et al. Valsartan, captopril, or both in myocardial infarction complicated by heart failure, left ventricular dysfunction, or both. *N Engl J Med* (2003). doi: 10.1056/NEJMoa032292
75. White HD, et al. Mortality and morbidity remain high despite captopril and/or valsartan therapy in elderly patients with left ventricular systolic dysfunction, heart failure, or both after acute myocardial infarction. *Circulation* (2005). doi: 10.1161/CIRCULATIONAHA.105.551143
76. Pitt B, et al. Eplerenone, a selective aldosterone blocker, in patients with left ventricular dysfunction after myocardial infarction. *N Engl J Med* (2003). doi: 10.1056/NEJMoa030207
77. Heart Protection Study Collaborative Group. MRC/BHF Heart Protection Study of cholesterol lowering with simvastatin in 20,536 high-risk individuals: a randomised placebo-controlled trial. *Lancet* (2002). doi: 10.1016/S0140-6736(11)61125-2
78. Shepherd J, et al. Pravastatin in elderly individuals at risk of vascular disease (PROSPER): a randomised controlled trial. *Lancet* (2002). doi: 10.1016/s0140-6736(02)11600-x
79. Schwartz GG, et al. Effects of atorvastatin on early recurrent ischemic events in acute coronary syndromes: the MIRACL study. *JAMA* (2001). PMID: 11428488
80. Cannon CP, et al. Intensive versus moderate lipid lowering with statins after acute coronary syndromes. *N Engl J Med* (2004). doi: 10.1056/NEJMoa040583

81. LimSY,etal.Effectonshort-andlong-termmajoradverse cardiac events of statin treatment in patients with acute myocardial infarction and renal dysfunction. *Am J Cardiol* (2012). doi: 10.1016/j.amjcard.2012.01.351
82. Cannon CP, et al. Ezetimibe added to statin therapy after acute coronary syndromes. *N Engl J Med* (2015). doi: 10.1056/NEJMoa1410489
83. Schwartz GG, et al. Alirocumab and cardiovascular outcomes after acute coronary syndrome. *N Engl J Med* (2018). doi: 10.1056/NEJMoa1801174
84. Sabatine MS, et al. Evolocumab and clinical outcomes in patients with cardiovascular disease. *N Engl J Med* (2017). doi: 10.1056/NEJMoa1615664
85. Nissen SE, et al. Bempedoic acid and cardiovascular outcomes in statin-intolerant patients. *N Engl J Med* (2023). doi: 10.1056/NEJMoa2215024
86. Bhatt DL, et al. Cardiovascular risk reduction with icosapent ethyl for hypertriglyceridemia. *N Engl J Med* (2019). doi: 10.1056/NEJMoa1812792
87. Lloyd-Jones DM, et al. 2022 ACC expert consensus decision pathway on the role of nonstatin therapies for LDL-cholesterol lowering in the management of atherosclerotic cardiovascular disease: a report of the ACC Solution Set Oversight Committee. *J Am Coll Cardiol* (2022). doi: 10.1016/j.jacc.2022.07.006
88. Zinman B, et al. Empagliflozin, cardiovascular outcomes, and mortality in type 2 diabetes. *N Engl J Med* (2015). doi: 10.1056/NEJMc1600827
89. Neal B, et al. Canagliflozin and cardiovascular and renal events in type 2 diabetes. *N Engl J Med* (2017). doi: 10.1056/NEJMc1712572
90. Wiviott SD, et al. Dapagliflozin and cardiovascular outcomes in type 2 diabetes. *N Engl J Med* (2019). doi: 10.1056/NEJMoa1812389
91. Marso SP, et al. Liraglutide and cardiovascular outcomes in type 2 diabetes. *N Engl J Med* (2016). doi: 10.1056/NEJMoa1603827
92. Marso SP, et al. Semaglutide and cardiovascular outcomes in patients with type 2 diabetes. *N Engl J Med* (2016). doi: 10.1056/NEJMoa1607141
93. Lincoff AM, et al. Semaglutide and cardiovascular outcomes in obesity without diabetes. *N Engl J Med* (2023). doi: 10.1056/NEJMoa2307563
94. Gerstein HC, et al. Dulaglutide and cardiovascular outcomes in type 2 diabetes (REWIND): a double-blind, randomised placebo-controlled trial. *Lancet* (2019). doi: 10.1016/S0140-6736(19)31149-3
95. Chaitman BR. Ranolazine for the treatment of chronic angina and potential use in other cardiovascular conditions. *Circulation* (2006). doi: 10.1161/CIRCULATIONAHA.105.597500
96. Morrow DA, et al. Effects of ranolazine on recurrent cardiovascular events in patients with non-ST-elevation acute coronary syndromes: the MERLIN-TIMI 36 randomized trial. *JAMA* (2007). doi: 10.1001/jama.297.16.1775
97. Hine LK, et al. Meta-analytic evidence against prophylactic use of lidocaine in acute myocardial infarction. *Arch Intern Med* (1989). PMID: 2688587
98. Moss AJ, et al. Improved survival with an implanted defibrillator in patients with coronary disease at high risk for ventricular arrhythmia. MADIT trial investigators. *N Engl J Med* (1996). doi: 10.1056/NEJM199612263352601
99. Moss AJ, et al. Prophylactic implantation of a defibrillator in patients with myocardial infarction and reduced ejection fraction. *N Engl J Med* (2002). doi: 10.1056/NEJMoa013474
100. Hohnloser SH, et al. Prophylactic use of an implantable cardioverter-defibrillator after acute myocardial infarction. *N Engl J Med* (2004). doi: 10.1056/NEJMoa041489
101. Steinbeck G, et al. Defibrillator implantation early after myocardial infarction. *N Engl J Med* (2009). doi: 10.1056/NEJMoa0901889
102. Santangeli P, et al. Meta-analysis: age and effectiveness of prophylactic implantable cardioverter-defibrillators. *Ann Intern Med* (2010). doi: 10.7326/0003-4819-153-9-201011020-00009
103. Epstein AE, et al. 2012 ACCF/AHA/HRS focused update incorporated into the ACCF/AHA/HRS 2008 guidelines for device-based therapy of cardiac rhythm abnormalities. *J Am Coll Cardiol* (2013). doi: 10.1016/j.jacc.2012.11.007
104. Lampert R, et al. HRS expert consensus statement on the management of cardiovascular implantable electronic devices in patients nearing end of life or requesting withdrawal of therapy. *Heart Rhythm* (2010). doi: 10.1016/j.hrthm.2010.04.033
105. Olgin JE, et al. Wearable cardioverter-defibrillator after myocardial infarction. *N Engl J Med* (2018). doi: 10.1056/NEJMoa1800781
106. Shah P, et al. Outcomes and quality of life in patients ≥85 years of age with ST-elevation myocardial infarction. *Am J Cardiol* (2009). doi: 10.1016/j.amjcard.2008.08.051
107. Biscaglia S, et al. for the FIRE Trial Investigators. Complete or culprit-only PCI in older patients with myocardial infarction. *N Engl J Med* (2023). doi: 10.1056/NEJMoa2300468
108. Campo G, et al. Complete versus culprit-only revascularization in older patients with ST-segment elevation myocardial infarction: an individual patient meta-analysis. *Circulation* (2024). doi: 10.1161/CIRCULATIONAHA.124.071493
109. Fibrinolytic Therapy Trialists' (FTT) Collaborative Group. Indications for fibrinolytic therapy in suspected acute myocardial infarction: collaborative overview of early mortality and major morbidity results from all randomised trials of more than 1000 patients. *Lancet* (1994). PMID: 7905143
110. White HD. Thrombolytic therapy in the elderly. *Lancet* (2000). doi: 10.1016/S0140-6736(00)03397-3
111. Thiemann DR, et al. Lack of benefit for intravenous thrombolysis in patients with myocardial infarction who are older than 75 years. *Circulation* (2000). doi: 10.1161/01.cir.101.19.2239

112. Soumerai SB, et al. Effectiveness of thrombolytic therapy for acute myocardial infarction in the elderly: cause for concern in the old-old. *Arch Intern Med* (2002). doi: 10.1001/archinte.162.5.561
113. Stenestrand U, et al. Fibrinolytic therapy in patients 75 years and older with ST-segment-elevation myocardial infarction: one-year follow-up of a large prospective cohort. *Arch Intern Med* (2003). doi: 10.1001/archinte.163.8.965
114. Gruppo Italiano per lo Studio della Sopravvivenza nell'Infarto Miocardico. GISSI-2: a factorial randomised trial of alteplase versus streptokinase and heparin versus no heparin among 12490 patients with acute myocardial infarction. *Lancet* (1990). PMID: 1975321
115. The International Study Group. In-hospital mortality and clinical course of 20891 patients with suspected acute myocardial infarction ramdomised between alteplase and streptokinase with or without heparin. *Lancet* (1990). PMID: 1975322
116. ISIS-3 Collaborative Group. ISIS-3: a randomised comparison of streptokinase vs. tissue plasminogen activator vs. anistreplase and of aspirin plus heparin vs. aspirin alone among 41299 cases of suspected acute myocardial infarction. *Lancet* (1992). PMID: 1347801
117. The GUSTO Investigators. An international randomized trial comparing four thrombolytic strategies for acute myocardial infarction. *N Engl J Med* (1993). doi: 10.1056/NEJM199309023291001
118. White HD, et al. Age and outcome with contemporary thrombolytic therapy: results from the GUSTO-I trial. *Circulation* (1996). doi: 10.1161/01.cir.94.8.1826
119. The GUSTO III Investigators. A comparison of reteplase with alteplase for acute myocardial infarction. *N Engl J Med* (1997). doi: 10.1056/NEJM199710163371603
120. ASSENT-2 Investigators. Single-bolus tenecteplase compared with front-loaded alteplase in acute myocardial infarction: the ASSENT-2 double-blind randomised trial. *Lancet* (1999). doi: 10.1016/s0140-6736(99)07403-6
121. Anderson JL, et al. Older age and elevated blood pressure are risk factors for intracerebral hemorrhage after thrombolysis. *Am J Cardiol* (1991). doi: 10.1016/0002-9149(91)90738-7
122. Brass LM, et al. Intracranial hemorrhage associated with thrombolytic therapy for elderly patients with acute myocardial infarction: results from the cooperative cardiovascular project. *Stroke* (2000). doi: 10.1161/01.str.31.8.1802
123. Selker HP, et al. Presenting pulse pressure predicts thrombolytic therapy-related intracranial hemorrhage: Thrombolytic Predictive Instrument (TPI) project results. *Circulation* (1994). doi: 10.1161/01.cir.90.4.1657
124. Boersma E for The Primary Coronary Angioplasty vs. Thrombolysis Group. Does time matter? A pooled analysis of randomized clinical trials comparing primary percutaneous coronary intervention and in-hospital fibrinolysis in acute myocardial infarction patients. *Eur Heart J* (2006). doi: 10.1093/eurheartj/ehi810
125. Simari RD, et al. Coronary angioplasty in acute myocardial infarction: primary, immediate adjunctive, rescue, or deferred adjunctive approach? *Mayo Clin Proc* (1994). doi: 10.1016/s0025-6196(12)62220-4
126. deBoer MJ, et al. Reperfusion therapy in elderly patients with acute myocardial infarction: a randomized comparison of primary angioplasty and thrombolytic therapy. *J Am Coll Cardiol* (2002). doi: 10.1016/s0735-1097(02)01878-8
127. Goldenberg I, et al. Primary angioplasty with routine stenting compared with thrombolytic therapy in elderly patients with acute myocardial infarction. *Am Heart J* (2003). doi: 10.1016/S0002-8703(02)94709-5
128. Grines C. Senior PAMI: a prospective randomized trial of primary angioplasty and thrombolytic therapy in elderly patients with acute myocardial infarction. Presented at Transcatheter Cardiovascular Therapeutics, Washington DC, October 2005.
129. Marso SP, et al. Association between use of bleeding avoidance strategies and risk of periprocedural bleeding among patients undergoing percutaneous coronary intervention. *JAMA* (2010). doi: 10.1001/jama.2010.708
130. Feldman DN, et al. Adoption of radial access and comparison of outcomes to femoral access in percutaneous coronary intervention: an updated report from the NCDR (2007–2012). *Circulation* (2013). doi: 10.1161/CIRCULATIONAHA.112.000536
131. Dzavik V, et al. Early revascularization is associated with improved survival in elderly patients with acute myocardial infarction complicated by cardiogenic shock: a report from the SHOCK trial registry. *Eur Heart J* (2003). doi: 10.1016/s0195-668x(02)00844-8
132. Madsen JK, et al. Danish multicenter randomized study of invasive versus conservative treatment in patients with inducible ischemia after thrombolysis in acute myocardial infarction (DANAMI). *Circulation* (1997). doi: 10.1161/01.cir.96.3.748
133. Gershlick AH, et al. Rescue angioplasty after failed thrombolytic therapy for acute myocardial infarction. *N Engl J Med* (2005). doi: 10.1056/NEJMoa050849
134. Patel TN, et al. A meta-analysis of randomized trials of rescue percutaneous coronary intervention after failed fibrinolysis. *Am J Cardiol* (2006). doi: 10.1016/j.amjcard.2006.01.028
135. Mehta SR, et al. Routine vs selective invasive strategies in patients with acute coronary syndromes: a collaborative meta-analysis of randomized trials. *JAMA* (2005). doi: 10.1001/jama.293.23.2908
136. Bach RG, et al. The effect of routine, early invasive management on outcome for elderly patients with non-ST-segment elevation acute coronary syndromes. *Ann Intern Med* (2004). doi: 10.7326/0003-4819-141-3-200408030-00007

137. Tegn N, et al. Invasive versus conservative strategy in patients aged 80 years or older with non-ST-elevation myocardial infarction or unstable angina pectoris (After Eighty study): an open-label randomised controlled trial. *Lancet* (2016). doi: 10.1016/S0140-6736(15)01166-6
138. Alexander KP, et al. Outcomes of cardiac surgery in patients > or = 80 years: results from the National Cardiovascular Network. *J Am Coll Cardiol* (2000). doi: 10.1016/s0735-1097(99)00606-3
139. Newman MF, et al. Longitudinal assessment of neurocognitive function after coronary-artery bypass surgery. *N Engl J Med* (2001). doi: 10.1056/NEJM200102083440601
140. Mozaffarian D, et al. Heart disease and stroke statistics—2016 update: a report from the American Heart Association. *Circulation* (2016). doi: 10.1161/CIR.0000000000000350
141. Boden WE, et al. Optimal medical therapy with or without PCI for stable coronary disease. *N Engl J Med* (2007). doi: 10.1056/NEJMoa070829
142. Pfisterer M. Long-term outcome in elderly patients with chronic angina managed invasively versus by optimized medical therapy: four-year follow-up of the randomized trial of invasive versus medical therapy in elderly patients (TIME). *Circulation* (2004). doi: 10.1161/01.CIR.0000140983.69571.BA
143. Benedetto U, et al. Coronary artery bypass grafting versus drug-eluting stents in multivessel coronary disease. A meta-analysis on 24,268 patients. *Eur J Cardiothorac Surg* (2009). doi: 10.1016/j.ejcts.2009.03.012
144. Serruys PW, et al. Percutaneous coronary intervention versus coronary-artery bypass grafting for severe coronary artery disease. *N Engl J Med* (2009). doi: 10.1056/NEJMoa0804626
145. Ezekowitz JA, et al. Declining in-hospital mortality and increasing heart failure incidence in elderly patients with first myocardial infarction. *J Am Coll Cardiol* (2009). doi: 10.1016/j.jacc.2008.08.067
146. Rich MW. Epidemiology, pathophysiology, and etiology of congestive heart failure in older adults. *J Am Geriatr Soc* (1997). doi: 10.1111/j.1532-5415.1997.tb02968.x
147. Bayer AJ, et al. Changing presentation of myocardial infarction with increasing age. *J Am Geriatr Soc* (1986). doi: 10.1111/j.1532-5415.1986.tb04221.x
148. Kyriakides ZS, et al. Systolic functional response of normal older and younger adult left ventricles to dobutamine. *Am J Cardiol* (1986). doi: 10.1016/0002-9149(86)90360-7
149. Rich MW, et al. Inotropic response to dobutamine in elderly patients with decompensated heart failure. *Am J Cardiol* (1990). doi: 10.1016/0002-9149(90)90823-j
150. Silke B, et al. Comparative haemodynamic dose-response effects of dobutamine and amrinone in left ventricular failure complicating acute myocardial infarction. *J Cardiovasc Pharmacol* (1987). PMID: 2434789
151. Volpi A, et al. In-hospital prognosis of patients with acute myocardial infarction complicated by primary ventricular fibrillation. *N Engl J Med* (1987). doi: 10.1056/NEJM198707303170501
152. Patel KK, et al. Beyond warfarin: a patient-centered approach to selecting novel oral anticoagulants for stroke prevention in atrial fibrillation. *J Hosp Med* (2014). doi: 10.1002/jhm.2201
153. Link MS, et al. Part 7: Adult advanced cardiovascular life support, 2015 American Heart Association guidelines update for cardiopulmonary resuscitation and emergency cardiovascular care. *Circulation* (2015). doi: 10.1161/CIR.0000000000000261
154. O'Connor RE, et al. Part 9: Acute coronary syndromes, 2015 American Heart Association guidelines update for cardiopulmonary resuscitation and emergency cardiovascular care. *Circulation* (2015). doi: 10.1161/CIR.0000000000000263
155. Bueno H, et al. In-hospital outcome of elderly patients with acute inferior myocardial infarction and right ventricular involvement. *Circulation* (1997). doi: 10.1161/01.cir.96.2.436
156. Zehender M, et al. Right ventricular infarction as an independent predictor of prognosis after acute inferior myocardial infarction. *N Engl J Med* (1993). doi: 10.1056/NEJM199304083281401
157. Yip HK, et al. Cardiac rupture complicating acute myocardial infarction in the direct percutaneous coronary intervention reperfusion era. *Chest* (2003). doi: 10.1378/chest.124.2.565
158. Becker RC, et al. Fatal cardiac rupture among patients treated with fibrinolytic agents and adjunctive thrombin antagonists: observations from the thrombolysis and thrombin inhibition in myocardial infarction 9 study. *J Am Coll Cardiol* (1999). doi: 10.1016/s0735-1097(98)00582-8
159. Solodky A, et al. Comparison of incidence of cardiac rupture among patients with acute myocardial infarction treated by thrombolysis versus percutaneous transluminal coronary angioplasty. *Am J Cardiol* (2001). doi: 10.1016/s0002-9149(01)01471-0
160. Becker RC, et al. A composite view of cardiac rupture in the United States National Registry of Myocardial Infarction. *J Am Coll Cardiol* (1996). doi: 10.1016/0735-1097(96)00008-3
161. Oliva PB, et al. Cardiac rupture, a clinically predictable complication of acute myocardial infarction: report of 70 cases with clinicopathologic correlations. *J Am Coll Cardiol* (1993). doi: 10.1016/0735-1097(93)90182-z
162. Birnbaum Y, et al. Ventricular septal rupture after acute myocardial infarction. *N Engl J Med* (2002). doi: 10.1056/NEJMra020228
163. Figueras J, et al. Medical management of selected patients with left ventricular free wall rupture during acute myocardial infarction. *J Am Coll Cardiol* (1997). doi: 10.1016/s0735-1097(96)00542-6

164. Raitt MH, et al. Subacute ventricular free wall rupture complicating myocardial infarction. *Am Heart J* (1993). doi: 10.1016/0002-8703(93)90711-h
165. Menon V, et al. Management of cardiogenic shock complicating acute myocardial infarction. *Heart* (2002). doi: 10.1136/heart.88.5.531
166. Leor J, et al. Cardiogenic shock complicating acute myocardial infarction in patients without heart failure on admission: incidence, risk factors, and outcome. *Am J Med* (1993). doi: 10.1016/0002-9343(93)90058-w
167. Goldberg RJ, et al. Cardiogenic shock after acute myocardial infarction. incidence and mortality from a community-wide perspective, 1975 to 1988. *N Engl J Med* (1991). doi: 10.1056/NEJM199110173251601
168. Berger AK, et al. Cardiogenic shock complicating acute myocardial infarction in elderly patients: does admission to a tertiary center improve survival? *Am Heart J* (2002). doi: 10.1067/mhj.2002.122289
169. Hochman JS, et al. Early revascularization in acute myocardial infarction complicated by cardiogenic shock. SHOCK Investigators. *N Engl J Med* (1999). doi: 10.1056/NEJM199908263410901
170. Hochman JS, et al. Cardiogenic shock complicating acute myocardial infarction—etiologies, management, and outcome: a report from the SHOCK trial registry. *J Am Coll Cardiol* (2000). doi: 10.1016/s0735-1097(00)00879-2
171. Thiele H, et al. for the CULPRIT-SHOCK Investigators. PCI strategies with acute myocardial infarction and cardiogenic shock. *N Engl J Med* (2017). doi: 10.1056/NEJMc1802622
172. Anderson RD, et al. Use of intra-aortic balloon counterpulsation in patients presenting with cardiogenic shock: observations from the GUSTO-I Study. *J Am Coll Cardiol* (1997). doi: 10.1016/s0735-1097(97)00227-1
173. Seyfarth M, et al. A randomized clinical trial to evaluate the safety and efficacy of a percutaneous left ventricular assist device versus intra-aortic balloon pumping for treatment of cardiogenic shock caused by myocardial infarction. *J Am Coll Cardiol* (2008). doi: 10.1016/j.jacc.2008.05.065
174. Thiele H, et al. Intraaortic balloon support for myocardial infarction with cardiogenic shock. *N Engl J Med* (2012). doi: 10.1056/NEJMoa1208410
175. Dixon SR, et al. A prospective feasibility trial investigating the use of the Impella 2.5 system in patients undergoing high-risk percutaneous coronary intervention (The PROTECT I Trial): initial U.S. experience. *JACC Cardiovasc Interv* (2009). doi: 10.1016/j.jcin.2008.11.005
176. O'Neill WW, et al. A prospective, randomized clinical trial of hemodynamic support with Impella 2.5 versus intra-aortic balloon pump in patients undergoing high-risk percutaneous coronary intervention: the PROTECT II study. *Circulation* (2012). doi: 10.1161/CIRCULATIONAHA.112.098194
177. Klein A, et al. Treating older patients in cardiogenic shock with a microaxial flow pump: is it DANGERous? *J Am Coll Cardiol* (2025). doi: 10.1016/j.jacc.2024.11.003
178. Moller JE, et al. Microaxial flow pump or standard care in infarct-related cardiogenic shock. *N Engl J Med* (2024). doi: 10.1056/NEJMoa2312572
179. Norhammar A, et al. Glucose metabolism in patients with acute myocardial infarction and no previous diagnosis of diabetes mellitus: a prospective study. *Lancet* (2002). doi: 10.1016/S0140-6736(02)09089-X
180. Capes SE, et al. Stress hyperglycaemia and increased risk of death after myocardial infarction in patients with and without diabetes: a systematic overview. *Lancet* (2000). doi: 10.1016/S0140-6736(99)08415-9
181. Kosiborod M, et al. Admission glucose and mortality in elderly patients hospitalized with acute myocardial infarction: implications for patients with and without recognized diabetes. *Circulation* (2005). doi: 10.1161/CIRCULATIONAHA.104.517839
182. Stranders I, et al. Admission blood glucose level as risk indicator of death after myocardial infarction in patients with and without diabetes mellitus. *Arch Intern Med* (2004). doi: 10.1001/archinte.164.9.982
183. Malmberg K, et al. Randomized trial of insulin-glucose infusion followed by subcutaneous insulin treatment in diabetic patients with acute myocardial infarction (DIGAMI study): effects on mortality at 1 year. *J Am Coll Cardiol* (1995). doi: 10.1016/0735-1097(95)00126-k
184. Malmberg K, et al. Intense metabolic control by means of insulin in patients with diabetes mellitus and acute myocardial infarction (DIGAMI-2): effects on mortality and morbidity. *Eur Heart J* (2005). doi: 10.1093/eurheartj/ehi199
185. Najjar SS, et al. Intravenous erythropoietin in patients with ST-segment elevation myocardial infarction. REVEAL: a randomized controlled trial. *JAMA* (2011). doi: 10.1001/jama.2011.592
186. Gonzalez-Juanatey JR, et al. One-year major cardiovascular events after restrictive versus liberal blood transfusion strategy in patients with acute myocardial infarction and anemia: the REALITY randomized trial. *Circulation* (2022). doi: 10.1161/CIRCULATIONAHA.121.057909
187. Carson JL, et al. Restrictive or liberal transfusion strategy in myocardial infarction and anemia. *N Engl J Med* (2023). doi: 10.1056/NEJMoa2307983
188. Rogers WJ, et al. Trends in presenting characteristics and hospital mortality among patients with ST elevation and non-ST elevation myocardial infarction in the National Registry of Myocardial Infarction from 1990 to 2006. *Am Heart J* (2008). doi: 10.1016/j.ahj.2008.07.030
189. Thygesen K, et al. Third universal definition of myocardial infarction. *Eur Heart J* (2012). doi: 10.1093/eurheartj/ehy655

190. Berger CJ, et al. Prognosis after first myocardial infarction. Comparison of Q-wave and non-Q-wave myocardial infarction in the Framingham Heart Study. *JAMA* (1992). doi: 10.1001/jama.268.12.1545
191. Chung MK, et al. Prognosis of patients is ≥70 years of age with non-Q-wave acute myocardial infarction compared with younger patients with similar infarcts and with patients ≥70 years of age with Q-wave acute myocardial infarction. *Am J Cardiol* (1995). doi: 10.1016/s0002-9149(99)80519-0
192. Fragmin and Fast Revascularization during Instability in Coronary artery disease Investigators. Invasive compared with non-invasive treatment in unstable coronary-artery disease: FRISC II prospective randomised multicentre study. *Lancet* (1999). PMID: 10475181
193. Wallentin L, et al. Outcome at 1 year after an invasive compared with a non-invasive strategy in unstable coronary-artery disease: the FRISC II invasive randomized trial. *Lancet* (2000). doi: 10.1016/s0140-6736(00)02427-2
194. Cannon CP, et al. Comparison of early invasive and conservative strategies in patients with unstable coronary syndromes treated with the glycoprotein IIb/IIIa inhibitor tirofiban. *N Engl J Med* (2001). doi: 10.1056/NEJM200106213442501
195. Fox KA, et al. Interventional versus conservative treatment for patients with unstable angina or non-ST-elevation myocardial infarction: the British Heart Foundation RITA 3 randomised trial. *Lancet* (2002). doi: 10.1016/s0140-6736(02)09894-x
196. Spacek R, et al. Value of first day angiography/angioplasty in evolving non-ST segment elevation myocardial infarction: an open multicenter randomized trial. The VINO study. *Eur Heart J* (2002). doi: 10.1053/euhj.2001.2735
197. DeWinter RJ, et al. Early invasive versus selectively invasive management for acute coronary syndromes. *N Engl J Med* (2005). doi: 10.1056/NEJMoa044259
198. Bhatt DL, et al. Utilization of early invasive management strategies for high-risk patients with non-ST-segment elevation acute coronary syndromes: results from the CRUSADE quality improvement initiative. *JAMA* (2004). doi: 10.1001/jama.292.17.2096
199. Kleiger RE, et al. Decreased heart rate variability and its association with increased mortality after acute myocardial infarction. *Am J Cardiol* (1987). doi: 10.1016/0002-9149(87)90795-8
200. Toss H, et al. Prognostic influence of increased fibrinogen and C-reactive protein levels in unstable coronary artery disease. *Circulation* (1997). doi: 10.1161/01.cir.96.12.4204
201. Tommasi S, et al. C-reactive protein as a marker for cardiac ischemic events in the year after a first, uncomplicated myocardial infarction. *Am J Cardiol* (1999). doi: 10.1016/s0002-9149(99)00162-9
202. Antman EM, et al. The TIMI risk score for unstable angina/non-ST elevation MI: a method for prognostication and therapeutic decision making. *JAMA* (2000). doi: 10.1001/jama.284.7.835
203. Pollack CV, et al. Application of the TIMI risk score for unstable angina and non-ST elevation acute coronary syndrome to an unselected emergency department chest pain population. *Acad Emerg Med* (2006). doi: 10.1197/j.aem.2005.06.031
204. Scirica BM, et al. Validation of the Thrombolysis In Myocardial Infarction (TIMI) risk score for unstable angina pectoris and non-ST-elevation myocardial infarction in the TIMI III registry. *Am J Cardiol* (2002). doi: 10.1016/s0002-9149(02)02468-2
205. Chase M, et al. Prospective validation of the thrombolysis in myocardial infarction risk score in the emergency department chest pain population. *Ann Emerg Med* (2006). doi: 10.1016/j.annemergmed.2006.01.032
206. Ciaroni S, et al. Early exercise testing after acute myocardial infarction in the elderly: clinical evaluation and prognostic significance. *Am Heart J* (1993). doi: 10.1016/0002-8703(93)91044-f
207. Jain S, et al. Prognostic value of dipyridamole thallium imaging after acute myocardial infarction in older patients. *J Am Geriatr Soc* (1999). doi: 10.1111/j.1532-5415.1999.tb02992.x
208. de la Torre MM, et al. Prognostic power of dobutamine echocardiography after uncomplicated acute myocardial infarction in the elderly. *Chest* (2001). doi: 10.1378/chest.120.4.1200
209. Roman M, et al. Revascularization in frail patients with acute coronary syndromes: a retrospective longitudinal study. *Eur Heart J* (2024). doi: 10.1093/eurheartj/ehae755
210. Fihn SD, et al. 2012 ACCF/AHA/ACP/AATS/PCNA/SCAI/STS guideline for the diagnosis and management of patients with stable ischemic heart disease. *J Am Coll Cardiol* (2012). doi: 10.1016/j.jacc.2012.07.013
211. Spertus JA, et al. Prevalence, predictors, and outcomes of premature discontinuation of thienopyridine therapy after drug-eluting stent placement: results from the PREMIER registry. *Circulation* (2006). doi: 10.1161/CIRCULATIONAHA.106.618066
212. Witt BJ, et al. Cardiac rehabilitation after myocardial infarction in the community. *J Am Coll Cardiol* (2004). doi: 10.1016/j.jacc.2004.05.062
213. Grace SL, et al. Observing temporal trends in cardiac rehabilitation from 1996 to 2010 in Ontario: characteristics of referred patients, programme participation, and mortality rates. *BMJ Open* (2015). doi: 10.1136/bmjopen-2015-009523
214. Califf RM. Patient-centered outcomes composites: a glimpse of the future. *Circulation* (2014). doi: 10.1161/CIRCULATIONAHA.114.013135
215. Byrne RA, et al. 2023 European Guidelines for the management of acute coronary syndromes. *Eur Heart J* (2023). doi: 10.1093/eurheartj/ehad191

11

Management of the older patient after myocardial infarction

HARIS PATAIL, WILBERT S. ARONOW, AND HOWARD A. COOPER

Key points

- Following AMI, elderly patients should be treated with a meticulous and comprehensive approach that prioritizes both lifestyle modifications and pharmacological therapy.
- Smoking cessation, cholesterol optimization, and careful targeting of blood pressure and hemoglobin A1c levels are imperative to reduce residual cardiovascular risk. Further lifestyle interventions, including physical activity and weight loss, are recommended.
- Medical therapy, including ß-blockers, ACE inhibitors, SGLT2 inhibitors, and antiplatelet therapy (if indicated), should be initiated or continued if there are no absolute or relative contraindications.
- The risks and benefits of hormone replacement therapy should be tailored to the individual patients.
- Ultimately, shared decision-making among patients, family members, and medical providers should be prioritized for optimal post-AMI care for elderly patients.

INTRODUCTION

In 2010, the number of Americans aged ≥75 years was estimated to be 18.6 million, a number that is expected to double by 2050. The very elderly (i.e., those aged ≥85 years) is the fastest-growing segment of the population, expected to reach 19.5 million by 2040 (1). Heart disease is the leading killer of people worldwide, with most of these deaths occurring in the elderly (2). Despite a progressive decline in age-adjusted mortality in the United States, the total number of deaths from heart disease continues to rise, largely as a consequence of the aging of the US population. With advances in the initial treatment of acute myocardial infarction (AMI) over the last decades, in-hospital mortality rates have dramatically declined, resulting in a large and growing population of patients requiring post-MI treatment. Among Americans 65 years of age or older, a remarkable 29% are living with heart disease, and among those 75 and older this reaches 35% (3). The appropriate post-MI treatment of these older patients is therefore of paramount importance if death and disability from heart disease are to be significantly impacted. Although authoritative guidelines can direct much of the post-MI care across all age groups, the elderly have a greater burden of comorbidities, disability, and frailty, which may impact the appropriateness of certain therapies. In addition, older patients were systematically underrepresented in many of the trials that have informed post-MI treatment guidelines, and therefore there is greater uncertainty regarding the role of many interventions in this population. A thoughtful approach, taking

DOI: 10.1201/9781003568933-11

into account the unique characteristics of older patients, as well as a consideration of patient-centered outcomes in addition to mortality alone, is therefore required.

CONTROL OF CORONARY RISK FACTORS

The control of coronary risk factors for secondary prevention is a cornerstone of post-MI treatment, with the goal of limiting the progression of coronary heart disease (CHD) and avoiding subsequent events. Each of the modifiable risk factors is discussed in the following sections.

Cigarette smoking

The Chicago Stroke Study demonstrated that current cigarette smokers 65–74 years of age had a 52% higher mortality from coronary artery disease (CAD) than nonsmokers, ex-smokers, and pipe and cigar smokers (4). Ex-smokers who had stopped smoking for 1–5 years had a similar mortality from CAD as did nonsmokers (4). The Systolic Hypertension in the Elderly Program (SHEP) pilot project showed that smoking was a predictor of first cardiovascular event and MI/sudden death (5). At 30-year follow-up of persons 65 years of age and older in the Framingham Heart Study, cigarette smoking was not associated with the incidence of CAD in older men and women but was associated with mortality from CAD in older men and women (6).

At 12-year follow-up of men aged 65–74 years in the Honolulu Heart Program, cigarette smoking was an independent risk factor for nonfatal MI and fatal CAD (7). The absolute excess risk associated with cigarette smoking was 1.9 times higher in older men than in middle-aged men. At 5-year follow-up of 7178 persons 65 years of age or older in three communities, current cigarette smokers had a higher incidence of cardiovascular mortality than nonsmokers (relative risk = 2.0 for men and 1.6 for women) (8). The incidence of cardiovascular death in former smokers was similar to those who had never smoked (8). At 6-year follow-up of older men and women in the Coronary Artery Surgery Study registry, the relative risk of MI or death was 1.5 for persons aged 65–69 years and 2.9 for persons 70 years of age or older who continued smoking compared with those who quit during the year before study enrollment (9).

At 40-month follow-up of 664 older men, mean age 80 years, and at 48-month follow-up of 1488 older women, mean age 82 years, current cigarette smoking increased the relative risk of new coronary events (nonfatal or fatal MI or sudden cardiac death) 2.2 times in older men and 2.0 times in older women (Table 11.1) (10). It was also observed that cigarette smoking aggravates angina pectoris and precipitates silent myocardial ischemia in older persons with CAD. At 6-month follow-up of 2231 patients, a left ventricular ejection fraction (LVEF) ≤40% after MI, smoking cessation was associated with a significant reduction in all-cause mortality of 43%, in death or recurrent MI of 32%, and in death or heart failure hospitalization of 35% (11).

On the basis of the available data, older persons who smoke should be strongly encouraged to stop smoking in order to reduce cardiovascular and all-cause mortality after MI. The American College of Cardiology (ACC)/American Heart Association (AHA) 2013 guidelines recommend that patients should be counseled regarding smoking cessation during and following hospitalization (12). A smoking cessation program should be recommended to smokers. Patients should be advised at every office visit to avoid exposure to environmental tobacco smoke at work, at home, and at public places (13).

A recent placebo-controlled randomized trial examined the use of varenicline for smoking cessation among patients hospitalized for acute coronary syndrome (ACS).

Table 11.1 Risk factors for new coronary events in 664 older men and in 1488 older women

Risk factor	Relative risk of new coronary events	
	Men	Women
Age	1.04	1.03
Prior coronary artery disease	1.7	1.9
Cigarette smoking	2.2	2.0
Hypertension	2.0	1.6
Diabetes mellitus	1.9	1.8
Obesity	NS	NS
Serum total cholesterol	1.12[a]	1.12[a]
Serum HDL cholesterol	1.70[b]	1.95[b]
Serum triglycerides	NS	1.002

Abbreviations: HDL, high-density lipoprotein; NS, not significant.

[a] Per 10 mg/dL increase.

[b] Per 10 mg/dL decrease.

Among 302 patients treated for 12 weeks, varenicline treatment resulted in significantly increased abstinence rates (47.3% vs. 32.5%, $p = 0.012$). No increase in cardiovascular events was seen with varenicline treatment (14). Although the mean age of enrolled patients was only 55 years, pharmacokinetic studies have determined that varenicline appears to be safe and well-tolerated in elderly patients (dose adjustment is required in the setting of renal impairment) (15). Therefore, given the aforementioned benefits of smoking cessation in older patients following MI, the use of varenicline for this purpose appears to be warranted. Patients should be screened for signs and symptoms of depression before and during treatment with varenicline.

Hypertension

Hypertension is extremely common among older men and women, with a prevalence of approximately 70% in those ≥75 years of age (16).

Isolated systolic hypertension and diastolic hypertension are both associated with increased cardiovascular morbidity and mortality in older persons (15, 16). Isolated systolic hypertension occurred in 51% of 499 older persons with hypertension (17). Increased systolic blood pressure is a greater risk factor for cardiovascular morbidity and mortality than is increased diastolic blood pressure (16, 18).

At 30-year follow-up of persons aged 65 years and older in the Framingham study, systolic hypertension correlated with the incidence of CAD in older men and women (6). Diastolic hypertension correlated with CAD in older men but not in older women (6). At 40-month follow-up of older men and 48-month follow-up of older women, systolic or diastolic hypertension increased the relative risk of new coronary events 2.0 times in men and 1.6 times in women (Table 11.1) (10).

Antihypertensive drugs have been demonstrated to decrease new coronary events in older men and women with hypertension (Table 11.2) (19–24). Hypertension is present in 69% of patients with a first MI (25). A meta-analysis of 147 randomized trials including 464,000 persons with hypertension showed that β-blockers were the most beneficial drugs to use in patients after MI (26).

Patients with prior MI and hypertension should be treated with β-blockers and angiotensin-converting enzyme (ACE) inhibitors (16, 26–33). If a third drug is needed, aldosterone antagonists may be used based on the EPHESUS trial (34). In an observational prospective study of 1212 older men and women, mean age 80 years, with prior MI and hypertension treated with β-blockers, ACE inhibitors, diuretics, calcium channel blockers, or alpha-blockers, at 40-month follow-up the incidence of new coronary events in persons treated with one antihypertensive drug was lowest among those treated with β-blockers or ACE inhibitors (33). In older persons treated with two antihypertensive drugs, the incidence of new coronary events was lowest in those treated with β-blockers plus ACE inhibitors (33). ACE inhibitors or angiotensin receptor blockers (ARBs) should also be administered to persons with diabetes mellitus, renal insufficiency, or proteinuria (16, 35, 36).

Other comorbid conditions that favor the use of β-blockers for the treatment of hypertension in the elderly include complex ventricular arrhythmias (37, 38), congestive heart failure (CHF) with reduced LVEF (37), angina pectoris (39), myocardial ischemia (40), supraventricular tachyarrhythmias such as atrial fibrillation with a rapid ventricular rate (41), and hyperthyroidism (42). In older patients with hypertension and CHF who have persistent

Table 11.2 Decrease in new coronary events in older persons with hypertension treated with antihypertensive drugs versus placebo

Study	Follow-up	Results
European Working Party on High Blood Pressure in the Elderly (18) (age 60–97 years)	4.7 years	60% reduction in fatal MI and 47% reduction in cardiac death
Swedish Trial in Old Patients with Hypertension (19) (age 70–84 years)	25 months	25% reduction in fatal MI and 67% reduction in sudden death
Medical Research Council (19, 20) (age 65–74 years)	5.8 years	19% reduction in coronary events
Systolic Hypertension in the Elderly Program (21) (mean age 72 years)	4.5 years	27% decrease in nonfatal MI plus coronary deaths
Systolic Hypertension in Europe (22) (mean age 70 years)	2.0 years	26% reduction in fatal and nonfatal cardiac events
Hypertension in the Very Elderly Trial (22, 23) (mean age 83.6 years)	1.8 years	39% reduction in fatal stroke, 21% reduction in all-cause mortality, and 64% reduction in heart failure

Abbreviation: MI, myocardial infarction.

symptoms, maximal therapy can include β-blockers, ACE inhibitors or ARBs, aldosterone antagonists, and diuretics if there are no contraindications for these medications (34, 35, 43, 44).

The target blood pressure for older patients with established CHD is <130/80 mmHg (35). As older persons are likely to have reduced absorption, metabolism, and especially excretion of antihypertensive drugs, initiation and titration should proceed cautiously. Combinations of medications at low doses may provide increased efficacy with limitation of dose-dependent side effects (1).

Caution should be maintained not to lower the diastolic blood pressure excessively when attempting to lower the systolic blood pressure in older post-MI patients with isolated systolic hypertension. There is some suggestion that excessive lowering of the diastolic blood pressure (<70 mmHg) in patients with CAD can lower coronary perfusion pressure and thereby provoke ischemia (45, 46).

In addition, the recent ACC/AHA Guidelines recommend that in "older adults (≥65 years of age) with hypertension and a high burden of comorbidity and limited life expectancy, clinical judgment, patient preference, and a team-based approach to assess risk/benefit is reasonable for decisions regarding intensity of BP lowering and choice of antihypertensive drugs" (26).

Hypercholesterolemia

An elevated level of low-density lipoprotein cholesterol (LDL-C) is a major risk factor for recurrent cardiovascular events. This relationship remains strong in older persons (47, 48). As discussed later, there is overwhelming evidence from multiple randomized, controlled trials that lowering LDL-C with statins reduces cardiovascular events, including in older persons.

At 5.4-year median follow-up of 4444 men and women (1021 aged 65–70 years) with CAD and hypercholesterolemia in the Scandinavian Simvastatin Survival Study, compared with placebo, simvastatin 20–40 mg daily significantly decreased in patients aged 65–70 years total mortality by 34%, CAD mortality by 43%, major coronary events by 34%, nonfatal MI by 33%, any acute CAD-related endpoint by 33%, any atherosclerosis-related endpoint by 34%, and coronary revascularization procedures by 41% (Table 11.3). The absolute risk reduction for both all-cause mortality and CAD mortality was

Table 11.3 Effects of lowering increased serum low-density lipoprotein cholesterol levels by simvastatin and pravastatin versus placebo in older patients with coronary artery disease

Study	Follow-up (years)	Results
Scandinavian Simvastatin Survival Study (49) (4444 men and women, 1021 aged 65–70 years, with CAD and hypercholesterolemia)	5.4	In patients 65 years and older, compared with placebo, simvastatin decreased all-cause mortality by 34%, CAD mortality by 43%, major coronary events by 34%, nonfatal MI by 33%, any acute CAD-related event by 33%, any atherosclerosis-related endpoint by 34%, and coronary revascularization procedures by 41%
Cholesterol and Recurrent Events trial (50) (4159 men and women, 1283 aged 65–75 years, with MI and serum total cholesterol <240 mg/dL but serum LDL cholesterol ≥115 mg/dL)	5.0	Compared with placebo, pravastatin decreased CAD death by 45%, CAD death or nonfatal MI by 39%, major coronary events by 32%, coronary revascularization by 32%, stroke by 40%, and insignificantly decreased unstable angina by 8% and congestive heart failure by 23%
Long-Term Intervention with Pravastatin in Ischaemic Disease Study (51) (9014 men and women, 3514 aged 65–75 years, with MI or unstable angina and mean serum total cholesterol 218 mg/dL)	6.1	Compared with placebo, pravastatin reduced all-cause mortality by 22%, death from CAD by 24%, fatal and nonfatal MI by 29%, death from cardiovascular disease by 25%, need for coronary artery surgery by 22%, need for coronary angioplasty by 19%, hospitalization for unstable angina by 12%, and stroke by 19%
Heart Protection Study (52) (20,536 men and women, 10,697 aged 65–85 years, with CAD, occlusive arterial disease of noncoronary arteries, diabetes, or treated hypertension and no serum lipid requirement)	5.0	Compared with placebo, simvastatin reduced all-cause mortality by 13%, any vascular mortality by 17%, major coronary events by 27%, any stroke by 25%, any revascularization procedure by 24%, and any major vascular event by 24%

Abbreviations: CAD, coronary artery disease; LDL, low-density lipoprotein; MI, myocardial infarction.

approximately twice as great in persons 65–70 years of age at study entry as in those younger than 65 years (49).

At 5-year follow-up of 4159 men and women (1283 aged 65–75 years) with MI and serum total cholesterol levels below 240 mg/dL, but serum LDL-C levels ≥115 mg/dL in the Cholesterol and Recurrent Events trial, compared with placebo, pravastatin 40 mg daily significantly reduced in patients aged 65–75 years CAD death by 45%, CAD death or nonfatal MI by 39%, major coronary events by 32%, coronary revascularization by 32%, insignificantly reduced unstable angina pectoris by 8%, and CHF by 23% (Table 11.3). For every 1000 patients 65 years and older treated for 5 years with pravastatin, 225 cardiovascular hospitalizations would be prevented compared with prevention of 121 cardiovascular hospitalizations in 1000 patients younger than 65 years (50).

At 6.1-year mean follow-up of 9014 men and women (3514 of whom were aged 65–75 years) with MI (64%) or unstable angina pectoris (36%) and serum total cholesterol levels of 155–271 mg/dL in the Long-Term Intervention with Pravastatin in Ischaemic Disease Study, compared with placebo, pravastatin 40 mg daily significantly reduced all-cause mortality by 22%, death from CAD by 24%, fatal and nonfatal MI by 29%, death from cardiovascular disease by 25%, need for coronary artery bypass surgery by 22%, need for coronary angioplasty by 19%, hospitalization for unstable angina pectoris by 12%, and stroke by 19% (Table 11.3). The absolute benefits of treatment with pravastatin were greater in groups of persons at higher absolute risk for a major coronary event, such as older persons, those with a higher serum LDL-C level, those with a lower serum high-density lipoprotein-cholesterol (HDL-C) level, and those with a history of diabetes mellitus or smoking (51).

At 5-year follow-up of 20,536 British men and women (10,697 aged 65–80 years) with either CAD, occlusive arterial disease of noncoronary arteries, diabetes mellitus, or treated hypertension and no serum lipid requirement in the Heart Protection Study, compared with placebo, simvastatin 40 mg daily significantly reduced all-cause mortality by 13%, any vascular mortality by 17%, major coronary events by 27%, any stroke by 25%, any revascularization procedure by 24%, and any major vascular event by 24% (Table 11.3). In the 1263 persons aged 75–80 years at study entry and 80–85 years at follow-up, any major vascular event was significantly reduced by 28% by simvastatin. Lowering serum LDL-C from <116 mg/dL to <77 mg/dL by simvastatin caused a 25% significant reduction in vascular events (52).

In the Heart Protection Study, 3500 persons had initial serum LDL-C levels less than 100 mg/dL (52). A decrease of serum LDL-C from 97 mg/dL to 65 mg/dL by simvastatin in these persons caused a similar decrease in risk as did treating patients with higher serum LDL-C levels. The Heart Protection Study Investigators recommended treating persons at high risk for cardiovascular events with statins, regardless of the initial levels of serum lipids, age, or gender (52). In the Study Assessing Goals in the Elderly (SAGE), 893 ambulatory patients with CAD were randomized to atorvastatin 80 mg daily or to pravastatin 40 mg daily. At 1-year follow-up, compared with pravastatin, atorvastatin significantly reduced serum LDL-C and significantly reduced all-cause mortality by 67% (53).

Although older patients were underrepresented in many of these statin trials, meta-analysis has allowed for robust investigation of the role of statins in secondary prevention in this group. Afilalo et al. demonstrated that statin therapy was associated with a 22% reduction in all-cause mortality among 19,569 secondary-prevention patients aged 65–82 years. Substantial reductions in CHD mortality, nonfatal MI, revascularization, and stroke were also noted (54). The benefit of more intensive versus less intensive statin treatment was assessed in the Cholesterol Treatment Trialists' meta-analysis of 26 randomized, controlled trials including over 170,000 patients. Major vascular events were reduced by 22% in patients aged 66–75 years, and 16% among patients over the age of 75. Importantly, the absolute risk reduction was higher among the oldest patients (55).

The nonstatin drug ezetimibe lowers LDL-C by inhibiting intestinal absorption, and, when added to statin therapy, had a modest, beneficial effect on LDL-C and hard clinical outcomes among patients stabilized after an acute coronary syndrome. This benefit was particularly pronounced among those aged ≥75 years (56).

The 2013 ACC/AHA Guidelines on the treatment of blood cholesterol recommend high-intensity statin treatment for secondary prevention in patients ≤75 years of age. For those >75 years of age, moderate- or high-intensity statin treatment is recommended, taking into account patient preferences and conditions that may increase the risk of statin-related adverse effects (57). If further LDL-C reduction is required after statin treatment, the addition of ezetimibe appears to be safe and effective in older patients and may be considered (58).

Diabetes

The incidence and prevalence of diabetes increase with age, due to both increased insulin resistance (from adiposity and sarcopenia) and impaired insulin secretion (due to pancreatic islet cell dysfunction) (59). The prevalence of diabetes is expected to double by 2050, with the largest increase expected in those ≥75 years of age (60). In addition, older persons with both diabetes and CHD are an especially high-risk population. For example, among over 2000 elderly patients (mean age 80 ± 8 years), diabetes was associated with an increase in the relative risk of new coronary events 1.9 times in men and 1.8 times in women (10). Despite this, many elderly patients with diabetes go undiagnosed (61). Therefore, all older post-MI patients should be screened for the presence of diabetes.

Following an MI, older patients with diabetes should first be treated with lifestyle modification: medical nutrition therapy, weight reduction (if necessary), and exercise. In the Diabetes Prevention Program, older patients had better adherence to lifestyle interventions and demonstrated the greatest improvement in glycemia (62). In most patients, however, drug therapy will be required. Because hypoglycemia is often unrecognized in older patients, great care should be taken to avoid this complication. In part because of the low incidence of hypoglycemia, metformin is generally recommended as the initial drug to treat hyperglycemia in older patients (13, 63). For those with contraindications or intolerance to metformin, the short-acting sulfonylurea, glipizide, is a reasonable alternative. Insulin may be used as first-line therapy for patients with marked hyperglycemia or as an adjunct if oral agents are not successful in achieving target levels of glycemia. In a recent randomized, controlled trial, the glucagon-like peptide-1 analog liraglutide was shown to reduce the incidence of cardiovascular adverse events when added to standard therapy in high-risk patients with type 2 diabetes. The majority of enrolled patients were over the age of 60, and subgroup analysis did not reveal any loss of efficacy among older enrolled patients (64). Therefore, it is reasonable to add liraglutide to metformin if glycemic goals have not been met.

There is significant uncertainty regarding the appropriate hemoglobin A1C target for older patients with diabetes. Goals should be individualized based on fitness level, comorbidities, risk of polypharmacy, and life expectancy. For very healthy older adults, a goal of <7% HbA1C may be reasonable. For those with elements of frailty or with multiple comorbidities (which will be the case for many post-MI patients), a more lenient target of 7%–7.9% is recommended. Even more lenient targets may be reasonable for those with very limited life expectancy (65–68).

Obesity

As in the general US population, obesity (defined as body mass index [BMI] >30 kg/m^2) has increased dramatically among older persons in recent decades. According to estimates from the National Health and Nutrition Examination Survey, approximately 40% of those aged 65–74, and 27% of those over the age of 75, are obese. The predisposition to obesity in the elderly is related to age-related declines in metabolic rate and physical activity.

Obesity increases the risk of developing hypertension, hyperlipidemia, and diabetes (1). However, the relationship between BMI and adverse cardiovascular outcomes is complex. An observational study of nearly 1 million persons demonstrated that obesity was associated with a small increase in total mortality. However, the associated risk decreased with age, such that no increase in risk was seen in persons over the age of 85 (69). Systematic reviews and meta-analyses have demonstrated that, among all persons ≥65 years of age, small increases in all-cause and cardiovascular mortality are associated with BMIs in the moderately increased range. The threshold values at which BMI conferred an increased mortality risk were higher in the elderly than in younger adults. However, although the relative risk of mortality appears to decrease with advancing age, the mortality risk attributable to obesity remained substantially higher among older persons because of their higher overall risk (1, 70). Finally, however, among patients with established CHD across a broad age range, a systematic review found no association between BMI and increased total or cardiovascular mortality, even among those with severe obesity (71).

Furthermore, there is a lack of strong evidence demonstrating that intentional weight loss reduces adverse cardiovascular events among the elderly. Two randomized trials of dietary weight loss interventions among older persons showed no significant impact on mortality. However, in both studies, the weight loss interventions led to improved physical functioning with no deleterious effects. Given the importance of physical function among the elderly, guidelines currently recommend modest weight reduction for severely obese elderly patients (72).

Few intervention studies have assessed the feasibility of lifestyle modification to achieve meaningful weight loss among elderly patients. A series of small clinical trials by Villareal and colleagues demonstrated successful weight loss among frail, obese patients with an energy-restricted diet, behavioral modification, and exercise over the short term. In those with established CHD, the intervention group achieved greater weight and fat mass loss, greater improvement in blood pressure and glycemic control, and reduced levels of C-reactive protein. Functional status and aerobic endurance were also improved (73–75). Unfortunately, the majority of individuals who attempt to lose weight using lifestyle interventions do not achieve significant weight loss, and most of those who do eventually regain the weight (1).

Glucagon-like peptide-1 (GLP-1) agonists have been increasingly used for weight loss in patients with obesity, followed by several trials showing positive cardiovascular outcomes including reduction in MACE in adult patients (64, 76–78). These trials have not specifically targeted elderly patients ≥65 or ≥75 years of age, however. A meta-analysis from 2021 analyzed all GLP-1 cardiovascular-outcome trials, specifically assessing GLP-1 effects in elderly patients (79). The meta-analysis found a reduction of MACE and individual components of cardiovascular mortality, stroke, and MI in patients >65 and who were treated with GLP-1 agonists when compared to placebo. Additionally, elderly patients also had significantly lower hospitalizations for heart failure. These data, however, were relatively limited for patients >75 years of age given they were underrepresented in a majority of the trials.

Guidelines from the AHA/ACC/Obesity Society (79) recommend that physicians advise adults with a BMI ≥40 or BMI ≥35 with obesity-related comorbid conditions who are motivated to lose weight and who have not responded to behavioral treatment with or without pharmacotherapy with sufficient weight loss to achieve targeted health outcome goals that bariatric surgery may be an appropriate option to improve health and offer referral to an experienced bariatric surgeon for consultation and evaluation.

However, until recently, bariatric weight loss surgery was considered too risky to perform in the elderly, particularly in those with established CHD. However, recent advances in surgical and anesthesia techniques have allowed for the application of bariatric surgery in older patients. A recent systematic review found that outcomes and complication rates were similar for patients above the age of 60 when compared to younger patients (80). Therefore, it may be reasonable to consider bariatric surgery for stable post-MI older patients in whom the benefits of substantial weight loss are felt to exceed the risks.

Physical inactivity

Physical inactivity is well established as a risk factor for CHD, dating back to the seminal study by Morris et al. in 1953 (1, 81). Furthermore, physical inactivity is strongly associated with cardiovascular mortality (82). As a sedentary lifestyle is common among older persons, physical inactivity is a major concern in this population.

Among older adults, the benefits of increasing physical activity have been consistently demonstrated, with reductions in blood pressure, hyperlipidemia, glycemic control, neurocognitive function, and quality of life (1). In both observational studies and randomized trials, older patients with established CHD demonstrated benefit from increasing physical activity, including recurrent CHD events (1). For example, men between the ages of 71 and 93 enrolled in the Honolulu Heart Program who walked >1.5 miles per day had a >50% reduction in CHD events when compared to those who walked minimally (83).

For healthy adults, the American Heart Association currently recommends at least 30 minutes of moderate-intensity aerobic activity at least 5 days per week or at least 25 minutes of vigorous aerobic activity at least 3 days per week, in addition to moderate- to high-intensity muscle strengthening activity at least 2 days per week (84). For older post-MI patients, especially those who are frail and dealing with multiple comorbidities, goals need to be individualized. A symptom-limited exercise test is recommended before initiating an exercise program, in order to ascertain the safety of exercise and to guide the initial exercise prescription. For patients following an MI, the 2014 ACC/AHA Guidelines recommend referral to a comprehensive cardiac rehabilitation program (85).

MEDICAL THERAPY

Aspirin

Aspirin decreases the aggregation of platelets exposed to thrombogenic stimuli by inhibiting the cyclooxygenase enzyme reaction within the platelet and thereby blocking the synthesis of thromboxane A_2, a powerful stimulus to platelet aggregation and vasoconstriction (86). Randomized, placebo-controlled trials involving 20,006 patients showed that aspirin administered to patients after MI decreased the incidence of recurrent MI, stroke, or vascular death by 36 events per 1000 patients treated for 2 years (87). Data from the Multicenter Study of Myocardial Ischemia in 936 patients enrolled 1 to 6 months after an acute MI (70% of patients) or unstable angina pectoris (30% of patients) showed at 23-month follow-up that the cardiac mortality rate was 1.6% for aspirin users and 5.4% for nonusers of aspirin (88). Based on data such as these, aspirin is considered a cornerstone therapy for post-MI secondary prevention.

However, little data are available regarding post-MI aspirin therapy specifically among older patients. In the previously mentioned meta-analysis, among patients older than 65 years there was an absolute reduction in vascular events of 4.5% and the number needed to treat to prevent 1 death from any cause was 67 (87). Krumholz et al. performed an observational study of aspirin use at discharge following an acute MI in 5490 Medicare patients (minimum age 65, mean age 76 years). After controlling for potential confounders, the prescribed use of aspirin at discharge was associated with a 23% reduction in the odds ratio for death at 6 months (89).

Because post-MI mortality increases with age, the absolute benefit of aspirin therapy is likely to be greatest among older patients. However, the risks of aspirin, particularly with respect to gastrointestinal and intracranial bleeding, may also be greater (90). On the basis of the available data, current guidelines recommend low-dose aspirin (75–100 mg daily) for all patients following an acute MI (85).

Thienopyridines

The addition of a thienopyridine to aspirin in patients with acute coronary syndromes, particularly those who have received a stent, results in a greater reduction in cardiovascular events than aspirin alone, albeit with an increased risk of bleeding (91). For example, in the Clopidogrel in Unstable Angina to Prevent Recurrent Events (CURE) trial, in which patients were randomized to receive clopidogrel or placebo for up to 12 months following an ACS, the benefits of clopidogrel were similar in older and younger patients (92). The more potent drugs in this class, prasugrel and ticagrelor, both reduce ischemic events to a greater extent than clopidogrel, at the expense of increased bleeding. Therefore, clopidogrel is generally used in elderly post-MI patients with an increased risk of bleeding, and prasugrel is not recommended for use in patients over the age of 75 (85). Proton pump inhibitors reduce the risk of gastrointestinal bleeding in patients being treated with dual antiplatelet therapy, and therefore should be considered in elderly post-MI patients (93).

In the Clopidogrel Versus Ticagrelor or Prasugrel in Patients Aged 70 Years or Older with Non-ST-Elevation Acute Coronary Syndrome (POPular AGE) trial, patients ≥70 years of age were randomly assigned to receive either clopidogrel versus ticagrelor or prasugrel following non-ST-elevation acute coronary syndrome (94). The primary bleeding outcome (major or minor bleeding) was significantly lower in the clopidogrel group compared to ticagrelor or prasugrel (18% vs. 24%; hazard ratio, 0.71; 95% CI, 0.54 to 0.94; $p = 0.02$). Furthermore, the composite net clinical benefit, including all-cause death, MI, stroke, and major or minor bleeding after 12 months, showed non-inferiority for the clopidogrel strategy.

Anticoagulants

The role of routine anticoagulation following MI has been debated for decades. The persistent risk of ischemic events following an ACS is in part attributable to sustained thrombin generation, suggesting that prolonged anticoagulation might reduce the risk of recurrent events (96). Earlier studies with vitamin K antagonists added to aspirin alone resulted in significant reductions in fatal and nonfatal events, but at the expense of increased major bleeding (97). In the era of dual antiplatelet therapy (DAPT), routine use of so-called triple therapy with vitamin K antagonists is associated with unacceptable bleeding risks, particularly in the elderly (98).

The advent of direct oral anticoagulants has reignited interest in the use of anticoagulation for secondary prevention of MI. The Phase II dose-ranging RE-DEEM trial of dabigatran in patients with recent MI randomly assigned 1861 patients on DAPT to different doses of dabigatran. There was a dose-dependent increase in major and clinically relevant minor bleeding without evidence of clinical benefit. Similarly, the large Phase II APPRAISE-2 trial investigated the use of apixaban in addition to DAPT after an ACS. Among the 7392 patients enrolled, 59% were ≥65 years old. The study was stopped prematurely because of an increase in intracranial and fatal bleeding with no significant reduction in ischemic events (99).

Rivaroxaban (at a dose of either 2.5 mg or 5 mg twice daily) or placebo was added to DAPT in 15,526 patients with a recent ACS in the ATLAS ACS 2-TIMI 51 study. Among enrolled patients, 36.5% were ≥65 years old. After a mean treatment period of 13.1 months, both dosing regimens showed a significant reduction in the primary efficacy endpoint of cardiovascular death, MI, or stroke. In addition, a reduction in all-cause mortality was seen with the 2.5 mg dose. Rivaroxaban was associated with an increase in major and fatal bleeding, including a three-fold excess of major bleeding with the 2.5 mg dose (100). Although the use of rivaroxaban in acute coronary syndrome has not been approved by the US Food and Drug Administration, the recent guidelines of the European Society of Cardiology give the use of low-dose rivaroxaban a IIb (may be considered) recommendation in high-risk post-MI patients without a history of prior stroke and at low bleeding risk. Most elderly patients will not meet the low-bleeding risk criteria, and indeed specific caution is provided against use in patients over the age of 75 (101).

β-Blockers

β-Blockers are very effective antianginal and anti-ischemic agents. They decrease heart rate, contractility, and blood pressure resulting in a reduction in oxygen consumption. Clinically, β-blockers given in the setting of AMI decrease myocardial ischemia and the frequency of complex ventricular arrhythmias (102–104). The impact of β-blockers on short- and long-term mortality has been investigated in a multitude of clinical trials over many years (see Table 11.4 for a list of some of these trials).

The vast majority of the trials of β-blockers for treatment following acute MI were conducted prior to the era of aggressive revascularization, and therefore may no longer be relevant. One analysis from early trials of primary percutaneous coronary intervention in ST-elevation MI found that β-blockers were associated with lower 6-month mortality. This benefit was limited to patients with reduced ejection fraction (EF) and multivessel disease (111).

Current guidelines recommend long-term post-MI β-blocker therapy for stabilized patients with heart failure with reduced EF, using carvedilol, bisoprolol, or sustained-release metoprolol succinate (class I recommendation) and for all other patients (class IIa recommendation) (85).

The duration of treatment for secondary prevention in patients with normal LV systolic function is controversial, with little data to support continued use beyond 1 year (112). Recently, the Beta-Blockers after Myocardial Infarction and Preserved Ejection Fraction (REDUCE AMI) trial found no difference in composite death or new MI in patients with EF >50% who were either treated with β-blockers (metoprolol or bisoprolol) or placebo. Of note, this trial included adult patients of any age; however, the median age in both groups was 65 years (113). This finding has particular relevance for elderly patients following MI, many of whom are dealing with the issue of polypharmacy. Given the lack of data demonstrating the benefit of long-term β-blocker therapy in elderly patients, it seems reasonable to consider discontinuing these drugs

Table 11.4 Effect of β-blockers on mortality after myocardial infarction

Study	Follow-up	Results
Goteborg Trial (105)	90 days	Compared with placebo, metoprolol caused a 21% nonsignificant decrease in mortality in patients <65 years and a 45% significant decrease in mortality in patients 65–74 years
Norwegian Multicenter Study (106)	17 months	Compared with placebo, timolol caused a 31% significant reduction in mortality in persons <65 years and a 43% significant reduction in mortality in persons 65–74 years
Norwegian Multicenter Study (107)	61 months	Compared with placebo, timolol caused a 13% nonsignificant decrease in mortality in persons <65 years and a 19% significant decrease in mortality in persons 65–74 years
β-Blocker Heart Attack Trial (108)	25 months	Compared with placebo, propranolol caused a 19% nonsignificant reduction in mortality in persons <60 years and a 33% significant reduction in mortality in persons 60–69 years
CAPRICORN Trial (109)	1.3 years	In patients, mean age 63 years (range 25–90 years) with a left ventricular ejection fraction ≤40% after myocardial infarction, compared with placebo, carvedilol caused a 23% significant reduction in mortality
COMMIT/CCS-2 (110)	In-hospital	Compared with placebo, intravenous followed by oral metoprolol reduced reinfarction, increased cardiogenic shock, and had a neutral effect on in-hospital mortality

after 1 year in elderly post-MI patients with preserved EF and no angina. Moreover, a very recent national analysis of long-stay nursing home patients 65 years of age or older found that the use of β-blockers for secondary prevention following MI was associated with a survival benefit but also a significant functional decline among those with substantial cognitive or functional impairment. In this population of frail elders, the balance between quality and quantity of life should be carefully considered with respect to continued β-blocker prescription (114).

Angiotensin-converting enzyme inhibitors

Table 11.5 shows that many trials have established that long-term treatment with ACE inhibitors reduces mortality in patients after MI (115–119). A patient-level meta-analysis of three of these trials, including 12,763 patients with left ventricular dysfunction or heart failure following MI, found that treatment with an ACE inhibitor reduced the risk of MI, hospitalization for heart failure, and all-cause mortality (120). These benefits were apparent across all age strata, although the benefits appeared to be attenuated in those over the age of 75. There was an increase in both symptomatic hypotension and renal dysfunction in patients assigned to ACE inhibitors.

Current guidelines recommend that ACE inhibitors be started, and continued indefinitely, in post-MI patients with reduced EF, hypertension, diabetes, or stable chronic kidney disease (class I recommendation). Given the age-related prevalence of hypertension and chronic kidney disease, this recommendation will likely encompass most elderly patients following MI. The long-term use of ACE inhibitors for all other post-MI patients may be considered (class IIb recommendation). Among elderly patients, great care should be taken to avoid symptomatic hypotension, either resting or orthostatic, as this may lead to falls with severe attendant consequences. Renal function should be monitored frequently (85).

Aldosterone antagonists

At 16-month follow-up of 6632 patients after MI with an LVEF ≤40% and either CHF or diabetes mellitus treated with ACE inhibitors or ARBs and β-blockers in the EPHESUS trial, compared with placebo, patients randomized to eplerenone 50 mg daily had a significant 15% reduction in mortality and a 13% significant reduction in death from cardiovascular causes or hospitalization for cardiovascular events (121). The ACCF/AHA guidelines recommend an aldosterone antagonist in patients after MI treated with ACE inhibitors plus β-blockers if they have an LVEF ≤40% with either CHF or diabetes mellitus if they do not have significant renal dysfunction or hyperkalemia (85). Data are limited on the use of this therapy in the elderly. Although there was no statistically significant interaction between age and outcomes in the EPHESUS trial, the benefit of eplerenone appeared to be attenuated in those over the age of 75 years (122). This, coupled with the risks of hyperkalemia in patients with renal insufficiency co-treated with ACE inhibitors, suggests that extreme diligence should be exercised with respect to the monitoring of renal function and serum potassium levels in elderly post-MI patients treated with eplerenone.

Table 11.5 Effect of angiotensin-converting-enzyme inhibitors on mortality in patients after myocardial infarction

Study	Follow-up	Results
Survival and Ventricular Enlargement Trial (115)	42 months	In patients with MI and LVEF ≤40%, compared with placebo, captopril reduced mortality 8% in patients aged ≥55 years, 13% in patients aged 56–64 years, and 25% in patients aged ≥65 years
Acute Infarction Ramipril Efficacy Study (116)	15 months	In patients with MI and clinical evidence of CHF, compared with placebo, ramipril decreased mortality 2% in patients aged <65 years and 36% in patients aged ≥65 years
Survival of Myocardial Infarction Long-Term Evaluation Trial (117)	1 year	In patients with anterior MI, compared with placebo, zofenopril reduced mortality or severe CHF 32% in patients aged <65 years and 39% in patients aged ≥65 years
Trandolapril Cardiac Evaluation Study (118)	24–50 months	In patients, mean age 68 years, with LVEF ≤35%, compared with placebo, trandolapril reduced mortality 33% in patients with anterior MI and 14% in patients without anterior MI
Heart Outcomes Prevention Evaluation Study (28)	4.5 years	In patients aged ≥55 years with MI (53%), cardiovascular disease (88%), or diabetes (38%) but no CHF or abnormal LVEF, ramipril reduced MI, stroke, and cardiovascular death 22%
EUROPA study (119)	4.2 years	In patients, mean age 60 years, with prior MI, compared with placebo, perindopril significantly reduced cardiovascular death, MI, or cardiac arrest by 20%

Abbreviations: CHF, congestive heart failure; LVEF, left ventricular ejection fraction; MI, myocardial infarction.

Sodium-glucose cotransporter 2 (SGLT2) inhibitors

SGLT2 inhibitors have been increasingly used in patients typically with concomitant type 2 diabetes mellitus and cardiovascular disease after several trials have shown positive outcomes (123, 124). In the Dapagliflozin and Cardiovascular Outcomes in Type 2 Diabetes (DECLARE-TIMI 58) trial, a broad set of patients who had or were at risk of coronary artery disease showed lower rates of cardiovascular death or hospitalization for heart failure (4.9% vs. 5.8%; hazard ratio, 0.83; 95% CI, 0.73 to 0.95; p = 0.005) when compared to placebo (125). Though the trial included adults >40, both patients ≥65 or ≥75 years of age showed consistent results, including decreased cardiovascular death and hospitalizations for heart failure (126). In the prospective Empagliflozin in Acute Myocardial Infarction (EMPACT-MI) trial more than 6000 patients who were hospitalized for acute MI were randomly assigned to receive empagliflozin (10 mg daily) versus placebo (127). Patients hospitalized with acute MI (average age of 63 years) who were treated with empagliflozin did not show a significantly lower risk of composite heart failure rehospitalizations or death from any cause. The trial did, however, show a modestly reduced rate of first hospitalization of heart failure (3.6% vs. 4.7%; hazard ratio, 0.77; 95% CI, 0.60 to 0.98) in patients who were assigned to empagliflozin. Supplementary analysis of the data shows that more than 50% of patients enrolled were above the age of 65 years. Similarly, the Dapagliflozin in Myocardial Infarction Without Diabetes or Heart Failure (DAPA-MI) trial did not show a positive benefit of SGLT2 inhibitor therapy post-MI in regards to composite cardiovascular death or heart-failure-associated hospitalizations in all adult patients (128). Further data is required regarding SGLT2 inhibitor therapy for elderly patients with acute MI, especially those without concomitant type 2 diabetes or heart failure.

Hormone replacement therapy

The Heart Estrogen/Progestin Replacement Study (HERS) investigated in 2763 women with documented CAD the effect of hormonal replacement therapy versus double-blind placebo on coronary events. At 4.1-year follow-up, there were no significant differences between hormonal replacement therapy and placebo in the primary outcome (nonfatal MI or CAD death) or in any of the secondary cardiovascular outcomes. However, there was a 52% significantly higher incidence of nonfatal MI or death from CAD in the first year in patients treated with hormonal replacement therapy (relative hazard = 1.52; 95% CI, 1.01–2.29) compared to patients treated with placebo. Women on hormonal replacement therapy had a significantly higher incidence of venous thromboembolic events (relative hazard = 2.89, 95% CI, 1.50–5.58) and a significantly higher incidence of gallbladder disease requiring surgery (relative hazard = 1.38, 95% CI, 1.00–1.92) than women on placebo (129).

The Estrogen Replacement and Atherosclerosis trial randomized 309 postmenopausal women, mean age 66 years, with coronary angiographic evidence of significant

CAD to estrogen plus progestin, estrogen alone, or double-blind placebo (130). At 3.2-year follow-up, quantitative coronary angiography showed no between-group differences in progression of coronary atherosclerosis (130).

The estrogen plus progestin component of the Women's Health Initiative (WHI) study included 16,608 healthy postmenopausal women aged 50–79 years with an intact uterus who were randomized to estrogen plus progestin or to placebo. At 5.2-year follow-up, this component of the WHI study was prematurely discontinued because the excess risk of events included in the global index was 19 per 10,000 person-years. Absolute excess risks per 10,000 person-years included 7 more coronary events, 8 more strokes, 8 more episodes of pulmonary embolism, and 8 more invasive breast cancers, while absolute risk reductions per 10,000 person-years were 6 fewer colorectal cancers and 5 fewer hip fractures (131).

A recent Cochrane systematic review, including 19 trials with a total of 40,410 patients, found that hormone replacement therapy in both primary and secondary prevention conferred no protective effects for all-cause mortality, cardiovascular death, nonfatal MI, angina, or revascularization. However, there was an increased risk of stroke and venous thromboembolic disease on hormone replacement therapy relative to placebo (132).

On the basis of the available data, current guidelines give the following class III recommendation (harmful, should not be performed) for the use of hormone replacement therapy for secondary prevention in postmenopausal women: "Hormone therapy with estrogen plus progestin, or estrogen alone, should not be given as new drugs for secondary prevention of coronary events to postmenopausal women after [MI] and should not be continued in previous users unless the benefits outweigh the estimated risks" (85).

INFLUENZA VACCINATION

Evidence from cohort studies and a randomized clinical trial indicates that annual vaccination against seasonal influenza prevents cardiovascular morbidity and mortality in patients with cardiovascular disease (133). Current guidelines provide a class I recommendation for annual influenza immunization as part of secondary prevention in all persons with cardiovascular disease (13, 133).

IMPLANTABLE CARDIOVERTER-DEFIBRILLATOR

Life-threatening ventricular arrhythmias occurring more than 48 hours after an AMI portend a poor prognosis. Randomized controlled trials of secondary prevention have demonstrated a clear mortality benefit for implantable cardioverter-defibrillator (ICD) therapy in survivors of sustained ventricular tachycardia or ventricular fibrillation in this setting (134–138). For patients with significantly reduced EF following an AMI, primary prevention trials have demonstrated benefit only if the EF remains low for several weeks following hospital discharge. Therefore, reassessment of patients should occur at least 40 days after MI and at least 90 days after revascularization in order to determine eligibility (139).

The use of ICDs in elderly patients raises many clinical and ethical issues. The benefit of ICD therapy for primary prevention in patients over the age of 75 enrolled in clinical trials has been demonstrated in a meta-analysis of available data, with a relative risk reduction of 28% with respect to all-cause mortality (140). Advanced age does not appear to be associated with an increased risk of acute complications from device implantation (141). Data are very limited regarding long-term complications directly related to ICD implantation in elderly patients, and data from registries are mixed with respect to the risk of device-related complications in older versus younger patients (142, 143). Based on these data, current guidelines provide a class IIa recommendation ("is reasonable") for the use of an ICD for primary prevention in older patients who meet indications if meaningful survival for greater than 1 year is anticipated (139). Several risk scores for survival following ICD implantation have been developed and may be useful in determining if 1-year survival is likely (144).

Quality-of-life considerations are paramount when considering ICD therapy in an elderly patient. However, such data are sparse. A recent systematic review concluded that "it was not possible to elucidate any trends regarding the relationship between age and QoL in patients with an ICD" (145). The risk of anxiety and depression, particularly among elderly ICD patients who receive inappropriate shocks, can be substantial, and this distress can extend to family members as well (146). The role of quality of life in elderly patients being considered for ICD therapy merits further study.

CORONARY REVASCULARIZATION

Many older patients with AMI will have undergone coronary revascularization during the acute phase of their illness. The role of revascularization following the acute phase raises many challenges in the elderly. Among other considerations, advanced age adds complexity due to an increased incidence of multivessel disease, significant coronary calcification, peripheral arterial disease, renal insufficiency, and frailty (1). Outside of the acute setting, the only indications for revascularization are prolongation of life and relief of unacceptable symptoms despite optimal medical management (147). Improved survival in the nonacute setting has only been demonstrated in certain subsets of patients, including those with significant left main obstructive disease, multivessel disease involving the proximal left anterior descending artery, or significant disease in the left anterior descending artery in the presence of a large ischemic burden. In the COURAGE trial, in which patients with stable ischemic heart disease were randomly assigned to percutaneous coronary intervention (PCI) plus aggressive medical therapy or aggressive medical therapy alone, there were no significant differences in outcomes between the two treatment groups in the overall population or in the subgroup ≥65 years of age (148). Therefore, aggressive medical therapy without revascularization is likely to be the most appropriate treatment option in the majority of elderly patients following the acute phase of MI (149).

If a decision to proceed with revascularization is reached, consideration must be given to the choice between coronary artery bypass graft (CABG) and PCI. Revascularization by PCI or by CABG is extensively discussed elsewhere in this book. Complete assessment by a heart team, as well as considerations of patient preferences, is essential in order to provide the most appropriate care. If coronary revascularization is performed, aggressive medical therapy must be continued.

REFERENCES

1. Fleg JL, Forman DE, Berra K, Bittner V, Blumenthal JA, Chen MA, et al. Secondary prevention of atherosclerotic cardiovascular disease in older adults: a scientific statement from the American Heart Association. *Circulation* 2013;128(22):2422-46.
2. Benjamin EJ, Blaha MJ, Chiuve SE, Cushman M, Das SR, Deo R, et al. Heart disease and stroke statistics-2017 update: a report from the American Heart Association. *Circulation* 2017;135(10):e146-e603.
3. Health, United States, 2016: with chartbook on long-term trends in health. 2017 May.
4. Jajich CL, Ostfeld AM, Freeman DH. Smoking and coronary heart disease mortality in the elderly. *JAMA* 1984;252(20):2831–4.
5. Siegel D, Kuller L, Lazarus NB, Black D, Feigal D, Hughes G, et al. Predictors of cardiovascular events and mortality in the Systolic Hypertension in the Elderly Program pilot project. *American Journal of Epidemiology* 1987;126(3):385–99.
6. Kannel WB, Vokonas PS. Primary risk factors for coronary heart disease in the elderly: The Framingham Study. In: Wenger NK, Furberg CD, Pitt B, eds. Coronary Heart Disease in the Elderly. New York: Elsevier Science Publishing Co, Inc, 1986:60–92.
7. Benfante R, Reed D, Frank J. Does cigarette smoking have an independent effect on coronary heart disease incidence in the elderly? *American Journal of Public Health* 1991;81(7):897–9.
8. LaCroix AZ, Lang J, Scherr P, Wallace RB, Cornoni-Huntley J, Berkman L, et al. Smoking and mortality among older men and women in three communities. *The New England Journal of Medicine* 1991;324(23):1619–25.
9. Hermanson B, Omenn GS, Kronmal RA, Gersh BJ. Beneficial six-year outcome of smoking cessation in older men and women with coronary artery disease. Results from the CASS registry. *The New England Journal of Medicine* 1988;319(21):1365–9.
10. Aronow WS, Ahn C. Risk factors for new coronary events in a large cohort of very elderly patients with and without coronary artery disease. *The American Journal of Cardiology* 1996;77(10):864–6.
11. Shah AM, Pfeffer MA, Hartley LH, Moyé LA, Gersh BJ, Rutherford JD, et al. Risk of all-cause mortality, recurrent myocardial infarction, and heart failure hospitalization associated with smoking status following myocardial infarction with left ventricular dysfunction. *The American Journal of Cardiology* 2010;106(7):911–16.
12. O'Gara PT, Kushner FG, Ascheim DD, Casey DE, Chung MK, de Lemos JA, et al. 2013 ACCF/AHA guideline for the management of ST-elevation myocardial infarction: a report of the American College of Cardiology Foundation/American Heart Association Task Force on Practice Guidelines. *Circulation* 2013;127(4):e78-e140.
13. Smith SC, Benjamin EJ, Bonow RO, Braun LT, Creager MA, Franklin BA, et al. AHA/ACCF secondary prevention and risk reduction therapy for patients with coronary and other atherosclerotic vascular disease: 2011 update: a guideline from the American Heart Association and American College of Cardiology Foundation. *Circulation* 2011;124(22):2432–46.
14. Eisenberg MJ, Windle SB, Roy N, Old W, Grondin FR, Bata I, et al. Varenicline for smoking cessation in hospitalized patients with acute coronary syndrome. *Circulation* 2016;133(1):21-30.
15. Burstein AH, Fullerton T, Clark DJ, Faessel HM. Pharmacokinetics, safety, and tolerability after single and multiple oral doses of varenicline in elderly smokers. *Journal of Clinical Pharmacology* 2006;46(11):1234-40.
16. Aronow WS, Fleg JL, Pepine CJ, Artinian NT, Bakris G, Brown AS, et al. ACCF/AHA 2011 expert consensus document on hypertension in the elderly: a report of the American College of Cardiology Foundation Task Force on Clinical Expert Consensus Documents. *Circulation* 2011;123(21):2037–114.
17. Aronow WS, Ahn C, Kronzon I, Koenigsberg M. Congestive heart failure, coronary events and atherothrombotic brain infarction in elderly blacks and whites with systemic hypertension and with and without echocardiographic and electrocardiographic evidence of left ventricular hypertrophy. *The American Journal of Cardiology* 1991;67(4):295–9.
18. Applegate WB, Rutan GH. Advances in management of hypertension in older persons. *Journal of the American Geriatrics Society* 1992;40(11).

19. Amery A, Birkenhäger W, Brixko P, Bulpitt C, Clement D, Deruyttere M, et al. Mortality and morbidity results from the European Working Party on High Blood Pressure in the Elderly trial. *Lancet (London, England)* 1985;1(8442):1164–74.
20. Dahlöf B, Lindholm LH, Hansson L, Scherstén B, Ekbom T, Wester PO. Morbidity and mortality in the Swedish Trial in Old Patients with Hypertension (STOP-Hypertension). *Lancet (London, England)* 1991;338(8778):1281–5.
21. Medical Research Council trial of treatment of hypertension in older adults: principal results. MRC Working Party. *BMJ (Clinical research ed)* 1992;304(6824):405–12.
22. Prevention of stroke by antihypertensive drug treatment in older persons with isolated systolic hypertension. Final results of the Systolic Hypertension in the Elderly Program (SHEP). SHEP Cooperative Research Group. *JAMA* 1991;265(24):3255–64.
23. Staessen JA, Fagard R, Thijs L, Celis H, Arabidze GG, Birkenhäger WH, et al. Randomised double-blind comparison of placebo and active treatment for older patients with isolated systolic hypertension. The Systolic Hypertension in Europe (Syst-Eur) Trial Investigators. *Lancet (London, England)* 1997;350(9080):757–64.
24. Beckett NS, Peters R, Fletcher AE, Staessen JA, Liu L, Dumitrascu D, et al. Treatment of hypertension in patients 80 years of age or older. *The New England Journal of Medicine* 2008;358(18):1887–98.
25. Lloyd-Jones D, Adams R, Carnethon M, De Simone G, Ferguson TB, Flegal K, et al. Heart disease and stroke statistics 2009 update: a report from the American Heart Association Statistics Committee and Stroke Statistics Subcommittee. *Circulation* 2009;119(3):e21–e181.
26. Law MR, Morris JK, Wald NJ. Use of blood pressure lowering drugs in the prevention of cardiovascular disease: meta-analysis of 147 randomised trials in the context of expectations from prospective epidemiological studies. *BMJ (Clinical research ed)* 2009;338:b1665.
27. Smith SC, Allen J, Blair SN, Bonow RO, Brass LM, Fonarow GC, et al. AHA/ACC guidelines for secondary prevention for patients with coronary and other atherosclerotic vascular disease: 2006 update: endorsed by the National Heart, Lung, and Blood Institute. *Circulation* 2006;113(19):2363–72.
28. Yusuf S, Sleight P, Pogue J, Bosch J, Davies R, Dagenais G. Effects of an angiotensin-converting-enzyme inhibitor, ramipril, on cardiovascular events in high-risk patients. *The New England Journal of Medicine* 2000;342(3):145–53.
29. Aronow WS, Ahn C, Kronzon I. Effect of beta blockers alone, of angiotensin-converting enzyme inhibitors alone, and of beta blockers plus angiotensin-converting enzyme inhibitors on new coronary events and on congestive heart failure in older persons with healed myocardial infarcts and asymptomatic left ventricular systolic dysfunction. *The American Journal of Cardiology* 2001;88(11):1298–300.
30. Aronow WS, Ahn C. Effect of beta blockers on incidence of new coronary events in older persons with prior myocardial infarction and diabetes mellitus. *The American Journal of Cardiology* 2001;87(6):780–1.
31. Pahor M, Psaty BM, Alderman MH, Applegate WB, Williamson JD, Cavazzini C, et al. Health outcomes associated with calcium antagonists compared with other first-line antihypertensive therapies: a meta-analysis of randomised controlled trials. *Lancet (London, England)* 2000;356(9246):1949–54.
32. Major cardiovascular events in hypertensive patients randomized to doxazosin vs chlorthalidone: the antihypertensive and lipid-lowering treatment to prevent heart attack trial (ALLHAT). ALLHAT Collaborative Research Group. *JAMA* 2000;283(15):1967–75.
33. Aronow WS, Ahn C. Incidence of new coronary events in older persons with prior myocardial infarction and systemic hypertension treated with beta blockers, angiotensin-converting enzyme inhibitors, diuretics, calcium antagonists, and alpha blockers. *The American Journal of Cardiology* 2002;89(10):1207–9.
34. Pitt B, White H, Nicolau J, Martinez F, Gheorghiade M, Aschermann M, et al. Eplerenone reduces mortality 30 days after randomization following acute myocardial infarction in patients with left ventricular systolic dysfunction and heart failure. *Journal of the American College of Cardiology* 2005;46(3):425–31.
35. Whelton PK, Carey RM, Aronow WS, Casey DE, Collins KJ, Dennison HC, et al. 2017 ACC/AHA/AAPA/ABC/ACPM/AGS/APhA/ASH/ASPC/NMA/PCNA guideline for the prevention, detection, evaluation, and management of high blood pressure in adults: executive summary: a report of the American College of Cardiology/American Heart Association Task Force on Clinical Practice Guidelines. *Hypertension* (Dallas, Tex: 1979) 2018;71(6).
36. de Boer IH, Bangalore S, Benetos A, Davis AM, Michos ED, Muntner P, et al. Diabetes and hypertension: a position statement by the American Diabetes Association. *Diabetes Care* 2017;40(9):1273–84.
37. Effect of metoprolol CR/XL in chronic heart failure: Metoprolol CR/XL Randomised Intervention Trial in Congestive Heart Failure (MERIT-HF). *Lancet (London, England)* 1999;353(9169):2001–7.
38. Aronow WS, Ahn C, Kronzon I. Effect of propranolol versus no propranolol on total mortality plus nonfatal myocardial infarction in older patients with prior myocardial infarction, congestive heart

failure, and left ventricular ejection fraction > or = 40% treated with diuretics plus angiotensin-converting enzyme inhibitors. *The American Journal of Cardiology* 1997;80(2):207–9.
39. Aronow WS, Frishman WH. Angina in the elderly. In: *Cardiovascular Disease in the Elderly.* 4th Edition. CRC Press; 2008:269–92.
40. Aronow WS, Ahn C, Mercando AD, Epstein S, Kronzon I. Decrease in mortality by propranolol in patients with heart disease and complex ventricular arrhythmias is more an anti-ischemic than an antiarrhythmic effect. *The American Journal of Cardiology* 1994;74(6):613–15.
41. Aronow WS. Management of the older person with atrial fibrillation. *The Journals of Gerontology Series A, Biological Sciences and Medical Sciences* 2002;57(6):M352–63.
42. Aronow WS. The Heart and Thyroid Disease. Clinics in geriatric medicine. *Scientific Research Publishing* 1995;11:219–29.
43. Yancy CW, Jessup M, Bozkurt B, Butler J, Casey DE, Drazner MH, et al. 2013 ACCF/AHA guideline for the management of heart failure: a report of the American College of Cardiology Foundation/American Heart Association Task Force on Practice Guidelines. *Journal of the American College of Cardiology* 2013;62(16):e147–239.
44. Aronow WS. Epidemiology, pathophysiology, prognosis, and treatment of systolic and diastolic heart failure. *Cardiology in Review* 2006;14(3):108–24.
45. Waits GS, O'Neal WT, Sandesara PB, Li Y, Shah AJ, Soliman EZ. Association between low diastolic blood pressure and subclinical myocardial injury. *Clinical Research in Cardiology: Official Journal of the German Cardiac Society* 2018;107(4).
46. Somes GW, Pahor M, Shorr RI, Cushman WC, Applegate WB. The role of diastolic blood pressure when treating isolated systolic hypertension. *Archives of Internal Medicine* 1999;159(17):2004–9.
47. Wong ND, Wilson PW, Kannel WB. Serum cholesterol as a prognostic factor after myocardial infarction: the Framingham Study. *Annals of Internal Medicine* 1991;115(9):687–93.
48. Lewington S, Whitlock G, Clarke R, Sherliker P, Emberson J, Halsey J, et al. Blood cholesterol and vascular mortality by age, sex, and blood pressure: a meta-analysis of individual data from 61 prospective studies with 55,000 vascular deaths. *Lancet (London, England)* 2007;370(9602):1829–39.
49. Miettinen TA, Pyörälä K, Olsson AG, Musliner TA, Cook TJ, Faergeman O, et al. Cholesterol-lowering therapy in women and elderly patients with myocardial infarction or angina pectoris: findings from the Scandinavian Simvastatin Survival Study (4S). *Circulation* 1997;96(12):4211–18.
50. Lewis SJ, Moye LA, Sacks FM, Johnstone DE, Timmis G, Mitchell J, et al. Effect of pravastatin on cardiovascular events in older patients with myocardial infarction and cholesterol levels in the average range. Results of the Cholesterol and Recurrent Events (CARE) trial. *Annals of Internal Medicine* 1998;129(9):681–9.
51. Long-Term Intervention with Pravastatin in Ischaemic Disease (LIPID) Study Group. Prevention of cardiovascular events and death with pravastatin in patients with coronary heart disease and a broad range of initial cholesterol levels. *The New England Journal of Medicine* 1998;339(19):1349–57
52. Heart Protection Study Collaborative Group. MRC/BHF Heart Protection Study of cholesterol lowering with simvastatin in 20,536 high-risk individuals: a randomised placebo-controlled trial. *Lancet (London, England)* 2002;360(9326):7–22.
53. Deedwania P, Stone PH, Merz CNB, Cosin-Aguilar J, Koylan N, Luo D, et al. Effects of intensive versus moderate lipid-lowering therapy on myocardial ischemia in older patients with coronary heart disease: results of the Study Assessing Goals in the Elderly (SAGE). *Circulation* 2007;115(6).
54. Afilalo J, Duque G, Steele R, Jukema JW, de Craen AJ, Eisenberg MJ. Statins for secondary prevention in elderly patients: a hierarchical bayesian meta-analysis. *Journal of the American College of Cardiology* 2008;51(1):37–45.
55. Baigent C, Blackwell L, Emberson J, Holland LE, Reith C, Bhala N, et al. Efficacy and safety of more intensive lowering of LDL cholesterol: a meta-analysis of data from 170,000 participants in 26 randomised trials. *Lancet (London, England)* 2010;376(9753).
56. Cannon CP, Blazing MA, Giugliano RP, McCagg A, White JA, Theroux P, et al. Ezetimibe added to statin therapy after acute coronary syndromes. *The New England Journal of Medicine* 2015;372(25):2387–97.
57. Stone NJ, Robinson JG, Lichtenstein AH, Cn BM, Blum CB, Eckel RH, et al. 2013 ACC/AHA guideline on the treatment of blood cholesterol to reduce atherosclerotic cardiovascular risk in adults: a report of the American College of Cardiology/American Heart Association Task Force on Practice Guidelines. *Journal of the American College of Cardiology* 2014;63(25 Pt B):2889–934.
58. Pearson T, Denke M, McBride P, Battisti WP, Brady WE, Palmisano J. Effectiveness of the addition of ezetimibe to ongoing statin therapy in modifying lipid profiles and attaining low-density lipoprotein cholesterol goals in older and elderly patients: subanalyses of data from a randomized, double-blind, placebo-controlled trial. *The American Journal of Geriatric Pharmacotherapy* 2005;3(4):218–28.

59. Scheen AJ. Diabetes mellitus in the elderly: insulin resistance and/or impaired insulin secretion? *Diabetes & Metabolism* 2005;31 Spec No 2.
60. Mozaffarian D, Benjamin EJ, Go AS, Arnett DK, Blaha MJ, Cushman M, et al. Heart disease and stroke statistics—2015 update: a report from the American Heart Association. *Circulation* 2015;131(4):e29–e322.
61. Selvin E, Coresh J, Brancati FL. The burden and treatment of diabetes in elderly individuals in the U.S. *Diabetes Care* 2006;29(11):2415–19.
62. Wing RR, Hamman RF, Bray GA, Delahanty L, Edelstein SL, Hill JO, et al. Achieving weight and activity goals among diabetes prevention program lifestyle participants. *Obesity Research* 2004;12(9):1426–34.
63. Qaseem A, Barry MJ, Humphrey LL, Forciea MA, Fitterman N, Horwitch C, et al. Oral pharmacologic treatment of type 2 diabetes mellitus: a clinical practice guideline update from the American College of Physicians. *Annals of Internal Medicine* 2017;166(4):218–31.
64. Marso SP, Daniels GH, Brown-Frandsen K, Kristensen P, Mann JF, Nauck MA, et al. Liraglutide and cardiovascular outcomes in type 2 diabetes. *The New England Journal of Medicine* 2016;375(4):311–22.
65. Damluji AA, Ramireddy A, Otalvaro L, Forman DE. Secondary cardiovascular prevention in older adults: an evidence based review. *Journal of Geriatric Cardiology: JGC* 2015;12(5):459–64.
66. Kirkman MS, Briscoe VJ, Clark N, Florez H, Haas LB, Halter JB, et al. Diabetes in older adults. *Diabetes Care* 2012;35(12):2650–64.
67. Ismail-Beigi F, Moghissi E, Tiktin M, Hirsch IB, Inzucchi SE, Genuth S. Individualizing glycemic targets in type 2 diabetes mellitus: implications of recent clinical trials. *Annals of Internal Medicine* 2011;154(8):554–9.
68. Moreno G, Mangione CM, Kimbro L, Vaisberg E. Guidelines abstracted from the American Geriatrics Society Guidelines for improving the care of older adults with diabetes mellitus: 2013 update. *Journal of the American Geriatrics Society* 2013;61(11):2020–6.
69. Stevens J, Cai J, Pamuk ER, Williamson DF, Thun MJ, Wood JL. The effect of age on the association between body-mass index and mortality. *The New England Journal of Medicine* 1998;338(1):1–7.
70. Mathus-Vliegen EM. Obesity and the elderly. *Journal of Clinical Gastroenterology* 2012;46(7):533–44.
71. Romero-Corral A, Montori VM, Somers VK, Korinek J, Thomas RJ, Allison TG, et al. Association of bodyweight with total mortality and with cardiovascular events in coronary artery disease: a systematic review of cohort studies. *Lancet (London, England)* 2006;368(9536):666–78.
72. Villareal DT, Apovian CM, Kushner RF, Klein S. Obesity in older adults: technical review and position statement of the American Society for Nutrition and NAASO, The Obesity Society. *The American Journal of Clinical Nutrition* 2005;82(5):923–34.
73. Villareal DT, Miller BV, Banks M, Fontana L, Sinacore DR, Klein S. Effect of lifestyle intervention on metabolic coronary heart disease risk factors in obese older adults. *The American Journal of Clinical Nutrition* 2006;84(6):1317–23.
74. Villareal DT, Banks M, Sinacore DR, Siener C, Klein S. Effect of weight loss and exercise on frailty in obese older adults. *Archives of Internal Medicine* 2006;166(8):860–6.
75. Villareal DT, Banks MR, Patterson BW, Polonsky KS, Klein S. Weight loss therapy improves pancreatic endocrine function in obese older adults. *Obesity* (Silver Spring, Md) 2008;16(6):1349–54.
76. Villareal DT, Shah K, Banks MR, Sinacore DR, Klein S. Effect of weight loss and exercise therapy on bone metabolism and mass in obese older adults: a one-year randomized controlled trial. *The Journal of Clinical Endocrinology and Metabolism* 2008;93(6):2181–8.
77. Villareal DT, Chode S, Parimi N, Sinacore DR, Hilton T, Armamento-Villareal R, et al. Weight loss, exercise, or both and physical function in obese older adults. *The New England Journal of Medicine* 2011;364(13):1218–29.
78. MacMillan M, Cummins K, Fujioka K. What weight loss treatment options do geriatric patients with overweight and obesity want to consider? *Obesity Science & Practice* 2016;2(4):477–82.
79. Jensen, Ryan DH, Apovian CM, Ard JD, Comuzzie AG, Donato KA, et al. 2013 AHA/ACC/TOS guideline for the management of overweight and obesity in adults: a report of the American College of Cardiology/American Heart Association Task Force on Practice Guidelines and The Obesity Society. *Circulation* 2014;129(25 Suppl 2).
80. Giordano S, Victorzon M. Bariatric surgery in elderly patients: a systematic review. *Clinical Interventions in Aging* 2015;10:1627–35.
81. Morris JN, Heady JA, Raffle PA, Roberts CG, Parks JW. Coronary heart-disease and physical activity of work. *Lancet (London, England)* 1953;262(6795):1111–20.
82. Thompson PD, Buchner D, Pina IL, Balady GJ, Williams MA, Marcus BH, et al. Exercise and physical activity in the prevention and treatment of atherosclerotic cardiovascular disease: a statement from the Council on Clinical Cardiology (Subcommittee on Exercise, Rehabilitation, and Prevention) and the Council on Nutrition, Physical Activity, and Metabolism (Subcommittee on Physical Activity). *Circulation* 2003;107(24):3109–16.

83. Hakim AA, Curb JD, Petrovitch H, Rodriguez BL, Yano K, Ross GW, et al. Effects of walking on coronary heart disease in elderly men: the Honolulu Heart Program. *Circulation* 1999;100(1):9–13.
84. Haskell WL, Lee IM, Pate RR, Powell KE, Blair SN, Franklin BA, et al. Physical activity and public health: updated recommendation for adults from the American College of Sports Medicine and the American Heart Association. *Medicine and Science in Sports and Exercise* 2007;39(8):1081–93.
85. Amsterdam EA, Wenger NK, Brindis RG, Casey DE, Ganiats TG, Holmes DR, et al. 2014 AHA/ACC guideline for the management of patients with non-ST-elevation acute coronary syndromes: a report of the American College of Cardiology/American Heart Association Task Force on Practice Guidelines. *Journal of the American College of Cardiology* 2014;64(24):e139–e228.
86. Théroux P. Antithrombotic treatment of acute coronary syndromes. *The Canadian Journal of Cardiology* 1998;114 (Suppl):611S–33S.
87. Antithrombotic Trialists' Collaboration. Collaborative meta-analysis of randomised trials of antiplatelet therapy for prevention of death, myocardial infarction, and stroke in high risk patients. *BMJ (Clinical research ed)* 2002;324(7329):71–86.
88. Goldstein RE, Andrews M, Hall WJ, Moss AJ. Marked reduction in long-term cardiac deaths with aspirin after a coronary event. Multicenter Myocardial Ischemia Research Group. *Journal of the American College of Cardiology* 1996;28(2):326–30.
89. Krumholz HM, Radford MJ, Ellerbeck EF, Hennen J, Meehan TP, Petrillo M, et al. Aspirin for secondary prevention after acute myocardial infarction in the elderly: prescribed use and outcomes. *Annals of Internal Medicine* 1996;124(3):292–8.
90. Mahé I, Leizorovicz A, Caulin C, Bergmann JF. Aspirin for the prevention of cardiovascular events in the elderly. *Drugs & Aging* 2003;20(13):999–1010.
91. Fleg JL, Aronow WS, Frishman WH. Cardiovascular drug therapy in the elderly: benefits and challenges. *Nature Reviews Cardiology* 2011;8(1):13–28.
92. Yusuf S, Zhao F, Mehta SR, Chrolavicius S, Tognoni G, Fox KK. Effects of clopidogrel in addition to aspirin in patients with acute coronary syndromes without ST-segment elevation. *The New England Journal of Medicine* 2001;345(7):494–502.
93. Bhatt DL, Cryer BL, Contant CF, Cohen M, Lanas A, Schnitzer TJ, et al. Clopidogrel with or without omeprazole in coronary artery disease. *The New England Journal of Medicine* 2010;363(20):1909–17.
94. Gimbel M, Qaderdan K, Willemsen L, Hermanides R, Bergmeijer T, de Vrey E, et al. Clopidogrel versus ticagrelor or prasugrel in patients aged 70 years or older with non-ST-elevation acute coronary syndrome (POPular AGE): the randomised, open-label, non-inferiority trial. *Lancet (London, England)* 2020;395(10233).
95. Qaderdan K, Ishak M, Heestermans AA, de Vrey E, Jukema JW, Voskuil M, et al. Ticagrelor or prasugrel versus clopidogrel in elderly patients with an acute coronary syndrome: optimization of antiplatelet treatment in patients 70 years and older—rationale and design of the POPular AGE study. *American Heart Journal* 2015;170(5):981–5.
96. Moon JY, Nagaraju D, Franchi F, Rollini F, Angiolillo DJ. The role of oral anticoagulant therapy in patients with acute coronary syndrome. *Therapeutic Advances in Hematology* 2017 Oct 13;8(12):353–66.
97. Andreotti F, Testa L, Biondi-Zoccai GG, Crea F. Aspirin plus warfarin compared to aspirin alone after acute coronary syndromes: an updated and comprehensive meta-analysis of 25,307 patients. *European Heart Journal* 2006;27(5):519–26.
98. Lamberts M, Olesen JB, Ruwald MH, Hansen CM, Karasoy D, Kristensen SL, et al. Bleeding after initiation of multiple antithrombotic drugs, including triple therapy, in atrial fibrillation patients following myocardial infarction and coronary intervention: a nationwide cohort study. *Circulation* 2012;126(10):1185–93.
99. Alexander JH, Lopes RD, James S, Kilaru R, He Y, Mohan P, et al. Apixaban with antiplatelet therapy after acute coronary syndrome. *The New England Journal of Medicine* 2011;365(8):699–708.
100. Mega JL, Braunwald E, Wiviott SD, Bassand JP, Bhatt DL, Bode C, et al. Rivaroxaban in patients with a recent acute coronary syndrome. *The New England Journal of Medicine* 2012 Jan 5;366(1):9–19.
101. Steg PG, James SK, Atar D, Badano LP, Blömstrom-Lundqvist C, Borger MA, et al. ESC Guidelines for the management of acute myocardial infarction in patients presenting with ST-segment elevation. *European Heart Journal* 2012;33(20):2569–619.
102. Furberg CD, Hawkins CM, Lichstein E. Effect of propranolol in postinfarction patients with mechanical or electrical complications. *Circulation* 1984;69(4):761–5.
103. Kennedy HL, Brooks MM, Barker AH, Bergstrand R, Huther ML, Beanlands DS, et al. Beta-blocker therapy in the Cardiac Arrhythmia Suppression Trial. CAST Investigators. *The American Journal of Cardiology* 1994;74(7):674–80.
104. Aronow WS, Ahn C, Mercando AD, Epstein S, Kronzon I. Effect of propranolol versus no antiarrhythmic drug on sudden cardiac death, total cardiac death, and total death in patients > or = 62 years of age with heart disease, complex ventricular arrhythmias, and left ventricular ejection fraction > or = 40%. *The American Journal of Cardiology* 1994;74(3):267–70.

105. Hjalmarson A, Elmfeldt D, Herlitz J, Holmberg S, Málek I, Nyberg G, et al. Effect on mortality of metoprolol in acute myocardial infarction. A double-blind randomised trial. *Lancet (London, England)* 1981;2(8251):823–7.
106. Gundersen T, Abrahamsen AM, Kjekshus J, Rønnevik PK. Timolol-related reduction in mortality and reinfarction in patients ages 65-75 years surviving acute myocardial infarction. Prepared for the Norwegian Multicentre Study Group. *Circulation* 1982;66(6):1179–84.
107. Pedersen TR. Six-year follow-up of the Norwegian Multicenter Study on timolol after acute myocardial infarction. *The New England Journal of Medicine* 1985;313(17):1055–8.
108. A randomized trial of propranolol in patients with acute myocardial infarction. I. Mortality results. *JAMA* 1982;247(12):1707–14.
109. Dargie HJ. Effect of carvedilol on outcome after myocardial infarction in patients with left-ventricular dysfunction: the CAPRICORN randomised trial. *Lancet (London, England)* 2001;357(9266):1385–90.
110. Chen ZM, Pan HC, Chen YP, Peto R, Collins R, Jiang LX, et al. Early intravenous then oral metoprolol in 45,852 patients with acute myocardial infarction: randomised placebo-controlled trial. *Lancet (London, England)* 2005;366(9497):1622–32.
111. Kernis SJ, Harjai KJ, Stone GW, Grines LL, Boura JA, O'Neill WW, et al. Does beta-blocker therapy improve clinical outcomes of acute myocardial infarction after successful primary angioplasty? *Journal of the American College of Cardiology* 2004;43(10):1773–9.
112. Kezerashvili A, Marzo K, De Leon J. Beta blocker use after acute myocardial infarction in the patient with normal systolic function: when is it "ok" to discontinue? *Current Cardiology Reviews* 2012;8(1):77–84.
113. Yndigegn T, Lindahl B, Mars K, Alfredsson J, Benatar J, Brandin L, et al. Beta-blockers after myocardial infarction and preserved ejection fraction. *The New England Journal of Medicine* 2024;390(15).
114. Steinman MA, Zullo AR, Lee Y, Daiello LA, Boscardin WJ, Dore DD, et al. Association of β-Blockers with functional outcomes, death, and rehospitalization in older nursing home residents after acute myocardial infarction. *JAMA Internal Medicine* 2017;177(2):254–62.
115. Pfeffer MA, Braunwald E, Moyé LA, Basta L, Brown EJ, Cuddy TE, et al. Effect of captopril on mortality and morbidity in patients with left ventricular dysfunction after myocardial infarction. Results of the survival and ventricular enlargement trial. The SAVE Investigators. *The New England Journal of Medicine* 1992 Sep 3;327(10):669–77.
116. Effect of ramipril on mortality and morbidity of survivors of acute myocardial infarction with clinical evidence of heart failure. The Acute Infarction Ramipril Efficacy (AIRE) Study Investigators. *Lancet (London, England)* 1993;342(8875).
117. Ambrosioni E, Borghi C, Magnani B. The effect of the angiotensin-converting-enzyme inhibitor zofenopril on mortality and morbidity after anterior myocardial infarction. The Survival of Myocardial Infarction Long-Term Evaluation (SMILE) Study Investigators. *The New England Journal of Medicine* 1995;332(2):80–5.
118. Køber L, Torp-Pedersen C, Carlsen JE, Bagger H, Eliasen P, Lyngborg K, et al. A clinical trial of the angiotensin-converting-enzyme inhibitor trandolapril in patients with left ventricular dysfunction after myocardial infarction. Trandolapril Cardiac Evaluation (TRACE) Study Group. *The New England Journal of Medicine* 1995;333(25):1670–6.
119. Fox KM. Efficacy of perindopril in reduction of cardiovascular events among patients with stable coronary artery disease: randomised, double-blind, placebo-controlled, multicentre trial (the EUROPA study). *Lancet (London, England)* 2003;362(9386):782–8.
120. Flather, Yusuf S, Køber L, Pfeffer M, Hall A, Murray G, et al. Long-term ACE-inhibitor therapy in patients with heart failure or left-ventricular dysfunction: a systematic overview of data from individual patients. ACE-Inhibitor Myocardial Infarction Collaborative Group. *Lancet (London, England)* 2000;355(9215):1575–81.
121. Pitt B, Remme W, Zannad F, Neaton J, Martinez F, Roniker B, et al. Eplerenone, a selective aldosterone blocker, in patients with left ventricular dysfunction after myocardial infarction. *The New England Journal of Medicine* 2003;348(14):1309–21.
122. Pitt B, Williams G, Remme W, Martinez F, Lopez-Sendon J, Zannad F, et al. The EPHESUS trial: eplerenone in patients with heart failure due to systolic dysfunction complicating acute myocardial infarction. Eplerenone Post-AMI Heart Failure Efficacy and Survival Study. *Cardiovascular Drugs and Therapy* 2001;15(1).
123. Zinman B, Wanner C, Lachin JM, Fitchett D, Bluhmki E, Hantel S, et al. Empagliflozin, cardiovascular outcomes, and mortality in type 2 diabetes. *The New England Journal of Medicine* 2015;373(22).
124. Neal B, Perkovic V, Mahaffey KW, de Zeeuw D, Fulcher G, Erondu N, et al. Canagliflozin and cardiovascular and renal events in type 2 diabetes. *The New England Journal of Medicine* 2017;377(7).
125. Wiviott SD, Raz I, Bonaca MP, Mosenzon O, Kato ET, Cahn A, et al. Dapagliflozin and cardiovascular outcomes in type 2 diabetes. *The New England Journal of Medicine* 2019;380(4).

126. Cahn A, Mosenzon O, Wiviott SD, Rozenberg A, Yanuv I, Goodrich EL, et al. Efficacy and safety of Dapagliflozin in the elderly: analysis from the DECLARE-TIMI 58 study. *Diabetes Care* 2020;43(2).
127. Butler J, Jones WS, Udell JA, Anker SD, Petrie MC, Harrington J, et al. Empagliflozin after acute myocardial infarction. *The New England Journal of Medicine* 2024;390(16).
128. James S, Erlinge D, Storey RF, McGuire DK, de Belder M, Eriksson N, et al. Dapagliflozin in myocardial infarction without diabetes or heart failure. *NEJM Evidence* 2024;3(2).
129. Hulley S, Furberg C, Barrett-Connor E, Cauley J, Grady D, Haskell W, et al. Noncardiovascular disease outcomes during 6.8 years of hormone therapy: Heart and Estrogen/progestin Replacement Study follow-up (HERS II). *JAMA* 2002;288(1):58–66.
130. Herrington DM, Reboussin DM, Brosnihan KB, Sharp PC, Shumaker SA, Snyder TE, et al. Effects of estrogen replacement on the progression of coronary-artery atherosclerosis. *The New England Journal of Medicine* 2000;343(8):522–9.
131. Rossouw JE, Anderson GL, Prentice RL, LaCroix AZ, Kooperberg C, Stefanick ML, et al. Risks and benefits of estrogen plus progestin in healthy postmenopausal women: principal results From the Women's Health Initiative randomized controlled trial. *JAMA* 2002;288(3):321.
132. Boardman HM, Hartley L, Eisinga A, Main C, Roqué i Figuls M, Bonfill CX, et al. Hormone therapy for preventing cardiovascular disease in postmenopausal women. *The Cochrane Database of Systematic Reviews* 2015;2015(3):CD002229.
133. Davis MM, Taubert K, Benin AL, Brown DW, Mensah GA, Baddour LM, et al. Influenza vaccination as secondary prevention for cardiovascular disease: a science advisory from the American Heart Association/American College of Cardiology. *Journal of the American College of Cardiology* 2006;48(7).
134. Siebels J, Kuck KH. Implantable cardioverter defibrillator compared with antiarrhythmic drug treatment in cardiac arrest survivors (the Cardiac Arrest Study Hamburg). *American Heart Journal* 1994;127(4 Pt 2):1139–44.
135. Connolly SJ, Hallstrom AP, Cappato R, Schron EB, Kuck KH, Zipes DP, et al. Meta-analysis of the implantable cardioverter defibrillator secondary prevention trials. AVID, CASH and CIDS studies. Antiarrhythmics vs Implantable Defibrillator study. Cardiac Arrest Study Hamburg. Canadian Implantable Defibrillator Study. *European Heart Journal* 2000;21(24):2071–8.
136. Antiarrhythmics versus Implantable Defibrillators (AVID) Investigators. A comparison of antiarrhythmic-drug therapy with implantable defibrillators in patients resuscitated from near-fatal ventricular arrhythmias. *The New England Journal of Medicine* 1997;337(22):1576–83.
137. Connolly SJ, Gent M, Roberts RS, Dorian P, Roy D, Sheldon RS, et al. Canadian implantable defibrillator study (CIDS): a randomized trial of the implantable cardioverter defibrillator against amiodarone. *Circulation* 2000;101(11):1297–1302.
138. Epstein AE, DiMarco JP, Ellenbogen KA, Estes NA, Freedman RA, Gettes LS, et al. ACC/AHA/HRS 2008 Guidelines for Device-Based Therapy of Cardiac Rhythm Abnormalities: a report of the American College of Cardiology/American Heart Association Task Force on Practice Guidelines (Writing Committee to Revise the ACC/AHA/NASPE 2002 Guideline Update for Implantation of Cardiac Pacemakers and Antiarrhythmia Devices) developed in collaboration with the American Association for Thoracic Surgery and Society of Thoracic Surgeons. *Journal of the American College of Cardiology* 2008;51(21):e1–62.
139. Al-Khatib SM, Stevenson WG, Ackerman MJ, Bryant WJ, Callans DJ, Curtis AB, et al. 2017 AHA/ACC/HRS guideline for management of patients with ventricular arrhythmias and the prevention of sudden cardiac death: executive summary: a report of the American College of Cardiology/American Heart Association Task Force on Clinical Practice Guidelines and the Heart Rhythm Society. *Circulation* 2018;138(13).
140. Kusumoto FM, Bailey KR, Chaouki AS, Deshmukh AJ, Gautam S, Kim RJ, et al. Systematic review for the 2017 AHA/ACC/HRS guideline for management of patients with ventricular arrhythmias and the prevention of sudden cardiac death: a report of the American College of Cardiology/American Heart Association Task Force on Clinical Practice Guidelines and the Heart Rhythm Society. *Journal of the American College of Cardiology* 2018;72(14).
141. Kong MH, Al-Khatib SM, Sanders GD, Hasselblad V, Peterson ED. Use of implantable cardioverter-defibrillators for primary prevention in older patients: a systematic literature review and meta-analysis. *Cardiology Journal* 2011;18(5):503–14.
142. Grimm W, Stula A, Sharkova J, Alter P, Maisch B. Outcomes of elderly recipients of implantable cardioverter defibrillators. *Pacing and Clinical Electrophysiology: PACE* 2007;30 Suppl 1:S134–8.
143. Suleiman M, Goldenberg I, Haim M, Schliamser JE, Boulos M, Ilan M, et al. Clinical characteristics and outcomes of elderly patients treated with an implantable cardioverter-defibrillator or cardiac resynchronization therapy in a real-world setting: data from the Israeli ICD Registry. *Heart Rhythm* 2014;11(3):435–41.

144. Barra S, Providência R, Paiva L, Heck P, Agarwal S. Implantable cardioverter-defibrillators in the elderly: rationale and specific age-related considerations. *Europace: European Pacing, Arrhythmias, and Cardiac Electrophysiology: Journal of the Working Groups on Cardiac Pacing, Arrhythmias, and Cardiac Cellular Electrophysiology of the European Society of Cardiology* 2015;17(2):174–86.
145. Tomzik J, Koltermann KC, Zabel M, Willich SN, Reinhold T. Quality of life in patients with an implantable cardioverter defibrillator: a systematic review. *Frontiers in Cardiovascular Medicine* 2015;2:1–11.
146. Den Broek KC Van, Heijmans N, Van Assen MA. Anxiety and depression in patients with an implantable cardioverter defibrillator and their partners: a longitudinal study. *Pacing and Clinical Electrophysiology: PACE* 2013;36(3):362–71.
147. Stemmer EA, Aronow WS. Surgical management of coronary arterial disease in the elderly. *Coronary Artery Disease* 1998;9(5):351–85.
148. Maron DJ, Spertus JA, Mancini GB, Hartigan PM, Sedlis SP, Bates ER, et al. Impact of an initial strategy of medical therapy without percutaneous coronary intervention in high-risk patients from the Clinical Outcomes Utilizing Revascularization and Aggressive DruG Evaluation (COURAGE) trial. *The American Journal of Cardiology* 2009;104(8):1055–62.
149. Fihn SD, Gardin JM, Abrams J, Berra K, Blankenship JC, Dallas AP, et al. 2012 ACCF/AHA/ACP/AATS/PCNA/SCAI/STS guideline for the diagnosis and management of patients with stable ischemic heart disease: a report of the American College of Cardiology Foundation/American Heart Association task force on practice guidelines, and the American College of Physicians, American Association for Thoracic Surgery, Preventive Cardiovascular Nurses Association, Society for Cardiovascular Angiography and Interventions, and Society of Thoracic Surgeons. *Circulation* 2012;126(25):e44–164.

12

Coronary artery revascularization in the older adult population

PATRICK BERCHIE, JENNIFER S. LAWTON, MICHAEL G. NANNA, AND ABDULLA A. DAMLUJI

Key points

- Population aging, age-related vascular changes, and an increase in cardiovascular risk factors with age are fueling a progressively rising burden of atherosclerotic cardiovascular disease, including coronary artery disease (CAD), among older adults.
- Older adults with CAD often have more severe and more diffuse disease than younger adults, with more complex anatomy and more left main coronary disease.
- Management of older adults with CAD is complicated by the high prevalence of multimorbidity and geriatric syndromes that impact procedural risks, complication rates, and clinical outcomes.
- Clinical trials and practice guidelines for coronary revascularization have focused primarily on younger patients, leaving significant gaps for the more complex older adult population.
- Despite these limitations, both percutaneous coronary interventions and coronary artery bypass surgery are highly effective in alleviating symptoms and improving clinical outcomes in appropriately selected older patients, including those over 90 years of age.

INTRODUCTION

According to the US Census Bureau 2017 National Population Projections, the population aged ≥65 years is projected to nearly double from approximately 56 million (2020) to 95 million by 2060. This underpins the predicted "demographic shift."[1] Chronological age is a major risk factor for cardiovascular disease (CVD). Advancing age is associated with structural and functional changes in the cardiovascular system.[2] These changes include endothelial dysfunction, arterial stiffness, and decreased vascular elasticity. These changes in turn result in increased incidence of hypertension, atherosclerosis, and inflammation. Taken together, these factors foster a progressively rising burden of CVD in the older adult population.[2]

DOI: 10.1201/9781003568933-12

Adults ≥75 years constitute about 30%–40% of all patients hospitalized for acute coronary syndromes (ACS) and related complications. Approximately 720,000 Americans experience an acute myocardial infarction (AMI) or coronary artery disease (CAD)-related death each year.[1] The older adult population is disproportionately affected and typically presents with complex anatomy. They tend to have a heavy atherosclerotic plaque burden and complex vessel anatomy, including tortuosity, proximal disease, and calcifications. Additionally, concomitant geriatric syndromes may complicate their clinical course. Frailty, multimorbidity, cognitive impairment, and functional decline portend a worse prognosis. It is therefore important to consider both cardiovascular and geriatric risks when choosing a coronary artery revascularization strategy.[3]

PHYSIOLOGY OF CARDIOVASCULAR AGING AND INFLUENCE ON PROCEDURAL OUTCOMES

Aging was historically defined based on chronological age, but most recent works have focused on studying biological aging.[4] Chronological aging refers to the number of years that have elapsed since an individual's birth. However, patients of the same chronological age may have differences in CVD burden that are not explained by chronological age alone. Conversely, biological aging describes the process of aging that is affected by epigenetics, genomics, cellular function, environmental factors, and chronic diseases.[4,5] In this regard, biological aging more accurately reflects disease burden, progression, and risk for future events.[4] The cardiovascular system undergoes changes in response to mechanical and metabolic stress.[5] Over time, this leads to a higher burden of cellular dysfunction and maladaptive processes that culminate in biological aging. Genomic instability, telomere attrition, epigenetic changes, loss of proteostasis, disabled macroautophagy, dysregulated nutrient-sensing, mitochondrial dysfunction, cell senescence, stem cell exhaustion, dysregulated neurohormonal signaling, dysbiosis, and inflammation have been named as the 12 biological hallmarks of aging (Figure 12.1).[5,6] These processes are closely interconnected; small changes in one component can lead to substantial changes in others. Inflammation, also called "inflammaging," has been increasingly recognized as a risk factor playing a key role in the cardiovascular aging process.[4]

With further study of biological age in individuals with premature CVD, factors that accelerate aging versus those that promote longevity have been identified. This has led to efforts to develop biomarkers focused on identifying predictors of cardiovascular aging. Additional work has explored tracking inflammatory markers to

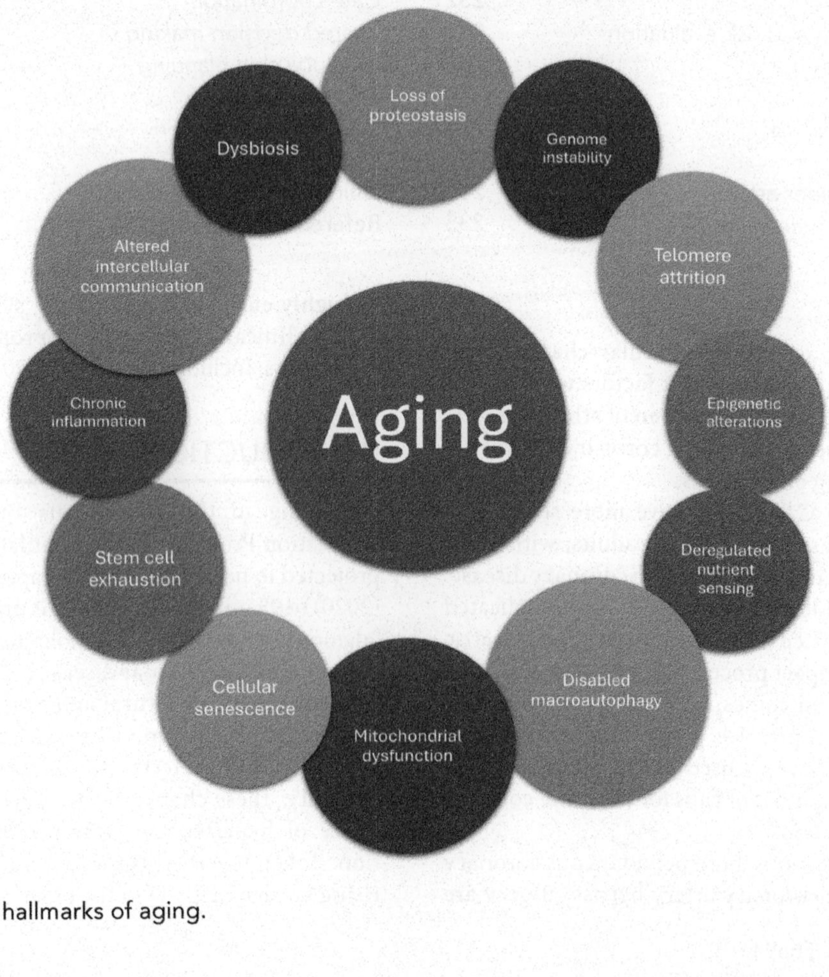

Figure 12.1 The 12 hallmarks of aging.

develop an inflammatory aging clock aimed at improving the prediction of inflammation-related cardiovascular disease morbidity and mortality.[7] As the initial changes associated with biological aging begin at the cellular level, early identification of physiologic and pathologic aging is both challenging and important. Furthermore, cardiovascular risk factors like uncontrolled diabetes mellitus and hypertension have been associated with an increased inflammatory milieu beyond that related to chronological aging.[8] Risk factor modification at the macroscopic level is therefore a key component of preventive care for CVD.

GERIATRIC SYNDROMES AND INVASIVE CARDIOVASCULAR CARE

Older adults of the same chronological age may have different physiologic responses to stressors, resulting in differences in risk, recovery, and survival.[1] Thus, it is important for the interventional cardiologist or cardiac surgeon to consider the physiological changes that occur with aging with a particular focus on geriatric syndromes (see Chapter 3 for additional discussion). These syndromes may not all be directly germane to invasive care but may still influence decisions and procedural outcomes. The framework of the 5 Ms of Geriatrics,[9] developed by Tinetti et al., encapsulates the aspects of aging that are relevant to invasive cardiovascular care for older adults (Table 12.1).

MATTERS MOST

Recognizing what matters most to older adults is a central tenet of patient-centered care when considering revascularization procedures. In a U.S. based study, Bernacki et al. reported that patients undergoing transcatheter aortic valve replacement (TAVR) often had their Do Not Resuscitate (DNR) code status automatically revoked and reverted to full code status.[10] This default approach may conflict with patient preferences, especially when a palliative care strategy or limited resuscitation aligns better with their goals.[10] Patient-priority care requires clinicians to move away from outcomes such as 30-day mortality and work towards patient-centered outcomes such as days alive out of the hospital/at home, alive to a particular milestone, or simply the possibility of relief of symptoms, without a change in life expectancy.[11] Decision-making frameworks such as the GOOD framework[12] which considers Goals, Options, Opinions, and the "Consider, Listen, Decide" model for stable ischemic heart disease can help structure these conversations.[13,14] A palliative approach may be appropriate to alleviate symptoms in the face of competing comorbidities like end-stage renal disease or advanced lung disease.

MEDICATIONS

There are multiple physiologic changes associated with the aging process that impact medication effects. These

Table 12.1 The 5Ms of Geriatrics: Framework for integrating geriatric principles in cardiovascular care pathways

5Ms framework component	Description
What Matters	Routinely elicit, document, and revisit each patient's individual goals, values, and care preferences using a Patient Priorities Care paradigm. Ensure treatment plans reflect what matters most to the patient. Central to all shared decision-making and a cornerstone of Age-Friendly Health Systems.
Medication	Perform comprehensive medication reconciliation at every encounter. Minimize polypharmacy, deprescribe potentially inappropriate medications using tools like the Beers criteria, consider age-related pharmacologic changes, and simplify regimens for better adherence.
Mentation	Screen systematically for cognitive impairment (Mini-Cog, AD8, MoCA if needed), delirium (especially in hospitalized patients with b-CAM or 4AT), and manage depression and anxiety, which are common in older adults with cardiovascular disease.
Mobility	Assess gait speed, balance, fall risk, and functional status (ADLs, IADLs). Encourage safe physical activity, refer to personalized exercise programs, and implement fall prevention strategies.
Multicomplexity	Manage multiple chronic conditions holistically. Consider disease interactions, cumulative burden, and the patient's overall treatment workload to guide care planning.

Abbreviations: AD8, ascertain dementia 8-item assessment questionnaire; ADLs, activities of daily living; CAM, confusion assessment method; 4AT, 4AT delirium assessment tool; IADLs, instrumental activities of daily living; MoCA, Montreal cognitive assessment.

Source: Modified from Tinetti et al., *J Am Geriatr Soc*, 65, 2115, 2017.[9]

include changes in weight, muscle composition, and adipose tissue mass that affect pharmacokinetics and pharmacodynamics. Additional factors include changes in hepatic and renal function that affect first-pass metabolism, bioavailability, and drug clearance.[15] Furthermore, renal dysfunction may be underestimated in older adults due to inaccurate calculations based on equations developed in younger cohorts.[16] These changes can result in decreased or increased drug efficacy in older patients, and increased risk of adverse events such as bleeding. Strategies that mitigate bleeding risk should be evaluated.[1] Additionally, many older adults take multiple medications with a potential for drug–drug interactions during the periprocedural period. Polypharmacy is common among older adults and puts them at increased risk of falls and changes in mental status.[17]

MIND

Mild cognitive impairment and dementia are common in older adults and remain underdiagnosed.[18] Ascertainment of cognitive function is important for obtaining adequate informed consent for any procedure (see Chapter 29). Cognitive impairment necessitates the engagement of a family member, caregiver, or designated healthcare proxy for healthcare-related decisions and support for older patients. Recognizing baseline cognitive dysfunction also helps in identifying those at risk for delirium. Delirium is common in hospitalized older adults, especially those who are critically ill. There are multiple triggers, including, but not limited to, hospitalization, change in medications, alterations in eating and sleeping patterns, and invasive cardiovascular care.[19] Delirium is often underdiagnosed resulting in significant healthcare costs, increased risk of postprocedural complications, morbidity, and mortality.[20]

Mental health disorders are also commonly underdiagnosed conditions in older adults.[21] Anxiety and depression are prevalent in this population and, when present, are associated with increased risk of complications following invasive cardiac procedures.[22] In patients with dementia, while the diagnosis alone should not lead to withholding care, it presents an important opportunity to evaluate the appropriateness of any intervention in the context of the stage of the illness and life goals.[23]

MOBILITY

Maximal functional capacity declines at varying rates with aging.[24] Functional status before an invasive procedure can help predict recovery after the procedure.[25] The addition of gait speed[26] and other indicators of physical function to preoperative risk scores has been shown to significantly improve the prediction of procedural complications.[27–29] Sarcopenia, defined as a decrease in muscle mass, quality, and function, is common in older adults.[30] Sarcopenia can help stratify operative risk and postprocedural length of stay.[30,31] Incorporating physical therapy and rehabilitation services may help decrease some of these risks and improve functional status and overall mobility.[32–34]

MULTICOMPLEXITY

Aging leads to physiologic changes in all organ systems that increase the risk of multimorbidity and complicate acute cardiovascular care.[35] Older adults often have multiple coexisting medical conditions beyond CVD, with high rates of multimorbidity (≥2 chronic conditions).[36] These conditions contribute to frailty with associated poor outcomes following stressors such as an acute myocardial infarction.[37] Frailty, a syndrome of vulnerability to stressors, has been conceptualized in the context of deficit accumulation across multiple systems.[38] Physical frailty, however, can be assessed using the five-item Fried physical frailty phenotype, shown in Table 12.2, which evaluates gait speed, grip strength, exhaustion, weight loss, and physical activity.[39,40] Regardless of the assessment method, frailty consistently predicts cardiovascular events and increased risk after invasive cardiac procedures.[41]

PROCEDURAL ASSESSMENT AND RISK EVALUATION

Older adults undergoing revascularization procedures face higher periprocedural risk than younger patients, which highlights the need for a comprehensive risk assessment to guide periprocedural planning, preventive strategies, and shared decision-making with patients and their families.[3,13,42–44] Traditionally, preprocedural risk assessment was limited to anatomic/technical risks, clinical considerations such as comorbidities, and the hemodynamic status of patients. More recently, the addition of a fourth domain, namely, geriatric syndromes, has been proposed when evaluating older adults.[3,44] The four pillars of risk are briefly reviewed next.

Table 12.2 The Fried physical frailty phenotype

Criteria	Definition
Weight loss	Unintentional weight loss ≥10 pounds in the past year
Exhaustion	Self-reported feeling of exhaustion or fatigue
Weakness	Measured by grip strength
Slowness	Measured by gait speed Slower walking speed may indicate frailty
Low physical activity	Measured through weekly energy expenditure questionnaires

Table 12.3 Models to estimate cardiovascular or major adverse cardiovascular event risk in older patients presenting with acute coronary syndromes

Model	Purpose	Key variables	Outcome predicted	Population	Scoring
GRACE[157]	ACS risk stratification	Age, HR, SBP, creatinine, cardiac arrest, ST deviation, elevated cardiac biomarkers	In-hospital and 6-month mortality, MI	ACS (UA/NSTEMI, STEMI)	0–372 points (higher score = higher risk)
TIMI[158]	ACS (UA/NSTEMI) risk stratification	Age ≥65, ≥3 CAD risk factors, prior stenosis, ST deviation, aspirin use, elevated biomarkers	14-day death/MI/urgent revascularization	UA/NSTEMI	0–7 points (higher score = higher risk)
CRUSADE[45]	Bleeding risk in NSTEMI	Age, sex, BMI, prior bleeding, creatinine clearance, HR, SBP, heart failure, diabetes	In-hospital major bleeding	NSTEMI	1–100 (higher score = higher bleeding risk)
EuroScore II[50]	Cardiac surgery mortality risk	Age, sex, serum creatinine, LV function, recent MI, pulmonary hypertension, urgency of surgery	In-hospital mortality post cardiac surgery	Patients undergoing cardiac surgery	% Mortality risk (0%–100%)
STS-PROM[159]	Cardiac surgery risk prediction	Age, sex, comorbidities (e.g., diabetes, COPD), LVEF, renal function, procedure type	30-day mortality, stroke, renal failure	Patients undergoing CABG/valve surgery	% Risk (0%–100%)
PRECISE-DAPT[160]	Bleeding risk on DAPT	Age, hemoglobin, white cell count, creatinine clearance, prior bleeding	Major bleeding risk during DAPT (1 year)	Post-PCI patients on DAPT	0–100 (≥25 = high bleeding risk)

Abbreviations: ACS, acute coronary syndrome; BMI, body mass index; CABG, coronary artery bypass graft; CAD, coronary artery disease; COPD, chronic obstructive pulmonary disease; DAPT, dual antiplatelet therapy; HR, heart rate; LV, left ventricular; LVEF, left ventricular ejection fraction; MI, myocardial infarction; NSTEMI, non-ST elevation myocardial infarction; SBP, systolic blood pressure; STEMI, ST-elevation myocardial infarction; UA, unstable angina.

Clinical risk assessment

Most of the same demographic, clinical, and diagnostic characteristics that impact the risk of coronary revascularization in younger populations apply to older adults.[4] Given the greater burden of comorbidities and the prominent contribution of chronological age as a driver of procedural risk in existing risk models, older adults are expected to have a higher periprocedural risk compared to younger populations using commonly available risk tools (Table 12.3).[3] For example, validated cardiovascular models such as the GRACE and the TIMI risk scores provide prognostic information in younger populations evaluated for revascularization procedures. Most older adults, however, are categorized as high risk under these models, limiting their discriminative utility in this population. Major bleeding, a critical outcome in older adults and a strong risk factor for other adverse outcomes, is captured by the CRUSADE score.[45] The strongest predictive models for in-hospital mortality for older adults undergoing percutaneous coronary intervention (PCI) are derived from the National Cardiovascular Data Registry (NCDR), which combines demographic, clinical, and diagnostic predictors with some of the hemodynamic, anatomic, and procedural characteristics with excellent performance.[46,47]

When considering older patients for coronary artery bypass grafting (CABG), use of the Society of Thoracic Surgeons Predicted Risk of Mortality (STS PROM) is recommended.[48] However, the STS PROM does not take into account frailty, biological age, or other technical aspects that are relevant to the consideration of CABG in the older patient, as shown in Figure 12.2. The original EuroSCORE and its updated versions provide accurate prediction of early mortality postsurgery for individuals undergoing cardiac surgery.[49,50] There is a need for models that take into account more geriatric-specific predictors

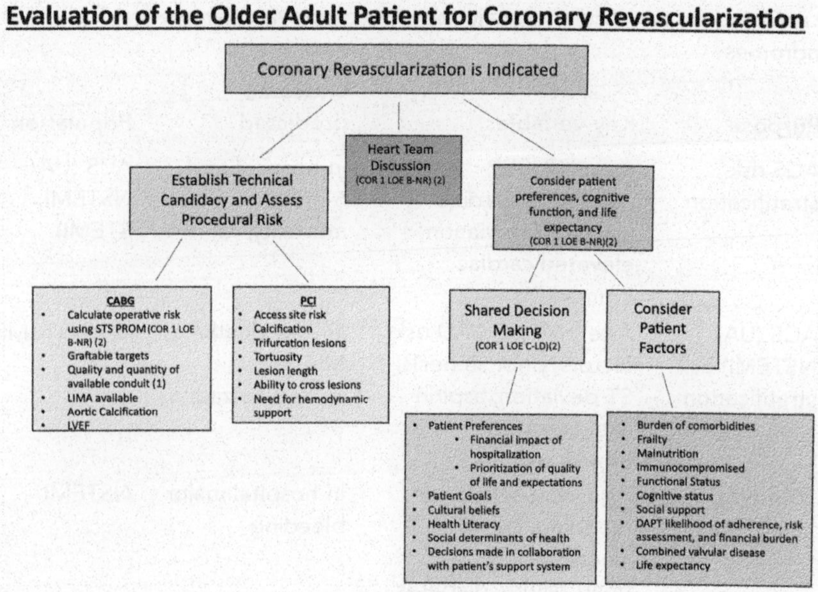

Figure 12.2 Algorithm for the evaluation of the older patient for coronary revascularization. The coronary anatomy has been defined, and the diagnostic workup has been completed. Emergent treatment for STEMI or NSTEMI may have already been completed for culprit vessel per guidelines. Revascularization has been deemed indicated. Class of recommendation (COR) and level of evidence (LOE) correspond to the 2021 ACC/AHA/SCAI Guideline for Coronary Artery Revascularization. *Abbreviations*: CABG, coronary artery bypass grafting; COR, class of recommendation; DAPT, dual antiplatelet therapy; LD, limited data; LIMA, left internal mammary artery; LOE, level of evidence; LVEF, left ventricular ejection fraction; NR, non-randomized; PCI, percutaneous coronary intervention; PROM, predicted risk of mortality; STS, Society of Thoracic Surgeons.

and outcomes to optimize risk stratification for older adults undergoing revascularization.

Hemodynamic risk

Hemodynamic status is a major contributor to periprocedural risk across the age spectrum.[51] The mortality rate of older adults presenting with AMI and cardiogenic shock exceeds 40% in those undergoing revascularization and is more than 50% in those who do not.[52–57] Factors that predict a poor prognosis and high risk for both subsequent complications and mortality include cardiac arrest at presentation,[58] acute heart failure,[59] severe valvular disease,[60] electrical instability,[61] and mechanical complications.[62] In the NCDR model, the presence of cardiogenic shock and "salvage" PCI are the strongest predictors of periprocedural risk.[46,47]

In patients undergoing surgical revascularization, emergent (ongoing refractory cardiac compromise not responsive to any form of therapy) and salvage (cardiopulmonary resuscitation (CPR) en route to the operating suite or ongoing extracorporeal membrane oxygenation (ECMO) to maintain life) procedures are associated with high mortality and morbidity rates.[63]

Anatomic and technical risk

Older adults tend to present with advanced CAD, including high-risk anatomic features such as left main disease, multivessel disease, chronic total occlusions, and generally more diffuse disease.[46,47,64,65] The SYNTAX risk score, among others, was developed to quantify the complexity of CAD and guide the optimal revascularization approach.[66] Severe coronary calcification, which is more prevalent in older adults,[67] can introduce significant technical challenges for the delivery of equipment, stent expansion, and complications from aggressive techniques to modify calcium.[68] Calcium modification therapies like atherectomy may lead to a higher risk for complications and mortality in older adults than in younger populations. Vascular tortuosity also presents challenges for vascular access and successful PCI.[69,70] In patients with concurrent peripheral arterial disease (PAD) who require mechanical circulatory support, access to site options may be limited with accompanying increased risk for complications.[71]

Important technical considerations in patients undergoing CABG include the degree of coronary calcium burden, availability of conduits, degree of ascending aortic calcification, and left ventricular ejection fraction and dimensions (see Figure 12.2).

Geriatric risk

Geriatric syndromes have been strongly associated with a higher risk for adverse outcomes. Frailty in particular is associated with poor outcomes for both PCI and CABG surgery, including triple the odds of in-hospital mortality. Biological age, as quantified by deficits and functional impairments, is superior to chronological age in the prediction of mortality. Thus, the use of comprehensive geriatric risk assessment is recommended in addition to the clinical, hemodynamic, and anatomic/technical risk assessments required to inform a shared decision around revascularization. This should include, at a minimum, a functional assessment, assessment of activities of daily living (ADLs) and instrumental activities of daily living (IADLs), and goals of care. It may include further targeted geriatric measures of multimorbidity, polypharmacy, cognition, delirium, depression, frailty, hearing or vision impairment, mobility, sarcopenia, and social support. Eliciting the older patient's goals of care and priorities using a validated tool like the patient priorities care approach,[72] evaluating individual risk tolerance, and implementing a shared-decision framework should all be considered to ensure person-centered care.

REVASCULARIZATION IN OLDER ADULTS

Revascularization in ST-elevation MI (STEMI)

Older age is associated with increased morbidity and mortality in patients with STEMI. Older adults are more likely to present with atypical symptoms, longer time from symptom onset to first medical contact, and non-diagnostic electrocardiogram (ECG) findings, and to have preexisting medical conditions that adversely impact tolerance of the acute cardiac event and related medical interventions.[1,73–75]

In the Assessment of Pexelizumab in Acute MI trial, adults >75 years old were significantly less likely to achieve angiographic success after primary PCI (pPCI), had less frequent ST-segment resolution, and had higher rates of in-hospital bleeding and electrical and mechanical complications compared to those <65 years. Age was the strongest predictor of 90-day mortality.[75] Studies have consistently demonstrated that older adults are less likely to receive reperfusion and guideline-directed medical therapies.[76] There is also a much higher prevalence of cardiogenic shock (CS) among older adults with STEMI compared to the younger population. Older adults with CS tend to have a much lower chance of survival.[77]

Current guidelines recommend pPCI as the preferred reperfusion strategy in all patients, regardless of age, with acute STEMI who have symptom onset to first medical contact <12 hours presenting to a PCI-capable facility. A door-to-balloon time of <90 minutes or anticipated transfer-to-reperfusion time of <120 minutes is also recommended.[78,79] Although clinical trial data are limited, available evidence supports pPCI over fibrinolysis in older patients with net improvement in mortality, disabling stroke, and reinfarction.[80] Even among nonagenarians, observational studies have demonstrated that pPCI is safe and associated with reduced in-hospital and 30-day mortality compared to medical therapy alone.[81,82]

In older adults unable to undergo pPCI, fibrinolysis is recommended when appropriate.[78,79] Due to the increased risk of bleeding complications, especially intracranial hemorrhage, special considerations are needed. Evidence from the STREAM and STREAM-2 trials support the use of half-dose fibrinolytic therapy for reducing bleeding complications in patients >75 years old. This strategy in older patients presenting within 3 hours of symptom onset and for whom pPCI was unavailable within 1 hour had similar safety and efficacy compared to pPCI.[83,84] Also, clopidogrel should be considered the preferred adjunctive $P2Y_{12}$ receptor inhibitor in patients receiving fibrinolytic therapy, and patients >75 years should receive an initial dose of 75 mg followed by a maintenance dose of 75 mg daily.[78] Lastly, transradial artery access has been proven safe in older adults undergoing pPCI and should be the preferred access site. It is associated with a lower risk of bleeding and vascular complications, acute kidney injury, and mortality in patients with STEMI.[85–87]

The management of cardiogenic shock (CS) and multivessel disease (MVD) in older adults with STEMI remains controversial. While the SHOCK trial concluded that patients ≥75 years old did not benefit from early revascularization, with a 30-day mortality rate of 75% in the treatment arm, this was based on a subgroup analysis of only 24 older patients of whom only 20 underwent PCI.[88] The SHOCK registry showed that for patients ≥75 years who received early revascularization, there was an adjusted survival benefit compared to those with delayed or no revascularization, with a similar relative benefit across age groups.[53] The use of microaxial flow pumps is also controversial in older patients. Recent data from the DanGer Shock trial demonstrated that older patients with STEMI complicated by CS experience high mortality and may not attain the same benefit from microaxial flow pump insertion compared to younger patients.[89] Future clinical trials are needed to better inform the safety and efficacy of revascularization with or without microaxial flow pumps in older adults with STEMI complicated by CS.[90] Among patients with STEMI who have MVD, complete revascularization has been proven safe and effective in lowering major adverse cardiac events (MACE) and is recommended by guidelines for all appropriately selected patients.[79,91] Among patients with STEMI and MVD in hemodynamically stable condition, immediate multivessel PCI was noninferior to staged multivessel PCI with respect to the risk of death from any cause, nonfatal myocardial infarction, stroke, unplanned ischemia-driven revascularization, or hospitalization for heart failure at 1 year based on data from the MULTISTARS AMI trial.[92]

CABG has a role in patients with STEMI with a large area of myocardium at risk when PCI is infeasible or unsuccessful[48,93,94] and in selected patients with complex multivessel non-infarct disease after successful primary PCI to reduce the risk of future cardiac events.

Revascularization in non-ST-elevation MI (NSTEMI)

Four out of the six randomized controlled trials investigating an invasive strategy in older NSTEMI patients have shown no benefit over conservative management. Two of these trials, however, demonstrated reduced recurrent MI and urgent revascularization.[95–98] The After Eighty trial,[99] which assessed patients aged ≥80 with NSTEMI or unstable angina, demonstrated significant benefit from invasive treatment in reducing a composite outcome of MI, urgent revascularization, stroke, and death.

The SENIOR-RITA trial[100] randomized patients aged ≥75 with type 1 NSTEMI and relatively high comorbidity burden to invasive or conservative management.[100] The published results showed no benefit with the invasive strategy in reducing the risk of cardiovascular death or myocardial infarction versus conservative therapy alone. However, similar to other small trials, there was a lower incidence of recurrent myocardial infarction in the invasive group.[100] SENIOR-RITA requires nuanced interpretation for several reasons.[101] Early revascularization drives improved outcomes from invasive management, but only half of the patients assigned to the invasive strategy underwent coronary angiography within 5 days of presentation, and only half of the patients in this arm underwent revascularization. Further, 24% of the patients in the conservative-strategy group crossed over to coronary angiography, and more than half of those underwent revascularization. These issues potentially diluted the treatment effects of the invasive strategy. In addition, nonrandomized data from SENIOR-RITA suggested a survival benefit for patients >80 years managed invasively. A recent meta-analysis in patients aged ≥75 with NSTE-ACS found that an early invasive strategy significantly reduced the composite of death or MI compared to conservative management, and was associated with lower rates of repeat revascularization and MI. This benefit was achieved without an increase in bleeding risk.[102] Thus, the evidence suggests that an invasive approach likely reduces MI and revascularization rates in patients ≥75, but its effect on mortality remains unclear. The benefits of an invasive strategy also appear to be dependent on patient profile and clinical characteristics. Further studies are needed in this population.[1,4]

CABG should be considered in older patients with NSTE-ACS who have failed PCI and have ongoing ischemia, hemodynamic compromise, or threatened occlusion of an artery supplying a substantial amount of myocardium, as well as in patients with NSTE-ACS who are initially stabilized and found to have multivessel disease appropriate for CABG.[48,103–108]

PCI versus CABG

Older patients with significant CAD that warrants revascularization are often excluded from randomized controlled trials comparing PCI and CABG. However, older patients who undergo indicated coronary revascularization derive significant benefits, including relief of symptoms, reduced risk for future MI, and improved survival. In retrospective studies,[109] retrospective studies with propensity score modeling[110] and meta-analyses,[111] older patients undergoing CABG have been found to have improved survival, lower risk of repeat revascularization, lower risk of subsequent MI, and higher periprocedural mortality compared to PCI; these findings are similar to those in younger patients. Comparable outcomes between PCI and CABG were noted in a subgroup analysis and extended follow-up of the SYNTAX trial.[112] A meta-analysis of three CABG versus PCI trials (BEST, PRECOMBAT, and SYNTAX) included 1079 patients aged 70–89 years (550 CABG vs. 529 PCI) and demonstrated that CABG was associated with a lower risk of all-cause mortality, MI, stroke, or repeat revascularization in older participants.[113] There was also a consistent point estimate for benefit with CABG in the 131 participants >80 years. Taken together, these findings are reassuring that CABG can provide consistent benefits and acceptable safety in selected older adults with left main or multivessel CAD.

CABG is often preferred in older patients with multivessel CAD, complex left main stenosis, diabetes, low left ventricular ejection fraction, contraindication to dual antiplatelet therapy (DAPT), and severe in-stent restenosis (Table 12.4). PCI is often more appropriate in patients

Table 12.4 Factors that may favor one revascularization strategy over another in older adults

Favors CABG	Favors PCI
Multivessel coronary artery disease	Advanced age, reduced life expectancy
Complex left main stenosis	Severe left ventricular dysfunction
Diabetes	Frailty, poor functional status, poor cognitive status
Low left ventricular ejection fraction	Multiple comorbidities
Contraindication, nonadherence, or high risk with DAPT therapy	Porcelain aorta
Severe in-stent restenosis	Poor conduits or lack of targets

Abbreviations: CABG, coronary artery bypass grafting; DAPT, dual antiplatelet therapy; PCI, percutaneous coronary intervention.

with advanced age or reduced life expectancy, severe left ventricular dysfunction, frailty, poor functional status, poor cognitive status, multimorbidity, severely calcified aorta, poor bypass conduits, or lack of bypass targets. These observations are consistent with findings in patients with three-vessel or left main disease who underwent PCI after they were deemed ineligible for CABG following a heart team discussion. The most common reasons for CABG ineligibility were poor conduits, severe systolic dysfunction, advanced age, severe cerebrovascular disease, severe lung disease, renal impairment, malignancy, severe PAD, morbid obesity, and cachexia.[114]

COMPLETE VERSUS CULPRIT-ONLY REVASCULARIZATION IN OLDER ADULTS

There have been several trials that have investigated culprit-only versus complete revascularization in patients with ACS. Most of these trials, however, excluded patients aged ≥75.[115,116] The FIRE trial addressed this gap by enrolling patients with STEMI or NSTEMI who had multivessel disease with at least one non-culprit lesion and who underwent successful PCI of the culprit lesion.[91] After successful culprit-only PCI, patients were randomized to receive either ongoing culprit-only treatment or physiology-guided complete revascularization. The physiology-guided complete revascularization group underwent PCI of all functionally significant non-culprit lesions. All individual components of the primary outcome (composite of death, MI, stroke, or ischemia-driven coronary revascularization at 1 year) were lower in the physiology-guided complete revascularization group, except for stroke. The secondary outcomes included a composite endpoint of cardiovascular death or MI at 1 year. This was also reduced with a physiology-guided complete revascularization strategy compared to a culprit-only one.

There was no difference between the two groups in the incidence of a composite of contrast-associated acute kidney injury, stroke, or bleeding at 1 year. This trial has provided insights into the safety and efficacy of physiology-guided complete revascularization in older adults with ACS and multivessel disease. Similarly, a meta-analysis including older adults evaluating complete versus culprit-only revascularization found that complete revascularization was associated with reduced MACE without a significant increase in acute kidney injury or major bleeding.[117]

TAVR AND REVASCULARIZATION IN THE OLDER ADULT POPULATION

Aging is not only associated with CAD but also with increased incidence of severe symptomatic aortic stenosis. For the older adult population, the advent of TAVR has offered a less invasive treatment option for severe aortic stenosis. TAVR is especially beneficial for older adults with high or inoperable risk for surgical aortic valve replacement (SAVR).[118] Compared to medical management, the PARTNER trial showed a significant mortality benefit associated with TAVR in older adults (mean 83 years) with prohibitive risk for surgical AVR.[119]

The symptoms of CAD and aortic stenosis tend to overlap. Additionally, 15%–80% of older patients with one of these conditions also have the other condition.[118] The 2020 ACC/AHA Guideline for the Management of Patients with Valvular Heart Disease recommends an individualized approach to the treatment of CAD prior to TAVR. Revascularization should be discussed prior to TAVR in patients with significant left main or proximal CAD.[118] In the NOTION-3 trial, patients with concomitant CAD and severe aortic stenosis who underwent PCI had a significantly lower incidence of MACE compared to those who received conservative treatment only for CAD. PCI was also associated with an increased risk of bleeding.[120] Some patients may need TAVR followed by reassessment of symptoms to guide the decision to proceed with PCI.[121] This is especially relevant in older patients for whom revascularization and postprocedure DAPT carry additional bleeding risk and management considerations.

For patients with an indication for coronary revascularization, there are higher associated risks in the setting of severe aortic stenosis that necessitate procedural planning and risk assessment. Timing of intervention is key.[122] The risks and benefits of staged versus combined procedures must be critically considered. For older adults with chronic kidney disease, it may be prudent to stage the PCI and TAVR rather than combining both procedures. For those with high-risk coronary anatomy or anticipated difficulty accessing the coronaries after TAVR, revascularization prior to TAVR may be beneficial. On the other hand, for a patient with critical aortic stenosis, TAVR must be prioritized. Overall, revascularization around the time of TAVR should be individualized while weighing the unique patient-specific clinical and anatomic risks versus the benefits of revascularization. The utilization of multidisciplinary heart teams involving interventional cardiologists, cardiac surgeons, cardiac anesthesiologists, geriatricians, palliative care, and advanced practice clinicians can facilitate optimal patient-centered treatment decisions in older adults with severe comorbidities, advanced frailty, and other geriatric syndromes.[123]

Patients with severe aortic stenosis and significant CAD (complex bifurcation left main and/or MV CAD with high SYNTAX score), SAVR + CABG is reasonable and preferred over TAVR + PCI.[118] In addition, CABG is reasonable for select patients undergoing valve repair or replacement with significant proximal CAD or left main CAD.[118]

PHARMACOTHERAPY IN PATIENTS UNDERGOING CORONARY REVASCULARIZATION

It is important to consider age-related pharmacokinetic and pharmacodynamic changes when choosing procedural medications for revascularization in older adults. Reduction in renal and/or hepatic function, along with changes in body composition, can prolong drug action, alter drug distribution, and modify receptor sensitivity, which ultimately impact medication responses.[15]

Conscious sedation is commonly used during PCI. For older adults, the use of opioid-based regimens without benzodiazepines has been proposed to mitigate delirium. However, in $P2Y_{12}$ inhibitor naïve patients, this approach may delay the onset of antiplatelet therapy.[124] The Society for Cardiovascular Angiography and Interventions recommends using lower initial doses of sedatives and analgesic medications to better balance patients' comfort and safety.

DAPT is the mainstay of therapy to prevent thrombotic events in patients undergoing PCI. It is important to consider the agent selected, clinical presentation, timing of angiography, concomitant medications, and risk of thrombotic and adverse events when selecting an oral $P2Y_{12}$ inhibitor for older patients. For patients with chronic coronary disease undergoing PCI, current guidelines recommend clopidogrel in addition to aspirin regardless of age. When coronary anatomy is not known, routine pretreatment prior to angiography may present challenges due to delays in surgical revascularization if the patient is found to have complex multivessel disease.[79]

Evidence on choice of oral $P2Y_{12}$ inhibitor in older adults undergoing PCI has been mixed. In the PLATO trial, the efficacy and safety of ticagrelor versus clopidogrel favored ticagrelor and findings were similar among patients ≥75 compared to those <75 years.[125] The POPular AGE trial showed significantly fewer bleeding events in the clopidogrel group without an increase in the composite ischemic endpoint in patients ≥70 years who were randomized to clopidogrel versus ticagrelor or prasugrel.[126] Guidelines recommend cautious use of prasugrel in patients ≥75 years[48] based on data from the TRITON trial, which used a 10 mg daily maintenance dose of prasugrel and showed higher rates of bleeding in patients ≥75 years with no net clinical benefit of prasugrel versus clopidogrel.[127]

The routine use of intravenous antiplatelet medications during PCI is not recommended by ACC/AHA guidelines.[48] There is a recommendation for the use of glycoprotein IIb/IIIa antagonists in patients undergoing PCI who have a large thrombus or no/slow reflow; cangrelor is reasonable in oral $P2Y_{12}$ inhibitor naïve patients.[48] There was no increased risk of major bleeding associated with cangrelor versus clopidogrel in patients ≥75 years; efficacy was similar based on a subanalysis of the CHAMPION PHOENIX trial.[128]

Given the concern about bleeding risk with longer-term DAPT in older adults post-PCI, recent strategies such as abbreviated DAPT and antiplatelet de-escalation (either early discontinuation of aspirin or changing from ticagrelor or prasugrel to clopidogrel after 1 to 3 months with or without the guidance of genotyping or platelet function testing) have been studied in an attempt to balance bleeding and ischemic risk.[129] In a recent systematic review, abbreviated DAPT durations were associated with lower bleeding rates without an increase in the rates of MACE.[130] Although studies of de-escalation strategies have shown reduced bleeding risk with no increased ischemic events, most of the studies were conducted in patients of East Asian descent, and their generalizability to other populations is uncertain.[129]

In the United States, unfractionated heparin (UFH) is the most commonly used anticoagulant during PCI. This is supported by the class I guideline recommendation to reduce ischemic events.[48,131] Bivalirudin has class I and 2b recommendations to reduce bleeding risk for patients with STEMI and NSTE-ACS, respectively, undergoing PCI.[131] A subanalysis of patients ≥75 years enrolled in the VALIDATE-SWEEDEHEART trial reported no difference in ischemic or bleeding risk between the UFH and bivalirudin groups, suggesting bivalirudin may be a safe alternative to UFH in this population undergoing PCI.[132] Intravenous enoxaparin at the time of PCI for ACS has a class 2b recommendation as an alternative to UFH to reduce ischemic events.[131]

In general, a heart team discussion should be considered when making medication choices during preoperative planning for older adults undergoing CABG. For these patients, the guidelines give a class I recommendation for the use of an intraoperative insulin infusion to maintain serum glucose of <180 mg/dL to reduce the risk of sternal wound infection.[48] For patients taking aspirin preoperatively, there is a class I recommendation for continuation until the time of surgery. Due to the increased risk of bleeding in older adults, there is a class 2a recommendation for those undergoing elective CABG on an oral $P2Y_{12}$ inhibitor to discontinue ticagrelor for 3 days, clopidogrel for 5 days, and prasugrel for 7 days before CABG.[48] There is a class 3 recommendation (i.e., not recommended) for initiating aspirin in the immediate preoperative period in patients undergoing elective CABG who were not previously on aspirin.

NONINTERVENTIONAL CONSIDERATIONS

Achieving a patient-centered approach in older adults considered for revascularization requires a multidisciplinary team, patient education, and shared decision-making.[133]

Patient-centered care in geriatric cardiology integrates clinical expertise and the latest evidence with the patient's health priorities, life goals, preferences, values, and beliefs.[134,135] Older adults are more likely to prioritize the ability to remain independent, with a focus on maintaining mobility, functional status, and quality of life rather than longevity.[24]

Care coordination

In view of the greater prevalence of geriatric syndromes and higher symptom burden in older adults, continuity of care when transitioning from hospital to home or a rehabilitation facility is imperative.[24] Decisions may need to be made for appropriate level of care, advanced care (e.g., surgical intervention), and multidisciplinary care coordination (e.g., primary care physicians, advanced practice providers, palliative care).[134] To achieve optimal coordination of care, a multidisciplinary team of physicians, nurses, geriatrics providers, physical therapists, dietitians, social workers, and the patient's support network is essential.[1] Geriatrics comanagement entails care for complex older adults that includes a designated geriatrician or geriatrics-trained nurse who provides concurrent care alongside the cardiologist and/or surgeon.[136]

Shared decision-making

Shared decision-making is defined as a communication process by which patients and clinicians collaborate to choose tests, treatments, and care that most align with the individual patient's preferences and values.[137] This is critical to personalized and holistic care of older adults. Through shared decision-making clinicians provide evidence-based information about reasonable options while the patient provides expertise on their personal situation, values, preferences, and attitude toward risk.[138] The evidence base from clinical trials to facilitate shared decision-making is sparse in older adults because of underrepresentation or deliberate exclusion based on age/comorbidities. Thus, limited data are available on patient-centered outcomes such as symptoms, function, or quality of life in this patient population.[139]

The sharing of medical information with older adults may be impeded by common challenges including cognitive impairment, hearing or visual impairment, and low health literacy.[138] Additional factors such as multimorbidity, frailty, and social determinants of health (SDoH) also pose a challenge to shared decision-making. Situational complexity and SDoH may also influence disease burden, access to care, the choice of revascularization strategy, and health outcomes.[139] Input from relevant multidisciplinary team members enhances the shared decision-making process with older adults and their support network.[138] There is evidence to support the use of patient decision aids when treatment decisions have no single best choice. These decision aids result in improved knowledge, accurate risk perceptions, and active role decision-making.[140]

Advance care planning

Advance care planning and advance directives are a common and important form of shared decision-making that helps patients and their families understand the risks and benefits of treatments in advanced CVD and to express their wishes regarding care choices (see also Chapter 29).[137] The intent of palliative care is to improve quality of life and reduce suffering among patients with serious illness. The guidelines suggest that care planning and decision-making processes, including discussions concerning goals of care, post-discharge needs, options, and resources, should be patient-directed and patient-centered. These processes should be conducted in consultation with the patient's surrogate decision-makers, family caregivers, and professionals responsible for the patient's care including palliative care generalists and specialists as needed.[141]

Patient education

There is a dearth of educational interventions for secondary prevention or structure for education delivery for older adults with CVD. However, there is evidence to support improvement in self-reported health behaviors in patients with CAD when education for secondary prevention is employed in various modes and intensities.[142] Patient education has also been reported to reduce anxiety and depressive symptoms in CAD patients.[143] Nurses are the main champions of educational interventions at hospital discharge and outpatient care. They deliver patient education on management of CVD risk factors, nutrition counseling, psychosocial interventions, and smoking cessation in collaboration with other healthcare providers through nurse-led cardiac rehabilitation programs.[144]

Cardiac rehabilitation

The ACC/AHA gives a class I recommendation for referral to an outpatient center-based cardiac rehabilitation (CR) program before hospital discharge for patients who have had ACS and for those who have undergone revascularization by PCI or CABG.[131] Structured CR has been shown to reduce death, MI, hospital readmissions, and improve functional status and quality of life (QOL).[131] CR is a multifaceted and comprehensive outpatient intervention that is considered the standard of care for secondary prevention of CVD.[131] This is achieved through a combination of monitored exercise training, health and nutrition education, psychological support, and personalized patient assessment, including medication optimization.[131] It has been found to be particularly beneficial in older adults, a group at higher risk for losing independence and function following hospitalization for a cardiac event or procedure.[145–147]

CR is particularly important for older patients following CABG. CR is associated with better clinical outcomes and provides social interactions for patients following CABG. However, older patients face multiple barriers that may prevent participation in CR. The probability of being discharged to a nursing home, rehabilitation center, or long-term care facility after CABG increases with age.[148–150] Older patients may also experience delays in their return to independent living and ability to attend CR due to weight-lifting and driving restrictions and incisional pain from sternal wound healing. These considerations are a vital part of shared decision-making prior to coronary revascularization.

An important aspect of CR for older adults is that it provides an opportunity to develop personalized approaches to cardiovascular health for older patients' aggregate health challenges.[151,152] Using a center-based approach, it fosters socialization among older adults who otherwise may have limited social interactions.[153] Through direct observation, CR also provides an opportunity for assessing tolerance to medications during supervised exercise allowing for a patient-centered approach to optimize medical therapy while reducing risks of adverse events, especially falls.[152]

Common barriers to center-based cardiac rehabilitation (CBCR) among older adults include a lack of understanding of its value among patients and clinicians, prohibitive logistics given that many older adults do not drive, unaffordable copayments for patients on fixed incomes, and lack of flexibility in format to achieve personalized approaches that are tailored to their wide range of needs and circumstances.[151]

Home-based cardiac rehabilitation (HBCR) or hybrid CR models have been developed to help address the aforementioned barriers to CBCR. HBCR comprises the core components of CBCR but is delivered through regular contact with healthcare professionals via telephone calls, videoconferencing, or mobile technology. These HBCR programs have been shown to have similar short-term safety and clinical outcomes (e.g., improvements in exercise capacity, quality of life, blood pressure) compared to CBCR.[131,154–156] Efficacy of HBCR is still uncertain for older adults who are frail, prone to falls, and/or cognitively impaired.[154]

CONCLUSION

Traditional reliance on chronological age is inadequate for risk stratification in older adults. Biological aging, characterized by hallmarks such as inflammaging, mitochondrial dysfunction, impaired proteostasis, and others, is closely associated with cardiovascular disease progression and procedural outcomes. Emerging research into aging biomarkers and inflammatory clocks offers promise for refining risk prediction models. Geriatric syndromes (frailty, cognitive impairment, polypharmacy, and sarcopenia) significantly impact morbidity and mortality after revascularization. These conditions are not captured in conventional risk models (e.g., GRACE, TIMI) and require systematic incorporation into preprocedural assessments to inform therapeutic decisions, particularly for patients undergoing PCI or CABG.

Evidence supports primary PCI over fibrinolysis in STEMI across age groups, including older adults, with additional safety from strategies like radial access and half-dose fibrinolytics for patients aged 75 years and older. In NSTEMI, trial heterogeneity highlights the need to tailor invasive strategies based on functional status and geriatric burden rather than age alone. In older patients with concomitant CAD and aortic stenosis, procedural sequencing (PCI vs. TAVR-first) must balance bleeding risks, coronary accessibility post-TAVR, and symptom attribution. Current evidence supports revascularization in select patients, but the strategy should be individualized with input from the heart team and geriatric assessment. Age-related changes in pharmacokinetics and pharmacodynamics necessitate the cautious use of antiplatelet and anticoagulant medications. Data favor clopidogrel over ticagrelor and prasugrel in reducing bleeding risk without compromising ischemic outcomes in older adults. De-escalation and abbreviated DAPT strategies are emerging as safe and effective for this population, although generalizability remains limited.

Compared to younger patients, older patients often have a higher burden of comorbidities that may impact preferences regarding treatment for CAD. In selected older patients, surgical coronary revascularization is associated with relief of symptoms, reduced future myocardial infarction, and improved survival. Similar to younger patients, CABG is often more appropriate in older patients with multivessel CAD, complex left main stenosis, diabetes, low left ventricular ejection fraction, contraindication to DAPT therapy, and severe in-stent restenosis. However, older patients represent a complex group that requires careful and individualized consideration of coronary artery revascularization strategies utilizing a heart team. Finally, in older patients with significant CAD and severe aortic stenosis, concomitant SAVR + CABG may be reasonable in the presence of severe proximal CAD or left main disease when the STS PROM is acceptable and after a heart team assessment and shared decision-making discussion with the patient.

GUIDELINE RECOMMENDATIONS

From the 2025 ACC/AHA[131] guidelines for the management of patients with acute coronary syndromes (ACS):

- In older adults presenting with ACS, use of risk stratification tools such as GRACE, TIMI, and PRECISE-DAPT is recommended to assess ischemic and bleeding risks.

- Frailty, multimorbidity, and renal function should be considered when determining treatment strategies in older adults with ACS.
- De-escalation strategies, such as switching to clopidogrel or transitioning to single antiplatelet therapy, are recommended for high-risk patients to reduce bleeding risks.
- Shortened DAPT duration (e.g., 1–6 months) may be appropriate for older adults with high bleeding risk.
- Multivessel PCI is recommended for stable older adults with STEMI and significant non-culprit lesions, while CABG may be preferred for complex coronary disease.
- Annual influenza vaccination is strongly recommended to reduce cardiovascular events and mortality.

From the 2021 ACC/AHA/SCAI[79] guideline for coronary revascularization:

- In patients who require coronary revascularization, treatment decisions should be based on clinical indications, regardless of sex, race, or ethnicity, and efforts to reduce disparities in care are warranted.
- In patients undergoing revascularization, decisions should be patient-centered—that is, considerate of the patient's preferences and goals, cultural beliefs, health literacy, and social determinants of health—and made in collaboration with the patient's support system.
- In patients undergoing coronary angiography or revascularization, adequate information about benefits, risks, therapeutic consequences, and potential alternatives in the performance of percutaneous and surgical myocardial revascularization should be given, when feasible, with sufficient time for informed decision-making to improve clinical outcomes.
- In patients for whom the optimal treatment is unclear, a heart team approach that includes representatives from interventional cardiology, cardiac surgery, and clinical cardiology is recommended to improve patient outcomes.
- In patients who are being considered for CABG, calculation of the STS risk score is recommended to help stratify patient risk.
- In older adults, as in all patients, the treatment strategy for CAD should be based on an individual patient's preferences, cognitive function, and life expectancy.

REFERENCES

1. Damluji AA, Forman DE, Wang TY, Chikwe J, Kunadian V, Rich MW, Young BA, Page RL, 2nd, DeVon HA, Alexander KP, et al. Management of Acute Coronary Syndrome in the Older Adult Population: A Scientific Statement From the American Heart Association. *Circulation*. 2023;147:e32–e62. doi: 10.1161/CIR.0000000000001112
2. Schmanske N, Ngo JM, Kalra K, Nanna MG, Damluji AA. Healthy Ageing in Older Adults with Cardiovascular Disease. *European Heart Journal*. 2025:ehaf231. doi: 10.1093/eurheartj/ehaf231
3. Nanna MG, Sutton NR, Kochar A, Rymer JA, Lowenstern AM, Gackenbach G, Hummel SL, Goyal P, Rich MW, Kirkpatrick JN, et al. Assessment and Management of Older Adults Undergoing PCI, Part 1: A JACC: Advances Expert Panel. *JACC Adv*. 2023;2. doi: 10.1016/j.jacadv.2023.100389
4. Damluji AA, Nanna MG, Rymer J, Kochar A, Lowenstern A, Baron SJ, Narins CR, Alkhouli M. Chronological vs Biological Age in Interventional Cardiology: A Comprehensive Approach to Care for Older Adults: JACC Family Series. *JACC Cardiovasc Interv*. 2024;17:961–978. doi: 10.1016/j.jcin.2024.01.284
5. Schmanske N, Ngo JM, Kalra K, Nanna MG, Damluji AA. Healthy Ageing in Older Adults with Cardiovascular Disease. *Eur Heart J*. 2025. doi: 10.1093/eurheartj/ehaf231
6. Abdellatif M, Rainer PP, Sedej S, Kroemer G. Hallmarks of Cardiovascular Ageing. *Nat Rev Cardiol*. 2023;20:754–777. doi: 10.1038/s41569-023-00881-3
7. Liberale L, Badimon L, Montecucco F, Luscher TF, Libby P, Camici GG. Inflammation, Aging, and Cardiovascular Disease: JACC Review Topic of the Week. *J Am Coll Cardiol*. 2022;79:837–847. doi: 10.1016/j.jacc.2021.12.017
8. Butkowski EG, Jelinek HF. Hyperglycaemia, Oxidative Stress and Inflammatory Markers. *Redox Rep*. 2017;22:257–264. doi: 10.1080/13510002.2016.1215643
9. Tinetti M, Huang A, Molnar F. The Geriatrics 5M's: A New Way of Communicating What We Do. *J Am Geriatr Soc*. 2017;65:2115. doi: 10.1111/jgs.14979
10. Bernacki GM, Starks H, Krishnaswami A, Steiner JM, Allen MB, Batchelor WB, Yang E, Wyman J, Kirkpatrick JN. Peri-procedural Code Status for Transcatheter Aortic Valve Replacement: Absence of Program Policies and Standard Practices. *J Am Geriatr Soc*. 2022;70:3378–3389. doi: 10.1111/jgs.17980
11. Sullivan MF, Kirkpatrick JN. Palliative Cardiovascular Care: The Right Patient at the Right Time. *Clin Cardiol*. 2020;43:205–212. doi: 10.1002/clc.23307
12. Smetana GW, Ho JE, Orkaby AR, Reynolds EE. How Would You Manage This Patient With Heart Failure With Preserved Ejection Fraction?: Grand Rounds Discussion From Beth Israel Deaconess Medical Center. *Ann Intern Med*. 2023;176:1656–1665. doi: 10.7326/M23-2384
13. Nanna MG, Wang SY, Damluji AA. Management of Stable Angina in the Older Adult Population. *Circ Cardiovasc Interv*. 2023;16:e012438. doi: 10.1161/CIRCINTERVENTIONS.122.012438

14. Goyal P, Nanna MG. Stable Coronary Artery Disease in the Age of Geriatric Cardiology. *J Am Coll Cardiol.* 2023;81:1710–1713. doi: 10.1016/j.jacc.2023.03.378
15. Mangoni AA, Jackson SH. Age-related Changes in Pharmacokinetics and Pharmacodynamics: Basic Principles and Practical Applications. *Br J Clin Pharmacol.* 2004;57:6–14. doi: 10.1046/j.1365-2125.2003.02007.x
16. Raman M, Middleton RJ, Kalra PA, Green D. Estimating Renal Function in Old People: An In-depth Review. *Int Urol Nephrol.* 2017;49:1979–1988. doi: 10.1007/s11255-017-1682-z
17. Charlesworth CJ, Smit E, Lee DS, Alramadhan F, Odden MC. Polypharmacy Among Adults Aged 65 Years and Older in the United States: 1988–2010. *J Gerontol A Biol Sci Med Sci.* 2015;70:989–995. doi: 10.1093/gerona/glv013
18. Tahami Monfared AA, Byrnes MJ, White LA, Zhang Q. Alzheimer's Disease: Epidemiology and Clinical Progression. *Neurol Ther.* 2022;11:553–569. doi: 10.1007/s40120-022-00338-8
19. Marcantonio ER. Delirium in Hospitalized Older Adults. *N Engl J Med.* 2017;377:1456–1466. doi: 10.1056/NEJMcp1605501
20. Gou RY, Hshieh TT, Marcantonio ER, Cooper Z, Jones RN, Travison TG, Fong TG, Abdeen A, Lange J, Earp B, et al. One-Year Medicare Costs Associated With Delirium in Older Patients Undergoing Major Elective Surgery. *JAMA Surg.* 2021;156:430–442. doi: 10.1001/jamasurg.2020.7260
21. Kok RM, Reynolds CF, 3rd. Management of Depression in Older Adults: A Review. *JAMA.* 2017;317:2114–2122. doi: 10.1001/jama.2017.5706
22. Zhang WY, Nan N, Song XT, Tian JF, Yang XY. Impact of Depression on Clinical Outcomes Following Percutaneous Coronary Intervention: A Systematic Review and Meta-analysis. *BMJ Open.* 2019;9:e026445. doi: 10.1136/bmjopen-2018-026445
23. Inohara T, Vemulapalli S, Kohsaka S, Yashima F, Watanabe Y, Shirai S, Tada N, Araki M, Naganuma T, Yamanaka F, et al. Appropriateness of Transcatheter Aortic Valve Replacement: Insight From the OCEAN-TAVI Registry. *Circ Cardiovasc Qual Outcomes.* 2020;13:e006146. doi: 10.1161/CIRCOUTCOMES.119.006146
24. Forman DE, Arena R, Boxer R, Dolansky MA, Eng JJ, Fleg JL, Haykowsky M, Jahangir A, Kaminsky LA, Kitzman DW, et al. Prioritizing Functional Capacity as a Principal End Point for Therapies Oriented to Older Adults With Cardiovascular Disease: A Scientific Statement for Healthcare Professionals From the American Heart Association. *Circulation.* 2017;135:e894–e918. doi: 10.1161/CIR.0000000000000483
25. Kim DH, Afilalo J, Shi SM, Popma JJ, Khabbaz KR, Laham RJ, Grodstein F, Guibone K, Lux E, Lipsitz LA. Evaluation of Changes in Functional Status in the Year After Aortic Valve Replacement. *JAMA Intern Med.* 2019;179:383–391. doi: 10.1001/jamainternmed.2018.6738
26. James K, Schwartz AW, Orkaby AR. Mobility Assessment in Older Adults. *N Engl J Med.* 2021;385:e22. doi: 10.1056/NEJMvcm2009406
27. Afilalo J, Eisenberg MJ, Morin JF, Bergman H, Monette J, Noiseux N, Perrault LP, Alexander KP, Langlois Y, Dendukuri N, et al. Gait Speed as an Incremental Predictor of Mortality and Major Morbidity in Elderly Patients Undergoing Cardiac Surgery. *J Am Coll Cardiol.* 2010;56:1668–1676. doi: 10.1016/j.jacc.2010.06.039
28. Afilalo J, Mottillo S, Eisenberg MJ, Alexander KP, Noiseux N, Perrault LP, Morin JF, Langlois Y, Ohayon SM, Monette J, et al. Addition of Frailty and Disability to Cardiac Surgery Risk Scores Identifies Elderly Patients at High Risk of Mortality or Major Morbidity. *Circ Cardiovasc Qual Outcomes.* 2012;5:222–228. doi: 10.1161/CIRCOUTCOMES.111.963157
29. Dodson JA, Arnold SV, Gosch KL, Gill TM, Spertus JA, Krumholz HM, Rich MW, Chaudhry SI, Forman DE, Masoudi FA, et al. Slow Gait Speed and Risk of Mortality or Hospital Readmission After Myocardial Infarction in the Translational Research Investigating Underlying Disparities in Recovery from Acute Myocardial Infarction: Patients' Health Status Registry. *J Am Geriatr Soc.* 2016;64:596–601. doi: 10.1111/jgs.14016
30. Damluji AA, Alfaraidhy M, AlHajri N, Rohant NN, Kumar M, Al Malouf C, Bahrainy S, Ji Kwak M, Batchelor WB, Forman DE, et al. Sarcopenia and Cardiovascular Diseases. *Circulation.* 2023;147:1534–1553. doi: 10.1161/CIRCULATIONAHA.123.064071
31. Zuckerman J, Ades M, Mullie L, Trnkus A, Morin JF, Langlois Y, Ma F, Levental M, Morais JA, Afilalo J. Psoas Muscle Area and Length of Stay in Older Adults Undergoing Cardiac Operations. *Ann Thorac Surg.* 2017;103:1498–1504. doi: 10.1016/j.athoracsur.2016.09.005
32. Baldasseroni S, Silverii MV, Pratesi A, Burgisser C, Orso F, Lucarelli G, Turrin G, Ungar A, Marchionni N, Fattirolli F. Cardiac Rehabilitation in Advanced aGE after PCI for Acute Coronary Syndromes: Predictors of Exercise Capacity Improvement in the CR-AGE ACS Study. *Aging Clin Exp Res.* 2022;34:2195–2203. doi: 10.1007/s40520-022-02130-y
33. Kitzman DW, Whellan DJ, Duncan P, Pastva AM, Mentz RJ, Reeves GR, Nelson MB, Chen H, Upadhya B, Reed SD, et al. Physical Rehabilitation for Older Patients Hospitalized for Heart Failure. *N Engl J Med.* 2021;385:203–216. doi: 10.1056/NEJMoa2026141

34. Rich MW, Chyun DA, Skolnick AH, Alexander KP, Forman DE, Kitzman DW, Maurer MS, McClurken JB, Resnick BM, Shen WK, et al. Knowledge Gaps in Cardiovascular Care of the Older Adult Population: A Scientific Statement From the American Heart Association, American College of Cardiology, and American Geriatrics Society. *Circulation.* 2016;133:2103–2122. doi: 10.1161/CIR.0000000000000380
35. Forman DE, Maurer MS, Boyd C, Brindis R, Salive ME, Horne FM, Bell SP, Fulmer T, Reuben DB, Zieman S, et al. Multimorbidity in Older Adults With Cardiovascular Disease. *J Am Coll Cardiol.* 2018;71:2149–2161. doi: 10.1016/j.jacc.2018.03.022
36. Salive ME. Multimorbidity in Older Adults. *Epidemiol Rev.* 2013;35:75–83. doi: 10.1093/epirev/mxs009
37. Clegg A, Young J, Iliffe S, Rikkert MO, Rockwood K. Frailty in Elderly People. *Lancet.* 2013;381:752–762. doi: 10.1016/S0140-6736(12)62167-9
38. Kim DH, Rockwood K. Frailty in Older Adults. *N Engl J Med.* 2024;391:538–548. doi: 10.1056/NEJMra2301292
39. Damluji AA, Chung SE, Xue QL, Hasan RK, Moscucci M, Forman DE, Bandeen-Roche K, Batchelor W, Walston JD, Resar JR, et al. Frailty and Cardiovascular Outcomes in the National Health and Aging Trends Study. *Eur Heart J.* 2021;42:3856–3865. doi: 10.1093/eurheartj/ehab468
40. Ijaz N, Buta B, Xue QL, Mohess DT, Bushan A, Tran H, Batchelor W, deFilippi CR, Walston JD, Bandeen-Roche K, et al. Interventions for Frailty Among Older Adults With Cardiovascular Disease: JACC State-of-the-Art Review. *J Am Coll Cardiol.* 2022;79:482–503. doi: 10.1016/j.jacc.2021.11.029
41. Hoogendijk EO, Afilalo J, Ensrud KE, Kowal P, Onder G, Fried LP. Frailty: Implications for Clinical Practice and Public Health. *Lancet.* 2019;394:1365–1375. doi: 10.1016/S0140-6736(19)31786-6
42. Hanna JM, Wang SY, Kochar A, Park DY, Damluji AA, Henry GA, Ahmad Y, Curtis JP, Nanna MG. Complex Percutaneous Coronary Intervention Outcomes in Older Adults. *J Am Heart Assoc.* 2023;12:e029057. doi: 10.1161/JAHA.122.029057
43. Park DY, Hanna JM, Kadian S, Kadian M, Jones WS, Damluji AA, Kochar A, Curtis JP, Nanna MG. In-hospital Outcomes and Readmission in Older Adults Treated with Percutaneous Coronary Intervention for Stable Ischemic Heart Disease. *J Geriatr Cardiol.* 2022;19:631–642. doi: 10.11909/j.issn.1671-5411.2022.09.006
44. Nanna MG, Sutton NR, Kochar A, Rymer JA, Lowenstern AM, Gackenbach G, Hummel SL, Goyal P, Rich MW, Kirkpatrick JN, et al. A Geriatric Approach to Percutaneous Coronary Interventions in Older Adults, Part II: A JACC: Advances Expert Panel. *JACC Adv.* 2023;2. doi: 10.1016/j.jacadv.2023.100421
45. Subherwal S, Bach RG, Chen AY, Gage BF, Rao SV, Newby LK, Wang TY, Gibler WB, Ohman EM, Roe MT, et al. Baseline Risk of Major Bleeding in Non-ST-Segment-Elevation Myocardial Infarction: The CRUSADE (Can Rapid risk stratification of Unstable angina patients Suppress ADverse outcomes with Early implementation of the ACC/AHA Guidelines) Bleeding Score. *Circulation.* 2009;119:1873–1882. doi: 10.1161/CIRCULATIONAHA.108.828541
46. Castro-Dominguez YS, Wang Y, Minges KE, McNamara RL, Spertus JA, Dehmer GJ, Messenger JC, Lavin K, Anderson C, Blankinship K, et al. Predicting In-Hospital Mortality in Patients Undergoing Percutaneous Coronary Intervention. *J Am Coll Cardiol.* 2021;78:216–229. doi: 10.1016/j.jacc.2021.04.067
47. Protty M, Sharp ASP, Gallagher S, Farooq V, Spratt JC, Ludman P, Anderson R, McEntegart MM, Hanratty C, Walsh S, et al. Defining Percutaneous Coronary Intervention Complexity and Risk: An Analysis of the United Kingdom BCIS Database 2006-2016. *JACC Cardiovasc Interv.* 2022;15:39–49. doi: 10.1016/j.jcin.2021.09.039
48. Lawton JS, Tamis-Holland JE, Bangalore S, Bates ER, Beckie TM, Bischoff JM, Bittl JA, Cohen MG, DiMaio JM, Don CW, et al. 2021 ACC/AHA/SCAI Guideline for Coronary Artery Revascularization: Executive Summary: A Report of the American College of Cardiology/American Heart Association Joint Committee on Clinical Practice Guidelines. *Circulation.* 2022;145:e4–e17. doi: 10.1161/CIR.0000000000001039
49. Nashef SA, Roques F, Michel P, Gauducheau E, Lemeshow S, Salamon R. European System for Cardiac Operative Risk Evaluation (EuroSCORE). *Eur J Cardiothorac Surg.* 1999;16:9–13. doi: 10.1016/s1010-7940(99)00134-7
50. Nashef SA, Roques F, Sharples LD, Nilsson J, Smith C, Goldstone AR, Lockowandt U. EuroSCORE II. *Eur J Cardiothorac Surg.* 2012;41:734–744; discussion 744–735. doi: 10.1093/ejcts/ezs043
51. Tehrani BN, Truesdell AG, Psotka MA, Rosner C, Singh R, Sinha SS, Damluji AA, Batchelor WB. A Standardized and Comprehensive Approach to the Management of Cardiogenic Shock. *JACC Heart Fail.* 2020;8:879–891. doi: 10.1016/j.jchf.2020.09.005
52. Damluji AA, Bandeen-Roche K, Berkower C, Boyd CM, Al-Damluji MS, Cohen MG, Forman DE, Chaudhary R, Gerstenblith G, Walston JD, et al. Percutaneous Coronary Intervention in Older Patients With ST-Segment Elevation Myocardial Infarction and Cardiogenic Shock. *J Am Coll Cardiol.* 2019;73:1890–1900. doi: 10.1016/j.jacc.2019.01.055

53. Dzavik V, Sleeper LA, Picard MH, Sanborn TA, Lowe AM, Gin K, Saucedo J, Webb JG, Menon V, Slater JN, et al. Outcome of Patients Aged >or=75 Years in the SHould We Emergently Revascularize Occluded Coronaries in Cardiogenic ShocK (SHOCK) Trial: Do Elderly Patients with Acute Myocardial Infarction Complicated by Cardiogenic Shock Respond Differently to Emergent Revascularization? *Am Heart J.* 2005;149:1128–1134. doi: 10.1016/j.ahj.2005.03.045
54. Lim HS, Farouque O, Andrianopoulos N, Yan BP, Lim CC, Brennan AL, Reid CM, Freeman M, Charter K, Black A, et al. Survival of Elderly Patients Undergoing Percutaneous Coronary Intervention for Acute Myocardial Infarction Complicated by Cardiogenic Shock. *JACC Cardiovasc Interv.* 2009;2:146–152. doi: 10.1016/j.jcin.2008.11.006
55. Migliorini A, Moschi G, Valenti R, Parodi G, Dovellini EV, Carrabba N, Buonamici P, Antoniucci D. Routine Percutaneous Coronary Intervention in Elderly Patients with Cardiogenic Shock Complicating Acute Myocardial Infarction. *Am Heart J.* 2006;152:903–908. doi: 10.1016/j.ahj.2005.12.030
56. Ratcovich HL, Josiassen J, Helgestad OKL, Linde L, Jensen LO, Ravn HB, Joshi FR, Engstrom T, Schmidt H, Hassager C, et al. Outcome in Elderly Patients With Cardiogenic Shock Complicating Acute Myocardial Infarction. *Shock.* 2022;57:327–335. doi: 10.1097/SHK.0000000000001837
57. Thiele H, Zeymer U, Neumann FJ, Ferenc M, Olbrich HG, Hausleiter J, Richardt G, Hennersdorf M, Empen K, Fuernau G, et al. Intraaortic Balloon Support for Myocardial Infarction with Cardiogenic Shock. *N Engl J Med.* 2012;367:1287–1296. doi: 10.1056/NEJMoa1208410
58. Kim C, Becker L, Eisenberg MS. Out-of-hospital Cardiac Arrest in Octogenarians and Nonagenarians. *Arch Intern Med.* 2000;160:3439–3443. doi: 10.1001/archinte.160.22.3439
59. Pasala S, Cooper LB, Psotka MA, Sinha SS, deFilippi CR, Tran H, Tehrani B, Sherwood M, Epps K, Batchelor W, et al. The Influence of Heart Failure on Clinical and Economic Outcomes among Older Adults >/=75 Years of Age with Acute Myocardial Infarction. *Am Heart J.* 2022;246:65–73. doi: 10.1016/j.ahj.2021.11.021
60. Goel SS, Agarwal S, Tuzcu EM, Ellis SG, Svensson LG, Zaman T, Bajaj N, Joseph L, Patel NS, Aksoy O, et al. Percutaneous Coronary Intervention in Patients with Severe Aortic Stenosis: Implications for Transcatheter Aortic Valve Replacement. *Circulation.* 2012;125:1005–1013. doi: 10.1161/CIRCULATIONAHA.111.039180
61. Collet JP, Thiele H, Barbato E, Barthelemy O, Bauersachs J, Bhatt DL, Dendale P, Dorobantu M, Edvardsen T, Folliguet T, et al. 2020 ESC Guidelines for the Management of Acute Coronary Syndromes in Patients Presenting without Persistent ST-segment Elevation. *Eur Heart J.* 2021;42:1289–1367. doi: 10.1093/eurheartj/ehaa575
62. Damluji AA, van Diepen S, Katz JN, Menon V, Tamis-Holland JE, Bakitas M, Cohen MG, Balsam LB, Chikwe J, American Heart Association Council on Clinical C, et al. Mechanical Complications of Acute Myocardial Infarction: A Scientific Statement From the American Heart Association. *Circulation.* 2021;144:e16–e35. doi: 10.1161/CIR.0000000000000985
63. Keeling WB, Binongo J, Wei J, Leshnower BG, Farrington W, Halkos ME. National Trends in Emergency Coronary Artery Bypass Grafting. *Eur J Cardiothorac Surg.* 2023;64. doi: 10.1093/ejcts/ezad352
64. Hannan EL, Farrell LS, Walford G, Jacobs AK, Berger PB, Holmes DR, Jr., Stamato NJ, Sharma S, King SB, 3rd. The New York State Risk Score for Predicting in-hospital/30-day Mortality Following Percutaneous Coronary Intervention. *JACC Cardiovasc Interv.* 2013;6:614–622. doi: 10.1016/j.jcin.2013.02.015
65. Singh M, Gulati R, Lewis BR, Zhou Z, Alkhouli M, Friedman P, Bell MR. Multimorbidity and Mortality Models to Predict Complications Following Percutaneous Coronary Interventions. *Circ Cardiovasc Interv.* 2022;15:e011540. doi: 10.1161/CIRCINTERVENTIONS.121.011540
66. Mohr FW, Morice MC, Kappetein AP, Feldman TE, Stahle E, Colombo A, Mack MJ, Holmes DR, Jr., Morel MA, Van Dyck N, et al. Coronary Artery Bypass Graft Surgery versus Percutaneous Coronary Intervention in Patients with Three-vessel Disease and Left Main Coronary Disease: 5-year Follow-up of the Randomised, Clinical SYNTAX Trial. *Lancet.* 2013;381:629–638. doi: 10.1016/S0140-6736(13)60141-5
67. Madhavan MV, Tarigopula M, Mintz GS, Maehara A, Stone GW, Genereux P. Coronary Artery Calcification: Pathogenesis and Prognostic Implications. *J Am Coll Cardiol.* 2014;63:1703–1714. doi: 10.1016/j.jacc.2014.01.017
68. Genereux P, Madhavan MV, Mintz GS, Maehara A, Palmerini T, Lasalle L, Xu K, McAndrew T, Kirtane A, Lansky AJ, et al. Ischemic Outcomes after Coronary Intervention of Calcified Vessels in Acute Coronary Syndromes. Pooled Analysis from the HORIZONS-AMI (Harmonizing Outcomes With Revascularization and Stents in Acute Myocardial Infarction) and ACUITY (Acute Catheterization and Urgent Intervention Triage Strategy) TRIALS. *J Am Coll Cardiol.* 2014;63:1845–1854. doi: 10.1016/j.jacc.2014.01.034
69. Ciurica S, Lopez-Sublet M, Loeys BL, Radhouani I, Natarajan N, Vikkula M, Maas A, Adlam D, Persu

A. Arterial Tortuosity. *Hypertension.* 2019;73:951–960. doi: 10.1161/HYPERTENSIONAHA.118.11647
70. Damluji AA, Tehrani B, Sinha SS, Samsky MD, Henry TD, Thiele H, West NEJ, Senatore FF, Truesdell AG, Dangas GD, et al. Position Statement on Vascular Access Safety for Percutaneous Devices in AMI Complicated by Cardiogenic Shock. *JACC Cardiovasc Interv.* 2022;15:2003–2019. doi: 10.1016/j.jcin.2022.08.041
71. Mihatov N, Mosarla RC, Kirtane AJ, Parikh SA, Rosenfield K, Chen S, Song Y, Yeh RW, Secemsky EA. Outcomes Associated With Peripheral Artery Disease in Myocardial Infarction With Cardiogenic Shock. *J Am Coll Cardiol.* 2022;79:1223–1235. doi: 10.1016/j.jacc.2022.01.037
72. Boyd C, Smith CD, Masoudi FA, Blaum CS, Dodson JA, Green AR, Kelley A, Matlock D, Ouellet J, Rich MW, et al. Decision Making for Older Adults With Multiple Chronic Conditions: Executive Summary for the American Geriatrics Society Guiding Principles on the Care of Older Adults With Multimorbidity. *J Am Geriatr Soc.* 2019;67:665–673. doi: 10.1111/jgs.15809
73. Alexander KP, Newby LK, Armstrong PW, Cannon CP, Gibler WB, Rich MW, Van de Werf F, White HD, Weaver WD, Naylor MD, et al. Acute Coronary Care in the Elderly, Part II: ST-segment-elevation Myocardial Infarction: A Scientific Statement for Healthcare Professionals from the American Heart Association Council on Clinical Cardiology: In collaboration with the Society of Geriatric Cardiology. *Circulation.* 2007;115:2570–2589. doi: 10.1161/CIRCULATIONAHA.107.182616
74. Dai X, Busby-Whitehead J, Alexander KP. Acute Coronary Syndrome in the Older Adults. *J Geriatr Cardiol.* 2016;13:101–108. doi: 10.11909/j.issn.1671-5411.2016.02.012
75. Gharacholou SM, Lopes RD, Alexander KP, Mehta RH, Stebbins AL, Pieper KS, James SK, Armstrong PW, Granger CB. Age and Outcomes in ST-segment Elevation Myocardial Infarction Treated with Primary Percutaneous Coronary Intervention: Findings from the APEX-AMI Trial. *Arch Intern Med.* 2011;171:559–567. doi: 10.1001/archinternmed.2011.36
76. Lawless M, Damluji A, Dirjayanto VJ, Mills G, Pompei G, Rubino F, Kunadian V. Differences in Treatment and Clinical Outcomes in Patients Aged >/=75 Years Compared with those Aged </=74 Years Following Acute Coronary Syndromes: A Prospective Multicentre Study. *Open Heart.* 2023;10. doi: 10.1136/openhrt-2023-002418
77. Kanwar M, Thayer KL, Garan AR, Hernandez-Montfort J, Whitehead E, Mahr C, Sinha SS, Vorovich E, Harwani NM, Zweck E, et al. Impact of Age on Outcomes in Patients With Cardiogenic Shock. *Front Cardiovasc Med.* 2021;8:688098. doi: 10.3389/fcvm.2021.688098
78. Ibanez B, James S, Agewall S, Antunes MJ, Bucciarelli-Ducci C, Bueno H, Caforio ALP, Crea F, Goudevenos JA, Halvorsen S, et al. 2017 ESC Guidelines for the Management of Acute Myocardial Infarction in Patients Presenting with ST-segment Elevation: The Task Force for the Management of Acute Myocardial Infarction in Patients Presenting with ST-segment Elevation of the European Society of Cardiology (ESC). *Eur Heart J.* 2018;39:119–177. doi: 10.1093/eurheartj/ehx393
79. Lawton JS, Tamis-Holland JE, Bangalore S, Bates ER, Beckie TM, Bischoff JM, Bittl JA, Cohen MG, DiMaio JM, Don CW, et al. 2021 ACC/AHA/SCAI Guideline for Coronary Artery Revascularization: A Report of the American College of Cardiology/American Heart Association Joint Committee on Clinical Practice Guidelines. *Circulation.* 2022;145:e18–e114. doi: 10.1161/CIR.0000000000001038
80. Bueno H, Betriu A, Heras M, Alonso JJ, Cequier A, Garcia EJ, Lopez-Sendon JL, Macaya C, Hernandez-Antolin R, Investigators T. Primary Angioplasty vs. Fibrinolysis in Very Old Patients with Acute Myocardial Infarction: TRIANA (TRatamiento del Infarto Agudo de miocardio eN Ancianos) Randomized Trial and Pooled Analysis with Previous Studies. *Eur Heart J.* 2011;32:51–60. doi: 10.1093/eurheartj/ehq375
81. Ismayl M, Machanahalli Balakrishna A, Walters RW, Pajjuru VS, Goldsweig AM, Aboeata A. In-hospital Mortality and Readmission after ST-Elevation Myocardial Infarction in Nonagenarians: A Nationwide Analysis from the United States. *Catheter Cardiovasc Interv.* 2022;100:5–16. doi: 10.1002/ccd.30227
82. Sheldon M, Blankenship JC. STEMI in Nonagenarians: Never Too Old. *Catheter Cardiovasc Interv.* 2022;100:17–18. doi: 10.1002/ccd.30306
83. Armstrong PW, Gershlick AH, Goldstein P, Wilcox R, Danays T, Lambert Y, Sulimov V, Rosell Ortiz F, Ostojic M, Welsh RC, et al. Fibrinolysis or Primary PCI in ST-segment Elevation Myocardial Infarction. *N Engl J Med.* 2013;368:1379–1387. doi: 10.1056/NEJMoa1301092
84. Van de Werf F, Ristic AD, Averkov OV, Arias-Mendoza A, Lambert Y, Kerr Saraiva JF, Sepulveda P, Rosell-Ortiz F, French JK, Music LB, et al. STREAM-2: Half-Dose Tenecteplase or Primary Percutaneous Coronary Intervention in Older Patients with ST-Segment-Elevation Myocardial Infarction: A Randomized, Open-Label Trial. *Circulation.* 2023;148:753–764. doi: 10.1161/CIRCULATIONAHA.123.064521
85. Jolly SS, Yusuf S, Cairns J, Niemela K, Xavier D, Widimsky P, Budaj A, Niemela M, Valentin V,

Lewis BS, et al. Radial versus Femoral Access for Coronary Angiography and Intervention in Patients with Acute Coronary Syndromes (RIVAL): A Randomised, Parallel Group, Multicentre Trial. *Lancet.* 2011;377:1409–1420. doi: 10.1016/S0140-6736(11)60404-2

86. Romagnoli E, Biondi-Zoccai G, Sciahbasi A, Politi L, Rigattieri S, Pendenza G, Summaria F, Patrizi R, Borghi A, Di Russo C, et al. Radial versus Femoral Randomized Investigation in ST-segment Elevation Acute Coronary Syndrome: The RIFLE-STEACS (Radial Versus Femoral Randomized Investigation in ST-Elevation Acute Coronary Syndrome) Study. *J Am Coll Cardiol.* 2012;60:2481–2489. doi: 10.1016/j.jacc.2012.06.017
87. Valgimigli M, Gagnor A, Calabro P, Frigoli E, Leonardi S, Zaro T, Rubartelli P, Briguori C, Ando G, Repetto A, et al. Radial versus Femoral Access in Patients with Acute Coronary Syndromes Undergoing Invasive Management: A Randomised Multicentre Trial. *Lancet.* 2015;385:2465–2476. doi: 10.1016/S0140-6736(15)60292-6
88. Hochman JS, Sleeper LA, Godfrey E, McKinlay SM, Sanborn T, Col J, LeJemtel T. SHould We Emergently Revascularize Occluded Coronaries for Cardiogenic ShocK: An International Randomized Trial of Emergency PTCA/CABG-trial Design. The SHOCK Trial Study Group. *Am Heart J.* 1999;137:313–321. doi: 10.1053/hj.1999.v137.95352
89. Klein A, Beske RP, Hassager C, Jensen LO, Eiskjær H, Mangner N, Linke A, Polzin A, Schulze PC, Skurk C, et al. Treating Older Patients in Cardiogenic Shock With a Microaxial Flow Pump: Is it DANGERous? *Journal of the American College of Cardiology.* 2025;85:595–603. doi: https://doi.org/10.1016/j.jacc.2024.11.003
90. Kumar S, McDaniel M, Samady H, Forouzandeh F. Contemporary Revascularization Dilemmas in Older Adults. *J Am Heart Assoc.* 2020;9:e014477. doi: 10.1161/JAHA.119.014477
91. Biscaglia S, Guiducci V, Escaned J, Moreno R, Lanzilotti V, Santarelli A, Cerrato E, Sacchetta G, Jurado-Roman A, Menozzi A, et al. Complete or Culprit-Only PCI in Older Patients with Myocardial Infarction. *N Engl J Med.* 2023;389:889–898. doi: 10.1056/NEJMoa2300468
92. Stahli BE, Varbella F, Linke A, Schwarz B, Felix SB, Seiffert M, Kesterke R, Nordbeck P, Witzenbichler B, Lang IM, et al. Timing of Complete Revascularization with Multivessel PCI for Myocardial Infarction. *N Engl J Med.* 2023;389:1368–1379. doi: 10.1056/NEJMoa2307823
93. Pi Y, Roe MT, Holmes DN, Chiswell K, Garvey JL, Fonarow GC, de Lemos JA, Garratt KN, Xian Y. Utilization, Characteristics, and In-Hospital Outcomes of Coronary Artery Bypass Grafting in Patients With ST-Segment-Elevation Myocardial Infarction: Results From the National Cardiovascular Data Registry Acute Coronary Treatment and Intervention Outcomes Network Registry-Get With The Guidelines. *Circ Cardiovasc Qual Outcomes.* 2017;10. doi: 10.1161/CIRCOUTCOMES.116.003490
94. Grothusen C, Friedrich C, Loehr J, Meinert J, Ohnewald E, Ulbricht U, Attmann T, Haneya A, Huenges K, Freitag-Wolf S, et al. Outcome of Stable Patients With Acute Myocardial Infarction and Coronary Artery Bypass Surgery Within 48 Hours: A Single-Center, Retrospective Experience. *J Am Heart Assoc.* 2017;6. doi: 10.1161/JAHA.117.005498
95. de Belder A, Myat A, Blaxill J, Haworth P, O'Kane PD, Hatrick R, Aggarwal RK, Davie A, Smith W, Gerber R, et al. Revascularisation or Medical Therapy in Elderly Patients with Acute Anginal Syndromes: The RINCAL Randomised Trial. *EuroIntervention.* 2021;17:67–74. doi: 10.4244/EIJ-D-20-00975
96. Hirlekar G, Libungan B, Karlsson T, Back M, Herlitz J, Albertsson P. Percutaneous Coronary Intervention in the Very Elderly with NSTE-ACS: The Randomized 80+ Study. *Scand Cardiovasc J.* 2020;54:315–321. doi: 10.1080/14017431.2020.1781243
97. Sanchis J, Nunez E, Barrabes JA, Marin F, Consuegra-Sanchez L, Ventura S, Valero E, Roque M, Bayes-Genis A, Del Blanco BG, et al. Randomized Comparison between the Invasive and Conservative Strategies in Comorbid Elderly Patients with Non-ST Elevation Myocardial Infarction. *Eur J Intern Med.* 2016;35:89–94. doi: 10.1016/j.ejim.2016.07.003
98. Savonitto S, Cavallini C, Petronio AS, Murena E, Antonicelli R, Sacco A, Steffenino G, Bonechi F, Mossuti E, Manari A, et al. Early Aggressive versus Initially Conservative Treatment in Elderly Patients with Non-ST-segment Elevation Acute Coronary Syndrome: A Randomized Controlled Trial. *JACC Cardiovasc Interv.* 2012;5:906–916. doi: 10.1016/j.jcin.2012.06.008
99. Tegn N, Abdelnoor M, Aaberge L, Endresen K, Smith P, Aakhus S, Gjertsen E, Dahl-Hofseth O, Ranhoff AH, Gullestad L, et al. Invasive versus Conservative Strategy in Patients Aged 80 Years or Older with Non-ST-elevation Myocardial Infarction or Unstable Angina Pectoris (After Eighty study): An Open-label Randomised Controlled Trial. *Lancet.* 2016;387:1057–1065. doi: 10.1016/S0140-6736(15)01166-6
100. Kunadian V, Mossop H, Shields C, Bardgett M, Watts P, Teare MD, Pritchard J, Adams-Hall J, Runnett C, Ripley DP, et al. Invasive Treatment Strategy for Older Patients with Myocardial Infarction. *N Engl J Med.* 2024;391:1673–1684. doi: 10.1056/NEJMoa2407791
101. Nanna MG, Kochar A, Damluji AA. Invasive Strategy for Older Patients with MI. *N Engl J Med.* 2025;392:516–517. doi: 10.1056/NEJMc2415597

102. Rout A, Moumneh MB, Kalra K, Singh S, Garg A, Kunadian V, Biscaglia S, Alkhouli MA, Rymer JA, Batchelor WB, et al. Invasive Versus Conservative Strategy in Older Adults >/=75 Years of Age With Non-ST-segment-Elevation Acute Coronary Syndrome: A Systematic Review and Meta-Analysis of Randomized Controlled Trials. *J Am Heart Assoc.* 2024;13:e036151. doi: 10.1161/JAHA.124.036151
103. Jobs A, Mehta SR, Montalescot G, Vicaut E, Van't Hof AWJ, Badings EA, Neumann FJ, Kastrati A, Sciahbasi A, Reuter PG, et al. Optimal Timing of an Invasive Strategy in Patients with Non-ST-elevation Acute Coronary Syndrome: A Meta-analysis of Randomised Trials. *Lancet.* 2017;390:737–746. doi: 10.1016/S0140-6736(17)31490-3
104. Kofoed KF, Kelbaek H, Hansen PR, Torp-Pedersen C, Hofsten D, Klovgaard L, Holmvang L, Helqvist S, Jorgensen E, Galatius S, et al. Early Versus Standard Care Invasive Examination and Treatment of Patients With Non-ST-Segment Elevation Acute Coronary Syndrome. *Circulation.* 2018;138:2741–2750. doi: 10.1161/CIRCULATIONAHA.118.037152
105. Milosevic A, Vasiljevic-Pokrajcic Z, Milasinovic D, Marinkovic J, Vukcevic V, Stefanovic B, Asanin M, Dikic M, Stankovic S, Stankovic G. Immediate Versus Delayed Invasive Intervention for Non-STEMI Patients: The RIDDLE-NSTEMI Study. *JACC Cardiovasc Interv.* 2016;9:541–549. doi: 10.1016/j.jcin.2015.11.018
106. Reuter PG, Rouchy C, Cattan S, Benamer H, Jullien T, Beruben A, Montely JM, Assez N, Raphael V, Hennequin B, et al. Early Invasive Strategy in High-risk Acute Coronary Syndrome without ST-segment Elevation. The Sisca Randomized Trial. *Int J Cardiol.* 2015;182:414–418. doi: 10.1016/j.ijcard.2014.12.089
107. Deharo P, Ducrocq G, Bode C, Cohen M, Cuisset T, Mehta SR, Pollack C, Jr., Wiviott SD, Elbez Y, Sabatine MS, et al. Timing of Angiography and Outcomes in High-Risk Patients With Non-ST-Segment-Elevation Myocardial Infarction Managed Invasively: Insights From the TAO Trial (Treatment of Acute Coronary Syndrome With Otamixaban). *Circulation.* 2017;136:1895–1907. doi: 10.1161/CIRCULATIONAHA.117.029779
108. Mehta SR, Granger CB, Boden WE, Steg PG, Bassand JP, Faxon DP, Afzal R, Chrolavicius S, Jolly SS, Widimsky P, et al. Early versus Delayed Invasive Intervention in Acute Coronary Syndromes. *N Engl J Med.* 2009;360:2165–2175. doi: 10.1056/NEJMoa0807986
109. Hara H, Watanabe H, Esaki J, Hori Y, Hirao S, Kanemitsu N, Morimoto T, Komiya T, Minatoya K, Kimura T, et al. Five-year Outcomes after Coronary Artery Bypass Grafting and Percutaneous Coronary Intervention in Octogenarians with Complex Coronary Artery Disease. *Gen Thorac Cardiovasc Surg.* 2022;70:419–429. doi: 10.1007/s11748-021-01711-4
110. Shah AI, Alabaster A, Dontsi M, Rana JS, Solomon MD, Krishnaswami A. Comparison of Coronary Revascularization Strategies in Older Adults Presenting with Acute Coronary Syndromes. *J Am Geriatr Soc.* 2022;70:2235–2245. doi: 10.1111/jgs.17794
111. Kirov H, Caldonazo T, Riedel LL, Tasoudis P, Moschovas A, Diab M, Farber G, Doenst T. Comparing Outcomes between Coronary artery Bypass Grafting and Percutaneous Coronary Intervention in Octogenarians with Left Main or Multivessel Disease. *Sci Rep.* 2023;13:22323. doi: 10.1038/s41598-023-49069-2
112. Ono M, Serruys PW, Hara H, Kawashima H, Gao C, Wang R, Takahashi K, O'Leary N, Wykrzykowska JJ, Sharif F, et al. 10-Year Follow-Up After Revascularization in Elderly Patients With Complex Coronary Artery Disease. *J Am Coll Cardiol.* 2021;77:2761–2773. doi: 10.1016/j.jacc.2021.04.016
113. Chang M, Lee CW, Ahn JM, Cavalcante R, Sotomi Y, Onuma Y, Park DW, Kang SJ, Lee SW, Kim YH, et al. Outcomes of Coronary Artery Bypass Graft Surgery Versus Drug-Eluting Stents in Older Adults. *J Am Geriatr Soc.* 2017;65:625–630. doi: 10.1111/jgs.14780
114. Koshy AN, Stone GW, Sartori S, Dhulipala V, Giustino G, Spirito A, Farhan S, Smith KF, Feng Y, Vinayak M, et al. Outcomes Following Percutaneous Coronary Intervention in Patients With Multivessel Disease Who Were Recommended for But Declined Coronary Artery Bypass Graft Surgery. *J Am Heart Assoc.* 2024;13:e033931. doi: 10.1161/JAHA.123.033931
115. Bohm F, Mogensen B, Engstrom T, Stankovic G, Srdanovic I, Lonborg J, Zwackman S, Hamid M, Kellerth T, Lauermann J, et al. FFR-Guided Complete or Culprit-Only PCI in Patients with Myocardial Infarction. *N Engl J Med.* 2024;390:1481–1492. doi: 10.1056/NEJMoa2314149
116. Mehta SR, Wood DA, Storey RF, Mehran R, Bainey KR, Nguyen H, Meeks B, Di Pasquale G, Lopez-Sendon J, Faxon DP, et al. Complete Revascularization with Multivessel PCI for Myocardial Infarction. *N Engl J Med.* 2019;381:1411–1421. doi: 10.1056/NEJMoa1907775
117. Park DY, Hu JR, Frampton J, Rymer J, Al Damluji A, Nanna MG. Complete Revascularization versus Culprit-only Revascularization in Older Adults with ST-elevation Myocardial Infarction: Systematic Review and Meta-analysis of Randomized Controlled Trials. *J Am Geriatr Soc.* 2025;73:874–880. doi: 10.1111/jgs.19295
118. Writing Committee M, Otto CM, Nishimura RA, Bonow RO, Carabello BA, Erwin JP, 3rd, Gentile F, Jneid H, Krieger EV, Mack M, et al. 2020 ACC/AHA Guideline for the Management of Patients With

Valvular Heart Disease: A Report of the American College of Cardiology/American Heart Association Joint Committee on Clinical Practice Guidelines. *J Am Coll Cardiol.* 2021;77:e25–e197. doi: 10.1016/j.jacc.2020.11.018

119. Leon MB, Smith CR, Mack M, Miller DC, Moses JW, Svensson LG, Tuzcu EM, Webb JG, Fontana GP, Makkar RR, et al. Transcatheter Aortic-valve Implantation for Aortic Stenosis in Patients Who Cannot Undergo Surgery. *N Engl J Med.* 2010;363:1597–1607. doi: 10.1056/NEJMoa1008232
120. Lonborg J, Jabbari R, Sabbah M, Veien KT, Niemela M, Freeman P, Linder R, Ioanes D, Terkelsen CJ, Kajander OA, et al. PCI in Patients Undergoing Transcatheter Aortic-Valve Implantation. *N Engl J Med.* 2024;391:2189–2200. doi: 10.1056/NEJMoa2401513
121. Persits I, Layoun H, Kondoleon NP, Spilias N, Badwan O, Sipko J, Yun JJ, Kalra A, Dykun I, Tereshchenko LG, et al. Impact of Untreated Chronic Obstructive Coronary Artery Disease on Outcomes after Transcatheter Aortic Valve Replacement. *Eur Heart J.* 2024;45:1890–1900. doi: 10.1093/eurheartj/ehae019
122. Park DY, Simonato M, Ahmad Y, Banks AZ, Lowenstern A, Nanna MG. Insight Into the Optimal Timing of Percutaneous Coronary Intervention and Transcatheter Aortic Valve Replacement. *Curr Probl Cardiol.* 2024;49:102050. doi: 10.1016/j.cpcardiol.2023.102050
123. Batchelor Wayne B, Anwaruddin S, Wang Dee D, Perpetua Elizabeth M, Krishnaswami A, Velagapudi P, Wyman Janet F, Fullerton D, Keegan P, Phillips A, et al. The Multidisciplinary Heart Team in Cardiovascular Medicine. *JACC: Advances.* 2023;2:100160. doi: 10.1016/j.jacadv.2022.100160
124. Bangalore S, Barsness GW, Dangas GD, Kern MJ, Rao SV, Shore-Lesserson L, Tamis-Holland JE. Evidence-Based Practices in the Cardiac Catheterization Laboratory: A Scientific Statement From the American Heart Association. *Circulation.* 2021;144:e107–e119. doi: 10.1161/CIR.0000000000000996
125. Husted S, James S, Becker RC, Horrow J, Katus H, Storey RF, Cannon CP, Heras M, Lopes RD, Morais J, et al. Ticagrelor versus Clopidogrel in Elderly Patients with Acute Coronary Syndromes: A Substudy from the Prospective Randomized PLATelet Inhibition and Patient Outcomes (PLATO) Trial. *Circ Cardiovasc Qual Outcomes.* 2012;5:680–688. doi: 10.1161/CIRCOUTCOMES.111.964395
126. Gimbel M, Qaderdan K, Willemsen L, Hermanides R, Bergmeijer T, de Vrey E, Heestermans T, Tjon Joe Gin M, Waalewijn R, Hofma S, et al. Clopidogrel versus Ticagrelor or Prasugrel in Patients Aged 70 Years or Older with Non-ST-elevation Acute Coronary Syndrome (POPular AGE): The Randomised, Open-label, Non-inferiority Trial. *Lancet.* 2020;395:1374–1381. doi: 10.1016/S0140-6736(20)30325-1
127. Wiviott SD, Braunwald E, McCabe CH, Montalescot G, Ruzyllo W, Gottlieb S, Neumann FJ, Ardissino D, De Servi S, Murphy SA, et al. Prasugrel versus Clopidogrel in Patients with Acute Coronary Syndromes. *N Engl J Med.* 2007;357:2001–2015. doi: 10.1056/NEJMoa0706482
128. Cavender MA, Bhatt DL, Stone GW, Steg PG, Gibson CM, Hamm CW, Price MJ, Prats J, Elkin S, Deliargyris EN, et al. Cangrelor in Older Patients Undergoing Percutaneous Coronary Intervention: Findings From CHAMPION PHOENIX. *Circ Cardiovasc Interv.* 2017;10. doi: 10.1161/CIRCINTERVENTIONS.117.005257
129. Gorog DA, Ferreiro JL, Ahrens I, Ako J, Geisler T, Halvorsen S, Huber K, Jeong YH, Navarese EP, Rubboli A, et al. De-escalation or Abbreviation of Dual Antiplatelet Therapy in Acute Coronary Syndromes and Percutaneous Coronary Intervention: A Consensus Statement from an International Expert Panel on Coronary Thrombosis. *Nat Rev Cardiol.* 2023;20:830–844. doi: 10.1038/s41569-023-00901-2
130. Park DY, Hu JR, Jamil Y, Kelsey MD, Jones WS, Frampton J, Kochar A, Aronow WS, Damluji AA, Nanna MG. Shorter Dual Antiplatelet Therapy for Older Adults After Percutaneous Coronary Intervention: A Systematic Review and Network Meta-Analysis. *JAMA Netw Open.* 2024;7:e244000. doi: 10.1001/jamanetworkopen.2024.4000
131. Rao SV, O'Donoghue ML, Ruel M, Rab T, Tamis-Holland JE, Alexander JH, Baber U, Baker H, Cohen MG, Cruz-Ruiz M, et al. 2025 ACC/AHA/ACEP/NAEMSP/SCAI Guideline for the Management of Patients With Acute Coronary Syndromes: A Report of the American College of Cardiology/American Heart Association Joint Committee on Clinical Practice Guidelines. *J Am Coll Cardiol.* 2025. doi: 10.1016/j.jacc.2024.11.009
132. Wester A, Attar R, Mohammad MA, Isma N, James S, Omerovic E, Erlinge D, Koul S. Bivalirudin Versus Heparin Monotherapy in Elderly Patients With Myocardial Infarction: A Prespecified Subgroup Analysis of the VALIDATE-SWEDEHEART Trial. *Circ Cardiovasc Interv.* 2020;13:e008671. doi: 10.1161/CIRCINTERVENTIONS.119.008671
133. Virani SS, Newby LK, Arnold SV, Bittner V, Brewer LC, Demeter SH, Dixon DL, Fearon WF, Hess B, Johnson HM, et al. 2023 AHA/ACC/ACCP/ASPC/NLA/PCNA Guideline for the Management of Patients With Chronic Coronary Disease: A Report of the American Heart Association/American College of Cardiology Joint Committee on Clinical Practice Guidelines. *Circulation.* 2023;148:e9–e119. doi: 10.1161/CIR.0000000000001168

134. Goldfarb MJ, Saylor MA, Bozkurt B, Code J, Di Palo KE, Durante A, Flanary K, Masterson Creber R, Ogunniyi MO, Rodriguez F, et al. Patient-Centered Adult Cardiovascular Care: A Scientific Statement From the American Heart Association. *Circulation.* 2024;149:e1176–e1188. doi: 10.1161/CIR.0000000000001233
135. Goldwater D, Wenger NK. Patient-centered Care in Geriatric Cardiology. *Trends Cardiovasc Med.* 2023;33:13–20. doi: 10.1016/j.tcm.2021.11.001
136. Goyal P, Kwak MJ, Al Malouf C, Kumar M, Rohant N, Damluji AA, Denfeld QE, Bircher KK, Krishnaswami A, Alexander KP, et al. Geriatric Cardiology: Coming of Age. *JACC Adv.* 2022;1. doi: 10.1016/j.jacadv.2022.100070
137. Dennison Himmelfarb CR, Beckie TM, Allen LA, Commodore-Mensah Y, Davidson PM, Lin G, Lutz B, Spatz ES, American Heart Association Council on C, Stroke N, et al. Shared Decision-Making and Cardiovascular Health: A Scientific Statement From the American Heart Association. *Circulation.* 2023;148:912–931. doi: 10.1161/CIR.0000000000001162
138. Backman WD, Levine SA, Wenger NK, Harold JG. Shared Decision-making for Older Adults with Cardiovascular Disease. *Clin Cardiol.* 2020;43:196–204. doi: 10.1002/clc.23267
139. Vervoort D, Sud M, Zeis TM, Haouzi AA, An KR, Rocha R, Eikelboom R, Fremes SE, Tamis-Holland JE. Do the Few Dictate Care for the Many? Revascularisation Considerations That Go Beyond the Guidelines. *Can J Cardiol.* 2024;40:275–289. doi: 10.1016/j.cjca.2023.11.007
140. Stacey D, Lewis KB, Smith M, Carley M, Volk R, Douglas EE, Pacheco-Brousseau L, Finderup J, Gunderson J, Barry MJ, et al. Decision Aids for People Facing Health Treatment or Screening Decisions. *Cochrane Database Syst Rev.* 2024;1:CD001431. doi: 10.1002/14651858.CD001431.pub6
141. Braun LT, Grady KL, Kutner JS, Adler E, Berlinger N, Boss R, Butler J, Enguidanos S, Friebert S, Gardner TJ, et al. Palliative Care and Cardiovascular Disease and Stroke: A Policy Statement From the American Heart Association/American Stroke Association. *Circulation.* 2016;134:e198–225. doi: 10.1161/CIR.0000000000000438
142. Shi W, Ghisi GLM, Zhang L, Hyun K, Pakosh M, Gallagher R. Systematic Review, Meta-analysis and Meta-regression to Determine the Effects of Patient Education on Health Behaviour Change in Adults Diagnosed with Coronary Heart Sisease. *J Clin Nurs.* 2023;32:5300–5327. doi: 10.1111/jocn.16519
143. Shi W, Ghisi GLM, Zhang L, Hyun K, Pakosh M, Gallagher R. A Systematic Review, Meta-analysis, and Meta-regression of Patient Education for Secondary Prevention in Patients with Coronary Heart Disease: Impact on Psychological Outcomes. *Eur J Cardiovasc Nurs.* 2022;21:643–654. doi: 10.1093/eurjcn/zvac001
144. Su JJ, Yu DS. Effects of a Nurse-led eHealth Cardiac Rehabilitation Programme on Health Outcomes of Patients with Coronary Heart Disease: A Randomised Controlled Trial. *Int J Nurs Stud.* 2021;122:104040. doi: 10.1016/j.ijnurstu.2021.104040
145. Williams MA, Maresh CM, Esterbrooks DJ, Harbrecht JJ, Sketch MH. Early Exercise Training in Patients Older than Age 65 Years Compared with that in Younger Patients after Acute Myocardial Infarction or Coronary Artery Bypass Grafting. *Am J Cardiol.* 1985;55:263–266. doi: 10.1016/0002-9149(85)90357-1
146. Lavie CJ, Milani RV. Effects of Cardiac Rehabilitation Programs on Exercise Capacity, Coronary Risk Factors, Behavioral Characteristics, and Quality of Life in a Large Elderly Cohort. *Am J Cardiol.* 1995;76:177–179. doi: 10.1016/s0002-9149(99)80054-x
147. Stahle A, Mattsson E, Ryden L, Unden A, Nordlander R. Improved Physical Fitness and Quality of Life Following Training of Elderly Patients after Acute Coronary Events. A 1 Year Follow-up Randomized Controlled Study. *Eur Heart J.* 1999;20:1475–1484. doi: 10.1053/euhj.1999.1581
148. Edgerton J, Filardo G, Ryan WH, Brinkman WT, Smith RL, Hebeler RF, Jr., Hamman B, Sass DM, Harbor JP, Mack MJ. Risk of not Being Discharged Home after Isolated Coronary Artery Bypass Graft Operations. *Ann Thorac Surg.* 2013;96:1287–1292. doi: 10.1016/j.athoracsur.2013.05.042
149. Nallamothu BK, Rogers MA, Saint S, McMahon LJ, Jr., Fries BE, Kaufman SR, Langa KM. Skilled Care Requirements for Elderly Patients after Coronary Artery Bypass Grafting. *J Am Geriatr Soc.* 2005;53:1133–1137. doi: 10.1111/j.1532-5415.2005.53356.x
150. Chang DC, Joyce DL, Shoher A, Yuh DD. Simple Index to Predict Likelihood of Skilled Nursing Facility Admission after Coronary Artery Bypass Grafting among Older Patients. *Ann Thorac Surg.* 2007;84:829–834; discussion 834–825. doi: 10.1016/j.athoracsur.2007.04.079
151. Beckie TM. Utility of Home-Based Cardiac Rehabilitation for Older Adults. *Clin Geriatr Med.* 2019;35:499–516. doi: 10.1016/j.cger.2019.07.003
152. O'Neill D, Forman DE. Never Too Old for Cardiac Rehabilitation. *Clin Geriatr Med.* 2019;35:407–421. doi: 10.1016/j.cger.2019.07.001
153. Lutz AH, Forman DE. Cardiac Rehabilitation in Older Adults: Apropos Yet Significantly Underutilized. *Prog Cardiovasc Dis.* 2022;70:94–101. doi: 10.1016/j.pcad.2022.01.001
154. Thomas RJ, Beatty AL, Beckie TM, Brewer LC, Brown TM, Forman DE, Franklin BA, Keteyian SJ, Kitzman DW, Regensteiner JG, et al. Home-Based

Cardiac Rehabilitation: A Scientific Statement From the American Association of Cardiovascular and Pulmonary Rehabilitation, the American Heart Association, and the American College of Cardiology. *Circulation*. 2019;140:e69–e89. doi: 10.1161/CIR.0000000000000663
155. Nkonde-Price C, Reynolds K, Najem M, Yang SJ, Batiste C, Cotter T, Lahti D, Gin N, Funahashi T. Comparison of Home-Based vs Center-Based Cardiac Rehabilitation in Hospitalization, Medication Adherence, and Risk Factor Control Among Patients With Cardiovascular Disease. *JAMA Netw Open*. 2022;5:e2228720. doi: 10.1001/jamanetworkopen.2022.28720
156. Huang K, Liu W, He D, Huang B, Xiao D, Peng Y, He Y, Hu H, Chen M, Huang D. Telehealth Interventions versus Center-based Cardiac Rehabilitation of Coronary Artery Disease: A Systematic Review and Meta-analysis. *Eur J Prev Cardiol*. 2015;22:959–971. doi: 10.1177/2047487314561168
157. Eagle KA, Lim MJ, Dabbous OH, Pieper KS, Goldberg RJ, Van de Werf F, Goodman SG, Granger CB, Steg PG, Gore JM, et al. A Validated Prediction Model for all Forms of Acute Coronary Syndrome: Estimating the Risk of 6-month Postdischarge Death in an International Registry. *JAMA*. 2004;291:2727–2733. doi: 10.1001/jama.291.22.2727
158. Antman EM, Cohen M, Bernink PJ, McCabe CH, Horacek T, Papuchis G, Mautner B, Corbalan R, Radley D, Braunwald E. The TIMI Risk Score for Unstable Angina/Non-ST Elevation MI: A Method for Prognostication and Therapeutic Decision Making. *JAMA*. 2000;284:835–842. doi: 10.1001/jama.284.7.835
159. Shahian DM, Jacobs JP, Badhwar V, Kurlansky PA, Furnary AP, Cleveland JC, Jr., Lobdell KW, Vassileva C, Wyler von Ballmoos MC, Thourani VH, et al. The Society of Thoracic Surgeons 2018 Adult Cardiac Surgery Risk Models: Part 1-Background, Design Considerations, and Model Development. *Ann Thorac Surg*. 2018;105:1411–1418. doi: 10.1016/j.athoracsur.2018.03.002
160. Costa F, van Klaveren D, James S, Heg D, Raber L, Feres F, Pilgrim T, Hong MK, Kim HS, Colombo A, et al. Derivation and Validation of the Predicting Bleeding Complications in Patients Undergoing Stent Implantation and Subsequent Dual Antiplatelet Therapy (PRECISE-DAPT) Score: A Pooled Analysis of Individual-patient Datasets from Clinical Trials. *Lancet*. 2017;389:1025–1034. doi: 10.1016/S0140-6736(17)30397-5

after coronary bypass grafting (CABG), and those with HF. A separate analysis of Medicare data assessed the relationship between the number of sessions of CR completed and 4-year risk of death or MI (14). Patients who attended 36 sessions had a 14% lower risk of death and a 12% lower risk of MI than those who attended 24 sessions and a 47% lower risk of death and a 31% lower risk of MI than those who attended just 1 session, suggesting a strong dose–response relationship. Finally, a large observational study, the British Regional Heart Study of almost 6000 men with established coronary heart disease (CHD), found that regular light to moderate physical activity was associated with a lower 5-year all-cause mortality (15).

CR and CVD risk factors

In older populations, CR has well-defined metabolic benefits that include improved blood lipid values, decreased body fat, improved glucose tolerance, and lower blood pressure (3, 16). Cardiac rehabilitation programs have been described as "secondary prevention centers" (3) and thus can function as a location to systematically measure and treat coronary risk factors with both lifestyle approaches (exercise and diet) and pharmacological therapy. For example, at the baseline medical evaluation, medication review for lipid and antiplatelet management can be reviewed; similarly, blood pressure monitoring and treatment, and obesity assessment and treatment should also be reviewed and coordinated in the CR setting. Cardiac rehabilitation participation has been linked with better medication adherence and lower downstream cardiovascular risk using the Medicare database in a dose–response relationship (17).

Cardiac rehabilitation also addresses the growing prevalence of obesity in older adults with CVD. From 1996 to 2006, body weight increased from 84.7 to 88.5 kg among individuals entering CR (18). For many individuals, the accomplishment of weight reduction will significantly lower the burden of coronary risk factors. An exercise program in CR that emphasizes daily longer distance walking to maximize caloric expenditure, associated with behavioral weight loss dietary counseling, has been shown to accomplish significant weight reduction associated with a comprehensive reduction of coronary risk factors (19).

For those with frailty and sarcopenia, weight loss can be a challenging endeavor; CR, therefore, can provide a multifaceted approach to address exercise, diet, and other elements of care to help facilitate weight loss in a healthy manner (20). Similarly, there has been a rise in the use of glucose-like peptide (GLP)-agonists to assist with weight loss, but these drugs may lead to a disproportionate loss of lean muscle mass, further complicating matters in older adults. CR can help counteract these effects by focusing on strength training and nutrition to help adapt to these clinical challenges (21).

The magnitude of exercise-related effects on blood lipid measures depends, in part, on associated weight loss. In a study of CR without weight loss, lipid effects were relatively modest with high-density lipoprotein (HDL) cholesterol increasing by 8%, but no significant effects on low-density lipoprotein (LDL) cholesterol, triglyceride levels, or glucose levels (3). On the other hand, when exercise was associated with 10 pounds of exercise-induced weight loss, favorable effects were noted on serum triglycerides (–24%), HDL cholesterol (+7%), on the atherogenic ratio (total cholesterol/HDL cholesterol [–14%]), and fasting serum insulin levels (–22%) (19). Even among individuals who are not deemed overweight or obese, there is still valuable benefit of CR in lowering lipids, as reductions in LDL cholesterol have been shown to reduce the risk of a recurrent cardiac event as well as lower the risk of stroke and peripheral arterial disease (3).

Exercise effects of CR have been associated with a reduction in indices of systemic inflammation, such as white blood cell count, fibrinogen, and interleukin-6 (22). Inflammatory biomarkers, such as high-sensitivity C-reactive protein (hsCRP), are risk markers for CHD, and studies have shown that exercise lowers hsCRP (22). Additionally, the benefits of lipid lowering, smoking cessation, angiotensin-converting enzyme inhibition, antiplatelet agents, and β-adrenergic blockade have all been demonstrated in both younger and older adults (3, 16).

CR to address geriatric intricacies of care

A unique aspect of CR is the opportunity it provides to address geriatric healthcare domains that tend to overlap with CVD. In particular, CR is useful for adults with frailty who may be less inclined to be physically active due to associated vulnerabilities to weakness, fatigability, falls, and fear. Frailty is a syndrome of decreased reserve and vulnerability to stressors, and a physical frailty phenotype is commonly characterized in terms of unintentional weight loss; weakness or poor handgrip strength; self-reported exhaustion; slow walking speed; and low physical activity (9). Cardiac rehabilitation provides the distinctive opportunity to integrate strength, aerobic, and balance training, in combination with dietary enrichment, to slow, reverse, or even prevent frailty and downstream disablement (23). A growing body of literature highlights the value of CR in modifying frailty, and underscores the utility of CR in advancing physical function in frail adults who are particularly susceptible to progressive functional decline (24, 25).

Depression and social isolation are also widespread among adults >65 years, and among older adults with CVD, depression is two to three times more common than in the age-matched general public (26). Roughly half of patients who suffer an acute cardiac event also experience anxiety and will self-limit physical activity due to fear, which predisposes them to loneliness, social

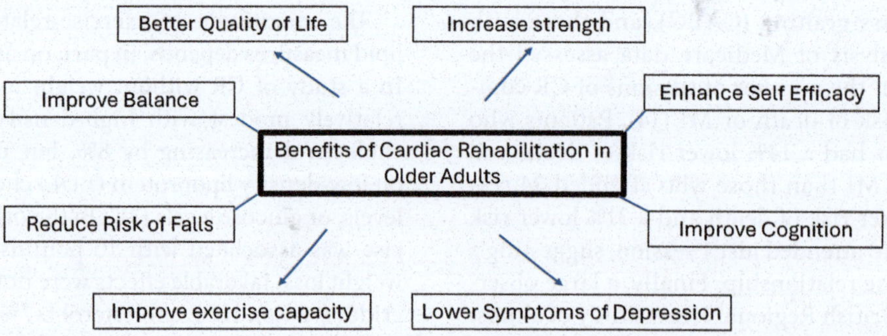

Figure 13.2 Benefits of CR.

isolation, and functional declines (27). Hospitalization associated with the principal cardiac event (especially for patients treated in the intensive care unit) often magnifies risks of deconditioning, frailty, malnutrition, and confusion, and thereby adds to risks of subsequent isolation, depression, and anxiety (1, 2). All these vulnerabilities may be improved by CR, by the effects of exercise training, enhanced nutrition, care coordination, and even by the social dynamics between patients and clinicians (3).

Debilitating effects of polypharmacy have become a major issue for older adults with CVD in the context of multimorbidity, affecting 40%–50% of older adults (28). CR can serve as an opportunity to address this with care coordination. Upon entry to CR and typically at each session, medications are reviewed by the staff with the patient, thus providing an opportunity to avoid redundancies and to consider deprescribing medications that are potentially detrimental. Ultimately, this helps to improve adherence to medications with clear benefits. The ACTION-Registry-GWTG examined close to 12,000 adults post-MI and >65 years of age who participated in CR and found that a higher number of CR sessions attended was improved with medication adherence; each five-session increase in participation was associated with lower mortality and lower risk of an adverse cardiac event (17). Cardiac rehabilitation provides numerous benefits that are specifically applicable to older patients (Figure 13.2).

IMPLEMENTATION OF CR

Prior to exercise, careful screening is a priority. Typically, this involves a clinical review of past medical problems, as well as musculoskeletal conditions, neuropsychologic function, and social challenges, which are common in older patients. To assess functional status, various assessment tools may be used, as listed in Table 13.1 (29–33); this information provides a basis for tailoring the individualized exercise prescription. Additionally, strength assessment is fundamental as well as screening for depression and/or anxiety, as these also have a direct bearing on CR management and goals. Family circumstances, transportation, and supports are also key (3, 10).

Exercise modalities include aerobic, resistance, balance, and flexibility exercise options. Aerobic choices include treadmills, a walking course, cycles, and rowers. Aerobic exercise is often guided by an exercise heart rate (HR) range and/or scales of perceived exertion such as the Borg scale. A gradual increment of exercise HR from 60% to 75% of maximal attained or predicted HR to higher levels of up to 85% is balanced against the greater risk of injury at higher levels and past demonstration of measurable benefits even with low levels of exercise (34). It has been observed that older CVD patients are less likely to exercise to a physiological maximum at their baseline exercise test than younger patients, often lowering the intensity of exercise prescription thereafter. Research is underway to better determine exercise testing strategies that can optimize exercise prescription and CR benefits in older adults (NCT05925634).

Duration of the exercise stimulus can begin with very brief, intermittent bouts of exercise, gradually increasing to 20–25 minutes or longer. Special considerations for older adults include that training regimens often need to be adjusted to accommodate limitations imposed by comorbidities (35). For example, patients with hip or knee arthritis may do better with cycling or rowing exercises to avoid the weight bearing of treadmill walking. However, walking is generally a preferred modality because of its direct relevance to daily activities. Finally, it should be noted that for many older adults, flexibility, or lack thereof, can be an exercise-limiting factor. Flexibility exercises can be as simple as 5–10 minutes of stretching per day to more complex protocols of yoga and tai chi.

Balance training is especially important for patients who are typically weakened (both aerobically and in respect to muscle strength), and further destabilized by medications affecting hemodynamics, neuroautonomic function, and gait, along with neuropathy, peripheral edema, vision impairments, and other common comorbidities (35, 36).

AEROBIC TRAINING

In middle-aged CVD patients and in patients with HF, reduced cardiovascular fitness (peak oxygen uptake

Table 13.1 Functional assessments

Assessment tool	Description	Utilization
Short Physical Performance Battery (29)	This is measured by a series of three timed physical performance tests (gait speed, chair rises, and tandem balance). Each is scored 0 to 4, composite score of 12.	• Assesses slowness, weakness, and balance • Measures physical frailty
5 m Gait Speed Test (30)	Measures the individual's ability to walk 5 meters at a usual pace without assistance or sitting.	• Used to evaluation mobility and potential fall risk
Six-Minute Walk Test (6MWT) (31)	Measures the distance a patient can walk on a flat, hard surface over 6 minutes. Patients are asked to walk as fast as possible back and forth along a fixed path (usually 25 meters) for 6 minutes. Assistive devices (cane, walker) can be used while performing the test. Individuals are allowed to rest if needed; however, the clock is not stopped.	• Assesses endurance and submaximal aerobic capacity • Widely utilized to assess the effect of an intervention and as an outcome measure • Is especially useful to discriminate differences in function if SPPB is ≥10 • Can be an index for a patient's ability to perform ADLs
Grip strength (32)	Measured by single hand dynamometer. Individuals are asked to squeeze the dynamometer as hard and as long as they can. Repeat the trial on each hand, alternating. The score is the average of three trials from both hands.	• Assesses upper body strength • Associated with other strength tests that measure upper- and lower-body strength (1RM testing) • Correlates strongly with physical function and disability
30 Second Sit-to-Stand Test (33)	Measures leg strength by counting how many times a person can stand up from a seated position in 30 seconds.	• Assesses lower extremity strength and endurance

[VO_2]) is a primary clinical predictor of impaired physical function and of survival (37, 38). Furthermore, favorable training-induced changes in peak aerobic capacity are associated with a lower mortality for patients with the greatest training effect (39). Meta-analyses of randomized trials of CR, including over 4000 patients, document a 25% decrease in mortality over an average follow-up of 3 years (40, 41). These studies are limited, however, by the inclusion of relatively few patients over the age of 65 years (42–45).

The CR literature supports the safety and efficacy of exercise training regimens in older patients with CVD (1, 4, 42–45). Compared with younger patients, older adults are typically less fit at entry into a rehabilitation (1, 46) (Figure 13.2). In a cross-sectional analysis of cardiac patients between ages 40 and 80 years, peak aerobic capacity decreased by 40% in men and 33% in women in comparisons of younger men and women versus older men and women (46) (Figure 13.3).

Moderate intensity continuous exercise training (MICT) has served as the foundation for exercise in CR; however, attention has recently focused on high intensity interval aerobic training (HIIT) as an alternative to MICT because it not only improves aerobic fitness to a greater extent but is also relatively safe and feasible for older adults enrolled in CR (47, 48).

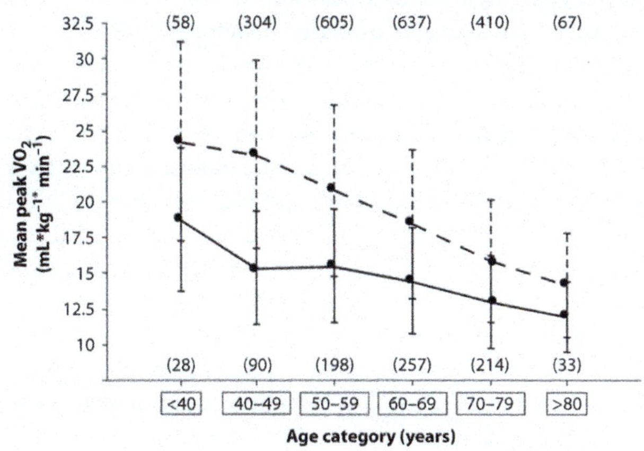

Figure 13.3 Peak aerobic capacity (peak VO_2) by age and gender entering cardiac rehabilitation. Dashed lines represent men; solid lines represent women. *Abbreviation*: VO_2, oxygen uptake. (From Ades PA et al., *Circulation*, 113, 2706–2712, 2006.)

The duration and ratio of high-intensity and low-intensity intervals are key aspects that distinguish HIIT from MICT. When implementing HIIT for older adults, high intensity is usually defined as 85%–95% of peak HR/peak VO_2 or RPE 15–17 followed by low intensity defined as 50%–75% of peak HR/peak VO_2 or RPE 12–14 (48). While prior studies have shown safety to be somewhat

Table 13.2 Implementing exercise in older adults with CVD

- Optimally performed in the cardiac rehabilitation setting
- Intensity of exercise generally based on an exercise tolerance test
- In severely disabled patients, forego exercise test and begin with low-level interval training on a treadmill and/or cycle
- Resistance training is always important, and sometimes must precede aerobic training to achieve sufficient capacity for aerobic activity
- Advance intensity actively
- Clarify long-term goals

similar between MICT and HIIT, HIIT may result in lower adherence, especially in home-based strategies of training (49).

Peak VO_2 or peak HR are widely used for prescribing exercise intensity; however, this information may not be readily available for some CR programs. Given that older adults often have musculoskeletal concerns or additional comorbidities, subjective methods to prescribe exercise, such as the ratings of perceived exertion (RPE) or dyspnea on exertion, can also be used.

Irrespective of the exercise intensity, older adults with CVD participating in CR derive a similar or greater relative training benefit as younger patients and thereby lessen mobility limitations and disability (1). Training programs have been extended to a year and longer with long-term maintenance of exercise-related benefits (44, 48).

Practical issues related to the implementation of exercise training programs in older coronary patients include the frequent need for training regimens to be adjusted to accommodate the presence of comorbidities such as arthritis, diabetes, and peripheral vascular disease (Table 13.2). The least fit individuals are often unable to sustain exercise for extended periods and do well with repeated intermittent brief bouts of exercise (often termed "interval training") that are gradually extended. Some authors recommend long-term exercise programs for older adults, partly related to their low baseline functional capacity (48). It should be noted, however, that even patients who use canes and walkers can perform an exercise test and can train on a treadmill with surround bars or on a cycle ergometer.

RESISTANCE TRAINING

Resistance training (RT) is a particularly important intervention in older adults with CVD (50, 51). In frail and deconditioned adults enrolling in CR it is often necessary to initiate RT before aerobic training can be considered to achieve rudimentary functional capacity.

First and foremost, even "normal" aging is associated with a significant loss of muscle mass and strength, related both to diminished activity profiles and to decreased rates of muscle protein synthesis (52, 53). Furthermore, in older populations ranging from healthy community living dwellers to those who are institutionalized, RT has been demonstrated to improve walking endurance, muscle mass, and strength (54–56). In CVD patients, aging-related musculoskeletal abnormalities are superimposed upon activity restrictions related to chronic disease (57), and diminished muscle mass and strength, termed "sarcopenia," is even more severe.

In a study that focused on resistance training in older CVD patients who had recently suffered a MI, relative increases in strength were found to be similar to increases seen in younger patients (50). In older women with chronic CVD, where the negative effects of age, gender, and chronic disease all conspire to result in a severe loss of strength and function, the effects of RT have been carefully studied (58, 59). Brochu et al. assessed the effects of 6 months of RT on strength, endurance, and on a physical performance test designed to assess physical function during practical household activities in 30 older women, mean age 71 ± 5 years (59). Compared with patients randomized to a control group, strength-trained women increased strength, endurance, and capacity to perform a wide range of household activities such as carrying groceries, doing household activities, and climbing stairs. The increase in strength after RT correlated with improvements in the overall physical function score (Figure 13.4) (60).

Resistance training is especially important for stable patients with HF due to the well-described skeletal muscle abnormalities (fiber atrophy, diminished oxidative capacity) (61). Pu et al. found that 10 weeks of strength training in women with HF led to increased strength and

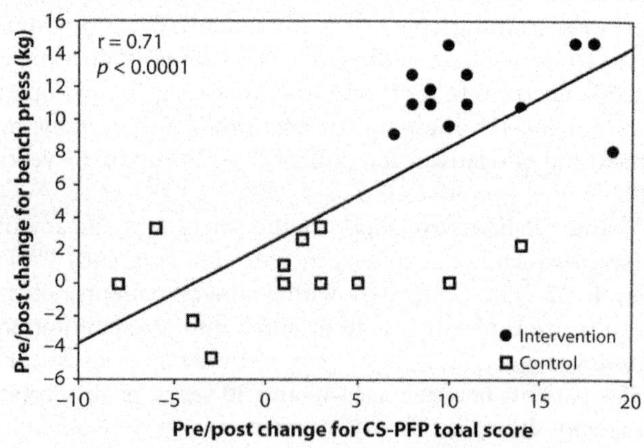

Figure 13.4 Association between percent changes in total continuous-scale physical functional performance test score (CS-PFP) and percent changes in maximal strength on the bench press before and after strength training in older women with CHD. *Abbreviations:* CS-PFP, continuous-scale physical functional performance test score; CHD, coronary heart disease. (Adapted from Fiatorone MA et al., *JAMA*, 263, 3029–3034, 1990.)

6-minute walk distance, and was supported by increases in skeletal muscle fiber area and oxidative capacity (62).

From a practical point of view, the onset of upper-body RT must be delayed after coronary bypass surgery to allow for full sternal healing (usually 3 months), while it can commence as soon as 2–4 weeks after MI after performance of a satisfactory baseline exercise tolerance test. Ideal RT programs include training of the leg extensor muscles to assist with walking, stair climbing, and fall prevention, and upper-body training to aid in the lifting and pushing required for the performance of daily household activities. Training intensity is usually based on the performance of a single-repetition maximal (1-RM) lift supplemented by a Borg scale for perceived exertion (63). Patients begin their resistance training with 8–10 repetitions of each exercise at 40%–50% of their 1-RM for a given exercise and gradually increase exercise intensity, as tolerated, to 50%–80% of updated 1-RMs.

Power training focuses on both strength and speed with the goal of moving resistance weight quickly; this type of exercise entails quick weight shifts and bursts of movement, which can mitigate falls by improving stability and reaction time, particularly in the lower body (49, 52, 55).

EXERCISE TRAINING IN OLDER ADULTS WITH HEART FAILURE

Heart failure is common in older adults and its prevalence is increasing both in the United States and around the world (63). Over 75% of HF patients are aged 65 years or older. These patients are at a particularly high risk of disability and have an exercise capacity that is 25%–70% below normal levels (64). Systematic reviews and meta-analyses of studies of exercise training for stable patients with HF demonstrate reductions in cardiac mortality and hospitalizations, whereas single individual trials are less conclusive (65–67). The single largest trial of exercise training in HF with reduced ejection fraction (HFrEF), HF-ACTION (Heart Failure: A Controlled Trial Investigating Outcomes of Exercise Training), found a lower combined endpoint of total mortality and hospitalizations (reduced by 11%; $p < 0.053$) when results were adjusted by prespecified predictors of mortality (67). This same study found a significantly improved quality of life versus control subjects, and virtually all studies show improved exercise capacity in intervention patients versus controls.

Facility-based CR provides a process to initiate exercise training and lifestyle modification that is supervised, which many regard as especially well-suited for older adults with HF. Nonetheless, studies have demonstrated home based CR to be safe and effective in well-screened patients. Cardiac rehabilitation exercise training has also been shown to be beneficial in the setting of HF with preserved ejection fraction (HFpEF), although CMS does not yet provide insurance coverage for CR with this condition (68, 69).

Barriers to CR participation and potential solutions

Despite the benefits of CR, it remains underutilized particularly among older adults and more so in women (70); only 24.4% participated in CR. Participation decreased with increasing age, was particularly lower in women compared to men, and varied by geographic region as well as qualifying event type (71).

Lack of referral, either due to physician bias or systematic issues, contributes to low participation rates. Often, patients are transferred from an initial hospitalization to a skilled nursing facility (SNF), and then discharged home. In the discharge from SNF to home, few older adults are referred to outpatient Phase 2 CR despite the typical need for continued functional and clinical improvement (72).

The type of qualifying cardiac event influences CR participation. Notably, those with an indication of CABG are much more likely to receive a referral and attend CR compared to those who underwent a percutaneous coronary intervention (PCI). This is pertinent given that as the population is aging and experiencing more comorbidities, older patients are more likely to undergo PCI rather than CABG (73). Additionally, referral rates are even lower for patients with HF compared to CHD patients. In a study of 106 patients >65 years of age hospitalized for HF, only 21% were referred upon discharge, even though 72% reported interest in CR participation (74).

Older coronary patients are far less likely than younger patients to participate in CR (75, 76). Our data documented a 21% participation rate in CR for patients with CHD over the age of 62 years, who recently suffered a coronary event and who lived within 1 hour driving time of the CR center, compared with a 42% participation rate in younger patients (72). Older cardiac patients perceive greater barriers to CR participation than do younger patients (77). Kinesiophobia (fear of exercise), low health literacy, transportation difficulty, and lack of self-efficacy are commonly reported by older adults as challenges for CR enrollment (73).

Various evidence-based solutions have been reported to improve CR engagement. By far, the most powerful predictor of CR participation in the clinical setting is the strength of the primary physician's recommendation for participation. In 1992, Ades et al. assessed the strength of physician's recommendation using a 5-point Likert scale with options ranging from 1 (recommend against CR), 2 (do not remember), 3 (mentioned but not recommended), 4 (mentioned and recommended), or 5 (mentioned and strongly recommended) (75). When the recommendation was weak (a score of 1–3), a 2% participation rate was noted, compared with a rate of 66% when it was strong (a score of 4–5). Twenty-eight years later, this still holds true (70). Among 294 hospitalized patients who were eligible for CR, strength of physician recommendation was found to be an independent predictor for CR participation. With increasing utilization of electronic medical records, computerized "automatic" referral of appropriate patients to CR at hospital discharge can partly help overcome the lack of CR endorsement and has shown great promise as a means to increase CR referral and participation (78).

GENDER DISPARITY

Even among older adults, there is a gender disparity regarding CR engagement and CR performance. While women tend to live longer than men, they also experience more episodes of HFpEF and increased frailty, in part due to lower strength and muscle mass, as well as lower levels of habitual physical activity and physical function (9, 79). While CR can potentially be utilized to address these distinctive challenges pertaining to women, CR enrollment remains disproportionately lower in women than men (80–82).

Notably, women are less likely to be referred to CR than men, prominently contributing to lower participation as seen by Ades et al. (15% vs. 25%; $p = 0.06$) (83). Older women with CVD also tend to limit physical activity overall because of apprehensions related to frailty and fear. Other factors undercutting participation of older women in CR include greater barriers related to transportation, comorbid conditions, and responsibilities to a dependent spouse at home. This distinction may relate, in part, to the older age of women with CVD, compared with men.

Ades et al. show that older women participating in CR increase their fitness (measured by peak VO_2) to a lesser degree than men (13% in women compared with 17% by men) (84). However, older women make similar improvements in muscular strength compared with men (85).

VARIOUS MODES OF CR DELIVERY

The growing availability of home-based CR in the United States is an important opportunity for older adults. In general, home-based CR is a means to widen access and increase participation, and many see it as a useful strategy to overcome logistic barriers that often limit older adults from participating in facility-based CR (86).

There are many factors that make home-based CR especially appealing and effective. The rapid evolution of telehealth technologies includes increasingly sophisticated smart devices, apps that recreate the basic elements of CR (e.g., exercise, education, nutrition, and healthful behaviors), as well as captivating websites that enable patients to track and compare progress, and to foster connections to clinicians and other patients (86). In addition, wearable tracking and communication devices enable meticulous monitoring, better clinician–patient engagement, and opportunities to better tailor care (87, 88).

A recent Cochrane review on home-based versus facility-based CR analyzed 23 trials, including 2890 patients with acute MI, revascularization, or HF, found no difference in outcomes between home and site-based CR formats (89). Several smaller studies have highlighted the potential of smartphone apps to recreate CR using technology, again highlighting overall efficacy and perhaps even superior clinician–patient engagement (90).

It is often assumed that mobile technology may not be widely adopted in older adults, but data from 2016 showed that among adults >65 years old in the US, 42% already owned a smartphone (91), and a 2020 survey from AARP indicated smartphone use had reached 62% in adults aged ≥70 years (92). Many companies have developed smartphone apps to facilitate CR. Nonetheless, the size of devices may still be challenging for older adults who are visually impaired or who have limited physical dexterity. Still, the evolving availability and sophistication of smartphones and wearables raise many thoughts about their value and utility to enhance participation of older adults in CR in home or community environments (91).

In an attempt to better assess mobile CR among older adults, the Rehabilitation at Home Using Mobile Health in Older Adults After Hospitalization for Ischemic Heart Disease (RESILIENT) trial was conducted from 2020 to 2024. This was a multicenter randomized controlled trial consisting of 400 adults aged 65 years or older with ischemic heart disease; no differences were seen in functional capacity as assessed by a 6-minute walk test for those assigned to mobile health CR versus usual care. While this trial demonstrated the feasibility of utilizing virtual CR platforms for older adults, the primary outcome of a 6-minute walk test may not be an ideal form of assessment for functional capacity, and, furthermore, the technological aspects of the program weren't necessarily tailored to address limited digital health literacy (93). More research is needed to explore ways to tailor technology for this specific population.

The majority of research showing efficacy of home-based CR pertains to younger adults, and/or subsets of older adults who are initially screened to include only those with low- to moderate-risk profiles and who are deemed by clinicians to be safe to continue at home. Older CR candidates include many with age-related health complexities that significantly compound challenges and risks. Frailty, multimorbidity, cognitive impairments, fall risks, neuropathy, and pain, as well as vision and hearing impairments are among the many comorbidities of aging that confound many aspects of CR process and safety (94). Even low-intensity activity regimens may amount to high-intensity for someone severely deconditioned and frail, and their capacity to follow critical directions may be less reliable. Typically, apprehension among patients and their families is also heightened by the thought of training.

One small study focused on CHD patients aged ≥65 years (mean age 74.7) (95) and showed similar gains in peak VO_2 or 6-minute walk distance with overall safety. However, this study included home visits by a physiotherapist who took steps to specifically lay out the training program and optimize safety. Such provision of direct contact as part of care may be especially important as part of home-based CR for adults who are more frail and complex.

Community-based CR programs may be another option that logically extends from a literature showing efficacy of community physical activity (PA) programs to reduce disability and frailty, to increase function, and to improve quality of life. The conceptual advantage of community-based formats in a centralized site (e.g., fitness or community center) is that several individuals can exercise together, providing opportunities to arrange supervision (i.e., reinforce monitoring and safety) and offering social reinforcement that has been demonstrated to augment adherence and satisfaction. The Lifestyle Interventions and Independence for Elders (LIFE) study was designed to assess the role of a community-based PA intervention (walking plus strength, balance, and flexibility training) in preventing or delaying development of major mobility disability (MMD) in older community-dwelling adults (95). MMD occurred in 30.1% of the PA group versus 35.5% of a control (education only) group ($p = 0.03$). Serious adverse events did not differ between the groups. The implications of LIFE are reinforced by related analyses showing that its utility persisted in subjects who were frail and that the improvements in PA were also associated with reduced cardiovascular risks (96, 97). Subsequent trials of community-based interventions have since augmented PA therapies with nutritional supplementation and other components of healthfulness that target interventions as integral dimensions of effective CR care for the expanding demographic of aging cardiovascular patients (96).

FUTURE DIRECTIONS

As the older adult demographic continues to grow in size, the role of CR is increasingly important as a vital means to address the CVD that is endemic in this population. Older adults have high susceptibility to both disease with vulnerabilities that are compounded by comorbidity, frailty, polypharmacy, and other complexities associated with age. Both aerobic and resistance training protocols have distinctive benefits in relation to age, but further study is merited to achieve better standards of dosing, progression, and long-term adherence. Greater emphasis on balance and flexibility exercises can also help minimize fall risk and improve quality of life. Diet is also of key importance in a population prone to adiposity, diabetes, hypertension, sarcopenia, and frailty. Goals to mitigate disability in pre-frail and frail adults are of key importance, with related goals to improve CR effectiveness for adults who are already frail. Finally, whether training regimens can affect the economics of healthcare is crucial, especially if costly hospitalizations, institutionalization, and/or home care services can be minimized.

CONCLUSION

Older patients with CVD are a particularly vulnerable group, yet quite heterogeneous as to physical functioning and disease severity. CR training programs have been demonstrated to be safe and to improve physical function, quality of life, and CVD management. It provides a key opportunity to optimize performance and well-being that are tailored for each older patient's circumstances and goals, extending to value in reversing or preventing disability. Expanding its utilization may involve greater physician endorsement as well as the expansion of hybrid and community options, including consideration of mobile health technologies.

ACKNOWLEDGMENTS

The authors acknowledge Dr. Philip A. Ades for his prior contributions to this chapter and for his excellence in advancing the field of cardiac rehabilitation.

REFERENCES

1. Ades PA, Grunvald MH. Cardiopulmonary exercise testing before and after conditioning in older coronary patients. *Am Heart J* 1990; *120*: 585–589.
2. Sugiura M, Hiraoka K, Ohkawa S. Severity of coronary sclerosis in the aged: A pathological study of 968 consecutive autopsy cases. *Jpn Heart J* 1976; *17*: 471–478.
3. Brown TM, Pack QR, Beregg EA et al. Core components of cardiac rehabilitation programs: 2024 update: A scientific statement from the American Heart Association and the American Association of Cardiovascular and Pulmonary Rehabilitation: Endorsed by the American College of Cardiology. *J Cardiopulm Rehabil Prev.* Published online November 18, 2024.
4. Forman DE, Arena R, Boxer R et al. Prioritizing functional capacity as a principal end point for therapies oriented to older adults with cardiovascular disease: A scientific statement for healthcare professionals from the American Heart Association. *Circulation* 2017; *135*: e894–e918.
5. Pinsky JL, Jette AM, Branch LG et al. The Framingham Disability Study: Relationship of various coronary heart disease manifestations to disability in older persons living in the community. *Am J Public Health* 1990; *80*: 1363–1368.
6. Triposkiadis F, Xanthopoulos A, Butler J. Cardiovascular aging and heart failure: JACC review topic of the week. *J Am Coll Cardiol* 2019; *74*(6): 804–813.
7. Bøtker MT, Stengaard C, Andersen MS et al. Dyspnea, a high-risk symptom in patients suspected of myocardial infarction in the ambulance? A population-based follow-up study. *Scand J Trauma Resusc Emerg Med* 2016; *24*: 15.
8. James K, Jamil Y, Kumar M et al. Frailty and cardiovascular health. *J Am Heart Assoc* 2024; *13*: e031736.
9. Damluji AA, Huang J, Bandeen-Roche K et al. Frailty among older adults with acute myocardial infarction and outcomes from percutaneous

coronary interventions. *J Am Heart Assoc* 2019; *8*: e013686.
10. Menezes AR, Lavie CJ, Forman DE et al. Cardiac rehabilitation in the elderly. *Prog Cardiovasc Dis* 2014; *57*: 152–159.
11. Balady GJ, Jette D, Scheer J et al. Changes in exercise capacity following cardiac rehabilitation in patients stratified according to age and gender. Results of the Massachusetts Association of Cardiovascular and Pulmonary Rehabilitation Multicenter Database. *J Cardiopulm Rehabil* 1996; *16(1)*: 38–46.
12. Lavie CJ, Milani RV. Effects of cardiac rehabilitation and exercise training programs in patients > or = 75 years of age. *Am J Cardiol* 1996; *78*: 675–677.
13. Suaya JA, Stason WB, Ades PA et al. Cardiac rehabilitation and survival in older coronary patients. *J Am Coll Cardiol* 2009; *54*: 25–33.
14. Hammill BG, Curtis LH, Schulman KA et al. Relationship between cardiac rehabilitation and long-term risks of death and myocardial infarction among elderly Medicare beneficiaries. *Circulation* 2010; *121*: 63–70.
15. Wannamethee SG, Shaper AG, Walker M. Physical activity and mortality in older men with diagnosed coronary heart disease. *Circulation* 2000; *102*: 1358–1363.
16. Fleg JL, Forman DE, Berra K et al. Secondary prevention of atherosclerotic cardiovascular disease in older adults: A scientific statement from the American Heart Association. *Circulation* 2013; *128*: 2422–2446.
17. Doll JA, Hellkamp A, Thomas L et al. Effectiveness of cardiac rehabilitation among older patients after acute myocardial infarction. *Am Heart J* 2015; *170*: 855–864.
18. Audelin MC, Savage PD, Ades PA. Changing clinical profile of patients entering cardiac rehabilitation/secondary prevention programs: 1996 to 2006. *J Cardiopulm Rehabil Prev* 2008; *28(5)*: 299–306.
19. Ades PA, Savage PD, Toth MJ et al. High-caloric expenditure exercise: A new approach to cardiac rehabilitation for overweight coronary patients. *Circulation* 2009; *119*: 2671–2678.
20. Prado CM, Batsis JA, Donini LM et al. Sarcopenic obesity in older adults: A clinical overview. *Nat Rev Endocrinol* 2024; *20*: 261–277.
21. Khadanga S, Barrett K, Sheahan KH et al. Novel therapeutics for type 2 diabetes, obesity, and heart failure: A review and practical recommendations for cardiac rehabilitation. *J Cardiopulm Rehabil Prev* 2023; *43*: 1–7.
22. Lavie CJ, Church TS, Milani RV et al. Impact of physical activity, cardiorespiratory fitness, and exercise training on markers of inflammation. *J Cardiopulm Rehabil Prev* 2011; *31*: 137–145.
23. Flint KM, Stevens-Lapsley J, Forman DE. Cardiac rehabilitation in frail older adults with cardiovascular disease: A new diagnostic and treatment paradigm. *J Cardiopulm Rehabil Prev* 2020; *40*: 72–78.
24. Ushijima A, Morita N, Hama T et al. Effects of cardiac rehabilitation on physical function and exercise capacity in elderly cardiovascular patients with frailty. *J Cardiol* 2021; *77*: 424–431.
25. Khadanga S, Savage PD, Ades PA. Resistance training for older adults in cardiac rehabilitation. *Clin Geriatr Med* 2019; *35*: 459–468.
26. Ades PA, Ballor DL, Ashikaga T et al. Weight training improves walking endurance in the healthy elderly. *Ann Intern Med* 1996; *124*: 568–572.
27. Ahlund K, Back M, Sernert N. Fear-avoidance beliefs and cardiac rehabilitation in patients with first-time myocardial infarction. *J Rehabil Med* 2013; *45*: 1028–1033.
28. Morin L, Johnell K, Laroche ML, Fastbom J, Wastesson JW. The epidemiology of polypharmacy in older adults: Register-based prospective cohort study. *Clin Epidemiol* 2018; *10*: 289–298.
29. Guralnik JM, Simonsick EM, Ferrucci L et al. A short physical performance battery assessing lower extremity function: Association with self-reported disability and prediction of mortality and nursing home admission. *J Gerontol* 1994; *49*: M85–M94.
30. Muñoz-Mendoza CL, Cabañero-Martínez MJ, Millán-Calenti JC et al. Reliability of 4-m and 6-m walking speed tests in elderly people with cognitive impairment. *Arch Gerontol Geriatr* 2011; *52*: e67–e70.
31. Bautmans I, Lambert M, Mets T. The six-minute walk test in community dwelling elderly: Influence of health status. *BMC Geriatr* 2004; *4*: 6. Published 2004 Jul 23.
32. Roberts H, Denison H, Martin H et al. A review of the measurement of grip strength in clinical and epidemiological studies: Towards a standardised approach. *Age and Ageing* 2011; *40*: 423–429.
33. Jones CJ, Rikli RE, Beam WC. A 30-s chair-stand test as a measure of lower body strength in community-residing older adults. *Res Q Exerc Sport* 1999; *70*: 113–119.
34. Lee JY, Jensen BE, Oberman A et al. Adherence in the training levels comparison trial. *Med Sci Sports Exerc* 1996; *28*: 47–52.
35. Afilalo J. Evaluating and treating frailty in cardiac rehabilitation. *Clin Geriatr Med* 2019; *35*: 445–457.
36. Ijaz N, Buta B, Xue QL et al. Interventions for frailty among older adults with cardiovascular disease: JACC State-of-the-Art review. *J Am Coll Cardiol* 2022; *79*: 482–503.
37. McNeer J, Margolis J, Lee K et al. The role of the exercise test in the evaluation of patients for ischemic heart disease. *Circulation* 1978; *57*: 64–70.
38. Mancini D, Eisen H, Kussmaul W et al. Value of peak oxygen consumption for optimal timing of cardiac transplantation in ambulatory patients with heart failure. *Circulation* 1991; *83*: 778–786.

39. Vanhees L, Fagard R, Thijs L et al. Prognostic value of training-induced change in peak exercise capacity in patients with myocardial infarcts and patients with coronary bypass surgery. *Am J Cardiol* 1995; *76*: 1014–1019.
40. Heran BS, Chen JM, Ebrahim S et al. Exercise-based cardiac rehabilitation for coronary heart disease. *Cochrane Database Syst Rev* 2011; *7*: CD001800.
41. Jolliffe J, Rees K, Taylor R et al. Exercise-based rehabilitation for coronary heart disease. *Cochrane Database Syst Rev* 2001: CD001800.
42. Williams MA, Maresh CM, Esterbrooks DJ et al. Early exercise training in patients older than age 65 years compared with that in younger patients after acute myocardial infarction of coronary bypass grafting. *Am J Cardiol* 1985; *55*: 263–266.
43. Ades PA, Hanson JS, Gunther PG et al. Exercise conditioning in the elderly coronary patient. *J Am Geriatr Soc* 1987; *35*: 121–124.
44. Ades PA, Waldmann ML, Gillespie C. A controlled trial of exercise training in older coronary patients. *J Gerontol* 1995; *50*: M7–M11.
45. Lavie CJ, Milani RV, Littman AB. Benefits of cardiac rehabilitation and exercise training in secondary coronary prevention in the elderly. *J Am Coll Cardiol* 1993; *22*: 678–683.
46. Ades PA, Savage PD, Brawner CA et al. Aerobic capacity in patients entering cardiac rehabilitation. *Circulation* 2006; *113*: 2706–2712.
47. Wewege MA, Ahn D, Yu J, Liou K, Keech A. High-intensity interval training for patients with cardiovascular disease-is it safe? A systematic review. *J Am Heart Assoc* 2018; *7(21)*: e009305.
48. Dun Y, Smith JR, Liu S, Olson TP. High-intensity interval training in cardiac rehabilitation. *Clin Geriatr Med* 2019; *35(4)*: 469–487.
49. Mueller S, Winzer EB, Duvinage A et al. Effect of high-intensity interval training, moderate continuous training, or guideline-based physical activity advice on peak oxygen consumption in patients with heart failure with preserved ejection fraction: A randomized clinical trial. *JAMA* 2021; *325(6)*: 542–551.
50. Fragnoli-Munn K, Savage P, Ades P. Combined resistive-aerobic training in older coronary patients early after myocardial infarction. *J Cardiopulm Rehabil* 1998; *18*: 416–420.
51. Squires RW, Muri AJ, Anderson LJ et al. Weight training during phase II (early outpatient) cardiac rehabilitation: Heart rate and blood pressure responses. *J Cardiopulm Rehabil* 1991; *11*: 360–364.
52. Frontera W, Meredith CN, O'Reilly KP et al. Strength conditioning in older men: Skeletal muscle hypertrophy and improved function. *J Appl Physiol* 1988; *64*: 1038–1044.
53. Balagopal P, Rooyackers O, Adey D et al. Effects of aging on in-vivo synthesis of skeletal muscle myosin heavy chain and sarcoplasmic protein in humans. *Am J Physiol* 1997; *273*: E790–E800.
54. Frontera WR, Meridith CN, O'Reilly KP et al. Strength training and determinants of VO2 max. *J Appl Physiol* 1990; *68*: 329–333.
55. Ades PA, Ballor DL, Ashikaga T et al. Weight training improves walking endurance in the healthy elderly. *Ann Intern Med* 1996; *124*: 568–572.
56. Fiatorone MA, Marks EC, Ryan ND et al. High intensity strength training in nonagenarians: Effects on skeletal muscle. *JAMA* 1990; *263*: 3029–3034.
57. Neill WA, Branch LG, DeJong G. Cardiac disability: The impact of coronary disease on patients' daily activities. *Arch Intern Med* 1981; *145*: 1642–1647.
58. Ades PA, Savage P, Cress ME, Brochu M, Lee NM, Poehlman ET. Resistance training on physical performance in disabled older female cardiac patients. *Med Sci Sports Exerc* 2003; *35(8)*: 1265–1270.
59. Brochu M, Savage P, Lee N et al. Effects of resistance training on physical function in older disabled women with coronary heart disease. *J Appl Physiol* 2002; *92*: 672–678.
60. Fiatarone MA, Marks EC, Ryan ND, Meredith CN, Lipsitz LA, Evans WJ. High-intensity strength training in nonagenarians. Effects on skeletal muscle. *JAMA* 1990; *263*: 3029–3034.
61. Middlekauff HR. Making the case for skeletal myopathy as the major limitation of exercise capacity in heart failure. *Circ Heart Fail* 2010; *3*: 537–546.
62. Pu CT, Johnson MT, Forman DE et al. Randomized trial of progressive resistance training to counteract the myopathy of chronic heart failure. *J Appl Physiol* 2001; *90*: 2341–2350.
63. Borg GA. Perceived exertion: A note on history and methods. *Med Sci Sports* 1973; *5*: 90–93.
64. Kitzman DW, Little WC, Brubaker PH et al. Pathophysiological characterization of isolated diastolic heart failure in comparison to systolic heart failure. *JAMA* 2002; *288*: 2144–2150.
65. Piepoli MF, Davos C, Francis DP et al. ExTraMATCH Collaborative. Exercise training meta-analysis of trials in patients with chronic heart failure (ExTraMATCH). *BMJ* 2004; *328(7433)*: 189.
66. Davies EJ, Moxham T, Rees K et al. Exercise based rehabilitation for heart failure. *Cochrane Database Syst Rev* 2010: CD003331.
67. O'Connor CM, Whellan DJ, Lee KL et al. Efficacy and safety of exercise training in patients with chronic heart failure: HF-ACTION randomized controlled trial. *JAMA* 2009; *01*: 1439–1450.
68. Pandey A, Kitzman DW, Brubaker P et al. Response to endurance exercise training in older adults with heart failure with preserved or reduced ejection fraction. *J Am Geriatr Soc* 2017; *65*: 1698–1704.
69. Kitzman DW, Whellan DJ, Duncan P et al. Physical rehabilitation for older patients hospitalized for heart failure. *N Engl J Med* 2021; *385(3)*: 203–216.
70. Khadanga S, Savage PD, Gaalema DE, Ades PA. Predictors of cardiac rehabilitation participation:

Opportunities to increase enrollment. *J Cardiopulm Rehabil Prev* 2021; *41(5)*: 322–327.
71. Ritchey MD, Maresh S, McNeely J et al. Tracking cardiac rehabilitation participation and completion among Medicare beneficiaries to inform the efforts of a national initiative. *Circ Cardiovasc Qual Outcomes* 2020; *13*: e005902.
72. Dolansky MA, Zullo MD, Hassanein S et al. Cardiac rehabilitation in skilled nursing facilities: A missed opportunity. *Heart Lung* 2012; *41*: 115–124.
73. Alfaraidhy MA, Regan C, Forman DE. Cardiac rehabilitation for older adults: Current evidence and future potential. *Expert Rev Cardiovasc Ther* 2022; *20*: 13–34.
74. Buttery GC-W AK, Martin FC, Glaser K et al. Cardiac rehabilitation for heart failure: Do older people want to attend and are they referred? *Eur Geriatric Med* 2014; *5(4)*: 246–251.
75. Ades PA, Waldmann ML, McCann W et al. Predictors of cardiac rehabilitation participation in older coronary patients. *Arch Intern Med* 1992; *152*: 1033–1035.
76. Parashar S, Spertus JA, Tang F et al. Predictors of early and late enrollment in cardiac rehabilitation, among those referred, after acute myocardial infarction. *Circulation* 2012; *126*: 1587–1595.
77. Grace SL, Shanmugasegaram S, Gravely-Witte S et al. Barriers to cardiac rehabilitation: Does age make a difference? *J Cardiopulm Rehabil Prev* 2009; *29*: 183–187.
78. Grace SL, Russell KL, Reid RD et al. Effect of cardiac rehabilitation referral strategies on utilization rates: A prospective, controlled study. *Arch Intern Med* 2011; *171*: 235–241.
79. Reaven PD, McPhillips JB, Barrett-Connor EL et al. Leisure time exercise and lipid and lipoprotein levels in an older population. *J Am Geriatr Soc* 1990; *38*: 847–854.
80. Khadanga S, Gaalema DE, Savage P, Ades PA. Underutilization of cardiac rehabilitation in women: Barriers and solutions. *J Cardiopulm Rehabil Prev* 2021; *41*: 207–213.
81. Khadanga S, Savage P, Keteyian S, Yant B, Gaalema D, Ades P. Cardiac rehabilitation: The gateway for secondary prevention. *Heart* 2024; *110*: 1427–1436.
82. Supervía M, Medina-Inojosa JR, Yeung C et al. Cardiac rehabilitation for women: A systematic review of barriers and solutions. *Mayo Clin Proc* 2017; S0025–6196: 30026–5.
83. Ades PA, Waldmann ML, Polk D et al. Referral patterns and exercise response in the rehabilitation of female coronary patients aged ≥62 years. *Am J Cardiol* 1992; *69*: 1422–1425.
84. Rengo JL, Khadanga S, Savage PD, Ades PA. Response to exercise training during cardiac rehabilitation differs by sex. *J Cardiopulm Rehabil Prev* 2020; *40*: 319–324.
85. Fragnoli-Munn K, Savage P, Ades P. Combined resistive-aerobic training in older coronary patients early after myocardial infarction. *J Cardiopulm Rehabil* 1998; *18*: 416–420.
86. Schopfer DW, Krishnamurthi N, Shen H et al. Association of veterans health administration home-based programs with access to and participation in cardiac rehabilitation. *JAMA Intern Med* 2018; *178*: 715–717.
87. Suaya JA, Shepard DS, Normand SL et al. Use of cardiac rehabilitation by Medicare beneficiaries after myocardial infarction or coronary bypass surgery. *Circulation* 2007; *116(15)*: 1653–1662.
88. Schopfer DW, Forman DE. Cardiac rehabilitation in older adults. *Can J Cardiol* 2016; *32*: 1088–1096.
89. Anderson L, Sharp GA, Norton RJ et al. Home-based versus centre-based cardiac rehabilitation. *Cochrane Database Syst Rev* 2017; *6*: CD007130.
90. Forman DE, LaFond K, Panch T et al. Utility and efficacy of a smartphone application to enhance the learning and behavior goals of traditional cardiac rehabilitation: A feasibility study. *J Cardiopulm Rehabil Prev* 2014; *34*: 327–334.
91. Redfern J. Can older adults benefit from smart devices, wearables, and other digital health options to enhance cardiac rehabilitation? *Clin Geriatr Med* 2019; *35(4)*: 489–497.
92. Kakulla B. Older adults keep pace on tech usage. *AARP*, https://www.aarp.org/pri/topics/technology/internet-media-devices/2020-technology-trends-older-americans/. Accessed Feb 2, 2025.
93. Dodson JA, Adhikari S, Schoenthaler A et al. Rehabilitation at home using mobile health for older adults hospitalized for ischemic heart disease: The RESILIENT randomized clinical trial. *JAMA Netw Open* 2025; 8: e2453499.
94. Bell SP, Orr NM, Dodson JA et al. What to expect from the evolving field of geriatric cardiology. *J Am Coll Cardiol* 2015; *66*: 1286–1299.
95. Pahor M, Guralnik JM, Ambrosius WT et al. Effect of structured physical activity on prevention of major mobility disability in older adults: The LIFE study randomized clinical trial. *JAMA* 2014; *311*: 2387–2396.
96. Romera-Liebana L, Orfila F, Segura JM et al. Effects of a primary-care based multifactorial intervention on physical and cognitive function in frail, elderly individuals: A randomized controlled trial. *Gerontol A Biol Sci Med Sci* 2018; *73(12)*: 1688–1674.
97. Brochu M, Poehlman ET, Savage P et al. Modest effects of exercise training alone on coronary risk factors and body composition in coronary patients. *J Cardiopulm Rehabil* 2000; *20*: 180–188.

14

Aortic valve disease in older persons

WILBERT S. ARONOW AND AAQUIB H. MALIK

Key points

- The prevalence of both aortic stenosis (AS) and aortic regurgitation (AR) increases with age.
- Transcatheter aortic valve replacement (TAVR) is performed more frequently than surgical aortic valve replacement (SAVR) in older persons with severe AS.
- Older persons with TAVR may need oral anticoagulation, most commonly because of the presence of atrial fibrillation.
- In older persons without a need for oral anticoagulation, single antiplatelet therapy such as aspirin is recommended.
- Currently, SAVR is recommended for older persons with severe chronic AR.
- A randomized trial of treating severe chronic AR with the JenaValve versus SAVR is in progress.

AORTIC STENOSIS

Etiology and prevalence

Valvular aortic stenosis (AS) in older patients is usually due to degenerative changes leading to stiffening, scarring, and calcification of the aortic valve leaflets. This is different from postinflammatory or rheumatic AS in which the commissural fusion is common. Calcific deposits in the aortic valve are common in elderly patients and may lead to valvular AS (1–5). Aortic cusp calcium was present in 295 of 752 men (36%), mean age 80 years, and in 672 of 1663 women (40%), mean age 82 years (4). Of 2358 patients, mean age 81 years, 378 (16%) of them had valvular AS, 981 (42%) had valvular aortic sclerosis (thickening of or calcific deposits on the aortic valve cusps with a peak flow velocity across the aortic valve $\leq$1.5 m/s), and 999 (42%) had no valvular AS or aortic sclerosis (5).

The frequency of a calcific aortic valve increases with age. In the Helsinki Aging Study, calcification of the aortic valve was diagnosed by Doppler echocardiography in 28% of 76 patients aged 55–71 years, in 48% of 197 patients aged 75–76 years, in 55% of 155 patients aged 80–81 years, and in 75% of 124 patients aged 85–86 years (3). Valvular AS diagnosed by Doppler echocardiography was present in 141 of 924 men (15%), mean age 80 years, and in 322 of 1881 women (17%), mean age 81 years (6). In this study, severe valvular AS (peak gradient across aortic valve of $\geq$50 mmHg or aortic valve area <0.75 cm^2) was diagnosed in 62 of 2805 elderly patients (2%); moderate valvular AS (peak gradient across aortic valve of 26–49 mmHg or aortic valve area of 0.75–1.49 cm^2) was present in 149 of 2805 elderly patients (5%); and mild valvular AS (peak gradient across aortic valve of 10–25 mmHg or

DOI: 10.1201/9781003568933-14

aortic valve area ≥1.50 cm²) occurred in 25 of 2805 older patients (9%) (6). In 501 unselected patients aged 75–86 years in the Helsinki Aging Study, critical AS was present in 3% and moderate to severe AS in 5% of the 501 older patients (3).

Calcific AS in the aging population was once thought of as a passive, degenerative condition in association with calcium accumulation (7). More recently, it is becoming clear that the disease process is regulated and shares risk factors with atherosclerosis (7–10). Otto et al. (7) demonstrated that the early lesion of degenerative AS is an active inflammatory process with some similarities to atherosclerosis, including lipid deposition, macrophage and T-cell infiltration, and basement membrane disruption. In 5201 patients older than 65 years of age in the Cardiovascular Health Study, independent clinical factors that were associated with degenerative aortic valve disease included age, male gender, smoking, history of hypertension, height, and high lipoprotein(a) (Lp[a]) and low-density lipoprotein (LDL) cholesterol levels (8). In a prospective study of 571 patients with a mean age of 82 years, 292 patients (51%) had calcified or thickened aortic cusps or root (9). A serum total cholesterol ≥200 mg/dL, a history of hypertension, diabetes mellitus, and a serum high-density lipoprotein (HDL) cholesterol <35 mg/dL were more prevalent in elderly patients with calcified or thickened aortic cusps or root than in elderly patients with normal aortic cusps and root (9). In the Helsinki Aging Study, age, hypertension, and a low body mass index were independent predictors of aortic valve calcification (10). Furthermore, genetic variants of LPA, mediated by Lp(a) levels, are also shown to be associated with AS (11). Chen et al. (11) reported in a case–control study that two genetic variants of LPA (rs10455872, rs3798220) were associated with a higher risk of AS. The risk for AS was greatest in individuals aged 55–64 years and declined with age (mean age of study population was 74.6 years).

Given the overlap of risk factors between atherosclerotic vascular disease and AS, it is not surprising that many of the older patients with AS also have vascular disease. In 1275 elderly patients, mean age 81 years, AS was present in 52 of 202 patients (26%) with 40%–100% extracranial carotid arterial disease (ECAD) and in 162 of 1073 patients (15%) with 0%–39% ECAD (12). In 2987 older patients, mean age 81 years, symptomatic peripheral arterial disease was present in 193 of 462 patients (42%) with AS and in 639 of 2525 patients (25%) without AS (13). Along with the vascular disease, calcification of the aortic valve and mitral annular calcification (MAC) frequently coexist and may also be associated with the progression of AS (14). In 290 patients, mean age 79 years, with valvular AS who had follow-up Doppler echocardiograms, elderly patients with MAC had a greater reduction in aortic valve area/year than elderly patients without MAC (15). Significant independent risk factors for progression of valvular AS in 102 patients, mean age 76 years, who had follow-up Doppler echocardiograms were cigarette smoking and hypercholesterolemia (16). A retrospective analysis of 180 older patients with mild AS who had follow-up Doppler echocardiograms at ≥2 years showed that significant independent predictors of the progression of AS were male gender, cigarette smoking, hypertension, diabetes mellitus, a serum LDL cholesterol ≥125 mg/dL, and a serum HDL cholesterol <35 mg/dL (17). These and other data suggest that aortic valve calcium, MAC, and coronary atherosclerosis in older patients have similar predisposing factors (7–13,15–17).

Older patients with AS have a higher prevalence of atherosclerotic risk factors, and since these risk factors seem to be associated with progression of AS, the use of statin to possibly reduce the progression of AS was hypothesized. Several retrospective studies indicated a reduction in the rate of progression of AS with the use of statin (17–19). However, the results from randomized clinical trials have been disappointing (20,21). Given this data, American College of Cardiology/American Heart Association (ACC/AHA) guidelines indicate statin therapy as a class III recommendation for prevention of hemodynamic progression of AS in patients with mild to moderate calcific AS (22).

Pathophysiology

In valvular AS, there is resistance to ejection of blood from the left ventricle (LV) into the aorta, with a pressure gradient across the aortic valve during systole and an increase in LV systolic pressure. The pressure overload on the LV initially leads to concentric LV hypertrophy, with an increase in LV wall thickness and mass. This compensatory mechanism attempts to normalize systolic wall stress and maintain normal LV ejection fraction and cardiac output. However, the hypertrophic LV also leads to abnormal LV compliance, LV diastolic dysfunction with reduced LV diastolic filling, and increased LV end-diastolic pressure. As such, atrial systole becomes an important factor for diastolic filling of the LV in patients with AS. Loss of effective atrial contraction (e.g., in atrial fibrillation) may cause immediate clinical deterioration in patients with severe AS. It is important to note that older patients with a comparable degree of AS have more impairment of LV diastolic function as compared to younger patients (23), and therefore may have more severe hemodynamic deterioration in atrial fibrillation. A compensated hyperdynamic response is common in older women (24).

Sustained LV hypertrophy eventually leads to LV chamber dilatation with decreased LV ejection fraction and, ultimately, congestive heart failure (CHF). The stroke volume and cardiac output decrease, the mean left atrial and pulmonary capillary pressures increase, and pulmonary hypertension occurs. Older patients with both obstructive and nonobstructive coronary artery disease (CAD) have an increased incidence of LV enlargement and LV systolic dysfunction (25). In some patients, the CHF is mainly from the diastolic dysfunction, and the systolic ejection fractions remain normal. In 48 older patients with CHF associated with unoperated severe valvular AS, the LV ejection fraction was normal in 30 patients (63%) (26). The prognosis of patients with AS and LV diastolic dysfunction is usually better than that of patients with AS and LV systolic dysfunction, but is worse than that of patients without LV diastolic dysfunction (26,27).

Symptoms

Angina pectoris, syncope or near syncope, and CHF are the three classic manifestations of severe AS. CHF, syncope, or angina pectoris was present in 36 of 40 older patients (90%) with severe AS, in 66 of 96 elderly patients (69%) with moderate valvular AS, and in 45 of 165 elderly patients (27%) with mild valvular AS (28).

Angina pectoris is the most common symptom associated with AS in older patients. Although coexistent CAD is frequently present in older patients with AS (4,5,28), angina pectoris may occur in the absence of CAD as a result of an increase in myocardial oxygen demand with a reduction in myocardial oxygen supply at the subendocardial level. Myocardial ischemia in patients with severe AS and normal coronary arteries is due to inadequate LV hypertrophy with increased LV systolic and diastolic wall stresses causing decreased coronary flow reserve (29).

Syncope in patients with AS may be caused by reduced cerebral perfusion following exertion when arterial pressure drops because of systemic vasodilatation in the presence of a fixed outflow obstruction. LV failure with a decrease in cardiac output may also cause syncope. In addition, syncope at rest may be caused by a marked reduction in cardiac output secondary to transient arrhythmia (such as ventricular fibrillation, atrial fibrillation [AF], or atrioventricular block) related to extension of the valve calcification into the conduction system. Coexistent cerebrovascular disease (12) with transient cerebral ischemia may contribute to syncope in elderly patients with AS.

Exertional dyspnea, paroxysmal nocturnal dyspnea, orthopnea, and pulmonary edema may be caused by pulmonary venous hypertension associated with AS. Coexistent CAD and hypertension may contribute to CHF in elderly patients with AS. Cardiac arrhythmias may also precipitate CHF in these patients. Small cohort studies have also demonstrated a higher prevalence of sleep-related breathing disorders (obstructive and central sleep apnea) in older patients with severe AS (30). Sleep-related breathing disorders may be associated with increased perioperative risk. Furthermore, a causal relationship may exist between severe AS and central sleep apnea, as some studies report a significant improvement in central sleep apnea after TAVR (30).

Sudden death occurs mainly in symptomatic valvular AS patients (26,28,31). It may also occur in 3%–5% of asymptomatic patients with AS (31). Marked fatigue and peripheral cyanosis in patients with AS may be caused by a low cardiac output. Older patients with AS are at higher risk for cerebral emboli causing stroke or transient cerebral ischemic attack, bacterial endocarditis, and gastrointestinal bleeding (due to angiodysplasia in the GI tract [32]).

Signs

A systolic ejection murmur heard in the second right intercostal space, down the left sternal border toward the apex or at the apex is classified as an aortic systolic ejection murmur (ASEM) (1,2,33). An ASEM is commonly heard in older patients (1), occurring in 265 of 565 unselected elderly patients (47%) (1). Of 220 elderly patients with an ASEM and technically adequate M-mode and two-dimensional echocardiograms of the aortic valve, 207 (94%) had aortic cuspal or root calcification or thickening (1). Of 75 older patients with an ASEM, valvular AS was diagnosed by continuous-wave Doppler echocardiography in 42 patients (56%) (33).

Table 14.1 shows that an ASEM was heard in 100% of 19 older patients with severe AS, in 100% of 49 elderly patients with moderate AS and in 95% of 74 older patients

Table 14.1 Correlation of physical signs of valvular aortic stenosis with the severity of aortic stenosis in older patients

	Severity of aortic stenosis		
Physical sign	**Mild (*n* = 74)%**	**Moderate (*n* = 49)%**	**Severe (*n* = 19)%**
ASEM	95	100	100
Prolonged duration ASEM	3	63	84
Late-peaking ASEM	3	63	84
Prolonged carotid upstroke time	3	33	53
A_2 absent	0	10	16
A_2 decreased or absent	5	49	74

Source: Aronow WS, Kronzon I, *Am J Cardiol*, 67, 776–777, 1991.
Abbreviations: ASEM, aortic systolic ejection murmur; A_2, aortic component of second heart sound.

with mild AS (2). However, the ASEM may become softer or absent in patients with CHF associated with severe AS because of a low cardiac output. The intensity and maximal location of the ASEM and transmission of the ASEM to the right carotid artery do not differentiate among mild, moderate, and severe AS (1,2,33). The ASEM may be heard only at the apex in some older patients with AS. The apical systolic ejection murmur may also be louder and more musical than the basal systolic ejection murmur in some older patients with AS. The intensity of the ASEM in valvular AS increases with squatting and by inhalation of amyl nitrite and decreases during the Valsalva maneuver.

Prolonged duration of the ASEM and late peaking of the ASEM best differentiate severe AS from mild AS (1,2,33). However, the physical signs do not distinguish between severe and moderate AS (Table 14.1) (2,33).

Some of the physical signs of AS may be diminished or masked in older patients due to hardened arteries with reduced elasticity. For example, stiff noncompliant arteries may mask a prolonged carotid upstroke time in older patients with severe AS. A prolonged carotid upstroke time does not differentiate between severe and moderate AS in older patients (2). A prolonged carotid upstroke time was palpable in 3% of older patients with mild AS, in 33% of older patients with moderate AS, and in 53% of older patients with severe AS (Table 14.1) (2). The pulse pressure may also be normal or wide rather than narrow in older patients with severe AS because of loss of vascular elasticity. Similarly, an aortic ejection click is rare in older patients with severe AS because of loss of vascular elasticity and immobile valve cusps (2,33).

An absent or decreased A_2 occurs more frequently in older patients with severe or moderate AS than in patients with mild AS (Table 14.1) (2,33). However, an absent or decreased A_2 does not differentiate between severe and moderate AS (2,33). The presence of AF, reversed splitting of S_2, or an audible fourth heart sound at the apex also does not differentiate between severe and moderate AS in elderly patients (33). The presence of a third heart sound in older patients with AS usually indicates the presence of LV systolic dysfunction and elevated LV filling pressure (34).

Electrocardiography and chest X-ray

Electrocardiogram in patients with AS may depict LV strain and LV hypertrophy patterns. These patterns may be indicators of poor prognosis. In the Simvastatin and Ezetimibe in Aortic Stenosis study of 1533 patients with asymptomatic AS, electrocardiographic LVH was associated with a 5.8 times increase in heart failure, 2.0 times increase in AVR, and 2.5 times increase in myocardial infarction, heart failure, or cardiovascular death (35). LV strain was associated with a 3.1 times increase in myocardial infarction (35). Echocardiography is more sensitive than electrocardiography in detecting LV hypertrophy in an older person with AS, as shown in Table 14.2 (2).

Conduction abnormalities are commonly associated with aortic valve disease, likely due to the involvement of the conduction system by calcific deposits. The most common conduction abnormalities seen in AS are left anterior hemiblock and left bundle branch block (36), likely due to its approximation to the left conducting system tract. Complex ventricular arrhythmias may be detected by 24-hour ambulatory electrocardiograms in patients with AS. Older patients with complex ventricular arrhythmias associated with AS have a higher incidence of new coronary events than elderly patients with AS and no complex ventricular arrhythmias (37).

Chest X-ray may reveal rounding of the LV border and apex as a result of concentric LV hypertrophy. Poststenotic dilatation of the ascending aorta is commonly seen.

Echocardiography and Doppler echocardiography

Transthoracic echocardiography (including M-mode, two-dimensional echocardiography, and Doppler echocardiography) is the first-line diagnostic test in patients with signs, symptoms, or suspicion of AS, since clinical diagnosis may be missed in a significant number of patients. Echocardiography can detect thickening, calcification, and reduced excursion of aortic valve leaflets (1). LV hypertrophy is best diagnosed by echocardiography (2). Echocardiographic measurements of chamber dimensions and LV end-systolic and end-diastolic volumes, LV

Table 14.2 Prevalence of electrocardiographic and echocardiographic left ventricular hypertrophy in elderly patients with mild, moderate, and severe valvular aortic stenosis

	Severity of valvular aortic stenosis		
	Mild (*n* = 74)%	**Moderate (*n* = 49)%**	**Severe (*n* = 19)%**
Electrocardiographic LVH	11	31	58
Echocardiographic LVH	74	96	100

Source: Aronow WS, Kronzon I, *Am J Cardiol*, 67, 776–777, 1991.
Abbreviation: LVH, left ventricular hypertrophy.

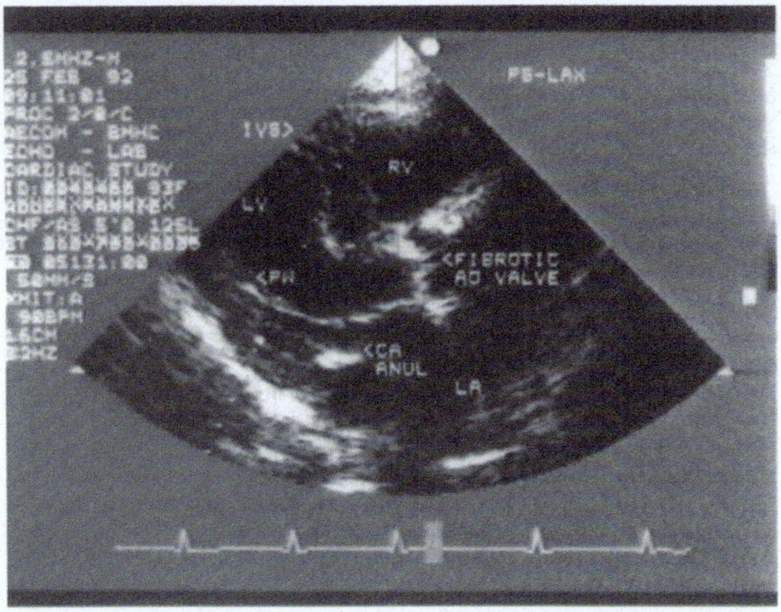

Figure 14.1 Two-dimensional echocardiographic image from a parasternal long-axis view of a 93-year-old female with aortic stenosis and moderately depressed left ventricular function showing a fibrotic aortic valve and mitral annular calcification. *Abbreviations*: PS-LAX, parasternal long-axis view; RV, right ventricular cavity; LV, left ventricular cavity; IVS, interventricular septum; PW, posterior wall; CA ANUL, mitral annulus calcification; LA, left atrium; AO, aorta.

ejection fraction, and assessment of global and regional LV wall motion give important information on LV systolic function.

Doppler echocardiography is used to measure peak and mean transvalvular gradients across the aortic valve and to assess the severity of the valve lesion. The aortic valve area can be calculated by the continuity equation using pulsed Doppler echocardiography to measure LV outflow tract velocity, continuous-wave Doppler echocardiography to measure transvalvular flow velocity, and a two-dimensional long-axis view to measure LV outflow tract area (38). The aortic valve area can be reliably detected by the continuity equation in elderly patients with AS. Figures 14.1 through 14.5 illustrate two-dimensional echocardiographic findings (Figures 14.1 and 14.3), continuous-wave Doppler echocardiographic findings (Figures 14.2 and 14.4), and simultaneous LV and femoral arterial pressure tracings (Figure 14.5) in older patients with severe valvular AS.

In most patients, Doppler echocardiography can reliably define the severity of the stenotic lesion and has been shown to have good correlation with invasive evaluation via cardiac catheterization. Shah and Graham (39) reported that the agreement in quantitation of the severity of AS between Doppler echocardiography and cardiac catheterization was greater than 95%. Patients with a peak jet velocity ≥4.5 m/s had critical AS, and those with a peak jet velocity <3.0 m/s had noncritical AS. In 75 patients, mean age 76 years, with valvular AS, the Bland–Altman plot showed that 4 of the 75 patients (5%) had disagreement between cardiac catheterization and Doppler echocardiography that was outside the 95% confidence limits (40). In a study (41) to determine the agreement between Doppler and catheterization, 105 patients in whom Doppler demonstrated critical AS (aortic valve area ≤0.75 cm^2 or a peak jet velocity ≥4.5 m/s) underwent cardiac catheterization. Doppler echocardiography was 97% accurate in this subgroup. Similarly, cardiac catheterization was performed in 133 patients with noncritical AS, in which Doppler echocardiography was 95% accurate. Doppler echocardiography can be obtained in most patients with AS; however, the severity of AS can be under- or overestimated in some patients. When there is a discrepancy between clinical manifestation and echocardiography data, or if the noninvasive data is nondiagnostic, an invasive evaluation with cardiac catheterization should be performed (ACC/AHA class I recommendation) (22). Simultaneous LV and aortic pressure measurements should be performed, and transaortic pressure gradients should be recorded for measurement of the mean transaortic gradient. The aortic valve area should be calculated with the Gorlin formula, using a Fick or thermodilution cardiac output measurement. Patients in whom Doppler echocardiography shows a peak jet velocity between 3.6 and 4.4 m/s and an aortic valve area >0.8 cm^2 should undergo cardiac catheterization if they have cardiac symptoms attributable to AS (38).

Furthermore, cardiac catheterization to determine coronary anatomy is indicated before valve intervention in most elderly patients with AS, given the high prevalence of atherosclerosis in this population. Knowledge of coronary anatomy facilitates risk stratification and

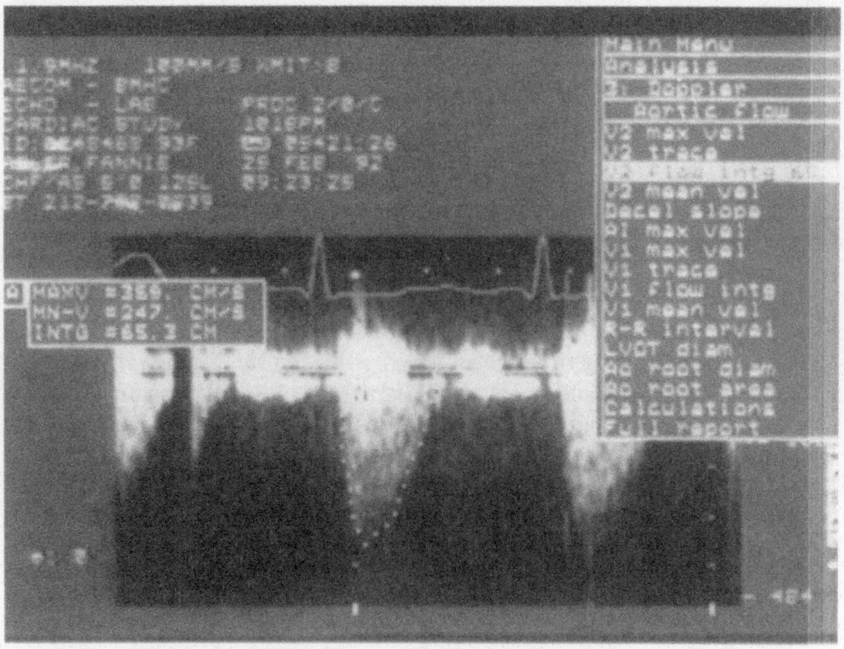

Figure 14.2 Continuous-wave Doppler recording of the velocity profile across the aortic valve in the same patient shown in Figure 14.1. A 52 mmHg gradient across the aortic valve is measured using the Bernoulli equation. Indexed aortic valve area is measured by the continuity equation using Doppler data = 0.5 cm^2/m^2.

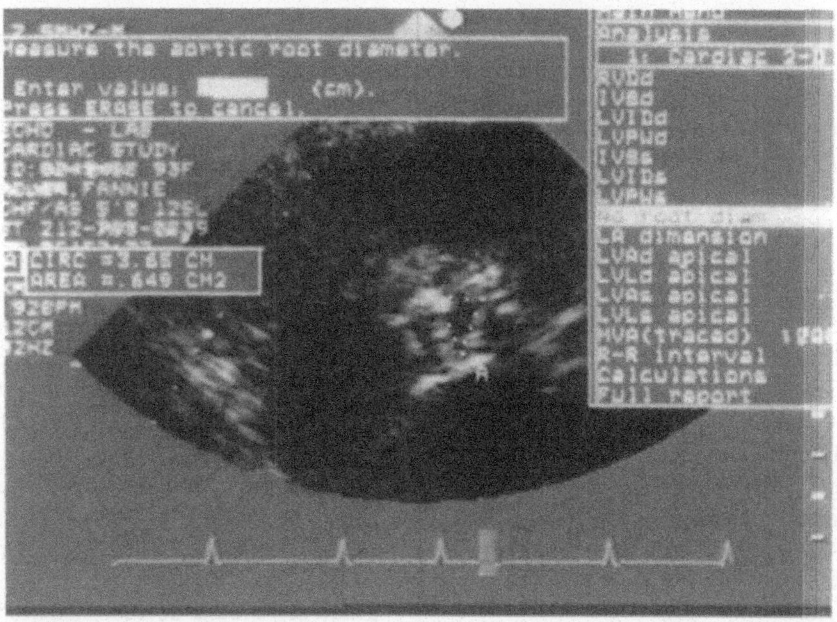

Figure 14.3 Two-dimensional echocardiographic image obtained in the same patient in Figures 14.1 and 14.2 from a short-axis parasternal view in which the aortic valve orifice is mapped, yielding an indexed area of 0.4 cm^2/m^2.

determines if concomitant coronary revascularization is needed.

Natural history

The prognosis of AS is, in the main, dictated by the severity of AS and symptom progression. It has been widely known that severe AS predicts high risk of death once the cardiac symptoms appear (28,31), whereas the prognosis is relatively better as long as the patient remains symptom free (41,42).

In a prospective study, at 19-month follow-up (range 2–36 months), 90% of 30 patients with CHF associated with unoperated severe AS and a normal LV ejection fraction were dead (26). At 13-month follow-up (range 2–24 months), 100% of 18 patients with CHF associated with

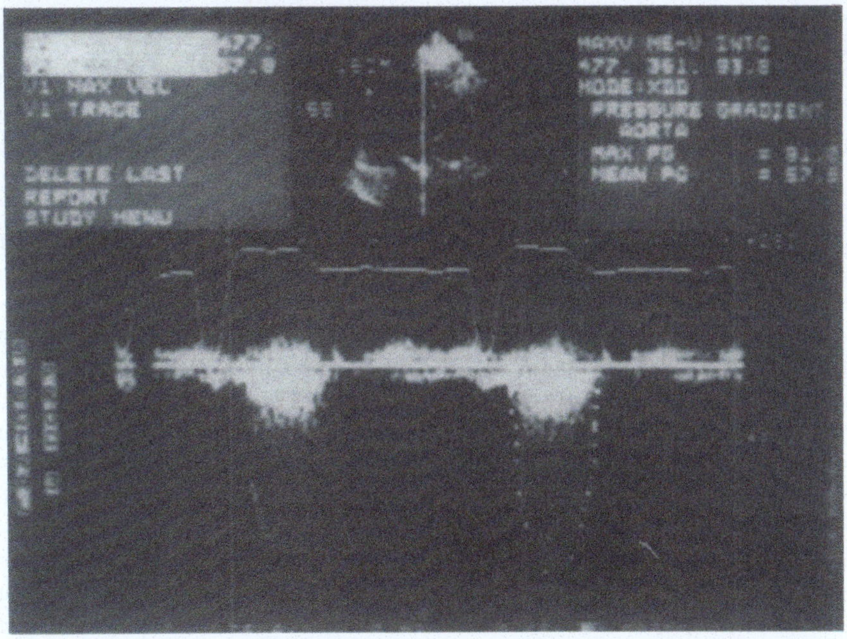

Figure 14.4 Continuous-wave Doppler recording of the velocity profile across the aortic valve in an elderly patient with aortic stenosis and normal left ventricular systolic function. The indexed aortic valve area is 0.5 cm^2/m^2 by both Gorlin's formula and the Doppler continuity equation. The peak gradient across the aortic valve by Bernoulli's equation is 81 mmHg, a value higher than that recorded in Figure 14.2 for the same indexed aortic valve area.

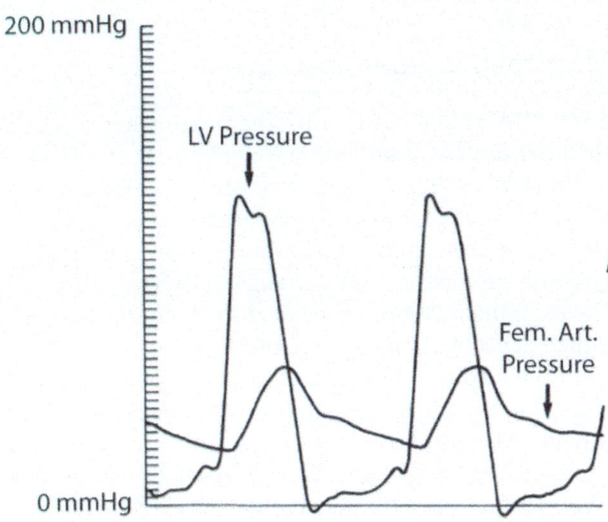

Figure 14.5 Simultaneous left ventricular and femoral artery pressure recordings obtained in the same patient in Figure 14.4, confirming a large gradient across the aortic valve with a maximum value of 81 mmHg (instantaneous pressure). *Abbreviations*: Fem. Art., femoral artery pressure tracing; LV, left ventricular pressure tracing.

unoperated severe AS and an abnormal LV ejection fraction were dead (26).

Studies have demonstrated that patients with asymptomatic severe AS are at low risk for death and can be followed until symptoms develop (43). However, these patients soon deteriorate and develop symptoms requiring therapy. Kelly et al. (43) followed 51 asymptomatic patients with severe AS. During 17-month follow-up, 21 (41%) of the patients became symptomatic. Only 2 of the 51 patients (4%) died of cardiac causes. In both patients, death was preceded by the development of angina pectoris or CHF. Pellikka et al. (41) observed that 113 of 143 patients (79%), mean age 72 years, with asymptomatic severe AS were not initially referred for AVR or percutaneous aortic balloon valvuloplasty. During 20-month follow-up, 37 of 113 patients (33%) became symptomatic. The actuarial probability of remaining free of cardiac events associated with AS, including cardiac death and aortic valve surgery, was 95% at 6 months, 93% at 1 year, and 74% at 2 years. No asymptomatic person with severe AS developed sudden death while asymptomatic.

Rosenheck et al. (42) followed 126 patients with asymptomatic severe AS for 22 months. Eight patients died, and 59 patients developed symptoms necessitating AVR. Event-free survival was 67% at 1 year, 56% at 2 years, and 33% at 4 years. Five of the six deaths from cardiac disease were preceded by symptoms. Of the patients with moderately or severely calcified aortic valves whose aortic jet velocity increased by 0.3 m/s or more within 1 year, 79% underwent AVR or died within 2 years of the observed increase.

Due to these observations, current ACC/AHA guidelines recommend a longer time period for routine follow-up in asymptomatic severe AS patients. Transthoracic echocardiogram (TTE) for reevaluation of asymptomatic patients with AS with normal LV systolic function who have no change in signs or symptoms is performed at intervals of 6 months to 1 year when aortic velocity is ≥4.0

m/s (stage C), 1 to 2 years when aortic velocity is between 3.0 m/s and 3.9 m/s (stage B), and 3–5 years when aortic velocity is 2.0 m/s to 2.9 m/s (stage B) (22).

Mild to moderate AS, on the other hand, was thought to have a more benign course. However, mild to moderate AS as well as aortic sclerosis (without increased gradients) also seem to have worse outcomes than commonly assumed. At 4-year follow-up of patients aged 75–86 years in the Helsinki Aging Study, the incidence of cardiovascular mortality was 62% in patients with severe AS and 35% in patients with moderate AS (44). At 4-year follow-up the incidence of total mortality was 76% in patients with severe AS and 50% in patients with moderate AS (44). Some of the factors that may determine the prognosis include valve calcification, CAD, and rate of progression. In a prospective study of 981 patients, mean age 82 years, with aortic sclerosis and of 999 patients, mean age 80 years, without valvular aortic sclerosis, older patients with aortic sclerosis had at 46-month follow-up a 1.8 times higher chance of developing a new coronary event than those without valvular aortic sclerosis (5). Otto et al. (45) also reported in 5621 men and women ≥65 years of age that AS and aortic sclerosis significantly increased cardiovascular morbidity and mortality.

Similar to severe AS, the prognosis in mild to moderate AS also seems worse if the cardiac symptoms (such as CHF, syncope, or angina pectoris) are present as compared to the asymptomatic patients. Results from a study prospectively comparing the incidence of new coronary events in older patients with no, mild, moderate, and severe AS are shown in Table 14.3 (28). Independent risk factors for new coronary events in this study were prior myocardial infarction, AS, male gender, and increasing age (28). In this prospective study, at 20-month follow-up of 40 older patients with severe AS, CHF, syncope, or angina pectoris was present in 36 of 37 patients (97%) who developed new coronary events and in none of the 3 patients (0%) without new coronary events (28). At 32-month follow-up of 96 older patients with moderate valvular AS, CHF, syncope, or angina pectoris was present in 65 of 77 patients (84%) who developed new coronary events and in 1 of 19 patients (5%) without new coronary events (28). At 52-month follow-up of 165 older patients with mild AS, CHF, syncope, or angina pectoris was present in 40 of 103 patients (39%) who developed new coronary events and in 5 of 62 patients (8%) without new coronary events (28).

Similar to new coronary events, the rate of death among symptomatic patients with moderate AS is worse compared to minimally symptomatic patients with moderate AS. Kennedy et al. (46) followed 66 patients with moderate AS diagnosed by cardiac catheterization (aortic valve area 0.7–1.2 cm^2). In 38 patients with symptomatic moderate AS and 28 patients with minimally symptomatic moderate AS, the probabilities of avoiding death from AS were 0.86 for symptomatic patients and 1.0 for patients with minimally symptomatic moderate AS at 1-year follow-up, 0.77 for patients with symptomatic AS and 1.0 for patients with minimally symptomatic AS at 2 years, 0.77 for patients with symptomatic AS and 0.96 for patients with minimally symptomatic AS at 3 years, and 0.70 for patients with symptomatic AS and 0.90 for patients with minimally symptomatic AS at 4 years (46).

When patients with low-gradient AS due to abnormal LV ejection fraction are considered for AVR, failure to respond to dobutamine and large preoperative LV end-systolic and end-diastolic volumes are poor prognostic signs (47). The ACC/AHA guidelines state that dobutamine stress echocardiography is reasonable to evaluate patients with low-flow/low-gradient AS and abnormal LV ejection fraction (22).

Medical management

ACC/AHA guidelines classify the progression of valvular heart diseases into four stages (A to D) (Table 14.4), and in case of AS, dependent on the presence of symptoms, severity of stenosis, hemodynamic effect on the left ventricle to the volume or pressure overload, effect on the systemic circulation, and a change in heart rhythm (22). The recommendations of medical/interventional therapy is then dependent on the stage of AS.

Initial medical therapy in older patients with AS is the same as in the general population with AS. Hypertension in patients with AS is associated with increased ischemic cardiovascular events and mortality rates (48). Hypertension in asymptomatic patients with AS (stages A, B, and C) should be treated according to standard goal-directed medical therapy. Optimal blood pressure targets in this population are not well defined, and overly aggressive blood pressure reduction may lead to adverse

Table 14.3 Incidence of new coronary events in older persons with no, mild, moderate, and severe valvular aortic stenosis

	No AS (*n* = 1496)	Mild AS (*n* = 165)	Moderate AS (*n* = 96)	Severe AS (*n* = 40)
Age (years)	81	84	85	85
Follow-up (months)	49	52	32	20
New coronary events (%)	41	62	80	93

Source: Aronow WS et al., *Am J Cardiol*, 81, 647–649, 1998.
Abbreviation: AS, aortic stenosis.

Table 14.4 Stages of valvular aortic stenosis

Stage	Definition	Valve anatomy	Valve hemodynamics	Hemodynamic changes	Symptoms
A	At risk of AS	• Bicuspid aortic valve (or other congenital valve anomaly) • Aortic valve sclerosis	Aortic Vmax <2 m/s	None	None
B	Progressive AS	• Mild to moderate leaflet calcification of a bicuspid or trileaflet valve with some reduction in systolic motion or rheumatic valve changes with commissural fusion	• Mild AS: Aortic Vmax 2.0–2.9 m/s or mean ΔP <20 mmHg • Moderate AS: Aortic Vmax 3.0–3.9 m/s or mean ΔP 20–39 mm Hg	• Early LV diastolic dysfunction may be present • Normal LVEF	None
C1	Asymptomatic severe AS	Severe leaflet calcification or congenital stenosis with severely reduced leaflet opening	• Aortic Vmax ≥4 m/s or mean ΔP ≥40 mmHg • AVA typically is ≤1 cm^2 (or AVAi ≤0.6 cm^2/m^2) • Very severe AS is an aortic Vmax ≥5 m/s, or mean ΔP ≥60 mmHg	• LV diastolic dysfunction • Mild LV hypertrophy • Normal LVEF	None; exercise testing is reasonable to confirm symptom status
C2	Asymptomatic severe AS with LV dysfunction	Severe leaflet calcification or congenital stenosis with severely reduced leaflet opening	• Aortic Vmax ≥ 4 m/s or mean ΔP ≥40 mmHg • AVA typically is ≤1 cm^2 (or AVAi ≤ 0.6 cm^2/m^2)	LVEF <50%	None
D1	Symptomatic severe high-gradient AS	Severe leaflet calcification or congenital stenosis with severely reduced leaflet opening	• Aortic Vmax ≥4 m/s, or mean Δ P ≥40 mmHg • AVA typically is ≤1 cm^2 (or AVAi ≤ 0.6 cm^2/m^2), but may be larger with mixed	• LV diastolic dysfunction • LV hypertrophy • Pulmonary hypertension may be present	• Exertional dyspnea or decreased exercise tolerance = Exertional angina • Exertional syncope or presyncope
D2	Symptomatic severe low-flow/low-gradient AS with reduced LVEF AS/AR	Severe leaflet calcification with severely reduced leaflet motion	• AVA ≤1 cm^2 with resting aortic Vmax <4 m/s or mean Δ P <40 mmHg • Dobutamine stress echo shows AVA ≤1 cm^2 with Vmax ≥4 m/s at any flow rate	• LV diastolic dysfunction • LV hypertrophy • LVEF <50% rate	• HF • Angina • Syncope or presyncope
D3	Symptomatic severe low-gradient AS with normal LVEF or paradoxical low-flow severe AS	Severe leaflet calcification with severely reduced leaflet motion	• AVA ≤1 cm^2 with aortic Vmax <4 m/s, or mean Δ P <40 mmHg • Indexed AVA ≤0.6 cm^2/m^2 • Stroke volume index <35 mL/m^2 • Measured when the patient is normotensive (systolic BP <140 mmHg)	• Increased LV relative wall thickness • Small LV chamber with low-stroke volume • Restrictive diastolic filling • LVEF ≥50%	• HF • Angina • Syncope or presyncope

Source: Nishimura RA et al., *J Am Coll Cardiol*, 63, 2438–2488, 2014.
Abbreviations: AS, aortic stenosis; LV, left ventricular; LVEF, left ventricular ejection fraction; P, pressure; AVA, aortic valve area.

effects. Nitrates should be used with caution in patients with angina pectoris and AS to prevent the occurrence of orthostatic hypotension and syncope. Diuretics should be used with caution in patients with CHF to prevent a decrease in cardiac output and hypotension. Vasodilators may be reasonable in the acute management of patients who present with severe AS and New York Heart Association (NYHA) class IV heart failure; however, invasive monitoring of LV filling pressures, cardiac output, and systemic vascular resistance is essential as a sudden decline in systemic vascular resistance may lead to a decline in cardiac output (22). Digitalis should not be used in patients with CHF and a normal LV ejection fraction unless needed to control a rapid ventricular rate associated with AF.

Prophylactic antibiotics are not recommended to prevent bacterial endocarditis in patients with AS regardless of the severity, according to updated ACC/AHA guidelines (22). Patients with CHF, exertional syncope, or angina pectoris associated with moderate or severe AS should undergo AVR promptly. Valvular replacement is the only definitive therapy in these older patients (22). Medical therapy does not relieve the mechanical obstruction to LV outflow and does not relieve symptoms or halt the progression of the disorder.

Aortic valve replacement

Current recommendations for performing AVR in patients with AS are listed in Table 14.5 (22). AVR is a class I indication for symptomatic elderly patients with severe AS. It is also a class I indication to perform AVR in elderly patients with severe asymptomatic AS with an LV ejection fraction <50%, and in patients undergoing other cardiac surgeries (such as CABG, aortic surgery, or surgery on other heart valves) (22).

Based on previous data, a watchful waiting approach for asymptomatic patients with severe AS has been demonstrated to be safe (40,42,43,46). Monitoring of these patients should be targeted at identifying the development of symptoms, reduction in LV ejection fraction, and for the development of critical AS. Transthoracic echocardiography is recommended in patients with AS who develop any changes in signs or symptoms. Asymptomatic patients with normal LV systolic function who have no change in signs or symptoms should be evaluated with TTE at intervals of 6 months to 1 year (22).

Most patients with asymptomatic severe AS will ultimately have disease progression and develop symptoms. Severe asymptomatic AS was present in 622 patients, mean age 72 years, at the Mayo Clinic (49). Of the 622 patients, 166 (27%) developed symptoms and underwent AVR. Another 97 patients (16%) had AVR in the absence of symptoms. At 3-year follow-up, 52% of the 622 patients had developed symptoms, undergone AVR, or died. The most important risk factor for 10-year mortality was absence of AVR (hazard ratio = 3.53, $p < 0.001$) (49).

Historical data demonstrate that the survival rate during the asymptomatic phase is similar to age-matched cohorts with a low risk of sudden cardiac death (22,40–43,46). In a prospective study of patients with asymptomatic AS, the rate of hemodynamic progression and clinical outcome was predicted by jet velocity at the time of diagnosis (50). In a prospective study of asymptomatic patients with AS, the likelihood of remaining alive without valve replacement at 2 years was 21 ± 18% for a jet velocity at entry >4.0 m/s, compared with 66 ± 13% for a velocity of 3.0–4.0 m/s. In the prospective follow-up study

Table 14.5 American College of Cardiology/American Heart Association class I and II indications for aortic valve replacement in persons with severe aortic stenosis

Recommendation	Class of recommendation
Severe symptomatic AS (stage D1)	Class I
Severe asymptomatic AS with reduced LVEF <50% (stage C2)	Class I
Severe asymptomatic AS undergoing other cardiac surgery (stage C or D)	Class I
Very severe asymptomatic AS (stage C1, aortic velocity ≥5 m/s) and low surgical risk (defined as an STS-PROM score of <4.0 in the absence of other comorbidities or advanced frailty; or operative mortality of <1.5%)	Class IIa
Severe asymptomatic AS and decreased exercise tolerance or an exercise fall in BP	Class IIa
Severe symptomatic AS with low flow/low gradient with reduced LVEF (stage D2) with a low-dose dobutamine stress study that shows an aortic velocity ≥4 m/s (or mean pressure gradient ≥40 mmHg) with a valve area ≤1.0 cm^2 at any dobutamine dose	Class IIa
Moderate AS (stage B; aortic velocity 3.0–3.9 m/s) who are undergoing other cardiac surgery	Class IIa
Severe asymptomatic AS (stage C1) with rapid disease progression and low surgical risk	Class IIb

Source: Nishimura RA et al., *J Am Coll Cardiol*, 63(22), 2438–2488, 2014.
Abbreviations: AS, aortic stenosis; LVEF, left ventricular ejection fraction; STS-PROM, Society of Thoracic Surgery Predicted Risk of Mortality.

by Rosenhek et al. (41), the presence of moderate–severe valve calcification was a risk factor for more rapid progression of disease in severe AS.

Recent data suggest that patients with asymptomatic severe AS may benefit from early AVR (49–53), especially in the era of catheter-based AVR. An observational study by Pai et al. (51) found that 99 of 338 patients (29%), mean age 71 years, with asymptomatic severe AS had AVR during 3.5-year follow-up. Survival at 1, 2, and 5 years was 67%, 56%, and 38%, respectively, for unoperated patients and 94%, 93%, and 90%, respectively, for those who had AVR. Current ACC/AHA guidelines recommend considering AVR in asymptomatic patients with severe and very severe AS who have a low surgical risk (22). Low surgical risk has been defined as an STS PROM (Society of Thoracic Surgeons Predicted Risk of Mortality) score of <4.0 in the absence of other comorbidities or advanced frailty; or operative mortality of <1.5%. In a study of 197 consecutive patients with asymptomatic severe AS, early AVR was performed in 102 patients (52%) (52). The estimated actuarial 6-year all-cause mortality rates were 2% for AVR and 32% for the conventional treatment group ($p < 0.001$) (87). A separate study of 73 patients with severe AS who did not undergo AVR, 15 (14%) died at 15-month follow-up (53). Of these 73 patients, symptoms were thought to be unrelated to the AS in 31 patients. Exercise stress tests for symptoms were performed in only 4% of the 42 asymptomatic patients (53).

Asymptomatic patients with low-gradient severe AS and normal LV ejection fraction with reduced stroke volume index had at 46-month follow-up aortic valve events similar to those with normal stroke volume index (54). Of 248 patients with severe AS and a normal LV ejection fraction, 94 had a low-gradient (<30 mmHg mean gradient) (group 1), 87 had a moderate gradient (30–40 mmHg mean gradient) (group 2), and 67 had a severe gradient (>40 mmHg mean gradient) (group 3) (55). Symptoms were present in 49% of group 1 patients, in 55% of group 2 patients, and in 60% of group 3 patients (p not significant). At 45- to 60-month follow-up, the incidence of AVR or death was 71% for group 1, 77% for group 2, and 76% for group 3 (p not significant). Kaplan–Meier survival curves for time to death in all three groups were significantly better for patients with AVR versus no AVR (55). $E/E^1_{lateral}$ was an independent predictor of time to death in patients who did not receive AVR (56).

The bioprosthesis is preferred over a mechanical prosthetic valve in older patients (>70 years of age) due to decreased life expectancy and the ability to avoid anticoagulation (22,56,57). Patients with mechanical prostheses need anticoagulant therapy indefinitely (with a vitamin K antagonist agent such as Coumadin), which may be problematic in elderly patients who are frail and may have a higher bleeding risk. Patients with bioprosthesis may be treated with aspirin in a dose of 75–100 mg daily unless the patient has AF, abnormal LV ejection fraction, previous thromboembolism, or a hypercoagulable condition (22,57). Table 14.6 lists the current ACC/AHA guideline recommendations for anticoagulant therapy in patients with AVR (22).

A UK heart valve registry observed in 1100 patients aged >80 years (56% women) who underwent AVR that the 30-day mortality was 6.6% (58). The actuarial survival was 89% at 1 year, 79% at 3 years, 69% at 5 years, and 46% at 8 years. In 242 patients, mean age 83 years, with AS who had AVR, actuarial survival was 92% at 1 year and 66% at 5 years (59). Concomitant CABGS did not affect late survival (59).

Paroxysmal or chronic AF is a risk factor for mortality in patients with severe AS and an LV ejection fraction <35% undergoing AVR (60). Of 83 patients, mean age 70 years, with severe AS and an LV ejection fraction <35%, 29 (35%) had paroxysmal or chronic AF (101). The perioperative mortality was 24% in the AF group versus 5.5% in the non-AF group ($p = 0.03$) (60).

Table 14.6 Indications for anticoagulant therapy in patients with aortic valve replacement

Recommendation	Class
Anticoagulation with vitamin K antagonist (VKA) for all patients with mechanical AVR	I
Anticoagulation with VKA to maintain INR of 2.5 in patients with mechanical AVR (bileaflet or current-generation single tilting disc) and no risk factors for thromboembolism	I
Anticoagulation with VKA to maintain INR of 3.0 in patients with mechanical AVR (bileaflet or current-generation single tilting disc) and risk factors for thromboembolism (AF, previous thromboembolism, LV dysfunction, or hypercoagulable conditions) or an older generation of mechanical valve	I
Aspirin 75 mg–100 mg daily is recommended in addition to anticoagulation with a VKA in patients with a mechanical valve prosthesis	I
Anticoagulation, with a VKA, to achieve an INR of 2.5 may be reasonable for the first 3 months after bioprosthetic AVR	IIb

Source: Nishimura RA et al., *J Am Coll Cardiol*, 63(22), 2438–2488, 2014.

Abbreviations: VKA, vitamin K antagonist; AVR, aortic valve replacement; INR, international normalized ratio; AF, atrial fibrillation; LV, left ventricular.

AVR is associated with a reduction in LV mass and an improvement in LV diastolic filling (61,62). Hoffman and Burckhardt (63) performed a prospective study in 100 patients who had AVR. At 41-month follow-up, the yearly cardiac mortality rate was 8% in patients with electrocardiographic LV hypertrophy and repetitive ventricular premature complexes >2 couplets per 24 hours during 24-hour ambulatory monitoring and 0.6% in patients without either of these findings (63).

If LV systolic dysfunction in patients with severe AS is associated with critical narrowing of the aortic valve rather than myocardial fibrosis, it often improves after successful AVR (64). In 154 patients, mean age 73 years, with AS and an LV ejection fraction <35% who underwent AVR, the 30-day mortality was 9%. The 5-year survival was 69% in patients without significant CAD and 39% in patients with significant CAD. NYHA functional class III or IV was present in 58% of patients before surgery versus 7% of patients after surgery. Postoperative LV ejection fraction was measured in 76% of survivors at a mean of 14 months after surgery. Improvement in LV ejection fraction was found in 76% of patients (64).

Balloon aortic valvuloplasty

AVR is the procedure of choice for symptomatic older patients with severe AS, but balloon aortic valvuloplasty (BAV) can be considered as a treatment option in selected groups of patients. In a Mayo Clinic study, the actuarial survival of 50 older patients, mean age 77 years, with symptomatic severe AS in whom AVR was refused (45 patients) or deferred (5 patients) was 57% at 1 year, 37% at 2 years, and 25% at 3 years (65). Because of the poor survival in this group of patients, BAV should be considered when operative intervention is refused or deferred. Additionally, BAV should be considered for older patients with symptomatic severe AS who are not candidates for AVR and possibly for patients with severe LV dysfunction as a bridge to subsequent valve replacement (66).

Transcatheter intervention for AS

Percutaneous TAVR is becoming more widely available worldwide with >400 sites and >50,000 TAVRs performed in the United States by the end of 2015 (67). Over the past decade, TAVR has emerged as a less invasive alternative to surgical aortic valve replacement (SAVR). The advent of TAVR has widened the management options for older patients who meet the criteria for AVR, initially being approved for patients who were prohibitive or at high risk to undergo surgical AVR (68,69). TAVR has also been approved for patients who are considered at intermediate risk for SAVR.

In randomized trials, TAVR has been shown to be superior to medical therapy alone for patients at prohibitive surgical risk, and non-inferior to SAVR for patients at high surgical risk. One of the landmark trials in this arena has been the Placement of Aortic Transcatheter Valves (PARTNER) trial, which evaluated two primary cohorts: inoperable and high surgical risk patients (68–70).

In the inoperative cohort of the PARTNER trial (deemed to be at prohibitive risk for SAVR), 358 patients (mean age 83 years, mean STS score 11.7%) were randomized to TAVR or standard medical care alone. At 1-year follow-up, all-cause mortality was 30.7% in the TAVR group, as compared to 50.7% in the medical therapy group ($p < 0.001$) (68). Compared to medical therapy alone, TAVR caused significant improvements in the rate of cardiac symptoms and health-related quality of life maintained for at least 1 year (68,71). At 30 days, TAVR was associated with a higher incidence of major strokes (5.0% vs. 1.1%, $p = 0.06$) and major vascular complications (16.2% vs. 1.1%, $p < 0.001$) as compared to those managed medically (67). At 3 years, the mortality rate was 54.1% in the TAVR group versus 80.9% with standard medical therapy ($p < 0.001$). The improvement in NYHA class symptoms was sustained at 3 years. The incidence of stroke at 3-year follow-up was 15.7% in the TAVR group versus 5.5% in the standard therapy group (72).

At 5-year follow-up, only 1 patient out of 179 in the standard therapy group survived as compared to 28% (49 out of 179) in the TAVR group (73).

In the high surgical risk cohort, 699 patients with severe AS were enrolled, mean age 84 years, and randomized to SAVR or TAVR (70). All-cause mortality was 3.4% for the TAVR group versus 6.5% for the SAVR group at 30 days (p = NS) and 24.2% for the TAVR group versus 26.8% for the SAVR group at 1 year (p = NS). Major stroke was 3.8% for the TAVR group versus 2.1% for the SAVR group at 30 days (p = NS) and 5.1% for the TAVR group versus 2.4% for the SAVR group at 1 year (p = NS). Major vascular complications at 30 days were 11.0% for the TAVR group versus 3.2% for the SAVR group ($p < 0.001$). At 1-year follow-up, there were similar improvements in cardiac symptoms for both groups (74).

Published follow-up data from the PARTNER trial include 2-year and 5-year outcomes in patients who are at increased surgical risk (75,76). At 5 years, risk of death was 67.8% in the TAVR group compared with 62.4% in the SAVR group (hazard ratio 1.04, 95% confidence interval [CI] 0.86–1.24; $p = 0.76$). However, moderate or severe AR occurred in 40 (14%) of 280 patients in the TAVR group and 2 (1%) of 228 in the SAVR group ($p < 0.0001$), and was associated with increased 5-year risk of mortality in the TAVR group (72.4% for moderate or severe AR vs. 56.6% for those with mild AR or less; $p = 0.003$) (76).

The PARTNER data demonstrate that TAVR is superior to standard medical therapy for the treatment of inoperable AS. The ACC/AHA valvular guidelines now give a class I indication for TAVR in symptomatic patients with severe AS and a prohibitive risk for surgical AVR (77).

More recently, randomized trials have shown TAVR to be non-inferior to SAVR with respect to death and disabling stroke in patients at intermediate risk for SAVR

(78,79). Each procedure carries a unique set of risks and benefits. Patients undergoing SAVR more often suffer acute kidney injury (AKI) and AF postoperatively, whereas patients receiving TAVR have higher rates of perivalvular AR and require permanent pacemaker implantation (79).

Due to the beneficial data of TAVR in high-risk and intermediate-risk populations, some clinicians may also argue that patients older than 80 years should only get TAVR. For this reason, a study retrospectively looked at 1028 octogenarians who underwent isolated AVR (306 TAVR and 722 SAVR), regardless of their surgical risk. The TAVR group had more comorbidities and had higher STS-PROM scores. After adjusting for confounders, TAVR had comparable mortality as compared to SAVR (80).

Risk factors for AS are similar to those for atherosclerosis, and concomitant CAD is often found in older patients presenting with severe AS. The association of CAD with the outcomes in patients undergoing TAVR is conflicting. There are studies that show that the presence of prior CAD (CABG or PCI) negatively impacts the procedural outcomes and long-term survival in patients undergoing TAVR (81). A study of 445 patients who underwent TAVR stratified the CAD severity according to the SYNTAX score (SS). They found that the greater CAD severity (defined as an SS >22) was associated with a higher rate of the combined primary endpoint compared with patients with less severe CAD (SS of 0–22) and no CAD. Although after multivariable analysis, this relationship was not statistically significant (82). Other studies have failed to show the negative impact of CAD on outcomes after TAVR. A pooled analysis of 2472 patients showed that the presence of CAD did not change the odds of death in patients who underwent TAVR (83).

Traditionally, SAVR and concomitant CABG have been the standard management for patients with severe AS and CAD. In patients undergoing TAVR, the general approach has been for complete revascularization by PCI prior to TAVR. The rationale for this is based on mirroring the historic standard of care: SAVR with CABG. Also, it is felt that patients who are revascularized are at lower risk for ischemic complications in the setting of rapid pacing for BAV or valve deployment during TAVR.

The PARTNER trial excluded patients with untreated clinically significant CAD requiring revascularization.

Data are limited and somewhat conflicting as to the benefit of percutaneous revascularization prior to TAVR (84,85). In data collected from the Nationwide Inpatient Sample, 608 patients who underwent TAVR and PCI in the same hospitalization showed higher rates of mortality (10.7% vs. 4.6%; $p < 0.001$) and vascular injury requiring surgery (8.2% vs. 4.2%; $p < 0.001$) (85).

The best management of CAD and AS in TAVR candidates requires individualized attention and should be based on the amount of myocardium at risk and the risk of complications from PCI (primarily vascular injury and renal impairment).

When considering a TAVR in an older patient, certain other topics require special attention. AKI following a TAVI procedure has been described to occur in 8.3%–57% of patients (86). The variability in incidence could be due to different definitions used to define AKI. Regardless, AKI has been associated with increased length of hospital stay, in-hospital mortality, 30-day mortality, and long-term mortality (86,87). Although age has not been reported a factor, baseline renal function or chronic kidney disease (which is prevalent in an older population) has been significantly associated to the risk of post-TAVR AKI (86,87).

Another factor to be mindful of when evaluating elderly patients for TAVR is the risk of developing conduction abnormalities requiring pacemaker implantation after TAVR. In a recent meta-analysis, preprocedural factors predicting the need for pacemaker after TAVR include male gender, first-degree atrioventricular block, left anterior hemiblock and right bundle branch block, calcifications of aortic valve, left ventricular outflow tract (LVOT), and mitral annulus. Procedural factors that increase the risk of pacemaker after TAVR include use of self-expandable prosthesis and a deep prosthesis implant relative to the anatomic annular plane (88).

After TAVR, treatment with clopidogrel for 3 months in addition to aspirin is widely practiced. However, a small study of 161 patients randomized to clopidogrel for 3 months (a loading dose of 300 mg on the day before TAVR followed by 75 mg daily) plus aspirin 100 mg daily or aspirin 100 mg daily alone showed no significant difference in major adverse cardiac and cerebrovascular events at 30 days and at 6 months (89). The benefit of dual antiplatelet therapy (DAPT) after TAVR is primarily to prevent leaflet thrombosis in the implanted valve. It does not appear that DAPT provides protection from leaflet thrombosis, and full anticoagulation (with warfarin or novel oral anticoagulant [NOAC]) in the immediate post-TAVR period to mitigate this risk. The rate of leaflet thrombosis is higher in TAVR valves as compared to surgically implanted bioprosthetic valves. Leaflet thrombosis manifests as high transvalvular gradients and decreased leaflet motion on TTE, and as leaflet thickening on CT scan. Leaflet thrombosis should be treated with 3 months of full anticoagulation, at which time repeat imaging should be performed. Additional data are required to identify which patients are at highest risk for leaflet thrombosis and the best methods for prophylaxis and treatment of these events.

AORTIC REGURGITATION

Etiology and prevalence

AR results from abnormalities of the aortic leaflets, their supporting structures (aortic root and annulus), or both.

Acute AR in older patients may be due to infective endocarditis, rheumatic fever, aortic dissection, trauma following prosthetic valve surgery, or rupture of the sinus of Valsalva, and it causes sudden severe LV failure. Chronic AR in older patients may be caused by valve leaflet disease (secondary to any cause of AS, infective endocarditis, rheumatic fever, congenital heart disease, rheumatoid arthritis, ankylosing spondylitis, following prosthetic valve surgery, or myxomatous degeneration of the valve) or by aortic root disease. Examples of aortic root disease causing chronic AR in elderly patients include association with systemic hypertension, syphilitic aortitis, cystic medial necrosis of the aorta, ankylosing spondylitis, rheumatoid arthritis, Reiter's disease, systemic lupus erythematosus, Ehler–Danlos syndrome, and pseudoxanthoma elasticum. Mild or moderate AR was also diagnosed by Doppler echocardiography in 9 of 29 patients (31%) with hypertrophic cardiomyopathy (90). The prevalence of AR increases with age (91,92). In a prospective study of 118 patients with color flow imaging, AR was present in 11% of patients younger than 50 years of age versus 100% of patients older than 50 (92).

In a prospective study of 450 unselected patients, mean age 82 years, AR was diagnosed by pulsed Doppler echocardiography in 39 of 114 men (34%) and in 92 of 336 women (27%) (91). Severe or moderate AR was diagnosed in 74 of 450 elderly patients (16%). Mild AR was diagnosed in 57 of 450 elderly patients (13%). In a prospective study of 924 men, mean age 80 years, and 1881 women, mean age 82 years, valvular AR was diagnosed by pulsed Doppler recordings of the aortic valve in 282 men (31%) and in 542 women (29%) (6).

Pathophysiology

The primary determinants of AR volume are the regurgitant orifice area, the transvalvular pressure gradient, and the duration of diastole (93). Chronic AR increases LV ventricular end-diastolic volume. The largest LV end-diastolic volumes are seen in patients with chronic severe AR. LV stroke volume increases to maintain the forward stroke volume. The increased preload causes an increase in LV diastolic stress and the addition of sarcomeres in series. This results in an increase in the ratio of the LV chamber size to wall thickness. This pattern of LV hypertrophy is called eccentric LV hypertrophy.

Primary myocardial abnormalities or ischemia due to coexistent CAD depresses the contractile state. LV diastolic compliance decreases, LV end-systolic volume increases, LV end-diastolic pressure rises, left atrial pressure increases, and pulmonary venous hypertension results. When the LV end-diastolic radius-to-wall thickness ratio rises, LV systolic wall stress increases abnormally because of the preload and afterload mismatch. Additional stress then decreases the LV ejection fraction response to exercise (94). Eventually, the LV ejection fraction, forward stroke volume, and effective cardiac output are decreased at rest. We demonstrated that an abnormal resting LV ejection fraction occurred in 8 of 25 older patients (32%) with CHF associated with chronic severe AR (95).

In patients with acute severe AR, the LV cannot adapt to the increased volume overload. Forward stroke volume falls, LV end-diastolic pressure increases rapidly to high levels, and pulmonary hypertension and pulmonary edema result. The rapid rise of the LV end-diastolic pressure to exceed the left atrial pressure in early diastole causes premature closure of the mitral valve (96). This prevents backward transmission of the elevated LV end-diastolic pressure to the pulmonary venous bed.

Symptoms

Patients with acute AR develop symptoms due to the sudden onset of CHF, with marked dyspnea and weakness. Patients with chronic AR may remain asymptomatic for many years. Mild dyspnea on exertion and palpitations, especially on lying down, may occur. Exertional dyspnea, orthopnea, paroxysmal nocturnal dyspnea, fatigue, and edema are common clinical symptoms when LV failure occurs. Syncope is rare. Angina pectoris occurs less often in patients with AR as compared to patients with AS and may be due to coexistent CAD. Patients with chronic AR have also been shown to have reduced coronary reserve, which may result in angina (97). However, nocturnal angina pectoris, often accompanied by flushing, diaphoresis, and palpitations, may develop when the heart rate slows and the arterial diastolic pressure falls to very low levels. Most patients with severe AR who do not have surgery die within 2 years of developing heart failure symptoms (98).

Signs

The AR murmur is typically a high-pitched blowing diastolic murmur that begins immediately after A_2. The diastolic murmur is best heard along the left sternal border in the third and fourth intercostal spaces when AR is due to valvular disease. The murmur is best heard along the right sternal border when AR is due to dilatation of the ascending aorta. The diastolic murmur is best heard with the diaphragm of the stethoscope with the person sitting up, leaning forward, and holding the breath in deep expiration. The severity of AR correlates with the duration of the diastolic murmur, not with the intensity of the murmur.

Table 14.7 shows that an AR murmur was heard in 95% of 74 elderly patients with severe or moderate AR diagnosed by pulsed Doppler echocardiography, in 61% of 57 elderly patients with mild AR, and in 3% of 319 elderly patients with no AR (91).

In patients with chronic severe AR, the LV apical impulse is diffuse, hyperdynamic, and displaced laterally and inferiorly. A rumbling diastolic murmur

Table 14.7 Correlation of aortic regurgitation murmur with severity of aortic regurgitation in elderly patients with chronic aortic regurgitation

	AR murmur (%)
Severe or moderate AR (*n* = 74)	95
Mild AR (*n* = 57)	61
No AR (*n* = 319)	3

Source: Aronow WS, Kronzon I, *Am J Cardiol*, 63, 128–129, 1989.
Abbreviation: AR, aortic regurgitation.

(Austin Flint) may be heard at the apex, with its intensity decreased by inhalation of amyl nitrite. A short basal systolic ejection murmur is heard. A palpable LV rapid filling wave and an audible S_3 at the apex are usually found. Physical findings due to a large LV stroke volume and a rapid diastolic runoff in patients with severe AR include a wide pulse pressure with an increased systolic arterial pressure and an abnormally low diastolic arterial pressure; an arterial pulse that abruptly rises and collapses; a bisferiens pulse; bobbing of the head with each heartbeat; booming systolic and diastolic sounds heard over the femoral artery, capillary pulsations, and systolic; and diastolic murmurs heard over the femoral artery when compressing it proximally and distally.

Electrocardiography and chest X-ray

The electrocardiogram may initially be normal in patients with acute severe AR. Roberts and Day (99) showed that in 30 necropsy patients with chronic severe AR, the electrocardiogram did not accurately predict the severity of AR or cardiac weight. Using various electrocardiographic criteria, the prevalence of LV hypertrophy varied from 30% ($RV_6 > RV_5$) to 90% (total 12-lead QRS voltage >175 mm). The P–R interval was prolonged in 28% of patients, and the QRS duration was ≥0.12 seconds in 20% of patients (99).

The chest X-ray in patients with acute severe AR may show a normal heart size and pulmonary edema. The chest X-ray in patients with chronic severe AR usually shows a dilated LV, with elongation of the apex inferiorly and posteriorly and a dilated aorta. Aneurysmal dilatation of the aorta suggests that aortic root disease is causing the AR. Linear calcifications in the wall of the ascending aorta are seen in syphilitic AR and in degenerative disease.

Echocardiography and Doppler echocardiography

M-mode and two-dimensional echocardiography and Doppler echocardiography are very useful in the diagnosis of AR. Two-dimensional echocardiography can provide information showing the etiology of the AR and measurements of LV function. Eccentric LV hypertrophy is diagnosed by echocardiography if the LV mass index is increased with a relative wall thickness <0.45 (100). Echocardiographic measurements reported to predict an unfavorable response to AVR in patients with chronic AR include an LV end-systolic dimension >55 mm (101), an LV shortening fraction <25% (101), an LV diastolic radius-to-wall thickness ratio >3.8 (102), an LV end-diastolic dimension index >38 mm/m^2 (101,102), and an LV ventricular end-systolic dimension index >26 mm/m^2 (101,102).

Continuous wave Doppler echocardiography has also been shown to be very useful in diagnosing and quantitating AR (103). AR is best assessed by color flow Doppler imaging (104). Figure 14.6 illustrates two-dimensional echocardiographic and color Doppler findings in an elderly patient with chronic severe AR. Figure 14.7 illustrates continuous-wave Doppler findings in the older patient with chronic severe AR shown in Figure 14.6.

In patients with suboptimal echocardiographic images, cardiac MRI can be used. In current ACC/AHA guidelines, cardiac magnetic resonance (CMR) has been given a class I indication in patients with moderate to severe AR and suboptimal echocardiographic assessment (22). Over the past decade, there have been significant advancements in the field of CMR specifically in the assessment of the intracardiac flow. CMR flow and velocity map imaging can provide volumetric, anatomical, functional, and flow information during the entire cardiac cycle. CMR velocity mapping can directly quantify AR with high accuracy and reproducibility (105).

Natural history

The natural history of acute and chronic AR differs significantly. Patients with acute AR should have immediate AVR because death may occur within hours to days. The morbidity and mortality associated with chronic AR is much more benign in comparison to acute AR. Of patients with moderate to severe chronic AR, 50% were alive at 10 years after diagnosis (106,107). The 10-year survival rate for patients with mild to moderate chronic AR was reported to be 85%–95% (106,107).

Similar to the natural history of AS, the prognosis of patients with chronic AR worsens once symptoms develop. In another study of 14 patients with chronic severe AR who did not have surgery, 13 (93%) died within 2 years of developing CHF (98). The mean survival time after the onset of angina pectoris is 5 years (106).

During 8-year follow-up of 104 asymptomatic patients with chronic severe AR and normal LV ejection fraction, 2 patients (2%) died suddenly and 23 patients (22%) had AVR (108). Of the 104 patients, 19 (18%) had AVR because of cardiac symptoms and 4 patients (4%) had AVR because of the development of LV systolic dysfunction in the absence of cardiac symptoms. Multivariate analysis

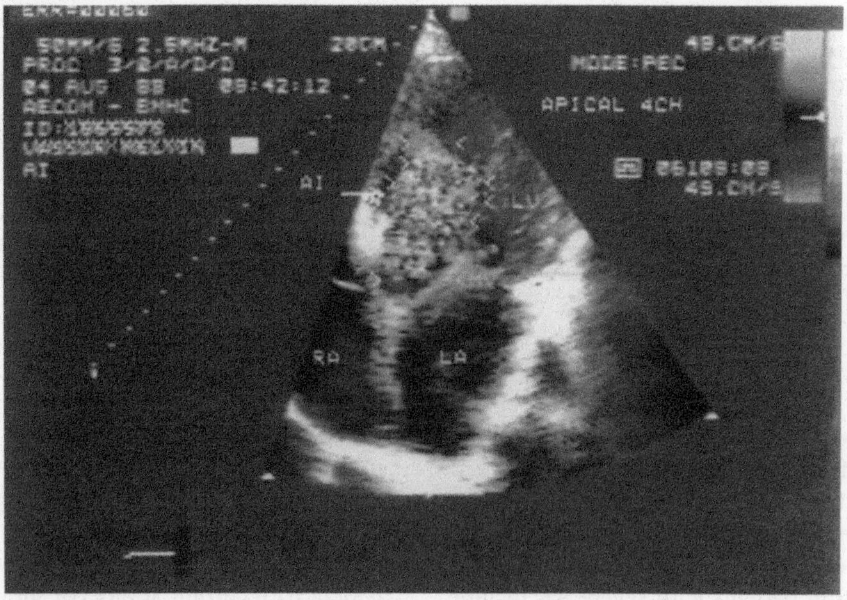

Figure 14.6 Two-dimensional echocardiographic image from an apical four-chamber view in an elderly patient with severe aortic insufficiency, showing a large diastolic aliasing color Doppler jet in the left ventricular outflow tract. *Abbreviations*: AI, aortic insufficiency; LV, left ventricular cavity; MV, mitral valve leaflets; LA, left atrium; RA, right atrium.

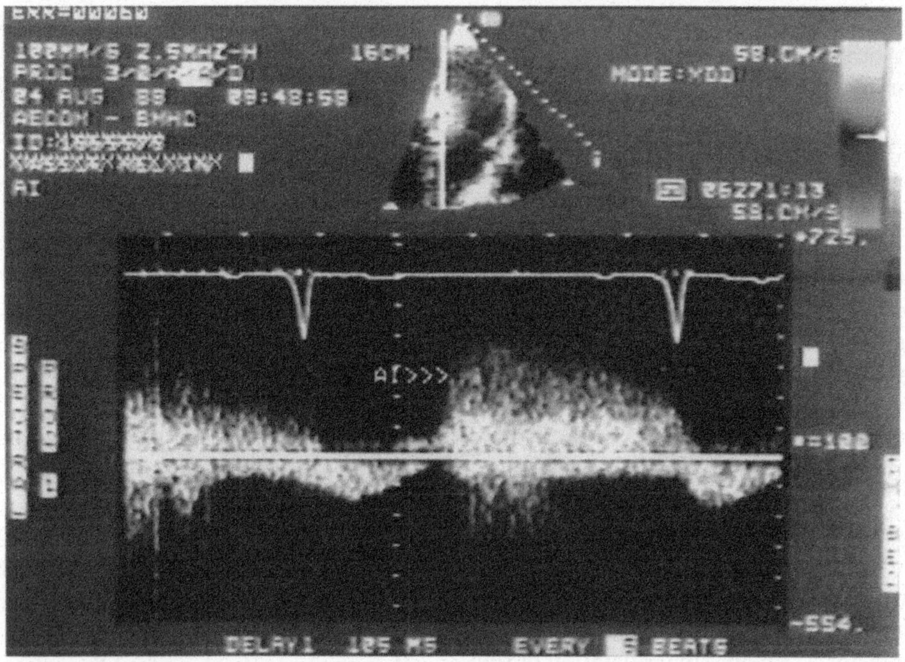

Figure 14.7 Continuous-wave Doppler recording of the velocity profile across the aortic valve in the same patient shown in Figure 14.6. A holosystolic decrescendo high-velocity profile is recorded from the left ventricular outflow tract, characteristic of aortic insufficiency. *Abbreviations*: AI, aortic insufficiency.

showed that age, initial end-systolic dimension, and rate of change in end-systolic dimension and resting LV ejection fraction during serial studies predicted the outcome.

Similarly, in a prospective study, prognosis of chronic AR with CHF associated with abnormal LV ejection fraction was worse as compared to patients with normal LV function. At 24-month follow-up (range 7–55 months) of 17 patients, mean age 83 years, with CHF associated with unoperated severe chronic AR and a normal LV ejection fraction, 15 patients (88%) were dead (95). At 15-month follow-up (range 8–21 months) of 8 patients, mean age 85 years, with CHF associated with unoperated severe chronic AR and an abnormal LV ejection fraction, 8 patients (100%) were dead (95).

Pulmonary artery hypertension also seems to increase the risk of mortality. The overall 15-year mortality for AR in 1156 patients was 74% and increased 1.94 times in patients with moderate or greater pulmonary artery systolic hypertension (109).

Medical and surgical management

As mentioned earlier, the clinical presentation and natural history of acute and chronic AR differ significantly and so do the treatment strategies. Since the presentation of acute AR can be catastrophic, leading to acute LV failure and death, early surgical management is imperative. Several studies have shown that emergent surgical AVR can be performed with reduction in in-hospital and long-term mortality (110). Based on above evidence, current ACC/AHA guidelines also recommend prompt surgical intervention for acute AR (22). While waiting for surgery, medical treatment may be necessary to temporarily stabilize the patient. Vasodilators and inotropes may be helpful; however, caution to their use is advised. Beta-blockers are recommended treatment for aortic dissection; however, their use in acute severe AR can be detrimental. Beta-blockers increase the length of diastole, therefore worsening AR; they also block the compensatory tachycardia needed to maintain cardiac output, contributing to circulatory collapse. Intra-aortic balloon counterpulsation device is contraindicated in severe AR because it augments peripheral resistance in diastole, worsening AR. Antibiotics should be started immediately after blood cultures if the acute AR is due to endocarditis. If the patient is hemodynamically stable, surgical intervention may be delayed for 5–7 days of aggressive antibiotic therapy if severe AR is due to active infective endocarditis. However, surgical intervention should be pursued at any signs of hemodynamic instability (111). Other indications for AVR in patients with AR due to bacterial endocarditis are CHF, uncontrolled infection, myocardial or valvular ring abscess, prosthetic valve dysfunction or dehiscence, and multiple embolic episodes (112,113). Patients with AR due to syphilitic aortitis should receive a course of penicillin therapy.

Chronic AR, in contrast to acute AR, tends to be free of major cardiovascular symptoms until relatively late in the course of the disease. Current ACC/AHA guidelines on valvular heart disease classify the progression of AR into four stages (stages A–D), as shown in Table 14.8 (22). Management of patients with AR depends on accurate diagnosis of the cause and stage of the disease process. Prophylactic antibiotics are not recommended to prevent bacterial endocarditis in patients with AR according to updated ACC/AHA guidelines (22). Echocardiographic evaluation of LV end-systolic dimension should be performed yearly if the measurement is less than 50 mm, but every 3–6 months if the LV end-systolic dimension is 50–54 mm. AVR should also be considered when the LV ejection fraction approaches 50% before the decompensated state (93).

The regurgitant volume in AR is determined by the regurgitant orifice area, diastolic pressure gradient across the valve, and duration of diastolic flow. The orifice area is relatively fixed and the diastolic pressure is already low in AR, thus medical therapy is not able to modify these variables. Therefore, the main aim of medical therapy is to reduce the systolic blood pressure to reduce LV wall stress, improve LV function, and improve forward flow (114). Hypertension (systolic blood pressure >140 mmHg) should be tightly controlled in asymptomatic patients with AR (stages B and C). However, routine use of vasodilators in asymptomatic chronic AR has no recommendations in current guidelines (22). This is because randomized clinical trials are not definitive and inconclusive whether vasodilators change the natural history of asymptomatic chronic AR with normal LV function. Several vasodilators have been studied in chronic AR with inconsistent results. Some of the drugs that have been studied include hydralazine, nifedipine, and angiotensin-converting enzyme (ACE) inhibitors (115–117). Only a single, randomized, placebo-controlled trial with nifedipine has shown significant reductions in LV end-diastolic diameter and increase in LV ejection fraction (116). Another small randomized trial showed that nifedipine delayed the need for surgery as compared to digoxin (115). Unfortunately these studies have small sample size and the results are not consistent. Another randomized study of 95 patients looked at long-term therapy with nifedipine and enalapril versus placebo in patients with asymptomatic severe AR and did not show that nifedipine or enalapril reduce or delay AVR (118). Current ACC/AHA guidelines recommend the use of dihydropyridine calcium channel blocker or ACE inhibitors/angiotensin receptor blockers (ARBs) as class I for the treatment of hypertension (systolic blood pressure >140) in asymptomatic chronic AR (stages B and C) and as a class II indication in symptomatic chronic AR with/or without LV dysfunction (stages C2 and D) when surgery is not able to performed due to comorbidities (22). There are no recommendations for routine use of vasodilators in asymptomatic chronic AR with normal LV function. Short-term medical therapy can also be used presurgically to improve the hemodynamic profile of symptomatic severe AR patients with severe LV dysfunction. Post-AVR, vasodilator therapy should be continued on a long-term basis only if LV systolic dysfunction persists after AVR. Beta-blockers and ARBs should be considered in patients with significant aortic root dilation owing to cystic medial necrosis and Marfan-related syndromes to slow the rate of aortic root enlargement (119,120).

Drugs that depress LV function should not be used, and arrhythmias should be treated according to guidelines. CHF should be treated with sodium restriction, diuretics, digoxin if the LV ejection fraction is abnormal,

Table 14.8 Stages of chronic aortic regurgitation

Stage	Definition	Valve anatomy	Valve hemodynamics	Hemodynamic changes	Symptoms
A	At risk of AR	• Bicuspid aortic valve (or other congenital valve anomaly) • Aortic valve sclerosis • Diseases of the aortic sinuses or ascending aorta • History of rheumatic fever or known rheumatic heart disease • IE	AR severity: none or trace	None	None
B	Progressive AR	• Mild to moderate calcification of a trileaflet valve bicuspid aortic valve (or other congenital valve anomaly) • Dilated aortic sinuses • Rheumatic valve changes • Previous IE	• **Mild AR** • Jet width <25% of LVOT • Vena contracta <0.3 cm • RVol <30 mL/beat; • RF <30% • ERO <0.10 cm^2 • Angiography grade 1+ • **Moderate AR** • Jet width 25%–64% of LVOT • Vena contracta 0.3–0.6 cm • RVol 30–59 mL/beat • RF 30%–49% • ERO 0.10–0.29 cm^2 • Angiography grade 2+	• Normal LV systolic function • Normal LV volume or mild LV dilation	None
C1	Asymptomatic severe AR	Calcific aortic valve disease • Bicuspid valve (or other congenital abnormality) • Dilated aortic sinuses or ascending aorta • Rheumatic valve changes • IE with abnormal leaflet closure or perforation	Severe AR • Jet width ≥65% of LVOT • Vena contracta >0.6 cm • Holodiastolic flow reversal in the proximal abdominal aorta • RVol ≥60 mL/beat • RF ≥50% • ERO ≥0.3 cm^2 • Angiography grade 3+ to 4+ • In addition, diagnosis of chronic severe AR requires evidence of LV dilation	Normal LVEF (≥50%) and mild to moderate LV dilation (LVESD ≤50 mm)	• None; exercise testing is reasonable to confirm symptom status

(Continued)

Table 14.8 (Continued) Stages of chronic aortic regurgitation

Stage	Definition	Valve anatomy	Valve hemodynamics	Hemodynamic changes	Symptoms
C2	Asymptomatic severe AR with LV dysfunction	Calcific aortic valve disease • Bicuspid valve (or other congenital abnormality) • Dilated aortic sinuses or ascending aorta • Rheumatic valve changes • IE with abnormal leaflet closure or perforation	Severe AR • Jet width ≥65% of LVOT • Vena contracta >0.6 cm • Holodiastolic flow reversal in the *proximal abdominal aorta* • RVol ≥60 mL/beat • RF ≥50% • ERO ≥0.3 cm^2 • Angiography grade 3+ to 4+ • In addition, diagnosis of chronic severe AR requires evidence of LV dilation	Abnormal LV systolic function with depressed LVEF (<50%) or severe LV dilatation (LVESD >50 mm *or* indexed LVESD >25 mm/m^2)	None; exercise testing is reasonable to confirm symptom status
D	Symptomatic severe AR	• Calcific valve disease • Bicuspid valve (or other congenital abnormality) • Dilated aortic sinuses or ascending aorta • Rheumatic valve changes • Previous IE with abnormal leaflet closure or perforation	Severe AR • Jet width ≥65% of LVOT • Vena contracta >0.6 cm • Holodiastolic flow reversal in the proximal abdominal aorta • RVol ≥60 mL/beat • RF ≥50%; • ERO ≥0.3 cm^2 • Angiography grade 3+ to 4+ • In addition, diagnosis of chronic severe AR requires evidence of LV dilation	Symptomatic severe AR may occur with normal systolic function (LVEF ≥50%), mild to moderate LV dysfunction (LVEF 40% to 50%), or severe LV dysfunction (LVEF <40%) • Moderate to severe LV dilation is present.	Exertional dyspnea or angina or more severe HF symptoms

Source: Nishimura RA et al., *J Am Coll Cardiol*, 63, 2438–2488, 2014.

Abbreviations: AR, aortic regurgitation; IE, infective endocarditis; LVOT, left ventricular outflow tract; R vol, regurgitant volume; RF, regurgitant fraction; ERO, effective regurgitant orifice; LVOT, left ventricular outflow tract; LV, left ventricular; LVEF, left ventricular ejection fraction; LVESD, left ventricular end-systolic dimension.

Table 14.9 American College of Cardiology/American Heart Association indications for aortic valve replacement in persons with chronic severe aortic regurgitation

Recommendation	Class
Symptomatic patients with severe AR (stage D) and normal or abnormal left ventricular ejection fraction	I
Asymptomatic patients with chronic severe AR and LV ejection fraction <50% at rest	I
Patients with severe AR (stage C or D) undergoing other cardiac surgery (e.g., coronary artery bypass surgery or surgery on the aorta or other heart valves)	I
Asymptomatic patients with severe AR with LV ejection fraction >50% but an LVESD >55 mm or indexed LVESD >25 mm/m^2 (stage C2)	IIa
Patients with moderate AR (stage B) who are undergoing other cardiac surgery	IIa
Asymptomatic patients with severe AR and normal LV function (LVEF ≥50%) (stage C1) but with progressive LV dilation (LVEDD > 65 mm) if surgical risk is low	IIb

Source: Nishimura RA et al., *J Am Coll Cardiol*, 63, 2438–2488, 2014.
Abbreviations: AR, aortic regurgitation; LV, left ventricular; LVESD, left ventricular end-systolic dimension; LVEDD, left ventricular end-diastolic dimension.

vasodilator therapy, and AVR. Angina pectoris should be treated with nitrates. Infections should be treated promptly to avoid development of infective endocarditis.

Prophylactic aortic root replacement with concomitant AVR should be considered in patients with Marfan syndrome when the aortic root diameter exceeds 55 mm (121).

Table 14.9 shows class I and class II ACC/AHA indications for AVR in patients with chronic severe AR (22). The class I indications for AVR in patients with chronic severe AR include symptoms (such as CHF, angina pectoris, syncope) with an abnormal or normal LV ejection fraction, no symptoms but an LV ejection fraction <50% at rest, and asymptomatic patients undergoing CABGS or surgery on the aorta or other heart valves. The class IIa indication for AVR is asymptomatic patients with severe AR with an LV ejection fraction >50% but a dilated LV with an LV end-systolic dimension >55 mm.

The operative mortality in elderly patients undergoing AVR in all comers (AS and AR) have been shown to be acceptable and that concomitant surgical procedures (such as CABG, mitral valve replacement/repair, aneurysm repair) increase the operative risk in older patients (122). LV dysfunction and urgency of surgery also seem to increase the operative risk (122). Of 450 patients with severe AR, 273 (61%) had an LV ejection fraction >50%, 134 (30%) had an LV ejection fraction of 35%–50%, and 43 patients (10%) had an LV ejection fraction <35% (123). The operative mortality was 3.7% for patients with a normal LV ejection fraction, 6.7% for patients with an LV ejection fraction of 35%–50%, and 14% for patients with an LV ejection fraction <35% (124). At 10-year follow-up, survival rates were 70% for patients with a normal LV ejection fraction, 56% for patients with an LV ejection fraction of 35%–50%, and 41% for patients with an LV ejection fraction <35% (123). However, the Cleveland Clinic has reported that for the patient with AR and severe LV dysfunction, AVR is the preferred treatment and can be performed with acceptable risk and late survival (124).

The postoperative survival is significantly dependent on LV ejection fraction and end-systolic dimension (or volume). Outcomes are better with an LV ejection fraction >55% or an LV end-systolic dimension (LVESD) <55 mm (indexed LVSD <25 mm/m^2) (125). Older patients undergoing AVR for severe AR have an excellent postoperative survival if the preoperative LV ejection fraction is normal (126). If LV systolic dysfunction was present for less than 1 year, patients also did well postoperatively. However, if the person with severe AR has an abnormal LV ejection fraction and impaired exercise tolerance and/or the presence of LV systolic dysfunction was for longer than 1 year, postoperative survival is poor (126). After AVR, women exhibit an excess late mortality, suggesting that surgical correction of severe chronic AR should be considered at an earlier stage in women (127).

Bioprosthesis is preferable to the mechanical prosthetic valve for AVR in older patients with severe AR as in older patients with valvular AS (57,58). Patients with porcine bioprosthesis may be treated with antiplatelet therapy alone unless they have atrial fibrillation, abnormal LV ejection fraction, previous thromboembolism, or a hypercoagulable state (Table 14.6) (22).

The change in LV function and dimensions after AVR seem to be dependent on LVESD prior to surgery. In a prospective study of 38 patients with chronic severe AR, LV chamber size and mass normalized in two thirds of the patients who underwent AVR (128). At 9-month follow-up after AVR, 58% of patients had a normal LV end-diastolic dimension, and 50% of patients had a normal LV mass. During further follow-up (18–56 months postoperatively) 66% of patients had a normal LV end-diastolic dimension and 68% of patients had a normal LV mass. The LV end-diastolic dimension normalized in 86% of patients with a preoperative LVESD ≤55 mm. A preoperative LVESD >55 mm was present in 81% of patients with postoperative persistent LV dilatation (128). Similarly, in 171 patients undergoing AVR for severe chronic AR, preoperative indexed LV end-systolic and end-diastolic dimensions were independent predictors of restored LV systolic function (93).

Transcatheter interventions for chronic AR

Surgical AVR is the gold standard therapeutic option for patients needing intervention for chronic AR. However, only 20% of patients with severe AR and LV ejection fraction of between 30% and 50% are referred for surgery, and 3% of patients with LV ejection fraction <30% undergo AVR (129). As mentioned earlier for AS, with the advent and the extreme rapid advancements in transcatheter valvular interventions, TAVR has emerged as a treatment alternative for intermediate and high-risk patients with AS. Use of TAVR to treat predominant aortic regurgitations has been challenged because of anatomical complexities. Noncalcified valve and hence lack of anchoring material, need for larger valve sizes, and the management of associated aortic root disease are particular concerns. There have been several reports of TAVR being performed in native AR. A systematic review of 13 reports that included 237 patients with native pure AR undergoing TAVR showed that successful device implantation ranged between 74% and 100%, and 7% of patients required implantation of a second valve, with 6 (2.5%) patients requiring conversion to surgical AVR. All-cause mortality at 30 days was 7%, an acceptable risk of early mortality in these high-risk patients (130). There are several newer TAVR options in development and research that are specific to AR (131) and may provide a great alternative option in patients who cannot undergo surgery.

UPDATE ON AS

In 2019, the annual number of TAVRs surpassed isolated surgical valve replacements (132). The decision regarding TAVR or SAVR is based upon multidisciplinary heart team discussions that incorporate clinical status, anatomy, frailty, and patient preference. This also forms a key discussion regarding lifetime management of aortic valve disease with potential valve-in-valve interventions following initial valve failure. A nationwide database analysis of 74,995 octogenarians showed that in patients with AS and heart failure, the in-hospital mortality with TAVR was five times lower compared to SAVR (1.8% vs. 9.8%) (133).

Valve choice based on age

Goldstone et al. concluded in their retrospective report of 2017 that the benefit of mechanical AVR persisted until the age of 55 years of age (134). The use of mechanical AVR has declined significantly over the last couple of decades in an effort to avoid lifelong anticoagulation in patients. In older persons, factors such as patient preference, frailty, increasing age, porcelain aorta, and prior cardiac surgery tend to favor TAVR. The rate of structural valve deterioration decreases with increasing age, thereby making the choice of a bioprosthetic aortic valve much easier.

Landmark trials such as the Placement of Aortic Transcatheter Valves (PARTNER1B) showed superiority to medical therapy for severe AS. TAVR was found to be noninferior to SAVR in PARTNER 1A and was superior in the US CoreValve high-risk study. PARTNER2 and Surgical Replacement and Transcatheter Aortic Valve Implantation (SURTAVI) trials later also showed noninferiority of TAVR to SAVR in intermediate risk patients. Finally, the PARTNER3 and Evolut LR trials paved the way for TAVR being noninferior to SAVR in low risk patients.

In the intermediate group trial of PARTNER 2 and SURTAVI, the mean STS-PROM (Society of Thoracic Surgery Predicted Risk of Mortality) were 5.8% and 4.5%, respectively. In PARTNER 2 and SURTAVI, the 2-year all-cause mortality was 16.3% and 11.4%, respectively, with no difference to SAVR. The use of TAVR in low surgical risk patients (STS-PROM <4%) showed superiority of TAVR to SAVR for clinical outcomes at 1 year in both PARTNER3 and Evolut LR patients, and the outcomes are similar at 4 years of follow-up for Evolut and 5 years of follow-up for PARTNER3. The Nordic Aortic Valve Intervention (NOTION) trial offers the longest follow-up at 10 years showing no differences in all-cause mortality, stroke, or MI compared to SAVR, and, moreover, TAVR appears to show lower rates of structural valve deterioration and valve dysfunction. Most recently there has been some data in patients with asymptomatic severe AS in the form of a multicenter randomized trial EARLY TAVR (Evaluation of TAVR Compared to Surveillance for Patients With Asymptomatic Severe Aortic Stenosis) that randomized 901 patients into surveillance versus early intervention and showed significant improvement in primary outcome of death, stroke, or unplanned hospitalization of 26.8% in TAVR group versus 45.3% in the surveillance group over a median follow up of 3.8 years.

There are conflicting data on percutaneous revascularization for coronary artery disease in patients undergoing TAVR. The first trial on this topic, ACTIVATION (PercutAneous Coronary inTervention prIor to transcatheter aortic VAlve implantaTION), had a follow-up of 1 year and showed similar rates of deaths and rehospitalization in patients with or without PCI. Another propensity-matched study followed these patients for 2 years and found patients who required PCI had higher mortality of 10.7% versus 4.6%. However, the latest data from the NOTION-3 trial, which randomized 455 TAVR patients into PCI and non-PCI groups, showed at a median follow-up of 2 years that the PCI group had MACE, defined as death, myocardial infarction, or urgent revascularization, of 26% versus 36% for those who did not have PCI. However, bleeding was 28% in the PCI group versus 20% in the non-PCI group. Further data from the

TAVI PCI Trial (Optimal Timing of Transcatheter Aortic Valve Implantation and Percutaneous Coronary Intervention) and COMPLETE TAVR (Staged Complete Revascularization for Coronary Artery Disease vs Medical Management Alone in Patients With AS Undergoing Transcatheter Aortic Valve Replacement) are expected to shed more light on this topic (135,136).

Nearly one third of severe aortic stenosis patients have concomitant mitral regurgitation (MR), and the degree of MR often improves after TAVR. However, a staged percutaneous treatment of MR can be performed if it remains severe in a symptomatic patient. Transthyretin cardiac amyloidosis has been found with increasing frequency in patients undergoing TAVR in as many as 15% of patients. With higher mortality associated with these patients, small studies still show safety and efficacy of TAVR in these patients (137,138).

A significant number of older people have concomitant need for oral anticoagulation, most commonly due to atrial fibrillation. Management of anticoagulation post-TAVR involves anticoagulation management. The POPular PAUSE TAVI (Periprocedural Continuation Versus Interruption of Oral Anticoagulant Drugs During Transcatheter Aortic Valve Implantation) trial looked at this question of stopping anticoagulation versus continuation of anticoagulant therapy in patients undergoing TAVR, but it failed to reach non inferiority margin with composite outcome for death, stroke, myocardial infarction, and vascular complications or bleeding were 16.5% in patients who continued versus 14.8% who did not (139). There are limited data for anticoagulation after TAVR in patients without an indication for anticoagulation based upon the GALILEO (Global Study Comparing a Rivaroxaban-based Antithrombotic Strategy to an Antiplatelet-based Strategy After TAVR to Optimize Clinical Outcomes) trial where 1644 patients were given rivaroxaban 10 mg with aspirin or aspirin alone for the first 3 months. The trial was prematurely stopped due to high rates of death and thromboembolic events in the rivaroxaban group, with also an increased risk of bleeding. In the substudy of this trial, however, there were lower rates of subclinical leaflet motion abnormalities of 2.1% versus 10.9% compared to the antiplatelet group (140). In patients without the need for anticoagulation, the general recommendation is to use single antiplatelet therapy based upon the POPular TAVI (Antithrombotic Therapy After Transcatheter Aortic Valve Implantation in Patients With a Long-Term Indication for Oral Anticoagulation) trial that compared aspirin and clopidogrel with aspirin alone and showed 26.6% bleeding with DAPT compared to 15.1% with aspirin alone at 1 year (141).

UPDATE ON AR

AR occurs mostly due to dilatation of the ascending aorta and aortic root due to increasing age, hypertension, and aortic diseases. Approximately 13% of isolated native left-sided valvular heart disease patients have AR, and it comprises about 2% of persons above 70 years of age. The transcatheter therapies to treat AR are challenging due to difficulty in proper positioning and, most importantly, stability of the transcatheter heart valve that can lead to paravalvular leak, conduction disorder, valve embolization, or annular rupture. There have been off-label attempts to secure these prostheses by oversizing the valves by 10%–20% to increase radial strength. On-label devices use secured fixation via a clip or a clasper mechanism. In severe symptomatic AR, TAVR using the Trilogy transcatheter heart valve by the name of JenaValve was tested in a single-arm study that showed promising results. Cardiac mortality was 7.8% at 1 year and 15.4% at 2 years, with nondisabling stroke rates of 4.1% and disabling stroke rates of 1.7% at 1 year and 2.3% at 2 years. Valve hemodynamics remained promising with a preserved orifice area over 2 years and PVL dropping from 8.2% at 1 year to 4.4% at year 2. The randomized trial of this valve against surgery in the ARTIST trial is eagerly awaited. AR after TAVR can occur due to poor tolerance of volume overload due to severe left ventricular diastolic dysfunction that is associated with worse outcomes. A retrospective study of 164 patients compared SAVR with TAVR and found similar outcomes in patients with perivalvular regurgitation. Perivalvular regurgitation led to worse outcomes in patients with lower or intermediate STS-PROM risk scores but not in those with high risk (142,143).

REFERENCES

1. Aronow WS, Schwartz KS, Koenigsberg M. Correlation of aortic cuspal and aortic root disease with aortic systolic ejection murmurs and with mitral annular calcium in persons older than 62 years in a long-term health care facility. *Am J Cardiol* 1986; *58*: 651–652.
2. Aronow WS, Kronzon I. Prevalence and severity of valvular aortic stenosis determined by Doppler echocardiography and its association with echocardiographic and electrocardiographic left ventricular hypertrophy and physical signs of aortic stenosis in elderly patients. *Am J Cardiol* 1991; *67*: 776–777.
3. Lindroos M, Kupari M, Heikkila J et al. Prevalence of aortic valve abnormalities in the elderly: An echocardiographic study of a random population sample. *J Am Coll Cardiol* 1993; *21*: 1220–1225.
4. Aronow WS, Ahn C, Kronzon I. Association of mitral annular calcium and of aortic cuspal calcium with coronary artery disease in older patients. *Am J Cardiol* 1999; *84*: 1084–1085.
5. Aronow WS, Ahn C, Shirani J et al. Comparison of frequency of new coronary events in older subjects with and without valvular aortic sclerosis. *Am J Cardiol* 1999; *83*: 599–600.

6. Aronow WS, Ahn C, Kronzon I. Comparison of echocardiographic abnormalities in African-American, Hispanic, and white men and women aged >60 years. *Am J Cardiol* 2001; *87*: 1131–1133.
7. Otto CM, Kuusisto J, Reichenbach DD et al. Characterization of the early lesion of "degenerative" valvular aortic stenosis. *Circulation* 1994; *90*: 844–853.
8. Stewart BF, Siscovick D, Lind BK et al. Clinical factors associated with calcific aortic valve disease. *J Am Coll Cardiol* 1997; *29*: 630–634.
9. Aronow WS, Schwartz KS, Koenigsberg M. Correlation of serum lipids, calcium, and phosphorus, diabetes mellitus and history of systemic hypertension with presence or absence of calcified or thickened aortic cusps or root in elderly patients. *Am J Cardiol* 1987; *59*: 998–999.
10. Lindroos M, Kupari M, Valvanne J et al. Factors associated with calcific aortic valve degeneration in the elderly. *Eur Heart J* 1994; *15*: 865–870.
11. Chen HY, Dufresne L, Burr H et al. Association of LPA variants with aortic stenosis: A large-scale study using diagnostic and procedural codes from electronic health records. *JAMA Cardiol* 2018; *3*: 18–23.
12. Aronow WS, Kronzon I, Schoenfeld MR. Prevalence of extracranial carotid arterial disease and of valvular aortic stenosis and their association in the elderly. *Am J Cardiol* 1995; *75*: 304–305.
13. Aronow WS, Ahn C, Kronzon I. Association of valvular aortic stenosis with symptomatic peripheral arterial disease in older persons. *Am J Cardiol* 2001; *88*: 1046–1047.
14. Nair CK, Aronow WS, Stokke K et al. Cardiac conduction defects in patients older than 60 years with aortic stenosis with and without mitral annular calcium. *Am J Cardiol* 1984; *53*: 169–172.
15. Nassimiha D, Aronow WS, Ahn C et al. Rate of progression of valvular aortic stenosis in persons >60 years. *Am J Cardiol* 2001; *87*: 807–809.
16. Nassimiha D, Aronow WS, Ahn C et al. Association of coronary risk factors with progression of valvular aortic stenosis in older persons. *Am J Cardiol* 2001; *87*: 1313–1314.
17. Aronow WS, Ahn C, Kronzon I et al. Association of coronary risk factors and use of statins with progression of mild valvular aortic stenosis in older persons. *Am J Cardiol* 2001; *88*: 693–695.
18. Novaro GM, Tiong IY, Pearce GL et al. Effect of hydroxymethylglutaryl coenzyme A reductase inhibitors on the progression of calcific aortic stenosis. *Circulation* 2001; *104*: 2205–2209.
19. Bellamy MF, Pellikka PA, Klarich KW et al. Association of cholesterol levels, hydroxymethylglutaryl coenzyme-A reductase inhibitor treatment, and progression of aortic stenosis in the community. *J Am Coll Cardiol* 2002; *40*: 1723–1730.
20. Rossebo AB, Pedersen TR, Boman K et al. Intensive lipid lowering with simvastatin and ezetimibe in aortic stenosis. *N Engl J Med* 2008; *359*: 1343–1356.
21. Chan KL, Teo K, Dumesnil JG et al. Effect of Lipid lowering with rosuvastatin on progression of aortic stenosis: Results of the aortic stenosis progression observation: Measuring effects of rosuvastatin (ASTRONOMER) trial. *Circulation* 2010; *121*(*2*): 306–314.
22. Nishimura RA, Otto CM, Bonow RO et al. 2014 AHA/ACC guideline for the management of patients with valvular heart disease: A report of the American College of Cardiology/American Heart Association Task Force on Practice Guidelines. *J Am Coll Cardiol* 2014; *63*(*22*): 2438–2488.
23. Villari B, Vassalli G, Schneider J et al. Age dependency of left ventricular diastolic function in pressure overload hypertrophy. *J Am Coll Cardiol* 1997; *29*: 181–186.
24. Carroll JD, Carroll EP, Feldman T et al. Sex-associated differences in left ventricular function in aortic stenosis of the elderly. *Circulation* 1992; *86*: 1099–1107.
25. Vekshtein VI, Alexander RW, Yeung AC et al. Coronary atherosclerosis is associated with left ventricular dysfunction and dilatation in aortic stenosis. *Circulation* 1990; *82*: 2068–2074.
26. Aronow WS, Ahn C, Kronzon I et al. Prognosis of congestive heart failure in patients aged >62 years with unoperated severe valvular aortic stenosis. *Am J Cardiol* 1993; *72*: 846–848.
27. Hess OM, Villari B, Krayenbuehl HP. Diastolic dysfunction in aortic stenosis. *Circulation* 1993; *87*: 73–76.
28. Aronow WS, Ahn C, Shirani J et al. Comparison of frequency of new coronary events in older persons with mild, moderate, and severe valvular aortic stenosis with those without aortic stenosis. *Am J Cardiol* 1998; *81*: 647–649.
29. Julius BK, Spillmann M, Vassalli G et al. Angina pectoris in patients with aortic stenosis and normal coronary arteries. Mechanisms and pathophysiological concepts. *Circulation* 1997; *95*: 892–898.
30. Dimitriadis Z, Wiemer M, Scholtz W et al. Sleep-disordered breathing in patients undergoing transfemoral aortic valve implantation for severe aortic stenosis. *Clin Res Cardiol* 2013; *102*(*12*): 895–8903.
31. Braunwald E. On the natural history of severe aortic stenosis. *J Am Coll Cardiol* 1990; *15*: 1018–1020.
32. Loscalzo J. From clinical observation to mechanism–Heyde's syndrome. *N Engl J Med* 2012; *367*(*20*): 1954–196.
33. Aronow WS, Kronzon I. Correlation of prevalence and severity of valvular aortic stenosis determined by continuous-wave Doppler echocardiography with physical signs of aortic stenosis in patients aged 62 to 100 years with aortic systolic ejection murmurs. *Am J Cardiol* 1987; *60*: 399–401.

34. Folland ED, Kriegel BJ, Henderson WG et al. Implications of third heart sounds in patients with valvular heart disease. *N Engl J Med* 1992; *327*: 458–462.
35. Greve AM, Boman K, Gohlke-Baerwolf C et al. Clinical implications of electrocardiographic left ventricular strain and hypertrophy in asymptomatic patients with aortic stenosis. The Simvastatin and Ezetimibe in Aortic Stenosis study. *Circulation* 2012; *125*: 346–353.
36. Thompson R, Mitchell A, Ahmed M et al. Conduction defects in aortic valve disease. *Am Heart J* 1979; *98(1)*: 3–10.
37. Aronow WS, Epstein S, Koenigsberg M et al. Usefulness of echocardiographic abnormal left ventricular ejection fraction, paroxysmal ventricular tachycardia and complex ventricular arrhythmias in predicting new coronary events in patients over 62 years of age. *Am J Cardiol* 1988; *61*: 1349–1351.
38. Come PC, Riley MF, McKay RG et al. Echocardiographic assessment of aortic valve area in elderly patients with aortic stenosis and of changes of valve area after percutaneous balloon valvuloplasty. *J Am Coll Cardiol* 1987; *10*: 115–124.
39. Shah PM, Graham BM. Management of aortic stenosis: Is cardiac catheterization necessary? *Am J Cardiol* 1991; *67*: 1031–1032.
40. Nassimiha D, Aronow WS, Ahn C et al. Comparison of aortic valve area determined by Doppler echocardiography and cardiac catheterization in 75 older patients with valvular aortic stenosis. *Cardiovasc Rev and Reports* 2000; *21*: 507–509.
41. Pellikka PA, Nishimura RA, Bailey KR et al. The natural history of adults with asymptomatic hemodynamically significant aortic stenosis. *J Am Coll Cardiol* 1990; *15*: 1012–1017.
42. Rosenhek R, Binder T, Porenta G et al. Predictors of outcome in severe, asymptomatic aortic stenosis. *N Engl J Med* 2000; *343*: 611–617.
43. Kelly TA, Rothbart RM, Cooper CM et al. Comparison of outcome of asymptomatic to symptomatic patients older than 20 years of age with valvular aortic stenosis. *Am J Cardiol* 1988; *61*: 123–130.
44. Livanainen AM, Lindroos M, Tilvis R et al. Natural history of aortic valve stenosis of varying severity in the elderly. *Am J Cardiol* 1996; *78*: 97–101.
45. Otto CM, Lind BK, Kitzman DW et al. Association of aortic-valve sclerosis with cardiovascular mortality and morbidity in the elderly. *N Engl J Med* 1999; *341*: 142–147.
46. Kennedy KD, Nishimura RA, Holmes Dr Jr et al. Natural history of moderate aortic stenosis. *J Am Coll Cardiol* 1991; *17*: 313–319.
47. Monin J-L, Quere J-P, Monchi M et al. Low-gradient aortic stenosis. Operative risk stratification and predictors for long-term outcome: A multicenter study using dobutamine stress hemodynamics. *Circulation* 2003; *108*: 319–324.
48. Rieck ÅE, Cramariuc D, Boman K et al. Hypertension in aortic stenosis: Implications for left ventricular structure and cardiovascular events. *Hypertension* 2012; *60*: 90–97.
49. Brown ML, Pellikka PA, Schaff HV et al. The benefits of early valve replacement in asymptomatic patients with severe aortic stenosis. *J Thorac Cardiovasc Surg* 2008; *135*: 308–315.
50. Kearney LG, Ord M, Buxton BF et al. Progression of aortic stenosis in elderly patients over long-term follow up. *Int J Cardiol* 2013; *167(4)*: 1226.
51. Pai RG, Kapoor N, Bansal RC et al. Malignant natural history of asymptomatic severe aortic stenosis: Benefit of aortic valve replacement. *Ann Thorac Surg* 2006; *82*: 2116–2122.
52. Kang D-H, Park S-J, Rim JH et al. Early surgery versus conventional treatment in asymptomatic very severe aortic stenosis. *Circulation* 2010; *121*: 1502–1509.
53. Freed BH, Sugeng L, Furlong K et al. Reasons for nonadherence to guidelines for aortic valve replacement in patients with very severe aortic stenosis and potential solutions. *Am J Cardiol* 2010; *105*: 1339–1342.
54. Jander N, Minners J, Holme I et al. Outcome of patients with low-gradient "severe" aortic stenosis and preserved ejection fraction. *Circulation* 2011; *123*: 887–895.
55. Belkin RN, Khalique O, Aronow WS et al. Outcomes and survival with aortic valve replacement c compared with medical therapy in patients with low-, moderate-, and severe-gradient severe aortic stenosis and normal left ventricular ejection fraction. *Echocardiography* 2011; *28*: 378–387.
56. Hammermeister K, Sethi GK, Henderson WG et al. Outcomes 15 years after valve replacement with a mechanical versus a bioprosthetic valve: Final report of the Veterans Affairs Randomized Trial. *J Am Coll Cardiol* 2000; *36*: 1152–1158.
57. Huang G, Rahimtoola SH. Prosthetic heart valve. *Circulation* 2011; *123*: 2602–2605.
58. Asimakopoulos G, Edwards M-B, Taylor KM. Aortic valve replacement in patients 80 years of age and older. Survival and cause of death based on 1100 cases: Collective results from the UK Heart Valve Registry. *Circulation* 1997; *96*: 3403–3408.
59. Unic D, Leacche M, Paul S et al. Early and late results of isolated and combined heart valve surgery in patients >80 years of age. *Am J Cardiol* 2005; *95*: 1500–1503.
60. Levy F, Garayalde E, Quere JP et al. Prognostic value of preoperative atrial fibrillation in patients with aortic stenosis and low ejection fraction having aortic valve replacement. *Am J Cardiol* 2006; *98*: 809–811.

61. Villari B, Vassalli G, Monrad ES et al. Normalization of diastolic dysfunction in aortic stenosis late after valve replacement. *Circulation* 1995; *91*: 2353–2358.
62. Kuhl HP, Franke A, Puschmann D et al. Regression of left ventricular mass one year after aortic valve replacement for pure severe aortic stenosis. *Am J Cardiol* 2002; *89*: 408–413.
63. Hoffman A, Burckhardt D. Patients at risk for cardiac death late after aortic valve replacement. *Am Heart J* 1990; *120*: 1142–1147.
64. Connolly HM, Oh JK, Orszulak TA et al. Aortic valve replacement for aortic stenosis with severe left ventricular dysfunction. Prognostic indicators. *Circulation* 1997; *95*: 2395–2400.
65. O'Keefe JH Jr, Vlietstra RE, Bailey KR et al. Natural history of candidates for balloon aortic valvuloplasty. *Mayo Clin Proc* 1987; *62*: 986–991.
66. Cheitlin MD. Severe aortic stenosis in the sick octogenarian. A clear indicator for balloon valvuloplasty as the initial procedure. *Circulation* 1989; *80*: 1906–1908.
67. Casey T. ACC, STS provide updated results on TAVR procedures in the US. *Cardiovascular Business*. http://www.cardiovascularbusiness.com/topics/coronary-intervention-surgery/acc-sts-provide-updated-results-tavr-procedures-us. (Assessed December 13, 2016).
68. Leon MB, Smith CR, Mack M et al. Transcatheter aortic-valve implantation for aortic stenosis in patients who cannot undergo surgery: The PARTNER trial investigators. *N Engl J Med* 2010; *363*: 1597–1607.
69. Makkar RR, Fontana GP, Jilaihawi H et al. Transcatheter aortic-valve replacement for inoperable severe aortic stenosis: The PARTNER trial investigators. *N Engl J Med* 2012; *366*: 1696–1704.
70. Smith CR, Leon MB, Mack MJ et al. Transcatheter versus surgical aortic-valve replacement in high-risk patients: The PARTNER trial investigators. *N Engl J Med* 2011; *364*: 2187–2198.
71. Reynolds MR, Magnuson EA, Lei Y et al. Health-related quality of life after transcatheter aortic valve replacement in inoperable patients with severe aortic stenosis. *Circulation* 2011; *124*: 1964–1972.
72. Kapadia SR, Tuzcu EM, Makkar RR et al. Long-term outcomes of inoperable patients with aortic stenosis randomly assigned to transcatheter aortic valve replacement or standard therapy. *Circulation* 2014; *130(17)*: 1483–9142.
73. Kapadia SR, Leon MB, Makkar RR et al. 5-year outcomes of transcatheter aortic valve replacement compared with standard treatment for patients with inoperable aortic stenosis (PARTNER 1): A randomised controlled trial. *Lancet* 2015; *385(9986)*: 2485–2491.
74. Wenaweser P, Pilgrim T, Kadner A et al. Clinical outcomes of patients with severe aortic stenosis at increased surgical risk according to treatment modality. *J Am Coll Cardiol* 2011; *58*: 2151–2162.
75. Kodali SK, Williams MR, Smith CR et al. Two-year outcomes after transcatheter or surgical aortic-valve replacement. *N Engl J Med* 2012; *366*: 1686–1695.
76. Mack MJ, Leon MB, Smith CR et al. 5-year outcomes of transcatheter aortic valve replacement or surgical aortic valve replacement for high surgical risk patients with aortic stenosis (PARTNER 1): A randomised controlled trial. *Lancet* 2015; *385(9986)*: 2477–2484.
77. Nishimura RA, Otto CM, Bonow RO et al. 2017 AHA/ACC focused update of the 2014 AHA/ACC guideline for the management of patients with valvular heart disease: A report of the American College of Cardiology/American Heart Association Task Force on Clinical Practice Guidelines. *J Am Coll Cardiol* 2017; *70(2)*: 252–289.
78. Reardon MJ, Van Mieghem NM, Popma JJ et al. Surgical or transcatheter aortic-valve replacement in intermediate-risk patients. *N Engl J Med* 2017; *376*: 1321–1331.
79. Leon MB, Smith CR, Mack MJ et al. Transcatheter or surgical aortic-valve replacement in intermediate-risk patients. *N Engl J Med* 2016; *374*: 1609–1620.
80. Hirji SA, Ramirez-Del Val F, Kolkailah AA et al. Outcomes of surgical and transcatheter aortic valve replacement in the octogenarians-surgery still the gold standard? *Ann Cardiothorac Surg* 2017; *6(5)*: 453–462.
81. Sankaramangalam K, Banerjee K, Kandregula K et al. Impact of coronary artery disease on 30-day and 1-year mortality in patients undergoing transcatheter aortic valve replacement: A meta-analysis. *J Am Heart Assoc* 2017; *6(10)*: e006092.
82. Stefanini GG, Stortecky S, Cao D et al. Coronary artery disease severity and aortic stenosis: Clinical outcomes according to SYNTAX score in patients undergoing transcatheter aortic valve implantation. *Eur Heart J* 2014; *35*: 2530–2540.
83. D'Ascenzo F, Conrotto F, Giordana F et al. Mid-term prognostic value of coronary artery disease in patients undergoing transcatheter aortic valve implantation: A meta-analysis of adjusted observational results. *Int J Cardiol* 2013; *168*: 2528–2532.
84. Chakravarty T, Sharma R, Abramowitz Y et al. Outcomes in patients with transcatheter aortic valve replacement and left main stenting. *J Am Coll Cardiol* 2016; *67*: 951–960.
85. Singh V, Rodriguez AP, Thakkar B et al. Comparison of outcomes of transcatheter aortic valve replacement plus percutaneous coronary intervention versus transcatheter aortic valve replacement alone in the United States. *Am J Cardiol* 2016; *118*: 1698–1704.
86. Elhmidi Y, Bleiziffer S, Deutsch MA et al. Acute kidney injury after transcatheter aortic valve

implantation: Incidence, predictors and impact on mortality. *Arch Cardiovasc Dis* 2014; *107(2)*: 133–139.
87. Gupta T, Goel K, Kolte D et al. Association of chronic kidney disease with in-hospital outcomes of transcatheter aortic valve replacement. *JACC Cardiovasc Interv* 2017; *10(20)*: 2050–2060.
88. Siontis GC, Jüni P, Pilgrim T et al. Predictors of permanent pacemaker implantation in patients with severe aortic stenosis undergoing TAVR: A meta-analysis. *J Am Coll Cardiol* 2014; *64*: 129–140.
89. Ussia GP, Scarabelli M, Mule M et al. Dual antiplatelet therapy versus aspirin alone in patients undergoing transcatheter aortic valve implantation. *Am J Cardiol* 2011; *108*: 1772–1776.
90. Theard MA, Bhatia SJ, Plappert T et al. Doppler echocardiographic study of the frequency and severity of aortic regurgitation in hypertrophic cardiomyopathy. *Am J Cardiol* 1987; *60*: 1143–1147.
91. Aronow WS, Kronzon I. Correlation of prevalence and severity of aortic regurgitation detected by pulsed Doppler echocardiography with the murmur of aortic regurgitation in elderly patients in a long-term health care facility. *Am J Cardiol* 1989; *63*: 128–129.
92. Klein AL, Burstow DJ, Tajik AJ et al. Age-related prevalence of valvular regurgitation in normal subjects: A comprehensive color flow examination of 118 volunteers. *J Am Soc Echocardiogr* 1990; *3(1)*: 54–63.
93. Gaasch WH, Sundaram M, Meyer TE. Managing asymptomatic patients with chronic aortic regurgitation. *Chest* 1997; *111*: 1702–1709.
94. Greenberg B, Massie B, Thomas D et al. Association between the exercise ejection fraction response and systolic wall stress in patients with chronic aortic insufficiency. *Circulation* 1985; *71*: 458–465.
95. Aronow WS, Ahn C, Kronzon I et al. Prognosis of patients with heart failure and unoperated severe aortic valvular regurgitation and relation to ejection fraction. *Am J Cardiol* 1994; *74*: 286–288.
96. Mann T, McLaurin LP, Grossman W et al. Assessing the hemodynamic severity of acute aortic regurgitation due to infective endocarditis. *N Engl J Med* 1975; *293*: 108–113.
97. Nitenberg A, Foult JM, Antony I et al. Coronary flow and resistance reserve in patients with chronic aortic regurgitation, angina pectoris and normal coronary arteries. *J Am Coll Cardiol* 1988; *11(3)*: 478–486.
98. Massell BF, Amezcua FJ, Czoniczer G. Prognosis of patients with pure or predominant aortic regurgitation in the absence of surgery (abstract). *Circulation* 1966; *34*: 164.
99. Roberts WC, Day PJ. Electrocardiographic observations in clinically isolated, pure, chronic, severe aortic regurgitation: Analysis of 30 necropsy patients aged 19 to 65 years. *Am J Cardiol* 1985; *55*: 431–438.
100. Aronow WS, Ahn C, Kronzon I et al. Congestive heart failure, coronary events, and atherothrombotic brain infarction in elderly blacks and whites with systemic hypertension and with and without echocardiographic and electrocardiographic evidence of left ventricular hypertrophy. *Am J Cardiol* 1991; *67*: 295–299.
101. Henry WL, Bonow RO, Borer JS et al. Observations on the optimum time for operative intervention for aortic regurgitation. I. Evaluation of the results of aortic valve replacement in symptomatic patients. *Circulation* 1980; *61*: 471–483.
102. Gaasch WH, Carroll JD, Levine HJ et al. Chronic aortic regurgitation: Prognostic value of left ventricular end-systolic dimension and end-diastolic radius/thickness ratio. *J Am Coll Cardiol* 1983; *1*: 775–782.
103. Beyer RW, Ramirez M, Josephson MA et al. Correlation of continuous-wave assessment of chronic aortic regurgitation with hemodynamics and angiography. *Am J Cardiol* 1987; *60*: 852–856.
104. Perry GJ, Helmcke F, Nanda NC et al. Evaluation of aortic insufficiency by Doppler color flow mapping. *J Am Coll Cardiol* 1987; *9*: 952–959.
105. Sondergaard L, Lindvig K, Hildebrandt P et al. Quantification of aortic regurgitation by magnetic resonance velocity mapping. *Am Heart J* 1993; *125*: 1081–1090.
106. Dexter L. Evaluation of the results of cardiac surgery. In: Jones AM, ed. *Modern Trends in Cardiology*, Vol. 2. New York: Appleton-Century-Crofts, 1969: pp. 311–333.
107. Hegglin R, Scheu H, Rothlin M. Aortic insufficiency. *Circulation* 1968; *38*: 77–92.
108. Bonow RO, Lakatos E, Maron BJ et al. Serial long-term assessment of the natural history of asymptomatic patients with chronic aortic regurgitation and normal left ventricular systolic function. *Circulation* 1991; *84*: 1625–1635.
109. Parker MVV, Mittleman MA, Waksmonski CA et al. Pulmonary hypertension and long-term mortality in aortic and mitral regurgitation. *Am J Med* 2010; *123*: 1043–1048.
110. Lalani T, Cabell CH, Benjamin DK et al. Analysis of the impact of early surgery on in-hospital mortality of native valve endocarditis: Use of propensity score and instrumental variable methods to adjust for treatment-selection bias. *Circulation* 2010; *121*: 1005–1013.
111. Otto C, Bonow RO. Valvular heart disease. In: Mann DL et al., eds. *Braunwald's Heart Disease: A Textbook of Cardiovascular Medicine*, 10th ed. Philadelphia, PA: Elsevier Saunders, 2015: pp. 1446–1523.

112. Alsip SG, Blackstone EH, Kirklin JW et al. Indications for cardiac surgery in patients with active infective endocarditis. *Am J Med* 1985; *78*: 138–148.
113. Karp RB. Role of surgery in infective endocarditis. *Cardiovasc Clin* 1987; *17*: 141–162.
114. Grayburn PA. Vasodilator therapy for chronic aortic and mitral regurgitation. *Am J Med Sci* 2000; *320*: 202–208.
115. Scognamiglio R, Rahimtoola SH, Fasoli G et al. Nifedipine in asymptomatic patients with severe aortic regurgitation and normal left ventricular function. *N Engl J Med* 1994; *331*: 689–694.
116. Scognamiglio R, Fasoli G, Ponchia A et al. Long-term nifedipine unloading therapy in asymptomatic patients with chronic severe aortic regurgitation. *J Am Coll Cardiol* 1990; *16*: 424–429.
117. Elder DH, Wei L, Szwejkowski BR et al. The impact of renin-angiotensin-aldosterone system blockade on heart failure outcomes and mortality in patients identified to have aortic regurgitation: A large population cohort study. *J Am Coll Cardiol* 2011; *58*: 2084–2091.
118. Evangelista A, Tornos P, Sambola A et al. Long-term vasodilator therapy in patients with severe aortic regurgitation. *N Engl J Med* 2005; *353*: 1342–1349.
119. Shores J, Berger KR, Murphy EA et al. Progression of aortic dilatation and the benefit of long-term β-adrenergic blockade in Marfan's syndrome. *N Engl J Med* 1994; *330*: 1335–1341.
120. Brooke BS, Habashi JP, Judge DP et al. Angiotensin II blockade and aortic-root dilation in Marfan's syndrome. *N Engl J Med* 2008; *358*: 2787–2795.
121. McDonald GR, Schaff HV, Pyeritz RE et al. Surgical management of patients with the Marfan syndrome and dilatation of the ascending aorta. *J Thorac Cardiovasc Surg* 1981; *81*: 180–186.
122. Freeman WK, Schaff HV, O'Brien PC et al. Cardiac surgery in the octogenarian: Perioperative outcome and clinical follow-up. *J Am Coll Cardiol* 1991; *18*(*1*): 29–35.
123. Chaliki HP, Mohty D, Avierinos JF et al. Outcomes after aortic valve replacement in patients with severe aortic regurgitation and markedly reduced left ventricular function. *Circulation* 2002; *106*: 2687–2693.
124. Bhudia SK, McCarthy PM, Kumpati GS et al. Improved outcomes after aortic valve surgery for chronic aortic regurgitation with severe left ventricular dysfunction. *J Am Coll Cardiol* 2007; *49*: 1465–1471.
125. Dujardin KS, Enriquez-Sarano M, Schaff HV et al. Mortality and morbidity of aortic regurgitation in clinical practice: A long-term follow-up study. *Circulation* 1999; *99*: 1851–1857.
126. Turina J, Milincic J, Seifert B et al. Valve replacement in chronic aortic regurgitation. True predictors of survival after extended follow-up. *Circulation* 1998; *98*: II100–II107.
127. Klodas E, Enriquez-Sarano M, Tajik AJ et al. Surgery for aortic regurgitation in women. Contrasting indications and outcomes compared with men. *Circulation* 1996; *94*: 2472–2478.
128. Roman MJ, Klein L, Devereux RB et al. Reversal of left ventricular dilatation, hypertrophy, and dysfunction by valve replacement in aortic regurgitation. *Am Heart J* 1989; *118*: 553–563.
129. Iung B, Baron G, Butchart EG et al. A prospective survey of patients with valvular heart disease in Europe: The Euro Heart Survey on valvular heart disease. *Eur Heart J* 2003; *24*: 1231–1243.
130. Franzone A, Piccolo R, Siontis GC et al. Transcatheter aortic valve replacement for the treatment of pure native aortic valve regurgitation: A systematic review. *JACC Cardiovasc Interv* 2016; *9*: 2308–2317.
131. Webb JG, Htun N. Transcatheter options for the treatment of noncalcified aortic regurgitation. *JACC Cardiovasc Interv* 2015; *8*(*14*): 1850–1853.
132. Carroll JD, Mack MJ, Vemulapalli S et al. STS-ACC TVT registry of transcatheter aortic valve replacement. *J Am Coll Cardiol* 2020; *76*: 2492–2516.
133. Sattar Y, Song D, Almas T et al. Cardiovascular outcomes and trends of Transcatheter vs. Surgical aortic valve replacement among octogenarians with heart failure: A Propensity Matched national cohort analysis. *IJC Heart & Vasc* 2022; *42*: 101119.
134. Goldstone AB, Chiu P, Baiocchi M et al. Mechanical or biologic prostheses for aortic-valve and mitral-valve replacement. *N Engl J Med* 2017; *377*: 1847–1857.
135. Ito S, Oh JK. Aortic stenosis: New insights in diagnosis, treatment, and prevention. *Korean Circ J* 2022; *52*: 721–736.
136. Caminiti R, Ielasi A, Vetta G et al. Percutaneous coronary intervention before or after transcatheter aortic valve replacement: A systematic review and meta-analysis involving 1531 patients. *J Clin Med* 2024; *13*: 3521.
137. Ferruzzi GJ, Silverio A, Giordano A et al. Prognostic impact of mitral regurgitation before and after transcatheter aortic valve replacement in patients with severe low-flow, low-gradient aortic stenosis. *J Am Heart Assoc* 2023; *12*: e029553.
138. Terentes-Printzios D, Antonopoulos AS, Omer M et al. Cardiac amyloidosis remains significantly underdiagnosed in patients undergoing TAVR: Analysis of National Inpatient Sample. *Amyloid* 2023; *30*: 246–247.
139. van Ginkel DJ, Bor WL, Aarts HM et al.. Continuation versus Interruption of Oral Anticoagulation during TAVI. *N Engl J Med* 2024; online ahead of print.
140. Dangas GD, Tijssen JG, Wöhrle J et al. A controlled trial of rivaroxaban after transcatheter aortic-valve replacement. *N Engl J Med* 2020; *382*: 120–129.
141. Brouwer J, Nijenhuis VJ, Delewi R et al. Aspirin with or without clopidogrel after transcatheter

aortic-valve implantation. *N Engl J Med* 2020; *38*: 1447–1457.

142. Liu R, Fu Z, Jiang Z et al. Transcatheter aortic valve replacement for aortic regurgitation: A systematic review and meta-analysis. *ESC Heart Fail* 2024. online ahead of print.

143. Vahl TP, Thourani VH, Makkar RR et al. Transcatheter aortic valve implantation in patients with high-risk symptomatic native aortic regurgitation (ALIGN-AR): A prospective, multicentre, single-arm study. *The Lancet* 2024; *403(10435)*: 1451–1459.

15

Mitral regurgitation, mitral stenosis, mitral annular calcification, and tricuspid disease in older persons

WILBERT S. ARONOW, YASSER RADWAN, AND HASAN AHMAD

Key points

- Management strategies for severe MS involve anticoagulation therapy for patients with AF, percutaneous balloon mitral valvuloplasty for suitable cases, and mitral valve replacement or transcatheter mitral valve replacement for high-risk surgical candidates.
- MAC is most frequently seen in the elderly patient, is probably a marker for vascular atherosclerosis, and is an independent predictor of adverse cardiovascular events such as myocardial infarction and stroke.
- Primary MR is a disease of the mitral valve apparatus itself, and secondary MR results from left ventricular dysfunction.
- Severe TR may be treated by transcatheter edge-to-edge repair with the TriClip device to improve the severity of TR with associated improvement in quality of life.

DOI: 10.1201/9781003568933-15

INTRODUCTION

Mitral valve disease in the elderly differs from that in the younger patients in several ways. Since rheumatic fever is now uncommon in North America and Western Europe, most rheumatic heart disease is seen in younger patients not born in the United States or in older patients. In patients born in North America or Western Europe, mitral stenosis (MS) is predominantly seen in patients over the age of 50–60 years, many of whom have had one or more surgical or balloon valvuloplasties. At present, balloon valvuloplasty is the procedure of choice, even in the elderly and even in patients who have had previously undergone valvulotomy and who now have mitral restenosis. Mitral regurgitation (MR) has many etiologies, the most common of which are degenerative or mitral valve prolapse, functional MR due to ischemia, or cardiomyopathy. In patients with grade I or II ischemic MR, revascularization alone can reduce or eliminate the MR. With grade III or IV ischemic MR, revascularization and concomitant annuloplasty or valve replacement can markedly reduce the degree of MR and result in better outcomes. With mitral valve disease, atrial fibrillation (AF) is a common complication, and if valve surgery is indicated, consideration should be given to a concomitant Maze procedure or ablation for AF. Mitral annular calcification (MAC) is most frequently seen in the elderly patient, is probably a marker for vascular atherosclerosis, and is an independent predictor of adverse cardiovascular events such as myocardial infarction and stroke. The American Heart Association recommendations for antibiotic prophylaxis for valvular disease have been markedly altered so that now prophylaxis is no longer recommended for valvular regurgitation. However, many physicians still prescribe antibiotic prophylaxis for their patients with valve disease.

ETIOLOGY

Mitral stenosis

The etiology of MS in the elderly, as in the young patient, is chronic rheumatic heart disease. There is a small incidence of MAC with exuberant atherosclerotic encroachment from the annulus into the base of the left ventricle such that the mitral orifice is decreased, producing some degree of MS, most often not severe. Reduced anterior leaflet mobility seems to be necessary to produce obstruction sufficient for a gradient of greater than 5 mmHg.

With the marked decrease in the incidence of acute rheumatic fever in the United States over the last half century, the prevalence of MS in those people under the age of 40 years, born and raised in the United States with chronic rheumatic heart disease and MS or mitral regurgitation (MR) has markedly decreased, so that MS in this population is seen predominantly in the elderly patient, frequently the older patient who has had earlier mitral valve surgery. Since rheumatic fever is still very common in Eastern Europe, Asia, Latin and South America, and Africa, most of the younger patients with MS in the United States were born and raised in these countries.

MITRAL REGURGITATION

In the elderly patient, mitral valve disease, especially MR, is more frequently seen than aortic valve disease, although aortic stenosis is much more often the reason for valve surgery in this age group. MR has numerous etiologies (Table 15.1) (1). The most frequent etiologies in elderly patients are myxomatous degeneration (mitral valve prolapse), functional MR due to left ventricular dilatation, coronary artery disease, rheumatic heart disease, and MAC. Since MAC is seen predominantly in the elderly patient and poses problems beyond those related to volume overload, a detailed discussion of this topic will be presented separately at the end of this chapter.

Anorexigenic drugs (fenfluramine and benfluorex, which have been withdrawn from most markets), possibly related to serotonergic medications that are agonists at the 5-hydroxytryptamine 2B (5-HT2B) receptor, have been shown to produce valvulopathy similar to that seen in carcinoid valve disease. Ergot-derived dopamine receptor agonists (pergolide and cabergoline), often used in Parkinson's disease, have been associated with increased risk of valvular regurgitation.

Table 15.1 Etiologies of mitral regurgitation

1. Rheumatic heart disease
2. Mitral valve prolapse (myxomatous degeneration)[a]
3. Infective endocarditis[a]
4. Left ventricular dilatation (left ventricular failure)
5. Idiopathic rupture of chordae tendinae[a]
6. Trauma, penetrating and nonpenetrating[a]
7. Coronary artery disease
   a. Transient ischemia[a]
   b. Myocardial infarction
   c. Ruptured papillary muscle[a]
8. Connective tissue diseases (lupus erythematosus, Marfan disease)
9. Mitral annular calcification
10. Post mitral valvotomy[a]
11. Valve dehiscence[a]
12. Paraprosthetic mitral regurgitation
13. Degeneration of a bioprosthetic valve
14. Drug-associated valvulopathy (fenfluramine, pergolide)
15. Hypertrophic cardiomyopathy

[a] Etiologies where clinical picture may be that of acute mitral regurgitation.

PATHOPHYSIOLOGY

Mitral stenosis

The major pathology of MS is that of commissural fusion, and fusion and shortening of the chordae tendineae. Later, there is increasing fibrosis and calcification of the valve leaflets. Therefore, the obstruction to diastolic flow across the mitral valve can be due to the narrowed mitral orifice caused by commissural fusion and to the thickening and calcification of the leaflets so that they do not open without a pressure gradient in spite of open commissures, or to obstruction due to a subvalvular component caused by fused, shortened chordae tendineae. In these latter two instances, commissurotomy will not relieve the obstruction, and valve replacement is necessary.

The normal mitral valve orifice is approximately 5.0 cm^2. With a normal stroke volume there is no obstruction to diastolic flow until the valve area is reduced to approximately 2.0 cm^2. When the valve area reaches about 1.0 cm^2, there is sufficient obstruction at resting flow rates to result in a diastolic gradient across the mitral valve, so the left atrial pressure as well as pulmonary venous and pulmonary capillary pressures rise enough to cause pulmonary congestive symptoms.

The obstruction and pressure gradient between the left atrium and left ventricle in diastole accelerate the blood through the narrowed orifice, causing the turbulence and vortex formation that generate the characteristic low-frequency diastolic murmur. The loudness of the murmur is related to the magnitude of the pressure gradient and to the volume of blood accelerated across the obstructed valve as well as to the nearness of the chamber in which the murmur is generated (here the left ventricle) to the ear. Since the left ventricular apex pushes the chest wall in systole creating the point of maximal impulse (PMI), this is where the murmur is best heard. In the elderly, the anteroposterior (AP) diameter of the chest may be increased, so that the left ventricular apex no longer contacts the chest wall and the low-pitched murmur of MS may be inaudible.

As left atrial pressure rises, pulmonary capillary pressure rises and overcomes the colloid osmotic pressure in the pulmonary capillary bed, leading to increasing congestion in the interstitial areas of the lung and finally to pulmonary edema. As left atrial pressure rises, there is a *pari passu* rise in right ventricular systolic pressure, increasing afterload on the right ventricle, right ventricular hypertrophy, and finally resulting in right ventricular failure. In 10%–15% of cases, there is a marked increase in pulmonary artery pressure and pulmonary vascular resistance due to edema pressure on the interstitial small arteries and vasoconstriction probably mediated by pulmonary artery endothelial release of vasoconstrictive amines such as endothelin. Eventually, with right ventricular failure, there is a decrease in cardiac output and signs of right ventricular failure with increased central venous pressure, edema, and even ascites.

As left atrial pressure rises, the left atrium enlarges resulting in atrial fibrillation (AF), which may occur relatively early in the course of MS. With AF, stasis of blood, especially in the left atrial appendage, as well as endocardial changes that promote platelet activation and release of thrombogenic substances result in atrial clotting and form the basis for the high incidence of systemic thromboemboli, the most important of which is embolic stroke that is common in MS (2).

Hemoptysis occurs in these patients as pulmonary venous pressure increases, opening collaterals for runoff to the bronchial veins. These protrude into the lumen of the bronchi and, when rupture occurs, cause hemoptysis. Ortner's syndrome (paralysis of the left vocal cord) can occur with the recurrent laryngeal nerve, which hooks around the ligamentum arteriosus being stretched by the enlarging left pulmonary artery and left atrium.

Mitral regurgitation

MECHANISM OF REGURGITANT ORIFICE FORMATION

The development of MR depends on the formation during systole of a regurgitant orifice. There are a number of mechanisms by which this can occur. Dilatation of the left ventricular opening snap (OS) (including the mitral annulus) is seen in any cause of ventricular failure with left ventricular dilatation. The valve itself remains normal, but the area of the mitral opening is too great to be closed by coaptation of the leaflets. There is also displacement of the papillary muscles and more lateral tension in systole on the leaflet edges, thus restricting leaflet motion (3). A similar problem occurs with ischemia and myocardial fibrosis where the mural leaflet is held from coapting with the anterior leaflet. Other mechanisms of regurgitant orifice formation are loss of leaflet tissue and fibrosis, retraction of leaflet tissue as is seen in rheumatic heart disease, or tearing of the leaflet as in infective endocarditis, seen also in penetrating and nonpenetrating trauma. With hypertrophic obstructive cardiomyopathy, a regurgitant orifice is formed by the displacement of the anterior leaflet to the septum during systole. Finally, there can be loss of intravalvular support as seen in chordal and papillary muscle rupture.

With myxomatous leaflets, mitral valve prolapse occurs where there may be coaptation of the leaflets early in systole, but as the left ventricle empties and becomes smaller, the redundant leaflet is displaced back above the mitral annulus into the left atrium, and at some point a regurgitant orifice is created. With myocardial infarction and fibrosis of the papillary muscle and its origin from the left ventricular wall, as systole progresses, the mitral valve leaflets prolapse toward the left atrium and a regurgitant orifice forms. With annular calcification, the OS of the left ventricle is prevented from constricting during systole and the mural leaflet can be immobilized, preventing it from coapting with the anterior leaflet.

PATHOPHYSIOLOGY-CAUSING SYMPTOMS

Acute mitral regurgitation

The pathophysiology of MR depends on the severity of the leak (regurgitant volume) and the rapidity with which the MR occurs. With sudden chordal or leaflet rupture or valve dehiscence, a sudden low-resistance runoff in systole from the left ventricle develops. If the regurgitant orifice is large, the regurgitant volume will be large. The total left ventricular stroke volume is now divided into the stroke volume going out of the aorta (effective forward stroke volume) and the blood regurgitating back into the left atrium (regurgitant volume). The left ventricle in this situation empties rapidly during systole. Since much of the regurgitant volume goes into the left atrium against low resistance, the left ventricle faces a decreased afterload early in systole, permitting it to empty more easily and achieving a smaller end-systolic volume and a higher ejection fraction (EF).

The increased blood coming into the left atrium during systole results in a higher V wave. With the next diastole, the blood coming from the pulmonary veins adds to the regurgitant blood, thus increasing the left ventricular end-diastolic volume (LVEDV). The Frank–Starling mechanism increases the next left ventricular stroke volume so that the regurgitant volume can be maintained as well as the effective forward stroke volume. In acute MR, the sudden increase in LVEDV, resisted by the unprepared left ventricle and unstretched pericardium, results in a marked rise in left ventricular filling pressure. With the increased filling pressure, the left atrial and pulmonary capillary pressure are increased causing pulmonary congestion and pulmonary edema. With the rise in left atrial pressure there is a sudden increase in afterload on the right ventricle, which may dilate and rapidly fail.

Chronic mitral regurgitation

With gradually increasing regurgitant volume, there is stimulus and time for remodeling of the left ventricle and eccentric hypertrophy to occur. As the ventricle dilates, left ventricular hypertrophy (LVH) occurs so that the wall does not become thinner, preventing an increase in left ventricular wall tension. The ventricle remains compliant, and the pericardium stretches to keep the left ventricular filling pressure and the left atrial pressure normal. The dilated, more compliant left atrium limits the height of the V wave to 30–35 mmHg. The left ventricular filling pressure remains normal until the left ventricle fails, at which time the filling pressure rises. Since the left ventricle is contracting against a lower afterload, the EF remains normal or even higher than normal. As the left ventricular end-diastolic diameter increases, eventually the wall tension and afterload increase, and the EF begins to fall. At this stage, even with the EF still "within normal limits," there is a decrease in myocardial contractility. When the left atrial mean pressure rises, there is increased afterload on the right ventricle, which eventually leads to right ventricular failure. Here, right ventricular failure is very late in the course of the natural history.

Age modifies the pathophysiology of mitral regurgitation

In the elderly there is decreased compliance of the left ventricle as well as LVH, which leads to a further, more rapid increase in left ventricular filling pressure given the volume load present in MR. With the increased aortic stiffness present in the elderly (4), there is increased left ventricular impedance to ejection and increased left ventricular afterload leading to earlier decompensation of the left ventricle in MR.

CLINICAL PICTURE

Mitral stenosis

SYMPTOMS

Patients may remain asymptomatic for many years. In the elderly, many patients have had a previous intervention, either surgical or balloon valvotomy. In elderly patients, pulmonary congestion almost always results in progressive dyspnea on exertion and eventually orthopnea and paroxysmal nocturnal dyspnea (PND). Wall tension and enlargement of the left atrium lead to the development of AF and the increased danger of systemic emboli, especially stroke. Frequently the first symptoms occur with the onset of AF or, in the young patient, during the course of pregnancy, secondary to the increased cardiac output and diastolic flow across the mitral valve, usually in the late second or third trimester. With decreasing right ventricular function, the patient may have fewer symptoms and signs of pulmonary congestion and more problems with decreased exercise tolerance. Eventually, the clinical picture is dominated by the signs and symptoms of right heart failure, pedal edema, engorged neck veins, and finally ascites and the stasis cyanosis of low cardiac output.

SIGNS

The murmur of MS is a characteristic low-pitched, rumbling diastolic murmur best heard at the apex. With flexible valve leaflets, the first heart sound is loud and even palpable and there is an opening snap after the S_2 in early diastole. The second heart sound may be increased and even palpable if the pulmonary artery pressure is elevated. With severe pulmonary hypertension, a diastolic blowing murmur of pulmonic insufficiency may be heard along the left-sternal border, indistinguishable from the murmur of aortic regurgitation (Graham–Steele murmur). With right ventricular hypertrophy, there may be a precordial lift. With right heart failure, a systolic murmur along the left sternal border of tricuspid regurgitation may be present, as well as an elevated central venous pressure, hepatomegaly, edema, and even ascites.

Age modifies signs and symptoms of mitral stenosis

In the elderly, symptoms of MS may be far advanced before the patient recognizes them.

Elderly patients may accept shortness of breath and decreased exercise tolerance as an inevitable consequence of "getting older." In addition, accompanying comorbidities, such as chronic obstructive pulmonary disease, may be accepted as the cause of the increasing symptoms. In the elderly patient, the AP diameter of the chest is frequently increased so that the left ventricle no longer contacts the chest wall. Also, dilatation of the right ventricle may move the left ventricle posteriorly away from contact with the chest wall. Since the low-frequency murmur does not conduct well through the blood of the right ventricle, the murmur may be inaudible. Sometimes, rolling the patient into the left lateral position can bring the left ventricle into contact with the chest wall and make the murmur detectable with the bell of the stethoscope over the PMI. In addition, increasing the heart rate and cardiac output with exercise increases the diastolic gradient across the mitral valve and makes the murmur louder.

Since the elderly are more likely to have a fibrotic, calcified valve, the first heart sound may not be loud, and the opening snap may be absent. In these patients, the MS may be truly silent, and the patient simply looks like a patient with heart failure.

LABORATORY FINDINGS AND DIAGNOSIS

The classic findings on a chest X-ray are those of right ventricular dilatation and prominence of the pulmonary artery and pulmonary veins, especially with redistribution to the upper lung fields. There is also a double density behind the right cardiac silhouette protruding beyond the right heart border of left atrial enlargement, and a filling in below the main pulmonary artery segment in the PA view of the left atrial appendage. In the lateral film, at times, calcification of the mitral valve can be seen but better observed on fluoroscopy.

The classic findings on electrocardiogram (ECG) are left atrial abnormality and right ventricular hypertrophy. In the elderly, AF is common.

The restricted opening of the mitral valve can be seen in the two-dimensional echocardiogram, and the mitral orifice can be planimetered. The diastolic area of the open mitral valve can be accurately measured using magnetic resonance imaging (MRI). The increased diastolic velocity across the mitral valve is measured by Doppler echocardiography, and the diastolic gradient is calculated by the formula (5):

$$\text{Gradient} = 4V^2$$

The severity of the MS can be calculated from the diastolic half-time and the mitral orifice area from the continuity equation:

$$\text{Mitral valve area} = \text{LV outflow tract area} \times \text{Velocity}/\text{Velocity across mitral valve}$$

Or by the proximal isovelocity surface area (PISA) method:

$$\text{Mitral area} = \text{Flow}(2\pi r2)/\text{Velocity across mitral valve}$$

where r is determined from the Nyquist limit.

There are several echocardiographic scores (6), which by looking at the thickness and mobility of the leaflets, the degree of leaflet and commissural calcification, and subvalvular chordal fusion, can reliably identify those patients who will benefit from balloon or surgical valvotomy and those who should have valve replacement. Other imaging techniques such as MRI and computed angiographic tomography (CAT) scanning can demonstrate the pathophysiologic abnormalities in MS but generally do not contribute significantly to the more common laboratory studies and therefore are not generally indicated.

Mitral regurgitation

SYMPTOMS

Acute mitral regurgitation

With sudden development of severe MR, there is no time for compensatory eccentric hypertrophy or enlargement of the left atrium, so the patient frequently develops severe shortness of breath, orthopnea, PND, early pulmonary edema, and even right heart failure. Since the left atrium is not dilated, it is unusual for the patient to be in AF.

Chronic mitral regurgitation

The patient may remain asymptomatic for years. Eventually the earliest symptom may be a decrease in exercise tolerance rather than dyspnea on exertion since with left ventricular dysfunction, the forward stroke volume may decrease with exercise. Later, shortness of breath, orthopnea, PND, and left heart failure occur.

Finally, right heart failure is very late in the course of the disease.

The elderly patient may deny symptoms thinking that decreased exercise tolerance is due to aging and shortness of breath is due to pulmonary disease. In addition, with a gradual decrease in the patient's ability to exercise, symptoms may be avoided by decreasing the level of activity so that the patient may have very severe MR and still deny symptoms.

SIGNS

Acute mitral regurgitation

With acute MR the PMI may not be displaced but is hyperactive, especially compared with the radial pulse, and may be rapid rising and abbreviated. If the regurgitant orifice is very large, pressure in the left atrium and left ventricle may approach equality, in which case the murmur may be short or even absent. These patients are usually extremely dyspneic or in pulmonary edema. With posterior leaflet prolapse, the regurgitant jet may be directed anteriorly and superiorly so that the murmur may be heard well at the base as well as at the apex. With anterior leaflet prolapse, the jet is directed posteriorly and is well heard in the back.

The murmur of acute MR may be confused with that of aortic stenosis, but with a premature ventricular contraction, the postextrasystolic beat results in a murmur that does not get louder, unlike that of the postextrasystolic beat in aortic stenosis.

Chronic mitral regurgitation

With chronic MR, the left ventricle is dilated, and the PMI is displaced laterally and sustained. With the PMI and carotid pulse felt simultaneously, instead of the PMI collapsing before the carotid pulse, with LVH the PMI collapses after the carotid pulse. The pansystolic murmur of MR, best heard at the apex, is flat throughout systole.

Since the regurgitation continues throughout all of left ventricular systole, there are no isovolumic contraction or relaxation phases, and the murmur classically buries the first and second heart sounds. In patients where the regurgitant orifice does not form until the ventricle is ejecting, such as in mitral valve prolapse, nonejection click or clicks may be present as the leaflet prolapses and is suddenly stopped in its motion. Since the regurgitant orifice continues to enlarge as the ventricle empties, the murmur starts after the click, crescendos in loudness, and incorporates the second sound. With the marked increase in diastolic blood flow across the mitral valve, there may be a short diastolic rumble and an S_3 sound. AF is common in the elderly patient with significant MR.

Other signs and symptoms may be related to the etiology of the MR. For instance, with MR secondary to a dilated left ventricle, the findings of cardiomyopathy may be present with an S_3 and S_4 gallop. Fever and immunoembolic signs may be present in patients with infective endocarditis, physical signs of connective tissue diseases such as Marfan disease, or a history of trauma, angina, or acute myocardial infarction.

LABORATORY FINDINGS AND DIAGNOSIS

Chest X-ray

Since there is no time for atrial or ventricular remodeling, in acute MR the heart may not be enlarged on the chest X-ray. Pulmonary congestion and edema are commonly seen. With chronic severe MR, the left atrium and ventricle are dilated and appear enlarged on the chest X-ray. With chronic MR, occasionally the left atrium can become extremely dilated so that it touches the right lateral chest wall compressing the right lower lung.

Electrocardiogram

With acute MR, the ECG may be normal, except for sinus tachycardia, or have only nonspecific ST–T wave changes. With chronic MR, LVH, left atrial abnormality, and AF are common.

Echocardiography

The regurgitant volume and size of the regurgitant orifice can be estimated by Doppler echocardiography. The effect of the MR on the size and function of the cardiac chambers can also be evaluated. With acute severe MR, there is frequently pulmonary hypertension that can be estimated by identifying a tricuspid regurgitant jet, which allows estimation of the pulmonary artery systolic pressure. The direction of the MR regurgitant jet as well as multiple views on transesophageal echocardiogram (TEE) can reliably show which scallops of the mitral leaflets are prolapsing and define the anatomical and functional mechanism causing the MR; and it is necessary for planning the surgical procedure (7).

The severity of MR is more difficult to quantitate than the severity of MS. By Doppler echocardiography, the regurgitant jet by color-flow mapping is composed of a roughly hemispherical area of flow convergence resulting from serial aliasing (PISA), the regurgitant orifice, and the fully developed regurgitant jet. Multiple measurements have been used to quantitate the magnitude of MR. The jet area in proportion to the left atrial area, the width of the jet at the regurgitant orifice, the calculated regurgitant volume, the intensity of the continuous-wave MR signal, and the mitral inflow/pulmonary vein Doppler signs have all been used. Using PISA, it is possible to calculate the regurgitant volume and the effective orifice area. This measurement should be the best estimate of regurgitant severity, although the accuracy of the flow rate depends on many variables such as the shape of the PISA, the orifice geometry, and aliasing velocity, among others. All methods of measuring the severity of MR have limitations and should be used with other signs and measurements of regurgitant severity such as LV chamber size and pulmonary venous flow patterns.

Thomas and colleagues (8) developed an MR index using six echo-Doppler findings, three related to the regurgitant volume and three to the effect on the cardiac chambers. The index correlated well with regurgitant fraction and other measures of MR severity and identified patients with severe MR with a 90% sensitivity, a 88% specificity, and a 79% positive predictive value.

As in the case of MS, the imaging techniques of MRI and CAT scanning can demonstrate similar pathophysiologic abnormalities, but are generally not used clinically.

NATURAL HISTORY OF MITRAL STENOSIS AND MITRAL REGURGITATION IN THE ELDERLY

Mitral stenosis

A patient over the age of 65 years with MS who has not already had a commissurotomy will have had mild MS for many years or may have progressed to moderate MS. Others have progressed to severe MS by valvular fibrosis and calcification. Many have had MS diagnosed at an early age and, if symptomatic, had a valvotomy or valve replacement.

Once MS becomes symptomatic, the course usually is to become progressively more symptomatic, going through the pulmonary congestive phase, then the right heart failure phase, and finally the low-cardiac-output stage leading to death. Since valvotomy or valve replacement has been available for over half a century, it is unusual to see an elderly person with severe MS who has not had at least one attempt at valvotomy. It is mainly in newly arrived patients in the United States that we see the elderly with previously unrecognized severe MS.

Mitral regurgitation

The natural history of patients with MR depends on the acuteness of onset, severity, and etiology of MR. The presence of echocardiographic MR early after acute myocardial infarction is predictive of decreased survival (9). The prevalence of MR increases with age, diabetes, hypertension, and previous revascularization. However, mild or moderate MR may not be an independent prognostic predictor (8). In patients who have decreased ventricular function or heart failure after an acute myocardial infarction, increased MR at baseline was associated with larger LVEDV and left ventricular end-systolic volume (LVESV), increased sphericity index, and reduced EF. Moderate to severe MR is an independent predictor of total mortality, cardiovascular mortality, and hospitalization for heart failure on follow-up. If the severity of the MR progresses during the first month after myocardial infarction, patients are likely to die or develop heart failure (10). With MR caused by ischemia or myocardial infarction, the prognosis is poor unless there is minimal myocardial damage and the ischemic muscle can be revascularized and the valve made competent. In patients with MR at the time of revascularization, there is conflicting evidence that repair of the mitral valve alters long-term functional status or survival (11). In addition, there is good evidence that after coronary bypass surgery, the preoperative MR will decrease. In one study (12), 66% of 131 patients preoperatively had mild, 31% had moderate, and 3% had severe ischemic MR. On follow-up after coronary bypass surgery, 52% had no or mild, 27% had moderate, and 6% had severe MR. When endocarditis is the cause of the MR, the course depends on the infecting organism and the complications seen with infective endocarditis. If trauma is the etiology, the damage to the heart and other organs determines the course.

ACUTE MITRAL REGURGITATION

How large the regurgitant volume is when the acute MR occurs will determine the symptomatic state of the patient. In the elderly patient, the stiffer left ventricle results in a higher filling pressure for a given volume overload. With a single chord rupture, there may be minimal to moderate regurgitation and the patient may not exhibit the clinical picture of acute MR. With the rupture of several primary chords or of the papillary muscle tip, the patient exhibits the classic clinical picture of acute MR and frequently presents with pulmonary edema, culminating in early demise.

With the decrease in afterload, the ventricle empties in systole to a greater extent than normal and the EF increases. With myocardial dysfunction, the left ventricular end-diastolic and end-systolic volumes increase and the EF begins to fall, at times into the normal range. The decrease in EF in this case still identifies myocardial dysfunction that has a negative effect on prognosis even after surgical correction of the MR (13).

After a period of time, remodeling of the left atrium and left ventricle allows the filling pressure to fall and the effective forward stroke volume to be maintained. The patient may become less symptomatic and the clinical picture may become that of chronic MR.

CHRONIC MITRAL REGURGITATION

Patients with chronic MR can remain asymptomatic for many years with good exercise tolerance (14). At some point, the volume load on the left ventricle combined with increasing afterload due to the ventricle becoming more spherical and increasing its radius results in myocardial dysfunction. The course becomes that of increasing symptoms and death, usually from congestive heart failure.

TREATMENT OF MITRAL STENOSIS AND MITRAL REGURGITATION IN THE ELDERLY

Mitral stenosis

BALLOON VALVOTOMY FOR MITRAL STENOSIS

In elderly patients with mild to moderate MS who have good or acceptable exercise tolerance consistent with their age and not interfering with their life, the best approach is controlling volume overload, the ventricular rate if in AF, and anticoagulation with warfarin because of the high risk of systemic embolization. If the patient develops symptoms that do not respond to gentle diuresis and rate control with β-blockers or calcium channel blockers, valvotomy should be considered. If the valve is flexible, with minimal calcification, no left atrial thrombus, and no more than mild (grade 2 or less) MR, the patient is a candidate for valvotomy (15). Commissural calcification has an adverse effect on the results of balloon valvotomy with smaller increases in the mitral valve area as calcification increases and a smaller reduction in functional class after balloon mitral valvotomy (16). In evaluating 848 consecutive patients with MS in normal sinus rhythm by both transthoracic echocardiogram (TTE) and TEE, the prevalence of atrial thrombus was 6.6%. TEE is warranted when the individual is over the age of 44 years, the left atrial inferior–superior diameter is >6.9 cm, or the mean diastolic gradient is >18 mmHg. When spontaneous echo contrast is absent on TEE, thrombus is unlikely (17). At the present time with experienced operators, balloon valvotomy is the treatment of choice rather than open commissurotomy (18). With balloon valvotomy, the success rate of increasing the valve area to 1.5 cm^2 or greater, effectively doubling the valve area, is high—about 90%, even in valves with a high echo score (46). Preexisting MR is a risk factor predicting poor outcome (19). The presence of commissural calcium is related to the development of MR after balloon valvotomy, and with calcification of the valve there is less chance that the valve can be opened to greater than or equal to 1.5 cm^2 and less improvement in symptoms.

Iung and colleagues (20) reported results of balloon valvotomy in 1514 patients, 45 ± 15 years of age; of those, 25% had calcified valves. A good result, defined as opening the mitral valve to 1.5 cm^2 or more without creating 2+ or greater MR, was obtained in 1348 (89%) patients. Important predictors of a good result were of younger age, had an echo score less than or equal to 8, and had a relatively large predilation valve area. Palacios and colleagues (18) reported 327 patients with balloon valvotomy. There were seven in-hospital deaths. The follow-up period was 26 ± 12 months. The echo score, which evaluates the anatomical suitability for valvotomy using the Wilkins scoring system, was determined. Patients with an echo score greater than 8 compared with those less than or equal to 8 were older (64 ± 11 years vs. 48 ± 14 years) had more AF (65% vs. 40%), more valve calcification (81% vs. 29%), and more previous surgical commissurotomy (30% vs. 16%). Event-free survival was 79 ± 10% for those with an echo score less than 8 versus 39 ± 18% with an echo score greater than or equal to 8.

Fawzy reported the results of mitral valvuloplasty in 547 consecutive patients, mean age 31.5 years, followed for 1.5–19 years after valvotomy. Valve area increased from 0.92 cm^2 to 1.95 cm^2. Restenosis occurred in 169 (31%) patients; it was less common in those with echocardiographic scores of ≤8. Event-free survival at 10, 15, and 19 years was 89%, 60%, and 28%, respectively. Multivariate analysis identified an echocardiographic score of ≤8 and post-procedure valve area ≤1.8 cm^2 as predictors of restenosis. The long-term outcome can be predicted from the baseline characteristics of the mitral valve (21).

There is limited experience with valvotomy in patients older than 60–70 years. Remadi and colleagues (22) reported the immediate and late outcomes of balloon mitral valvotomy in 745 patients, 45 of whom were aged 60 years or older. They compared the immediate and late outcomes with those younger than 60. The baseline hemodynamic parameters were comparable in the two groups, as was the degree of mitral valve opening and favorable hemodynamic response. Complication rates, including the development of grade I and II MR, were also similar. After a mean of 43 months of follow-up, a good result was maintained in 60% of patients, even though some degree of restenosis occurred in 40% of the older patients, compared to 25% of the younger patients. Le Feuvre and colleagues (23) reported on 234 patients who had a balloon valvotomy, only 28 of whom (10%) were aged 70 years or older. Compared to younger patients, the older patients had a higher percentage of New York Heart Association (NYHA) class III and IV (84% vs. 67%) and higher echo scores (9.3 ± 2.1 vs. 8.0 ± 1.6), meaning they were less suitable for valvotomy. They also had more AF (61% vs. 36%), more complications (27% vs. 9%), and a higher 30-day mortality (12% vs. 0.8%). The success rate in opening the valve was similar in both groups.

Long-term survival without cardiac events (death, cerebrovascular accidents, another intervention) depends on the patient's age as well as comorbidity. In general, the older the patient and the more the comorbidity, the shorter the survival.

Meneveau and colleagues (24) reported 532 patients after balloon valvotomy (Table 15.2). The event-free survival was age dependent. The anatomical form of the mitral valve was the second most important factor in event-free survival. Given the fact that a calcified valve is unfavorable for valvotomy, balloon valvotomy can be palliative in those very symptomatic patients with calcified valves believed to be too great a risk for surgery, achieving

Table 15.2 Long-term follow-up of 532 patients with balloon valvotomy

Event-free survival	3 years	5 years	7.5 years
Entire group	84%	74%	52%
Age ≤65	80%	70%	45%
Age >65	52%	38%	17%
Favorable anatomy (echo score of 1)	92%	84%	70%
Intermediate anatomy	86%	73%	34%

Source: Meneveau N et al. *Heart*, 80, 359–364, 1998.
Note: The anatomic form of the mitral valve was the second important factor in event-free survival.

a moderate increase in valve area at low procedural risk and with improvement of symptoms in the majority of patients (25). Patients with echo scores that make them unsuitable for balloon valvotomy and who are rejected for surgery because of frailty or comorbidity can benefit from balloon valvotomy. Sutaria and colleagues (26) reported on 80 patients over 70 years of age, 55 of whom were considered unsuitable for surgery. There was a 95% success rate in opening the valve. One year later, 28 of the 55 unsuitable patients (51%) had improved at least one NYHA class and 14 (25%) at 5 years. Of the 25 with suitable valves, 16 (64%) had achieved this outcome at 1 year and 9 (36%) at 5 years. Shaw and colleagues (27) reported similar results in 20 patients 70 years of age and older. The absence of commissural calcification is a significant predictor of the frequency of achieving a mitral valve opening of 1.5 cm^2 without creating severe MR. Sutaria and colleagues (28) reported that calcification of one or more commissures predicts a less than 50% chance of achieving a valve area of greater than or equal to 1.5 cm^2. Its influence is greatest in valves with an echo score of less than or equal to 8. Patients with a commissural calcification grade of 0/1 had greater improvement in symptoms and achieved a valve area of 1.5 cm^2 (67%) compared to those with a grade of 2/3 (46%) (28). If the echo score is greater than 8, the degree of commissural calcification is less important.

Complications of balloon valvotomy reported in the literature are a mortality of 0.5%–1%, development of MR requiring surgery of 1.3%–3%, and cerebrovascular accident 0.5%–1%. These complications compare favorably with those reported after surgical commissurotomy. Restenosis after balloon valvotomy ranges from 4% to 70% depending on patient selection, morphology of the valve, and length of follow-up (29).

In patients age 80 and older, there is limited experience of balloon valvotomy. Sutaria and colleagues (30) reported 20 octogenarians (age range 80–89) with balloon valvuloplasty, all functional classes II–IV, and 14 among them were unfit for surgery. The mitral valve area was increased by 106% from 0.81 ± 0.3 cm^2 to 1.67 ± 0.8 cm^2. Eight patients attained a valve area of greater than or equal to 1.5 cm^2 and 16 an area greater than or equal to 1.2 cm^2; 80% improved at least one NYHA functional class.

Since many elderly patients with MS have had a previous surgical commissurotomy, the question arises whether balloon valvotomy could be successful if restenosis occurs. Iung and colleagues (31) reported the results of balloon valvotomy in 232 patients, mean age 47 ± 14 years, who had undergone a surgical commissurotomy 16 ± 8 years earlier. Eighty-one of these patients had valve calcification and bilateral commissural fusion. One patient died (0.4%), MR >2/4 developed in 4%, and 82% achieved an immediate valve area of greater than or equal to 1.5 cm^2 without significant MR. Predictors of a poor result were age ($p < 0.001$), smaller initial valve area ($p = 0.01$), and use of a double-balloon technique ($p = 0.015$), indicating that results in the elderly would not be as good. In the 175 patients with follow-up, 8-year survival without operation and in NYHA class I and II was 48% ± 5% and in those with good immediate results, 58% ± 6%.

Aslanabadi and colleagues (32) reported on 47 post-balloon valvotomy restenosis patients with unfavorable valve characteristics assigned either to repeat balloon valvotomy (25) or to mitral valve replacement (22). The mean follow-up was 41 months for the repeat valvotomy patients and 63 months for the mitral valve replacement patients. The 10-year survival was higher in the re-balloon patients than in the surgical patients, 96% versus 73%, respectively ($p < 0.05$), but the event-free survival was similar (52% vs. 50%) due to a high reintervention rate in the re-balloon group (48% vs. 18%; $p = 0.02$). Others have had similar results with re-balloon valvotomy in patients with restenosis and found that independent predictors of event-free survival were an echo score of <7 and absence of prior surgical commissurotomy (33).

The question of whether balloon valvotomy will prevent the later development of AF in the patient with MS or in the patient in normal sinus rhythm addresses the argument that early commissurotomy is necessary to avoid his complication. Eid Fawzy and colleagues (34) reported a retrospective analysis of 382 consecutive patients with severe MS in sinus rhythm who had successful balloon valvotomy and were followed for a mean of 5.6 years. Thirty-four (8.9%) patients developed AF compared with 348 (91.1%) who remained in sinus rhythm at follow-up. They compared these results with a reported series in the literature of patients with MS where AF occurred in 29% of patients with similar baseline characteristics who did not have an intervention. The baseline characteristics that were predictive of the late postvalvotomy development of AF were older age, larger left atrium, and a smaller mitral valve area at follow-up.

These findings differ from an earlier report by Krasuski and colleagues (35) of a prospective cohort of patients with MS and no history of atrial arrhythmias, who showed no decrease in AF after successful versus unsuccessful balloon valvotomy. Advanced age and left atrial dimension were the best predictors of AF at follow-up, whereas procedural success at balloon valvotomy and left trial pressure reduction did not have an impact on the incidence of late AF.

SURGICAL MANAGEMENT OF MITRAL VALVE DISEASE

The surgical management of mitral valve disease in the 65–75 age group is not much different than in younger patients, except that older patients have more comorbidity, which increases the mortality and morbidity of surgery. Over the age of 75 years, there is a marked increase in surgical mortality and morbidity related to limited cardiac, renal, and pulmonary reserves. Since prolongation of life is not as likely in this age group, other therapeutic goals must justify surgery, such as improvement in quality of life (QOL) and return to independent lifestyle (36). Surgery in an unacceptably symptomatic patient should not be denied on the basis of age alone, and a patient who is symptomatically doing well should not be subjected to surgery with its higher mortality and morbidity.

Mitral stenosis

Open commissurotomy should be considered when the valve is flexible enough to open when the commissures are released; when there is minimal MR but the subvalvular apparatus is obstructive; sand when there is thrombus in the left atrium, especially in the body of the left atrium, that remains after 2–3 months of anticoagulation, which would make balloon valvotomy hazardous (15). At surgery, the subvalvular structures can be separated, the commissures opened, and the valve preserved. If not, the valve can be replaced.

Cotrufo and colleagues (37) reported on 540 consecutive MS patients, 300 with mitral commissurotomy and 240 with a bileaflet valve replacement. The majority of patients were younger than 65 years of age at the time of surgery. Hospital mortality was 2% in each group (Table 15.3). With a 15-year follow-up, late mortality was lower in the open commissurotomy group (1%) than in the valve replacement group (3%). With the exception of a greater incidence of reoperation, long-term results were better in the open commissurotomy group. This observation is consistent with many other studies that found that mitral valve repair is preferable to replacement (38).

Table 15.3 Mitral commissurotomy versus mitral valve replacement

	Commissurotomy	Valve replacement
10-year survival rate	98.7 ± 1%	93.7 ± 3%
Freedom from reop	88.1 ± 2%	97.7 ± 1%
Freedom from emboli	93.7 ± 2%	83.9 ± 7%
Freedom from hemorrhage	99.3 ± 0.5%	98.4 ± 1%

Source: Cotrufo M et al., *Eur J Cardiothorac Surg*, 12, 335–339, 1997.

With balloon valvotomy available for most patients with MS, the incidence of open commissurotomy has decreased. With the operative technique of preserving the papillary muscle-chordal apparatus in mitral valve replacement, the long-term outcome has approached that of valve commissurotomy. Ismeno and colleagues (39) report on 313 patients with isolated MS who received either balloon valvulotomy, open commissurotomy, or valve replacement (Table 15.4). There was no difference in operative mortality or 7-year actuarial survival. Freedom from reoperation was significantly better in those with mitral valve replacement, and the mean functional class at the end of the follow-up period was lowest in those with open commissurotomy. At present, conservative techniques are the best, especially in the elderly. With the latest operative techniques, the late outcome after mitral valve replacement has markedly improved. Similar results have been reported in other studies (40).

Table 15.4 Outcome of mitral stenosis intervention

	BV	OC	VR
Number	111	82	120
7-year survival (%)	95.4	95.1	92.8 (p = NS)
Freedom from emboli (%)	95.8	98.8	92.5 ($p > 0.05$)
Freedom from reop (%)	84.4	96.4	97.7 ($p > 0.05$)
NYHA class at follow-up	1.39	1.14	1.41 ($p = 0.001$)

Source: Ismeno G et al., *Acta Cardiol*, 56, 155–161, 2001.
Abbreviations: BV, balloon valvulotomy; OC, open commissurotomy; VR, valve replacement; NS, not significant.

Mitral regurgitation

With the present techniques, most patients with MR (except those with extensive loss of flexible leaflet tissue) can have the valve repaired successfully, but the selection of patients and the expertise of the surgeon are critical factors for success (37, 41). MR due to rheumatic heart disease is characterized by fibrosis and retraction of the leaflet edges as well as chordal shortening and fusion (42). Repair is least successful in this group, and selection of the proper patients for repair is essential (42). Most MR in the elderly is caused by myxomatous redundant leaflets, and these are ideal candidates for valve repair (41). With ischemic MR or a dilated left ventricle and left ventricular OS, annuloplasty, with or without an annular ring, is frequently sufficient to create a competent valve (43, 44). However, restricted leaflet motion can make the repair less predictable.

Contraindications for repair are loss of leaflet area, extreme leaflet thickening, or calcification of leaflets or commissures (42). Some surgeons have suggested that calcification of the annulus or leaflets does not preclude successful valve repair (45). Grossi and colleagues (46) reported the results of mitral valve repair in 558 patients. Debridement of calcification in annulus and/or leaflets was necessary in 64 (11.5%) patients. Freedom from reoperation at 10 years was 88.1% for debrided patients and 82.6% for those who did not need debridement. When good annulus and leaflet mobility can be achieved in calcified valves, calcium debridement allows durable valve repair.

Patients with a small mitral annulus or multiple leaflet defects have a small probability of successful repair. Patients with small left ventricular cavities, most often seen in elderly women, have a high incidence of postoperative systolic anterior motion and left ventricular outflow tract obstruction (38). Patients with mitral valve prolapse involving the posterior leaflet have the most success with repair. However, although less successful than repair with mural leaflet prolapse, there have been reports of successful repair of anterior leaflet prolapse (47). For the best results, the patient needs a careful evaluation by TEE and an experienced surgeon.

Because the expected life span after surgery is shorter for the elderly patient at the time of surgery, there is an advantage of bioprosthetic valves over mechanical valves in older patients since anticoagulation is not necessary in the absence of AF. The frequency of AF in elderly patients with moderate to severe chronic MR lessens the advantage because these patients require anticoagulants to prevent systemic emboli (41). There is evidence that valve degeneration occurs much more slowly in elderly patients than in younger patients. In one study, the rate of primary structural deterioration in patients over the age of 65 years was 0.95% per patient-year (48). For this reason, in patients over 65 years of age, the prevailing opinion is that the preferred valve is a bioprosthetic one.

Chikwe and colleagues (49) reported on 322 octogenarian patients with MR, mean age 82.6 years, 70% undergoing mitral valve repair and 30% replacement. A propensity-adjusted analysis showed that elective mitral valve repair can be performed with low operative mortality and good long-term outcomes in patients with degenerative MR. In octogenarians with mitral valve prolapse, repair is associated with better survival than with replacement, although this is more questionable in patients with nondegenerative MR.

Dalrymple-Hay and colleagues (50) reported on 329 patients with MR due to myxomatous degeneration, mean age of 65.5 years; 169 had valve repair and 160 had valve replacement. Operative mortality occurred in 4 patients (1.2%), all in those with valve replacement. Actuarial survival at 1, 5, and 10 years was 94% ± 1.4%, 77% ± 2.9%, and 41% ± 5.8%, respectively, with survival in patients with repair significantly better ($p < 0.05$) than with valve replacement. Reoperation was required in 10 (6%) of those with valve repair and in 13 (8%) of those with valve replacement. Increased age, worse left ventricular function, the type of operation (repair vs. replacement), and left ventricular size were all significantly associated with poorer survival.

Gogbashian and colleagues (51) reported a 10-year experience with mitral valve repair versus replacement in 292 patients aged 70 years and over for MR due to mitral valve prolapse, including patients with concomitant revascularization. Comparing repair to replacement, in-hospital mortality was higher (0.7% vs. 13.9%), length of hospital stay was longer (8.7 vs. 9.6 days), and 5-year survival was greater (81% vs. 63%). The 10-year freedom from valve reoperation in the patients with repair was 93.9% and for repair plus coronary bypass surgery 98.2%. They concluded that the preferred option for elderly patients was mitral valve repair.

Daneshmand and colleagues (52) from Duke University followed 2064 patients with mitral valve surgery with and without coronary bypass surgery for a median of 5 years, with maximal follow-up of 20 years. Mitral valve repair had a better survival across all ages than mitral valve replacement. If replacement was required, mechanical valves achieved better outcomes than tissue valves, even in the elderly. The recommendation from this study was that in patients needing valve replacement, tissue valves should be reserved for those where anticoagulation is contraindicated.

Lee and colleagues (53) reported on 614 patients with valve surgery for severe MR, of whom 190 were aged 70 and older and 424 were younger than 70. In the older patients, there was significantly more myxomatous disease, coronary disease, worse left ventricular function, and worse NYHA class III–IV symptoms. Operative mortality in both young and old patients was low (3.5% vs. 3.7%). In the older patients, 7-year survival was lower than in the young (49% ± 6% vs. 72% ± 3%) as were overt heart failure (74 ± 3% vs. 44 ± 7%) and complication-related deaths (78

Table 15.5 Long-term survival after surgery for mitral regurgitation

	Gr 1	Gr 2	Gr 3
Number	284	504	556
5-year survival	57 ± 3%	73 ± 2%	85 ± 2% ($p < 0.001$)
Rate of observed/expected survival (for age)	83%	85%	88% (p = NS)

Source: Detaint D et al., *Circulation*, 114, 265–272, 2006.
Abbreviation: NS, not significant.

± 3% vs. 57 ± 7%). However, both young and old patients who were NYHA class I with an EF greater than 40% had the same freedom from complication-related death (93 ± 3% in the younger patients vs. 90 ± 7% in the elderly). These findings support the approach to early surgery once symptoms occur and before the EF begins to fall, especially if valve repair is possible.

There is good evidence that valve repair or replacement for MR improves QOL (36). Goldsmith and colleagues (54), in a prospective study of 61 consecutive patients with severe MR, mean age 64 ± 12 years, who had mitral valve repair (40) or replacement (21), obtained QOL scores using the short form 36 questionnaire before and 3 months after surgery. There was significant improvement in seven out of eight QOL parameters in those with repair and in three out of eight in those with valve replacement. Patients with an EF greater than or equal to 50% improved in seven out of eight parameters. Those with impaired function or end-systolic dimensions of greater than or equal to 45 mm showed no improvement in any of the parameters. These findings support the importance of early surgery before a decline in left ventricular function.

Grossi and colleagues (55) studied 278 patients with mitral valve repair aged 70 and older (mean age 75.2 years). Concomitant procedures were done in 72.3%, with over half having coronary revascularization. Mortality was lower in those with isolated mitral valve repair than in those with concomitant revascularization (6.5% vs. 17%). With an additional valve procedure, the mortality was 13.2%. Long-term survival was excellent, with freedom from cardiac death in 100% of those with isolated mitral valve repair and lower in those with a concomitant procedure (79.7%; $p = 0.006$), and freedom from reoperation in 91.2% patients.

Surgery for MR in octogenarians is usually reserved for patients who are very symptomatic despite optimal medical management. There is evidence of improvement in the results of surgery for MR in these elderly patients. DeTaint and colleagues (56) reported the results of surgery for MR performed from 1980 to 1995 in patients 75 years of age and older (group 1), 65–75 (group 2), and younger than 65 (group 3). Preoperatively, group 1 patients had a higher prevalence of functional class III–IV symptoms, more AF and coronary disease, increased creatinine, and higher comorbidity index. The temporal trend of operative mortality showed a decrease in each age group from 27% to 5% in group 1, 21% to 4% in group 2, and 7% to 2% in group 3. Over time, the feasibility of valve repair also increased in all groups from 30% to 54%, and in those with degenerative MR (mitral valve prolapse) from 31% to 93%. Multivariate analysis of relative survival showed no difference in restoration of life expectancy compared with younger patients (Table 15.5).

There are several reports of valve surgery in patients over the age of 75 years including reports in octogenarians that conclude that surgery can be performed with acceptable mortality and good long-term outcomes, including good QOL. All stress the importance of risk evaluation, avoidance of nonelective surgery whenever possible, and early surgery before moderate to severe symptoms develop (57, 58).

Present guidelines (15) recommend that surgery may be postponed safely in asymptomatic patients with severe MR, even if repair is possible, until the patient develops symptoms or AF, evidence of left ventricular dysfunction with EF falling below 60%, or left ventricular end-systolic dimension (LVESD) increases to 45 mm, or pulmonary hypertension becomes greater than 50 mmHg at rest or greater than 60 mmHg with exercise. Rosenheek and colleagues (14) reported on 132 such patients, 55 ± 15 years of age with severe MR due to mitral valve prolapse or flail leaflet. They underwent serial clinical and echocardiographic monitoring and were followed prospectively for 62 ± 26 months. They were referred for surgery for the above criteria. Only 30% of patients needed surgery by 5 years and fewer than half by 8 years. Symptoms were the most common indication for surgery. There was no operative mortality and the postoperative outcome was good with regard to survival, symptomatic status, and late left ventricular function.

The question of the timing of surgery in asymptomatic or mildly symptomatic patients with degenerative MR is addressed in the American College of Cardiology (ACC)/American Heart Association (AHA) guidelines (41) with the recommendation that surgery be done with the onset of symptoms or in asymptomatic patients, with EF <60% or left ventricular systolic diameter > 40 mm. Supporting these recommendations are the studies of Suri and colleagues (59) who reported on 204 patients with mitral valve prolapse and less than severe MR followed for a mean of 8.6 years. Over half of those patients developed left ventricular dysfunction or worsening MR. Despite optimal medical management, left ventricular dysfunction can develop in the absence of MR progression. Gillinov and colleagues (60) reviewed 4586 patients with surgery for degenerative mitral valve disease with repair in 93%. Thirty percent of the patients were asymptomatic and even the development of mild symptoms by the time of surgery was associated with deleterious changes in cardiac structure and function. Finally, in a cohort of 481 patients with severe degenerative mitral valve disease and one ACC/AHA indication for surgery, 168 patients were grouped into those with early surgery (<2 months from the development of the surgical indication), 94 who had late surgery (>2 months), and 219 who were managed medically. Follow-up time was 5.6 years. Those selected for early surgery had a hazard ratio of 0.54 compared to those with late surgery (61). These studies support the guidelines for early referral for surgery in patients with severe MR and the development of symptoms, enlarged left ventricular dimensions, or decreased EF, providing that repair is possible and the surgical mortality is low (≤1%). Optimal timing of surgery in asymptomatic patients with MR is crucial to avoid excess morbidity and mortality. In asymptomatic patients with severe MR, both elevation of brain-type natriuretic peptide (BNP) on serial measurements and pulmonary hypertension have been shown by multivariate analysis to independently predict early deterioration of left ventricular function or the onset of symptoms (62). The presence of pulmonary hypertension in the resting patient and the development of systolic pulmonary artery pressure ≥56 mm Hg on exercise has been shown to be a good predictor of symptom development in asymptomatic patients with degenerative MR (63).

Valve replacement is performed in more elderly patients for aortic valve than for mitral valve disease, most often calcific aortic stenosis, and operative mortality is lower than with mitral valve replacement (64). Helft and colleagues (48) reported on 110 patients, 65 and older (mean 73.4 years), with bioprosthetic valve replacement: 71 with aortic, 32 with mitral, and 7 with both. Follow-up was 8.5 years. At 5 years the actuarial survival was 79.6% and at 10 years 62.4%. Of the 44 patients who died, over half (52.3%) died from non-valve-related causes. Reoperation was needed in 13 patients (11.8%), 10 for structural deterioration, with 1 death (7.7%). Anticoagulation for AF was needed in 26%, with 6.4% developing severe bleeding (2.9% per patient-year). Similar results have been reported in octogenarians (65). In examining the reasons for a higher mortality in octogenarians with MR surgery compared to aortic valve surgery, it is probable that the higher mortality is related more to the patients' preoperative clinical state and comorbidities than to the type of surgery (65).

Ischemic MR results from ventricular remodeling related to the position and extent of the ischemic or infarcted left ventricular myocardium (66). With MR due to ischemia, operative and late mortality is higher than with MR due to myxomatous degeneration (8).

Operative mortality is also higher when the EF is 30% or lower. Hausmann and colleagues (67) reported on 337 patients with ischemic MR and mitral valve repair or replacement (Table 15.6). The goal of surgery in patients with ischemic MR is to reduce the MR to no more than grade 1. Schurr and colleagues (68) compared 196 patients with coronary bypass surgery alone with 102 patients with bypass surgery and mitral valve repair or replacement. Perioperative mortality was double in the patients with bypass surgery and mitral valve surgery (10.8% vs. 5.1%; $p < 0.05$). In patients with moderate to severe MR, postoperative echocardiography showed improvement in MR in 95% in those with bypass and mitral valve surgery and in 64% of only bypass surgery patients. With lesser degrees of MR, improvement rates were similar (74% vs. 69%, respectively). Significant predictors of postoperative mortality were renal insufficiency, older age, and NYHA class III–IV.

A frequent problem with ischemia and 1 to 3+ MR is whether to simply revascularize the patient or also make the mitral valve more competent, usually with an annuloplasty. Kang and colleagues (69) reported an observational study of 185 consecutive patients, age 63 ± 9 years, with significant ischemic MR, of whom 66 had percutaneous angioplasty (PCI) and 119 coronary bypass surgery. Of those with surgical revascularization, 68 had concomitant mitral annuloplasty. In a median of 54 months of follow-up, survival and cardiac mortality rates were similar between the two groups. For the 45 propensity score-matched pairs, the risk of cardiac events was significantly lower in the operative group (hazard ratio 0.499; 95% confidence interval [CI] 0.251–0.990, $p = 0.043$). Compared to those with bypass surgery alone, patients with concomitant annuloplasty had a significantly higher event-free survival rate. To evaluate the impact of moderate MR in

Table 15.6 Surgery for ischemic mitral regurgitation

			Op mort with EF		Actuarial survival rate		
Type of operation	*n*	Op mort	10%–30%	>30%	2 years	5 years	7 years
Valve repair	140	12.1%	33.3%	8.4%	75.4%	66.8%	61.7%
Valve replace	197	14.2%	30.3%	11.0%	78.6%	73.4%	67.2%
When MR reduced to grade 0–1 patient survival best					81.0%	78.4%	77.2%

Source: Hausmann H, *J Heart Valve Dis*, 8, 536–542, 1999.
Abbreviations: EF, ejection fraction; Op mort, operative mortality.

patients undergoing isolated coronary surgery, Grossi and colleagues (70) followed 2242 consecutive patients with no to moderate MR. They found that, independent of ventricular function, mild to moderate MR is associated with significantly decreased survival.

Tolis and colleagues (71) had 49 patients, mean age 66.3 years, with advanced ischemic heart disease, 1 to 3+ MR (62% had 2 to 3+ MR), and an EF of 10%–30% (mean 22.4%). In-hospital mortality was 2% and the mean degree of MR went from 1.73 down to 0.54 ($p < 0.05$). The NYHA class decreased from 3.3 to 1.8 ($p < 0.05$) and the EF rose from 22% to 31.5% ($p < 0.05$). The 1-, 3-, and 5-year survivals were 88%, 65%, and 50%, respectively. They concluded that in such patients revascularization was sufficient and that improvement in MR and EF occur from improved left ventricular function and size after revascularization.

Aklog and colleagues (43) reported on 136 patients, mean age 70.5 years with ischemic heart disease and more severe 3+ MR with a mean EF of 38.1% who had isolated coronary bypass surgery. Operative mortality was 2.9%. They found the intraoperative TEE underestimated the degree of MR and the postoperative TTE revealed that 40% of the patients still had 3+ MR, 51% improved to 2+ MR, and only 9% had 0 to 1+ MR. They concluded that ischemic MR required more than just revascularization, usually concomitant annuloplasty. Campwala and colleagues (72) reported the fate of MR following surgical revascularization in 523 patients, 92 of whom had 3 to 4+ MR on preoperative echocardiogram. Postsurgery, residual 3 to 4+ MR was present in 43 (47%) patients and was associated with a trend to increased mortality ($p = 0.3$) over a mean follow-up of 3.9 years. Other studies have reported benefit in terms of symptoms and improved survival in patients with severe left ventricular dysfunction and MR, not only due to coronary artery disease but also in patients with cardiomyopathy and chronic valvular regurgitation (73).

AF is common in patients with mitral valve disease, both MS and MR. At the time of surgery, consideration should be given to performing a Cox–Maze procedure with particular attention to isolating the entrance of the pulmonary veins. Saint and colleagues (74) reported on 101 patients who underwent the Cox–Maze IV procedure for lone AF and 99 concomitantly with mitral valve operations. Operative mortality was similar in both groups and at 1-year, freedom from AF and antiarrhythmic drugs was also similar in both groups (76% vs. 77%). In patients with mitral valve replacement and AF, the addition of the Maze procedure was associated with a reduction in thromboembolic events and better long-term event-free survival in patients with AF undergoing mechanical mitral valve replacement (75). Other studies showed that including radiofrequency ablation for AF in conjunction with mitral valve surgery was equally effective in restoring normal sinus rhythm (76).

Finally, there are constant innovations in cardiac surgery that should make surgery easier on the patient and possibly safer for elderly patients with multiple comorbidities. These include minimally invasive surgery compared to standard thoracotomy (77) and robotic surgery (78). Catheter interventions have also shown promise in relatively noninvasively repaired MR. Whitlow and colleagues reported on the acute and 1-year results of the Endovascular Valve Edge-to-Edge Repair (EVEREST II) study where the mitral valve is converted into a double orifice by clipping the edges of the two leaflets together using a percutaneous catheter (MitraClip device). Seventy-eight patients, mean age 77 years old, with 3-to-4+ MR who were high risk for surgery had the procedure. At 1 year, the patients had improvement in clinical symptoms and significant left ventricular reverse remodeling (79). Another innovative technique for performing a mitral annuloplasty by transcatheter implantation of a coronary sinus device has been developed. The 1-year results in 59 patients with MR grade ≥2 show a reduction in MR by ≥1 grade. However, there was coronary compression in 15 patients where the great cardiac vein passes over a coronary artery, so strategies for avoiding this occurrence must be developed before this becomes a useful technique (80).

MITRAL ANNULAR CALCIFICATION

MAC is a chronic degenerative process that is common in elderly persons, especially women. The amount of calcium may vary from a few spicules to a large mass behind the posterior cusp, often extending to form a ridge or ring encircling the mitral leaflets, occasionally lifting the leaflets toward the left atrium and protruding into the left ventricular cavity below the mural leaflet of the mitral valve. Sphincter function loss of the mitral annulus and mechanical stretching of the mitral leaflets can cause improper coaptation of the leaflets during systole, resulting in MR (47). Although the calcific mass may immobilize the mitral valve, actual calcification of the leaflets is rare. In persons with severe MAC, the calcification may extend inward to involve the underside of the leaflets. MS may result from severe calcific deposits within the mitral annulus protruding into the orifice (1), but the obstruction is rarely severe. Calcific deposits may extend from the mitral annulus into the membranous portions of the ventricular septum, involving the conduction system and causing rhythm and conduction disturbances. Although the annular calcium is covered with a layer of endothelium, ulceration of this lining can expose the underlying calcific deposits, which may serve as a nidus for platelet-fibrin aggregation and subsequent thromboembolic episodes. Rodriguez and colleagues (81) reported a substudy of the Cardiovascular Health Study involving 2680 subjects without a history of stroke or transient ischemic attacks who had an MRI head scan. The mean age was

Table 15.7 Prevalence of mitral annular calcium with increasing age in elderly men and elderly women

Age (years)	MAC Men		Women	
	n	%	*n*	%
62–70	4/22	18	7/35	20
71–80	13/42	31	40/116	34
81–90	44/75	59	146/226	65
91–100	19/22	86	56/63	89
101–103	—	—	3/3	100

Source: Adapted from Aronow WS et al., *Am J Cardiol*, 59, 1213– 1214, 1987.

74.5 years. They found an increased prevalence of covert brain infarcts in those with MAC, aortic annular or valve calcification, or aortic valve sclerosis. After adjusted analysis for known risk factors, the risk ratio was 1.24 and the severity of valvular calcification was directly related to the covert brain MRI findings. In patients with endocarditis associated with MAC, the avascular nature of the mitral annulus predisposes to periannular and myocardial abscesses (82).

Prevalence

MAC is a degenerative process that increases with age and occurs more frequently in women than in men. In an unselected multiethnic population of 6814 men and women aged 45–84 years, MAC was present by CT in 9%, highest in Caucasians (12%) and lowest in Chinese (5%) (83). In a prospective study of 1797 unselected elderly persons in a long-term health care facility, mean age 81 ± 8 years (range 60–103 years), with technically adequate M-mode and two-dimensional echocardiograms of the mitral valve, MAC was present in 665 of 1243 women (53%) and in 194 of 554 men (35%) (124). Table 15.7 shows the prevalence of MAC with increasing age in elderly men and elderly women (85).

Predisposing factors

Because calcific deposits in the mitral annulus, in the aortic valve cusps, and in the epicardial coronary arteries are commonly associated in elderly persons and have similar predisposing factors, MAC and aortic cuspal calcium are a form of atherosclerosis. MAC and aortic cuspal calcium may coexist (86). Breakdown of lipid deposits on the ventricular surface of the posterior mitral leaflet at or below the mitral annulus and on the aortic surfaces of the aortic valve cusps is probably responsible for the calcification. Increased left ventricular systolic pressure due to aortic valve stenosis increases stress on the mitral apparatus and may accelerate development of MAC (87). Tricuspid annular calcium and MAC may also coexist and have similar predisposing factors (88). MAC has been suggested as a time-averaged marker of atherosclerosis and is associated with coronary artery disease, stroke, and increased mortality. Consistent with this is the association of coronary risk factors including age, hypertension, diabetes, and smoking (83, 89). In a 27-year follow-up, the Framingham Offspring Study demonstrated that exposure to multiple atherosclerotic risk factors in early to mid-adulthood is associated with aortic and mitral valve calcification (89).

Systemic hypertension increases with age and predisposes to MAC (82, 84). Persons with diabetes mellitus also have a higher prevalence of MAC than nondiabetic persons (90). MAC occurs in the teens with serum total cholesterol levels greater than 500 mg/dL (91). Hypercholesterolemia predisposes to MAC. The prevalence of hypercholesterolemia with serum total cholesterol greater than 200 mg/dL was higher in elderly persons with MAC than in elderly persons without MAC (90). Yetkin and colleagues (92) reported on 484 consecutive patients, mean age 60 ± 10 years, undergoing coronary arteriography for suspected coronary artery disease, 20% of whom had MAC. There were no statistically significant differences between those with and without MAC with respect to body mass index, diabetes mellitus, hypercholesterolemia, or the presence of coronary artery disease.

Roberts and Waller (93) found that chronic hypercalcemia predisposes to MAC. Patients undergoing dialysis for chronic renal insufficiency have an increased prevalence of MAC (93, 94). MAC has also been found to be a marker of left ventricular dilatation and decreased left ventricular systolic function in patients with end-stage renal disease on peritoneal dialysis (95). Fox and colleagues (96) studying 3047 participants in the Framingham study of patients with chronic kidney disease, defined by a glomerular filtration rate less than 60 mL/min/1.73 m^2, found that the odds of having MAC was increased by 60% in those with chronic kidney disease. Aronow and colleagues (90) observed no significant difference in mean serum calcium, serum phosphorus, or product of serum calcium and phosphorus between elderly persons with and without MAC. By accelerating the rate of rise of left ventricular systolic pressure, hypertrophic cardiomyopathy predisposes to MAC. Motamed and Roberts (97) demonstrated MAC in 30 of 100 autopsy patients (30%) with hypertrophic cardiomyopathy older than 40 years and in none of 100 autopsy patients (0%) younger than 40 years with hypertrophic cardiomyopathy. Aronow and Kronzon (98) diagnosed MAC in 13 of 17 older persons (76%) with hypertrophic cardiomyopathy and in 176 of 362 older persons (49%) without hypertrophic cardiomyopathy.

Elderly men and women with MAC have a higher prevalence of coronary artery disease (99), peripheral arterial disease (100), extracranial carotid arterial disease (ECAD) (101), and aortic atherosclerotic disease (101) than elderly men and women without MAC.

Diagnosis

Calcific deposits in the mitral annulus are J-, C-, U-, or O-shaped and are visualized in the posterior third of the heart shadow. MAC may be diagnosed by chest X-ray films or by fluoroscopy and by computed tomography (89). However, the procedures of choice for diagnosing MAC are M-mode and two-dimensional echocardiography.

Posterior MAC (Figure 15.1) is diagnosed by M-mode echocardiography when a band of dense echoes is recorded anterior to the left ventricular posterior wall and moving parallel with it. These echoes end at the atrioventricular junction and merge with the left ventricular posterior wall on echocardiographic sweep from the aortic root to the left ventricular apex.

Anterior MAC (Figure 15.1) is diagnosed by M-mode echocardiography when a continuous band of dense echoes is observed at the level of the anterior mitral leaflet in both systole and diastole. These echoes are contiguous with the posterior wall of the aortic root. Calcification may extend from the mitral annulus throughout the base of the heart and into the mitral and aortic valves.

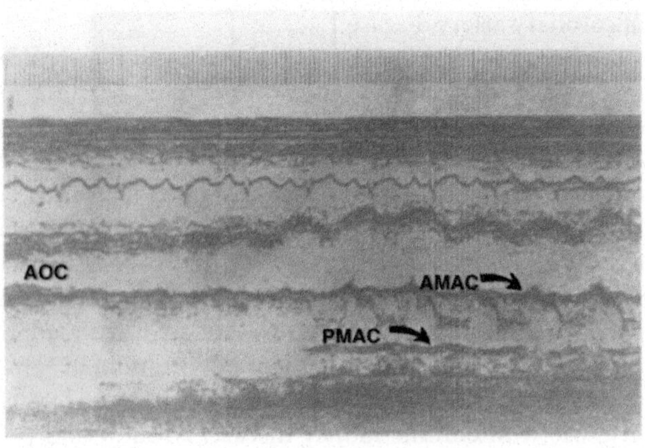

Figure 15.1 M-mode echocardiogram with scan from the aortic root to the left ventricular apex in a patient with both anterior and posterior mitral annular calcium. *Abbreviations*: AOC, aortic calcium; AMAC, anterior mitral annular calcium; PMAC, posterior mitral annular calcium.

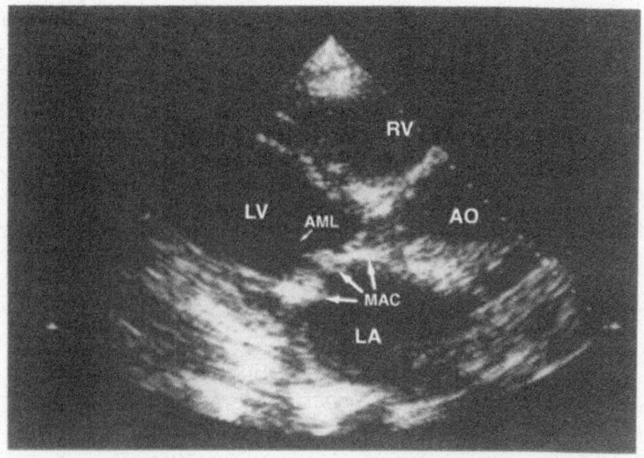

Figure 15.2 Two-dimensional echocardiogram long-axis view depicting MAC. *Abbreviations*: LA, left atrium; LV, left ventricle; RV, right ventricle; AO, aorta; AML, anterior mitral leaflet; MAC, mitral annular calcium.

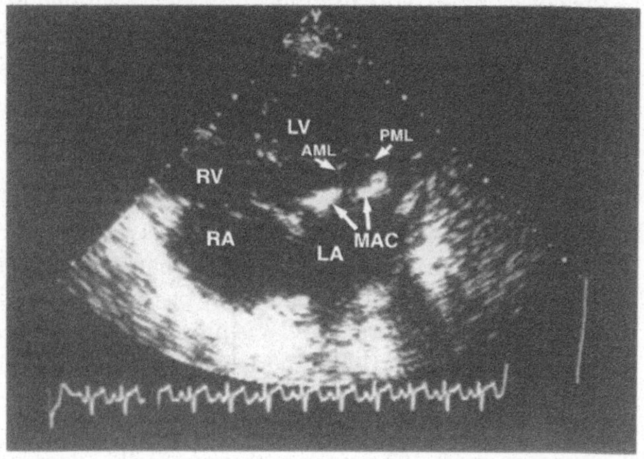

Figure 15.3 Two-dimensional echocardiogram four-chamber view of a patient with MAC. *Abbreviations*: LA, left atrium; RA, right atrium; RV, right ventricle; LV, left ventricle; AML, anterior mitral leaflet; PML, posterior mitral leaflet; MAC, mitral annular calcium.

Figures 15.2 and 15.3 are two-dimensional echocardiograms showing increased echogenicity and brightness of the mitral annulus characteristic of MAC. Using multiple echocardiographic views, MAC may be classified as mild, moderate, or severe. The echo densities in mild MAC involve less than one-third of the annular circumference (<3 mm in width) and are usually restricted to the angle between the posterior leaflet of the mitral valve and the left ventricular posterior wall. The echo densities in moderate MAC involve less than two-thirds of the annular circumference (3–5 mm in width). The echo densities in severe MAC involve more than two thirds of the annular circumference (>5 mm in width), usually extending beneath the entire posterior mitral leaflet with or without making a complete circle.

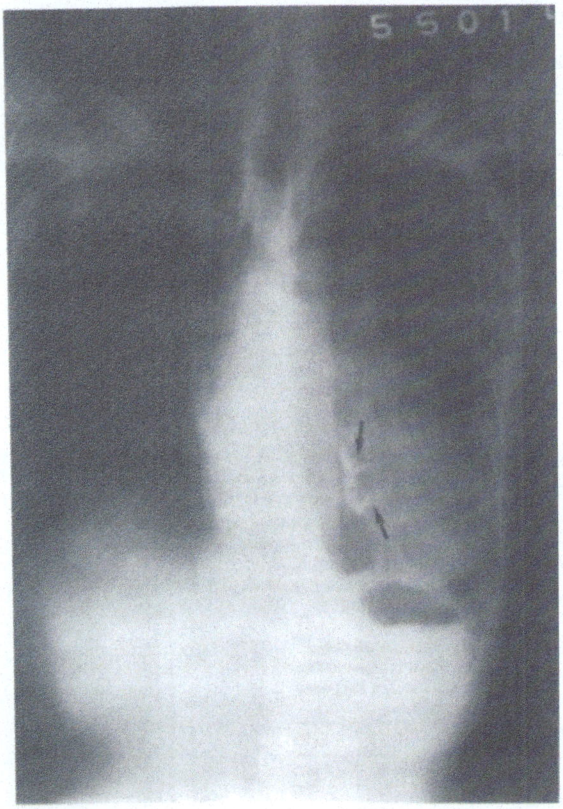

Figure 15.4 Posterior–anterior chest X-ray in a patient with C-shaped calcification of the mitral annulus (arrows).

In a blinded prospective study, MAC was diagnosed by M-mode and two-dimensional echocardiography in 55% of 604 unselected elderly patients in a long-term health care facility (102). The diagnosis of MAC by chest X-ray films using a lateral chest X-ray in addition to the posterior–anterior or anterior–posterior chest X-ray had a sensitivity of 12%, a specificity of 99%, a positive predictive value of 95%, and a negative predictive value of 47%. Patients with radiographic MAC were more likely than patients without radiographic MAC to have a more severe form of the disease, with significant MR, functional MS, or conduction defects. However, patients with echocardiographically severe MAC and significant MR, functional MS, or conduction defects may have no evidence of MAC on chest X-ray films. Figure 15.4 shows C-shaped calcification of the mitral annulus. Figure 15.5 illustrates J-shaped calcification of the mitral annulus.

Chamber size

Patients with MAC have a higher prevalence of left atrial enlargement (84, 85, 94) and left ventricular enlargement (94) than patients without MAC. In a prospective study of 976 elderly patients (526 with MAC and 450 without MAC), left atrial enlargement was 2.4 times more prevalent in patients with MAC than in the group without MAC (82).

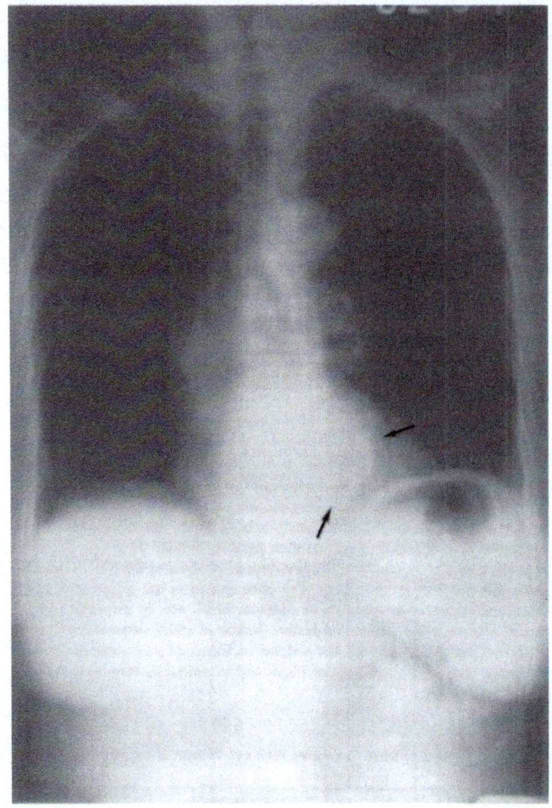

Figure 15.5 Posterior–anterior chest X-ray in a patient with J-shaped calcification of the mitral annulus (arrows).

Atrial fibrillation

Patients with MAC also have a higher prevalence of AF than patients without MAC (82, 85, 103). Table 15.8 shows that the prevalence of AF was increased 12, 5, and 2.8 times in patients with MAC than in patients without MAC (94, 103, 104).

Conduction defects

Because of the close proximity of the mitral annulus to the atrioventricular node and the bundle of His, patients with MAC have a higher prevalence of conduction defects, such as sinoatrial disease, atrioventricular block, bundle branch block, left anterior fascicular block, and intraventricular conduction defect than patients without MAC (87). The calcific deposits may also extend into the membranous portions of the interventricular septum involving the conduction system, or may even extend to the left atrium, interrupting interatrial and intra-atrial conduction. In addition, MAC may be associated with a sclerodegenerative process in the conduction system.

Mitral regurgitation

MAC is thought to generate systolic murmurs by the sphincter action loss of the annulus and the mechanical stretching of the mitral leaflets causing MR and from

Table 15.8 Prevalence of atrial fibrillation in patients with and without mitral annular calcium

	Atrial fibrillation				
	MAC		No MAC		Relative risk
	n	%	*n*	%	
Framingham study (104)	20/162	12	53/5532	1	12
Patients younger than 61 years (94)	11/107	10	2/107	2	5
Patients older than 60 years (mean age 81 + 8 years) (103)	225/1028	22	85/1120	8	2.8

Abbreviation: MAC, mitral annular calcium.

Table 15.9 Prevalence of apical systolic murmurs of mitral regurgitation in patients with mitral annular calcium

	Prevalence of mitral regurgitation murmur	
	n	%
Korn et al. (105)	14/14	100
Schott et al. (106)	10/14	71[a]
Savage et al. (104)	26/132	12
Nair et al. (94)	17/104	16
Aronow et al. (107)	129/293	44
Aronow et al. (108)	43/100	43

[a] MAC due to noninflammatory calcific disease.

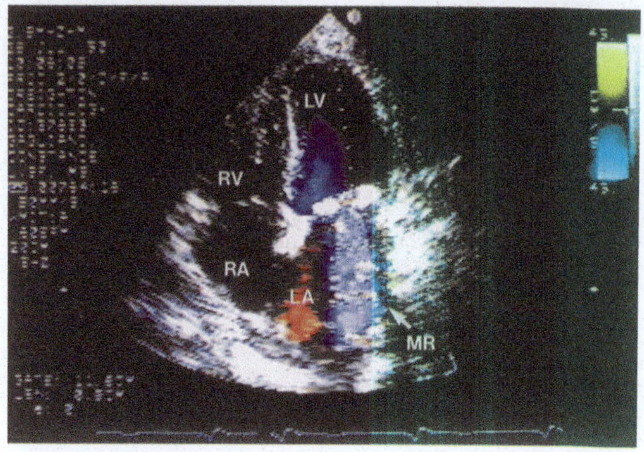

Figure 15.6 Color Doppler echocardiographic findings in a patient with mitral annular calcium and severe MR. *Abbreviations*: LA, left atrium; RA, right atrium; RV, right ventricle; LV, left ventricle; MR, mitral regurgitation.

vibration of the calcified ring or vortex formation around the annulus. Table 15.9 shows that the prevalence of apical systolic murmurs of MR in patients with MAC ranged from 12% to 100% in different studies (94, 104–108). Table 15.10 states the prevalence of MR diagnosed by Doppler echocardiography in patients with MAC (103, 108–110). The prevalence of MR associated with MAC ranged from 54% to 97% in the Doppler echocardiographic studies (108–110). Figure 15.6 illustrates severe MR due to MAC diagnosed by color Doppler echocardiography.

The greater the severity of MAC, the greater is the severity of MR associated with MAC. Moderate to severe MR was diagnosed by Doppler echocardiography in 33% of 51 patients with MAC by Labovitz and colleagues (110) and in 22% of 1028 patients with MAC by Aronow and colleagues (103). Kaul and colleagues (109) diagnosed severe MR in 7% of their 29 patients with MAC, and concluded that MR in patients with MAC is caused by a reduced sphincteric action of the mitral annulus, with MAC preventing the posterior annulus from contracting and assuming a flatter shape during systole.

Table 15.10 Prevalence of mitral regurgitation diagnosed by Doppler echocardiography in patients with mitral annular calcium

	MR		Moderate to severe MR	
	n	%	*n*	%
Labovitz et al. (110)	28/51	55	17/51	33
Aronow et al. (108)	54/100	54	18/100	18
Kaul et al. (109)	28/29	97[a]	—	
Aronow et al. (103)	—	—	24/1028	22

Abbreviation: MR, mitral regurgitation.
[a] Severe MR in 2 of 29 patients (7%).

Table 15.11 Prevalence of apical diastolic murmurs of mitral stenosis and of MS in patients with MAC

	Prevalence of MS by Doppler			
	Prevalence of MS murmur		Echocardiography	
	n	%	n	%
Korn et al. (105)	3/14	21	—	—
Schott et al. (106)	2/14	14[a]	—	—
Savage et al. (104)	2/132	2	—	—
Nair et al. (111)	7/104	7	—	—
Aronow et al. (107)	28/293	10	—	—
Labovitz et al. (110)	0/51	0	4/51	8
Aronow et al. (108)	6/100	6	6/100	6
Aronow et al. (103)	—	—	83/1028	8

Abbreviations: MS, mitral stenosis; MAC, mitral annular calcium.
[a] MAC due to noninflammatory calcific disease.

Mitral stenosis

An apical diastolic murmur may be heard in patients with MAC as a result of turbulent flow across the calcified and narrowed annulus (annular stenosis). Table 15.11 shows that the prevalence of apical diastolic murmurs of MS in patients with MAC ranged from 0% to 25% in different studies (103–108, 110, 111). Table 15.11 also indicates that MS associated with MAC was diagnosed by Doppler echocardiography in 8% of 51 patients by Labovitz and colleagues (110), in 6% of 100 patients by Aronow and Kronzon (108), and in 8% of 1028 patients by Aronow et al. (103). Figure 15.7 illustrates MS due to MAC diagnosed by Doppler echocardiography.

The reduction of mitral valve orifice in patients with MAC is due to the annular calcium and to decreased mitral excursion and mobility secondary to calcium at the base of the leaflets (108). The commissures are fused in rheumatic MS but are not fused in MS associated with MAC. The mitral leaflet margins in MAC may be thin and mobile, and the posterior mitral leaflet may move normally during diastole. However, Doppler echocardiographic recordings show increased transvalvular flow velocity and prolonged pressure half-time and, therefore, smaller mitral valve orifice in patients with MS, regardless of the etiology.

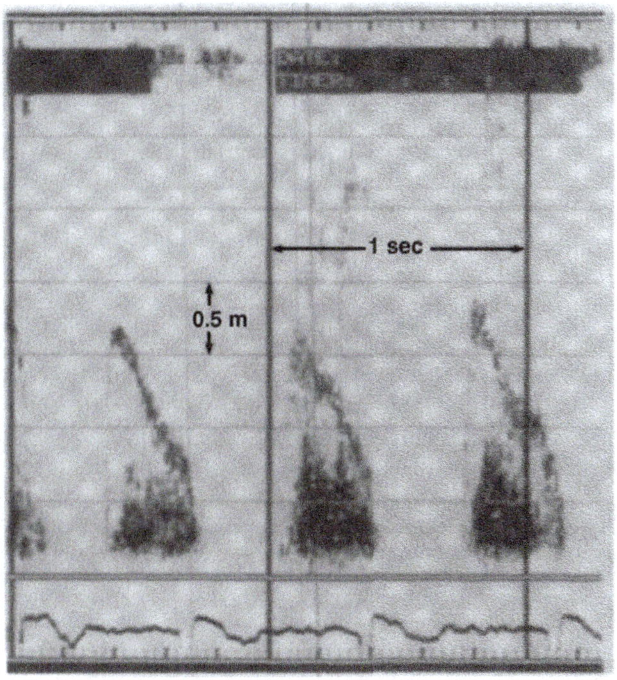

Figure 15.7 Continuous-wave Doppler tracing across a stenotic mitral valve orifice due to mitral annular calcium. Peak diastolic gradient = 12 mmHg. Pressure half-time = 200 ms. Mitral valve area = 1.1 cm^2.

Bacterial endocarditis

Bacterial endocarditis, with a high incidence of *Staphylococcus aureus* endocarditis, may complicate MAC (82, 88). Patients with MAC associated with chronic renal failure are especially at increased risk for developing bacterial endocarditis (106). The calcific mass erodes the endothelium under the mitral valve that is exposed to transient bacteremia. The avascular nature of the mitral annulus interferes with antibiotics reaching a nidus of bacteria, predisposing to periannular and myocardial abscesses and, consequently, to a poor prognosis. Nair and colleagues (111) observed at 4.4-year mean follow-up with no significant difference in incidence of bacterial endocarditis in 99 patients younger than 61 years with MAC compared to a control group of 101 patients. However, Aronow and colleagues (82) demonstrated at 39-month mean follow-up of 3% incidence of bacterial endocarditis in 526 elderly patients with MAC and a 1% incidence of bacterial endocarditis in 450 elderly patients without MAC.

Until 2007, prophylactic antibiotics were recommended to prevent bacterial endocarditis in patients with MAC, according to AHA guidelines (112). At that time, after reevaluating the evidence in the literature, the consensus was that the vast majority of cases of infective endocarditis were the result of bacteremia, which occurs extremely frequently as a result of daily activities such as vigorous chewing, brushing the teeth, and flossing and not from dental manipulations. Therefore, the present AHA recommendation is that antibiotic prophylaxis should be reserved for high-risk patients such as those with prosthetic valves, cyanotic and other high-risk congenital heart disease, patients with a previous episode of infective endocarditis, and cardiac transplant patients with valvulopathy (113). Despite the AHA recommendations, many physicians still prescribe antibiotic prophylaxis for their patients with valvular disease.

Cardiac events

The presence of MAC, a marker of atherosclerosis, is associated with an increase in cardiovascular events, including myocardial infarction, stroke, and death. Gondrie and colleagues (86), using a case-cohort design, evaluated 10,410 subjects undergoing chest CT, excluding patients referred for cardiovascular disease. The mean follow-up was 17 months, and there were 515 cardiovascular events in 1285 subjects. Patients with MAC compared to those without valve calcification had a risk ratio of 1.53 (95% CI 1.13–2.00).

In a prospective study of 107 patients (8 lost to follow-up) younger than 61 years with MAC and 107 (6 lost to follow-up) age- and sex-matched control subjects, Nair and colleagues (111) demonstrated at 4.4-year mean follow-up that patients with MAC had a higher incidence of new cardiac events than control subjects (Table 15.12). In a prospective study of 526 elderly patients with MAC and 450 elderly patients without MAC, Aronow and colleagues (82) found at 39-month mean follow-up that the incidence of new cardiac events (myocardial infarction, primary ventricular fibrillation, or sudden cardiac death) was also higher in elderly patients with MAC than in elderly patients without MAC.

Mitral valve replacement

Nair and colleagues (114) reported that mitral valve replacement could be accomplished in patients with MAC with morbidity and mortality similar to that in patients without MAC. Following mitral valve replacement, subsequent morbidity and mortality during 4.4-year mean follow-up were also similar in patients with and without MAC.

Cerebrovascular events

Although the increased prevalence of AF, MS, MR, left atrial enlargement, and congestive heart failure predisposes patients with MAC to thromboembolic stroke, some investigators consider MAC a marker of other vascular disease causing stroke rather the primary embolic source. Others believe that MAC with ulcerated endothelium and platelet agglutination is responsible for clinically silent brain infarcts. Rodriguez and colleagues (81) reported cerebral MRIs in 2680 Cardiovascular Health Study subjects without a clinical history of strokes or transient ischemic attacks. The mean age of the population was 75 ± 4.8 years. The presence of any left-sided valvular or annular calcification was associated with covert brain infarcts with a risk ratio of 1.24 (95% CI 1.05–1.47) compared to those with no calcification, and the severity of calcification was directly related to the presence of MRI findings. In a retrospective study of 110 elderly patients with chronic AF, 44 (40%) had documented thromboembolic stroke (115). In this study, the prevalence of MAC was not significantly different in elderly patients

Table 15.12 Incidence of new cardiac events in patients with and without mitral annular calcium

	Follow-up	Cardiac events				Relative risk
		MAC		No MAC		
		n	%	*n*	%	
Nair et al. (111)	4.4 years	31/99	31	2/101	2	15.5
Total cardiac death		12/99	12	1/101	1	12.0
Sudden cardiac death		41/99	41	6/101	6	6.8
Congestive heart failure; mitral or aortic valve replacement		9/99	9	0/101	0	—
Aronow et al. (82)	39 months					
Cardiac events[a] if: Atrial fibrillation		62/90	69	22/41	54	1.3
Sinus rhythm		157/436	36	106/409	26	1.4
All patients		219/526	42	128/450	28	1.5

Abbreviation: MAC, mitral annular calcium.
[a] Myocardial infarction, primary ventricular fibrillation, or sudden cardiac death.

Table 15.13 Incidence of new cerebrovascular events in patients with and without mitral annular calcium

	Follow-up	Cerebrovascular events				Relative risk
		MAC		No MAC		
			%		%	
Nair et al. (111)	4.4 years	10/99	10	2/101	2	5.0
TE cardiovascular events: Benjamin et al. (167)	8 years	22/160	14	51/999	5	2.7
Stroke: Aronow et al. (82)	39 months					
TE stroke if:		45/90	50	14/41	34	1.5
Atrial fibrillation						
Sinus rhythm		59/436	14	38/409	9	1.6
All patients		104/526	20	52/450	12	1.7
Boston Area Anticoagulation	2.2 years	10/129	8	5/291	2	4.0
Trial for Atrial Fibrillation (116)	45 months					
Ischemia stroke: Aronow et al. (117)						
TE stroke if:		52/101	51	16/49	33	1.5
40%–100% ECAD						
0%–39% ECAD		88/365	24	47/413	11	2.2
TIA if:		8/101	8	3/49	6	1.3
40%–100% ECAD						
0%–39% ECAD		11/365	3	3/413	1	3.0

Abbreviations: ECAD, extracranial carotid arterial disease; MAC, mitral annular calcium; TE, thromboembolic; TIA, cerebral transient ischemic attack.

with thromboembolic stroke (80%) or without thromboembolic stroke (65%) (relative risk = 1.2). However, six prospective studies have demonstrated an increased incidence of new cerebrovascular events in patients with MAC than in patients without MAC (Tables 15.13–15.15) (120) ranging from a relative risk of 1.5 up to 5.0.

Aronow and colleagues studied the incidence of new thromboembolic stroke at 44-month mean follow-up in 310 unselected elderly patients with chronic AF in a long-term healthcare facility (103) (Table 15.14). MS and the severity of MR were diagnosed by Doppler echocardiography in this study (103). In elderly persons with chronic AF, MAC increased the incidence of new thromboembolic stroke 2.1 times if MS was associated with MAC, 1.7 times if 2–4+ MR was associated with MAC, and 1.4 times if 0–1+ MR was present. Table 15.15 shows the incidence of new thromboembolic stroke at 44-month mean follow-up in 1838 unselected older persons, mean age 81 years, with sinus rhythm, in a long-term healthcare facility (103). In elderly persons with sinus rhythm, MAC increased the incidence of new thromboembolic stroke 3.6 times if MS was associated with MAC, 3.1 times if 2–4+ MR was associated with MAC, and 2.7 times if 0–1+ MR was present. Using the multivariate Cox regression model, independent risk factors for new thromboembolic stroke in this study were prior stroke (risk ratio = 2.4), MAC (risk ratio = 2.6), AF (risk ratio = 3.0), and male gender (risk ratio = 1.6).

There was a higher prevalence of MAC in elderly patients with 40%–100% ECAD (67% of 150 patients) than in elderly patients with 0%–39% ECAD (47% of 778 patients) (117). The increased prevalence of significant

Table 15.14 Incidence of new thromboembolic stroke at 44-month mean follow-up in elderly patients with chronic atrial fibrillation

	Thromboembolic stroke (%)
Atrial fibrillation, no MAC (*n* = 85)	35
Atrial fibrillation with MS due to MAC (*n* = 42)	74
Atrial fibrillation with MAC and 2–4+ MR (*n* = 90)	59
Atrial fibrillation with MAC and 0–1+ MR (*n* = 93)	48

Source: Aronow WS et al., *Am J Cardiol*, 81, 105–106, 1998.
Abbreviations: MAC, mitral annular calcium; MR, mitral regurgitation; MS, mitral stenosis.

Table 15.15 Incidence of new thromboembolic stroke at 44-month mean follow-up in elderly patients with sinus rhythm

	Thromboembolic stroke (%)
Sinus rhythm, no MAC (*n* = 1035)	9
Sinus rhythm with MS due to MAC (*n* = 41)	32
Sinus rhythm with MAC and 2–4+ MR (*n* = 134)	28
Sinus rhythm with MAC and 0–1+ MR (*n* = 625)	24

Source: Aronow WS et al., *Am J Cardiol*, 81, 105–106, 1998.
Abbreviations: MAC, mitral annular calcium; MR, mitral regurgitation; MS, mitral stenosis.

ECAD contributes to a higher stroke rate. Thrombi of the mitral annulus also contribute to thromboembolic stroke in elderly patients with MAC. In addition, MAC is associated with aortic atheromatous disease, complex intra-aortic debris (118), and thoracic aorta calcium that could contribute to thromboembolic stroke. Some patients with MAC who experienced thromboembolic events also had a mobile component that was associated with the thromboembolic events (119). There was no significant difference in the association of MAC with prior stroke between elderly Whites and elderly African Americans, between elderly Whites and elderly Hispanics, and between elderly African Americans and elderly Hispanics (120).

Kizer and colleagues (121), from the Strong Heart Study, followed 2723 American Indians without clinical cardiovascular disease and with baseline echocardiograms for 7 years. Eighty-six strokes occurred. The presence of MAC but not aortic valve sclerosis was a strong risk factor for incident stroke after extensive adjustment for other predictors. Since patients with MAC and AF or sinus rhythm have a higher incidence of thromboembolic stroke than patients without MAC, antithrombotic therapy should be considered in patients with MAC and no contraindications to antithrombotic therapy. In the Boston Area Anticoagulation Trial for Atrial Fibrillation study, warfarin reduced the incidence of thromboembolic stroke in patients with MAC by about 90% (122, 123).

Until data from prospective, randomized studies evaluating the efficacy and risk of antithrombotic therapy in patients with MAC are available, patients with MAC associated with either AF, MS, or moderate to severe MR should be considered for treatment with warfarin if they have no contraindications to anticoagulant therapy. The international normalized ratio should be maintained between 2.0 and 3.0. The efficacy of antiplatelet therapy in patients with MAC is unknown.

Percutaneous edge-to-edge mitral valve repair (MitraClip)

Percutaneous mitral valve edge-to-edge repair (E2E) for MR was developed based on the surgical technique of creating a double orifice valve by Alfieri (124) (Figure 15.8). The original surgical technique as reported by Alfieri involved creating a double orifice mitral valve by approximating the free edges of the leaflets at the site of regurgitation with a suture (124) in 260 patients. The majority of patients had degenerative MR (DMR) (80%), bileaflet or anterior leaflet prolapse (83%), and EF >45% (93%), and underwent associated annuloplasty (80%). Five-year survival was 94.4% and freedom from reoperation was 90%, but echocardiographic data on recurrent MR was not reported (124). A subsequent study of surgical E2E in 29 patients without annuloplasty reported a 5-year freedom from the combined endpoint of recurrent MR >2+ and reoperation of 90% (125).

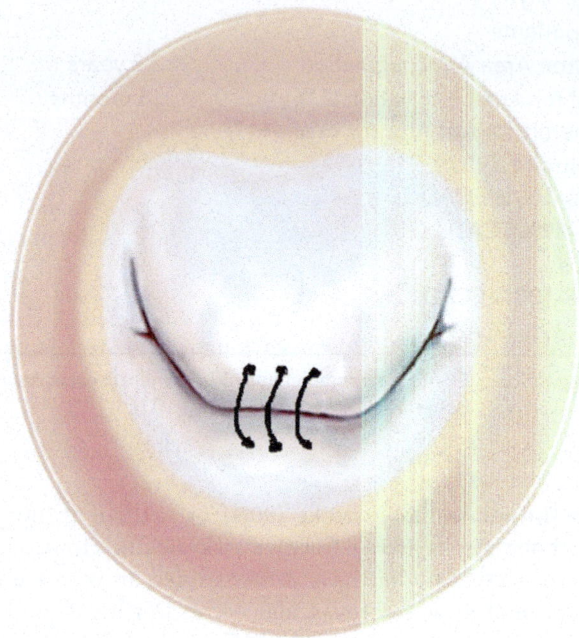

Figure 15.8 Percutaneous mitral valve edge-to-edge repair.

EVEREST II was a randomized comparison of MitraClip to mitral valve surgery with similar inclusion criteria, in which 279 patients with moderately severe or severe MR (71% DMR) were randomly assigned in a 2:1 ratio to undergo MitraClip or conventional surgical repair or replacement (126). The primary composite endpoint for efficacy was freedom from death, surgery for mitral valve dysfunction, and from grade 3+ or 4+ mitral regurgitation at 12 months. At 12 months, the rates of the primary endpoint for efficacy were 55% in the MitraClip group and 73% in the surgery group (p = 0.007) with similar mortality (6%). Compared to surgery, MitraClip patients had lower major adverse events (15% vs. 48% respectively), higher rates for surgery due to mitral valve dysfunction (20% vs. 2% respectively), and significantly less reduction in severity of MR. MitraClip also did not reduce MR below grade 3+ in 23% of patients (126).

At 5 years, the EVEREST II study showed the rate of the composite endpoint was 44.2% versus 64.3% in the MitraClip and surgical groups, respectively (p = 0.01). The difference was driven by increased rates of 3+ to 4+ MR (12.3% vs. 1.8%; p = 0.02) and surgery (27.9% vs. 8.9%; p = 0.003). However, in the MitraClip group 78% of surgeries occurred within the first 6 months, and past 6 months, rates of surgery and moderate to severe MR were comparable between groups. Five-year mortality rates were 20.8% and 26.8% (p = 0.4) for MitraClip and surgery, respectively. In multivariable analysis, treatment strategy was not associated with survival (127).

Real-world data from Europe in 567 patients from 14 countries showed that 97% had 3+ to 4+ MR, 70% had FMR, and 52% had LVEF <40%. At 12 months post MitraClip, 82% were alive, 6.3% required mitral valve surgery, 78.9% were free from MR >2+, and 71.4% of patients had NYHA functional class II or class I (128).

In a prohibitive surgical risk cohort from the EVEREST II trial of 127 DMR patients with an average age of 82, mortality at 1 year was 24%, but of the surviving patients, 83% had MR ≤2, 87% had NYHA class I or II, and a majority had improved quality of life and rehospitalization rates (129).

Data from the Society of Thoracic Surgery/American College of Cardiology Transcatheter Valve Therapy registry on patients commercially treated with MitraClip showed that 2952 patients were treated at 145 hospitals between November 2013 and September 2015 in the United States. These patients had a median age of 82, 94% of patients had 3+ or 4+ MR, 86% had DMR, and 64% had LVEF ≥50%. Clip implantation site was A2-P2 in 83%, more than one clip was implanted in 34% of patients, post-procedure MR ≤2 was achieved in 93% of patients, and in-hospital mortality was 2.7%. At 12 months, mortality was 25.8% and repeat hospitalization for heart failure was 20%. The cumulative incidences of mortality (24.7%), rehospitalization for heart failure (20.5%), and the combined endpoint for both of these two outcomes (35.7%) were lower for patients with DMR compared with FMR (31.2%, 32.6%, and 49.0%, respectively). Mortality and the rate of heart failure rehospitalization at 1 year were higher for patients who had residual MR grade 3 or 4 following MitraClip. The presence of higher LVEF was associated with a lower risk of death and heart failure rehospitalization (130).

MitraClip received CE Mark approval in Europe in 2008 for FMR or DMR. In the United States, it was approved in 2013 but only for severe DMR in patients who have been determined to be at prohibitive risk for mitral valve surgery by a heart team.

In summary, percutaneous E2E mitral valve repair with the MitraClip system can be successfully and safely performed in the vast majority of patients. Residual MR >3+ after MitraClip, FMR, lower EF, and severe tricuspid valve regurgitation are associated with worse outcomes (130). It is approved for DMR in the United States, but in current practice outside the United States, 70% of patients being treated have FMR (131). The use of MitraClip in FMR patients is being compared with guideline-directed medical therapy in two trials: COAPT Trial (Cardiovascular Outcomes Assessment of the MitraClip Percutaneous Therapy for Heart Failure Patients With Functional Mitral Regurgitation) and MITRA-FR (Multicentre Study of Percutaneous Mitral Valve Repair MitraClip Device in Patients with Severe Secondary MR).

UPDATE

MS is a significant valvular heart disease characterized by the narrowing of the mitral valve orifice, resulting in impaired blood flow from the left atrium to the left ventricle (132, 133). Globally, rheumatic fever remains the leading cause of MS, although degenerative or calcific changes are increasingly observed in developed countries, particularly among the elderly (133, 134). The condition often leads to complications such as left atrial enlargement, AF, and a heightened risk of thromboembolism (132, 135). Advances in imaging techniques, including echocardiography, have improved diagnostic accuracy, while treatment options now range from medical management to percutaneous interventions, such as balloon mitral valvuloplasty, and surgical valve repair or replacement, depending on the severity and patient characteristics (134, 136).

The ACC/AHA guidelines classify MS into four stages (137). Stage A includes patients at risk for MS but without valve obstructions. Stage B describes progressive MS with mild-to-moderate obstruction (mitral valve area [MVA] > 1.5 cm^2), usually asymptomatic. Stage C, or severe asymptomatic MS, is defined by significant valve obstruction (MVA ≤ 1.5 cm^2) and the presence of resting or exertional pulmonary hypertension. Stage D represents severe symptomatic MS, where patients experience debilitating symptoms during minimal exertion or rest, often accompanied by pulmonary hypertension.

Rheumatic heart disease (RHD) remains the most common etiology of MS in developing countries, with symptoms typically manifesting 10 to 15 years after an initial episode of rheumatic fever (138). In developed nations, rheumatic MS is more prevalent in immigrant populations and individuals with limited access to healthcare (138). AF is a common and severe complication, increasing the risk of thromboembolism and negatively impacting prognosis. Diagnostic tools include echocardiography, the gold standard for assessing valve anatomy and hemodynamics, as well as electrocardiograms for detecting AF and cardiac catheterization in select cases (139, 140). Computed tomography imaging may also assist in planning interventions. Management strategies involve anticoagulation therapy for patients with AF, percutaneous balloon mitral valvuloplasty for suitable cases, and mitral valve replacement or transcatheter mitral valve replacement for high-risk surgical candidates (140–142).

MR is the most common valvular heart disease, characterized by the backward flow of blood from the left ventricle to the left atrium during systole due to improper closure of the mitral valve (143). This condition can be classified into two main types: primary MR, which is a disease of the mitral valve apparatus itself, and secondary MR, which results from left ventricular dysfunction (143).

The management of mitral regurgitation has evolved significantly in recent years, with a growing emphasis on early intervention, particularly in asymptomatic patients with severe MR (144, 145). This approach is supported by guidelines and has shown promising outcomes in terms of safety and long-term results (144).

Diagnosis and management of MR require a structured approach that integrates findings from patient history, physical examination, and imaging studies (143). Echocardiography plays a crucial role in determining the etiology, severity of regurgitation, and its impact on left ventricular function (143). These factors, along with the potential for a durable valve repair, are key considerations in deciding the optimal timing for intervention (143).

Recent advances in both surgical and catheter-based therapies have led to recommendations for earlier intervention and the extension of treatment options to older and higher-risk patient populations (143). These developments aim to improve long-term outcomes and quality of life for patients with mitral regurgitation (145).

Acute MR is a severe cardiac condition characterized by the sudden onset of significant backward flow of blood from the left ventricle to the left atrium during systole. This occurs due to an abrupt failure of the mitral valve apparatus to close properly, leading to rapid hemodynamic deterioration and potentially life-threatening complications (146). The most common causes of acute severe MR include chordae tendineae rupture, papillary muscle rupture, and infective endocarditis. Chordal rupture in patients with floppy mitral valve or mitral valve prolapse is currently the most prevalent etiology. In cases of infective endocarditis, both native and prosthetic valves can be affected, resulting in leaflet perforation, ring detachment, or rupture of chordae tendineae or papillary muscles (146).

Diagnosis of acute MR requires a rapid and comprehensive evaluation. Echocardiography with Doppler imaging plays a crucial role in providing vital information about the underlying pathology and severity of regurgitation. However, it's important to note that echocardiographic findings in acute MR can differ from those seen in chronic MR due to the sudden elevation of left atrial and pulmonary artery pressures, coupled with a small left ventricle and atrium with low compliance (146, 147).

Initial medical management aims to stabilize the patient before definitive intervention. This may include the use of vasodilators, diuretics, and inotropic agents to improve hemodynamics and reduce pulmonary congestion. In many cases, mechanical circulatory support may be necessary to maintain adequate perfusion and oxygenation (146). While surgical correction has traditionally been the primary treatment for acute severe MR, many patients are considered high-risk surgical candidates due to their unstable condition or comorbidities. In recent years, transcatheter mitral valve repair, particularly using the MitraClip device, has emerged as a suitable therapy for these high-risk patients. This minimally invasive approach can provide rapid improvement in hemodynamics and symptoms, serving as a bridge to definitive treatment or as a standalone procedure in select cases (147). However, the decision for intervention should be individualized, and a multidisciplinary team approach is crucial in determining the optimal management strategy for each patient with acute MR (146).

Chronic primary MR is a progressive valvular heart disease characterized by the inadequate closure of the mitral valve during systole, leading to blood regurgitation from the left ventricle to the left atrium. This condition is primarily caused by structural abnormalities of the mitral valve apparatus, including leaflet prolapse, chordal rupture, or annular dilatation (148).

The AHA and ACC have defined four stages of chronic primary MR: Stage A (at risk), Stage B (progressive), Stage C (asymptomatic severe), and Stage D (symptomatic severe). Stage C is further divided into C1 (preserved left ventricular function) and C2 (reduced left ventricular function). This staging system helps guide management decisions and predict outcomes (149).

Diagnosis of chronic primary MR relies heavily on echocardiography, which remains the gold standard for assessment. Transthoracic echocardiography with Doppler imaging provides crucial information about the etiology, severity of regurgitation, and its impact on left ventricular function. Quantitative parameters such as effective regurgitant orifice area (EROA) $\geq$0.4 cm^2, regurgitant volume $\geq$60 mL, and regurgitant fraction $\geq$50% indicate severe MR. Additionally, cardiac magnetic resonance imaging may be used for more precise quantification of regurgitant volume and left ventricular function (148).

Follow-up of chronic primary MR depends on the severity and stage of the disease. For asymptomatic patients with severe MR (Stage C), guidelines recommend clinical and echocardiographic follow-up every 6–12 months. Patients with moderate MR should be followed every 1–2 years, while those with mild MR can be evaluated every 3–5 years. Regular monitoring is crucial to detect progression of MR, development of symptoms, or changes in left ventricular function that may warrant intervention (149).

Medical therapy for chronic primary MR is primarily supportive and does not alter the natural history of the disease. However, it plays a role in managing symptoms and comorbidities. Beta-blockers and ACE inhibitors may be considered in patients with heart failure symptoms or reduced left ventricular function. For patients with severe symptomatic MR (Stage D) or asymptomatic severe MR with left ventricular dysfunction (Stage C2), surgical intervention is the mainstay of treatment. Mitral valve repair is preferred over replacement when feasible, as it offers better long-term outcomes. In high-risk surgical candidates, the transcatheter mitral valve repair device, MitraClip, is a viable alternative, showing promising results in reducing MR and improving quality of life (144, 148).

Tricuspid valve regurgitation (TR) and stenosis can be treated medically but often require surgical repair of the valve. Percutaneous intervention or transcatheter valve repair may be used for nonsurgical candidates. TR can be primary coming from structural issues with the tricuspid valve or more commonly secondary due to conditions affecting the right ventricle or the pulmonary circulation (150). Severe TR may be treated by transcatheter edge-to-edge repair with the TriClip device to improve the severity of TR with associated improvement in quality of life (150).

REFERENCES

1. Cheitlin MD. Management of valve disease in the elderly. *Am J Geriatr Cardiol* 1996; *5*: 65–67.
2. Chiang CW, Lo SK, Kuo CT et al. Noninvasive predictors of systemic embolism in mitral stenosis. An echocardiographic and clinical study of 500 patients. *Chest* 1994; *106*: 396–399.
3. Otsuji Y, Handschumacher MD, Liel-Cohen N et al. Mechanism of ischemic mitral regurgitation with segmental left ventricular dysfunction: Three-dimensional echocardiographic studies in models of acute and chronic progressive regurgitation. *J Am Coll Cardiol* 2001; *37*: 641–648.
4. Vaitkevicius PV, Fleg JL, Engel JH et al. Effects of age and aerobic capacity on arterial stiffness in healthy adults. *Circulation* 1993; *88*: 1456–1462.
5. .Handshoe R, DeMaria AN. Doppler assessment of intracardiac pressures. *Echocardiogr Rev Cardiovasc Ultrasound* 1985; *2*: 127–139.
6. Padial LR, Freitas N, Sagie A et al. Echocardiography can predict which patients will develop severe mitral regurgitation after percutaneous mitral valvulotomy. *J Am Coll Cardiol* 1996; *27*: 1225–1231.
7. Grewal KS, Malkowski MJ, Kramer CM et al. Multiplane transesophageal echocardiographic identification of the involved scallop in patients with flail mitral valve leaflet: Intraoperative correlation. *J Am Soc Echocardiogr* 1998; *11*: 966–971.
8. Thomas L, Foster E, Hoffman JI et al. Prospective validation of an echocardiographic index for determining the severity of chronic mitral regurgitation. *Am J Cardiol* 2002; *90*: 607–612.
9. Zamorano J, Perez de Isla L, Oliveros L et al. Prognostic influence of mitral regurgitation prior to a first myocardial infarction. *Eur Heart J* 2005; *26*: 343–349.
10. Amigoni M, Meris A, Thune JJ et al. Mitral regurgitation in myocardial infarction complicated by heart failure, left ventricular dysfunction, or both: Prognostic significance and relation to ventricular size and function. *Eur Heart J* 2007; *28*: 326–333.
11. Mihaljevic T, Lam B-U, Rajeswaran J et al. Impact of mitral valve annuloplasty combined with revascularization in patients with functional ischemic mitral regurgitation. *J Am Coll Cardiol* 2007; *49*: 2191–2201.
12. Mustonen J, Suurmunne H, Kouri J et al. Impact of coronary artery bypass surgery on ischemic mitral regurgitation. *Scand J Surg* 2011; *100*: 114–119.
13. Ling LH, Enriquez-Sarano M, Seward JB et al. Clinical outcome of mitral regurgitation due to flail leaflet. *N Engl J Med* 1996; *335*: 1417–1423.
14. .Rosenhek R, Rader F, Klaar U et al. Outcome of watchful waiting in asymptomatic severe mitral regurgitation. *Circulation* 2006; *113*: 2238–2244.
15. Bonow RO, Carabello B, Chatterjee K et al. ACC/AHA 2006 guidelines for the management of patients with valvular heart disease. A report of the American College of Cardiology/American Heart Association Task Force on Practice Guidelines (writing Committee to Revise the 1998 guidelines on the management of patients with valvular heart disease): Developed in collaboration with the society of cardiovascular anesthesiologists: Endorsed by the society for cardiovascular angiography and interventions. *Circulation* 2006; *114*: e84–e231.
16. Wei T, Zeng C, Chen F et al. Influence of commissural calcification on the immediate outcomes of percutaneous balloon mitral valvuloplasty. *Acta Cardiol* 2003; *58*: 411–415.
17. Manjunath CN, Srinivasa KH, Panneerselvam A et al. Incidence and predictors of left atrial thrombus in patients with rheumatic mitral stenosis and sinus rhythm: A transesophageal echocardiographic study. *Echocardiography* 2011; *28*: 457–460.
18. Palacios IF, Tuzcu ME, Weyman AE et al. Clinical follow-up of patients undergoing percutaneous mitral balloon valvotomy. *Circulation* 1995; *91*: 671–676.
19. Iung B, Garbarz E, Doutrelant L et al. Late results of percutaneous mitral commissurotomy for calcific mitral stenosis. *Am J Cardiol* 2000; *85*: 1308–1314.
20. Iung B, Cormier B, Ducimetiere P et al. Immediate results of percutaneous mitral commissurotomy. A predictive model on a series of 1514 patients. *Circulation* 1996; *94*: 2124–2130.

21. Fawzy ME. Long-term results up to 19 years of mitral balloon valvuloplasty. *Asian Cardiovasc Thorac Ann* 2009; *17*: 627–633.
22. Remadi F, Boughzala E, Neffati E et al. Percutaneous mitral commissurotomy in patients aged 60 years and more. *Ann Cardiol Angeiol* 2006; *55*: 149–152.
23. Le Feuvre C, Bonan R, Lachurie ML et al. Balloon mitral commissurotomy in patients aged > or = 70 years. *Am J Cardiol* 1993; *71*: 233–236.
24. Meneveau N, Schiele F, Seronde MF et al. Predictors of event-free survival after percutaneous mitral commissurotomy. *Heart* 1998; *80*: 359–364.
25. Hildick-Smith DJ, Taylor GJ, Shapiro LM. Inoue balloon mitral valvuloplasty: Long-term clinical and echocardiographic follow-up of a predominantly unfavourable population. *Eur Heart J* 2000; *21*: 1690–1697.
26. Sutaria N, Elder AT, Shaw TR. Long term outcome of percutaneous mitral balloon valvotomy in patients aged 70 and over. *Heart* 2000; *83*: 433–438.
27. Shaw TR, Elder AT, Flapan AD et al. Mitral balloon valvuloplasty for patients aged over 70 years: An alternative to surgical treatment. *Age Ageing* 1991; *20*: 299–303.
28. Sutaria N, Northridge DB, Shaw TR. Significance of commissural calcification on outcome of mitral balloon valvotomy. *Heart* 2000; *84*: 398–402.
29. Fawzy ME. Percutaneous mitral balloon valvotomy. *Catheter Cardiovasc Interv* 2007; *69*: 313–321.
30. Sutaria N, Elder AT, Shaw TR. Mitral balloon valvotomy for the treatment of mitral stenosis in octogenarians. *J Am Geriatr Soc* 2000; *48*: 971–974.
31. Iung B, Garbarz E, Michaud P et al. Percutaneous mitral commissurotomy for restenosis after surgical commissurotomy: Late efficacy and implications for patient selection. *J Am Coll Cardiol* 2000; *35*: 1295–1302.
32. Aslanabadi N, Golmohammadi A, Sohrabi B et al. Repeat percutaneous balloon mitral valvotomy vs. mitral valve replacement in patients with restenosis after previous balloon mitral valvotomy and unfavorable valve characteristics. *Clin Cardiol* 2011; *34*: 401–406.
33. Chmielak Z, Klopotowski M, Kruk M et al. Repeat percutaneous mitral balloon valvuloplasty for patients with mitral valve restenosis. *Catheter Cardiovasc Interv* 2010; *76*: 986–992.
34. Eid Fawzy M, Shoukri M, Al Sergani H et al. Favorable effect of balloon mitral valvuloplasty on the incidence of atrial fibrillation in patients with severe mitral stenosis. *Catheter Cardiovasc Interv* 2006; *68*: 536–541.
35. Krasuski RA, Assar MD, Wang A et al. Usefulness of percutaneous balloon mitral commissurotomy in preventing the development of atrial fibrillation in patients with mitral stenosis. *Am J Cardiol* 2004; *93*: 936–939.
36. Rumsfeld JS. Valve surgery in the elderly. A question of quality (of Life)? *J Am Coll Cardiol* 2003; *42*: 1215–1217.
37. Cotrufo M, Renzulli A, Vitale N et al. Long-term follow-up of open commissurotomy versus bileaflet valve replacement for rheumatic mitral stenosis. *Eur J Cardiothorac Surg* 1997; *12*: 335–339.
38. Lawrie GM. Mitral valve repair vs. replacement. Current recommendations and long-term results. *Cardiol Clin* 1998; *16*: 437–448.
39. Ismeno G, Renzulli A, De Feo M et al. Surgery of rheumatic mitral stenosis: Comparison of different techniques. *Acta Cardiol* 2001; *56*: 155–161.
40. Ben Farhat M, Ayari M, Maatouk F et al. Percutaneous balloon versus surgical closed and open mitral commissurotomy seven-year follow-up results of a randomized trial. *Circulation* 1998; *97*: 245–250.
41. Nardi P, Pellegrino A, Scafuri A et al. Survival and durability of mitral valve repair surgery for degenerative mitral valve disease. *J Card Surg* 2011; *26*: 360–366.
42. Cheitlin MD, Sokolow M, Mcllroy MB. Valvular heart disease; mitral valve disease. In: Sokolow M, McIlroy MB, eds. *Clinical Cardiology*, 6th ed. New York: Appleton & Lange, 1997: 407–437.
43. Aklog L, Filsoufi F, Flores KQ et al. Does coronary artery bypass grafting alone correct moderate ischemic mitral regurgitation? *Circulation* 2001; *104*: 168–175.
44. Grossi EA, Woo YJ, Patel N et al. Outcomes of coronary artery bypass grafting and reduction annuloplasty for functional ischemic mitral regurgitation: A prospective multicenter study (Randomized evaluation of a surgical treatment for off-pump repair of the mitral valve). *J Thorac Cardiovasc Surg* 2011; *141*: 91–97.
45. Skoularigis J, Sinovich V, Joubert G et al. Evaluation of the long-term results of mitral valve repair in 254 young patients with rheumatic mitral regurgitation. *Circulation* 1994; *90*: II167–II174.
46. Grossi EA, Galloway AC, Steinberg BM et al. Severe calcification does not affect long-term outcome of mitral valve repair. *Ann Thorac Surg* 1994; *58*: 685–687.
47. Galloway AC, Grossi EA, Bizekis CS et al. Evolving techniques for mitral valve reconstruction. *Ann Surg* 2002; *236*: 288–293.
48. Helft G, Tabone X, Georges JL et al. Late results with bioprosthetic valves in the elderly. *J Card Surg* 1999; *14*: 252–258.
49. Chikwe J, Goldstone AB, Passage J et al. A propensity score-adjusted retrospective comparison of early and mid-term results of mitral valve repair versus replacement in octogenarians. *Eur Heart J* 2011; *32*: 618–626.

50. Dalrymple-Hay MJ, Bryant M, Jones RA et al. Degenerative mitral regurgitation: When should we operate? *Ann Thorac Surg* 1998; *66*: 1579–1584.
51. Gogbashian A, Sepic J, Soltesz EG et al. Operative and long-term survival of elderly is significantly improved by mitral valve repair. *Am Heart J* 2006; *151*: 1325–1333.
52. Daneshmand MA, Milano CA, Rankin JS et al. Influence of patient age on procedural selection in mitral valve surgery. *Ann Thorac Surg* 2010; *90*: 1479–1485.
53. Lee EM, Porter JN, Shapiro LM et al. Mitral valve surgery in the elderly. *J Heart Valve Dis* 1997; *6*: 22–31.
54. Goldsmith IR, Lip GY, Patel RL. A prospective study of changes in the quality of life of patients following mitral valve repair and replacement. *Eur J Cardiothorac Surg* 2001; *20*: 949–955.
55. Grossi EA, Zakow PK, Sussman M et al. Late results of mitral valve reconstruction in the elderly. *Ann Thorac Surg* 2000; *70*: 1224–1226.
56. Detaint D, Sundt TM, Nkomo VT et al. Surgical correction of mitral regurgitation in the elderly: Outcomes and recent improvements. *Circulation* 2006; *114*: 265–272.
57. Aoyagi S, Fukunaga S, Arinaga K et al. Heart valve surgery in octogenarians: Operative and long-term results. *Heart Vessels* 2010; *25*: 522–528.
58. Rizzoli G, Bejko J, Bottio T et al. Valve surgery in octogenarians: Does it prolong life? *Eur J Cardiothorac Surg* 2010; *37*: 1047–1055.
59. Suri RM, Aviernos JF, Dearani JA et al. Management of less-than-severe mitral regurgitation: Should guidelines recommend earlier surgical intervention? *Eur J Cardiothorac Surg* 2011; *40*: 496–502.
60. Gillinov AM, Mihaljevic T, Blackstone EH et al. Should patients with severe degenerative mitral regurgitation delay surgery until symptoms develop? *Ann Thorac Surg* 2010; *90*: 481–488.
61. Samad Z, Kaul P, Shaw LK et al. Impact of early surgery on survival of patients with severe mitral regurgitation. *Heart* 2011; *97*: 221–224.
62. Klaar U, Gabriel H, Bergler-Klein J et al. Prognostic value of serial B-type natriuretic peptide measurement in asymptomatic organic mitral regurgitation. *Eur J Heart Fail* 2011; *13*: 163–169.
63. Magne J, Lancellotti P, Piérard LA. Exercise pulmonary hypertension in asymptomatic degenerative mitral regurgitation. *Circulation* 2010; *122*: 33–41.
64. Ralph-Edwards AC, Robinson AG, Gordon RS et al. Valve surgery in octogenarians. *Can J Cardiol* 1999; *15*: 1113–1119.
65. Bossone E, Di Benedetto G, Frigiola A et al. Valve surgery in octogenarians: In-hospital and longterm outcomes. *Can J Cardiol* 2007; *23*: 223–237.
66. Fattouch K, Sampognaro R, Speziale G et al. Impact of moderate ischemic mitral regurgitation after isolated coronary artery bypass grafting. *Ann Thorac Surg* 2010; *90*: 1187–1194.
67. Hausmann H, Siniawski H, Hetzer R. Mitralvalve reconstruction and replacement for ischemic mitral insufficiency: Seven years follow-up. *J Heart Valve Dis* 1999; *8*: 536–542.
68. Schurr P, Boeken U, Limathe J et al. Impact of mitral valve repair in patients with mitral regurgitation undergoing coronary artery bypass grafting. *Acta Cardiol* 2010; *65*: 441–447.
69. Kang DH, Sun BJ, Kim DH et al. Percutaneous versus surgical revascularization in patients with ischemic mitral regurgitation. *Circulation* 2011; *124*: S156–S162.
70. Grossi EA, Crooke GA, DiGiorgi PL et al. Impact of moderate functional mitral insufficiency in patients undergoing surgical revascularization. *Circulation* 2006; *114*: I573–I576.
71. Tolis GA Jr, Korkolis DP, Kopf GS et al. Revascularization alone (without mitral valve repair) suffices in patients with advanced ischemic cardiomyopathy and mild-to-moderate mitral regurgitation. *Ann Thorac Surg* 2002; *74*: 1476–1480.
72. Campwala SZ, Bansal RC, Wang N et al. Factors affecting regression of mitral regurgitation following isolated coronary artery bypass surgery. *Eur J Cardiothorac Surg* 2005; *28*: 783–787.
73. De Bonis M, Lapenna E, La Canna G et al. Mitral valve repair for functional mitral regurgitation in end-stage dilated cardiomyopathy: Role of the "edge-to-edge" technique. *Circulation* 2005; *112*: I402–I408.
74. Saint LL, Bailey MS, Prasad S et al. Cox-Maze IV results for patients with lone atrial fibrillation versus concomitant mitral disease. *Ann Thorac Surg* 2012; *93*: 789–794.
75. Kim JB, Ju MH, Yun SC et al. Mitral valve replacement with or without a concomitant Maze procedure in patients with atrial fibrillation. *Heart* 2010; *96*: 1126–1131.
76. Wu M, Zhang S, Dong A et al. Long-term outcomes of maze procedure plus valve replacement in treating rheumatic valve disease resulting in atrial fibrillation. *Ann Thorac Surg* 2010; *89*: 1942–1949.
77. Holzhey DM, Shi W, Borger MA et al. Minimally invasive versus sternotomy approach for mitral valve surgery in patients greater than 70 years old: A propensity-matched comparison. *Ann Thorac Surg* 2011; *91*: 401–405.
78. Suri RM, Burkhart HM, Daly RC et al. Robotic mitral valve repair for all prolapse subsets using techniques identical to open valvuloplasty: Establishing the benchmark against which percutaneous interventions should be judged. *J Thorac Cardiovasc Surg* 2011; *142*: 970–979.
79. Whitlow PL, Feldman T, Pedersen WR et al. Acute and 12-month results with catheter-based mitral valve leaflet repair: The EVEREST II (Endovascular

valve edge-to-edge repair) high risk study. *J Am Coll Cardiol* 2012; *59*: 130–139.
80. Harnek J, Webb JG, Kuck KH et al. Transcatheter implantation of the MONARC coronary sinus device for mitral regurgitation: 1-year results from the EVOLUTION phase I study (Clinical Evaluation of the Edwards Lifesciences Percutaneous Mitral Annuloplasty System for the Treatment Of Mitral Regurgitation). *JACC Cardiovasc Interv* 2011; *4*: 115–122.
81. Rodriguez CJ, Bartz TM, Longstreth WT Jr et al. Association of annular calcification and aortic valve sclerosis with brain findings on magnetic resonance imaging in community dwelling older adults: The cardiovascular health study. *J Am Coll Cardiol* 2011; *57*: 2172–2180.
82. Aronow WS, Koenigsberg M, Kronzon I et al. Association of mitral anular calcium with new thromboembolic stroke and cardiac events at 39-month follow-up in elderly patients. *Am J Cardiol* 1990; *65*: 1511–1512.
83. Kanjanauthai S, Nasir K, Katz R et al. Relationships of mitral annular calcification to cardiovascular risk factors: The Multi-Ethnic Study of Atherosclerosis (MESA). *Atherosclerosis* 2010; *213*: 558–562.
84. Aronow WS, Ahn C, Kronzon I. Prevalence of echocardiographic findings in 554 men and in 1,243 women aged >60 years in a long-term health care facility. *Am J Cardiol* 1997; *79*: 379–380.
85. Aronow WS, Schwartz KS, Koenigsberg M. Correlation of atrial fibrillation with presence or absence of mitral anular calcium in 604 persons older than 60 years. *Am J Cardiol* 1987; *59*: 1213–1214.
86. Gondrie MJ, van der Graaf Y, Jacobs PC et al. The association of incidentally detected heart valve calcification with future cardiovascular events. *Eur Radiol* 2011; *21*: 963–973.
87. Nair CK, Sketch MH, Ahmed I et al. Calcific valvular aortic stenosis with and without mitral anular calcium. *Am J Cardiol* 1987; *60*: 865–870.
88. Aronow WS, Schwartz KS, Koenigsberg M. Prevalence of tricuspid anular calcium diagnosed by echocardiography in elderly patients. *Am J Noninvas Cardiol* 1987; *1*: 275–277..
89. Thanassoulis G, Massaro JM, Cury R et al. Associations of long-term and early adult atherosclerosis risk factors with aortic and mitral valve calcium. *J Am Coll Cardiol* 2010; *55*: 2491–2498.
90. Aronow WS, Schwartz KS, Koenigsberg M. Correlation of serum lipids, calcium and phosphorus, diabetes mellitus, aortic valve stenosis and history of systemic hypertension with presence or absence of mitral anular calcium in persons older than 62 years in a long-term health care facility. *Am J Cardiol* 1987; *59*: 381–382.
91. Sprecher DL, Schaefer EJ, Kent KM et al. Cardiovascular features of homozygous familial hypercholesterolemia: Analysis of 16 patients. *Am J Cardiol* 1984; *54*: 20–30.
92. Yetkin E, Yagmur C, Yagmur J et al. Evaluation of cardiovascular risk factors and bone mineral density in patients undergoing coronary angiography and relation of findings to mitral annular calcium. *Am J Cardiol* 2007; *99*: 159–162.
93. Roberts WC, Waller BF. Effect of chronic hypercalcemia on the heart: An analysis of 18 necropsy patients. *Am J Med* 1981; *71*: 371–384.
94. Aronow WS, Kronzon I. Prevalence of aortic valve calcium and mitral annular calcium in older persons with and without chronic renal insufficiency. *Cardiovasc Rev Rep* 2000; *21*: 623–624.
95. Huting J. Mitral valve calcification as an index of left ventricular dysfunction in patients with end stage renal disease on peritoneal dialysis. *Chest* 1994; *105*: 383–388.
96. Fox CS, Larson MG, Vasan RS et al. Cross-sectional association of kidney function with valvular and annular calcification: The Framingham Heart Study. *J Am Soc Nephrol* 2006; *17*: 521–527.
97. Motamed HE, Roberts WC. Frequency and significance of mitral anular calcium in hypertrophic cardiomyopathy: Analysis of 200 necropsy patients. *Am J Cardiol* 1987; *60*: 877–884.
98. Aronow WS, Kronzon I. Prevalence of hypertrophic cardiomyopathy and its association with mitral anular calcium in elderly patients. *Chest* 1988; *94*: 1295–1296.
99. Aronow WS, Ahm C, Kronzon I. Association of mitral annular calcium and of aortic cuspal calcium with coronary artery disease in older patients. *Am J Cardiol* 1999; *84*: 1084–1085.
100. Aronow WS, Ahn C, Kronzon I. Association of mitral annular calcium with symptomatic peripheral arterial disease in older persons. *Am J Cardiol* 2001; *88*: 333–334.
101. Seo Y, Ishimitsu T, Ishizu T et al. Relationship between mitral annular calcification and severity of carotid atherosclerosis in patients. *J Cardiol* 2005; *46*: 17–24.
102. Aronow WS, Schwartz KS, Koenigsberg M. Sensitivity, specificity, positive predictive value, and negative predictive value of mitral anular calcium detected by chest roentgenograms correlated with mitral anular calcium diagnosed by echocardiography in elderly patients. *Am J Noninvas Cardiol* 1987; *1*: 252–253.
103. Aronow WS, Ahn C, Kronzon I et al. Association of mitral annular calcium with new thromboembolic stroke at 44-month follow-up of 2,148 persons, mean age 81 years. *Am J Cardiol* 1998; *81*: 105–106.
104. Savage DD, Garrison RJ, Castelli WP et al. Prevalence of submitral (anular) calcium and its correlates in a general population-based sample (the Framingham Study). *Am J Cardiol* 1983; *51*: 1375–1378

105. Korn D, DeSanctis RW, Sell S. Massive calcification of the mitral annulus: A clinicopathologic study of fourteen cases. *N Engl J Med* 1962; *267*: 900–909.
106. Schott CR, Kotler MN, Parry WR et al. Mitral annular calcification: Clinical and echocardiography correlations. *Arch Intern Med* 1977; *137*: 1143–1150.
107. Aronow WS, Schwartz KS, Koenigsberg M. Correlation of murmurs of mitral stenosis and mitral regurgitation with presence or absence of mitral anular calcium in persons older than 62 years in a long-term health care facility. *Am J Cardiol* 1987; *59*: 181–182.
108. Aronow WS, Kronzon I. Correlation of prevalence and severity of mitral regurgitation and mitral stenosis determined by Doppler echocardiography with physical signs of mitral regurgitation and mitral stenosis in 100 patients aged 62 to 100 years with mitral anular calcium. *Am J Cardiol* 1997; *60*: 1189–1190.
109. Kaul S, Pearlman JD, Touchstone DA et al. Prevalence and mechanisms of mitral regurgitation in the absence of intrinsic abnormalities of the mitral leaflets. *Am Heart J* 1989; *118*: 963–972.
110. Labovitz AJ, Nelson JG, Windhorst DM et al. Frequency of mitral valve dysfunction from mitral anular calcium as detected by Doppler echocardiography. *Am J Cardiol* 1985; *55*: 133–137.
111. Nair CK, Thomson W, Ryschon K et al. Long-term follow-up of patients with echocardiographically detected mitral anular calcium and comparison with age- and sex-matched control subjects. *Am J Cardiol* 1989; *63*: 465–470.
112. Dajani AS, Taubert KA, Wilson W et al. Prevention of bacterial endocarditis. Recommendations by the American heart association. *Circulation* 1997; *96*: 358–366.
113. Wilson W, Taubert KA, Gewitz M et al. Prevention of infective endocarditis: Guidelines from the American Heart Association: A guideline from the American Heart Association rheumatic fever, endocarditis, and Kawasaki disease committee, council on cardiovascular disease in the young, and the council on clinical cardiology, council on cardiovascular surgery and anesthesia, and the quality of care outcomes research interdisciplinary working group. *Circulation* 2007; *116*: 1736–1754.
114. Nair CK, Biddle P, Kaneshige A et al. Mitral valve replacement in patients with mitral anular calcium (abstract). *Chest* 1991; *100*(Suppl): S109.
115. Aronow WS, Gutstein H, Hsieh FY. Risk factors for thromboembolic stroke in elderly patients with chronic atrial fibrillation. *Am J Cardiol* 1989; *63*: 366–367.
116. Boston Area Anticoagulation Trial for Atrial Fibrillation Investigators. The effect of low-dose warfarin on the risk of stroke in patients with nonrheumatic atrial fibrillation. *N Engl J Med* 1990; *323*: 1505–1511.
117. Aronow WS, Schoenfeld MR, Gutstein H. Frequency of thromboembolic stroke in persons ≥60 years of age with extracranial carotid arterial disease and/or mitral annular calcium. *Am J Cardiol* 1992; *70*: 123–124.
118. Rubin DC, Hawke MW, Plotnick GD. Relation between mitral annular calcium and complex intraaortic debris. *Am J Cardiol* 1993; *71*: 1251–1252.
119. Shohat-Zabarski R, Paz R, Adler Y et al. Mitral annulus calcification with a mobile component as a possible source of embolism. *Am J Geriatr Cardiol* 2001; *10*: 196–198.
120. Aronow WS, Ahn C, Kronzon I et al. Association of mitral annular calcium with prior thromboembolic stroke in older white, African American, and Hispanic men and women. *Am J Cardiol* 2000; *85*: 672–673.
121. Kizer JR, Wiebers DO, Whisnant JP et al. Mitral annular calcification, aortic valve sclerosis, and incident stroke in adults free of clinical cardiovascular disease: The strong heart study. *Stroke* 2005; *36*: 2533–2537.
122. Aronow WS. The effect of low-dose warfarin on the risk of non-rheumatic atrial fibrillation. Letter to the editor. *N Engl J Med* 1991; *325*: 130.
123. Singer DE, Hughes RA, Gress DR et al. The effect of low-dose warfarin on the risk of stroke in patients with nonrheumatic atrial fibrillation. *N Engl J Med* 1991; *325*: 131.
124. Alfieri O, Maisano F, DeBonis M et al. The edge-to-edge technique in mitral valve repair: A simple solution for complex problems. *J Thorac Cardiovasc Surg* 2001; *122*: 674–681.
125. Maisano F, Torracca L, Oppizzi M et al. The edge-to-edge technique: A simplified method to correct mitral insufficiency. *Eur J Cardiothorac Surg* 1998; *13*: 240–245.
126. Feldman T, Foster E, Glower DD et al. Percutaneous repair or surgery for mitral regurgitation. *N Engl J Med* 2011; *364*: 1395–1406.
127. Feldman T et al. Randomized comparison of percutaneous repair and surgery for mitral regurgitation: 5-Year results of EVEREST II. *J Am Coll Cardiol* 2015; *66*(25): 2844–2854. doi:10.1016/j.jacc.2015.
128. Maisano F et al. Percutaneous mitral valve interventions in the real world: Early and 1-year results from the ACCESS-EU, a prospective, multicenter, nonrandomized post-approval study of the MitraClip therapy in Europe. *J Am Coll Cardiol* 2013; *17, 62(12)*: 1052–1061.
129. Lim DS et al. Real world expanded multi-center study of the MitraClip system. *J Am Coll Cardiol* 2014; *64*: 181–192.
130. Sorajja P et al. Outcomes with transcatheter mitral valve repair in the United States: An STS/ACC TVT registry report. *J Am Coll Cardiol* 2017; *70(19)*: 2315–2327.

131. Nickenig G, Estevez-Loureiro R, Franzen O et al. Percutaneous mitral valve edge-to-edge repair. In-hospital results and 1-year follow-up of 628 patients of the 2011–2012 pilot European Sentinel Registry. *J Am Coll Cardiol* 2014; *64*: 875–884.
132. Al-Taweel A, Almahmoud MF, Khairandish Y, Ahmad M. Degenerative mitral valve stenosis: Diagnosis and management. *Echocardiography* 2019; *36*: 1901–1909.
133. Banovic M, DaCosta M. Degenerative mitral stenosis: From pathophysiology to challenging interventional treatment. *Curr Probl Cardiol* 2019; *44*: 10–35.
134. Giannini C, Mazzola M, Pugliese NR, Petronio AS. Mitral valve stenosis in the current era: A changing landscape. *J Cardiovasc Med (Hagerstown)* 2022; *23*: 701–709.
135. Islam H, Puttagunta SM, Islam R et al. Risk of stroke with mitral stenosis: The underlying mechanism, treatment, and prevention. *Cureus* 2022; *14*: e23784.
136. Galusko V, Ionescu A, Edwards A et al. Management of mitral stenosis: A systematic review of clinical practice guidelines and recommendations. *Eur Heart J Qual Care Clin Outcomes* 2022; *8*: 602–618.
137. Otto CM, Nishimura RA, Bonow RO et al. 2020 ACC/AHA guideline for the management of patients with valvular heart disease: A report of the American College of Cardiology/American Heart Association joint committee on clinical practice guidelines. *Circulation* 2021; *143*: e72–e227.
138. Brown KN, Ahmed I, Kanmanthareddy A. *Catheter management of mitral stenosis*. StatPearls. Treasure Island (FL): StatPearls Publishing. StatPearls Publishing LLC, 2024.
139. Iung B, Leenhardt A, Extramiana F. Management of atrial fibrillation in patients with rheumatic mitral stenosis. *Heart* 2018; *104*: 1062–1068.
140. Meneguz-Moreno RA, Costa JR, Jr., Gomes NL et al. Very long term follow-up after percutaneous balloon mitral valvuloplasty. *JACC Cardiovasc Interv* 2018; *11*: 1945–1952.
141. Itzhaki Ben Zadok O, Sagie A, Vaturi M et al. Long-term outcomes after mitral valve replacement and tricuspid annuloplasty in rheumatic patients. *Ann Thorac Surg* 2019; *107*: 539–545.
142. Zhai ME, Mao Y, Liu Y, Yang J. Transcatheter mitral valve replacement to treat severe calcified rheumatic native mitral stenosis: Role of three-dimensional printing-a case report. *Eur Heart J Case Rep* 2023; *7*: ytad434.
143. El Sabbagh A, Reddy YNV, Nishimura RA. Mitral valve regurgitation in the contemporary era: Insights into diagnosis, management, and future directions. *JACC Cardiovasc Imaging* 2018; *11*: 628–643.
144. Desai A, Thomas JD, Bonow RO et al. Asymptomatic degenerative mitral regurgitation repair: Validating guidelines for early intervention. *J Thorac Cardiovasc Surg* 2021; *161*: 981–994.e5.
145. Tomšič A, Hiemstra YL, van Hout FMA et al. Long-term results of mitral valve repair for severe mitral regurgitation in asymptomatic patients. *J Cardiol* 2018; *72*: 473–479.
146. Boudoulas KD, Triposkiadis F, Koenig S et al. Acute mitral regurgitation with and without acute heart failure. *Heart Fail Rev* 2023; *28*: 1201–1209.
147. Hayashi A, Mantha Y, Harada R. Acute mitral regurgitation and transcatheter mitral valve repair in an emergency case: Focus on the mechanical disorder of mitral valve complex. *Heart Fail Clin* 2020; *16*: 211–219.
148. Apostolidou E, Maslow AD, Poppas A. Primary mitral valve regurgitation: Update and review. *Glob Cardiol Sci Pract* 2017; *2017*: e201703.
149. Douedi S, Douedi H. *Mitral regurgitation*. StatPearls. Treasure Island (FL): StatPearls Publishing, StatPearls Publishing LLC, 2025.
150. Sharedalalois A, Zois A, Sharedalal P et al. Transcatheter intervention for management of tricuspid regurgitation using TriClip. *Cardiol Rev*. Published online ahead of print PMID 38934619

16

Infective endocarditis in older adults

HSINHUI HUA AND LONA MODY

Key points

- Age is a strong risk factor for infective endocarditis (IE), and older adults with IE tend to have more complications and a worse prognosis than younger individuals.
- The increasing use of cardiac implantable electronic devices and transcatheter valve procedures in older adults has led to a rising burden of device-associated IE with distinct microbiologic and clinical features.
- Diagnosis of IE in older adults is often delayed, the spectrum of causative organisms is broader, and there is higher incidence of aggressive pathogens.
- Management of IE in older adults requires a multidisciplinary team and should align with patients' goals of care.
- Additional research is needed to incorporate functional status, comorbidities, geriatric syndromes, and personal preferences into therapeutic strategies for IE in older adults.

DEFINITION

In 1835 Jean-Baptiste Bouillaud coined the term *endocardium* and described inflammation of this membranous tissue, calling it "endocarditis" [1]. He also noted that this lesion was frequently associated with acute inflammatory rheumatism (i.e., rheumatic fever). Rudolf Virchow described "small granules" on microscopy of these lesions, but it was not until 1869 when Emanuel Winge presented the findings of a patient with endocarditis in which he noted short rod-shaped bodies "similar to *Leptothrix*" on microscopy leading him to theorize that "parasitic organisms" may have entered the patient's body through a foot wound and later colonized the heart valve, thus providing the first description of infective endocarditis. Sir William Osler provided a comprehensive understanding of the disease, including an in-depth description for clinicians [2].

Infective endocarditis is a term that now refers to microbial infection of the endocardial surface of native heart valves as well as nonvalvular endocardial surfaces [3], but it is also widely used to indicate infection of prosthetic material that crosses heart valves and is embedded within endocardial tissues (e.g., pacemaker and ICD wires), as well as mechanical or bioprosthetic heart valves. Once considered a disease of young adults with rheumatic valvular abnormalities, studies now show additional risk factors that include degenerative valvulopathy, prosthetic valves, diabetes, and other healthcare exposures. These important distinctions have a great impact on classification, diagnosis, and treatment in older adults, as addressed in this chapter.

CLASSIFICATION

IE was traditionally classified either based on acuity level (acute, subacute, or chronic) or localization (left-sided, right-sided, or valve involved). However, given the evolving epidemiology, microbiology, and increased presence of cardiac devices and valve surgery, a classification involving a description of the valve involved and whether it is native or prosthetic valve endocarditis (PVE) is becoming more commonplace [4, 5]. IE may also be

DOI: 10.1201/9781003568933-16

Table 16.1 Microbiology of prosthetic valve endocarditis (PVE)

Pathogen	Early PVE (%)	Late PVE (%)
Methicillin-susceptible *Staphylococcus aureus*	15–30	10–22
Methicillin-resistant *S. aureus*	15-25	2–5
Coagulase-negative staphylococci	15–35	10–20
Viridans group streptococci	0–2	15–20
Enterococci	5–25	8–20
Gram-negative bacilli	2–15	1–7
Culture negative	3–15	3–15
Polymicrobial	2–7	2–7
Fungi	3-10	1–3

Sources: Adapted from Galar, A., et al., *Clin Microbiol Rev*, 32(2), e00041–18, 2019; Reisinger, M., et al., *Pathogens*, 13(7),543, 2024; Berisha, B., et al., *J Intern Med*, 292(3), 428–437, 2022.

classified according to the mode of acquisition into community-acquired, hospital-acquired, or intravenous drug abuse-associated IE [5, 6].

PVE is further divided into early PVE, usually defined as occurring within 12 months after implantation, versus late PVE, which occurs more than 12 months after surgery. This distinction is important since the causative agents vary substantially by PVE subclass. Most early PVE is due to acquisition of a pathogen during the index hospitalization either through surgical contamination or nosocomial bacteremia often from intravenous lines. Thus, coagulase-negative staphylococci, *Staphylococcus aureus* (including methicillin-resistant *S. aureus* [MRSA]), and hospital-acquired gram-negative rods are more common in early PVE than in late PVE or native valve IE (Table 16.1) [7–9]. In contrast, late PVE endocarditis is thought to primarily result from community-acquired bacteremia with seeding of the valve, and thus the microbiology resembles native valve disease [3].

With increasing use of invasive cardiac interventions, device-related IE subtypes have emerged. Surgical aortic valve replacement (SAVR)-IE and transcatheter aortic valve replacement (TAVR)-IE are both considered PVE. Further, the 2023 Duke-ISCVID criteria [4] formally recognize cardiac implantable electronic device (CIED) IE as a distinct entity within the broader IE classification. It refers to infections related to prosthetic devices such as pacemakers, implantable cardioverter-defibrillators (ICDs), and cardiac resynchronization therapy (CRT).

AGE, EPIDEMIOLOGIC FEATURES, RISK FACTORS, AND PROGNOSIS

Age remains one of the most significant risk factors for IE with a fivefold higher risk compared to the general adult population. As the world population ages, the burden of IE is anticipated to increase [5]. According to the Global Burden of Disease study, the age-standardized incidence of IE rose globally from 9.9 to 13.8 per 100,000 person-years between 1990 and 2019, with individuals aged 50 and above accounting for over 60% of new cases and nearly 80% of IE-related deaths [6]. In a US national inpatient analysis, the incidence increased from 10.2 to 14.4 per 100,000 between 1990 and 2019, highlighting a consistent upward trend in older populations [10].

The peak incidence is observed in men aged 75–79 years, reaching approximately 19.4 cases per 100,000 [6, 11]. According to the Global Burden of Disease 2019 study, the incidence and mortality rates of IE remain consistently higher in males than in females across global, regional, and national levels. Although both sexes experienced an increasing burden over the past three decades, the magnitude of increase was more pronounced among men [6]. However, the increase in mortality over 30 years was larger in women than in men [6, 11, 23]. This narrowing gap may reflect shifts in healthcare exposure, comorbidities, and device use among older women. Some studies have also suggested that women may experience higher mortality or complications, possibly due to later presentation or increased comorbidity burden [12, 13, 23].

Recent data suggest that community-acquired infective endocarditis (CA-IE) is on the rise, particularly in association with *Staphylococcus aureus* bacteremia (SAB). A nationwide Danish study conducted from 2010 to 2018 analyzed 13,040 patients with first-time SAB, categorizing them into community-acquired and healthcare-associated groups. The study found that 12.1% of patients with community-acquired SAB developed IE, compared to 6.6% in the healthcare-associated group. This indicates that community-acquired SAB may be associated with a higher risk of IE (odds ratio, 2.12; 95% confidence interval, 1.86–2.41) [14]. Interestingly, although early mortality (within 40 days) did not differ significantly between the two groups, longer-term mortality (41–365 days) was significantly lower in the community-acquired group (hazard ratio, 0.71; 95% CI, 0.53–0.95), likely reflecting a lower burden of comorbidity and more favorable treatment trajectories among CA-SAB cases.

Most reports suggest that IE in older patients is associated with a poor prognosis and high rate of complications attributed to insidious initial symptoms, delayed diagnosis, multimorbidity, and a higher incidence of more aggressive pathogens than occurs in young adults [15, 23]. Older age, clinical manifestations (heart failure, septic shock), evidence of valve obstruction on echocardiography, *Staphylococcus aureus* etiology, and negative blood cultures are risk factors for in-hospital mortality in those with IE [15–17]. However, many earlier analyses lacked adjustment for comorbidities, which are disproportionately prevalent in older patients. More recent multivariable models incorporating comorbidity burden show that the Charlson Comorbidity Index (CCI) >3 is an independent predictor of both in-hospital (OR 1.46, 95% CI 1.07–1.99) and 1-year mortality (HR 1.34, 95% CI 1.08–1.66) [15]. These findings underscore the importance of individualized prognostic assessment in geriatric patients. Comorbidities such as diabetes, chronic kidney disease, and malignancy are common and not only influence prognosis but may also influence the causative microorganisms (see "Microbiology" section) [18, 39]. For instance, patients with cancer, a population that has shown a rising incidence of IE, are frequently immunosuppressed and have long-term central venous catheters, both of which predispose to bloodstream infection and healthcare-associated IE [19]. Similarly, the presence of indwelling devices such as feeding tubes or urinary catheters in older patients is associated with increased mortality and reflects a population at higher risk for nosocomial infection [20–22].

Recent cohort studies show that infective endocarditis in older adults is overwhelmingly left-sided, with a predominance of mitral valve involvement. For example, Scheggi et al. (2023) found that 97.9% of octogenarian patients with IE had left-sided infection, versus 89.8% of younger patients [23]. Likewise, a 2022 review noted that elderly IE patients have "higher rates of mitral valve involvement" than younger adults [24]. In practice, this means older patients seldom present with tricuspid/right-sided IE (which is more common in IV drug users).

Older age is also associated with more prosthetic valve cases. In Scheggi's surgical series, 52.5% of IE cases in patients ≥80 were prosthetic-valve endocarditis, compared to 39.6% in those <80 [23]. In other words, over half of octogenarian IE occurred on a prosthetic device, whereas younger patients more often had native-valve IE. This likely reflects both the higher prevalence of valve replacements/implants in older adults and degenerative mitral disease in this group. Thus, TAVR-IE has emerged as a distinct clinical entity. In a national, multicenter cohort study, the incidence of infective endocarditis after TAVR was estimated at 1.0 events per 100 person-years, with 62.4% of cases occurring within the first year post-implantation. The median time from TAVR to infective endocarditis was 196 days (25% to 75%, interquartile range: 80 to 577 days) [23].

Although both SAVR-IE and TAVR-IE are associated with high morbidity and mortality, studies suggest that patients with TAVR-IE may have less surgical intervention and worse long-term outcomes due to advanced age and comorbidities [24, 36]. As TAVR expands into lower-risk populations, the burden of TAVR-IE is expected to rise, underscoring the need for careful postprocedural monitoring and preventive strategies in older adults.

Similarly, a higher frequency of pacemaker lead-associated IE has been noted in older patients [25]. According to one study of 3996 IE patients, 17.7% had a CIED, and CIED-related IE accounted for 10.6% of all cases. Patients in the CIED group were older, with a mean age of 73 ± 8 years, whereas patients without CIEDs were aged 68 ± 11 years [25]. Additionally, a study spanning from 1981 to 2020 revealed that the incidence of CIED-IE increased 4.5-fold, particularly among patients with ICDs and CRT devices. During this period, the median age of affected patients rose from 63 to 71 years, indicating a higher occurrence of CIED-IE in the older population [23].

MICROBIOLOGY

Contemporary reviews estimate that up to 80%–90% of IE cases are due to staphylococci, streptococci, or enterococci [11, 26, 27]. However, the microbiologic profile of IE has changed over the past decade due to changes in demographics, medical device usage, and healthcare exposures. Older patients increasingly develop healthcare-associated IE, and thus *Staphylococcus* species (especially MRSA and coagulase-negative staphylococci) and *Enterococcus* species are predominant among them [26]. In one referral center study (2007–2018), enterococci were responsible for 30% of IE cases in patients over age 75, a sharp increase from previous decades [28].

Culture-negative endocarditis remains an important consideration in older adults. Up to 5%-20% of IE cases have no organism grown in routine culture [29–33]. In a study comparing characteristics of culture-negative (CN-IE) versus culture-positive IE (CP-IE), CN-IE has been associated with higher short-term and long-term mortality, likely due to diagnostic delays and challenges in initiating appropriate therapy [34]. Advances in molecular diagnostics, such as 16S rRNA gene sequencing and PCR, have improved detection of pathogens such as *Coxiella burnetii*, *Bartonella* species, and *Tropheryma whipplei*, organisms that are particularly relevant in older or prosthesis-bearing patients [4, 57]. For all three pathogens, diagnosis is suggested by serologic testing and confirmed by polymerase chain reaction (PCR) of either blood or valvular material. Given the atypical presentation and diagnostic challenges, a high index of suspicion is essential. Management of these infections also differs significantly from typical IE treatment, often requiring prolonged, pathogen-specific antimicrobial regimens. Consultation with an infectious disease specialist is strongly recommended to guide appropriate therapy [33, 57].

S. aureus remains the most common pathogen globally in native IE, responsible for approximately 30%–40% of cases. It often presents acutely and is associated with high mortality (around 30%–37%), especially in cases involving methicillin resistance (MRSA) [34]. This is followed by viridans group streptococci (20%–30%) and enterococci (10%–15%) [8, 35]. However, this distribution varies substantially in older adults. Several studies have demonstrated that *Enterococcus faecalis* and *Streptococcus gallolyticus* are more prevalent in older populations, while the burden of methicillin-resistant *S. aureus* is also elevated in this age group, likely due to increased healthcare exposure and comorbidities [26, 27, 35].

PVE, including SAVR and TAVR, shows a microbiologic dominance of staphylococci, especially coagulase-negative staphylococci (CoNS) and *S. aureus*. In older SAVR patients, early-onset PVE is commonly caused by *S. aureus*, while CoNS and enterococci are seen more often with late PVE [10, 24, 27]. In one meta-analysis, staphylococci accounted for over 60% of SAVR-IE cases, with *S. aureus* more common in early cases and CoNS more prevalent in late-onset infections. Enterococci were identified in approximately 10%–15% of cases, typically associated with healthcare exposure or genitourinary procedures [36].

In contrast, TAVR-IE exhibits a distinct microbiological profile, primarily involving enterococci, *S. aureus*, and coagulase-negative staphylococci. Enterococci are implicated in over 25% of TAVR-IE cases, a markedly higher proportion compared to approximately 10% in SAVR-IE [36, 37, 39]. This may be attributed to their affinity for warm, moist environments (e.g., groin) and the frequent use of transfemoral access in TAVR. *S. aureus* follows closely, exhibiting heightened virulence, with significantly elevated in-hospital (47.8% vs. 26.9%) and 2-year mortality rates (71.5% vs. 49.6%) [38]. Coagulase-negative staphylococci account for >15% of cases, whereas streptococcal infections (6.9% vs. 21%) and culture-negative IE (~5% vs. 10%–20%) are less frequent in TAVR-IE than in SAVR-IE [36].

Infections associated with CIED share similar microbiologic features with early PVE. Recent studies demonstrate that *Staphylococcus* species predominate in the microbiology of CIED-IE, with coagulase-negative staphylococci (40%–45%) and *S. aureus* (22%–38%) as primary pathogens. CoNS is associated with localized infections, whereas *S. aureus*, including MRSA (3%–10%), is more often linked to systemic disease and increased mortality [23, 25, 40]. Enterococci and gram-negative organisms collectively account for fewer than 10% of cases. Notably, in two cohort studies from Denmark and China, *S. aureus* was more likely to cause early (typically within 6 months) rather than late infections after CIED-related procedures. Further, the highest incidence was in the first 3 months post-implant, especially with CRT and ICD devices [41, 42]. Regional differences are also evident, with a higher prevalence of CoNS reported in Asia (45.2%) [41].

Emerging and special pathogens

Several pathogens deserve further comment due to their increasing frequency, diagnostic requirements or therapeutic implications. *S. lugdunensis* is a coagulase-negative *Staphylococcus* recognized with increasing frequency in IE including device-associated IE [43–45]. Although it is a CoNS, it should never be dismissed as a contaminant. The organism is often aggressive, causing valve destruction or abscess, and surgical intervention/device removal is frequently required; in retrospective analysis, medical treatment alone was associated with increased mortality [43]. Although it accounts for only 1% of IE episodes, it carries a disproportionally high 30-day mortality rate, up to 20%–40% in some cohorts [45]. Unlike many other CoNS, the vast majority of *S. lugdunensis* are susceptible to β-lactams, with more than 80% susceptible to penicillin in one series of IE cases [43].

Culture-negative (CN) endocarditis has always been a vexing clinical problem and is often caused by previous antibiotic exposure or difficult-to-grow organisms such as the HACEK group (*Haemophilus*, *Aggregatibacter*, *Cardiobacterium*, *Eikenella corrodens*, *Kingella*), which cause about 3%–5% of cases [5, 35]. New culture techniques and media support the growth of HACEK organisms, so that this group is now a relatively rare cause of culture-negative IE. When culture-negative IE is encountered in the absence of prior antibiotics, specific pathogens should be suspected that often require special diagnostic studies.

As noted earlier, the most common causes of culture-negative IE include *Coxiella burnetii*, *Bartonella* species, and *Tropheryma whipplei* [33]. *Coxiella burnetii*, the causative agent of Q fever, is a zoonotic pathogen typically associated with animal contact. In its acute phase, infection often presents as a nonspecific, flu-like illness. However, if unrecognized or undertreated, *C. burnetii* can persist and progress to chronic Q fever endocarditis, especially in individuals with underlying valvular or vascular abnormalities [11, 46, 47]. In the largest prospective studies of blood CN-IE, *C. burnetii* was identified as the etiologic agent in 37% to 48% of confirmed cases. Diagnosis requires a high index of suspicion and is based on elevated phase I IgG titers (≥1:800) and confirmatory PCR testing from blood or excised valvular tissue [4, 33]. *Bartonella* species have been implicated as a cause of 12.4%–28.4% of CN-IE for several decades, primarily affecting younger adults, particularly homeless individuals since the major *Bartonella* species that causes IE, *B. quintana*, is louse-borne [33]. Although most literature regarding *B. quintana* endocarditis has originated from Europe and Africa, a resurgence of cases has been noted in North America over the past decade [48]. Other *Bartonella* species are carried by fleas/other vectors or can be transmitted by cat scratches/bites and have also been reported as a cause of IE [33, 49]. Recent reports of IE due to *Bartonella* have emerged in older patients with prosthetic valves and in device-associated IE [49, 50]. *T. whipplei*, the causative agent of Whipple's disease, is well recognized as a cause of CN-IE, and in a recent study of such patients, the organism was the fourth most common pathogen identified by PCR of surgical valve material (causing 2%–7% of cases) [51]. Of the 16 patients in that series, the aortic valve was affected in 13, the mitral valve in 3. A literature review identified 44 publications documenting 169 patients with Whipple's endocarditis. The average age was 57.1 years. There is a clear sex predominance, with 85% of cases being male [52]. Thus, *T. whipplei* may be a relatively common cause of CN-IE in older adults and appears to rarely present with classic signs of Whipple's disease.

Mycobacterium chimaera, a slow-growing nontuberculous *Mycobacterium* (NTM), has emerged globally as a rare but deadly cause of prosthetic valve endocarditis. It has been linked to contaminated heater–cooler devices used during cardiac surgery. The infection typically presents insidiously, months to years after surgery, with disseminated systemic symptoms such as fever, night sweats, and weight loss. Diagnosis is difficult and often delayed, requiring 16S rRNA gene sequencing or prolonged culture of tissue samples. Medical therapy involves multidrug regimens (e.g., macrolides, rifamycins, ethambutol) for more than 12 months. Outcomes are poor without surgical explantation, and mortality rates have been reported as high as 60% in case series, with many patients dying before a definitive diagnosis is made [53, 54].

Most instances of blood CN-IE are caused by fastidious or intracellular pathogens, however, a minority are due to non-infectious causes. In a large prospective French cohort study, Fournier et al. found non-infectious conditions in roughly 2.5% of blood CN-IE [33, 55]. These represented autoimmune disorders such as systemic lupus erythematosus (Libman–Sacks endocarditis), rheumatoid arthritis, and malignancy-associated nonbacterial thrombotic endocarditis (marantic endocarditis). Behçet's disease is also linked with valvular inflammation and endocarditis. Allergic reactions to porcine bioprosthetic valves are a rare but interesting etiology. There are several reports describing recurrent endocarditis-like presentations in pork-allergic individuals, necessitating replacement with non-porcine material [33, 56].

CLINICAL AND LABORATORY MANIFESTATIONS

The clinical presentation of infective endocarditis is diverse and nonspecific, which often leads to late diagnosis [24, 58]. The most common symptom is fever with chills (around 90%) anemia (around 50%), and cardiac murmur (about 85%). Patients may have malaise, headache, myalgias, arthralgia, night sweats, abdominal pain, and dyspnea. Splenomegaly or cutaneous manifestations, such as petechiae or splinter hemorrhages, are supportive signs [41, 58, 59]. The clinical presentation of older patients with IE is often atypical, such as lethargy, fatigue, malaise, anorexia, and weight loss. Delirium is a common clinical presentation in older patients and may occasionally be the sole manifestation of infective endocarditis. Sometimes fever can be absent in older patients [24, 41, 59, 60]. Further, older patients often have multiple comorbidities, and the symptoms of IE may be mistaken for worsening of underlying conditions. Endocarditis can also present in an acute deceptive clinical context, where endocardial infection arises amidst sudden and severe medical conditions, without overt signs indicative of a cardiac source [62].

In addition, some patients may have long-term extracardiac symptoms before IE is formally diagnosed. These may arise from infection, immune complex deposition, or embolic phenomena and include joint and muscle pain, weight loss, night sweats, splenomegaly or splenic pain, hematuria, renal dysfunction, ocular changes like Roth spots, and cutaneous manifestations such as Osler nodes and Janeway lesions [24, 61, 62]. These symptoms are not specific and can be mistaken for other conditions.

Heart murmurs are relatively common in older adults due to degenerative valve disease and calcification so IE in older adults may not present with the typical new or changing murmur [24, 41, 59]. Vascular and immune-mediated phenomena, including embolic events, splenomegaly, ocular and cutaneous manifestations, are also observed less commonly in older IE patients than in young adults [24, 58, 62]. Heart failure is another common clinical manifestation. Approximately 30% of IE patients develop clinical heart failure [63, 64]. In older adults, who have less cardiac reserve, acute valve failure (especially aortic or mitral regurgitation) can precipitate acute pulmonary edema or cardiogenic shock. Therefore, the development or worsening of heart failure in an older patient with an active infection should raise strong suspicion for IE. In fact, heart failure is the single strongest indication for surgery in IE and a leading cause of death (see "Surgical Therapy" section). Conversely, overt sepsis and septic shock are less common initial presentations in cases of subacute endocarditis. However, in acute staphylococcal IE, older adults may indeed present with septic shock or experience rapid clinical deterioration, both of which are associated with poor prognosis [58].

In some cases, IE may initially present as spondylodiscitis, particularly in older or immunocompromised individuals. This condition results from hematogenous spread of IE-associated pathogens to the intervertebral discs and adjacent vertebrae. Patients may present with severe back pain, stiffness, or neurological deficits due to spinal cord or nerve compression that can mask the underlying cardiac infection and delay diagnosis [62, 65].

Laboratory findings in IE are often nonspecific but can provide valuable diagnostic clues. For instance, elevated inflammatory markers and a normocytic, normochromic anemia may be present. Rheumatoid factor can be positive in a substantial proportion of cases. Urinalysis commonly shows microscopic hematuria and may also reveal red blood cell casts or pyuria, indicating renal involvement [58]. Imaging plays a critical role in diagnosis. Transesophageal echocardiography (TEE) is preferred over transthoracic echocardiography (TTE) due to superior sensitivity, especially in patients with prosthetic valves or CIEDs. Advanced imaging modalities, including 18F-FDG PET/CT and radio-labeled leukocyte SPECT/CT, have been incorporated into the 2023 Duke-ISCVID diagnostic criteria, particularly improving sensitivity for prosthetic valve endocarditis and detecting metastatic infectious foci [4].

DIAGNOSIS

The diagnosis of IE in older adults is frequently delayed due to atypical clinical presentations and difficulty interpreting echocardiographic findings. In a cohort study of IE, 74.5% of patients were diagnosed early (within 1 month of the first symptoms), while 25.5% experienced delayed diagnosis. Among those with early-diagnosed IE and known symptom onset dates, 70.2% were diagnosed within 7 days of symptom onset, 17.5% within 7–14 days, and 12.3% after more than 14 days. Notably, in the late-diagnosed group, 33.9% reported that their initial symptoms had occurred over 3 months before diagnosis. These findings highlight the potential for significant diagnostic delays, particularly among older adults, and suggest that such delays may contribute to their poorer prognosis [59].

Echocardiography remains the first-line imaging modality for detecting anatomic evidence of IE [33] and continues to be a critical Major Criterion in the 2023 Duke-ISCVID IE 2023 Criteria (Table 16.2) [4]. TTE, while noninvasive, often has reduced sensitivity in this population, particularly in detecting vegetations on prosthetic valves or in the presence of calcified structures. Conversely, TEE offers superior imaging quality and is more effective in identifying endocardial involvement, making it a preferred diagnostic tool in older patients with suspected IE [4, 24, 66]. For instance, Sekar et al. reported that TTE detected endocardial involvement in only 21% of cases, whereas TEE identified it in 86% of the same cohort, underscoring TEE's superior diagnostic capability [66]. However, the use of TEE must be balanced against potential risks, such as complications from sedation, especially in patients with cognitive impairment or multiple comorbidities [67].

Diagnosis is generally based on the 2023 modified Duke criteria (Table 16.2). The 2023 Duke-ISCVID diagnostic criteria introduced several key updates to enhance diagnostic sensitivity and reflect modern imaging and microbiologic techniques. Among the major changes is the incorporation of intraoperative findings (e.g., observed vegetations, abscesses), cardiac CT, PET/CT, and molecular tools such as 16S rRNA PCR as major criteria. Minor criteria were also refined, including more flexible blood culture timing, better-defined risk factors, and expanded recognition of fastidious and emerging pathogens [4].

Advanced imaging and molecular tools have significantly improved the diagnosis of IE, especially in older adults and prosthetic valve recipients. 18F-FDG PET/CT, now a major Duke-ISCVID criterion, demonstrates up to 90% sensitivity in prosthetic valve IE [68]. Cardiac CT is similarly effective in detecting perivalvular abscesses, with sensitivity exceeding 95% [69]. In culture-negative cases, 16S rRNA PCR and metagenomic sequencing offer valuable diagnostic yield, particularly when valve tissue is available [70, 71].

Compared with the 2000 version, there is a notable increase in diagnostic sensitivity, from 74.9% to 84.2%. This improvement is especially meaningful in detecting culture-negative endocarditis or atypical organisms, thus allowing earlier diagnosis and better alignment of medical and surgical management. The enhanced criteria support more timely intervention, particularly in cases where standard imaging or cultures are non-diagnostic [72].

TREATMENT

Older adults who are at risk for IE and have unexplained fever for more than 48 hours should have at least three sets of blood cultures obtained at 30-minute intervals prior to antibiotic therapy, each containing 10 mL of blood, with incubation in both aerobic and anaerobic atmospheres [4, 57]. In general, broad-spectrum empiric intravenous antibiotics should be initiated only *after* obtaining blood cultures. Antibiotics should then be adjusted based on microbiological data, antibiotic susceptibilities, and whether native valve or prosthetic valve endocarditis is being treated (Table 16.3). Among patients with no evidence of IE on admission or occurring within 60 days of a prior admission that was associated with a risk for bacteremia or IE, IE diagnosed more than 72 hours after hospital admission is considered to be healthcare acquired. In such cases, coverage for antibiotic-resistant organisms is recommended. Blood cultures should be repeated every 24–48 hours until clearance of bacteremia is documented. The first day of negative blood cultures "starts the clock" for the planned duration of antibiotic therapy, which typically lasts 4–6 weeks, depending on the valve type and pathogen.

Although an option for abbreviated courses of antibiotics with combination therapy of beta-lactams and an aminoglycoside can be used in young adults for penicillin-resistant viridians streptococci, this strategy is not favored in older adults due to their higher risk of renal dysfunction and ototoxicity. The 2023 ESC guidelines now explicitly advise against aminoglycoside use in staphylococcal native valve endocarditis (NVE) because clinical benefits have not been demonstrated [57].

When aminoglycosides are necessary (e.g., for treatment of enterococcal IE) close attention should be paid to

Table 16.2 Modified Duke criteria for diagnosis of infective endocarditis (IE)

Definitions of infective endocarditis

I. Definite endocarditis

A. Pathologic Criteria

(1) Microorganisms identified in the context of clinical signs of active endocarditis in a vegetation; from cardiac tissue; from an explanted prosthetic valve or sewing ring; from an ascending aortic graft (with concomitant evidence of valve involvement); from an endovascular intracardiac implantable electronic device (CIED); or from an arterial embolus

or

(2) Active endocarditis (may be acute or subacute/chronic) identified in or on a vegetation; from cardiac tissue; from an explanted prosthetic valve or sewing ring; from an ascending aortic graft (with concomitant evidence of valve involvement); from a CIED; or from an arterial embolus

B. Clinical Criteria

(1) 2 Major Criteria

or

(2) 1 Major Criterion and 3 Minor Criteria

or

(3) 5 Minor Criteria

II. Possible endocarditis

A. 1 Major Criterion and 1 Minor Criterion; or

B. 3 Minor Criteria

III. Rejected endocarditis

A. Firm alternate diagnosis explaining signs/symptoms

or

B. Lack of recurrence despite antibiotic therapy for less than 4 days

or

C. No pathologic or macroscopic evidence of IE at surgery or autopsy, with antibiotic therapy for less than 4 days

or

D. Does not meet criteria for possible IE, as above

Clinical criteria

I. Major Criteria

A. Microbiologic Major Criteria

(1) Positive blood cultures

i. Microorganisms that commonly cause IE isolated from 2 or more separate blood culture sets (Typical); or

ii. Microorganisms that occasionally or rarely cause IE isolated from 3 or more separate blood culture sets (Nontypical)

(2) Positive laboratory tests

i. Positive polymerase chain reaction (PCR) or other nucleic acid-based technique for *Coxiella burnetii*, *Bartonella* species, or *Tropheryma whipplei* from blood or

ii. *Coxiella burnetii* antiphase I immunoglobulin G (IgG) antibody titer >1:800, or isolated from a single blood culture or

iii. Indirect immunofluorescence assays (IFA) for detection of IgM and IgG antibodies to *Bartonella henselae* or *Bartonella quintana* with immunoglobulin G (IgG) titer ≥1:800

B. Imaging Major Criteria

(1) Echocardiography and cardiac computed tomography (CT) imaging

i. Echocardiography and/or cardiac CT showing vegetation, valvular/leaflet perforation, valvular/leaflet aneurysm, abscess, pseudoaneurysm, or intracardiac fistula or

ii. Significant new valvular regurgitation on echocardiography as compared with previous imaging; worsening or changing of preexisting regurgitation is not sufficient or

iii. New partial dehiscence of prosthetic valve as compared with previous imaging

(2) Positron emission computed tomography with 18F-fluorodeoxyglucose ([18F]FDG PET/CT imaging)

i. Abnormal metabolic activity involving a native or prosthetic valve, ascending aortic graft (with concomitant evidence of valve involvement), intracardiac device leads or other prosthetic material

C. Surgical Major Criteria

Evidence of IE documented by direct inspection during heart surgery, without meeting major imaging criteria or subsequent histologic or microbiologic confirmation

(Continued)

Table 16.2 (Continued) Modified Duke criteria for diagnosis of infective endocarditis (IE)

II. Minor Criteria
   A. Predisposition
      - Previous history of IE
      - Prosthetic valve
      - Previous valve repair
      - Congenital heart disease
      - More than mild regurgitation or stenosis of any etiology
      - Endovascular intracardiac implantable electronic device (CIED)
      - Hypertrophic obstructive cardiomyopathy
      - Injection drug use
   B. Fever: Documented temperature greater than 38.0°C (100.4°F)
   C. Vascular phenomena: Clinical or radiological evidence of arterial emboli, septic pulmonary infarcts, cerebral or splenic abscess, mycotic aneurysm, intracranial hemorrhage, conjunctival hemorrhage, Janeway lesions, purulent purpura
   D. Immunologic phenomena: Positive rheumatoid factor, Osler nodes, Roth spots, or immune complex-mediated glomerulonephriti
   E. Microbiologic evidence, falling short of a Major Criterion
      (1) Positive blood cultures for a microorganism consistent with IE but not meeting the requirements for Major Criterion or
      (2) Positive culture, PCR, or other nucleic acid based test (amplicon or shotgun sequencing, in situ hybridization) for an organism consistent with IE from a sterile body site other than cardiac tissue, cardiac prosthesis, or arterial embolus; or a single finding of a skin bacterium by PCR on a valve or wire without additional clinical or microbiological supporting evidence
   F. Imaging Criteria
      Abnormal metabolic activity as detected by [18F]FDG PET/CT within 3 months of implantation of prosthetic valve, ascending aortic graft (with concomitant evidence of valve involvement), intracardiac device leads or other prosthetic material
   G. Physical Examination Criteria
      New valvular regurgitation identified on auscultation if echocardiography is not available; worsening or changing of preexisting murmur not sufficient

Source: Adapted from Fowler, V.G., et al., *Clin Infect Dis*, 77(4), 518–526, 2023.

renal function and therapeutic drug level measurements in order to minimize toxicities. Some authors recommend audiometry at baseline and weekly to monitor for ototoxicity for all patients anticipated to receive aminoglycoside therapy for more than 2 weeks. Serum levels of aminoglycosides that are lower than levels generally considered "therapeutic" (i.e., peaks of 3–4 mcg/ml) are adequate for synergy when administered with cell wall-active agents [73] and are associated with reduced risk of toxicity.

A two-phase approach to IE treatment is now recognized in the 2023 ESC guidelines. After an initial inpatient phase—typically 2 weeks of intravenous therapy, during which surgery or device removal may be performed if indicated—selected stable patients may transition to outpatient parenteral antibiotic therapy (OPAT) or oral step-down regimens. This strategy, supported by the POET trial and OPAT-GAMES study, has been shown to be safe even in select PVE cases. OPAT should only begin after TEE confirms no complications such as abscess or severe valve dysfunction. Long-acting agents like dalbavancin or oritavancin may offer additional flexibility for outpatient care in stable patients [57].

SURGICAL THERAPY

Decisions on surgical intervention are complex and depend on many clinical and prognostic factors, including the infecting organism, vegetation size, presence of perivalvular infection, presence of embolism or heart failure, age, noncardiac comorbidities, and available surgical expertise [57, 74]. While surgical decision-making in infective endocarditis increasingly incorporates standardized criteria, including those outlined in the 2023 ESC guidelines (Table 16.4), there remains a paucity of high-level evidence to define the optimal timing of surgery in many clinical scenarios. These include heart failure due to valve dysfunction, uncontrolled infection with perivalvular extension, and embolic events associated with large vegetations [41]. Surgical timing is categorized into emergency (within 24 hours), urgent (within 3–5 days), or elective procedures depending on clinical stability and imaging findings.

Multiple studies have evaluated the impact of early surgical intervention on outcomes in IE patients with growing evidence supporting a survival benefit, particularly

Table 16.3 Antimicrobial therapy for common causes of infective endocarditis

Pathogen	Native valve endocarditis			Prosthetic valve endocarditis		
Penicillin-susceptible oral streptococci and *Streptococcus gallolyticus* group	Penicillin G	12–18 million U/day IV, either in 4–6 doses or continuously	4 weeks	Penicillin G	12–18 million U/day IV, either in 4–6 doses or continuously	6 weeks
	Amoxicillin	12 g/day IV in 4–6 doses		Amoxicillin	12 g/day IV in 4–6 doses	
	Ceftriaxone	2 g/day IV in 1 dose		Ceftriaxone	2 g/day IV in 1 dose	
	Non-complicated NVE (with normal renal function)			If allergy to beta-lactams		
	Gentamicin	3 mg/kg/day IV or IM in 1 dose	2 weeks	Vancomycin	30 mg/kg/day IV in 2 doses	6 weeks
	Plus one of the following					
	Penicillin G	12–18 million U/day IV, either in 4–6 doses or continuously	2 weeks			
	Amoxicillin	12 g/day IV in 4–6 doses				
	Ceftriaxone	2 g/day IV in 1 dose				
	If allergy to beta-lactams					
	Vancomycin	30 mg/kg/day IV in 2 doses	4 weeks			
Oral streptococci and *Streptococcus gallolyticus* group susceptible, increased exposure or resistant to penicillin	Penicillin G	24 million U/day IV, either in 4–6 doses or continuously	4 weeks	Penicillin G	24 million U/day IV, either in 4–6 doses or continuously	6 weeks
	Amoxicillin	12 g/day IV, in 4–6 doses		Amoxicillin	12 g/day IV, in 4–6 doses	
	Ceftriaxone	2 g/day IV, in 1 dose		Ceftriaxone	2 g/day IV, in 1 dose	
	Plus			Plus		
	Gentamicin	3 mg/kg/day IV, or IM in 1 dose	2 weeks	Gentamicin	3 mg/kg/day IV, or IM in 1 dose	2 weeks
	If allergy to beta-lactams			If allergy to beta-lactams		
	Vancomycin	30 mg/kg/day IV, in 2 doses	4 weeks	Vancomycin	30 mg/kg/day IV in 2 doses	6 weeks
				Plus		
				Gentamicin	3 mg/kg/day IV or IM in 1 dose	2 weeks
Methicillin-susceptible staphylococci	(Flu)cloxacillin	12 g/day IV in 4–6 divided doses	4–6 weeks	(Flu)cloxacillin	12 g/day IV in 4–6 doses	6 weeks
				Cefazolin	6 g/day IV in 3 doses	
				Plus		
	Cefazolin	6 g/day IV in 3 divided doses		Rifampin	900 mg/day IV or orally in 3 divided doses	6 weeks
				Plus		
				Gentamicin	3 mg/kg/day IV or IM (1 preferred or 2 doses)	2 weeks
	If allergy to beta-lactams			If allergy to beta-lactams		
	Cefazolin	6 g/day IV in 3 divided doses	4–6 weeks	Cefazolin	6 g/day IV in 3 doses **Plus**	6 weeks
				Rifampin	900 mg/day IV or orally in 3 divided doses **Plus**	
				Gentamicin	3 mg/kg/day IV or IM (1 preferred or 2 doses)	2 weeks

(Continued)

Table 16.3 (Continued) Antimicrobial therapy for common causes of infective endocarditis

Pathogen	Native valve endocarditis			Prosthetic valve endocarditis		
Methicillin-resistant staphylococci	Vancomycin	30–60 mg/kg/day IV, in 2–3 divided doses	4–6 weeks	Vancomycin	30–60 mg/kg/day IV, in 2–3 divided doses Plus	≥6 weeks
				Rifampin	900–1200 mg/day IV, or orally in 2–3 divided doses Plus	≥6 weeks
				Gentamicin	3 mg/kg/day IV, or IM, in 1 (preferred) or 2 doses	2 weeks
Non-HLAR (high-level aminoglycoside-resistant) *Enterococcus* species	Amoxicillin	12 g/day IV in 4–6 doses	Depends on which antibiotic with (2 or 6 weeks)	Amoxicillin	12 g/day IV in 4–6 doses	Depends on which antibiotic with (2 or 6 weeks)
	Ampicillin	12 g/day IV in 4–6 doses		Ampicillin	12 g/day IV in 4–6 doses	
	With one of the following			With one of the following		
	Ceftriaxone	4 g/day IV in 2 doses	6 weeks	Ceftriaxone	4 g/day IV in 2 doses	6 weeks
	Gentamicin	3 mg/kg/day IV or IM in 1 dose	2 weeks	Gentamicin	3 mg/kg/day IV or IM in 1 dose	2 weeks
HLAR *Enterococcus*	Amoxicillin	12 g/day IV in 4–6 doses	6 weeks	Amoxicillin	12 g/day IV in 4–6 doses	6 weeks
	Ampicillin	12 g/day IV in 4–6 doses		Ampicillin	12 g/day IV in 4–6 doses	
	Plus			Plus		
	Ceftriaxone	4 g/day IV or IM in 2 doses		Ceftriaxone	4 g/day IV or IM in 2 doses	
Beta-lactam resistant *Enterococcus* species	Vancomycin	30 mg/kg/day IV, in 2 doses	6 weeks	Vancomycin	30 mg/kg/day IV, in 2 doses	6 weeks
	Gentamicin	3 mg/kg/day IV, or IM in 1 dose	2 weeks	Gentamicin	3 mg/kg/day IV, or IM in 1 dose	2 weeks
Vancomycin-resistant *Enterococcus* species	Daptomycin	10–12 mg/kg/day IV, in 1 dose	≥8 weeks	Daptomycin	10–12 mg/kg/day IV, in 1 dose	≥8 weeks
	Plus one of the following			Plus one of the following		
	Ampicillin	12 g/day IV, in 4–6 doses		Ampicillin	12 g/day IV, in 4–6 doses	
	Fosfomycin	12 g/day IV, in 4 doses		Fosfomycin	12 g/day IV, in 4 doses	
	Ceftaroline	1800 mg/day IV, in 3 doses		Ceftaroline	1800 mg/day IV, in 3 doses	
	Ertapenem	2 g/day IV, or IM in 1 dose		Ertapenem	2 g/day IV, or IM in 1 dose	

Source: Adapted from Delgado, V., et al. *Eur Heart J*, 44(39), 3948–4042, 2023.
Abbreviations: HLAR, high-level aminoglycoside-resistant; IM, intramuscular; IV, intravenous.

Table 16.4 Class I indications for surgical intervention in infective endocarditis (IE)

Recommendations	Timing
Left-sided native valve endocarditis with: • Acute heart failure due to severe regurgitation, obstruction, or fistula (e.g., pulmonary edema, cardiogenic shock)	Emergency (within 24 h)
• Fungi or highly resistant organisms • Uncontrolled infection: perivalvular abscess, pseudoaneurysm, fistula, prosthesis dehiscence, or new conduction abnormalities • Evidence of persistent infection after the start of appropriate antimicrobial therapy • Severe valve regurgitation and mobile vegetations >10 mm	Urgent (within 3-5 days)
Right-sided valve endocarditis with: • Persistent bacteremia after at least 1 week of appropriate antibiotic therapy • Right ventricular dysfunction secondary to acute severe tricuspid regurgitation nonresponsive to diuretics • Tricuspid valve vegetations that are ≥20 mm in diameter after recurrent pulmonary emboli • Respiratory insufficiency requiring ventilatory support after recurrent pulmonary emboli • Involvement of left-sided structures	Individualized
Prosthetic valve endocarditis with: • Symptoms or signs of heart failure resulting from valve dehiscence, intracardiac fistula, or severe prosthetic valve dysfunction	Emergency
• Uncontrolled infection with perivalvular extension or persistent bacteremia • Infection with fungi or multidrug-resistant organisms • Mobile vegetations >10 mm • Same criteria as native valve endocarditis regarding embolism and hemodynamic instability	Urgent

Source: Adapted from Delgado, V., et al., *Eur Heart J*, 44(39), 3948–4042, 2023.

when performed within the first 2–3 weeks of diagnosis. A meta-analysis of 21 studies comparing early surgery (≤20 days) with conservative therapy reported a significant reduction in all-cause mortality, with an odds ratio of 0.61 in unmatched cohorts and 0.41 in propensity-matched cohorts ($p < 0.001$ for both) [75]. Subgroup analysis further demonstrated that surgery within 7 days was associated with the greatest mortality benefit (OR = 0.30, 95% CI = 0.16–0.54) compared to delayed surgery or medical treatment alone [75]. Similarly, a large US nationwide study using the National Inpatient Sample (2016–2020) found that early surgery (≤7 days) was associated with significantly lower risks of acute stroke, peripheral embolism, and intracranial/intraspinal abscesses, though no difference in in-hospital mortality was observed [76].

Additional meta-analyses have yielded mixed results. One meta-analysis of 16 cohort studies found early surgery significantly lowered both in-hospital (OR = 0.57) and long-term mortality (OR = 0.57), particularly in patients with native valve endocarditis, while no clear benefit was seen in prosthetic valve endocarditis [77]. Conversely, another meta-analysis including 15 cohort studies with over 2400 patients found no significant difference between early surgery (within 14 days) and delayed surgery in either in-hospital mortality (OR 1.08, 95% CI 0.80–1.46) or long-term mortality (OR 1.12, 95% CI 0.68–1.86) [78].

Importantly, the survival benefit of surgery extends to older adults. In one study stratified by age (<65 years [n = 230], 65–80 years [n = 173], and ≥80 years [n = 51]), octogenarians who met surgical criteria had markedly different outcomes depending on treatment approach. Those who underwent surgery had in-hospital mortality of just 6.3%, compared to 72.7% among those managed medically. Postoperative 3-year survival rates were similarly high across all age groups (93.7%, 89.9%, and 90.4%, respectively) [79]. Another study reported a 3-year survival rate of 75% in older adults undergoing surgery, comparable to their younger counterparts [80].

Taken together, these results support early surgery (within 7 to 14 days of hospitalization) in selected patients with IE, particularly those with NVE or high embolic risk, but delayed surgery may also be appropriate in some patients, particularly those requiring initial stabilization. The optimal timing remains individualized based on clinical stability, surgical indication, and comorbid conditions.

Despite the benefits of surgery, older adults are less likely to receive it. In a Swedish national registry of 2186 left-sided IE cases, only 6% of patients aged ≥80 underwent surgery, compared to 46% of those under 65 [81]. The lower rate of referral for surgery may be due to factors such as prevalent comorbidities, cognitive dysfunction, patient preferences, and the higher operative mortality reported in older adults (20%–30%) [82–84]. Nonetheless, several recent cohort studies have confirmed that age over 65 is an independent predictor of reduced likelihood of surgical intervention, even after adjusting for clinical severity, comorbidities, and infection characteristics [23, 81, 91]. This underutilization likely reflects a complex interplay of clinical and nonclinical factors, such as perceived limited long-term benefit and aversion to surgery.

Several scores are in use to predict early mortality after cardiac surgery [88–90]. These scoring systems, such as EuroSCORE II and the STS score, were developed for elective surgery and tend to underestimate risk in urgent IE cases, especially in older adults [88]. They also lack geriatric-specific factors such as frailty. Recent studies have shown that incorporating frailty measures, like the Clinical Frailty Scale or Hospital Frailty Risk Score, can significantly improve risk prediction [90]. A machine learning-based model tailored for IE surgery has also shown superior accuracy (AUC $\approx$ 0.81) compared to traditional tools, but these approaches still require broader validation before routine use [89, 90].

Older adults are more prone to perioperative complications such as prosthetic valve dysfunction, pericardial tamponade, acute kidney injury, arrhythmias (especially atrial fibrillation), and the need for reoperation [85, 92]. They are also at increased risk for post-operative delirium, cognitive dysfunction, functional decline, prolonged length of stay, and discharge to a transitional or long-term care facility. Nonetheless, multiple studies show that when surgery is performed in carefully selected older patients, outcomes can be excellent. These findings underscore that advanced age alone should not preclude surgical referral, and that careful risk–benefit assessment involving a multidisciplinary endocarditis team is essential [81–84]. Thus, the decision to operate and the timing of surgery in IE, especially in older adults, should be discussed by a multispecialty team with expertise in cardiology, imaging, cardiothoracic surgery, infectious disease, and geriatric medicine. These discussions should also incorporate the perspectives of the patient and family/caregivers to achieve consensus on the best course forward for the patient utilizing a shared decision-making process.

For older IE patients with advanced frailty, multimorbidity, or poor functional status, palliative care should be considered when surgery is not feasible or the patient declines surgery. Early integration of palliative care can support symptom management, clarify goals of care, and guide decisions about the intensity of treatment. Including palliative care on the multidisciplinary team helps ensure care aligns with the patient's values and maintains their quality of life.

COMPLICATIONS

Infective endocarditis in older patients is frequently accompanied by serious complications that worsen outcomes. In contemporary cohorts, roughly 30%–50% of patients develop one or more major complications from infective endocarditis [15, 24, 64, 91]. The most common are cardiovascular complications, especially acute heart failure, which occurs in roughly 14%–40% of cases [15, 63, 64]. In some patients, this progresses to cardiogenic shock (approximately 5%), a life-threatening condition with in-hospital mortality rates exceeding 50% [93]. Advanced age further increases the risk of these complications. Older patients with IE are more prone to hemodynamic instability due to age-related declines in cardiac reserve and preexisting valvular disease, making acute heart failure one of the most serious and frequent complications in this group [93].

Systemic embolization and neurologic complications are also common. Around 15%–20% of IE patients experience neurologic events such as ischemic stroke [15], which are often especially debilitating in older adults. These events can greatly worsen prognosis; cerebrovascular complications, for example, have been shown to increase the odds of in-hospital death by nearly 80% [63]. Interestingly, older patients may present with fewer overt embolic events than younger adults, possibly due to smaller vegetations or more subacute presentations [86, 87]. Despite this, some surgical and autopsy reports have noted a higher prevalence of local destructive complications, such as perivalvular abscesses, even when vegetations are small. However, large registry-based studies have found a lower diagnosed rate of abscesses in older patients, possibly reflecting less frequent use of transesophageal echocardiography or lower surgical referral rates in this group [81].

Perivalvular abscesses, when present, are serious complications associated with new-onset atrioventricular (AV) block, persistent bacteremia, and refractory heart failure. Their prevalence varies by cohort and diagnostic method, with reported rates ranging from 10% to over 30% in some surgical studies [94, 95]. Timely recognition is essential. The appearance of new conduction abnormalities on electrocardiogram (including first-degree AV block, higher degrees of AV block, and bundle branch block) should raise suspicion for abscess formation and prompt further evaluation, as surgical intervention is often necessary to prevent rupture, fistula, or uncontrolled sepsis [95].

Other embolic complications, such as splenic infarcts, renal or mesenteric ischemia, and limb emboli, are often underdiagnosed in older patients with IE, partly due to atypical symptoms or attribution to other age-related conditions [57, 62]. Recent studies reported splenic infarcts in up to 10%–20% of IE cases, with a higher risk of ICU admission and mortality among those affected [96]. Vertebral osteomyelitis, particularly associated with *S. aureus* or enterococcal IE, should be suspected in patients presenting with new or unexplained back pain. One 2025 study found vertebral infection in 12% of IE patients, most commonly in older patients and those with enterococcal disease [97]. Renal impairment is also a frequent complication, and is often multifactorial, resulting from embolic infarction, sepsis-associated acute kidney injury (AKI), or nephrotoxic antibiotics. In one large cohort, AKI occurred in 52.7% of patients with IE, with *S. aureus* infection being significantly associated with renal injury [98]. These findings highlight the need for clinicians to maintain a high index of suspicion and consider early monitoring of renal function, particularly in older patients whose clinical presentations may be muted or atypical.

With early diagnosis, targeted antibiotic therapy, and timely surgical evaluation, a significant proportion of older patients can survive and return to meaningful functional status. Prognostication should be personalized and multidimensional, incorporating medical, surgical, and geriatric considerations. Post-discharge planning and follow-up are essential to monitor for complications, manage valvular sequelae, and support long-term recovery [57].

PREVENTION

Prevention of IE relies on general infection control principles and targeted prophylaxis for high-risk individuals. Maintaining optimal oral hygiene and routine dental care are foundational measures because poor dental status is an independent risk factor for IE. Hand hygiene compliance, sterile technique during invasive procedures, and timely removal of unnecessary indwelling devices, such as urinary catheters, central lines, and feeding tubes, are essential to reduce bacteremia risk in hospitalized or immunocompromised patients [57]. The 2021 American Heart Association (AHA) Scientific Statement and the 2023 European Society of Cardiology (ESC) guidelines reiterate that antibiotic prophylaxis for dental procedures is recommended only in patients at highest risk of adverse IE outcomes, specifically, those with prosthetic valves (including TAVR), a history of IE, unrepaired cyanotic congenital heart disease, or cardiac transplant recipients with valvulopathy [57, 99]. For these individuals, oral amoxicillin 2 g, 30–60 minutes before dental treatment is recommended; clindamycin is no longer advised due to adverse event risk. For individuals who are allergic to penicillin, a single dose of cephalexin 2 g, doxycycline 100 mg, or azithromycin 500 mg is a suggested alternative. The ESC 2023 guidelines also consider prophylaxis for high-risk patients undergoing invasive genitourinary or gastrointestinal procedures on a case-by-case basis. While the presence of CIEDs does not always routinely require antibiotic prophylaxis for dental work, periprocedural prevention is critical. A single preoperative dose of cefazolin or vancomycin at implantation can reduce CIED-related IE. Strict aseptic technique is crucial, particularly to avoid hematoma, a major risk factor for infection, especially during pocket revisions. In some high-risk patients, it is important to prevent infection around the time of the procedure [57]. For TAVR patients, who are at high risk of developing enterococcal and staphylococcal IE, perioperative prophylaxis tailored to local flora and patient risk is strongly advised. In cancer patients and frail older adults, minimizing device days, enforcing sterile technique, and avoiding unnecessary catheterization are critical for IE prevention. Lastly, all guidelines emphasize the importance of antimicrobial stewardship, avoiding indiscriminate antibiotic use and instead targeting prevention strategies based on individual risk [57].

CONCLUSION

IE affects older adults at a much higher rate than young adults primarily due to higher prevalence of degenerative valve disease and wider use of prosthetic devices. Other factors include an increased number of procedures predisposing to bacteremia, poor dentition, comorbidities (such as diabetes or malignancy), higher incidence of other infections (especially urinary tract infections and pneumonia), diminished immune function due to immunosenescence, comorbid illnesses (e.g., cancer), nutritional deficits, and certain medications (e.g., prednisone and other immunosuppressants).

Key differences between IE in older versus young adults include the following:

- Nonspecific clinical presentations with lower rates of fever, chills, embolic events, and leukocytosis contribute to delayed diagnosis of IE in older adults.
- Higher rates of renal failure and heart failure on presentation, and a much higher burden of chronic disease/comorbidities that likely underlie age-associated increases in mortality.
- More likely to have *Staphylococcus aureus*, *Enterococcus faecalis*, and healthcare-associated pathogens due to frequent exposure to medical devices and procedures.
- The sensitivity of transthoracic echocardiography is often reduced in older adults due to calcified valvular structures or the presence of prosthetic material, whereas transesophageal echocardiography maintains high sensitivity and should be prioritized in this population.
- Older adults are less likely to undergo surgery for IE, even when meeting standard criteria. However, with timely and appropriate intervention, selected patients can achieve excellent outcomes.
- Careful use of nephrotoxic agents, particularly aminoglycosides, is warranted in older adults, with monitoring of audiometry and renal function when use of aminoglycosides is necessary.

In older patients with IE, functional and nutritional status are important predictors of outcomes. To optimize management decisions, the use of comprehensive geriatric assessments and individualized surgical risk stratification tools is increasingly recommended. Additionally, 2023 guidelines endorse a shift toward multimodal imaging, multidisciplinary management, and outpatient antibiotic strategies tailored to patient-specific risk. When feasible, management of IE in the older population should involve a multidisciplinary team including cardiologists, infectious disease specialists, cardiac surgeons, anesthesiologists, and geriatricians. Geriatricians can play a major role in ensuring compliance with treatment, managing potential drug interactions, facilitating shared decision-making, and maximizing quality of life.

REFERENCES

1. Contrepois, A., Notes on the early history of infective endocarditis and the development of an experimental model. *Clin Infect Dis*, 1995. 20(2): p. 461–466.
2. Pruitt, R.D., William Osler and his Gulstonian Lectures on malignant endocarditis. *Mayo Clin Proc*, 1982. 57(1): p. 4–9.
3. Mylonakis, E., et al., Infective endocarditis in adults. *N Engl J Med*, 2001. 345: p. 1318–1330.
4. Fowler, V.G., et al., The 2023 Duke-International Society for Cardiovascular Infectious Diseases criteria for infective endocarditis: updating the modified Duke criteria. *Clin Infect Dis*, 2023. 77(4): p. 518–526.
5. Tornos, P., et al., Infective endocarditis: the European viewpoint. *Curr Probl Cardiol*, 2011. 36(5): p. 175–222.
6. Chen, H., et al., The global, regional, and national burden and trends of infective endocarditis from 1990 to 2019: results from the global burden of disease study 2019. *Front Med (Lausanne)*, 2022. 9: p. 774224.
7. Galar, A., et al., Methicillin-resistant *Staphylococcus aureus* prosthetic valve endocarditis: pathophysiology, epidemiology, clinical presentation, diagnosis, and management. *Clin Microbiol Rev*, 2019. 32(2): e00041-18. doi:10.1128/CMR.00041-18.
8. Reisinger, M., Kachel, M., George, I., Emerging and re-emerging pathogens in valvular infective endocarditis: a review. *Pathogens*, 2024. 13(7): p. 543.
9. Berisha, B., et al., Microbiological etiology in prosthetic valve endocarditis: a nationwide registry study. *J Intern Med*, 2022. 292(3): p. 428–437. doi:10.1111/joim.13491.
10. Mettler, S.K., et al., Gender, age, and regional disparities in the incidence and mortality trends of infective endocarditis in the United States between 1990 and 2019. *Am J Cardiol*, 2023. 203: p. 128–135.
11. Selton-Suty, C., et al., Preeminence of *Staphylococcus aureus* in infective endocarditis: a 1-year population-based survey. *Clin Infect Dis*, 2012. 54(9): p. 1230–1239.
12. Ahtela, E., et al., Short- and long-term outcomes of infective endocarditis admission in adults: a population-based registry study in Finland. *PLoS One*, 2021. 16(7): p. e0254553.
13. Varela Barca, L., et al., Analysis of sex differences in the clinical presentation, management and prognosis of infective endocarditis in Spain. *Heart*, 2021. 107(21): p. 1717–1724.
14. García-Carretero, R., et al., Trends in infective endocarditis incidence, microbiology, and valve surgery in Spain: a nationwide population-based study (2001–2015). *Open Forum Infect Dis*, 2022. 9(12): p. ofac647.
15. Perez-Rivera, J.A., et al., Comorbidity and prognosis in octogenarians with infective endocarditis. *J Clin Med*, 2022. 11(13): p. 3774.
16. Marques, M., et al., Risk factors for in-hospital mortality in infective endocarditis. *Arq Bras Cardiol*, 2020. 114(1): p. 1–8.
17. Cresti, A., et al., Epidemiological and mortality trends in infective endocarditis, a 17-year population-based prospective study. *Cardiovasc Diagn Ther*, 2017. 7(1): p. 27–35.
18. Budea, C.M., et al., Clinical presentation and risk factors of infective endocarditis in the elderly: a systematic review. *J Pers Med*, 2023. 13(2): p. 296.
19. Chen, H., et al., Predictors of central line-associated bloodstream infections in cancer patients undergoing chemotherapy through implanted venous access ports: a retrospective, observational study. *Transl Cancer Res*, 2023. 12(12): p. 3538–3546.
20. Di Salvo, G., et al., Endocarditis in the elderly: clinical, echocardiographic, and prognostic features. *Eur Heart J*, 2003. 24: p. 1576–1583.
21. Musci, T., Grubitzsch, H., Healthcare-associated infective endocarditis—Surgical perspectives. *J Clin Med*, 2022. 11(17): p. 4957.
22. Shen, L., et al., 7295 elderly hospitalized patients with catheter-associated urinary tract infection: a case-control study. *BMC Infect Dis*, 2023. 23: p. 825.
23. Scheggi, V., et al., Infective endocarditis in octogenarians: a retrospective study in a single, high-volume surgical centre. *BMC Geriatr*, 2023. 23(1): p. 345.
24. Bea, C., Vela, S., García-Blas, S., Perez-Rivera, J.-A., Díez-Villanueva, P., de Gracia, A.I., Fuertes, E., Oltra, M.R., Ferrer, A., Belmonte, A., et al., Infective endocarditis in the elderly: challenges and strategies. *J Cardiovasc Dev Dis*, 2022. 9(6): p. 192.
25. Deharo, J.C., et al., Infective endocarditis in patients with cardiac implantable electronic devices: a nationwide study. *Europace*, 2020. 22(7): p. 1062–1069.
26. Rapti, V., Giannitsioti, E., Spernovasilis, N., Magiorakos, A.-P., Poulakou, G., The evolving landscape of infective endocarditis: difficult-to-treat

resistance bacteria and novel diagnostics at the foreground. *J Clin Med*, 2025. 14(6): p. 2087.

27. Østergaard, L., et al., Temporal changes, patient characteristics, and mortality, according to microbiological cause of infective endocarditis: a nationwide study. *J Am Heart Assoc*, 2022. 11(16): p. e025801.
28. Escolà-Vergé, L., Fernández-Hidalgo, N., Larrosa, M.N., Fernandez-Galera, R., Almirante, B., Secular trends in the epidemiology and clinical characteristics of Enterococcus faecalis infective endocarditis at a referral center (2007–2018). *Eur J Clin Microbiol Infect Dis*, 2021. 40(6): p. 1137–1148.
29. Di Salvo, G., et al., Endocarditis in the elderly: clinical, echocardiographic, and prognostic features. *Eur Heart J*, 2003. 24: p. 1576–1583.
30. Zamorano, J., et al., Better prognosis of elderly patients with infectious endocarditis in the era of routine echocardiography and nonrestrictive indications for valve surgery. *Soc Echocardiogr*, 2002. 15: p. 702–707.
31. de Isla, L., Zamorano, J., Lennie, V., Pérez negative blood culture infective endocarditis in the elderly: long-term follow-up. *Gerontology*, 2007. 53: p. 245–249.
32. Tackling, G., Lala, V., *Endocarditis antibiotic regimens*. StatPearls, 2023. [Online] Available at: https://www.ncbi.nlm.nih.gov/books/NBK542162/
33. McHugh, J., Abu Saleh, O., Updates in culture-negative endocarditis. *Pathogens*, 2023. 12(8): p. 1027.
34. Kong, W.K.F., et al., Outcomes of culture-negative vs. culture-positive infective endocarditis: the ESC-EORP EURO-ENDO registry. *Eur Heart J*, 2022. 43(29): p. 2770–2780.
35. Siddiqui, A.H., Koirala, J., *Methicillin-resistant Staphylococcus aureus*. StatPearls, 2023. [Online] Available at: https://www.ncbi.nlm.nih.gov/books/NBK482221/
36. Lamas, C.C., Eykyn, S.J., Native infective endocarditis: a state-of-the-art review. *Clin Microbiol Rev*, 2003. 16(3): p. 333–365.
37. Del Val, D., Panagides, V., Mestres, C.A., Miró, J.M., Rodés-Cabau, J., Infective endocarditis after transcatheter aortic valve replacement: JACC state-of-the-art review. *J Am Coll Cardiol*, 2023. 81(4): p. 394–412.
38. Del Val, D., Abdel-Wahab, M., Mangner, N., Durand, E., Ihlemann, N., Urena, M., Pellegrini, C., Giannini, F., Gasior, T., Wojakowski, W., et al., Infective endocarditis caused by *Staphylococcus aureus* after transcatheter aortic valve replacement. *Can J Cardiol*, 2022. 38(1): p. 102–112.
39. Tabata, N., Al-Kassou, B., Sugiura, A., Shamekhi, J., Sedaghat, A., Treede, H., Tsujita, K., Werner, N., Grube, E., Nickenig, G., Sinning, J.-M., Predictive factors and long-term prognosis of transcatheter aortic valve implantation-associated endocarditis. *Clin Res Cardiol*, 2020. 109(9): p. 1165–1176.
40. Baddour, L.M., et al., Update on cardiovascular implantable electronic device infections and their prevention, diagnosis, and management: a scientific statement from the American heart association. *Circulation*, 2024. 149(2): p. e201–e216.
41. Wang, R., et al., Microbiological characteristics and clinical features of cardiac implantable electronic device infections at a tertiary hospital in China. *Front Microbiol*, 2017. 8: p. 360.
42. Bengtsen, K.H., et al., Incidence of *Staphylococcus aureus* bacteremia in patients following implantation of cardiac implantable electronic devices: a Danish nationwide cohort study. *Open Forum Infect Dis*, 2024. 11(9): p. ofae515.
43. Liu, P.Y., et al., *Staphylococcus lugdunensis* infective endocarditis: a literature review and analysis of risk factors. *Immunol Infect*, 2010. 43: p. 478–484.
44. Tsao, Y.T., et al., Characterization of *Staphylococcus lugdunensis* endocarditis in patients with cardiac implantable electronic devices. *Int Dis*, 2012. 16: p. e464–e467.
45. Kyaw, H., et al., *Staphylococcus lugdunensis* endocarditis and cerebrovascular accident: a systemic review of risk factors and clinical outcome. *Cureus*, 2018. 10(4): p. e2469.
46. Neupane, K., Kaswan, D., Coxiella burnetii Infection. In: *StatPearls* [Internet]. Treasure Island (FL): StatPearls Publishing; 2025 Jan. [Updated 2023 May 22].
47. Fragner, M., et al., Atypical presentation of *Coxiella burnetii* endocarditis: diagnostic considerations and the importance of keeping a broad differential. *Cureus*, 2024. 16(7): p. e63659.
48. Lam, J.C., Fonseca, K., Pabbaraju, K., Meatherall, B.L., Case report: Bartonella quintana endocarditis outside of the Europe-African gradient: comprehensive review of cases within North America. *Am J Trop Med Hyg*, 2019. 100(5): p. 1125–1129.
49. Chaloner, G.L., Harrison, T.G., Birtles, R.J., Bartonella species as a cause of infective endocarditis in the UK. Epidemiol Infect, 2013. 141: p. 841–846.
50. Hajj-Chahine, J., Houmaida, H., Plouzeau, C., Bartonella as a cause of mechanical prosthetic aortic root endocarditis. *Ann Thorac Surg*, 2012. 93: p. e93–e95.
51. Fenollar, F., Célard, M., Lagier, J.-C., Lepidi, H., Fournier, P.-E., Raoult, D., Tropheryma whipplei endocarditis. *Emerging Infectious Diseases*, 2013. 19(11): p. 1721–1730.
52. McGee, M., et al., Tropheryma whipplei endocarditis: case presentation and review of the literature. *Open Forum Infect Dis*, 2019. 6(1): p. ofy330.
53. Schreiber, P.W., et al., Mycobacterium chimaera infections after cardiac surgery—lessons learned. *Clin Microbiol Infect*, 2018. 24(11): p. 1117–1118.

54. Trauth, J., et al., Blind spot in endocarditis guidelines: Mycobacterium chimaera prosthetic valve endocarditis after cardiac surgery—a case series. *Eur Heart J Case Rep*, 2023. 7(8): p. ytad400.
55. Fournier, P.E., et al., Comprehensive diagnostic strategy for blood culture-negative endocarditis: a prospective study of 819 new cases. *Clin Infect Dis*, 2010. 51(2): p. 131–140.
56. Loyens, M., et al. Link between endocarditis on porcine bioprosthetic valves and allergy to pork. *Int J Cardiol*, 2013. 167(2): p. 600–602.
57. Delgado, V., et al., 2023 ESC Guidelines for the management of endocarditis: developed by the task force on the management of endocarditis of the European Society of Cardiology (ESC) Endorsed by the European Association for Cardio-Thoracic Surgery (EACTS) and the European Association of Nuclear Medicine (EANM). *Eur Heart J*, 2023. 44(39): p. 3948–4042.
58. Cahill, T.J., Prendergast, B.D., Infective endocarditis. *Lancet*, 2016. 387(10021): p. 882–893.
59. N'Guyen, Y., et al. Time interval between infective endocarditis first symptoms and diagnosis: relationship to infective endocarditis characteristics, microorganisms and prognosis. *Ann Med*, 2017. 49(2): p. 117–125.
60. Wu, Z., Chen, Y., Xiao, T., Niu, T., Shi, Q., Xiao, Y. The clinical features and prognosis of infective endocarditis in the elderly from 2007 to 2016 in a tertiary hospital in China. *BMC Infectious Diseases*, 2019. 19: p. 937.
61. Elyoussfi, S., et al., Cutaneous dermatologic manifestations of cardiovascular diseases: a narrative review. *Cureus*, 2024. 16(4): p. e56284.
62. La Canna, G., Torracca, L., Barbone, A., Scarfò, I. Unexpected infective endocarditis: towards a new alert for clinicians. *J Clin Med*, 2024, 13(17): p. 5058.
63. Okamoto, H., et al., Trends in the clinical characteristics and outcome of infective endocarditis: a nationwide study from 2016 to 2021. *J Am Heart Assoc*, 2024. 13(1): p. e037188. doi:10.1161/JAHA.124.037188.
64. Mir, T., Uddin, M., Qureshi, W.T., Regmi, N., Tleyjeh, I.M., Saydain, G., Predictors of complications secondary to infective endocarditis and their associated outcomes: a large cohort study from the National Emergency Database (2016–2018). *Infect Dis Ther*, 2022. 11: p. 305–321.
65. Viezens, L., et al., Spontaneous spondylodiscitis and endocarditis: interdisciplinary experience from a tertiary institutional case series and proposal of a treatment algorithm. *Neurosurg Rev*, 2022. 45(2): p. 1335–1342.
66. Sekar, P., Johnson, J.R., Thurn, J.R., Drekonja, D.M., Morrison, V.A., Chandrashekhar, Y., Adabag, S., Kuskowski, M.A., Filice, G.A. Comparative sensitivity of transthoracic and transesophageal echocardiography in diagnosis of infective endocarditis among veterans with *Staphylococcus aureus* bacteremia. *Open Forum Infect Dis*, 2017. 4(2): p. ofx035.
67. Kersey, C.B., Medhane, F., Pattock, A.M., Liu, L., Huang, G., Lele, A.V., Kwon, Y. Cardiac arrest during transesophageal echocardiogram (TEE) due to acute right ventricular failure. *Case Rep Cardiol*, 2021. 2021: p. 7427127.
68. O'Gorman, P., et al. Meta-analysis assessing the sensitivity and specificity of ^{18}F-FDG PET/CT for the diagnosis of prosthetic valve endocarditis (PVE) using individual patient data (IPD). *Am Heart J*. 2023. 261: p. 21–34.
69. Ghanem-Zoubi, N., FDG PET/CT in Cardiac infection: does it matter? A narrative review. *Infect Dis Ther*. 2022. 11(5): p. 1769–1777.
70. Galli, A., Barbieri, R., Graziano, E., Dodi, C., Di Lella, F., Franceschi, M., et al. Molecular analysis with 16S rRNA PCR/Sanger sequencing and molecular antibiogram performed on DNA extracted from valve improve diagnosis and targeted therapy of infective endocarditis: a prospective study. *Clin Infect Dis*, 2023. 76(3): e1484.
71. Hong, H.L., Flurin, L., Greenwood-Quaintance, et al. 16S rRNA Gene PCR/sequencing of heart valves for diagnosis of infective endocarditis in routine clinical practice. *J Clin Microbiol*, 2023. 61(8): e00341–e00423.
72. Van Der Vaart, T.W., et al., External validation of the 2023 Duke–International Society for Cardiovascular Infectious Diseases diagnostic criteria for infective endocarditis. *Clin Infect Dis*, 2024. 78(6): p. 922–929.
73. Habib, G., et al., Guidelines on the prevention diagnosis and treatment of infective endocarditis (new version 2009): the Task Force on the Prevention Diagnosis and Treatment of Infective Endocarditis of the European Society of Cardiology (ESC). *Eur Heart J*. 2009. 30(19): p. 2369–413. PMID 19713420; doi: 10.1093/eurheartj/ehp285.
74. Iaccarino, A., Barbone, A., Basciu, A., et al., Surgical challenges in infective endocarditis: state of the art. *J Clin Med*, 2023. 12(18): p. 5891.
75. Narayanan, M.A., et al., Early versus late surgical intervention or medical management for infective endocarditis: a systematic review and meta-analysis. *Heart*, 2016. 102(12): p. 950–957.
76. Llah, S.T., Sharif, S., Ullah, S., Sheikh, S.A., Shah, M.A., Shafi, O.M., Dar, T., Infective endocarditis surgery timing. *Cardiovasc Revasc Med*, 2024. 58: p. 16–22.
77. Liang, F., et al., Optimal timing for early surgery in infective endocarditis: a meta-analysis. *Interact Cardiovasc Thorac Surg*, 2016. 22(3): p. 336–345.
78. Manikantan, P., Tao, M., Despotidis, G., Alkhalil, A., Parikh, P., Pyo, R., Optimal timing of surgery

for patients with infective endocarditis, European heart journal. *Acute Cardiovascular Care*, 2023. 12(Supplement_1), May: p. zuad036.148.

79. Oliver, L., et al., Infective endocarditis in octogenarians. *Heart*, 2017. 103(20): p. 1602–1609. doi:10.1136/heartjnl-2016-310853.
80. Lin, C.-Y., Lu, C.-H., Lee, H.-A., See, L.-C., Wu, M.-Y., Han, Y., Tseng, C.-N., Su, I.-L., Li, H.-Y., Tsai, F.-C., Elderly versus non-elderly patients undergoing surgery for left-sided native valve infective endocarditis: a 10-year institutional experience. *Sci Rep*, 2020. 10: p. 2690.
81. Ragnarsson, S., et al., Surgery is underused in elderly patients with left-sided infective endocarditis: a nationwide registry study. *J Am Heart Assoc*, 2021. 10(19): p. e020221.
82. Correspondence to: Ravi K. Ghanta, MD, Michael E. DeBakey Department of Surgery, Baylor College of Medicine, One Baylor Plaza, MC-390, Houston, TX 77030.
83. Hémar, V., et al. The Mortality of Infective Endocarditis with and without Surgery in Elderly (MoISE) Study. Clin Infect Dis, 2023. 77(10): p. 1440–1448.
84. Jussli-Melchers, J., et al. Mid- and long-term surgical outcomes due to infective endocarditis in elderly patients: a retrospective cohort study. *J Clin Med*, 2022. 11(22): p. 6693.
85. Lin, C.-Y., Lu, C.-H., Lee, H.-A., See, L.-C., Wu, M.-Y., Han, Y., Tseng, C.-N., Su, I.-L., Li, H.-Y., Tsai, F.-C., Elderly versus non-elderly patients undergoing surgery for left-sided native valve infective endocarditis: a 10-year institutional experience. *Sci Rep*, 2020. 10: p. 2690.
86. Lemos, L.H.B., et al. Infective endocarditis in the elderly: distinct characteristics. *Arq Bras Cardiol*, 2021. 117(4): p. 775–781.
87. Durante-Mangoni, E., et al. Current features of infective endocarditis in elderly patients: results of the international collaboration on endocarditis prospective cohort study. *Arch Intern Med*, 2008. 168(19): p. 2095–2103.
88. Patrat-Delon, S., et al. EuroSCORE II underestimates mortality after cardiac surgery for infective endocarditis. *Eur J Cardiothorac Surg*, 2016. 49(3): p. 944–951.
89. Luo, L., et al. Machine learning-based risk model for predicting early mortality after surgery for infective endocarditis. *J Am Heart Assoc*, 2022. 11(11): p. e025433.
90. Rizzo, V., et al. Infective endocarditis: do we have an effective risk score model? A systematic review. *Front Cardiovasc Med*, 2023. 10: p. 1093363.
91. Kiriyama, H., et al., Surgical treatment for infective endocarditis in the ageing society: a nationwide retrospective study in Japan. *Open Heart*, 2021. 8(1): p. e001627.
92. Hermanns, H., et al. Perioperative complications in infective endocarditis. *J Clin Med*, 2023. 12(17): p. 5762.
93. Pericàs, J.M., et al., Characteristics and outcome of acute heart failure in infective endocarditis: focus on cardiogenic shock. *Clin Infect Dis*, 2021. 73(5): p. 765–774.
94. Mahmoud, K., Hammouda, T., Kandil, H., Mashaal, M., Prevalence and predictors of aortic root abscess among patients with left-sided infective endocarditis: a cross-sectional comparative study. *Egypt Heart J*, 2020. 72: p. 62.
95. Blomjous, M.S.H., Budde, R.P.J., Infective endocarditis related abscess is an important complication and requires awareness on all imaging modalities. *J Nucl Cardiol*, 2023. 30(6): p. 2415–2417.
96. Yen, C.C., et al. Risk assessment and prognostic analysis of patients with splenic infarction in emergency department: a multicenter retrospective study. *Sci Rep*, 2021. 11(1): p. 21423.
97. Douiyeb, S., Sigaloff, K.C.E., Ulas, E.G., Duffels, M.G.J., Drexhage, O., Germans, T., Wagenaar, J.F.P., Buis, D.T.P., van der Vaart, T.W., van Werkhoven, C.H., Prins, J.M., Umans, V.A.W.M., Vertebral osteomyelitis in patients with infective endocarditis: prevalence, risk factors and mortality. *Eur J Clin Microbiol Infect Dis*, 2025 Apr. 44(4): p. 819–825. doi: 10.1007/s10096-025-05041-8. Epub 2025 Jan 21.
98. Von Tokarski, F., et al. Risk factors and outcomes of early acute kidney injury in infective endocarditis: a retrospective cohort study. *Int J Infect Dis*, 2020. 99: p. 421–427.
99. Lockhart, P.B., et al. The 2021 American Heart Association statement on prevention of infective endocarditis. *J Am Dent Assoc*, 2021. 152(11): p. 880–882.

17

Cardiomyopathies in older persons

NATHANIEL ABITTAN, SRIHARI S. NAIDU, AND WILBERT S. ARONOW

Key points

- Cardiomyopathy is the leading diagnosis for hospitalized patients in older persons in high-income countries.
- HFpEF is a heterogeneous multimorbid cardiomyopathy that is becoming increasingly more common in the elderly, but with limited treatment options.
- The diagnosis of TTR amyloidosis is sharply rising, with novel therapeutic agents being developed that can delay progression of the disease.
- The mortality for older patients with HCM is similar to age- and sex-matched controls. In symptomatic patients, myosin inhibitors improve symptoms and reduce obstructive gradients, as well as the need for invasive septal reduction therapies. However, percutaneous alcohol septal ablation is a reasonable option that carries low morbidity and mortality.

PREVALENCE

The true prevalence of cardiomyopathy in older adults may be underestimated because of the low sensitivity of the clinical criteria, particularly in milder cases. Current data suggests an incidence of 32.8 per 1000 person-years for older persons ages 75–79 years rising to 80.8 per 1000 person-years in those older than 85 years, with over half of all hospitalized patients having heart failure once >75 years, evenly distributed by sex.[1,2] Heart failure is the leading diagnosis for hospitalized patients in older adults in high-income countries.[1,3]

HEART FAILURE WITH PRESERVED EJECTION FRACTION (HFPEF)

HFpEF is especially prevalent in older persons and accounts for very high morbidity and mortality.[4] Of patients identified as having congestive failure by the Framingham study, more than 50% had a left ventricular (LV) ejection fraction greater than 50%.[5] Mortality and morbidity is now equal to patients with diminished ejection fraction and is four times greater than that of age- and sex-matched controls. Comparing three decades of Framingham study participants, Ramachandran et al. found that among those diagnosed with heart failure, there was a steady rise in the proportion of those diagnosed with HFpEF compared to HFrEF (heart failure with reduced ejection fraction), with over 56% of patients having a preserved EF.[6] In one large study of over 6000 older adults with heart failure, at least two thirds had a preserved ejection fraction.[7]

The pathophysiology of HFpEF is complex. Delayed relaxation, or more properly prolonged systolic contraction, can be induced by anything that will increase the pressure or volume load to the ventricle. While delayed relaxation represents a compensatory adjustment to loading phenomena, impaired relaxation with secondary reduction in ventricular filling constitutes active pathology that relates to specific underlying causes. Patients with HFpEF demonstrate blunted exercise-induced increases in chronotropy, contractility, and vasodilation that result in impaired ventricular–arterial coupling responses during exercise compared to both patients with hypertension

DOI: 10.1201/9781003568933-17

only and age- and sex-matched controls.[8] It is important to recognize that increasing ventricular stiffness is, to some extent, a function of aging per se, perhaps related to an increase in cellular apoptosis over time.[9] Increases in both LV end-systolic and end-diastolic elastance has been observed with aging despite improvement in afterload and a reduction in LV mass.[10] A tendency toward diastolic dysfunction with aging has been demonstrated to be reversible with exercise in an animal model.[11]

However, patients presenting with heart failure and preserved ejection fraction manifest ventricular systolic and arterial stiffening in excess of that associated with aging or hypertension.[12] Similarly, patients presenting with clinical HFpEF have been shown to have significant reductions in longitudinal strain when compared to age- and sex-matched hypertensive patients with echocardiographic evidence of diastolic dysfunction and healthy controls, hence confirming subclinical impairment.[13] As a result, the clinician must be able to differentiate between what could be a result of normal sedentary aging and abnormal deterioration in ventricular compliance.

Compared to patients with HFrEF, patients with HFpEF have a significant increase in the noncardiac comorbidities of chronic obstructive pulmonary disease (COPD), diabetes mellitus (DM), anemia, and obesity, each of which is associated with an increased inflammatory profile.[14] This observation, in concert with tissue findings in HFpEF hearts of abnormal intramyocardial signaling from endothelial cell-derived adhesion molecules, inflammatory cells, and an increase in nitrotyrosine content, has suggested to some that at least part of the pathophysiology of HFpEF is mediated by enhanced inflammation mediated by these comorbidities.[15,16] Although as many as 60% of older persons presenting with clinically significant diastolic dysfunction die of cardiovascular causes, with sudden cardiac death and heart failure being the most common, the overall prevalence of these modes of death remains lower in patients with HFpEF than in those with HFrEF.[17]

Pharmacologic therapies that have been investigated for patients with heart failure and preserved LV systolic function include inhibition of the renin–angiotensin–aldosterone system (RAAS), beta-blockade, statins, and sodium-glucose cotransporter 2 (SGLT2) inhibitors.[18–21] Although the SOLVD database suggested that enalapril therapy might modestly improve diastolic function in patients with reduced ejection fraction, the use of RAAS inhibitors has been demonstrated to be ineffective at reducing either mortality or prespecified morbidity endpoints in patients aged 60 or older with preserved ejection fraction and clinical heart failure.[22,23] Candesartan has been shown to have a very modest benefit on the frequency of hospitalization in this patient population, but has no effect on cardiovascular mortality.[24] Spironolactone has been studied in a small cohort of 30 patients with isolated diastolic dysfunction over the age of 60 years and has been found to improve echocardiographic indices of diastolic function.[25] A subsequent larger trial with 422 patients also showed an improvement in echocardiographic indices; however, symptoms, exercise capacity, and quality of life were unchanged.[26] An analysis of 492 older persons with HFpEF in the Medicare database similarly demonstrated no difference in either subsequent hospitalization or mortality associated with the use of aldosterone antagonists when compared to a matched cohort.[27] Recently, however, finerenone, a nonsteroidal mineralocorticoid receptor antagonist (MRA), was shown to be effective in reducing the primary outcome of heart failure events and cardiovascular death in patients with EF >40%. Subgroup analysis suggested though that the greatest benefit was in those aged ≤73 years.[28]

Beta-blockade with either nebivolol or carvedilol has similarly been demonstrated to have no effect on either frequency of hospitalization or mortality.[29,30] Statin therapy has been associated with a reduction in mortality, adverse cardiovascular outcomes, and hospitalizations in veterans with HFpEF and no ASCVD.[19] However, there has not yet been any randomized trial testing statin therapy in HFpEF. The only pharmacological therapy given at least a 2a recommendation by the most recent AHA/ACC/HFSA guidelines is SGLT2 inhibitors.[31] In the EMPEROR PRESERVED trial, patients with an EF >40 were randomized to receive empagliflozin or placebo. Those in the empagliflozin arm had a 21% reduction in the primary outcome of heart failure hospitalization or cardiovascular death, though the outcome was mainly driven by hospitalizations. In subgroup analysis, there appeared to be an even greater benefit in the primary outcome in those over 70 years old.[21]

Of the nonpharmacologic therapies that have been investigated, exercise training appears to consistently result in improved peak VO_2, 6-minute walk distance, anaerobic threshold, and quality-of-life scores; however, these results appear to primarily reflect skeletal muscle adaptation rather than any primary cardiac effect.[32,33] Finally, an intriguing option could be the use of cardiac resynchronization therapy (CRT) in patients with HFpEF, however, data supporting this remain sparse.[34,35]

RESTRICTIVE CARDIOMYOPATHY

Restrictive cardiomyopathy results from increased stiffness of the LV myocardium, generally as a result of infiltrative disease.[36] As the infiltrative disorder is often biventricular, right-sided signs often predominate. Disturbances in conduction as well as dysrhythmia can also be common.[37] Clinical findings are often similar to pericardial constriction, and care is required in order to establish the correct diagnosis.[38]

Etiology

In contrast to younger patients, idiopathic restrictive myopathy is not only rare in older adults but also carries a better prognosis.[39] Amyloidosis constitutes the most common etiology in older adults, followed by other infiltrative processes such as cardiac sarcoid, carcinoid, hemochromatosis, and systemic sclerosis.[9,40] The broader use of both chest radiotherapy and anthracyclines in older patients with cancer leaves these patients at risk of developing restrictive cardiomyopathy secondary to endomyocardial fibrosis.[41]

Amyloid infiltration of the atria is extremely common in older adults and has been documented in 91% of subjects of advanced age in a histological study.[42] Clinically significant cardiac amyloidosis, however, has previously been considered to be markedly less common. The incidence of cardiac amyloidosis was formerly estimated to be between 6.1 and 10.5 per million person-years with the median age of presentation to medical attention being roughly 74 years.[43] However, autopsy studies of patients presenting with HFpEF have revealed TTR amyloid deposits in 21% and that the prevalence was significantly greater in those 75 years old or older.[44]

Cardiac amyloid is currently classified as one of two types depending on its etiology. AL or light-chain amyloid is a result of overproduction of plasma cell clonal antibody with its associated misfolded protein light chains. Transthyretin (ATTR) amyloid results from misfolded transthyretin protein. It may be related to a mutation in the TTR protein, called "familial" or "variant" TTR (ATTRv) or appear in genetically normal patients, termed "wild-type" TTR (ATTRwt). Wild-type increases in frequency with age. Increased ventricular stiffness in AL amyloidosis may result directly from the presence of monoclonal immunoglobulins rather than requiring the presence of the amyloid deposit itself. Diastolic dysfunction similar to that observed in patients with cardiac involvement can be replicated in mice simply by the systemic infusion of light chains isolated from patients with AL cardiac amyloidosis.[45]

Morphologically, the ventricular cavities are generally normal or small in size; however, mild dilatation can be noted (Figure 17.1). The atria are characteristically dilated and in some cases may present with thrombi in their cavities or appendages.[41] Only 25% of patients with primary amyloidosis present with congestive heart failure, while about one sixth present with orthostatic hypotension.[40] Without treatment, median survival from diagnosis is 57 months for ATTRwt and 31 months for ATTRv. Prognosis is even worse with impaired renal function and/or elevated BNP levels.[46] Dysrhythmia associated with amyloidosis ranges from node dysfunction and bundle branch blocks to ventricular dysrhythmia; however, the most common rhythm abnormality is atrial fibrillation, noted in 40%–60% of patients at the time of diagnosis. Often, there is a controlled ventricular response despite the lack of AV nodal blockers due to underlying conduction disease.[47] Anticoagulation is recommended in these patients regardless of CHA_2DS_2-VASc score.[48]

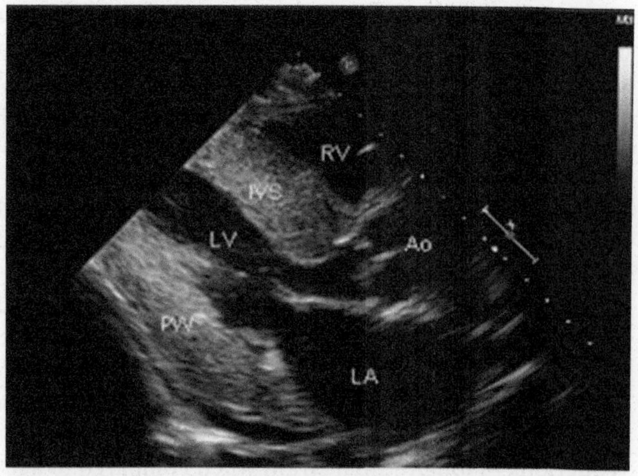

Figure 17.1 Two-dimensional echocardiogram from a parasternal long-axis view in a patient with cardiac amyloidosis shows a hypertrophic interventricular septum and posterior wall with the characteristic "speckling" appearance of myocardium. *Abbreviations*: RV, right ventricle; IVS, interventricular septum; AO, aorta; LA, left atrium; LV, left ventricle; PW, posterior wall.

Cardiac sarcoidosis is associated with interstitial inflammation resulting in abnormal diastolic function.[49] Incidence and prevalence of cardiac involvement remain largely unknown, with only a minority of patients presenting in their older ages. Cardiac involvement can apparently be frequently subclinical with studies demonstrating between five and eight times as many patients presenting with cardiac infiltration at necropsy as had been previously diagnosed clinically.[50] As many as half the patients presenting with sarcoidosis can have electrocardiographic abnormalities. Sudden death is the most common cause of mortality in patients presenting with cardiac sarcoid as a result of either complete heart block or malignant tachyarrhythmia.[51]

The mean age of patients presenting with carcinoid syndrome has been reported to be 64 years with a range extending up to 83 years.[52] Up to half of the cases present with carcinoid heart disease as a late complication.[53] The majority of cases present with tricuspid regurgitation with additional fibrotic involvement of the pulmonic valve and the right ventricular endocardium.

Presentation and diagnosis

Restrictive myopathies often present with generalized findings of fatigue, peripheral edema, paroxysmal nocturnal dyspnea, orthopnea, dyspnea, and occasionally ascites. Chest pain can occur in patients presenting with amyloidosis.[54] Similar clinical presentations require that this diagnosis be differentiated from pericardial constriction. This task is accomplished largely by a combination of clinical history with echocardiographic and Doppler findings, cardiac magnetic resonance imaging, and hemodynamic observations in the cardiac catheterization lab or on echocardiography. Similar to pericardial constriction, restrictive myopathy often presents with a prominent y descent in the jugular venous pulse, a positive Kussmaul's sign, an enlarged and pulsatile liver, ascites, and pedal edema. The presence of a third heart sound can serve to help differentiate restriction from constriction, which classically presents with a pericardial knock. The presence of pulmonary alveolar congestion on chest radiography favors restriction over constriction. Patients with cardiac amyloidosis may also have other associated features, including carpal tunnel syndrome, lumbar spinal stenosis, or aortic stenosis. In fact, many older patients undergoing transcatheter aortic valve replacement have subsequent positive cardiac scintigraphy scans for cardiac ATTR amyloidosis.[55]

The classic echocardiographic presentation of amyloid heart disease includes LVH with characteristic speckling of the myocardium.[56] Mitral inflow velocities in patients with diastolic dysfunction vary depending on the extent of the disease. E/A ratios in older persons customarily become less than one in most normal individuals. The first sign of diastolic dysfunction is often pseudonormalization of the Doppler spectral display in which the E/A ratio once again becomes greater than one associated with increasing prominence of the diastolic filling velocity in the pulmonary vein.[57] Active restrictive physiology results in a very steep, high-velocity mitral E wave with a short deceleration time, followed by a very small or absent A wave (Figure 17.2).[29] B-natriuretic peptide assay has been used to enhance the diagnosis of diastolic dysfunction in patients who present with normal systolic function on echocardiography.[58]

Thickening of the pericardium, which is common in pericardial constriction, is absent in patients with restrictive cardiomyopathy on cardiac magnetic resonance imaging. Nuclear isotope scanning has become an incredibly sensitive and specific method with which to diagnose ATTR amyloid, while urine and serum protein studies can be used for the diagnosis of AL amyloid.[59] At cardiac catheterization, the end-diastolic pressures can be equalized in both restrictive and constrictive physiology; however, it is rare for the pre-A pressure to fall toward zero in patients with restriction. Ventricular concordance is seen in restrictive cardiomyopathy, whereas discordance is seen in constrictive pericarditis and differentiates the two disease states. In some patients, endomyocardial biopsy may be necessary for diagnosis.[60]

Treatment

Drug therapy has been primarily aimed at the presumed cause of the disorder.[8] For those patients presenting with AL cardiac amyloid, advances in the chemotherapy of plasma cell dyscrasias have improved the cardiac prognosis significantly.[61] In the past, therapy for TTR amyloid was primarily focused on symptom management. Because patients with restrictive cardiomyopathy have a narrow euvolemic window, careful monitoring of volume status is necessary. Loop diuretics and MRAs are commonly used. Standard pharmacological therapy including beta-blockers and RAAS inhibition for heart failure is not routinely recommended. These patients are often dependent on heart rate to increase their stroke volume and are unable to augment their cardiac output in response to vasodilatation.[47]

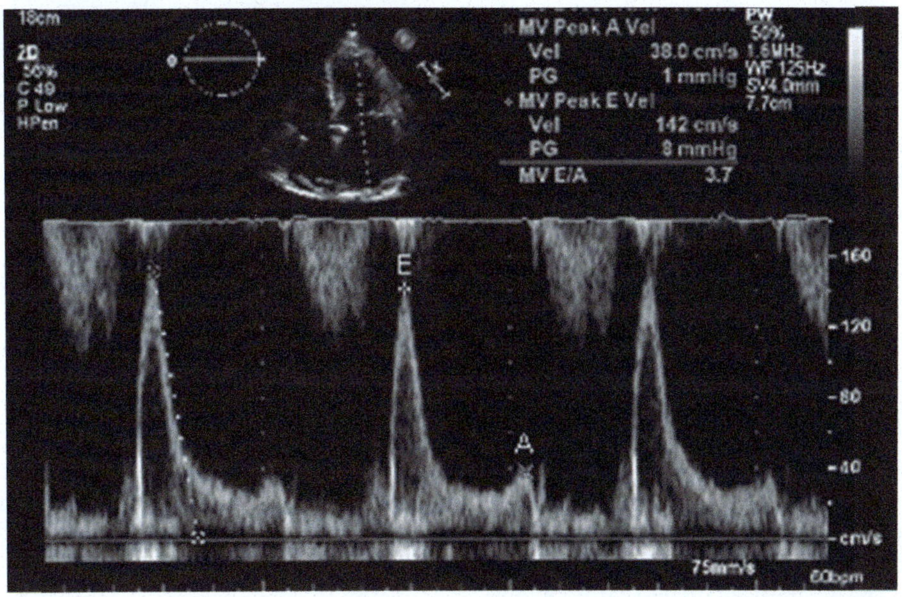

Figure 17.2 LV mitral inflow diastolic waveforms obtained with pulsed Doppler echocardiography in an older patient with cardiac amyloidosis show a substantial increase in the flow velocity of the early peak (E) and decreased maximal velocity of the late peak (A) that is characteristic of a marked increase in atrial pressure.

Although there is limited evidence, many experts suggest the use of antiarrhythmics in patients with atrial arrythmias to maintain sinus rhythm.[62] Permanent pacing is also commonly needed due to infiltration of the conduction system.[47] No studies have yet to show convincing benefit of ICD insertion in this population for prevention of ventricular arrythmias.[62,63]

In recent years, however, the treatment of ATTR amyloidosis has made tremendous strides. In the ATTR-ACT trial, treatment with tafamidis, a transthyretin tetramer stabilizer, in older patients with TTR amyloidosis led to improvement in survival, less frequent cardiovascular hospitalizations, a slower decline in functional status, and improvement in heart failure symptoms.[64] The number needed to treat with tafamidis to prevent one death at 30 months was eight, and four to prevent a cardiovascular hospitalization. Diflunisal, an NSAID with a similar chemical structure to tafamidis, may also prolong survival, but its evidence is from small, nonrandomized studies.[48,65] Additionally, as an NSAID, caution should be used in patients with impaired renal function, history of gastrointestinal bleeding, or recent heart failure hospitalizations. Vutrisiran, a subcutaneously administered RNA interference therapeutic agent that inhibits hepatic synthesis of both wild-type and variant *TTR* messenger RNA, has also been shown to be efficacious in the treatment of amyloidosis. In the HELIOS-B trial, there was a lower risk of death or cardiovascular events in the group randomized to receive vutrisiran compared to placebo. This effect was seen even while taking tafamidis.[66] The benefit of these medications seems to be highest when started earlier in the pathological process as indicated by less benefit when stratified by subgroups who are older or who are at a more advanced staged of heart failure.

Further studies with other pharmacological TTR stabilizers and TTR silencers, as well as with gene editing are ongoing.[48]

DILATED CARDIOMYOPATHY

Idiopathic dilated cardiomyopathy is primarily a disease of ventricular muscle, characterized by increased LV or biventricular volumes, without an appropriate increase in ventricular septal or free wall thickness, and with depression of LV systolic function.[67] Other etiological factors that can cause diffuse LV systolic dysfunction must be excluded. In a large cohort of 554 unselected men and 1243 women older than 60 years of age in a long-term health care facility, the prevalence of idiopathic dilated cardiomyopathy was 1% for both sexes.[68] In the same cohort, the prevalence of abnormal LV ejection fraction (<50%) was 29% in men and 21% in women. Approximately 10% of patients with dilated cardiomyopathy are older than 65 years of age.[69,70] The diagnosis of dilated cardiomyopathy can be confirmed by echocardiography (Figures 17.3 and 17.4). Coronary angiography should be considered in patients with dilated cardiomyopathy and chest pain

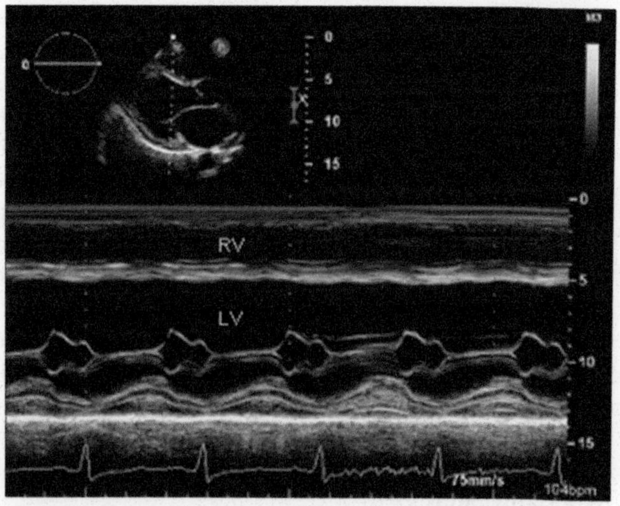

Figure 17.3 M-mode echocardiogram at the mitral valve level in an older patient with dilated cardiomyopathy shows thinning of the interventricular septum, a markedly dilated left ventricle cavity, and increased E point septal separation. *Abbreviations*: LV, left ventricle; RV, right ventricle.

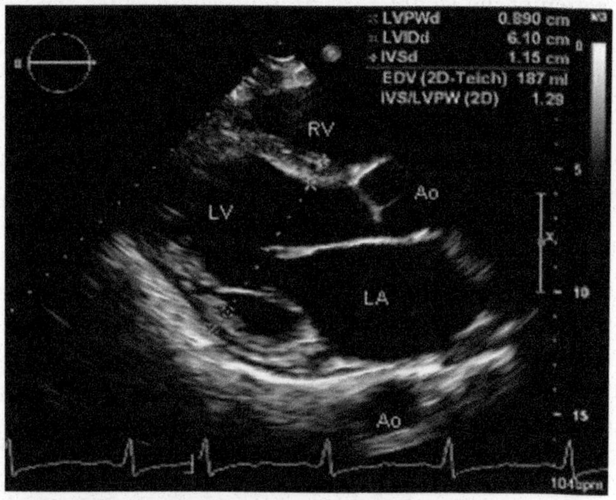

Figure 17.4 Diastolic frame of a two-dimensional echocardiogram from a parasternal long-axis view in an older patient with dilated cardiomyopathy shows thinning of the interventricular septum and a large left ventricular cavity with secondary enlargement of the left atrium and right ventricle. *Abbreviations*: AO, aorta; IVS, interventricular septum; LA, left atrium; LV, left ventricle; PW, posterior wall; RV, right ventricle.

to rule out ischemic cardiomyopathy or a mixed picture. Transthoracic coronary echocardiography has been proposed as a potentially useful method for distinguishing between ischemic and nonischemic dilated cardiomyopathy in some patients.[71] Magnetic resonance imaging is also helpful in the diagnosis of sarcoidosis, muscular dystrophy, myocarditis, and subclinical myocardial infarction, while MRI detected myocardial fibrosis has been shown to be an independent predictor of the risk for sudden cardiac death.[72]

Symptoms

Symptoms due to dilated cardiomyopathy include fatigue and weakness resulting from decreased cardiac output, exercise intolerance, dyspnea due to pulmonary congestion, chest pain, and syncope. Symptoms due to systemic or pulmonary emboli may also occur. Physical examination reveals moderate to severe cardiomegaly and audible third and fourth heart sounds. Signs of LV or biventricular failure may be present.

Fuster et al. reported 104 patients at the Mayo Clinic with idiopathic dilated cardiomyopathy followed for 6–20 years.[69] Of these 104 patients, 73% had congestive heart failure at the time of diagnosis, and 96% had congestive heart failure at follow-up. Systemic emboli were present in 4% of the patients at the time of diagnosis and in 18% of the patients at follow-up. Systemic thromboembolism developed in 8 of 24 patients (33%) with atrial fibrillation and in 11 of 80 patients (14%) with sinus rhythm (p = NS). Systemic thromboembolism developed in 18% of patients who did not receive anticoagulant therapy and in none of those who did ($p = 0.05$). Of 104 patients, 80 (77%) had died at follow-up, two thirds of the deaths having occurred within 2 years.

Roberts et al. reported that 148 of 152 necropsy patients (97%) with idiopathic dilated cardiomyopathy had clinical evidence of chronic congestive heart failure.[70] Sudden death was the initial manifestation in 114 of 152 patients (75%), and in most patients, ventricular dysrhythmia became intractable and caused death. The mean duration from the onset of chronic congestive heart failure to known death in 120 patients was 54 months. The cause of death was chronic congestive heart failure in 58% of patients, sudden death in 27% of patients, pulmonary emboli in 9% of patients, and other in 6% of patients. Clinical evidence of pulmonary emboli was present in 39% of patients. Clinical evidence of systemic emboli was present in 20% of patients. Of 131 patients, 79 (60%) had either clinical or necropsy evidence, or both, of pulmonary or systemic emboli.

Falk et al., studying 25 patients with nonischemic dilated cardiomyopathy who were not receiving anticoagulant therapy, demonstrated that a LV thrombus was present on initial echocardiogram in 11 patients (44%), developed during 21.5 months of follow-up in an additional 4 patients (16%), and disappeared in 2 patients (8%) during follow-up.[73] Systemic thromboembolism developed in 5 of 25 patients (20%) during follow-up. Of the five thromboembolic events, four occurred in patients with echocardiographic evidence of a LV thrombus.

Therapy

The past few decades have witnessed a significant improvement in the prognosis for older adults presenting with dilated cardiomyopathy, much of it driven by the increased use of beta-blockers, RAAS inhibitors or angiotensin receptor-neprilysin inhibitors (ARNIs), MRAs, and SGLT2 inhibitors.[74,75] Congestive heart failure in these patients should be treated with salt restriction, diuretics, and guideline-directed medical therapy.

Digoxin has been demonstrated to reduce the number of hospital admissions due to heart failure; however, its effect on total mortality appears to be neutral, and high levels may paradoxically increase mortality. In this regard care must be taken in older patients who have a higher prevalence of renal insufficiency that affects digoxin clearance.[76] An analysis of the effect of increasing age on patients in the Digitalis Investigation Group database, however, specifically found that advanced age per se was not associated with an increased risk for digoxin intoxication.[77] The withdrawal of digoxin therapy has been demonstrated to result in an increase in both heart failure hospitalization and in mortality even in patients concurrently maintained on therapy with ACE inhibition and diuretics.[78]

Beta-blockade has now been shown unequivocally to be associated with improvement in symptoms, quality of life, exercise capacity, ejection fraction, and survival.[79–82] Multivariate analysis has demonstrated that shorter duration of congestive symptoms and the use of beta-blockers are independently associated with reverse remodeling in patients older than 70 years of age with nonischemic cardiomyopathy.[83] This observation has been attributed to an increase in α_1-adrenergic receptor density, prolongation of the action potential with secondary increase in calcium influx, and induction of changes in gene expression.[84] Beta-blockade also enhances calcium release channel function in patients with heart failure.[85] In addition, beta-blockers have been demonstrated to improve contractile dyssynchrony in patients with heart failure who have narrow QRS complexes.[86]

Beneficial effects have also been observed in patients with heart failure treated with spironolactone and ACE inhibition, including ARNIs.[82,87] RAAS inhibition with ACE inhibitors, ARBs, or ARNIs have also been proven to be effective in improving mortality and morbidity in this population. In PARADIGM-HF, those treated with the ARNI sacubitril-valsartan had a 20% reduction in the primary outcomes of cardiovascular death and heart failure hospitalizations.[88] In retrospective cohorts, a beneficial effect was also seen in older adults.[89] However, in the subgroup analysis of the trial itself, the benefit wasn't seen in those older than 75. Most recently, SGLT2 inhibitors have been shown to decrease cardiovascular mortality and heart failure hospitalizations across all age subgroups.[90]

As noted earlier, there is evidence, both clinical and necropsy, for intracavitary thrombi and both pulmonary and systemic emboli in patients with dilated cardiomyopathy. However, in patients presenting with sinus rhythm and LV dysfunction, the use of warfarin therapy, although associated with a reduced incidence of thromboembolic strokes, is associated with an unacceptable risk of major bleeding events including intracranial hemorrhage.[91]

There is no evidence that antiarrhythmic drugs prolong life or prevent sudden cardiac death in patients with dilated cardiomyopathy; however, there is clearly increased survival associated with automatic implantable cardioverter-defibrillator (ICD) therapy in patients with dilated cardiomyopathy and a low ejection fraction.[92] Cardiac resynchronization therapy with biventricular pacing has been shown to be of value in reducing symptoms, improving exercise capacity, reducing complications, and reducing mortality in patients with advanced heart failure, a wide QRS complex, and evidence of contraction dyssynchrony.[93] Although prior small studies had suggested that biventricular pacing had the potential to improve symptoms and reverse remodeling in patients with heart failure, evidence of LV dyssynchrony on echocardiography, and narrow QRS complexes,[94] more recent randomized controlled data reveals no benefit in patients with a QRS duration of less than 130 msec as well as a possible increase in mortality in men.[95,96] Resynchronization therapy in concert with a cardioverter-defibrillator has been suggested as a means to decrease the risk of clinical heart failure in patients presenting with a low ejection fraction, a wide QRS complex, and no significant preexisting symptoms of heart failure.[97] Finally, the benefits of resynchronization appear to be identical across all age groups, making it an appropriate therapy for older adults with dilated cardiomyopathy.[98]

After multiple prior trials and meta-analyses of nesiritide for the treatment of decompensated heart failure suggested a possible increase in mortality with its use[99,100] as well as a decrease in renal function,[101] the ASCEND-HF trial demonstrated categorically that there was no associated change in mortality or rehospitalization, a nonsignificant effect on dyspnea, no change in renal function, but an increase in associated hypotension.[102] As such, there is little current use for this agent in addition to other proven therapies.

Finally, it has been observed that decreased mobility, disability, and dementia are independently associated with an increase in short- and long-term mortality in older persons with decreased ejection fractions that are admitted with heart failure.[103,104] Given that these conditions are generally not reversible, it is incumbent on the clinician and the health care system to employ a multidisciplinary disease-management program in order to maximize the support given to this ever-increasing patient population.[105]

HYPERTROPHIC CARDIOMYOPATHY (HCM)

HCM, with or without outflow tract obstruction, has an autosomal dominant inheritance pattern with many different mutations implicated in the pathogenesis, some of which appear to be specific to phenotypic expression at an older age.[106] Although disease severity can vary depending on the type of mutation, phenotypic expression varies to such a degree as to render the type of mutation a poor indicator of prognosis on a case-by-case basis.[107,108] The histological pattern of obstructive HCM has been demonstrated to be distinctly different from the hypertrophy associated with hypertension, with substantially more myocardial fiber disarray, hypertrophy, intramyocardial scar, and intramural small vessel coronary hyperplasia.[109,110]

Older patients diagnosed with HCM present with an increased severity of symptoms compared to younger individuals, partly explained by deconditioning and comorbidities; however, the progression of the disease appears to be slower with as many as 23% of older adult patients achieving a normal life expectancy.[111–113] The annual mortality for older adults with HCM has been reported to be only 3% and does not appear to be demonstrably different from that of age- and sex-matched controls.[114,115] Advanced NYHA functional class, increased left atrial size, and increased septal wall thickness are associated with increased incidence of HCM-related death.[114] A significant increase in baseline LV mass measured by either echocardiography or electrocardiography has been associated with a decrease in ejection fraction over time in a cohort of older adult patients.[116] More recent data of cardiac magnetic resonance has also linked a high scar burden, as demonstrated by late gadolinium enhancement, to the risk of sudden cardiac arrest as well as to the progression to an end-stage or "burnt out" phase of the disease, categorized by wall thinning, LV dilation, and systolic dysfunction.[117,118]

The predominant symptom noted by multiple authors is dyspnea, with between one third and one half of older patients presenting with chest pain.[111,112] Dyspnea in these patients is a result of diastolic heart failure and obstructive physiology, reducing cardiac output, with secondary effects of pulmonary hypertension and congestion, especially in older persons who have lived with their disease for decades. Chest pain in most HCM patients is due to microvascular ischemia from supply-demand mismatch and intramural coronary hyperplasia, with poor coronary flow reserve, but in older persons may also be due to epicardial atherosclerotic coronary disease, the presence of which further elevates mortality in HCM patients.[119,120] Between 20% and 30% of patients complain of syncope or presyncope, most commonly due to severe, dynamic LV outflow tract obstruction, while some authors report palpitations in as many as half of patients.[112–114] Presentation in NYHA class III or IV heart failure has been noted to increase the annual mortality rate to 36%.[114] It is important to note that in older patients, mitral annular calcification (MAC) may be a contributor to late development of outflow tract obstruction, as it potentiates a narrow outflow tract that promotes SAM. This is one of the reasons why previously quiescent or undiagnosed HCM may become clinically significant at advanced age.

Classic physical findings of HCM with obstruction include the presence of carotid pulsus bisferiens, a fourth heart sound, and a systolic ejection murmur at the left sternal margin that becomes more prominent with the Valsalva maneuver and less audible with isometric exercise.[121,122] The bisferiens pulse may be less noticeable in older patients as a result of increased atherosclerosis in the peripheral vasculature.[112,123] In addition to the classic heart sounds, older patients may have signs of pulmonary congestion, volume overload with peripheral edema, pulmonary hypertension, or the irregular pulse of atrial fibrillation, due to the chronicity of their disease and accumulated sequelae of long-standing cardiac dysfunction.

Both atrial fibrillation and hypertension have been reported to be more commonly associated with the diagnosis in older persons and are also associated with decreased survival.[115,124] Electrocardiographic presentation in the older adult includes the presence of atrial abnormality, LVH, and bundle branch block; however, the anterior Q waves that are typical of HCM in the young are only rarely seen.[115,125]

Echocardiographic findings in the older patient with HCM, like younger patients, include LVH, systolic anterior motion (SAM) of the anterior leaflet of the mitral valve, and increased LV outflow tract velocity (Figures 17.5–17.7).[123] LV cavity shape in older persons appears to be more oval than that of younger patients with HCM.[112]

In addition, and as previously mentioned, mitral annular calcification is much more common in older patients presenting with HCM, with prevalence rates reported to be anywhere between 30% and 100%.[126,127] As a result, the mechanism for outflow tract obstruction may depend more on the posterior displacement of the septum and less on the anterior displacement of the mitral apparatus than it does in younger patients.

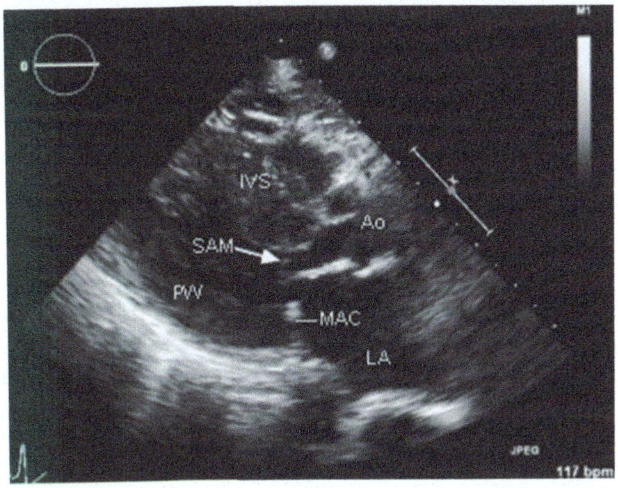

Figure 17.5 Early systolic frame from a two-dimensional parasternal long-axis view in a 75-year-old female with HCM showing a prominent septal bulge and systolic anterior motion of the mitral valve. *Abbreviations*: IVS, interventricular septum; Ao, aortic root; LA, left atrium; PW, posterior wall; MAC, mitral annular calcification; SAM, systolic anterior motion of the mitral valve leaflets.

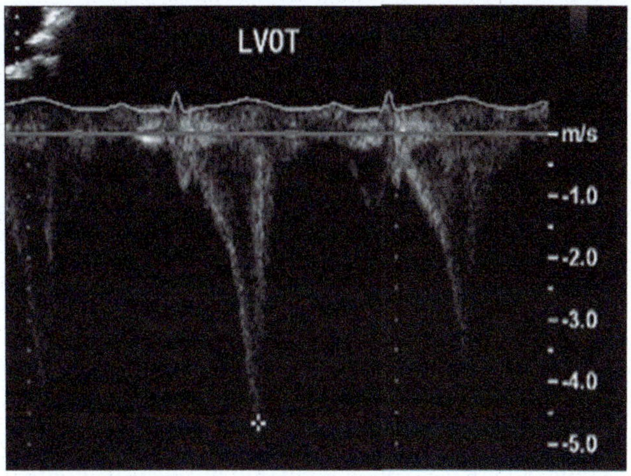

Figure 17.6 High PRF Doppler obtained from interrogation of the left ventricular outflow tract flow in the same patient shown in Figure 17.5, demonstrating a large increase of the outflow velocity (maximum = 5 m/sec) and a Bernoulli-derived gradient of 87 mmHg. The waveform demonstrates the dagger shape that is characteristic of obstructive hypertrophic cardiomyopathy with a late systolic peak. *Abbreviation*: LVOT, left ventricular outflow tract.

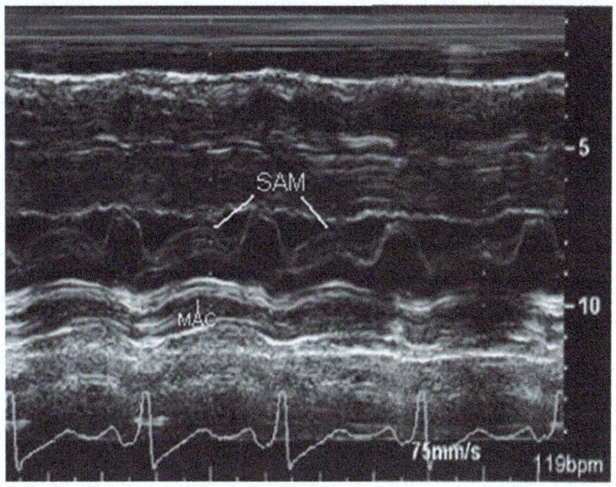

Figure 17.7 M-mode echocardiogram at the mitral valve level in the same patient illustrated in Figure 17.5. During mid-systole, a smooth anterior motion at the mitral valve is noted. The mitral valve assumes a flattened curve appearance as it approaches the septum, and the contact with the septum is facilitated by the posterior motion of the septum. Mitral annular calcification is present behind the posterior leaflet. *Abbreviations*: MAC, mitral annular calcification; SAM, systolic anterior motion of the mitral valve leaflets.

β-adrenergic blocking agents and nondihydropyridine calcium channel blockers, particularly verapamil, have been shown to reduce symptoms in patients with obstructive HCM; however, no clear effect on mortality has been documented.[121,128] As in patients with coronary disease, hypersensitivity to beta-adrenergic stimulation accompanied by precipitous clinical deterioration may occur in patients who are abruptly withdrawn from beta-blockers.[129] Patients who do not respond to beta-blockade can have a salutary response to relatively large doses of verapamil, although care must be taken to avoid paradoxical worsening of obstruction due to marked afterload-reducing effects at high doses in some patients.[130] Disopyramide has also been demonstrated to decrease symptoms in as many as 66% of patients, with a reduction in subaortic gradient of approximately 50% over 3 years, however, its vagolytic effects may lead to discontinuation in some patients.[131] It should not be given to those with prostate hypertrophy or open angle glaucoma. All these agents are relatively contraindicated in patients with conduction system disease in the absence of cardiac pacing, and disopyramide must be given concomitantly with other AV nodal blocking agents to prevent rapid conduction of atrial fibrillation.

Myosin inhibition has become a novel and effective option for persistent symptoms despite initial therapy. In EXPLORER-HCM, the addition of a myosin inhibitor, Mavacamten, increased peak VO_2 and improved NYHA functional class, and decreased LVOT gradients in comparison to placebo.[132] Adults older than 65 years of age comprised 33% of the studied cohort and subgroup analysis showed even more impressive results in that population. Similar results were seen in the subsequent SEQUOIA-HCM trial for Aficamten.[133] Myosin inhibitors are now given a class 1 recommendation in patients whose symptoms are not controlled with initial pharmacotherapy.[134] Positive inotropic agents such as digoxin are relatively contraindicated because of their ability to increase the gradient across the LV outflow tract. Additionally, afterload-reducing medications will potentiate obstruction in HCM patients, and therefore hydralazine, nitrates, ARBs, ACE inhibitors and alpha-one antagonists are all contraindicated, especially in older patients who may be more prone to balance issues and syncope.[134] However, as previously mentioned, patients with hypervolemia may require diuretic therapy.

Dysrhythmia requires special attention in this patient population. Atrial fibrillation is associated with worsening heart failure, stroke, and a diminished long-term prognosis and requires anticoagulation regardless of CHA_2DS_2-VASc score.[135] Older age is independently related to increased stroke and vascular events from atrial fibrillation in patients with HCM.[136] Additionally, stroke appears to be the most common mode of death in HCM patients >75 years of age.[137] It is therefore recommended to screen all patients with HCM at higher risk of developing AF, including the older adult population, with extended ambulatory monitoring as initiation of anticoagulation has been associated with a reduction in ischemic strokes in older adults with HCM and atrial fibrillation.[134,136]

Ventricular dysrhythmia poses a more vexing problem. One trial has demonstrated that ventricular tachycardia or fibrillation appears to be the primary mechanism for sudden death in patients carrying a diagnosis of HCM.[138] In these cases, ICDs were found to be efficacious in the treatment of these rhythms and the prevention of sudden death.[138] Mean age in this patient population, however, was 40 ± 16 years with more than half the sample size younger than 41 years. A subsequent trial demonstrated that LV wall thickness is directly and linearly related to the risk of sudden death and may, therefore, be an indicator of the need for automatic ICD placement.[139] Once again, however, the mean age was only 47 years with the mean age being youngest (31 years) for the patients with the thickest walls. As a result, it currently remains unclear how much relevance these data have for the older patient with obstructive myopathy, who more commonly has more meager basal septal focal hypertrophy and perhaps different underlying mutations. Consistent with this, data suggests that sudden death risk declines with age, with only a small minority of patients dying from sudden death in the older adult population.[140] Achieving older age in this disease may itself be declarative of a more favorable prognosis and therefore, the decision to place an ICD must be individualized.[134,140,141] Nonetheless, the appearance of complex ventricular dysrhythmia, especially when symptomatic, in older patients with HCM does, in fact, suggest a negative prognosis in comparison to patients in whom they do not appear, and these patients should be considered for ICD placement.

Dual-chamber pacing for patients with obstructive HCM who have not responded to medical therapy has been associated with variable results.[134,142] However, there is some evidence that RV pacing may be beneficial in improving functional capacity for those who are older than 65 years.[143] As such, pacing may be of some benefit to older adults with obstructive HCM who do not respond well to medical therapy, who have a pacemaker or ICD already in place for alternate indication, or who refuse or are not optimal candidates for septal myectomy or alcohol septal ablation.

In patients who continue to demonstrate class III or IV symptoms, or recurrent obstruction-related syncope/presyncope, despite first-line medical therapy, surgery or transcatheter alcohol septal ablation can be considered. The 2024 AHA/ACC/AMSSM/HRS/PACES/SCMR HCM guidelines support septal reduction therapy (SRT) with either surgical septal myectomy or percutaneous alcohol septal ablation in experienced HCM centers as a class 1 recommendation in those who have failed first line therapy.[134] Studies have described symptomatic improvement in as many as 80%–90% of patients older than 65 years undergoing surgical myectomy, with outcomes similar for alcohol septal ablation.[112,144] Operative mortality, however, has been observed to more than triple in patients older than 65 years when myectomy is combined with coronary artery bypass surgery.[145] The concurrent presence of severe mitral annular calcification may require mitral valve surgery as well.[126] Data from a six-patient subset of patients with obstructive HCM and mitral annular calcification undergoing myectomy (mean age 61 years) suggest that the myectomy alone may significantly reduce the amount of mitral regurgitation such that mitral surgery may be unnecessary.[146] Indeed, as mitral regurgitation is part of the pathophysiology of SAM and septal contact, most mitral regurgitation is improved after myectomy or alcohol septal ablation and does not require direct intervention. When there is concern about intrinsic mitral valve pathology that might not improve after relief of obstruction, a transesophageal echocardiogram may aid in determining whether mitral valve replacement should be considered at the time of myectomy.[134]

Alcohol septal ablation, due to lower morbidity, may be preferable in older patients, especially as their anatomy more commonly entails hypertrophy that is focal and not massive, and is supported in the guidelines for older patients.[134] Many older patients already have a pacemaker or ICD, making the procedure safer as well. Therefore, this procedure may be an ideal alternative to surgical intervention in older patients with comorbidities that elevate surgical risk, but also in younger patients with favorable anatomy who wish to avoid surgery with no other indication for surgery.[134] With the favorable outcomes of the VALOR-HCM trial showing a 59% absolute risk reduction in need for SRT at 12 weeks and persistent deferral of SRT at 1 year in follow up, the amount of older adults referred for SRT may decline.[147,148]

Hypertrophic obstructive cardiomyopathy and calcific aortic stenosis

As they age, HCM patients may develop calcific aortic stenosis. Indeed, the combination of both valvular and outflow tract stenosis is increasingly recognized. The diagnosis of both pathologic processes can be difficult on echocardiography, as the lesions occur in series. Meticulous invasive hemodynamic assessment may be necessary to determine the relative significance and contributions of both obstructive lesions. Surgical candidates should proceed with surgical aortic valve replacement with concomitant septal myectomy, while poor surgical or nonsurgical candidates might benefit from sequential alcohol septal ablation followed by transcutaneous aortic valve replacement (TAVR). This sequence, separated by about 3 months, is necessary to truly improve the outflow tract and thereby avoid severe obstructive physiology after TAVR, with profound hypotension, due to the acute relief of the increased afterload of the stenotic valve.[149]

REFERENCES

1. Curtis LH, Whellan DJ, Hammill BG et al. Incidence and prevalence of heart failure in elderly persons, 1994–2003. *Arch Intern Med.* 2008; 168(4): 418–424.
2. Chen J, Dharmarajan K, Wang Y et al. National trends in heart failure hospital stay rates, 2001 to 2009. *J Am Coll Cardiol* 2013 Mar 12; 61(10): 1078–1088.
3. Braunwald E. The war against heart failure: The Lancet lecture. *Lancet.* 2015; 385(9970): 812–824.
4. Gottdiener JS, McClelland RL, Marshall R et al. Outcome of congestive heart failure in elderly persons: Influence of left ventricular systolic function. *Ann Intern Med* 2002; 137: 631–639.
5. Vasan RS, Larson MG, Benjamin EJ et al. Defining diastolic heart failure: A call for standardized diagnostic criteria. *Circulation* 2000; 101: 2118.
6. Vasan RS, Xanthakis V, Lyass A et al. Epidemiology of left ventricular systolic dysfunction and heart failure in the Framingham study: An echocardiographic study over 3 decades. *JACC Cardiovasc Imaging* 2018; 11(1): 1–11.
7. Shah AM, Claggett B, Loehr LR et al. Heart failure stages among older adults in the community: The atherosclerosis risk in communities study. *Circulation* 2017; 135(3): 224–240.
8. Borlaug BA, Olson TP, Lam CSP et al. Global cardiovascular reserve dysfunction in heart failure with preserved ejection fraction. *J Am Coll Cardiol* 2010; 56: 845–854.
9. Backes RJ, Gersh BJ. Cardiomyopathies in the elderly. *Cardiovasc Clin* 1992; 22: 105–125.
10. Borlaug B, Redfield M, Melenovsky V et al. Longitudinal changes in left ventricular stiffness: A community-based study. *Circ Heart Fail* 2013; 6: 944–952.
11. Brenner DA, Apstein CS, Saupe KW. Exercise training attenuates age-associated diastolic dysfunction in rats. *Circulation* 2001; 104: 221–226.
12. Kawaguchi M, Hay I, Fetics B et al. Combined ventricular systolic and arterial stiffening in patients with heart failure and preserved ejection fraction: Implications for systolic and diastolic reserve limitations. *Circulation* 2003; 107: 714–720.
13. Kraigher-Krainer E, Shah AM, Gupta DK et al. Impaired systolic function by strain imaging in heart failure with preserved ejection fraction. *J Am Coll Cardiol* 2014; 63: 447–456.
14. Mentz RJ, Kelly JP, von Lueder TG et al. Noncardiac comorbidities in heart failure with reduced versus preserved ejection fraction. *J Am Coll Cardiol* 2014; 64: 2281–2293.
15. Westermann D, Lindner D, Kasner M et al. Cardiac inflammation contributes to changes in the extracellular matrix in patients with heart failure and normal ejection fraction. *Circ Heart Fail* 2011; 4: 44–52.
16. Paulus WJ, Carsten T. A novel paradigm for heart failure with preserved ejection fraction. *J Am Coll Cardiol* 2013; 62: 263–271.

17. Zile MR, Gaasch WH, Anand IS et al. Mode of death in patients with heart failure and a preserved ejection fraction: Results from the Irbesartan in heart failure with preserved ejection fraction study (I-Preserve) trial. *Circulation* 2010; 121: 1393–1405.
18. Kasama S, Toyama T, Kumakura H et al. Effects of candesartan on cardiac sympathetic nerve activity in patients with congestive heart failure and preserved left ventricular ejection fraction. *J Am Coll Cardiol* 2005; 45: 661–667.
19. Orkaby AR, Goyal P, Charest B et al. Initiation of statins for primary prevention in heart failure with preserved ejection fraction. *JACC Adv* 2024; 3(4): 100869. Published 2024 Feb 20.
20. Mottram PM, Haluska B, Leano R et al. Effect of aldosterone antagonism on myocardial dysfunction in hypertensive patients with diastolic heart failure. *Circulation* 2004; 110: 558–565.
21. Anker SD, Butler J, Filippatos G et al. Empagliflozin in heart failure with a preserved ejection fraction. *N Engl J Med* 2021; 385(16): 1451–1461.
22. Hayashida W, Van Eyll C, Rousseau MF et al. Regional remodeling and nonuniform changes in diastolic function in patients with left ventricular dysfunction: Modification by long-term enalapril treatment. *J Am Coll Cardiol* 1993; 22: 1403–1410.
23. Massie BM, Carson PE, McMurray JJ et al. Irbesartan in patients with heart failure and preserved ejection fraction. *N Engl J Med* 2008; 359: 2456–2467.
24. Yusuf S, Pfeffer MA, Swedberg K et al. CHARM investigators and committees. Effects of candesartan in patients with chronic heart failure and preserved left-ventricular ejection fraction: The CHARM-preserved trial. *Lancet* 2003; 362: 777–781.
25. Roongsritong C, Sutthiwan P, Bradley J et al. Spironolactone improves diastolic function in the elderly. *Clin Cardiol* 2005; 28: 484–487.
26. Edelmann F, Wachter R, Schmidt AG et al. Effect of spironolactone on diastolic function and exercise capacity in patients with heart failure with preserved ejection fraction: The Aldo-DHF randomized controlled trial. *JAMA* 2013; 309: 781–791.
27. Patel K, Fonarow GC, Kitzman DW et al. Aldosterone antagonists and outcomes in real-world older patients with heart failure and preserved ejection fraction. *JACC Heart Fail* 2013; 1: 40–47.
28. Solomon SD, McMurray JJV, Vaduganathan M et al. Finerenone in heart failure with mildly reduced or preserved ejection fraction. *N Engl J Med* 2024; 391(16): 1475–1485.
29. Conraads VM, Metra M, Kamp O et al. Effects of the long-term administration of nebivolol on the clinical symptoms, exercise capacity, and left ventricular function of patients with diastolic dysfunction: Results of the ELANDD study. *Eur J Heart Fail* 2012; 14: 219–225.
30. Yamamoto K, Origasa H, Hori M, J-DHF Investigators. Effects of carvedilol on heart failure with preserved ejection fraction: The Japanese diastolic heart failure study (J-DHF). *Eur J Heart Fail* 2013; 15: 110–118.
31. Writing Committee Members; ACC/AHA Joint Committee Members 2022 AHA/ACC/HFSA guideline for the management of heart failure. *J Card Fail* 2022; 28(5): e1–e167.
32. Pandey A, Parashar A, Kumbhani D et al. Exercise training in patients with heart failure and preserved ejection fraction: Meta-analysis of randomized control trials. *Circ Heart Fail* 2015; 8: 33–40.
33. Tucker WJ, Nelson MD, Beaudry R et al. Impact of exercise training on peak oxygen uptake and its determinants in heart failure with preserved ejection fraction. *Card Fail Rev* 2016; 2: 95–101.
34. Penicka M, Kocka V, Herman D et al. Cardiac resynchronization therapy for the causal treatment of heart failure with preserved ejection fraction: Insight from a pressure-volume loop analysis. *Eur J Heart Fail* 2010; 12: 634–636.
35. Wang YC, Yu CC, Chiu FC et al. Acute effects of biventricular pacing in heart failure patients with a normal ejection fraction and mechanical dyssynchrony. *Cardiology* 2015; 130: 112–119.
36. Zieman SJ, Fortuin NJ. Hypertrophic and restrictive cardiomyopathies in the elderly. *Cardiol Clin* 1999; 17: 159–172.
37. Child JS, Perloff JK. The restrictive cardiomyopathies. *Cardiol Clin* 1988; 6: 289–316.
38. Schoenfeld MH. The differentiation of restrictive cardiomyopathy from constrictive pericarditis. *Cardiol Clin* 1990; 8: 663–671.
39. Tresch DD, McGough MF. Heart failure with normal systolic function: A common disorder in older people. *J Am Geriatr Soc* 1995; 43: 1035–1042.
40. Falk RH, Comenzo RL, Skinner M. The systemic amyloidoses. *N Engl J Med* 1997; 337: 898–909.
41. Kushwaha SS, Fallen JT, Fuster V. Restrictive cardiomyopathy. *N Engl J Med* 1997; 336: 267–276.
42. Kawamura S, Takahashi M, Ishihara T et al. Incidence and distribution of isolated atrial amyloid: Histologic and immunohistochemical studies of 100 aging hearts. *Pathol Int* 1995; 45: 335–342.
43. Kyle RA, Linos A, Beard CM et al. Incidence and natural history of primary systemic amyloidosis in Olmsted County Minnesota 1950 through 1989. *Blood* 1992; 79: 1817–1822.
44. Mohammed SF, Mirzoyev SA, Edwards WD et al. Left ventricular amyloid deposition in patients with heart failure and preserved ejection fraction. *JACC Heart Fail* 2014; 2: 113–122.
45. Liao R, Jain M, Teller P et al. Infusion of light chains from patients with cardiac amyloidosis causes diastolic dysfunction in isolated mouse hearts. *Circulation* 2001; 104: 1594–1597.

46. Lane T, Fontana M, Martinez-Naharro A et al. Natural history, quality of life, and outcome in cardiac transthyretin amyloidosis. *Circulation* 2019; 140(1): 16–26.
47. Ruberg FL, Grogan M, Hanna M, Kelly JW, Maurer MS. Transthyretin amyloid cardiomyopathy: JACC state-of-the-art review. *J Am Coll Cardiol* 2019; 73(22): 2872–2891.
48. Kittleson MM, Ruberg FL et al. 2023 ACC Expert consensus decision pathway on comprehensive multidisciplinary care for the patient with cardiac amyloidosis: a report of the American college of *cardiology* solution set oversight committee. *J Am Coll Cardiol* 2023; 81(11): 1076–1126.
49. Angomachalelis N, Hourzamanis A, Vamvalis C et al. Doppler echocardiographic evaluation of left ventricular diastolic function in patients with systemic sarcoidosis. *Postgrad Med J* 1992; 68: S52–S56.
50. Roberts WC, McAllister HA, Ferrans VJ. Sarcoidosis of the heart. *Am J Med* 1977; 63: 86–108.
51. Mitchell DN, du Bois RM, Oldershaw PJ. Cardiac sarcoidosis: A potentially fatal condition that needs expert assessment. *Br Med J* 1997; 314: 320–321.
52. Ballantyne GH, Savoca PE, Flannery JT et al. Incidence and mortality of carcinoids of the colon: Data from the Connecticut tumor registry. *Cancer* 1992; 69: 2400–2405.
53. Pellikka PA, Tajik AJ, Khandheria BK et al. Carcinoid heart disease: Clinical and echocardiographic spectrum in 74 patients. *Circulation* 1993; 87: 1188–1196.
54. Hesse A, Altland K, Linke RP et al. Cardiac amyloidosis: A review and report of a new transthyretin (prealbumin) variant. *Br Heart J* 1993; 70: 111–115.
55. Castaño A, Narotsky DL, Hamid N et al. Unveiling transthyretin cardiac amyloidosis and its predictors among elderly patients with severe aortic stenosis undergoing transcatheter aortic valve replacement. *Eur Heart J* 2017; 38(38): 2879–2887.
56. Falk RH, Plehn JF, Deering T. Sensitivity and specificity of the echocardiographic features of cardiac amyloidosis. *Am J Cardiol* 1987; 59: 418–422.
57. Pai RG, Shah PM. Echo-Doppler evaluation of left ventricular diastolic function. *Am Coll Cardiol Curr J Rev* 1994; 3: 30–33.
58. Lubien E, DeMaria A, Krishnaswamy P et al. Utility of B-natriuretic peptide in detecting diastolic dysfunction: Comparison with Doppler velocity recordings. *Circulation* 2002; 105: 595–601.
59. Bokhari S, Castaño A, Pozniakoff T et al. 99mTc-pyrophosphate scintigraphy for differentiating light-chain cardiac amyloidosis from the transthyretin-related familial and senile cardiac amyloidoses. *Circ Cardiovasc Imaging* 2013; 6: 195–201.
60. Mason JW, O'Connell JB. Clinical merit of endomyocardial biopsy. *Circulation* 1989; 79: 971–979.
61. Dispenzieri A, Buadi F, Kumar SK et al. Treatment of immunoglobulin light chain amyloidosis: Mayo stratification of myeloma and risk-adapted therapy (mSMART) consensus statement. *Mayo Clin Proc* 2015; 90: 1054–1081.
62. Falk RH, Alexander KM, Liao R, Dorbala S. AL (Light-Chain) cardiac amyloidosis: a review of diagnosis and therapy. *J Am Coll Cardiol* 2016; 68(12): 1323–1341.
63. Hartnett J, Jaber W, Maurer M et al. Electrophysiological manifestations of cardiac amyloidosis: *JACC: CardioOncology* state-of-the-art review. *JACC CardioOncol* 2021; 3(4): 506–515. Published 2021 Oct 19.
64. Maurer MS, Schwartz JH, Gundapaneni B et al. Tafamidis treatment for patients with transthyretin amyloid cardiomyopathy. *N Engl J Med* 2018; 379(11): 1007–1016.
65. Siddiqi OK, Mints YY, Berk JL et al. Diflunisal treatment is associated with improved survival for patients with early stage wild-type transthyretin (ATTR) amyloid cardiomyopathy: The Boston University Amyloidosis Center experience. *Amyloid* 2022; 29(2): 71–78.
66. Fontana M, Berk JL, Gillmore JD et al. Vutrisiran in patients with transthyretin amyloidosis with cardiomyopathy. *N Engl J Med*. Published online August 30, 2024.
67. Stevenson LW, Perloff JK. The dilated cardiomyopathies: Clinical aspects. *Cardiol Clin* 1988; 6: 197–218.
68. Aronow WS, Ahn C, Kronzon I. Prevalence of echocardiographic findings in 554 men and in 1243 women aged >60 years in a long term health care facility. *Am J Cardiol* 1997; 79: 379–380.
69. Fuster V, Gersh BJ, Giuliani ER et al. The natural history of idiopathic dilated cardiomyopathy. *Am J Cardiol* 1981; 47: 525–531.
70. Roberts WC, Siegel RJ, McManus BM. Idiopathic dilated cardiomyopathy: Analysis of 152 necropsy patients. *Am J Cardiol* 1987; 60: 1340–1355.
71. Sawada SG, Ryan T, Segar D et al. Distinguishing ischemic cardiomyopathy from nonischemic dilated cardiomyopathy with coronary echocardiography. *J Am Coll Cardiol* 1992; 19: 1223–1228.
72. Japp AG, Gulati A, Cook SA et al. The diagnosis and evaluation of dilated cardiomyopathy. *J Am Coll Cardiol* 2016; 67: 2996–3010.
73. Falk RH, Foster E, Coats MH. Ventricular thrombi and thromboembolism in dilated cardiomyopathy: A prospective follow up study. *Am Heart J* 1992; 123: 136–142.
74. Matsumura Y, Takata J, Kitaoka H et al. Long-term prognosis of dilated cardiomyopathy revisited: An improvement in survival over the past 20 years. *Circ J* 2006; 70: 376–383.

75. Kubo T, Matsumura Y, Okawa M et al. Improvement in prognosis of dilated cardiomyopathy in the elderly over the past 20 years. *J Cardiol* 2008; 52: 111–117.
76. Van Veldhuisen DJ, de Graeff PA, Remme WJ et al. Value of digoxin in heart failure and sinus rhythm: New features of an old drug. *J Am Coll Cardiol* 1996; 28: 813–819.
77. Rich MW, McSherry F, Williford WO et al. Effect of age on mortality, hospitalizations and response to digoxin in patients with heart failure: The DIG study. *J Am Coll Cardiol* 2001; 38: 806–813.
78. Ahmed A, Gambassi G, Weaver MT et al. Effects of discontinuation of digoxin versus continuation at low serum digoxin concentrations in chronic heart failure. *Am J Cardiol* 2007; 100: 280–284.
79. Packer M, Bristow M, Cohn J et al. The effect of carvedilol on morbidity and mortality in patients with chronic heart failure. *N Engl J Med* 1996; 334: 1349–1355.
80. Sanderson JE, Chan SKW, Yip G et al. Beta-blockade in heart failure: A comparison of carvedilol with metoprolol. *J Am Coll Cardiol* 1999; 33: 1522–1528.
81. MERIT-HF Study Group. Effect of metoprolol CR/XL in chronic heart failure: Metoprolol CR/XL randomised intervention trial in congestive heart failure (MERIT-HF) . *Lancet* 1999; 353: 2001–2007.
82. Pitt B, Zannad F, Remme WJ et al. The effect of spironolactone on morbidity and mortality in patients with severe heart failure. *N Engl J Med* 1999; 341: 709–717.
83. Cioffi G, Tarantini L, DeFeo S et al. Pharmacological left ventricular reverse remodeling in elderly patients receiving optimal therapy for chronic heart failure. *Eur J Heart Fail* 2005; 7: 1040–1048.
84. Barry WH, Gilbert EM. How do β-blockers improve ventricular function in patients with congestive heart failure? *Circulation* 2003; 107: 2395–2397.
85. Reiken S, Wehrens XHT, Vest JA et al. β-Blockers restore calcium release channel function and improve cardiac muscle performance in human heart failure. *Circulation* 2003; 107: 2459–2466.
86. Takemoto Y, Hozumi T, Sugioka K et al. Beta-blocker therapy induces ventricular resynchronization in dilated cardiomyopathy with narrow QRS complex. *J Am Coll Cardiol* 2007; 49: 778–783.
87. Cohn JN, Tognoni G. A randomized trial of the angiotensin-receptor blocker valsartan in chronic heart failure. *N Engl J Med* 2001; 345: 1667–1675.
88. McMurray JJ, Packer M, Desai AS et al. Angiotensin-neprilysin inhibition versus enalapril in heart failure. *N Engl J Med* 2014; 371(11): 993–1004.
89. Desai RJ, Patorno E, Vaduganathan M et al. Effectiveness of angiotensin-neprilysin inhibitor treatment versus renin-angiotensin system blockade in older adults with heart failure in clinical care. *Heart* 2021; 107(17): 1407–1416.
90. Packer M, Anker SD, Butler J et al. Cardiovascular and renal outcomes with empagliflozin in heart failure. *N Engl J Med* 2020; 383(15): 1413–1424.
91. Mischie AN, Chioncel V, Droc I et al. Anticoagulation in patients with dilated cardiomyopathy, low ejection fraction, and sinus rhythm: Back to the drawing board. *Cardiovasc Ther* 2013; 31: 298–302.
92. Goldberger Z, Lampert R. Implantable cardioverter-defibrillators: Expanding indications and technologies. *JAMA* 2006; 295: 809–818.
93. Cleland JGF, Daubert J-C, Erdmann E et al. The effect of cardiac resynchronization on morbidity and mortality in heart failure. *N Engl J Med* 2005; 352: 1539–1549.
94. Bleeker GB, Holman ER, Steendijk P et al. Cardiac resynchronization therapy in patients with a narrow QRS complex. *J Am Coll Cardiol* 2006; 48: 2243–2250.
95. Ruschitzka F, Abraham WT, Singh JP et al. Cardiac-resynchronization therapy in heart failure with a narrow QRS complex. *N Engl J Med* 2013; 369: 1395–1405.
96. Steffel J, Varma N, Robertson M et al. Effect of gender on outcomes after cardiac resynchronization therapy in patients with a narrow QRS complex: A subgroup analysis of the EchoCRT trial. *Circ Arrhythm Electrophysiol* 2016; 9: e003924.
97. Moss AJ, Hall WJ, Cannom DS et al. Cardiac-resynchronization therapy for the prevention of heart failure events. *N Engl J Med* 2009; 361: 1329–1338.
98. Antonio N, Elvas L, Goncalves L, Providencia LA. Cardiac resynchronization therapy in the elderly: A realistic option for an increasing population? *Int J Cardiol* 2012; 155: 49–51.
99. Abraham WT, Adams KF, Fonarow GC et al. In-hospital mortality in patients with acute decompensated heart failure requiring intravenous vasoactive medications. *J Am Coll Cardiol* 2005; 46: 57–64.
100. Sackner-Bernstein JD, Kowalski M, Fox M et al. Short-term risk of death after treatment with nesiritide for decompensated heart failure: A pooled analysis of randomized controlled trials. *JAMA* 2005; 293: 1900–1905.
101. Sackner-Bernstein JD, Skopicki HA, Aaronson KD. Risk of worsening renal function with nesiritide in patients with acutely decompensated heart failure. *Circulation* 2005; 111: 1487–1491.
102. O'Connor CM, Starling RC, Hernandez AF et al. Effect of nesiritide in patients with acute decompensated heart failure. *N Engl J Med* 2011; 365: 32–43.
103. Chaudhry SI, Wang Y, Gill TM et al. Geriatric conditions and subsequent mortality in older patients with heart failure. *J Am Coll Cardiol* 2010; 55: 309–316.

104. Venkitachalam L, Spertus JA. Stepping outside of the heart: Using nontraditional patient characteristics to understand and improve outcomes. *J Am Coll Cardiol* 2010; 55: 317–319.
105. Heckman GA, McKelvie RS, Rockwood K. Individualizing the care of older heart failure patients. *Curr Opin Cardiol* 2017; 32: Epub ahead of print 4 December 2017.
106. Konno T, Shimizu M, Ino H et al. A novel missense mutation in the myosin binding protein-C gene is responsible for hypertrophic cardiomyopathy with left ventricular dysfunction and dilation in elderly patients. *J Am Coll Cardiol* 2003; 41: 781–786.
107. Seidman JG, Seidman C. The genetic basis for cardiomyopathy: From mutation identification to mechanistic paradigms. *Cell* 2001; 104: 557–567.
108. Ackerman MJ, VanDriest SL, Ommen SR et al. Prevalence and age-dependence of malignant mutations in the beta-myosin heavy chain and troponin T genes in hypertrophic cardiomyopathy. *J Am Coll Cardiol* 2002; 39: 2042–2048.
109. Davies MJ, McKenna WJ. Hypertrophic cardiomyopathy: An introduction to pathology and pathogenesis. *Br Heart J* 1994; 72: S2–S3.
110. Maron BJ, Roberts WC. Quantitative analysis of cardiac muscle cell disorganization in the ventricular septum of patients with hypertrophic cardiomyopathy. *Circulation* 1979; 59(4): 689–706.
111. Cannan CR, Reeder GS, Bailey KR et al. Natural history of hypertrophic cardiomyopathy: A population based study, 1976 through 1990. *Circulation* 1994; 92: 2488–2495.
112. Lewis JF, Maron BJ. Clinical and morphological expression of hypertrophic cardiomyopathy in patients > 65 years of age. *J Am Coll Cardiol* 1994; 73: 1105–1111.
113. Maron BJ, Casey S, Hauser RG et al. Clinical course of hypertrophic cardiomyopathy with survival to advanced age. *J Am Coll Cardiol* 2003; 42: 882–888.
114. Fay WP, Taliercio CP, Ilstrup DM et al. Natural history of hypertrophic cardiomyopathy in the elderly. *J Am Coll Cardiol* 1990; 16: 821–826.
115. McKenna W, Deanfield J, Faruqui A et al. Prognosis in hypertrophic cardiomyopathy: Role of age and clinical, electrocardiographic and hemodynamic features. *Am J Cardiol* 1981; 47: 532–538.
116. Drazner MH, Rame JE, Marino EK et al. Increased left ventricular mass is a risk factor for the development of a depressed left ventricular ejection fraction within five years. *J Am Coll Cardiol* 2004; 43: 2207–2215.
117. Biagini E, Coccolo F, Ferlito M et al. Dilated-hypokinetic evolution of hypertrophic cardiomyopathy: Prevalence, incidence, risk factors, and prognostic implications in pediatric and adult patients. *J Am Coll Cardiol* 2004; 46(8): 1543–1550.
118. Olivotto I, Maron BJ, Appelbaum E et al. Spectrum and clinical significance of systolic function and myocardial fibrosis assessed by cardiovascular magnetic resonance in hypertrophic cardiomyopathy. *Am J Cardiol* 2010; 106(2): 261–267.
119. Sorajja P, Ommen SR, Nishimura RA et al. Adverse prognosis of patients with hypertrophic cardiomyopathy who have epicardial coronary artery disease. *Circulation* 2003; 108: 2342–2348.
120. Maron BJ, Wolfson JK, Epstein SE et al. Intramural ("small vessel") coronary artery disease in hypertrophic cardiomyopathy. *J Am Coll Cardiol* 1986; 8: 545–557.
121. Wigle ED, Rakowski H, Kimball BP et al. Hypertrophic cardiomyopathy: Clinical spectrum and treatment. *Circulation* 1995; 92: 1680–1692.
122. Cassidy J, Aronow WS, Prakash R. The effect of isometric exercise on the systolic murmur of patients with idiopathic hypertrophic subaortic stenosis. *Chest* 1975; 67: 395–397.
123. Shenoy MM, Khanna A, Nejat M et al. Hypertrophic cardiomyopathy in the elderly: A frequently misdiagnosed disease. *Arch Intern Med* 1986; 146: 658–661.
124. Chikamori T, Doi YL, Dickie S et al. Comparison of clinical features in patients >60 years of age to those <40 years of age with hypertrophic cardiomyopathy. *Am J Cardiol* 1990; 66: 875–878.
125. Olivotto I, Cecchi F, Casey SA et al. Impact of atrial fibrillation on the clinical course of hypertrophic cardiomyopathy. *Circulation* 2001; 104: 2517–2524.
126. Aronow WS, Kronzon I. Prevalence of hypertrophic cardiomyopathy and its association with mitral annual calcium in elderly patients. *Chest* 1988; 94: 1295–1296.
127. Lewis JF, Maron BJ. Elderly patients with hypertrophic cardiomyopathy: A subset with distinctive left ventricular morphology and progressive clinical course late in life. *J Am Coll Cardiol* 1989; 13: 36–45.
128. Seiler C, Hess OM, Schoenbeck M et al. Long-term follow-up of medical versus surgical therapy for hypertrophic cardiomyopathy: A retrospective study. *J Am Coll Cardiol* 1991; 17: 634–642.
129. Gilligan DM, Chan WL, Stewart R et al. Adrenergic hypersensitivity after beta-blocker withdrawal in hypertrophic cardiomyopathy. *Am J Cardiol* 1991; 68: 766–772.
130. Rosing DR, Idanpaan-Heikkila U, Maron BJ et al. Use of calcium-channel blocking drugs in hypertrophic cardiomyopathy. *Am J Cardiol* 1985; 55: 185B–195B.
131. Sherrid MV, Barac I, McKenna WJ et al. Multicenter study of the efficacy and safety of disopyramide in obstructive hypertrophic cardiomyopathy. *J Am Coll Cardiol* 2005; 45: 1251.
132. Olivotto I, Oreziak A, Barriales-Villa R et al. Mavacamten for treatment of symptomatic

obstructive hypertrophic cardiomyopathy (EXPLORER-HCM): A randomised, double-blind, placebo-controlled, phase 3 trial. *Lancet* 2020; 396(10253): 759–769.

133. Maron MS, Masri A, Nassif ME et al. Aficamten for symptomatic obstructive hypertrophic cardiomyopathy. *N Engl J Med* 2024; 390(20): 1849–1861.
134. Ommen SR, Ho CY, Asif IM et al. 2024 AHA/ACC/AMSSM/HRS/PACES/SCMR Guideline for the Management of Hypertrophic Cardiomyopathy: A Report of the American Heart Association/American College of *Cardiology* Joint Committee on Clinical Practice Guidelines [published correction appears in]. *Circulation* 2024 Aug 20; 150(8): e198.
135. Maron BJ, Bonow RO, Cannon RO et al. Hypertrophic cardiomyopathy: Interrelations of clinical manifestations, pathophysiology, and therapy (second of two parts). *N Engl J Med* 1987; 316: 844–852.
136. Maron BJ, Olivotto I, Bellone P et al. Clinical profile of stroke in 900 patients with hypertrophic cardiomyopathy. *J Am Coll Cardiol* 2002; 39(2): 301–307.
137. Maron BJ, Olivotto I, Spirito P, Casey A, Bellone P, Gohman TE, Graham KJ, Burton DA, Cecchi F. Epidemiology of hypertrophic cardiomyopathy-related death: Revisited in a large non-referral based patient population. *Circulation* 2000. August 2022;102(8):858–64.
138. Maron BJ, Shen W, Link MS et al. Efficacy of implantable cardioverter-defibrillators for the prevention of sudden death in patients with hypertrophic cardiomyopathy. *N Engl J Med* 2000; 342: 365–373.
139. Spirito P, Bellone P, Harris KM et al. Magnitude of left ventricular hypertrophy and the risk of sudden death in hypertrophic cardiomyopathy. *N Engl J Med* 2000; 342: 1778–1785.
140. Maron BJ, Rowin EJ, Casey SA et al. Risk stratification and outcome of patients with hypertrophic cardiomyopathy >=60 years of age. *Circulation* 2013; 127(5): 585–593.
141. O'Mahony C, Jichi F, Pavlou M et al. Hypertrophic cardiomyopathy outcomes investigators, a novel clinical risk prediction model for sudden cardiac death in hypertrophic cardiomyopathy (HCM risk-SCD). *Eur Heart J* 2014; 35(30): 2010–2020.
142. Nishimura RA, Trusty JM, Hayes DL et al. Dual-chamber pacing for hypertrophic obstructive cardiomyopathy: A randomized, double-blind crossover trial. *J Am Coll Cardiol* 1997; 29: 435–441.
143. Maron BJ, Nishimura RA, McKenna WJ et al. Assessment of permanent dual-chamber pacing as a treatment for drug-refractory symptomatic patients with obstructive hypertrophic cardiomyopathy. *Circulation* 1999; 99: 2927–2933.
144. Sorajja P, Ommen SR, Holmes DR Jr et al. Survival after alcohol septal ablation for obstructive hypertrophic cardiomyopathy. *Circulation* 2012; 126(20): 2374–2380.
145. Cooper MM, McIntosh CL, Tucker E et al. Operation for hypertrophic subaortic stenosis in the aged. *Ann Thorac Surg* 1987; 44: 370–378.
146. Yu EHC, Omran AS, Wigle D et al. Mitral regurgitation in hypertrophic obstructive cardiomyopathy: Relationship to obstruction and relief with myectomy. *J Am Coll Cardiol* 2000; 36: 2219–2225.
147. Desai MY, Owens A, Geske JB et al. Myosin inhibition in patients with obstructive hypertrophic cardiomyopathy referred for septal reduction therapy. *J Am Coll Cardiol* 2022; 80(2): 95–108.
148. Desai MY, Owens A, Wolski K et al. Mavacamten in patients with hypertrophic cardiomyopathy referred for septal reduction: Week 56 results from the VALOR-HCM randomized clinical trial. *JAMA Cardiol* 2023; 8(10): 968–977.
149. Shenouda J, Silber D, Subramaniam M et al. Evaluation and management of concomitant hypertrophic obstructive cardiomyopathy and valvular aortic stenosis. *Curr Treat Options Cardiovasc Med* 2016; 18(3): 17.

18

Cancer and cardiovascular disease in older adults

RYLIE PIETROWICZ, DINA IOFFE, EFRAT DOTAN, AND EMAN HAMAD

Key points

- In older adults undergoing anticancer therapy, a comprehensive geriatric assessment in addition to care from a multidisciplinary geriatric cardio-oncology team can help to improve care and outcomes.
- Baseline assessment of cardiovascular risk prior to cancer treatment is important to help tailor and personalize cancer-related therapy.
- Serial evaluations, including physical examination, cardiac imaging, and cardiac biomarkers, can help to identify development of cancer therapy-related cardiotoxicity early, allowing for adjustment of cancer treatment and introduction of cardioprotective interventions in an effort to mitigate further damage.
- At the completion of anticancer therapy, it is important to identify those older adults at risk for development of cardiovascular disease and ensure close follow-up.

INTRODUCTION

Aging is an established risk factor for both cardiovascular diseases (CVD) and cancer, two of the leading causes of morbidity and mortality in older adults. As life expectancy increases, there is a growing prevalence of older patients facing both conditions simultaneously, complicating treatment approaches and overall patient care. Despite being two distinct entities, CVD and cancer have many similar risk factors including hypertension, obesity, diabetes mellitus, and smoking, among others.

DOI: 10.1201/9781003568933-18

This points to shared biology and pathophysiology. This chapter explores the intersection of oncology and cardiovascular disease in the aging population, highlighting overlaps in pathophysiological mechanisms, treatment challenges, and management strategies before, during, and after treatment.

EPIDEMIOLOGY

Cardiovascular disease and cancer are the two most prevalent chronic diseases in geriatric patients. Geriatric cardiology has long been described with origins dating to the early 1900s, but its importance has only increased exponentially given the shift in demographics [1].

In the current era, there are over 64 million people in the United States older than 65 years of age and that number is expected to increase to 95 million by 2060 [1,2]. According to the American Heart Association, nearly 70% of individuals over the age of 65 have some form of CVD, including hypertension, coronary artery disease (CAD), and heart failure. Among these, CAD is the leading cause of morbidity and mortality in older adults, followed by stroke and hypertensive heart disease [3].

Similarly, cancer is highly prevalent among older adults, with prostate, breast, lung, and colorectal cancers being the most common malignancies diagnosed in this population [4]. Lung cancer remains the leading cause of cancer-related mortality in both men and women, while prostate cancer and breast cancer account for the highest incidence rates among men and women, respectively [5].

Approximately 60% of all cancer diagnoses and 70% of cancer-related deaths occur in individuals aged 65 years and older [4]. Similarly, CVD remains the leading cause of death in this age group, with heart disease and stroke significantly contributing to mortality [3].

BIOLOGY AND PATHOPHYSIOLOGY

The coexistence of cancer and CVD in older adults results from overlapping biologic and pathophysiologic mechanisms. Cellular changes implicated in the development of cardiovascular disease are closely intertwined with those that occur during normal aging. Aging is considered one of the most complex biological processes with several factors implicated in observed cellular changes. Changes in vasculature associated with aging have significant implications for the development of cardiovascular disease. It has been observed that in aging vessels, generalized endothelial dysfunction mediated by increased oxidative stress and inflammatory properties lead to increased arterial stiffness, atherogenesis, and a prothrombotic state—all predisposing to cardiovascular disease [6]. Both cancer and cardiovascular disease are associated with impaired endothelial function, leading to decreased nitric oxide bioavailability and increased vascular stiffness [7,8].

With increasing age and the development of arteriosclerosis mediated by the above mechanisms, a myriad of downstream effects may develop including accumulation of atherosclerotic plaques, reduced arterial compliance, left ventricular hypertrophy, impaired relaxation of ventricular myocytes, and ventricular and atrial enlargement. These changes can lead to the development of clinical syndromes including diastolic and systolic heart failure, arrhythmias, hypertension, stroke, and valvular heart disease [6].

RISK FACTORS AND COMORBID CONDITIONS

Shared risk factors, including smoking, obesity, sedentary lifestyle, and chronic inflammation, contribute to the concurrent rise of CVD and cancer in aging individuals. Smoking is a major risk factor for both CVD and various cancers—lung, bladder, oral, and many others—as it leads to oxidative stress, inflammation, and endothelial dysfunction [9]. Excess adiposity leads to increased levels of inflammatory cytokines, insulin resistance, and hormonal imbalances, raising risks for breast, colorectal, and endometrial cancers as well as CVD [10]. Hyperglycemia and insulin resistance promote endothelial dysfunction, chronic inflammation, and abnormal cell growth leading to both CVD and cancer [11]. Chronic hypertension leads to vascular remodeling, increased oxidative stress, and higher risk for renal and colorectal cancers [11]. Excessive alcohol consumption increases the risk of hypertension, cardiomyopathy, liver disease, and cancers of the liver, esophagus, breast, mouth, and throat [12].

Air pollution, radiation, and carcinogens induce DNA damage and oxidative stress, thereby contributing to both diseases [11]. Some genetic predispositions and inherited mutations increase susceptibility to both conditions as well [13].

Older adults do not typically have cardiovascular disease in isolation but rather it is often accompanied by additional comorbid conditions. Coexistence of two or more conditions occurs in 30%–83% of older adults, with CVD conditions being the most reported. Other geriatric syndromes affecting older adults, including cognitive impairment, dementia, depression, and frailty exacerbate these medical conditions. Frailty is prevalent in at least 10% of older adults with polypharmacy present in 26%–40%. Frailty is predictive of all-cause and cardiovascular mortality in very old adults [14].

Therefore, cardiovascular disease in the older adult becomes increasingly more complex and necessitates care that not only considers medical treatment but accounts for factors such as polypharmacy, patient priorities, and social support [1]. In older adults with cardiovascular disease and cancer, a holistic approach with a focused geriatric assessment can help inform appropriate treatment for the individual (Table 18.1 [15–17] and Table 18.2).

Table 18.1 Geriatric domains, geriatric assessment tools, and potential interventions for older adults with cancer

Domain	Geriatric assessment tool(s)	Deficit	Potential interventions
Functional status [18]	Activities of Daily Living (ADLs): Katz Index [19] Instrumental Activities of Daily living (IADL): Lawton-Brody Scale [20]	Dependence with ADL and/or IADL	• Physical and/or occupational therapy • Promotes physical activity and exercise • Home safety evaluation • Consider cardiac rehabilitation in older adults with comorbid cardiovascular disease and/or risk factors
	Short Physical Performance Battery (SPPB) [21]	Combined score <=9	
	Timed Up and Go Test (TUG) [22]	TUG >13 seconds	
Comorbidities	Cumulative Illness Rating – Geriatrics (CIRS-G) [23]	Comorbid conditions, including hearing and/or visual impairment	• Treat and optimize comorbid conditions in coordination with other providers (e.g., primary care, geriatrician)
Polypharmacy [24]	Beers Criteria [25] Medication Appropriateness Index (MAI) Screening Tool to Alert Doctors to Right Treatment/Screening Tool of Older Person's Prescriptions (START/STOPP) [16]	Use of >5 prescribed medications and/or inappropriate medication use (e.g., misuse, overuse, duplication, unnecessary use)	• Close medication reconciliation including herbal supplements and over-the-counter medications • Review drug interactions and consider deprescribing at regular intervals • Assess use and indication of potentially inappropriate medications (e.g., long-acting benzodiazepines, anticholinergic drugs)
Cognition [26]	Mini-Cog Blessed Orientation Memory Concentration Test (BOMC)	Memory loss, confusion, abnormal screening (Mini-Cog score <4; BOMC score >=4)	• Assess decision-making capacity • Consider referrals to neuropsychiatry, geriatrics, neurology, psychiatry, and/or cognitive rehabilitation • Screen for potential confounders (e.g., depression, fatigue, polypharmacy, nutritional deficiency, endocrine dysfunction, substance use disorder)
Geriatric syndromes	Balducci Frailty Criteria [27]	Age >85 years, >3 comorbidities, dependence for >=1 ADL, >=1 geriatric syndrome	• Physical and/or occupational therapy • Home safety evaluation • Address potentially reversible or modifiable vulnerabilities
	Bone health screening (e.g., DEXA, FRAX)	Osteopenia, osteoporosis; high fracture risk	• Optimize bone health with vitamin D and calcium supplementation • Bone-modifying agents if indicated • Fall risk precautions
	Fall risk assessment	TUG score >13 seconds Gait speed <1 meter/second Repeated falls (>3 in past 6 months)	• Physical therapy • Home safety evaluation • Address polypharmacy and deprescribe psychotropic and/or sedating medications • Assess for potential underlying risk factors (e.g., orthostatic hypotension, cognitive impairment) • Fall risk precautions

(*Continued*)

Table 18.1 (Continued) Geriatric domains, geriatric assessment tools, and potential interventions for older adults with cancer

Domain	Geriatric assessment tool(s)	Deficit	Potential interventions
	Fatigue scale	Significant self-reported fatigue that does not resolve with sleep or rest (scale 0–10)	• Physical therapy and/exercise programs [28] • Optimize sleep hygiene, nutrition, pain control • Cognitive behavioral therapy • Stress management, and/or mindfulness programs
	Confusion Assessment Method (CAM) [29]	CAM positive: acute onset with fluctuating course and inattention, plus disorganized thinking or altered level of consciousness	• Address polypharmacy • Assess for and address potential underlying causes • Non-pharmacologic approaches are preferred
Nutrition	Mini Nutritional Assessment (MNA)	>3 kg unintentional weight loss in 3 months, body mass index <=21 or >=30	• Referral to registered dietician • Nutritional supplements and diet recommendations to prevent nutritional deficiencies, maintain a healthy weight, and optimize caloric intake • Address treatment-related toxicities such as mucositis, nausea, vomiting • Screen for food insecurity • Consider referral to speech pathology and/or occupational therapy if difficulty with swallowing, eating
Social support [30]	Assess primary caregiver(s) and support system, living conditions, financial concerns, transportation barriers	Lack of social, physical, psychological, and financial support and assistance	• Referral to social work and home health services • Home safety evaluation • Screen for elder abuse • Identify health care proxy, caregiver(s), emergency contact(s) • Advanced care planning • Consider counseling and/or peer support groups
Psychological distress	Geriatric Depression Scale (GDS) NCCN Distress Thermometer [31] Patient Health Questionnaires (PHQ-2, PHQ-9)	Depression, anxiety, adjustment disorder	• Further assessment for positive screen • Referral to psychosocial services and providers • Consider chaplain referral based on patient beliefs
Geriatric screening	G8 Geriatric Screening Tool [32]	Score <14 indicates vulnerability	Comprehensive geriatric assessment recommended
Risk for treatment-related toxicity	CARG Toxicity Prediction Tool [33] Chemotherapy Risk Assessment Scale for High-Age Patients (CRASH) [34]	Graded risk of treatment-related adverse effects	Consider dose modification and closer toxicity monitoring

Abbreviations: CARG, Cancer and Aging Research Group; DEXA, dual-energy x-ray absorptiometry; FRAX, Fracture Risk Assessment Tool; NCCN, National Comprehensive Cancer Network.

Table 18.2 Validated geriatric assessment screening tools

Geriatric assessment	Objective	Evaluated factors	Scoring		
G8 Geriatric Screening Tool [32, 35]	Identify patients who would benefit from a full geriatric assessment	Age, food intake, weight loss, mobility, neuropsychological problems, BMI, polypharmacy, perceived health status	<=14: Full geriatric evaluation recommended >14: Full geriatric evaluation not necessary		
Cancer and Aging Research Group Chemotherapy (CARG) Toxicity Tool [33, 35]	Predicts rates of grade >=3 treatment-related toxicity	Sex, age, cancer type, chemotherapy dose reduction, number of chemotherapy agents, hemoglobin, kidney function, hearing impairment, falls, assistance with medication management, mobility, social activity	0–5 6–9 10–23		30% risk (low) 52% risk (intermediate) 83% risk (high)
Chemotherapy Risk Assessment Scale for High-Age Patients (CRASH) [34, 35]	Predicts severe hematologic and non-hematologic treatment-related toxicity	ECOG performance status, cognition, nutritional status, IADL, chemotherapy risk (chemotox), diastolic blood pressure, lactate dehydrogenase	Hematologic score	0–1 2–3 4–5 >=6	Low Low-intermediate Intermediate-high High
			Non-hematologic score	0–2 3–4 5–6 >=7	Low Low-intermediate Intermediate-high High
			Combined score	0–3 4–6 7–9 >=10	Low Low-intermediate Intermediate-high High

Abbreviations: BMI, body mass index; ECOG, Eastern Cooperative Oncology Group; IADL, Instrumental Activities of Daily Living.

Geriatric assessment

Prospective data to guide the management of older adults with cancer are limited despite the rapidly aging population and growing number of older adults with cancer. Although 42% of the overall population with cancer is >70 years old, this age group comprised 24% of participants in US Food and Drug Administration (FDA)-registered studies and <10% of participants in National Cancer Institute (NCI)-sponsored studies [37]. The generalizability of most prospective oncology data is unclear as older adults enrolled in these studies are carefully selected and tend to be more robust than the average older patient with cancer, and geriatric-specific toxicity and efficacy data are not consistently reported. Eastern Cooperative Oncology Group (ECOG) performance status is often used to determine appropriateness for treatment for patients with cancer; however, this subjective measure of functional reserve can lead to biased assessments that often do not accurately capture fitness of older adults (Table 18.3 [36]). Aging is a heterogeneous biologic process that can affect cancer treatment tolerance and response in older adults in ways that cannot solely be predicted by chronologic age and performance status. As such, the management of older adults with cancer necessitates a holistic approach that appropriately balances the risks and benefits of cancer treatments, personalizes treatments to maximize efficacy while minimizing potential adverse effects, and maintains a good quality of life (QOL). This is particularly important to this patient population that often values QOL, preserved cognition, and functional independence over longevity [38].

Geriatric assessment tools offer a multidimensional assessment of a patient's overall health that is clinically relevant to older adults and can identify potentially modifiable deficits that are missed on routine oncologic evaluation [15]. These tools evaluate several domains affected by aging that are relevant to the management and outcomes

Table 18.3 Eastern Cooperative Oncology Group (ECOG) Performance Status

Grade	ECOG Performance Status (PS)
0	Fully active, able to carry on all pre-disease performance without restriction
1	Restricted in physically strenuous activity but ambulatory and able to carry out work of a light or sedentary nature, e.g., light housework, office work
2	Ambulatory and capable of all self-care but unable to carry out any work activities; up and about more than 50% of waking hours
3	Capable of only limited self-care; confined to bed or chair more than 50% of waking hours
4	Completely disabled; cannot carry on any self-care; totally confined to bed or chair
5	Dead

among older adults with cancer: functional status, comorbidities, polypharmacy, cognition, geriatric syndromes (e.g., falls, frailty, fatigue, osteoporosis), nutrition, social support, and psychological distress (Table 18.1) [39].

Functional status generally refers to physical activity level, mobility, strength, and degree of independence. It is highly variable and does not solely depend on chronologic age. ECOG performance status and chronologic age are frequently used as surrogates for functional status, though they are not accurate predictors of a patient's true biological age and do not take into account the significant heterogeneity in fitness and reserve between older adults of similar age [33, 40]. Assessing functional status and physical function, which can be predictive of treatment tolerability and outcomes, is a critical part of determining whether treatment is appropriate and if treatment modifications are indicated.

Older adults with cancer are more likely to have multiple comorbidities with increasing age compared to age-matched controls, including CVD, hypertension, diabetes, kidney disease, pulmonary disease, osteoporosis, and dementia. Comorbidities are associated with lower rates of cancer treatment, increased treatment-related toxicity, higher rates of hospitalization, more treatment modifications and/or delays, inferior QOL, and higher all-cause mortality [41, 42]. Importantly, comorbid conditions also represent a competing risk of death in older adults with cancer and their potential impact on life expectancy should be considered in formulating a treatment approach.

Assessing the severity of and interaction between comorbidities, as well as their impact on functional status, is critical in determining if cancer treatment is appropriate and in personalizing a treatment plan.

Polypharmacy has several definitions including the use of multiple (>5) medications and/or inappropriate medication use (e.g., misuse, overuse, duplication, unnecessary use). It tends to be more prevalent in older adults in the setting of several comorbidities requiring multiple drugs, as well as aging-related changes (e.g., impaired organ function) that affect drug metabolism [24]. This is particularly important for older adults with cancer, who are often prescribed multiple additional medications to manage cancer and cancer treatment-related symptoms, such as nausea, vomiting, diarrhea, constipation, and pain. There are several tools to assess polypharmacy, though none have been validated in patients with cancer. A comprehensive review of patient medications, including assessment of potential drug interactions, herbal therapies/supplements, and inappropriate medications for older adults (e.g., long-acting benzodiazepines, anticholinergic drugs) should be performed at regular intervals and deprescribing should be considered [43].

Cognitive impairment and dementia are more prevalent with age and are associated with changes in attention, memory, and information processing speed. Cancer and cancer-associated symptoms, including fatigue, sleep disturbance, pain, depression, and psychological distress, can contribute to cognitive impairment as well [44]. Baseline cognitive testing is recommended to identify which older adults would benefit from further assessment and to guide treatment decisions. Periodic assessment of cognitive function should also be performed during and after cancer treatment considering potential short- and long-term sequelae of these therapies on cognition.

Geriatric syndromes, such as frailty, fatigue, osteoporosis, incontinence, delirium, and falls, are clinical conditions related to accumulating impairments in multiple domains and/or systems that are more prevalent with increasing age. These clinical syndromes are more common in older adults with cancer and increase the risk of further functional decline and death [45]. Frailty is defined by decreased physiologic reserve leading to vulnerability, and is associated with falls, increased comorbidities, dependence with activities of daily living, decreased mobility, hospitalization, and death [45]. Cancer-related fatigue can be due to the underlying malignancy, pain, treatment side effects, medications, psychological or emotional distress, comorbidities (e.g., anemia), and/or poor sleep. Unlike typical fatigue, cancer-related fatigue does not resolve with rest or sleep and can be particularly distressing to older adults with cancer. It often affects functional status, increases fall risk, and can precipitate a loss of functional independence, as well as decline in other geriatric domains. Falls are a potentially serious health issue for older adults and fall risk can increase due to cancer, cancer treatments (e.g., fatigue, neuropathy), sarcopenia, or cognitive impairment [46]. Conversely, falls are associated with inferior treatment tolerability and survival in older adults with cancer. Asking older patients about falls at regular intervals is recommended and can shed light on other potentially modifiable impairments such as dizziness, weakness, and polypharmacy.

Osteoporosis increases the risk of fractures in older adults with cancer, particularly among those at risk for falls. Patients receiving treatments that affect muscle mass and/or bone density (e.g., steroids, hormone treatments) are at highest risk for these complications. Older adults with cancer are also at risk for delirium, an acute disturbance in attention, cognition, and/or behavior, which is often underrecognized. Those with preexisting cognitive impairment, multiple comorbidities, sensory impairments, and functional dependence are at increased risk. Delirium is most often multifactorial and can frequently be precipitated by polypharmacy, infection, dehydration, malnutrition, sleep disturbance, hospitalization, and cancer treatments, as well as supportive care medications [29].

Unintentional weight loss and malnutrition are common in older adults with cancer as malignancy often causes metabolic dysregulation and catabolism, leading to anorexia and cachexia. Poor nutritional status is often compounded by treatment-related side effects (e.g., nausea, mucositis, fatigue, weakness) and age-related sarcopenia, which often leads to frailty [47]. Geriatric syndromes, including cognitive impairment, falls, and depression, are independent risk factors for malnutrition [48]. Poor nutritional status is a significant risk factor for poor treatment tolerability, increased toxicity, decreased QOL, and increased mortality risk in older adults with cancer [49].

Adequate social support, defined as a network available to provide physical, psychological, and financial assistance, is another essential part of optimizing care delivery and improving treatment outcomes for older individuals with cancer [30].

Psychologic concerns, such as depression, anxiety, and adjustment disorder, are reported in 30%–40% of older adults with cancer and are higher among older patients with cancer compared to those with other comorbidities [50,51]. Depression in older adults with cancer is independently associated with impaired mobility and functional status, multiple comorbidities, polypharmacy, cognitive impairment, and inadequate social support [52]. Older adults with cancer and comorbid depression have more severe physical symptoms, increased risk of emergency room visits, hospitalizations and readmissions, inferior QOL, and reduced survival [46].

Cancer and cancer treatments can affect these interconnected geriatric domains, triggering a cascade that decreases functional status, increases frailty, affects treatment tolerability, and decreases survival. Conversely, vulnerabilities in these domains can affect eligibility for certain treatments and necessitate treatment modifications. A comprehensive geriatric assessment (CGA) consists of several validated tools that identify vulnerabilities in these domains and inform treatment decisions, as well as goals of care. CGA-based interventions and CGA-guided cancer care help assess appropriateness for treatment and treatment toxicity risk [53]. CGA-guided care is recommended by the American Society for Clinical Oncology (ASCO) and the National Comprehensive Cancer Network (NCCN) as it provides prognostic information, identifies potentially modifiable geriatric vulnerabilities, and supports a personalized, holistic treatment approach [16, 17]. Despite mounting evidence to support CGA-guided care for older adults with cancer, widespread adoption of CGA in clinical practice remains suboptimal, largely due to lack of awareness of these guideline recommendations, as well as time and personnel constraints [54]. While a comprehensive CGA may be time consuming, several screening tools and chemotherapy toxicity prediction calculators offer faster, simplified evaluations of older adults with cancer (Table 18.2). The G8 geriatric screening tool identifies who would benefit from a CGA, which remains the gold standard [32]. The Chemotherapy Risk Assessment Scale for High-Age Patients (CRASH) and Cancer and Aging Research Group Chemotherapy (CARG) toxicity tool are validated assessments that predict the risk of treatment-related toxicity in older adults with cancer [33, 55]. Most recently, ASCO, CARG, and the International Society for Geriatric Oncology (SIOG) developed the Practical Geriatric Assessment (https://www.mycarg.org/wp-content/uploads/2025/02/PGA-Final.pdf) to address implementation barriers by simplifying and consolidating several assessment tools into one easily accessible document [17].

The use of CGA and CGA screening tools at regular intervals along with prespecified interventions and multidisciplinary care is essential in optimizing treatment of older adults with cancer, providing holistic care, and improving clinical outcomes. In addition to interval assessment of geriatric domains before, during, and after cancer treatment, frequent consideration and discussion of competing risks of death and treatment tradeoffs (e.g., potentially life-prolonging cancer treatment may affect other domains or QOL) with patients is crucial. Shared decision-making is arguably the cornerstone of caring for older adults with cancer, particularly given the complexities and nuances in treatment management. Similarly, it is essential to regularly revisit the topic of "what matters" and patients' goals of care as patient priorities may change over time.

CARDIOPULMONARY EXERCISE TESTING IN CARDIO-ONCOLOGY RISK ASSESSMENT

With advancements in cancer therapy, older adults diagnosed with cancer have increased mortality and morbidity from noncancer-related causes, specifically cardiovascular disease [56]. Research has demonstrated that cardiorespiratory fitness is associated with mortality in the general population but especially in older adults diagnosed with cancer [57]. Those with higher fitness levels as demonstrated by protocolized cardiopulmonary exercise testing had increased survival following cancer diagnosis [58]. Therefore, supervised exercise programs and high-intensity interval training can be implemented to improve the cardiovascular fitness of older adults before, during and after cancer treatment. Additionally, in patients with decreased physical activity and multiple comorbidities, cardiopulmonary exercise testing can be used to distinguish between cardiovascular causes versus non-cardiovascular causes during and following treatment [59]. However, maximal cardiopulmonary exercise testing coupled with gas exchange and/or invasive hemodynamics may not be feasible for older adults with multiple comorbidities and geriatric syndromes, and providers should therefore consider objective methods of assessing submaximal aerobic capacity including 6-minute walk testing or other validated methods, such as the University of Northern Colorado Cancer Rehabilitation Institute treadmill protocol [60, 61].

Cardiotoxic cancer treatments

There is a growing body of literature describing cardiotoxic effects of many different classes of anticancer treatment with a scarcity of data and knowledge on cardiotoxic effects in older adults. Here we outline a select group of cardiotoxic anticancer therapies and known considerations when using them to treat older adults with cancer. A summary of cardiotoxic chemotherapies can be found in Table 18.4. Cardiotoxic effects can be described as type 1 cardiotoxicity (irreversible cardiac injury due to damage of cardiac myocytes) or type 2 cardiotoxicity (impairment of cardiac myocytes by anticancer agents that can be at least partially reversible) [62].

ANTHRACYCLINES

Anthracyclines directly cause DNA strand breaks and inhibit DNA transcription and replication. This class of drugs, including doxorubicin, daunorubicin, epirubicin, and idarubicin, has a wide variety of uses as anticancer therapy and is primarily used to treat hematologic malignancies such as Hodgkin's and non-Hodgkin's lymphomas in addition to solid cancers like breast and bladder. Anthracyclines are known to cause acute and chronic cardiomyopathies, arrhythmias, and pericardial diseases. Effects of anthracyclines on myocardial cells can be seen immediately with release of troponin shortly after infusion of the medication. A large meta-analysis demonstrated a significant decline in LVEF in 6% of patients receiving anthracyclines with subclinical effects in another 18% [89]. The risk of heart failure increases on a dose-dependent basis and increases with increasing age; however, additional patient-specific and disease-specific risk factors can mitigate or accentuate the effects of anthracyclines. For example, those with low cumulative anthracycline doses (<300 mg/m^2) may have more profound cardiovascular toxicity if the patient also has genetic predisposition, concomitant radiation therapy, or advanced age [90]. Alternative formulations including liposomal doxorubicin have been shown to have a more favorable cardiotoxic risk profile [91].

FLUOROPYRIMIDINES

Fluoropyrimidines such as 5-FU and its oral prodrug capecitabine are primarily used to treat head and neck cancers in addition to metastatic breast cancers and GI malignancies. Associated cardiovascular risks include coronary vasospasm, acute coronary syndromes, and very rarely cardiac arrest [92].

ANTI-HER2 THERAPIES

Trastuzumab and Pertuzumab are two anti-HER2 monoclonal antibodies used to treat certain breast cancers, colorectal cancers, and other malignancies expressing the HER-2 protein. Anti-HER2 therapies are known to cause decreased systolic function and in rare cases severe cardiomyopathy and heart failure. Cardiotoxic risk is thought to be proportional to treatment duration and is often reversible upon discontinuation of anti-HER2 therapy. Additionally, sequential use of Anti-HER2 therapy and anthracyclines increases risk of cardiotoxicity [93, 94].

VEGF INHIBITORS

Vascular endothelial growth factor, or VEGF, is associated with cancer development by stimulating angiogenesis. VEGF inhibitors are used to treat many cancer subtypes including non-small cell lung, ovarian, cervical, and colorectal cancers. Given that VEGF inhibitors affect vascular endothelia, hypertension and coronary artery disease are the two most common cardiotoxicities within this class, which can also rarely lead to cardiomyopathy. Cardiotoxic effects can often be reversed with cessation of the VEGF inhibitor. Additional rare risks include venous or arterial thromboembolism, bleeding complications, and poor wound healing [11, 95].

MULTIKINASE INHIBITORS

Protein kinase inhibition is used to treat a variety of cancer subtypes by targeting signals that regulate cell growth, apoptosis, and angiogenesis. Most of these agents target multiple kinases and present a broad range of activity, with efficacy in many cancer subtypes at the expense of significant cardiotoxic risks. Some tyrosine kinase inhibitors have anti-VEGF activity and can lead to hypertension

Table 18.4 Cancer treatments and associated cardiovascular concerns for older adults

Treatment [General indications]	Associated cardiovascular toxicity and risk in older adults	Recommendations for modifications and monitoring
Doxorubicin, Daunorubicin, Idarubicin [Multiple cancers: acute lymphoblastic leukemia, bladder, breast, lymphomas, sarcomas]	Acute CM (<5%) • Arrhythmias, acute HF, myocarditis, and/or pericarditis • Chronic CM (<5%) • Arrhythmias, chronic HF, dilated CM • Dose-dependent Risk of HF increases with time and age (~5%) [63]	Two-dimensional echocardiogram within 1 year of completing anthracycline therapy (high cumulative dose or a low cumulative dose + >1 risk factor for HF) [64] Pegylated liposomal doxorubicin (PLD) has a better cardiac toxicity profile without decreased anti-cancer efficacy [65, 66]
Fluorouracil (5-FU) [GI malignancies, advanced head and neck cancers] Capecitabine (oral pro-drug of 5-FU) [GI and metastatic breast cancers; radiosensitizer with radiation therapy]	Chest pain, coronary vasospasm, palpitations (<5%) MI, cardiac arrest (<2%) [67] Cardiotoxicity is rare and does not increase based on age alone [68, 69]	Screen for CVD and CV risk factors CGA-based dose modification and interventions for patient selection and to improve planned treatment completion rates without increased toxicity [70, 71]
Trastuzumab [HER2-positive breast, colorectal, GEJ, gastric cancers]	Decreased LVEF (2%–5%), severe cardiotoxicity <1% [72] Cardiotoxicity risk is similar in older adults and proportional to treatment duration	Consider primary prevention with lisinopril or carvedilol during treatment with trastuzumab + anthracycline [73] • Does not decrease rates of cardiotoxicity; associated with decreased treatment interruptions with trastuzumab alone Optimize borderline LVEF and other CV risk factors Baseline echocardiogram and monitoring ~12 weeks during treatment, followed by echocardiogram every 3 months for at least 2 years after completing HER-2 therapy [74] Use with caution in older adults who have previously received anthracyclines or who have significant vulnerabilities on CGA
Pertuzumab [HER2-positive breast cancer in combination with trastuzumab]	No increased toxicity compared to trastuzumab alone [75]	Screen for CVD and CV risk factors Use with caution in older adults due to increased risk of diarrhea, fatigue [76]
Trastuzumab Emtansine (T-DM1) [HER2-positive metastatic breast cancer]	Decreased LVEF (<2%) [77] No increased cardiotoxicity based on age	Screen for CVD and CV risk factors Use with caution in older adults due to increased risk of fatigue, nausea, diarrhea, skin changes [77]
Trastuzumab Deruxtecan (T-DXd) [HER2-positive breast, GEJ, gastric cancers]	Decreased LVEF (2%–5%), severe LV dysfunction 0.5% [78, 79]*	Use with caution with underlying lung disease or other pulmonary comorbidities
VEGF inhibitors (Bevacizumab, Ramucirumab) [Multiple cancers: cervical, colorectal, glioblastoma, hepatocellular, non-small cell lung, ovarian, renal cell]	HTN most common; arterial and venous thromboembolism less common; CM rare [80] No increased cardiotoxicity based on age [81, 82]	Close blood pressure monitoring and management

(Continued)

Table 18.4 (Continued) Cancer treatments and associated cardiovascular concerns for older adults

Treatment [General indications]	Associated cardiovascular toxicity and risk in older adults	Recommendations for modifications and monitoring
Protein kinase inhibitors [Multiple cancers: chronic lymphocytic leukemia, chronic myeloid leukemia, hepatocellular, prostate, renal cell]	HTN, arrhythmias, arterial and venous thromboembolism, bleeding (frequency varies based on drug, dose, and disease) No increased cardiotoxicity based on age*	Blood pressure monitoring, periodic electrocardiogram based on drug toxicity profile Tailor therapy and monitoring based on individual patients and CGA
Androgen deprivation therapy (ADT): Abiraterone, Darolutamide, Apalutamide, Enazluatamide [Prostate cancer]	HTN, acute coronary syndrome, CAD, atrial fibrillation (rare) [83–85] No increased cardiotoxicity based on age*	Screen for CVD and CV risk factors; blood pressure monitoring Consider alternatives to abiraterone, which requires concomitant low-dose steroid use [83, 84] Close monitoring for osteoporosis and sarcopenia Darolutamide is not associated with a higher risk of falls, fractures, or seizures
Aromatase Inhibitors (e.g., Anastrozole) [Hormone receptor-positive breast cancer]	HF, venous thromboembolism, myocardial infarction rare (<2%) [86] No increased cardiotoxicity based on age	Screen for CVD and CV risk factors Close monitoring for osteoporosis, sarcopenia
Immune checkpoint inhibitors [Multiple cancers: colorectal, hepatocellular, melanoma, non-small cell lung, renal cell]	Arrhythmias myocarditis; CM, HF, pericardial disease are rare No increased cardiotoxicity based on age*	Consider other IO-related toxicities if CV IO toxicity suspected Use high-dose steroids with caution in older adults when treating IO-related toxicity
Chimeric antigen receptor (CAR) T-cell therapy [lymphoma, multiple myeloma]	Mixed results on cardiotoxicity risk in older adults compared to younger patients*	Cardiac evaluation and optimization in all patients
Radiation therapy (RT) [Multiple cancers]	CAD, aortic regurgitation, aortic stenosis, non-ischemic CM, pericardial disease Risk of cardiotoxicity increases with time from RT and increasing age [87]	Modification and toxicity management depend on dose and radiation field; consider intensity-modulated RT (IMRT) Avoid adjuvant RT for patients with breast cancer >70 years old [88]

Abbreviations: CAD, coronary artery disease; CGA, comprehensive geriatric assessment; CM, cardiomyopathy; CV, cardiovascular; CVD, cardiovascular disease; GEJ, gastroesophageal junction; GI, gastrointestinal; HF, heart failure; HTN, hypertension; IO, immunotherapy; LVEF, left ventricular ejection fraction; OA, older adults.

* Limited or no age-specific cardiotoxicity data available.

and cardiac ischemia as noted earlier. One kinase inhibitor with anti-VEGF properties, vandetanib, has a black box warning for torsades de pointes and sudden cardiac death [96]. Multikinase inhibitors can be associated with systemic and pulmonary hypertension, cardiac ischemia, arrhythmias, and thrombotic and bleeding complications [97]. Kinase inhibition has become a mainstay of treatment for chronic myeloid leukemia, and these therapies are prescribed as oral medications, perhaps raising the possibility that patients are seen less in an office setting. Thus, monitoring must be scheduled regularly to ensure early identification of cardiovascular toxicity.

ENDOCRINE THERAPIES

Often when treating prostate cancer, androgen deprivation therapy is implemented using agents such as darolutamide, apalutamide, and abiraterone. These agents are associated with increased risk of hypertension, coronary artery disease and acute coronary syndromes (ACS), and atrial fibrillation [98]. Other endocrine-based therapies, such as aromatase inhibitors used to treat certain breast cancers, raise the risk of heart failure, coronary artery disease, ACS, and venous thromboembolism [86].

IMMUNE CHECKPOINT INHIBITORS

Immune checkpoint inhibitors (ICIs) harness the body's immune system to target and bind to receptors on the surface of malignant cells, treating several different cancers including melanoma, lung cancers, and gastrointestinal cancers. Cardiotoxicity due to immune checkpoint inhibitors is distinctly different from cardiotoxicity of other chemotherapeutic agents, and the primary insult to the cardiovascular system is due to the immune-system activation and the overwhelming inflammatory response caused by the ICI [99]. Adverse events due to immune checkpoint inhibitors are common and reported in nearly 75% of patients, with severe, symptomatic adverse events occurring in 13%–23% [100]. In certain cancers, patients are prescribed dual immune checkpoint inhibition, a treatment associated with adverse events in upwards of 90% of patients, making the potential for cardiotoxicity higher than in patients treated with a single ICI [99]. The most worrisome cardiotoxic effect is myocarditis, occurring in under 2% of patients taking an ICI but with mortality rates as high as 50%. ICI myocarditis typically develops 1-2 months after initiation of therapy and leads to critical illness and severe cardiomyopathy. Immunosuppression with high doses of corticosteroids is the mainstay of treatment, but if the response is suboptimal, more aggressive forms of immunosuppression such as antithymocyte globulin, mycophenolate, and tocilizumab can be initiated. Additionally, less common cardiotoxicities associated with immune checkpoint inhibitors include supraventricular and ventricular arrhythmias, pericarditis, vasculitis, and acute coronary syndrome [101, 102].

CELLULAR THERAPY

The development of T-cell therapies such as chimeric antigen receptor T-cell (CAR-T), tumor-infiltrating lymphocyte (TIL), and bispecific T-cell engager (BITE) therapies aimed at altering a patient's immune cells to attack cancer cells has been monumental in cancer treatment. Though each with different mechanisms, this therapy stimulates a T-cell-mediated systemic immune response and often cytokine release syndrome (CRS). Mechanisms of cardiotoxicity are thought to be related to CRS and/or an inadvertent T-cell attack on an antigen other than its intended tumor antigen. Cardiotoxic effects can be variable, ranging from atrial arrhythmias and pericardial effusions to cardiomyopathy, heart failure, and sudden cardiac death. Typically, cardiotoxic effects are seen within 2–14 days after infusion with T-cell therapy and in patients with Grade 2–4 CRS, as defined by the American Society for Transplantation and Cellular Therapy [103].

RADIATION THERAPY AND CARDIOVASCULAR RISK

Radiation therapy is a key component of cancer treatment, used in over half of all cancer patients [104]. While it offers significant benefits, it also carries risks, particularly for cardiovascular health. Among cancer survivors, cardiovascular disease is the leading cause of noncancer-related death, with prior thoracic radiation substantially increasing this risk [105]. Patients with lymphoma, esophageal, breast, thymomas, and lung cancers are most vulnerable due to the heart's proximity to the radiation field [106]. Radiation can affect all cardiac structures, including the coronary arteries, valves, myocardium, and pericardium [107]. Recognizing and managing these complications are essential to optimizing patient outcomes.

Several factors influence the development of radiation-induced cardiovascular disease, including radiation dose, location, concurrent use of cardiotoxic chemotherapy, and preexisting heart conditions. Younger patients and women appear to be at higher risk [108]. Research has demonstrated a direct correlation between radiation dose and cardiovascular complications, with one study by Darby et al. reporting a 6.4% increase in coronary events per gray (Gy) unit of radiation [109]. Radiation exposure to the left breast, compared to the right, also significantly increases cardiovascular risk. Proper management of preexisting conditions—such as hypertension, hyperlipidemia, diabetes, smoking, and alcohol use—is crucial in patients undergoing radiation therapy [109]. For patients who have completed thoracic radiation therapy, initial screening transthoracic echocardiography is recommended to be done at 5–10 years after radiation based on the patient's risk level. High-risk patients are also recommended to have noninvasive coronary assessment 5–10 years after radiation exposure and every 5 years thereafter to assess for asymptomatic but clinically significant myocardial ischemia or scarring [110].

As cancer survival rates improve, awareness of radiation-induced cardiovascular disease is increasingly important. Early detection and aggressive management of cardiovascular risk factors are essential to improving outcomes in this high-risk population. Tailored strategies, including dose optimization, cardioprotective interventions, and long-term cardiac surveillance, are critical in mitigating radiation-associated cardiac complications.

Coronary artery disease

Coronary artery disease (CAD) is the most common radiation-related cardiovascular complication. Up to 85% of patients treated with thoracic radiation for Hodgkin's lymphoma develop CAD, with an average onset of 9 years post-treatment [111, 112]. This population also faces a 2.5-fold increased risk of fatal myocardial infarction [113]. Radiation-induced endothelial injury and inflammation accelerate stenosis and atherosclerosis, often resulting in diffuse, multivessel disease. These patients are generally poor candidates for coronary artery bypass grafting (CABG) due to fibrosis of graft vessels, atherosclerosis of the thoracic aorta, and impaired wound healing [114]. Studies indicate worse post-CABG outcomes, making percutaneous coronary intervention the preferred approach [110].

Pericardial disease

Pericardial complications are also common following thoracic radiation. Acute manifestations include pericardial effusion, cardiac tamponade, and pericarditis, while chronic effects include pericardial fibrosis, calcification, and pericardial constriction. Radiation-induced inflammation leads to collagen and fibrin deposition, causing pericardial stiffening. Impaired venous drainage can further contribute to effusion and tamponade [115]. A study of esophageal cancer patients found that 35% developed pericardial effusions, while autopsy reports suggest pericardial disease in up to 70% of those with prior thoracic radiation [116]. Many cases remain asymptomatic, suggesting the true prevalence may be underestimated [117].

Valvular heart disease

Aortic valve disease is another well-documented consequence of thoracic radiation. Chronic inflammation leads to thickening and fibrosis of the aortic valve, with regurgitation being more common than stenosis due to high-pressure circulation through a damaged valve [118]. While mild cases often require no intervention, severe aortic stenosis is best managed with transcatheter aortic valve replacement (TAVR) rather than surgical aortic valve replacement (SAVR), as per 2020 ACC/AHA guidelines, due to higher surgical mortality in this population [114, 119].

Conduction system disease

Radiation can also affect the heart's electrical conduction system, either through direct injury or secondary ischemia and fibrosis. More than 75% of patients exposed to >40 Gy of thoracic radiation develop electrocardiographic abnormalities, including prolonged QT intervals, sinus node dysfunction, atrioventricular block, or fascicular block [120]. While some may experience transient arrhythmias within the first year, permanent conduction defects often appear a decade after treatment, frequently in conjunction with coronary artery disease or cardiomyopathy [106].

Cardiomyopathy and heart failure

Radiation significantly increases the risk of nonischemic cardiomyopathy, affecting approximately 10% of patients who undergo radiation therapy [121]. High radiation doses lead to myocardial inflammation, injury, and fibrosis, resulting in ventricular stiffening and diastolic dysfunction. Additionally, radiation-induced endothelial damage and coronary stenosis can contribute to myocardial ischemia and cardiomyopathy [122]. Early management involves guideline-directed medical therapy (GDMT), while advanced cases may require heart transplantation. However, post-transplant survival is lower in these patients due to impaired wound healing and increased postoperative complications [123].

CARDIOVASCULAR CONSIDERATIONS BEFORE, DURING, AND AFTER CANCER TREATMENT

Cardiovascular screening before cancer treatment

Older adults with cancer often have concomitant clinical or subclinical cardiovascular disease due to shared risk factors. Identifying cardiovascular disease and risk for cardiovascular disease ahead of cancer treatment is imperative, especially in older adults, to properly inform care. Current guidelines recommend cardiovascular screening in all older adults undergoing cancer-directed treatment with the goal to target modifiable cardiovascular risk factors and establish baseline cardiovascular health ahead of potential cardiotoxic treatments using screening algorithms [11]. It is important to take a patient-centered and individualized approach when focusing on older adults (Figure 18.1).

For baseline risk stratification, all patients should undergo a comprehensive review of past medical history for risk factors that increase the risk of developing cardiotoxicities. The significance of each risk factor is based on the proposed treatment regimen. These risk factors include smoking history, elevated BMI, history of arrhythmia, heart failure, history of CAD, hyperlipidemia, hypertension, diabetes, and history of prior exposure to cancer treatment regimens. Full examination with vital signs and laboratory studies is necessary to evaluate the presence of risk factors and the degree of optimization necessary before cancer treatment [11]. As highlighted in Figure 18.1, these clinical variables need to be taken into consideration along with other aspects including frailty, polypharmacy, nutrition, and social support. In addition, collaboration between cardiologists and oncologists is central to patient care before, during, and after cancer therapy.

Attention to the cardiovascular physical examination is important to identify murmurs, elevation in jugular venous pressure, pulmonary crackles, or lower extremity edema. It is imperative for a 12-lead ECG to be performed ahead of cancer treatment as a screening tool for arrhythmias, potential structural heart disease, and measurement of the QTc interval [124].

Using information obtained during a baseline cardiovascular risk assessment can guide the need for further testing, such as an echocardiogram or ischemic evaluation, in patients with elevated risk factors or concerns for structural or valvular heart disease. This will be decided based on the patient risk factors and the proposed treatment regimen. An echocardiogram should include measurement of left ventricular ejection fraction as well as global longitudinal strain (GLS), a parameter utilizing

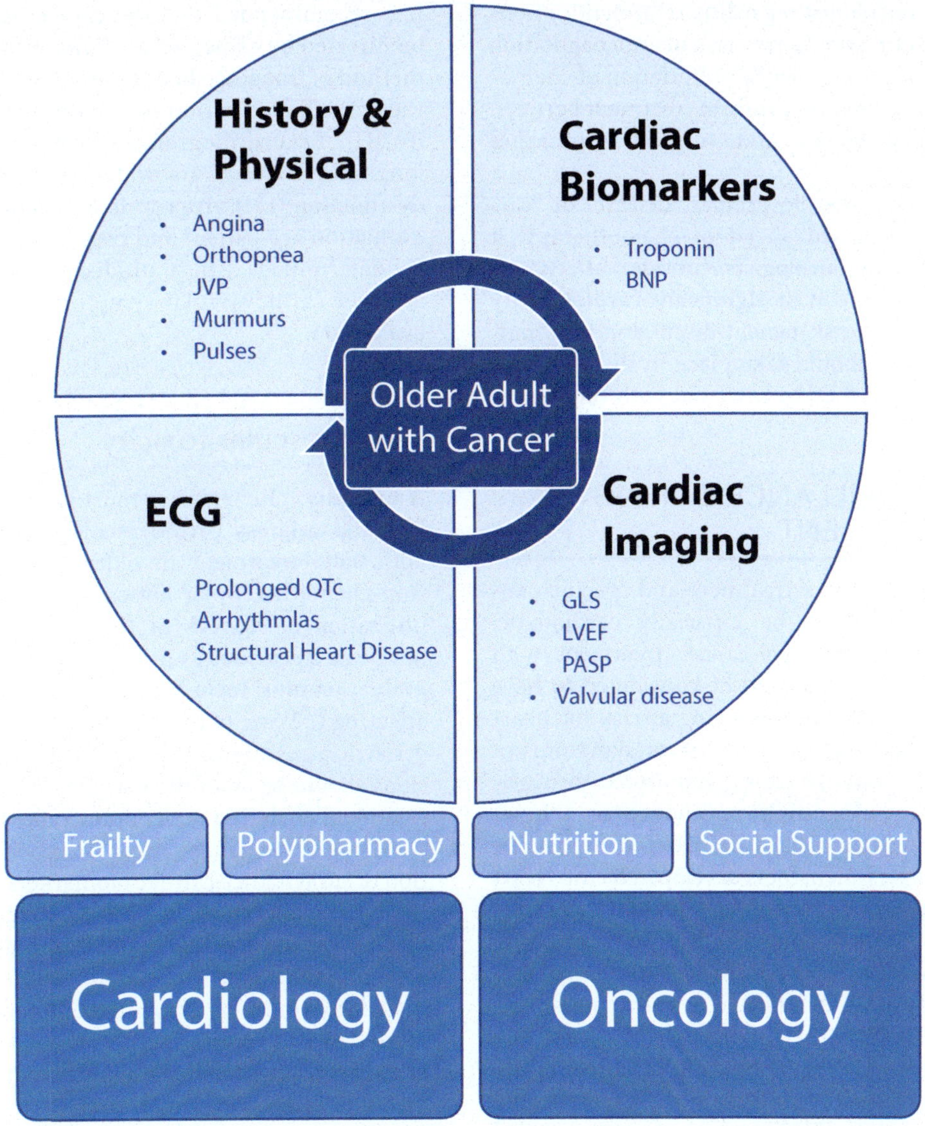

Figure 18.1 Cardiovascular evaluation in older patients undergoing treatment for cancer. *Abbreviations*: BNP, brain-natriuretic peptide; GLS, global longitudinal strain; JVP, jugular venous pressure; LVEF, left ventricular ejection fraction; PASP, pulmonary artery systolic pressure.

speckle tracking to quantify longitudinal shortening of left ventricular myocardium as a percentage when compared to baseline length. If technical limitations preclude assessment of these findings, cardiac magnetic resonance imaging (MRI) can be considered as an alternative. Patients expected to receive cancer treatments known to be cardiotoxic should undergo cardiac imaging with a transthoracic echocardiogram or cardiac MRI regardless of risk assessment. Additionally, it is recommended to obtain baseline cardiac biomarkers including high-sensitivity troponin and brain natriuretic peptide (or NT-proBNP) in patients with known cardiovascular disease and/or ahead of cardiotoxic chemotherapy [125].

Prior to initiation of cancer treatment that is known to be cardiotoxic in a patient deemed to have high cardiovascular risk, it is recommended to consider cardioprotective therapies [126]. For example, if screening identified elevated troponin or BNP prior to the initiation of a cardiotoxic chemotherapeutic agent, like anthracycline or anti-HER2 agents, there is evidence to suggest treatment with beta-blockers and angiotensin receptor blockers can mitigate further cardiac damage [126]. Evidence suggests that treatment with neurohormonal blockade in conjunction with anthracyclines can mitigate reductions in left ventricular ejection fraction, but further studies are ongoing to determine if this also translates to reduced incidence of clinical heart failure [11]. Alterations in the dosing, infusion rates, or coadministered medications may help to attenuate cardiac damage as well [11, 127].

Separate from routine screening noted earlier, patients who are symptomatic from a cardiovascular perspective should have an individualized treatment approach. For those with angina or valvular disease necessitating intervention, shared decision-making between patient, cardiologist, and oncologist regarding treatment options is imperative. Careful attention to risk of anticoagulation or antiplatelet agents and urgency of initiation of chemotherapy is needed, as that may inform treatment between percutaneous interventions and surgical approaches [124].

Should significant cardiovascular disease or cardiomyopathy be identified ahead of chemotherapy, it is recommended that oncologists consider alternative treatments without known or significant cardiotoxicity as first-line therapy. A risk–benefit discussion in a multidisciplinary setting should take place to discuss these options, which should then be reviewed with the patient in full transparency.

CARDIAC SURVEILLANCE DURING CANCER TREATMENT

As previously noted, cancer treatment and specific cancer-directed therapies can be especially cardiotoxic. Patients planning to undergo cancer treatment with known cardiotoxic effects should be considered to have Stage A heart failure, defined as being at risk for heart failure without structural heart disease or symptoms of heart failure, and should be closely monitored throughout treatment. Many older adults may have Stage B heart failure if structural changes like LVH are seen on baseline assessment. Risk assessment tools developed by the Heart Failure Association International Cardio-Oncology Society (HFA-ICOS) use patient-specific factors including prior cardiac history, age, chronic kidney disease, diabetes, and prior exposures, in addition to anticipated treatments to define risk [128, 129].

First and foremost, care focused on modifiable cardiovascular risk factors identified in the pretreatment phase must be maintained. This may include structured nutrition and exercise plans for those who are diabetic or obese, or monitoring of lipid-lowering therapy for those with elevated total cholesterol or low-density lipoprotein [126]. Similarly, common cardiovascular diseases like hypertension should be monitored for adequate control throughout cancer therapy.

Surveillance throughout cancer therapy is imperative for recognizing early signs or symptoms of developing cardiovascular disease. A careful history, physical exam, and cardiac serum biomarkers like BNP or NT-proBNP and troponin can help to identify cardiovascular disease early and enable treatment adjustments. Importantly, reference values for these biomarkers have not been identified in the context of chemotherapy or cancer-directed treatment and therefore interpretation of the results should be done with careful consideration of symptoms, physical exam, and other cardiovascular risk factors [130]. In addition, cardiac imaging plays a crucial role in serial monitoring of patients undergoing cancer treatment. Transthoracic echocardiography and cardiac MRI can help to identify and facilitate early cardiac diagnoses. It is recommended that the choice of imaging modality be directed by center accessibility and expertise and that method of imaging should remain consistent throughout the surveillance period to avoid intertechnique variability [11]. Echocardiograms should deploy use of global longitudinal strain to evaluate subclinical myocardial dysfunction [131]. Appropriate intervals between cardiac evaluation are patient and treatment specific and should be determined with multidisciplinary discussion, but any new cardiovascular symptom should prompt timely evaluation.

Diagnosis and management of cardiovascular toxicity

A multidisciplinary team must be implemented to identify and address cardiovascular complications during anticancer treatment in older adults. The decision to stop chemotherapy or anticancer treatments may mean utilization of second- or third-line therapies that may not be as efficacious as first-line therapies for cancer. The evaluation must include a holistic review of all the factors affecting the care of the patient through a comprehensive geriatric assessment. The risks and benefits of these decisions should be carefully considered in conjunction with treatment goals and patient preferences.

While undergoing cancer treatment, if the combination of surveillance cardiac biomarkers and cardiac imaging raises concern for subclinical cardiotoxicity, further assessment must be conducted. In older adults who are asymptomatic with only mild cardiotoxicity, it is suggested to continue anticancer therapy but implement more frequent screening intervals in addition to starting cardioprotective medications such as beta-blockers and/or angiotensin-converting enzyme (ACE) inhibitors or angiotensin receptor blockers (ARBs). This is dependent on the treatment regimen as anti-HER2 treatment regimen type 2 cardiotoxicities are more likely to be reversible compared to doxorubicin type 1. The ESC 2022 guidelines have identified an algorithm for resumption of treatment based on level of toxicity and agent used [11].

In patients with more severe or symptomatic cardiotoxicity, a multidisciplinary team should be involved to decide on appropriateness of interrupting anticancer therapy [11].

Specifically in older adults, development of cardiac disease while undergoing anticancer treatment may be attributable to cardiotoxic therapy, but it is imperative to consider more common forms of cardiovascular disease. For instance, new systolic dysfunction detected on a routine surveillance echocardiogram may be attributable to coronary artery disease in an older adult, or accelerating hypertension may be related to acute on chronic kidney disease. Given the complexities in managing older adults with comorbidities, it is imperative to have serial assessments by all members of a multidisciplinary team.

Cancer therapy-related cardiac dysfunction (CTRCD)

Cancer therapy-related cardiac dysfunction, or CTRCD, is a broad term aimed at capturing the variable presentations and etiologies of cardiomyopathy and cardiac injury in patients undergoing cancer treatment. Patients can have symptomatic or asymptomatic CTRCD and the range of symptoms combined with the severity of effect helps to determine next steps in oncologic and cardiac care. CTRCD is defined as a new elevation in cardiac biomarkers including troponin and natriuretic peptide, a decline in global longitudinal strain, or a decrease in LVEF with or without symptoms of heart failure [132]. In asymptomatic patients, severe CTRCD is defined as an LVEF less than 40%, while mild CTRCD is diagnosed when patients have an LVEF of >50% but a fall in GLS by >15% from their baseline and/or a rise in cardiac biomarkers. Those with moderate asymptomatic CTRCD will have a reduction in their LVEF with or without change in GLS or cardiac biomarkers. Symptomatic CTRCD is a clinical syndrome diagnosed when patients present with typical signs and symptoms of heart failure. Those with mild or moderate symptomatic CTRCD will have mild symptoms necessitating outpatient diuretic therapy or outpatient intensification of HF therapy, whereas those with severe or very severe CTRCD will be hospitalized perhaps even necessitating mechanical circulatory devices for support of cardiogenic shock [133].

Development of cardiomyopathy and systolic dysfunction are known side effects of several chemotherapeutic agents including anthracyclines and anti-HER2 therapies. Surveillance cardiac imaging either by transthoracic echocardiogram or cardiac MRI as noted previously can help to detect early manifestations of cardiotoxicity, while serial assessments by oncology and cardiology teams can detect development of heart failure symptoms.

In scenarios in which cardiomyopathy develops, severity of cardiotoxic effects and symptoms drive decisions to interrupt anticancer therapies. In the vast majority of cases of cancer treatment-related cardiotoxicity, it is subclinical or asymptomatic cardiomyopathy that is detected. In these scenarios, early initiation of guideline-directed medical therapy using beta-blockers, ACE inhibitors, ARBs, and mineralocorticoid antagonists is recommended to mitigate further cardiotoxic effects.

In all cases of symptomatic CTRCD, guideline-directed heart failure medications should be started including beta-blockers, RAAS inhibitors, mineralocorticoid antagonists, and SGLT-2 inhibitors. Generally, in severe cases of CTRCD in which patients are hospitalized due to heart failure symptoms, anticancer treatment, commonly anthracyclines, should be discontinued. In those with mild-moderate symptomatic CTRCD, multidisciplinary discussions should be held to determine the appropriateness of interruption of anticancer treatment. The decision to restart chemotherapy in patients with CTRCD can be considered after recovery of LVEF and improvement in symptoms with strategies in place to mitigate further cardiac damage including up-titration of GDMT and minimizing the dose of anticancer treatment. During reinitiation of treatment, patients should undergo cardiac evaluation after each session to ensure no signs or symptoms of heart failure develop.

IMMUNE CHECKPOINT INHIBITOR MYOCARDITIS

ICI myocarditis is a rare but potentially fatal cardiotoxicity that might first present with signs and symptoms of heart failure. In patients undergoing anti-cancer treatment with an immune checkpoint inhibitor, such as pembrolizumab, signs and symptoms of heart failure must raise suspicion for myocarditis [134]. Though rare, early detection and a high index of suspicion are key as immune checkpoint myocarditis is estimated to be fatal in over half of cases and can lead to cardiovascular events even after recovery [102]. ICI myocarditis is diagnosed in patients with heart failure symptoms, rise in cardiac troponin, and arrhythmias. After acute coronary syndrome and other etiologies of myocarditis are ruled out, the diagnosis of ICI myocarditis can be made. Diagnosis can be confirmed or further supported with cardiac imaging such as an echocardiogram or cardiac MRI, or even an endomyocardial biopsy when suspicion is high but alternative testing is inconclusive [135]. ICI myocarditis can present either as a fulminant or non-fulminant condition and in all cases requires discontinuation of ICI. In those with severe, hemodynamically unstable myocarditis, prompt treatment with high dose steroids is imperative with close monitoring in an intensive care unit. In rare cases, ICI myocarditis may be refractory to a 3-day course of steroids and the patient may progress to cardiogenic shock despite treatment, in which case mechanical circulatory support should be considered as well as second-line immunosuppressive agents such as mycophenolate, IV immunoglobulins, tocilizumab, or antithymocyte globulin [11]. In older adults receiving high-dose steroids, careful attention should be paid to potential side effects, including gastrointestinal bleeding and hyperglycemia [11]. After recovery, multidisciplinary discussions should be undertaken to decide on further treatment with immune checkpoint inhibitors. However, given its high fatality rate, resumption of ICI therapy is generally not recommended [136, 137].

HYPERTENSION

Cancer and hypertension often coexist in older adults, but hypertension can be exacerbated by anticancer therapies, namely, antiandrogens, anti-VEGF, and multikinase inhibitors [95, 97, 98]. Ongoing uncontrolled hypertension during cancer treatment is a risk factor for development of other cancer treatment-related cardiotoxicities like heart failure necessitating close monitoring and prompt treatment. The primary goal of treatment of hypertension is to prevent end-organ damage such as cardiomyopathy or renal dysfunction especially as development of these may limit cancer therapies. It is reasonable to use beta-blockers, ACE inhibitors, and ARBs as first-line agents to treat cancer therapy-related hypertension given the evidence that they may reduce incidence of cardiomyopathy, e.g., in patients being treated with anti-HER2 therapies [138]. In older adults specifically, diuretics should be prescribed with caution given considerable risk of dehydration with cancer-related early satiety, anorexia, and nausea and vomiting. Orthostatic vital signs should be monitored in older adults with these symptoms, and individually tailored approaches to hypertension management should consider risk of hypovolemia and orthostatic syncope.

CORONARY ARTERY DISEASE

Coronary artery disease is more prevalent in older adults due to accumulation of risk factors over several decades. In older adults undergoing anticancer treatment with cardiotoxic agents, development of coronary artery disease may be accelerated [139]. In older adults, symptoms of acute coronary syndrome can be atypical and include nausea, vomiting, or fatigue. In those undergoing anticancer treatment, especially with agents such as VEGF inhibitors or 5-FU, these symptoms may be masked or mistaken for side effects of the anticancer regimen; therefore, a high index of suspicion for acute coronary syndrome must be maintained in older adults presenting with new, vague symptoms.

Management of acute coronary syndromes can be challenging in older adults with cancer, especially considering common comorbid conditions like frailty. It is necessary to consider individual risk factors for anticoagulants and antiplatelets, in addition to patient preference in regard to invasive procedures, in those presenting with ACS. In older adults with good cancer prognosis and high-risk presentation of ST-elevation myocardial infarction (STEMI) or non-STEMI, it is reasonable to pursue percutaneous coronary intervention as studies have demonstrated overall reduction in major adverse cardiac events (MACE) [140]. Due to the potential for higher bleeding risk, especially in patients with gastrointestinal or hematologic cancers, careful attention to reduce necessary time on antiplatelet agents and anticoagulants is important when considering treatment of ACS. In select older adults with coronary artery disease necessitating coronary artery bypass grafting, a multidisciplinary approach is necessary, taking into consideration cancer prognosis, nutritional status, frailty, and social support to ensure optimal outcomes following major surgery.

After treatment and recovery following acute coronary syndrome, careful review of anticancer therapies should be conducted and possible offending agents or agents increasing thrombotic risk should be discontinued where appropriate in conjunction with the multidisciplinary cardio-oncology team. If ACS was thought to be provoked by an anticancer agent, such as 5-FU or an anti-VEGF agent, oncologists should consider alternative treatment agents as appropriate.

ARRHYTHMIAS

Atrial fibrillation is a common cardiac arrhythmia, increasing in prevalence with age, with approximately 50% of patients with atrial fibrillation being older than age 75. A cancer diagnosis increases the risk for development of atrial fibrillation perhaps due to shared risk factors, anticancer therapies including surgeries, autonomic nervous system imbalances, paraneoplastic syndromes, and chronic inflammation [141]. Important in the identification of atrial fibrillation in older adults with cancer is risk stratification for thromboembolic complications and bleeding. Traditional risk stratification tools like the CHA2DS2-VASc score have not been validated in older adults with cancer and do not include thrombotic risks associated with cancer diagnosis. Instead, older adults with cancer should be considered elevated risk for stroke and systemic embolic events and this should be weighed carefully against individualized bleeding risk, taking into consideration platelet count, type of malignancy, location of metastasis, renal function, and bleeding scores such as HAS-BLED. Importantly, patient preferences should play a key role as often bleeding risk factors and thrombotic risk factors coexist in these older adults [11].

PROLONGED QT

Prolonged QT and QTc intervals can increase the risk for ventricular arrhythmias, namely, polymorphic ventricular tachycardia, or torsades de pointes. Many medications and electrolyte abnormalities contribute to prolongation of QTc, including anticancer therapies like arsenic trioxide. In older adults undergoing cancer treatment, common side effects like nausea and vomiting can further exacerbate nutritional deficiencies leading to hypokalemia and hypomagnesemia. When treated with antiemetics like ondansetron, there is increased risk of dangerous QTc prolongation. When QTc prolongation greater than 500 ms is detected on surveillance ECG, a careful medication reconciliation is necessary to minimize and substitute for medications that have potential to increase QTc, and hospitalization for monitoring should be considered on a case-by-case basis [133]. Should QTc remain above 500 ms or if torsades de pointes is detected after addressing reversible causes, anticancer therapies known to prolong QTc should be interrupted, and multidisciplinary decision-making should be used to determine the best course of treatment [11].

CARDIAC IMPLANTABLE ELECTRONIC DEVICES (CIEDS)

It is estimated that greater than 50% of patients with cancer will undergo radiation therapy. Ionizing radiation can damage cardiac implantable electronic devices (CIEDs), which are present more often among older patients. Careful consideration should be taken prior to performing radiation therapy in patients with pacemakers or defibrillators [138]. Risks of radiation and electromagnetic interference include inappropriate pacing inhibition, leading to asystole, inappropriate antitachycardia therapies, and damage to CIEDs [142]. Patients should be evaluated by both an electrophysiologist and a radiation oncologist to determine patient- and treatment-specific risk. Patients who are pacemaker dependent, have an ICD, or are scheduled to undergo radiation ≥5 Gy at or near the site of implant are at elevated risk of device malfunction. Those at elevated risk should have careful cardiovascular monitoring during radiation therapy and regularly planned CIED interrogations throughout radiation treatment. In rare cases in which the risk of radiation is extremely high, relocation of the CIED can be considered by a multidisciplinary team [143].

PERIPHERAL ARTERIAL DISEASE (PAD)

Peripheral arterial disease (PAD) commonly affects older adults and certain anticancer treatments can provoke or worsen arterial disease. Treatments including radiation, VEGF inhibitors, and multikinase inhibitors have been demonstrated to lead to arterial remodeling, arterial stiffness, and development of PAD. Those with diabetes, chronic kidney disease, hypertension, or preexisting PAD are at the highest risk and should undergo pretreatment screening for PAD [11]. There is growing evidence to suggest that antiplatelet agents or anticoagulation should be considered for prevention of this complication in patients thought to be at elevated risk. In older adults with multiple comorbidities, it is even more important to consider antithrombotic agents as preventive strategies after carefully weighing risks of bleeding.

Peripheral arterial disease may present as neuropathy, lower extremity skin changes, or pain and claudication. The diagnosis can be made with noninvasive methods including arterial–brachial indices, and further evaluation can be pursued with computed tomography arteriography or invasive angiography. Peripheral arterial disease caused by anticancer treatments, such as tyrosine kinase inhibitors, can be rapidly progressive, preferentially affect small vessels in the lower extremities, and cause critical limb ischemia, necessitating urgent intervention with stenting or bypass [144]. In situations in which peripheral arterial disease is symptomatic and severe despite treatment, multidisciplinary discussions should be held to consider transition to an alternative anticancer agent, even within the same class with lesser risk of PAD [11].

SURGICAL PLANNING AND PREOPERATIVE CARDIAC EVALUATION

Cardiovascular risk assessment prior to noncardiac surgery falls under the risk assessment guidelines outlined by major medical societies including the ACC and AHA [145]. Risk stratification in older adults considers comorbid conditions, urgency of surgical intervention, exclusion of acute unstable cardiovascular conditions, and functional capacity and frailty of the patient [146]. Prior exposure to cardiotoxic cancer treatment is not included in risk scores; therefore, it is important for providers to take a careful history and make note of prior treatments to assess individual risks. In those with a prior history of radiation exposure to the chest, pre-test probability for coronary artery disease, valvular disease, and pericardial disease is higher, and therefore additional preoperative cardiac testing may be warranted to help inform risk. Older adults with limited functional capacity are at increased risk for perioperative cardiac events regardless of disability, but preoperative revascularization has not been efficacious in reducing risk of major adverse cardiovascular events such as heart attack, heart failure, stroke, or cardiac death [146]. Therefore, preoperative testing should be aimed at identifying those with signs or symptoms concerning for angina, severe valvular disease, or heart failure. In asymptomatic patients at elevated risk, serum biomarkers like BNP/NT pro-BNP are recommended to further stratify risk and inform need for further testing. Identification of prior cardiotoxic treatments and their effects, like anthracyclines and cardiomyopathy or radiation and valvular disease, can help inform providers of patient-specific risks, allowing individualized preoperative evaluation, usually in consultation with a cardiologist.

SURVIVORSHIP

Cardiovascular risk assessment at end of cancer therapy

At the completion of anti-cancer therapy, several factors indicate an increased risk for future cardiovascular disease. High-risk conditions include a high or very high baseline cardiovascular toxicity risk based on the HFA-ICOS assessment [129]. Specific anticancer treatments associated with a high risk of long-term cardiovascular complications include doxorubicin at a cumulative dose of ≥250 mg/m², radiation therapy (RT) with a mean heart dose (MHD) exceeding 15 Gy, or a combination of doxorubicin (≥100 mg/m²) and RT with an MHD between 5 and 15 Gy [147]. Other concerning factors include moderate or severe cancer therapy-related cardiovascular toxicity during treatment, particularly cancer therapy-related cardiac dysfunction, immune checkpoint inhibitor-related myocarditis, cardiac arrhythmias, or severe vascular toxicities such as acute coronary syndrome, stroke, or peripheral vascular disease [148]. Finally, new cardiovascular symptoms or newly detected asymptomatic abnormalities by echocardiography and/or cardiac serum biomarkers at the end of therapy also signal an increased risk for future cardiovascular disease [149].

All patients who have completed potentially cardiotoxic anticancer therapy should have a formal cardiovascular risk assessment within the first year after finishing treatment [11]. Risk assessment should include an updated assessment of left ventricular function and cardiac serum biomarkers including natriuretic peptide and troponin. Studies have demonstrated that elevations in cardiac biomarkers can predict those at risk for future cardiac events who may benefit from cardioprotective therapy and close follow-up with their cardiologist [130, 150]. Additionally, anthracycline-induced cardiomyopathy is usually discovered within 12 months after treatment completion, and those with preserved left ventricular function within 12 months are at lower risk of cardiomyopathy thereafter [149]. Those with prior cancer treatment-related cardiotoxicity and those with high-risk features at end-of-treatment reassessment are at high cardiovascular risk and require long-term cardiovascular follow-up and/or treatment.

Annual risk assessment to include ECG, cardiac biomarkers, and reassessment of new or worsening cardiac risk factors should be performed in all adults who received cardiotoxic therapy [11, 151, 152]. Long-term cancer survivorship is an emerging field with special implications among older adults. When managing older adults following cancer treatment, special attention should be paid to those at high risk in the first 5 years post-treatment, rather than risk over a much longer time horizon. Cancer survivors with high or very high baseline risk as defined by HFA-ICOS criteria are at risk for developing cardiotoxicity early on. Therefore, frequent monitoring by a multidisciplinary team should be implemented for these patients [129].

CONCLUSION

Cardiovascular disease and cancer share common biological pathways and risk factors, and the overlap between patients with cancer and cardiovascular disease is expected to increase, especially among older adults [153]. Therefore, development and implementation of a multidisciplinary approach to evaluation and care in these individuals is imperative to ensure the safety of their care, improve quality of life, manage comorbidities, and maximize survival. Assessment of cardiovascular risk of the patient in addition to awareness of the cardiovascular risk of the anticipated anticancer treatment is paramount to inform decisions on monitoring throughout treatment, while structured assessment and follow-up can help to identify evolving cardiovascular toxicities. As the population ages and advancements in cancer treatment and cardiovascular disease progress, geriatric cardio-oncology will become even more critical for the care of these patients.

GUIDELINE RECOMMENDATIONS

Adapted from the 2022 European Society of Cardiology Cardio-Oncology Guidelines [11]:

- Cancer patients share several common risk factors with cardiovascular disease, such as hypertension, diabetes, smoking, and obesity. These shared risk factors should be carefully managed to reduce both cancer treatment-related cardiotoxicity and the risk of cardiovascular events.
- Cardiotoxicity from chemotherapy agents such as anthracyclines, trastuzumab, and others should be anticipated, and cardiac monitoring should be performed throughout the treatment course to detect early signs of heart failure, with dosage adjustments, initiation of guideline-directed medical therapy, and treatment modifications implemented as needed.
- Long-term survivors of cancer, particularly those who have received cardiotoxic therapies, should undergo regular cardiac surveillance with clinical assessment and imaging, such as echocardiography or magnetic resonance imaging as indicated, to monitor for late-onset cardiotoxicity.

REFERENCES

1. Goyal, P., et al., Geriatric cardiology: coming of age. *JACC Adv*, 2022 Aug 26. **1**(3): 100070. doi: 10.1016/j.jacadv.2022.100070.
2. Vespa, J.E., D.M. Armstrong, and L. Medina, *Demographic turning points for the United States: population projections for 2020 to 2060*. US Department of Commerce, Economics and Statistics Administration, 2018.
3. Martin, S.S., et al., 2025 heart disease and stroke statistics: a report of US and global data from the American Heart Association. *Circulation*, 2025. **15**(8): p. e41–e660. https://doi.org/10.1161/CIR.0000000000001303
4. Siegel, R.L., et al., Cancer statistics, 2023. *CA Cancer J Clin*, 2023. **73**(1): p. 17–48.
5. Sung, H., et al., Global cancer statistics 2020: GLOBOCAN estimates of incidence and mortality worldwide for 36 cancers in 185 countries. *CA Cancer J Clin*, 2021. **71**(3): p. 209–49.
6. Paneni, F., et al., The aging cardiovascular system: understanding it at the cellular and clinical levels. *J Am Coll Cardiol*, 2017. **69**(15): p. 1952–67.
7. Koene, R.J., et al., Shared risk factors in cardiovascular disease and cancer. *Circulation*, 2016. **133**(11): p. 1104–14.

8. Liberale, L., et al., Inflammation, aging, and cardiovascular disease: JACC review topic of the week. *J Am Coll Cardiol*, 2022. **79**(8): p. 837–47.
9. Khan, S.S., et al., Novel prediction equations for absolute risk assessment of total cardiovascular disease incorporating cardiovascular-kidney-metabolic health: a scientific statement from the American Aeart Association. *Circulation*, 2023. **148**(24): p. 1982–2004.
10. Kalaoja, M., et al., The role of inflammatory cytokines as intermediates in the pathway from increased adiposity to disease. *Obesity (Silver Spring)*, 2021. **29**(2): p. 428–37.
11. Lyon, A.R., et al., 2022 ESC guidelines on cardio-oncology developed in collaboration with the European Hematology Association (EHA), the European Society for Therapeutic Radiology and Oncology (ESTRO) and the International Cardio-Oncology Society (IC-OS). *Eur Heart J*, 2022. **43**(41): p. 4229–361.
12. Islami, F., et al., National and state estimates of lost earnings from cancer deaths in the United States. *JAMA Oncol*, 2019. **5**(9): p. e191460.
13. Arnold, M., et al., Global burden of 5 major types of gastrointestinal cancer. *Gastroenterology*, 2020. **159**(1): p. 335–49 e15.
14. Aidoud, A., et al., High prevalence of geriatric conditions among older adults with cardiovascular disease. *J Am Heart Assoc*, 2023. **12**(2): p. e026850.
15. Wildiers, H., et al., International society of geriatric oncology consensus on geriatric assessment in older patients with cancer. *J Clin Oncol*, 2014. **32**(24): p. 2595–603.
16. Dotan, E., et al., NCCN Clinical Practical Guidelines in Oncology®: older adult oncology, version 1.2025. *J Natl Compr Canc Netw*, 2025. **19**(9): p. 1006–19. https://doi.org/10.6004/jnccn.2021.0043.
17. Dale, W., et al., Practical assessment and management of vulnerabilities in older patients receiving systemic cancer therapy: ASCO guideline update. *J Clin Oncol*, 2023. **41**(26): p. 4293–312.
18. Verweij, N.M., et al., Physical performance measures for predicting outcome in cancer patients: a systematic review. *Acta Oncologica*, 2016. **55**(12): p. 1386–91.
19. Katz, S., et al., Studies of illness in the aged: the index of ADL: a standardized measure of biological and psychosocial function. *JAMA*, 1963. **185**(12): p. 914–19.
20. Lawton, M.P. and E.M. Brody, Assessment of older people: self-maintaining and instrumental activities of daily living. *Gerontologist*, 1969. **9**(3): p. 179–86.
21. Almugbel, F.A., et al., The role of grip strength and short physical performance battery test in predicting chemotherapy-related outcomes in older adults with cancer. *J Geriatr Oncol*, 2022. **13**(3): p. 318–24.
22. Podsiadlo, D. and S. Richardson, The timed "Up & Go": a test of basic functional mobility for frail elderly persons. *J Am Geriatr Soc*, 1991. **39**(2): p. 142–8.
23. Extermann, M., Measuring comorbidity in older cancer patients. *Eur J Cancer*, 2000. **36**(4): p. 453–71.
24. Miller, M.G., et al., Identifying potentially inappropriate medication (PIM) use in geriatric oncology. *J Geriatr Oncol*, 2021. **12**(1): p. 34–40.
25. 2023 American Geriatrics Society Beers Criteria Update Expert Panel, American Geriatrics Society 2023 updated AGS Beers Criteria® for potentially inappropriate medication use in older adults. *J Am Geriatr Soc*, 2023. **71**(7): p. 2052–81.
26. Magnuson, A., S. Mohile, and M. Janelsins, Cognition and cognitive impairment in older adults with cancer. *Curr Geriatr Rep*, 2016. **5**(3): p. 213–19.
27. Balducci, L. and M. Extermann, Management of cancer in the older person: a practical approach. *Oncologist*, 2000. **5**(3): p. 224–37.
28. Bower, J.E., et al., Management of fatigue in adult survivors of cancer: ASCO–society for integrative oncology guideline update. *J Clin Oncol*, 2024. **42**(20): p. 2456–87.
29. Wei, L.A., et al., The confusion assessment method: a systematic review of current usage. *J Am Geriatr Soc*, 2008. **56**(5): p. 823–30.
30. Kadambi, S., et al., Social support for older adults with cancer: young international society of geriatric oncology review paper. *J Geriatr Oncol*, 2020. **11**(2): p. 217–24.
31. Riba, M.B., et al., NCCN Clinical Practical Guidelines in Oncology®: distress management, version 1.2025. *J Natl Compr Canc Netw*, 2025.
32. Bellera, C.A., et al., Screening older cancer patients: first evaluation of the G-8 geriatric screening tool. *Ann Oncol*, 2012. **23**(8): p. 2166–72.
33. Hurria, A., et al., Predicting chemotherapy toxicity in older adults with cancer: a prospective multicenter study. *J Clin Oncol*, 2011. **29**(25): p. 3457–65.
34. Extermann, M., et al., Predicting the risk of chemotherapy toxicity in older patients: the Chemotherapy Risk Assessment Scale for High-Age Patients (CRASH) score. *Cancer*, 2012. **118**(13): p. 3377–86.
35. Hurria A, Mohile S, Gajra A, et al. Validation of a Prediction Tool for Chemotherapy Toxicity in Older Adults With Cancer. *J Clin Oncol*. 2016;34(20):2366-2371. doi:10.1200/JCO.2015.65.4327.
36. Oken, M.M., et al., Toxicity and response criteria of the Eastern Cooperative Oncology Group. *Am J Clin Oncol*, 1982. **5**(6): p. 649–55.
37. Sedrak, M.S., et al., Older adult participation in cancer clinical trials: a systematic review of barriers and interventions. *CA Cancer J Clin*, 2021. **71**(1): p. 78–92.
38. Celis, E.S.P.D., et al., Patient-defined goals and preferences among older adults with cancer starting chemotherapy (CT). *J Clin Oncol*, 2018. **36**(15_suppl): p. 10009.

39. Paillaud, E., et al., Optimal management of elderly cancer patients: usefulness of the comprehensive geriatric assessment. *Clin Interv Aging*, 2014. **9**: p. 1645–60. https://doi.org/10.2147/CIA.S57849.
40. Broderick, J.M., et al., Patients over 65 years are assigned lower ECOG PS scores than younger patients, although objectively measured physical activity is no different. *J Geriatr Oncol*, 2014. **5**(1): p. 49–56.
41. Williams, G.R., et al., Comorbidity in older adults with cancer. *J Geriatr Oncol*, 2016. **7**(4): p. 249–57.
42. Lee, L., et al., Impact of comorbidity on chemotherapy use and outcomes in solid tumors: a systematic review. *J Clin Oncol*, 2011. **29**(1): p. 106–17.
43. Sharma, M., et al., Polypharmacy and potentially inappropriate medication use in geriatric oncology. *J Geriatr Oncol*, 2016. 7(5): p. 346–53.
44. Magnuson, A., et al., Cognitive function in older adults with cancer: assessment, management, and research opportunities. *J Clin Oncol*, 2021. **39**(19): p. 2138–49.
45. Mohile, S.G., et al., Association of cancer with geriatric syndromes in older Medicare beneficiaries. *J Clin Oncol*, 2011. **29**(11): p. 1458–64.
46. Magnuson, A., et al., A practical guide to geriatric syndromes in older adults with cancer: a focus on falls, cognition, polypharmacy, and depression. *Am Soc Clin Oncol Educ Book*, 2019. **39**: p. e96–e109.
47. Meza-Valderrama, D., et al., Sarcopenia, malnutrition, and cachexia: adapting definitions and terminology of nutritional disorders in older people with cancer. *Nutrients*, 2021. **13**(3).
48. Paillaud, E., et al., Geriatric syndromes increased the nutritional risk in elderly cancer patients independently from tumour site and metastatic status. The ELCAPA-05 cohort study. *Clin Nutr*, 2014. **33**(2): p. 330–5.
49. Presley, C.J., et al., Gaps in nutritional research among older adults with cancer. *J Geriatr Oncol*, 2016. **7**(4): p. 281–92.
50. Hurria, A., et al., Distress in older patients with cancer. *J Clin Oncol*, 2009. **27**(26): p. 4346–51.
51. Kumar Pal, S., V. Katheria, and A. Hurria, Evaluating the older patient with cancer: understanding frailty and the geriatric assessment. *CA Cancer J Clin*, 2010. **60**(2): p. 120–32.
52. Canoui-Poitrine, F., et al., Geriatric assessment findings independently associated with clinical depression in 1092 older patients with cancer: the ELCAPA cohort study. *Psychooncology*, 2016. **25**(1): p. 104–11.
53. Magnuson, A., et al., Geriatric assessment for the practicing clinician: the why, what, and how. *CA Cancer J Clin*, 2024. **74**(6): p. 496–518.
54. Dale, W., et al., How is geriatric assessment used in clinical practice for older adults with cancer? A survey of cancer providers by the American Society of Clinical Oncology. *JCO Oncol Pract*, 2021. **17**(6): p. 336–44.
55. Extermann, M., et al., Predicting the risk of chemotherapy toxicity in older patients: the Chemotherapy Risk Assessment Scale for High-Age Patients (CRASH) score. *Cancer*, 2012. **118**(13): p. 3377–86.
56. Gilchrist, S.C., et al., Cardio-oncology rehabilitation to manage cardiovascular outcomes in cancer patients and survivors: a scientific statement from the American Heart Association. *Circulation*, 2019. **139**(21): p. e997–e1012.
57. Groarke, J.D., et al., Association of post-diagnosis cardiorespiratory fitness with cause-specific mortality in cancer. *Eur Heart J Qual Care Clin Outcomes*, 2020. **6**(4): p. 315–22.
58. Fardman, A., et al., Cardiorespiratory fitness and survival following cancer diagnosis. *Eur J Prev Cardiol*, 2021. **28**(11): p. 1242–49.
59. Smarż, K., et al., Cardiopulmonary exercise testing in adult cardiology: expert opinion of the Working Group of Cardiac Rehabilitation and Exercise Physiology of the Polish Cardiac Society. *Kardiol Pol (Polish Heart Journal)*, 2019. **77**(7–8): p. 730–56.
60. Wilson, R.L., et al., Incorporating exercise training into cardio-oncology care: current evidence and opportunities: JACC: CardioOncology state-of-the-art review. *JACC CardioOncol*, 2023. **5**(5): p. 553–69.
61. Peterson, B.M., University of Northern Colorado Cancer Rehabilitation Institute treadmill protocol accurately measures VO2peak in cancer survivors. *Int J Phys Med Rehabil*, 2017. **5**(6): p. 1.
62. Morelli, M.B., et al., Cardiotoxicity of anticancer drugs: molecular mechanisms and strategies for cardioprotection. *Front Cardiovasc Med*, 2022. **9**: p. 847012.
63. Du, X.L., et al., Cardiac toxicity associated with anthracycline-containing chemotherapy in older women with breast cancer. *Cancer*, 2009. **115**(22): p. 5296–308.
64. Sanft, T., et al., NCCN guidelines® insights: survivorship, version 1.2023. *J Natl Compr Canc Netw*, 2023. **21**(8): p. 792–803. https://doi.org/10.6004/jnccn.2023.0041.
65. Gil-Gil, M.J., et al., Long-term cardiac safety and survival outcomes of neoadjuvant pegylated liposomal doxorubicin in elderly patients or prone to cardiotoxicity and triple negative breast cancer. Final results of the multicentre phase II CAPRICE study. *Front Oncol*, 2021. **11**: p. 645026.
66. Coltelli, L., et al., Cardiac safety of adjuvant non-pegylated liposomal doxorubicin combined with cyclophosphamide and followed by paclitaxel in older breast cancer patients. *The Breast*, 2017. **31**: p. 186–91.
67. Polk, A., et al., Cardiotoxicity in cancer patients treated with 5-fluorouracil or capecitabine: a systematic review of incidence, manifestations and predisposing factors. *Cancer Treat Rev*, 2013. **39**(8): p. 974–84.

68. Cunningham, D., et al., Bevacizumab plus capecitabine versus capecitabine alone in elderly patients with previously untreated metastatic colorectal cancer (AVEX): an open-label, randomised phase 3 trial. *Lancet Oncol*, 2013. **14**(11): p. 1077–85.
69. Lonardi, S., et al., Initial panitumumab plus FOLFOX or 5-FU/LV in elderly patients with RAS and BRAF wild-type metastatic colorectal cancer: the PANDA trial by GONO Foundation. *J Clin Oncol*, 2023. **41**(34): p. 5263–73. https://doi.org/10.1200/JCO.23.00506.
70. Antonio, M., et al., Geriatric assessment predicts survival and competing mortality in elderly patients with early colorectal cancer: can it help in adjuvant therapy decision-making? *The Oncologist*, 2017. **22**(8): p. 934–43.
71. Lund, C.M., et al., The effect of geriatric intervention in frail older patients receiving chemotherapy for colorectal cancer: a randomised trial (GERICO). *Br J Cancer*, 2021. **124**(12): p. 1949–58.
72. Advani, P.P., et al., Long-term cardiac safety analysis of NCCTG N9831 (alliance) adjuvant trastuzumab trial. *J Clin Oncol*, 2016. **34**(6): p. 581–7.
73. Guglin, M., et al., Randomized trial of lisinopril versus carvedilol to prevent trastuzumab cardiotoxicity in patients with breast cancer. *J Am Coll Cardiol*, 2019. **73**(22): p. 2859–68.
74. Blaes, A., C. Manisty, and A. Barac, How to follow, manage and treat cardiac dysfunction in patients with Her2+ breast cancer. *JACC CardioOncol*, 2020. *2*(4): p. 661–5.
75. Swain, S.M., et al., Pertuzumab, trastuzumab, and docetaxel for HER2-positive metastatic breast cancer (CLEOPATRA): end-of-study results from a double-blind, randomised, placebo-controlled, phase 3 study. *Lancet Oncol*, 2020. **21**(4): p. 519–30.
76. Miles, D., et al., Treatment of older patients with HER2-positive metastatic breast cancer with pertuzumab, trastuzumab, and docetaxel: subgroup analyses from a randomized, double-blind, placebo-controlled phase III trial (CLEOPATRA). *Breast Cancer Res Treat*, 2013. **142**(1): p. 89–99.
77. Barrios, C.H., et al., Safety of trastuzumab emtansine (T-DM1) in 373 patients 65 years or older with HER2-positive advanced breast cancer: a subgroup analysis of the Kamilla study. *J Clin Oncol*, 2015. **33**(15_suppl): p. 603–3.
78. Cortés, J., et al., Trastuzumab deruxtecan versus trastuzumab emtansine for breast cancer. *N Engl J Med*, 2022. **386**(12): p. 1143–54.
79. Modi, S., et al., Trastuzumab deruxtecan in previously treated HER2-low advanced breast cancer. *N Engl J Med*, 2022. **387**(1): p. 9–20.
80. Bair, S.M., T.K. Choueiri, and J. Moslehi, Cardiovascular complications associated with novel angiogenesis inhibitors: emerging evidence and evolving perspectives. *Trends Cardiovasc Med*, 2013. **23**(4): p. 104–13.
81. Sclafani, F. and D. Cunningham, Bevacizumab in elderly patients with metastatic colorectal cancer. *J Geriatr Oncol*, 2014. **5**(1): p. 78–88.
82. Amadio, G., et al., ToleRability of BevacizUmab in elderly Ovarian cancer patients (TURBO study): a case-control study of a real-life experience. *J Gynecol Oncol*, 2020. **31**(1): p. e6. https://doi.org/10.3802/jgo.2020.31.e6.
83. Chi, K.N., et al., Apalutamide for metastatic, castration-sensitive prostate cancer. *N Engl J Med*, 2019. **381**(1): p. 13–24.
84. Fizazi, K., et al., Darolutamide in nonmetastatic, castration-resistant prostate cancer. *N Engl J Med*, 2019. **380**(13): p. 1235–46.
85. Iacovelli, R., et al., The cardiovascular toxicity of abiraterone and enzalutamide in prostate cancer. *Clin Genitourin Cancer*, 2018. **16**(3): p. e645–53.
86. Khosrow-Khavar, F., et al., Aromatase inhibitors and the risk of cardiovascular outcomes in women with breast cancer. *Circulation*, 2020. **141**(7): p. 549–59.
87. Darby, S.C., et al., Risk of ischemic heart disease in women after radiotherapy for breast cancer. *N Engl J Med*, 2013. **368**(11): p. 987–98.
88. Kunkler, I.H., et al., Breast-conserving surgery with or without irradiation in early breast cancer. *N Engl J Med*, 2023. **388**(7): p. 585–94.
89. Cardinale, D., et al., Left ventricular dysfunction predicted by early troponin I release after high-dose chemotherapy. *J Am Coll Cardiol*, 2000. **36**(2): p. 517–22.
90. Camilli, M., et al., Anthracycline cardiotoxicity in adult cancer patients: *JACC: CardioOncology* state-of-the-art review. *JACC CardioOncol*, 2024. **6**(5): p. 655–77.
91. Cardinale, D., F. Iacopo, and C.M. Cipolla, Cardiotoxicity of anthracyclines. *Front Cardiovasc Med*, 2020. **7**: p. 26.
92. Polk, A., et al., Cardiotoxicity in cancer patients treated with 5-fluorouracil or capecitabine: a systematic review of incidence, manifestations and predisposing factors. *Cancer Treat Rev*, 2013. **39**(8): p. 974–84.
93. Chavez-MacGregor, M., et al., Trastuzumab-related cardiotoxicity among older patients with breast cancer. *J Clin Oncol*, 2013. **31**(33): p. 4222–8.
94. Chen, J., et al., Incidence of heart failure or cardiomyopathy after adjuvant trastuzumab therapy for breast cancer. *J Am Coll Cardiol*, 2012. **60**(24): p. 2504–12.

95. Touyz, R.M. and J. Herrmann, Cardiotoxicity with vascular endothelial growth factor inhibitor therapy. *NPJ Precis Oncol*, 2018. **2**: p. 13.
96. CAPRELSA (vandetanib) [package insert]. Cambridge, MA: Genzyme Corporation, 2022.
97. Shyam Sunder, S., U.C. Sharma, and S. Pokharel, Adverse effects of tyrosine kinase inhibitors in cancer therapy: pathophysiology, mechanisms and clinical management. *Signal Transduct Target Ther*, 2023. **8**(1): p. 262.
98. Hu, J.R., et al., Cardiovascular effects of androgen deprivation therapy in prostate cancer: contemporary meta-analyses. *Arterioscler Thromb Vasc Biol*, 2020. **40**(3): p. e55–e64.
99. Brahmer, J.R., et al., Society for Immunotherapy of Cancer (SITC) clinical practice guideline on immune checkpoint inhibitor-related adverse events. *J Immunother Cancer*, 2021. 9(6): p. e002435. https://doi.org/10.1136/jitc-2021-002435.
100. Ball, S., et al., Cardiovascular toxicities of immune checkpoint inhibitors: JACC review topic of the week. *J Am Coll Cardiol*, 2019. **74**(13): p. 1714–27.
101. Achim, A., K. Liblik, and S. Gevaert, Immune checkpoint inhibitors – the revolutionary cancer immunotherapy comes with a cardiotoxic price. *Trends Cardiovasc Med*, 2024. **34**(2): p. 71–77.
102. Dolladille, C., et al., Late cardiac adverse events in patients with cancer treated with immune checkpoint inhibitors. *J Immunother Cancer*, 2020. **8**(1): p. e000261. https://doi.org/10.1136/jitc-2019-000261.
103. Ganatra, S., et al., Cardiotoxicity of T-cell antineoplastic therapies. *JACC CardioOncol*, 2022. **4**(5): p. 616–23.
104. Groarke, J.D., et al., Cardiovascular complications of radiation therapy for thoracic malignancies: the role for non-invasive imaging for detection of cardiovascular disease. *Eur Heart J*, 2014. **35**(10): p. 612–23.
105. Ramin, C., et al., All-cause and cardiovascular disease mortality among breast cancer survivors in CLUE II, a long-standing community-based cohort. *J Natl Cancer Inst*, 2021. **113**(2): p. 137–45.
106. Hufnagle, J.J., S.N. Andersen, and E.V. Maani, *Radiation-induced cardiac toxicity*. Treasure Island (FL): StatPearls, 2025.
107. Belzile-Dugas, E. and M.J. Eisenberg, Radiation-induced cardiovascular disease: review of an underrecognized pathology. *J Am Heart Assoc*, 2021. **10**(18): p. e021686.
108. Khalid, Y., et al., Gender disparity in cardiovascular mortality following radiation therapy for Hodgkin's lymphoma: a systematic review. *Cardiooncology*, 2020. **6**: p. 12. https://doi.org/10.1186/s40959-020-00067-7.
109. Darby, S.C., et al., Risk of ischemic heart disease in women after radiotherapy for breast cancer. *N Engl J Med*, 2013. **368**(11): p. 987–98.
110. Donnellan, E., et al., Radiation-induced heart disease: a practical guide to diagnosis and management. *Cleve Clin J Med*, 2016. **83**(12): p. 914–22.
111. Chang, H.M., et al., Cardiovascular complications of cancer therapy: best practices in diagnosis, prevention, and management: part 2. *J Am Coll Cardiol*, 2017. **70**(20): p. 2552–65.
112. Hull, M.C., et al., Valvular dysfunction and carotid, subclavian, and coronary artery disease in survivors of Hodgkin lymphoma treated with radiation therapy. *JAMA*, 2003. **290**(21): p. 2831–7.
113. Heidenreich, P.A., et al., Diastolic dysfunction after mediastinal irradiation. *Am Heart J*, 2005. **150**(5): p. 977–82.
114. Wu, W., et al., Long-term survival of patients with radiation heart disease undergoing cardiac surgery: a cohort study. *Circulation*, 2013. **127**(14): p. 1476–85.
115. Veinot, J.P. and W.D. Edwards, Pathology of radiation-induced heart disease: a surgical and autopsy study of 27 cases. *Hum Pathol*, 1996. **27**(8): p. 766–73.
116. Fukada, J., et al., Symptomatic pericardial effusion after chemoradiation therapy in esophageal cancer patients. *Int J Radiat Oncol Biol Phys*, 2013. **87**(3): p. 487–93.
117. Ghosh, A.K., et al., Pericardial disease in cancer patients. *Curr Treat Options Cardiovasc Med*, 2018. **20**(7): p. 60.
118. Lee, P.J. and R. Mallik, Cardiovascular effects of radiation therapy: practical approach to radiation therapy-induced heart disease. *Cardiol Rev*, 2005. **13**(2): p. 80–6.
119. Zhang, D., et al., Outcomes of patients with severe symptomatic aortic valve stenosis after chest radiation: transcatheter versus surgical aortic valve replacement. *J Am Heart Assoc*, 2019. **8**(10): p. e012110.
120. Adams, M.J., et al., Radiation-associated cardiovascular disease. *Crit Rev Oncol Hematol*, 2003. **45**(1): p. 55–75.
121. Belzile-Dugas, E. and M.J. Eisenberg, Radiation-induced cardiovascular disease: review of an underrecognized pathology. *J Am Heart Assoc*, 2021. **10**(18): p. e021686.
122. Liu, X.C. and P.K. Zhou, Tissue reactions and mechanism in cardiovascular diseases induced by radiation. *Int J Mol Sci*, 2022. *23*(23): p. 14786. https://doi.org/10.3390/ijms232314786.
123. Al-Kindi, S.G. and G.H. Oliveira, Heart transplantation outcomes in radiation-induced restrictive cardiomyopathy. *J Card Fail*, 2016. **22**(6): p. 475–8.
124. Raisi-Estabragh, Z., et al., Cardiovascular considerations before cancer therapy: gaps in evidence and JACC: CardioOncology expert panel recommendations. *JACC CardioOncol*, 2024. **6**(5): p. 631–54.

125. Ioffe, D., et al., Cardiovascular concerns, cancer treatment, and biological and chronological aging in cancer: JACC family series. *JACC CardioOncol*, 2024. **6**(2): p. 143–58.
126. Omland, T., S.L. Heck, and G. Gulati, The role of cardioprotection in cancer therapy cardiotoxicity: JACC: CardioOncology state-of-the-art review. *JACC CardioOncol*, 2022. **4**(1): p. 19–37.
127. Shapira, J., et al., Reduced cardiotoxicity of doxorubicin by a 6-hour infusion regimen. A prospective randomized evaluation. *Cancer*, 1990. **65**(4): p. 870–3.
128. Battisti, N.M.L., et al., Incidence of cardiotoxicity and validation of the heart failure association-international cardio-oncology society risk stratification tool in patients treated with trastuzumab for HER2-positive early breast cancer. *Breast Cancer Res Treat*, 2021. **188**: p. 149–63.
129. Lyon, A.R., et al., Baseline cardiovascular risk assessment in cancer patients scheduled to receive cardiotoxic cancer therapies: a position statement and new risk assessment tools from the Cardio-Oncology Study Group of the Heart Failure Association of the European Society of Cardiology in collaboration with the International Cardio-Oncology Society. *Eur J Heart Fail*, 2020. **22**(11): p. 1945–60.
130. Pudil, R., et al., Role of serum biomarkers in cancer patients receiving cardiotoxic cancer therapies: a position statement from the Cardio-Oncology Study Group of the Heart Failure Association and the Cardio-Oncology Council of the European Society of Cardiology. *Eur J Heart Fail*, 2020. **22**(11): p. 1966–83.
131. Liu, J.E., et al., Strain imaging in cardio-oncology. *JACC CardioOncol*, 2020. **2**(5): p. 677–89.
132. Mecinaj, A., et al., Impact of the ESC cardio-oncology guidelines biomarker criteria on incidence of cancer therapy–related cardiac dysfunction. *JACC CardioOncol*, 2024. 6(1): p. 83–95.
133. Herrmann, J., et al., Defining cardiovascular toxicities of cancer therapies: an International Cardio-Oncology Society (IC-OS) consensus statement. *Eur Heart J*, 2022. **43**(4): p. 280–99.
134. Salem, J.E., et al., Cardiovascular toxicities associated with immune checkpoint inhibitors: an observational, retrospective, pharmacovigilance study. *Lancet Oncol*, 2018. **19**(12): p. 1579–89.
135. Palaskas, N.L., et al., Immune checkpoint inhibitor myocarditis: elucidating the spectrum of disease through endomyocardial biopsy. *Eur J Heart Fail*, 2021. **23**(10): p. 1725–35.
136. Dolladille, C., et al., Immune checkpoint inhibitor rechallenge after immune-related adverse events in patients with cancer. *JAMA Oncol*, 2020. **6**(6): p. 865–71.
137. Thuny, F., et al., Management of immune checkpoint inhibitor-induced myocarditis: the french working group's plea for a pragmatic approach. *JACC CardioOncol*, 2021. **3**(1): p. 157–61.
138. Yeh, E.T. and C.L. Bickford, Cardiovascular complications of cancer therapy: incidence, pathogenesis, diagnosis, and management. *J Am Coll Cardiol*, 2009. **53**(24): p. 2231–47.
139. Zhou, F., et al., Coronary atherosclerosis and chemotherapy: from bench to bedside. *Front Cardiovasc Med*, 2023. **10**: p. 1118002.
140. Mohamed, M.O., et al., Effect of primary percutaneous coronary intervention on in-hospital outcomes among active cancer patients presenting with ST-elevation myocardial infarction: a propensity score matching analysis. *Eur Heart J Acute Cardiovasc Care*, 2021. **10**(8): p. 829–39.
141. Yun, J.P., et al., Risk of atrial fibrillation according to cancer type: a nationwide population-based study. *JACC CardioOncol*, 2021. **3**(2): p. 221–32.
142. Zecchin, M., et al., Management of patients with cardiac implantable electronic devices (CIED) undergoing radiotherapy: a consensus document from Associazione Italiana Aritmologia e Cardiostimolazione (AIAC), Associazione Italiana Radioterapia Oncologica (AIRO), Associazione Italiana Fisica Medica (AIFM). *Int J Cardiol*, 2018. **255**: p. 175–83.
143. Fradley, M.G., et al., How to manage patients with cardiac implantable electronic devices undergoing radiation therapy. *JACC CardioOncol*, 2021. **3**(3): p. 447–51.
144. Aichberger, K.J., et al., Progressive peripheral arterial occlusive disease and other vascular events during nilotinib therapy in CML. *Am J Hematol*, 2011. **86**(7): p. 533–9.
145. Thompson, A., et al., 2024 AHA/ACC/ACS/ASNC/HRS/SCA/SCCT/SCMR/SVM guideline for perioperative cardiovascular management for noncardiac surgery: a report of the American college of cardiology/American heart association joint committee on clinical practice guidelines. *Circulation*, 2024. **150**(19): p. e351–e442.
146. Thompson, A., et al., 2024 AHA/ACC/ACS/ASNC/HRS/SCA/SCCT/SCMR/SVM guideline for perioperative cardiovascular management for noncardiac surgery. *J Am Coll Cardiol*, 2024. **84**(19): p. 1869–969.
147. Armenian, S.H., C. Lacchetti, and D. Lenihan, Prevention and monitoring of cardiac dysfunction in survivors of adult cancers: American Society of Clinical Oncology clinical practice guideline summary. *J Oncol Pract*, 2017. **13**(4): p. 270–5.
148. Lopez-Sendon, J., et al., Classification, prevalence, and outcomes of anticancer therapy-induced cardiotoxicity: the CARDIOTOX registry. *Eur Heart J*, 2020. **41**(18): p. 1720–9.

149. Cardinale, D., et al., Early detection of anthracycline cardiotoxicity and improvement with heart failure therapy. *Circulation*, 2015. **131**(22): p. 1981–8.
150. Ananthan, K. and A.R. Lyon, The role of biomarkers in cardio-oncology. *J Cardiovasc Transl Res*, 2020. **13**(3): p. 431–50.
151. Hershman, D.L., et al., Association of cardiovascular risk factors with cardiac events and survival outcomes among patients with breast cancer enrolled in SWOG clinical trials. *J Clin Oncol*, 2018. **36**(26): p. 2710–17.
152. Tromp, J., et al., Long-term survivors of early breast cancer treated with chemotherapy are characterized by a pro-inflammatory biomarker profile compared to matched controls. *Eur J Heart Fail*, 2020. **22**(7): p. 1239–46.
153. Reddy, P., C. Shenoy, and A.H. Blaes, Cardio-oncology in the older adult. *J Geriatr Oncol*, 2017. **8**(4): p. 308–14.

19

Heart failure with reduced ejection fraction in older adults

ALI AHMED AND JEROME L. FLEG

Key points

- Heart failure (HF) is primarily a disorder of older adults and is the leading cause for hospital admission in this age group.
- Major causes of HF in older adults include hypertension, diabetes, coronary artery disease, valvular disease, and atrial fibrillation, all of which increase in prevalence with age.
- Heart failure with preserved ejection fraction (HFpEF) accounts for half or more of prevalent HF cases in older adults, especially older women.
- The four pillars of treatment for heart failure with reduced ejection fraction (HFrEF) in both older and younger adults include angiotensin system antagonists, beta-blockers, mineralocorticoid antagonists, and sodium glucose cotransporter-2 inhibitors, plus diuretics as required.
- Cardiac resynchronization therapy, implantable cardioverter-defibrillators, and left ventricular assist devices have shown similar clinical benefits across adult age groups.
- Selected older patients with HFrEF appear to benefit from coronary revascularization, surgical or percutaneous aortic or mitral valve replacement, and cardiac transplantation.
- Older patients with end-stage HFrEF should be considered for referral to palliative care and possibly hospice, where they can receive appropriate end-of-life care.

EPIDEMIOLOGY AND RISK FACTORS

Heart failure (HF) is a geriatric syndrome. Geriatric syndromes are a heterogeneous group of disorders that are characterized by multiple etiologies and pathogenetic pathways, a high prevalence in older adults, and a substantial adverse impact on quality of life, morbidity, and mortality (Figure 19.1) (1). An estimated 6.7 million or 2.3% of Americans ≥20 years of age have HF, which is projected to reach more than 8 million or 3.0% by 2030 (2). The prevalence of HF increases with age, reaching 7.1% and 10.9% among men and women 80 years or older (2). Among Medicare beneficiaries at risk for HF, the incidence of HF was 26.5 cases per 1000 beneficiaries (2). Findings from all cohorts of the Framingham Heart Study show that during the 25 years (1990–2014) HFrEF developed

DOI: 10.1201/9781003568933-19

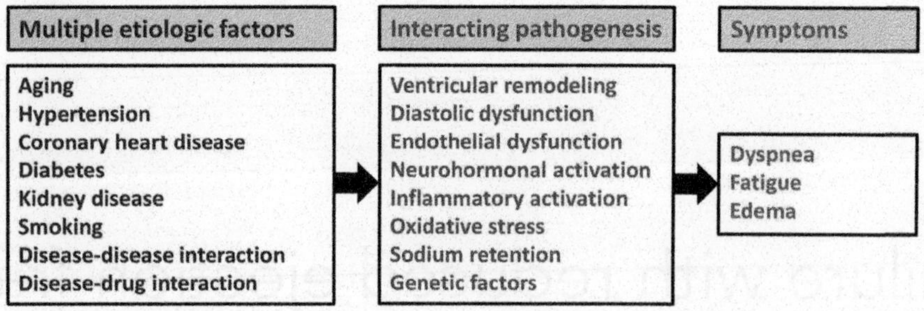

Figure 19.1 Geriatric syndrome model of heart failure in older adults: Multiple etiologic factors and interactive pathogenetic pathways leading to common symptoms and signs of geriatric heart failure. (Adopted from Inouye SK et al., *J Am Geriatr Soc*, 55, 780–791, 2007.)

in 338 patients (incidence rate, 3.33 per 1000 person-years), while HFpEF developed in 429 patients (incidence rate, 2.63 per 1000 person-years), with corresponding mean age at onset of 76.1 (SD 9.6) in men and 80.4 (SD 8.8) in women for HFrEF, and 81 (SD 8.4) years for HFpEF for both men and women (3). In 2022, HF was the contributing cause in 457,212 deaths and was responsible for 13.9% of all deaths. Findings from community-based cohorts suggest that mortality in patients with HFrEF was higher (459/10,000 person-years) than in HFpEF (394/10,000 person-years) (2).

Like most geriatric syndromes, HF has multiple etiologies (Figure 19.1). Findings from the Cardiovascular Health Study (CHS) sponsored by the National Heart, Lung, and Blood Institute (NHLBI) provide information about risk factors for development and progression of HF in older adults. The CHS recruited 5201 community-dwelling older adults aged ≥65 years during 1989–1990, which was later supplemented in 1992–1993 by 687 African American participants. CHS participants were seen annually in the clinic and contacted by phone biannually for outcomes, which included predetermined cardiovascular events including incident HF, which was later centrally adjudicated. Findings from CHS have demonstrated that hypertension, coronary artery disease, and diabetes are major traditional risk factors for HF (4).

The CHS collected data on left ventricular ejection fraction (LVEF) at baseline but not during follow-up, making it difficult to ascertain the risk of HFrEF separately from that of HFpEF. However, considering that the most common risk factors for HF, such as age, obesity, smoking, hypertension, diabetes mellitus, and coronary artery disease, are risk factors for both HFrEF and HFpEF, findings from CHS provide insights into the risk of HFrEF in older adults. As such, smoking cessation, physical activity, and control of blood pressure may play important roles in the prevention of both types of HF. Findings from the CHS suggest that a third of HF in older adults could be prevented if hypertension, diabetes, and coronary artery disease were eliminated from an older adult population (4). Among the CHS participants with hypertension, systolic blood pressure (SBP) ≥140 mmHg was associated with a significant 39% higher risk of incident HF. Hypertension in older adults is predominantly isolated systolic hypertension (ISH). ISH, defined as SBP ≥140 mmHg and DBP <90 mmHg, was present in 38% of CHS participants and was associated with a significant 26% increased risk of incident HF (5). ISH is a manifestation of increased arterial stiffness of large conduit arteries, which explains the wide pulse pressure and low diastolic blood pressure (DBP). In the CHS, about 18% of the participants had isolated diastolic hypotension (IDH), defined as DBP <60 mmHg and SBP ≥100 mmHg, and IDH was associated with a 33% higher risk of developing new-onset HF when compared with no IDH (6).

The CHS also provides insights into many other risk factors and predictors of incident HF in older adults. Diabetes mellitus, valvular heart disease, and peripheral arterial disease are associated with a significantly higher risk of incident HF (7). Adverse left ventricular (LV) remodeling, LV hypertrophy, and asymptomatic LV systolic dysfunction are strong predictors of incident HF in older adults (8). CHS participants with estimated glomerular filtration rate (eGFR) <45 ml/min/1.73 m^2 were at a 44% significantly higher risk of incident HF, whereas those with eGFR 45 to 59 ml/min/1.73 m^2 were not (9). Elevated serum uric acid levels, low serum albumin levels, orthostatic hypotension, and impaired activities of daily living have emerged as potential nontraditional risk factors for incident HF in older adults (10–14).

Among sociodemographic and lifestyle risk factors, both current smoking and heavy smoking in the past have been associated with a higher risk of incident HF in older adults (15). However, moderate alcohol consumption, on the other hand, has been associated with a lower risk of incident HF (16). Older adults with low income may be at increased risk of developing HF (17). Although physical activity is associated with a lower risk of cardiovascular events, a higher degree of physical activity is needed for such association with HF in older adults (18).

Findings from CHS and other population-based studies suggest that more than half of older HF patients have HFpEF (19). Findings from these studies indicate that the typical profile of a HF patient in the community is that of an older woman with HFpEF and a history of systolic hypertension

Table 19.1 Heart failure in older versus middle-aged adults

Characteristic	Older adults	Middle-aged adults
Prevalence	6%–18%	<1%
Gender	Predominantly women	Predominantly men
Etiology	Hypertension	Coronary heart disease
Left ventricular systolic function	Normal	Impaired
Left ventricular diastolic function	Impaired	Normal or mildly impaired
Comorbidities	Multiple	Few

(Table 19.1) (19). Older patients with HFpEF are often clinically indistinguishable from those with HFrEF. Both types of HF share similar risk factors. Biomarkers of elevated LV wall stress, endothelial dysfunction, and inflammation have also been linked to a higher risk of HFrEF, while natriuretic peptides and urinary albumin to creatinine ratio link to HFpEF (20). Chapter 20 will focus on HFpEF in older adults.

PATHOPHYSIOLOGY

As a geriatric syndrome, the development of HF in older adults involves multiple etiologies and pathogenetic pathways (Figure 19.1) (1). Aging is associated with multiple cardiovascular and non-cardiovascular structural and functional changes (21, 22). These age-related changes, along with various other etiologies and pathogenetic pathways present in older adults and interact with each other, thus increasing the risk of incident HF. For example, normal aging is associated with increased arterial stiffness, concentric remodeling of the LV myocardium, and reduced early diastolic relaxation and filling rates (23, 24). Aging is also associated with reduced chronotropic, inotropic, and vasodilator responses to beta-adrenergic stimulation (22, 25). Reduced maximal stroke volume, reflecting reduced inotropic and lusitropic reserves, may contribute to HF in some older individuals, though not generally in those screened to exclude occult coronary artery disease (26).

Despite these pathophysiological age differences in the substrate for HF, relatively few studies have specifically compared younger versus older HF patients in this regard. Neurohormonal activation plays an important role in the pathophysiology of HFrEF. In a study that compared ambulatory younger (<65 years) versus older (>75 years) adults with HFrEF, plasma norepinephrine levels were higher in older HF patients (1191, ±80 pg/ml) and older adults without HF (958, ±84 pg/ml) than younger HF patients (620, ±67 pg/ml) (27). In that study, except for serum aldosterone level, which was higher in older HF patients, serum levels of other neurohormones, such as atrial natriuretic peptide, renin activity, and angiotensin II, were higher in younger HF patients (27). Aging is also associated with elevated myocardial and serum norepinephrine levels, which are associated with downregulation of beta-1 receptors (28).

DIAGNOSIS AND CLINICAL FINDINGS

Because no single test or procedure can definitively diagnose or rule out HF, the diagnosis of HF is based on a constellation of clinical findings (29). The syndrome of HF is characterized by dyspnea, fatigue, and fluid retention, which are manifestations of a reduced cardiac output and compensatory renal and neurohormonal adaptations. A clinical diagnosis of HF should preferably be made before ordering an echocardiogram, considering that a diagnosis of HF in older adults should not be ruled out because of normal left ventricular EF. There are many diagnostic criteria for HF for use in clinical and population settings, but none is perfect or universally accepted. Orthopnea and paroxysmal nocturnal dyspnea (PND) are two major criteria for the diagnosis of HF according to modified Framingham Heart Study criteria (30); the presence of two major criteria is expected to establish a definite diagnosis of HF. However, findings from CHS suggest that many older adults with both orthopnea and PND do not have HF (31). In that study, 7% (388/5771) of the community-dwelling adults ≥65 years had both orthopnea and PND, yet only 20% (76/388) of these individuals had centrally adjudicated HF. Because HF is a clinical syndrome by definition, all newly diagnosed HF patients are symptomatic and usually have fluid retention and an elevated jugular venous pressure (JVP). However, patients with chronic HF may be euvolemic and may not have classic symptoms and signs. An elevated JVP, another major Framingham Heart Study criterion for HF, is the most specific sign of fluid retention in HF and is likely the most important physical finding for the diagnosis of HF in older adults. Both internal jugular vein and external jugular vein can be used to estimate JVP.

Establishing a diagnosis of HF in older adults may be challenging, as many of the symptoms and signs of HF can also be found in various non-HF disorders, such as pulmonary conditions, deconditioning, and depression. Older adults often attribute their HF symptoms to aging, thus delaying presentation until symptoms are more advanced, which may paradoxically make the diagnosis easier. The diagnosis of HF in older adults may also be delayed due to inadequate history because of cognitive or sensory impairments. However, objective determination of an elevated JVP may be particularly helpful in establishing a new diagnosis of HF when historical data are insufficient. B-type natriuretic peptide (BNP) and N-terminal pro-BNP (NT-proBNP) are neurohormones that are secreted by the failing ventricle in HF in response to myocardial wall stress. Several studies have suggested serum levels of these neurohormones may assist in the diagnosis of HF (32, 33). However, currently there are no standard cutoffs for these neurohormones to confirm or rule out HF in general, and even less is known about their usefulness in older adults. Furthermore, the accuracy of diagnosis or treatment of HF in real-world settings has not been shown to be significantly improved by BNP levels (34).

Following establishment of an HF diagnosis, the next most important step is to determine its etiology. Just as a clinical diagnosis of fever is incomplete without a search for the underlying cause, a clinical diagnosis of HF is incomplete without a search for an underlying etiology. The sequence of steps in evaluation of HF can be conveniently remembered by the mnemonic DEFEAT: Diagnosis, Etiology, Fluid volume, Ejection fraction, And Treatment (35). Although a direct causal association is difficult to establish, the presence of common risk factors such as hypertension, coronary heart disease, or diabetes suggests that they may have played a role in the multifactorial causal pathways leading to incident HF in older adults. After an appropriate fluid volume assessment, the next most important step in the workup for HF diagnosis is to determine LVEF, as this has both prognostic and therapeutic implications (29). Because life-prolonging therapies for HF are available only for HFrEF, it is important to make this determination expeditiously. Echocardiography is the most convenient, noninvasive, and cost-effective way to estimate LVEF, which also provide additional insights about potential HF etiologies such as prior myocardial infarction or valvular heart disease.

PROGNOSIS

HF presages a poor prognosis, especially in older adults (36). Of the 5795 Medicare-eligible community-dwelling adults ≥65 years in the CHS, 274 (4.7%) had centrally-adjudicated HF at baseline; their mean age was 75 (±6) years, 52% were women, 22% were African American, and 46% had multiple hospitalizations (37). In a study of over 9000 patients hospitalized with HF, predictors of death in older patients were reduced LVEF, obstructive lung disease, pulmonary hypertension, and mitral regurgitation (38). Of note, the mode of death in HF changes with disease progression (39, 40), and HFrEF in older adults is more likely to be more advanced and of longer duration than in younger patients. Thus, older HFrEF patients are more likely to die from progressive pump failure than fatal arrhythmias.

Although older age and male sex are predictors of poor outcomes in HF patients, the role of race is less clear (41–44). Functional class and aerobic capacity are strong predictors of mortality in both older and younger HF patients (45–47). Prognosis of HF also varies by LVEF (48, 49) as well as right ventricular EF (50). Patients with HF accompanied by comorbidities such as diabetes, atrial fibrillation, coronary heart disease, or chronic kidney disease have higher mortality (51, 52). When CKD is defined using Kidney Disease: Improving Global Outcomes (KDIGO) guideline criteria that require the presence of abnormal kidney structure or function for >3 months with implications for health, even mild CKD with an estimated glomerular filtration rate is associated with a higher risk of death and hospitalization (53). CKD was associated with 16%, 19%, and 26% higher risks for death and 31%, 33%, and 32% higher risks for HF hospitalization in patients with HFpEF, HFmrEF (HF with mildly reduced ejection fraction), and HFrEF, respectively (54). Hypokalemia is common in HF and is associated with poor outcomes in ambulatory patients (55, 56), but may not be in hospitalized patients (57). Mild hyperkalemia, on the other hand, is less common, and although it has unadjusted association with mortality, there appears to be no independent association with this endpoint (58). Older HF patients with serum magnesium level ≤2 mEq/L may be at higher risk for cardiovascular mortality, but not for cardiovascular hospitalization (59). Older HF patients with higher levels of New York Heart Association (NYHA) class symptoms were at higher risk for mortality but not for hospitalization (46, 47). Low gait speed, a marker of frailty, is independently associated with a higher risk of death, HF hospitalization, and all-cause hospitalization in older patients with HFrEF (60). HF is also a risk factor for incident driving cessation among community-dwelling older adults (61). HF has also been shown to be associated with a higher risk of residential relocation to a new home address (62).

TREATMENT: GENERAL APPROACH

The treatment goals of HF can be classified into three broad categories: (1) general approach, including lifestyle modifications such as salt and fluid restriction or system-based interventions such as multidisciplinary HF management programs; (2) pharmacotherapy; and (3) device-based therapy. Pharmacotherapy can be divided into two categories: symptom-relieving therapy and life-prolonging therapy. Life-prolonging therapy using neurohormonal blockade, on the other hand, has been demonstrated only in HFrEF patients. Although the evidence for their benefit is derived from randomized clinical trials (RCTs) of mostly younger HFrEF patients (Table 19.2), the findings are generalized to older patients with HFrEF. Currently, the favorable effects of device-based therapies are also restricted to patients with HFrEF.

DIET

As described earlier, nonadherence to a salt- and fluid-restricted diet may precipitate acute decompensation of

Table 19.2 Mean age of real-world HF patient in HF registries versus HF patients enrolled in randomized clinical trials

HF studies	Number of patients	Age, mean (±SD)
Registries of hospitalized HF patients		
ADHERE – Adams KF Jr. et al., *Am Heart J*, 2005	105,388	72 (±14)
OPTIMIZE-HF – Fonarow GC et al., *JACC*, 2007	48,612	73 (±14)
Alabama HF Project – Feller M et al., *Int J Cardiol*, 2012	8049	76 (±11)
National HF Project – Vidan MT et al., *Euro J Heart Fail*, 2010	56,924	80 (±23)
Registries of hospitalized HFrEF patients		
CHAMP-HF – Greene SJ et al., *J Am Coll Cardiol*, 2018	3518	66 (±13)
Randomized trials of ambulatory HFrEF patients		
SOLVD-Treatment (Angiotensin-converting enzyme inhibitor) – The SOLVD Investigators, *N Engl J Med*, 1991	2569	60 (±10)
CHARM-Alternative (Angiotensin receptor blocker) – Granger CB et al., *Lancet*, 2003	2028	67 (±11)
DIG-Main (Digoxin) – The DIG Investigators, *N Engl J Med*, 1997	6800	64 (±11)
COPERNICUS (Beta-blocker) – Packer M et al., *N Engl J Med*, 2001	2298	58 (±11)
MERIT-HF (Beta-blocker) – The MERIT-HF Investigators, *Lancet*, 1999	3991	64 (±10)
RALES (Mineralocorticoid receptor antagonist) – Pitt B et al., *N Engl J Med*, 1999	1663	65 (±12)
EMPHASIS-HF (Mineralocorticoid receptor antagonist) – Zannad F et al., *N Engl J Med*, 2011	2737	69 (±8)
PARADIGM-HF (Angiotensin receptor-neprilysin inhibitors) – McMurray JJV et al., *N Engl J Med*, 2014	8422	64 (±11)
DAPA-HF (Sodium-glucose cotransporter 2 inhibitor) – McMurray JJV et al., *New Engl J Med*, 2019	4744	66 (±11)

chronic HF. It is generally accepted that sodium intake should be restricted to <2 grams per day, and fluid intake should be restricted to <2 liters per day. However, there is little prospective data on the role of sodium and fluid intake on HF exacerbations (63). Hyponatremia is associated with poor outcomes in HF (64). Chronic HF patients with hyponatremia often require a more severe albeit temporary fluid restriction. Most older HF patients do not need to monitor their dietary intake of potassium unless they have substantial renal dysfunction, especially if taking mineralocorticoid antagonists. However, those with hyperkalemia may need to limit their intake of potassium-rich foods, such as tomatoes, bananas, and orange juice. Although obesity is associated with a higher risk of incident HF (65, 66), obesity has been shown to confer survival benefit to older HFrEF patients (67); thus, intentional weight loss may not be desirable except to improve physical function in obese individuals.

PHYSICAL ACTIVITY

Higher levels of physical activity are associated with reduced risk of HF (68, 69), and HF is characterized by exertional fatigue and exercise intolerance. Therefore, physical activity would be expected to improve outcomes and quality of life of older HF patients. Aerobic exercise has been shown to improve peak VO_2 and other physiological parameters in younger patients with HFrEF (70). In one study of 200 HFrEF patients, mean age 72 years (range 60–89 years), combined aerobic and low-resistance strength training exercise for 24 weeks improved health-related quality of life, NYHA class, and 6-minute walk distance (71).

Although single-center trials have suggested reduced mortality and HF hospitalizations after exercise training, none has been adequately powered for these endpoints. In the multicenter Heart Failure: A Controlled Trial Investigating Outcomes of Exercise Training (HF-ACTION) trial, 2331 chronic HFrEF patients were randomized to usual care plus aerobic exercise training (36 supervised sessions followed by home-based practice) versus usual care alone and followed for a median of 30 months (72). Patients had a median age of 59 years, median LVEF of 25%, 28% were women, 37% had NYHA class III–IV symptoms, and 51% had ischemic heart disease. The composite primary endpoint of all-cause mortality or hospitalization occurred in 759 patients (65%) in the exercise training group and 796 patients (68%) in the usual care group (hazard ratio = 0.93; 95% confidence interval = 0.84–1.02; p = 0.13) (72). The modest benefits of training in this largest and most comprehensive study of exercise training in mild to moderate HFrEF patients were likely related to low adherence, but suggested that exercise training modestly improved self-reported health status and depressive symptoms (73, 74). Post hoc analyses of HF-ACTION suggest that exercise was more effective in lowering the risk of all-cause hospitalization but not mortality in patients with baseline frailty (75).

PATIENT EDUCATION

Like other chronic conditions, a great deal of proper HF care depends on patients themselves. Patient participation thus is important for achieving optimal outcomes, and patient education is essential in this regard. Older HF patients should be informed of their diagnosis, including their LVEF, and its prognostic and therapeutic implications. They also should be educated about the role of fluid retention in precipitating or exacerbating HF warning symptoms and signs. Patients should be encouraged to record their weight daily, generally in the morning, after emptying the bladder and wearing similar clothes. They may be advised to take an extra dose of diuretic for 3 to 5 days if they gain 3–5 pounds within a week. If the baseline weight is not achieved in 3–5 days, they should be advised to consult their health care providers. To prevent overdiuresis, patients should be reassured that daily fluctuation in weight by 1 or 2 pounds is not uncommon in HF and does not require extra diuretics. Patients should avoid high ambient temperature and humidity. A rule of thumb is to stay indoors when the sum of outdoor temperature (in Fahrenheit) and humidity exceeds 160.

DISEASE MANAGEMENT PROGRAMS

Because much of HF care involves non-drug interventions that require patient and family participation, it would be expected that programs supporting patients and families would improve outcomes, especially hospital admission and readmission. Although such programs have generally improved quality of life and reduced hospital readmissions, telephone monitoring and dedicated HF clinics have not been associated with improved outcomes (76). The efficacy of pulmonary artery pressure monitoring via an implantable sensor has shown mixed results in reducing HF readmissions, although a recent meta-analysis found significant reductions in both HF hospitalizations and mortality (77).

TREATMENT: PHARMACOTHERAPY FOR HFREF

Prior to the 1980s, therapy for HFrEF was directed solely toward symptom control using diuretics to control fluid retention and improving cardiac function using digitalis. Despite their temporarily beneficial hemodynamic actions, long-term therapy with more potent inotropes was associated with increased morbidity and mortality (78, 79). The understanding that HFrEF is characterized by activation of the renin–angiotensin system (RAS) and sympathetic nervous system (80, 81) led to clinical trials showing that their suppression with drugs such as angiotensin-converting enzyme (ACE) inhibitors (82), angiotensin receptor blockers (ARB) alone (83) or combined with a neprilysin inhibitor (84), beta-adrenergic receptor blockers (85, 86), and aldosterone antagonists (87, 88) reduced mortality and morbidity.

Drug therapy for HFrEF may be divided into two broad categories: (1) diuretics to improve symptoms of volume overload and (2) neurohormonal antagonists of the sympathetic nervous system and renin–angiotensin–aldosterone system to improve symptoms and clinical outcomes. It is important to understand the HF care extends well beyond the appropriate use of evidence-based pharmacotherapy. A 79-year-old man with HFrEF receiving evidence-based life-prolonging therapy with enalapril 10 mg twice a day, carvedilol 12.5 mg twice a day, and spironolactone 12.5 mg daily may still have frequent decompensations, hospital admissions, and poor quality of life. Therefore, careful attention to fluid volume status and symptoms during follow-up visits remains important. Clinicians should consider avoiding overzealous implementation of evidence-based guidelines in older HFrEF patients, especially among frail older HF patients, who were often excluded from pivotal clinical trials (89). For example, in the Studies Of Left Ventricular Dysfunction (SOLVD)-Treatment trial, 36% of the HFrEF patients were ≥65 years, and none ≥81 years of age (82). Similarly, none of the HFrEF patients in the MERIT-HF trial were ≥81 years (86). The mean age of real-world patients in HF registries and those enrolled in major RCTs are displayed in Table 19.2. The 10–15 year younger age of patients in large pivotal HF trials versus real-world HF patients is noteworthy.

DIURETICS

Nearly all symptomatic HFrEF patients with fluid retention require diuretics to achieve and maintain euvolemia (90). This is generally achieved by loop diuretics, furosemide, torsemide, or bumetanide. Despite their nearly universal use, there is no RCT data on the long-term effects of chronic therapy with loop diuretics on clinical outcomes in HF. Findings from a propensity-matched study suggest that loop diuretic use is associated with a lower risk of 30-day all-cause mortality and 30-day HF hospitalization (Figure 19.2) (91). Findings from the subgroup analysis of that study shows this association was similar for both HFrEF and HFpEF and that it was numerically stronger in the subgroup ≥80 years of age (91). Although the use of loop diuretic had no association with either outcome during longer follow-up, in the subgroup with evidence of fluid retention, there was a lower risk of associated HF hospitalization, while the risk was higher in the group without (92).

A potential explanation for adverse long-term effects of diuretics in the absence of fluid retention is that the use of loop diuretics is associated with electrolyte imbalance and neurohormonal activation, both associated with poor outcomes, especially among ambulatory patients (55–57). Therefore, after euvolemia has been achieved, patients

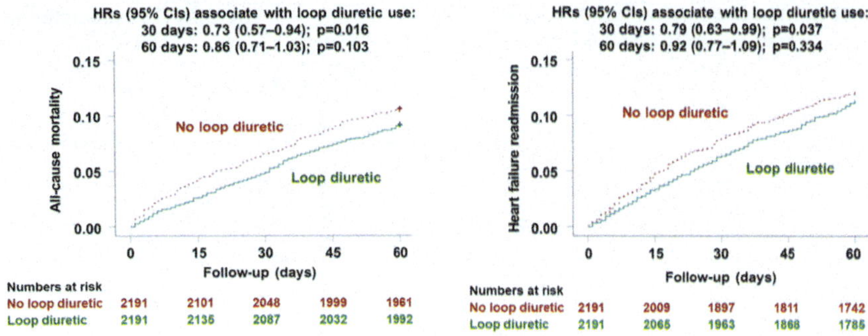

Figure 19.2 Association of loop diuretic use with risk of short-term death and hospitalization in older patients with HF. (From Faselis C. et al., *J Am Coll Cardiol*, 76, 669–679, 2020.)

should be encouraged to restrict their salt and fluid intake so that the lower doses of diuretics are needed to maintain euvolemia. Serum potassium levels should be closely monitored and maintained between 4 and 5 mEq/L. Hypokalemia should be corrected with potassium supplements. When patients require chronic therapy with potassium supplements to maintain normokalemia, an aldosterone antagonist should be considered before starting potassium supplements.

Torsemide and bumetanide are less frequently used than furosemide but were thought to be possibly associated with less neurohormonal activation and better outcomes (93). However, the recent large Torsemide Comparison With Furosemide for Management of Heart Failure (TRANSFORM-HF) trial showed no significant difference in the primary endpoint of death or the secondary endpoint of all-cause hospitalization between furosemide and torsemide (94). Although the findings from subgroup analyses need to be interpreted with caution, subgroup analyses from that study suggest that torsemide may be more beneficial in older adults, but less beneficial in those with HFrEF.

Generally speaking, torsemide 20 mg and bumetanide 1 mg are equivalent to furosemide 40 mg. Because older HF patients may suffer from diuretic-related overactive bladder symptoms (95), it is preferable to use diuretics as a single morning dose. Larger doses may be given twice daily, with the afternoon dose around 2 pm to avoid nighttime diuresis. Patients resistant to high doses of loop diuretics may respond to a lower dose of furosemide combined with a small dose of metolazone, a thiazide-like diuretic that works primarily at the distal convoluted tubule. Older HF patients resistant to high doses of furosemide may also respond to other loop diuretics such as torsemide or bumetanide.

ANGIOTENSIN-CONVERTING ENZYME (ACE) INHIBITORS

Multiple RCTs have conclusively demonstrated the efficacy of ACE inhibitors to prolong survival and improve symptoms in patients with HFrEF. A subgroup analysis based on the public-use copy of the SOLVD data suggests that ACE inhibitors may be beneficial in older HFrEF patients, though the effect may be more modest in those patients. However, in the SOLVD-Treatment trial, only eight patients were 80 years of age and none were ≥81 years old (82). Findings from propensity-matched studies suggest that ACE inhibitors are also effective in older patients with HFrEF, including those with CKD (96, 97).

Despite their benefits in improving survival and reducing symptoms, ACE inhibitors have several side effects that are particularly relevant to older adults. These include worsening kidney function, hypotension, and hyperkalemia, all of which are dose related and may be avoided if ACE inhibitors are used in lower doses. However, findings from a propensity score-matched cohort of older patients with HFrEF shows the use ACE inhibitors in higher target doses is associated with a lower risk of death and kidney failure (Figure 19.3) (98).

ANGIOTENSIN-RECEPTOR BLOCKERS (ARBS)

ARBs, like ACE inhibitors, also antagonize the RAS system. However, in RCTs of ARBs, most of which were conducted in more contemporary HFrEF patients receiving beta-blockers, there was no mortality reduction, and evidence of their benefits is based mainly on a significant reduction in combined endpoints (83). Findings from subgroup analysis of a propensity score-matched cohort of octogenarian patients with HFrEF receiving RAS inhibitors show that the greater effectiveness of higher target doses was similar for ACE inhibitors and ARBs (98).

ANGIOTENSIN RECEPTOR-NEPRILYSIN INHIBITOR (ARNI)

In the Prospective Comparison of ARNI With ACEI to Determine Impact on Global Mortality and Morbidity in Heart Failure (PARADIGM-HF) trial, 8442 patients with HFrEF were randomly assigned to combined therapy with sacubitril (a neprilysin inhibitor) and valsartan (an ARB) versus enalapril. During 27 months of median follow-up, ARNI therapy significantly reduced the risk of the primary outcome of cardiovascular death or HF hospitalization by

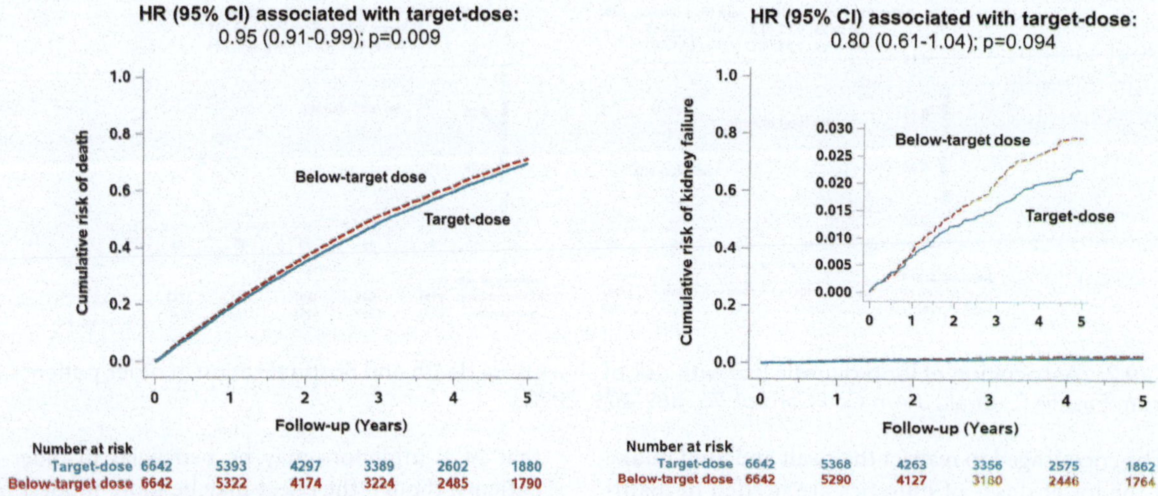

Figure 19.3 Association of higher target dose ACE inhibitor or ARB with death and kidney failure in octogenarian patients with HFrEF. (From Sin M. et al., *Am J Med*, 2025; 138: 639–649.e4.)

20% (84). Findings from PARADIGM-HF suggest that the efficacy of ARNI is similar among those <55, 55–64, 65–74, and ≥75 years of age (99).

BETA-ADRENERGIC BLOCKERS

Evidence for the benefit of beta-blockers in older HFrEF patients is extrapolated from RCTs of much younger HF patients (Table 19.2). Findings from a subgroup analysis of the MERIT-HF trial suggest that metoprolol succinate extended release was equally effective in older and younger HFrEF patients (100). Older HFrEF patients without contraindications should be prescribed one of three beta-blockers with RCT evidence of proven benefit. These include carvedilol, metoprolol succinate extended release, and bisoprolol (90). Based on the findings of the COMET trial, when prescribing metoprolol in HFrEF, long-acting metoprolol succinate should be preferred over short-acting metoprolol tartrate (101).

MINERALOCORTICOID RECEPTOR ANTAGONISTS (MRAS)

MRAs, also known as aldosterone antagonists, have emerged as a powerful tool to improve outcomes in HFrEF (87, 88). In the Randomized Aldactone Evaluation Study (RALES) of patients with severe HFrEF, spironolactone reduced the primary outcome of all-cause death by 30% and hospitalization for HF by 35%, and clinical benefits were similar for younger and older patients (87). Findings from the Eplerenone in Mild Patients Hospitalization and Survival Study in Heart Failure (EMPHASIS-HF) trial suggest that this selective aldosterone antagonist is beneficial in contemporary patients with mild to moderate HFrEF (88). A subgroup analysis of EMPHASIS-HF provides further evidence that this class of drugs is equally effective in younger and older HFrEF patients, although it is not clear how many of the older subset were octogenarians. A meta-analysis that included individual patient data from the RALES, EMPHASIS, and TOPCAT trials showed a 26% reduction in the composite endpoint of cardiovascular death, or HF hospitalization with MRAs without significant heterogeneity by age ≥75 years versus younger patients (102). However, studies of MRAs in the real world suggest no or weak clinical effectiveness (74).

Spironolactone should be considered for older HFrEF patients without renal insufficiency and should be started low with 12.5 mg daily and increased to 25 mg daily if tolerated. Serum potassium should be closely monitored and kept between 4 and 5 mEq/L. Male patients with painful gynecomastia should be prescribed eplerenone. In older patients, eplerenone should be started at 25 mg daily and increased to 50 mg daily if tolerated.

HYDRALAZINE AND ISOSORBIDE DINITRATE

Findings from the African-American Heart Failure Trial (A-HeFT) demonstrated that combined therapy with hydralazine and isosorbide dinitrate may improve outcomes in African American HFrEF patients (mean age 57 years) receiving ACE inhibitors and beta-blockers (103). Minimal data on the efficacy and safety of this therapy exist for older African Americans.

DIGOXIN

The DIG trial demonstrated that digoxin significantly reduced HF hospitalizations but had no effect on total mortality (104). Findings from a post hoc analysis of DIG data suggest that at lower serum digoxin concentrations (0.5–0.9 ng/ml), digoxin use may be associated with a lower risk of death (105). Digoxin use is associated with a lower risk of 30-day all-cause readmission (106, 107). In a propensity-matched sample of 316 long-term care residents (mean age 83 years), digoxin had no association with all-cause death, HF readmission, or a combined endpoint of all-cause death or readmission (108). Given that only 5% of the DIG participants were ≥80 years of age, digoxin should be used with caution in frail older patients. In older HF patients, digoxin should generally be prescribed as 0.125 mg daily (109).

Implementing recommendations for the use of contemporary guideline-directed medical therapy (GDMT) in older HFrEF patients may lead to polypharmacy. Discontinuation of digoxin may be considered in older HFrEF patients receiving the full complement of RAS inhibitors (an ACE inhibitor, ARB or ARNI), a beta-blocker, an MRA, and a sodium-glucose cotransporter 2 (SGLT2) inhibitor, along with diuretics, which most patients need to remain euvolemic. Although discontinuation of digoxin therapy has been shown to be associated with poor outcomes in older HFrEF patients (110), this may be attenuated in patients who are on beta-blockers (Figure 19.4) (111).

OTHER INOTROPES

The long-term use of oral phosphodiesterase inhibitors, such as amrinone, milrinone, and vesnarinone, is associated with increased mortality (78, 79); thus, these drugs are not be used. Intravenous milrinone is also not associated with significant mortality benefit (112). The calcium-sensitizing phosphodiesterase inhibitor levosimendan has been shown to improve hemodynamic function and symptoms in younger patients with decompensated HF (113), but it does not have a mortality benefit compared with dobutamine (114). Synthetic catecholamines such as dobutamine or dopamine may also be used intravenously to treat refractory HF symptoms, although older HFrEF patients may derive smaller hemodynamic benefits (115).

SODIUM-GLUCOSE COTRANSPORTER (SGLT2) INHIBITORS

In the past few years, several trials of SGLT2 inhibitors have shown significant reduction in HF hospitalizations and cardiovascular death in patients with HFrEF. These drugs reduce glucose and sodium absorption in the proximal renal tubule, producing an osmotic diuresis. In the Dapagliflozin and Prevention of Adverse Outcomes in Heart Failure (DAPA-HF) trial, dapagliflozin, an SGLT2 inhibitor, significantly reduced the risk of worsening heart failure or death from cardiovascular causes in patients with HFrEF as well as the risk of total mortality (116). In the Empagliflozin Outcome Trial in Patients with Chronic Heart Failure and a Reduced Ejection Fraction (EMPEROR-Reduced) trial, empagliflozin, another SGLT2 inhibitor, significantly reduced the risk of the primary outcome, a composite endpoint of cardiovascular death or heart failure hospitalization, but there was no significant effect on total mortality or cardiovascular mortality (117). Findings from a meta-analysis of both trials suggest that the efficacy of SGLT2 inhibitors is unaffected by age (118). As mentioned earlier, SGLT2 inhibitors are now considered a component of GDMT for HFrEF (90).

NEWER THERAPIES

Other relatively recent advances in drug therapy for HFrEF include vericiguat, an oral guanylate cyclase stimulator causing vasodilatory, antifibrotic, and anti-inflammatory effects, and omencantiv, a selective cardiac myosin activator (119). In the Vericiguat Global Study in Subjects with Heart Failure with Reduced Ejection Fraction (VICTORIA) trial, vericiguat, a novel oral soluble guanylate cyclase stimulator, reduced the composite endpoint of cardiovascular death or first heart failure hospitalization in high-risk HFrEF patients by

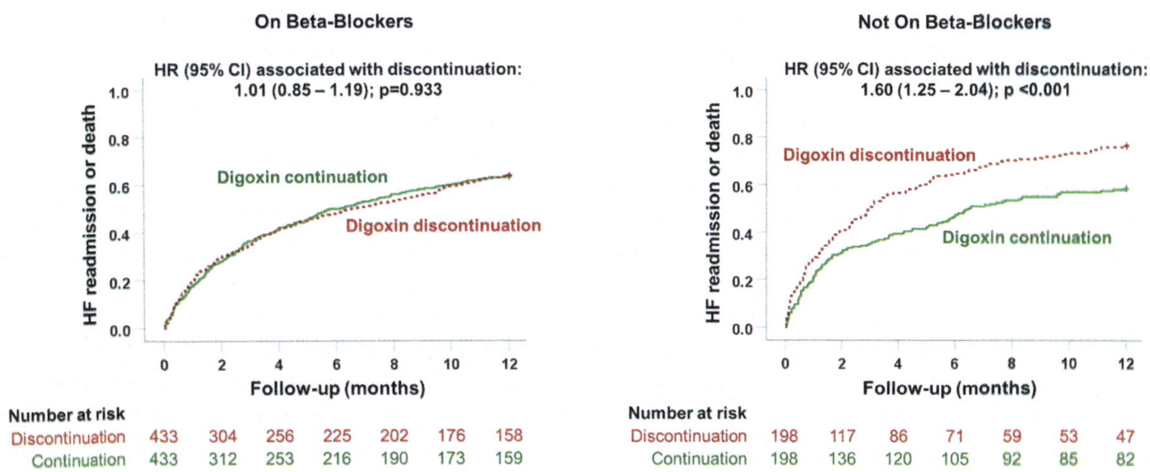

Figure 19.4 Association of discontinuation of digoxin and outcomes in older patients with HFrEF, receiving and not receiving beta-blockers. (From Lam PH et al., *Am J Med*, 2025; 138: 495–503.e1.)

10% over a median 10.8 month follow-up (120). In the Global Approach to Lowering Adverse Cardiac Outcomes through Improving Contractility in Heart Failure (GALACTIC-HF) trial, omencantiv mecarbil, a selective cardiac myosin activator, reduced the risk of the primary composite endpoint of heart-failure event (hospitalization or urgent visit for heart failure) or cardiovascular death in patients with HFrEF but had no significant effect on total mortality or cardiovascular mortality (121).

Ivabradine reduces heart rate by inhibiting the I_f current but has no effect on contractility. In the Systolic Heart Failure Treatment with I_f Inhibitor Trial (SHIFT), at 30 months of follow-up, compared to placebo, ivabradine reduced the primary composite endpoint of cardiovascular death or HF hospitalization but not of mortality (122). Significant benefit was found across age groups though risk reduction was greater in patients <53 years (HR = 0.62) than in those >69 years (HR = 0.84). Despite elevated endothelin levels in HF, RCTs have failed to demonstrate the clinical benefit of endothelin receptor antagonists in chronic HFrEF (123).

Most older HF patients have lower hemoglobin levels without evidence of iron deficiency. In the recent IRONMAN trial of 1137 patients with chronic HFrEF and iron deficiency (mean age 73 years), intravenous ferric derisomaltose reduced the composite primary endpoint of cardiovascular death or HF hospitalization by 18% over 2.7 years ($p = 0.07$) with a significant 17% decrease in the secondary endpoint of cardiovascular death or hospital admission for stroke, myocardial infarction, or heart failure ($p = 0.045$) (124). Based on these results and similar findings in other recent trials, intravenous iron should be considered for older HFrEF patients with iron deficiency.

TREATMENT: DEVICES AND SURGERY FOR HFREF

Devices

The high morbidity and mortality associated with HFrEF despite maximal medical therapy has led to the pursuit of additional interventions using devices and surgery in this population. Dyssynchrony in intraventricular conduction, which manifests as a wide QRS complex on electrocardiogram, is not uncommon in HFrEF and is associated with poor outcomes. Atrial-synchronized biventricular pacing, also known as cardiac resynchronization therapy (CRT), can synchronize intraventricular conduction and coordinate contraction between the left and right ventricles. Randomized trials have shown that CRT can improve LV function and enhance functional capacity, quality of life, and survival in HFrEF patients with a wide (>120 milliseconds) QRS complex (125, 126). Although no randomized trial has specifically addressed the role of CRT in older adults, subgroup analyses of those RCTs suggest that the benefit of CRT is similar in older versus younger patients. A recent patient-level meta-analysis using age as a continuous variable found that older patients had a greater reduction in the composite endpoint of HF hospitalization or all-cause death (127). Thus, CRT should be considered in older patients with HFrEF, though with caution in those ≥80 years of age.

Given the nearly exponential increase in the risk of sudden cardiac death as LVEF decreases below 30%, it is not surprising that several studies have shown a benefit of an implantable cardioverter-defibrillator (ICD) in patients with systolic HF. In the Multicenter Automatic Defibrillator Implantation Trial II (MADIT II), prophylactic implantation of an ICD in patients with a prior myocardial infarction and LVEF <30% reduced all-cause mortality from 20% to 14% over a 20-month mean follow-up (128). Although HF was not required for study entry and the baseline history of HF was not reported, approximately 75% of patients were receiving diuretics.

The effect of ICD therapy in a more specific HF population was tested in the Sudden Cardiac Death in Heart Failure Trial (SCD-HeFT). In SCD-HFT, 2521 HFrEF patients (52% ischemic etiology) with NYHA class II–III symptoms (70% class II), median age 60 years, and median LVEF 25%, were randomized to conventional therapy plus placebo ($n = 847$), conventional therapy plus amiodarone ($n = 845$), or conventional therapy plus a conservatively programmed, shock-only, single-lead ICD ($n = 829$) (129). During a median follow-up of 46 months, the primary endpoint of all-cause mortality occurred in 29% of patients in the placebo group, 28% of those in the amiodarone group, and 22% in the ICD group (129). Although there was no interaction between age and ICD benefit in SCD-HeFT, the ICD-associated mortality benefit (versus placebo) was somewhat more favorable among patients <65 years (HR = 0.68; 95% CI = 0.50–0.93) versus those ≥65 years (HR = 0.86; 95% CI = 0.62–1.18). In SCD-HeFT patients who received an ICD shock, a quality-of-life assessment within 1 month after shock revealed a significant decrease in perceived general health, physical and emotional functioning, social functioning, and self-rated health, although this perception tended to attenuate with passage of time (130).

The effect of ICD on outcomes in 229 HFrEF patients with nonischemic dilated cardiomyopathy was examined in the Defibrillators in Non-Ischemic Cardiomyopathy Treatment Evaluation (DEFINITE) trial. During a mean follow-up of 29 months, the primary endpoint of all-cause mortality occurred in 17% and 9% of patients in the control and ICD groups, respectively ($p = 0.08$), which was similar for those <65 years and ≥65 years (131). In DEFINITE, 18% and 21% of patients received appropriate and inappropriate ICD shocks, respectively (131).

The role of CRT alone or combined with ICD was examined in the Comparison of Medical Therapy, Pacing, and Defibrillation in Heart Failure (COMPANION) trial, in which 1520 HFrEF patients (mean age 67 years) with wide QRS (≥120 milliseconds), NYHA class III–IV symptoms, and mean LVEF of 22% were randomized to receive optimal medical therapy alone, additional CRT, or additional CRT plus ICD (126). The risk of the 12-month primary composite endpoint of all-cause death or all-cause hospitalization was similarly reduced in the CRT alone (19%) and CRT plus-ICD groups (20%) (126). In COMPANION, CRT use was associated with improvement in symptoms and quality of life and a reduction in hospitalizations. These benefits were similar in younger and older (>65 years) patients, though the proportion of ≥80 years in the study was not reported.

The left ventricular assist device (LVAD) has become an important intervention for patients with end-stage HFrEF. Although LVADs were initially developed as a temporary bridge to cardiac transplantation, in recent years LVADs have become increasingly used as destination therapy in patients who are not transplant candidates. In the Randomized Evaluation of Mechanical Assistance for the Treatment of Congestive Heart Failure (REMATCH) trial, 129 patients with end-stage heart failure who were ineligible for cardiac transplantation were randomly assigned to receive a pulsatile flow LVAD (n = 68) or optimal medical management (n = 61). During a 2-year follow-up, there was a significant 48% reduction in the risk of death in the LVAD group (132). Data from the Mechanical Circulatory Support Research Network (MCSRN) registry demonstrate that of 1149 recipients of continuous-flow LVADs, 1-year mortality occurred in 25% (40/163) of patients ≥70 years and 16% (158/986) of patients <70 years. However, age ≥70 years had no significant independent association with 1-year mortality (HR, 0.94; 95% CI, 0.70–1.26; p = 0.67). Compared with patients <70 years, older patients had similar 1-year rates of device thrombosis and stroke, but higher rates of gastrointestinal bleeding (133). Findings from the Multicenter Study of MagLev Technology in Patients Undergoing Mechanical Circulatory Support Therapy with HeartMate 3 (MOMENTUM 3) trial show that a fully magnetically levitated centrifugal-flow LVAD reduced the risk of the composite primary endpoint of 2-year disabling stroke-free survival or reoperation to replace or remove a malfunctioning device from 40% to 25% when compared with an axial-flow LVAD, and this effect was similar in younger and older (≥65 years) patients (134).

Surgery

Selected older patients with HFrEF may derive major benefits from cardiac surgery. Although surgical aortic valve replacement was the treatment of choice for older adults with HF secondary to severe calcific aortic stenosis (135), transcatheter aortic valve replacement is now available for those considered inoperable as well as those with moderate or high surgical risk, with similar survival and lower morbidity (136–138). Findings from the Cardiovascular Outcomes Assessment of the MitraClip Percutaneous Therapy for Heart Failure Patients with Functional Mitral Regurgitation (COAPT) trial show that in patients with HFrEF (mean age 72 years; mean EF 31%) who had moderate-to-severe or severe secondary mitral regurgitation and were symptomatic despite optimal GDMT, transcatheter mitral valve repair reduced the annualized risk of hospitalization for heart failure from 68% to 36% and all-cause death from 46% to 29% over 24 months (139).

Coronary revascularization has been considered to ameliorate HF symptoms in selected older HFrEF patients with substantial amounts of viable but ischemic myocardium due to coronary artery disease. Although the multicenter Surgical Treatment for Ischemic Heart Failure (STICH) trial initially failed to show a survival benefit from coronary artery bypass graft (CABG) surgery (140), extended follow-up over 9.8 years showed a significant 16% lower all-cause mortality and 21% lower cardiovascular mortality versus medical therapy (141). However, no significant mortality benefit was seen in the subset aged 60 years and older. Therefore, consideration for CABG should be carefully individualized in eligible older HFrEF patients with ongoing myocardial ischemia who are refractory to optimal medical and device therapy.

Cardiac transplantation has been successfully employed to treat end-stage HF in carefully selected patients in their seventh and eighth decades. In a recent series, patients ≥70 years old increased from 3.7% before 2018 to 4.5% after the US change its heart allocation policy in 2018. Of note, the 90-day and 1-year survival was similar in older and younger patients before 2018, but from 2018 onward, the older group had comparable 90-day but lower 1-year survival, 86.5% versus 90.9% (142). The shortage of donors and the high likelihood of medical contraindications, such as intrinsic renal or cerebrovascular disease in this age group, limit the use of cardiac transplantation in older adults.

TREATMENT: ACUTE DECOMPENSATED HFREF

Acute decompensated heart failure (ADHF) accounted for 1.2 million hospitalizations among 949,075 unique individuals in the US in 2021 at an estimated $32 billion in direct costs (cost of HF-related treatment) and $14 billion in indirect costs (lost economic productivity) (143). The median age of patients admitted with ADHF declined from 74 to 71 years between 2008 and 2018. Although HF signs and symptoms generally improve with treatment, rehospitalization and mortality occur in up to 30% and 15%, respectively, within 60–90 days after discharge, and are generally higher in the elderly. Whereas acute treatment varies with the underlying precipitant, common goals are stabilizing hemodynamics and relieving clinical congestion. Intensive diuretic administration is therefore a cornerstone of therapy.

In the Diuretic Optimization Strategies Evaluation (DOSE) trial, furosemide at higher doses relieved congestion more rapidly than at lower doses, and there was no significant difference between bolus and continuous infusion (144). Although elevated levels of blood vasopressin are common in ADHF, the vasopressin antagonist tolvaptan did not reduce hospital stay or mortality in hospitalized patients with HFrEF (145). Similarly, the synthetic natriuretic peptide nesiritide had no significant effect on death or rehospitalization due to heart failure, including in subgroups with HFrEF (146). Serelaxin, a recombinant human relaxin-2 vasoactive peptide hormone, improved dyspnea, was well tolerated, and reduced 180-day mortality but had no effect on cardiovascular death heart failure readmissions in older adults with ADHF (147).

TREATMENT: END-OF-LIFE CARE FOR HFREF

Patients with HFrEF who are symptomatic at rest despite optimal medical therapy are considered to have end-stage HF (90). Because HF symptoms are often associated with fluid retention, euvolemia should be achieved with proper doses of diuretics. Near the end of life, HF patients may have dyspnea despite euvolemia, and small doses of opioids may be useful (148). These drugs may also alleviate other symptoms such as cough, pain, and anxiety that may be seen in end-of-life situations. Therapy may be initiated with a short-acting opioid on an as-needed basis, and titrated and given around the clock as needed and tolerated. Commonly prescribed short-acting opioids such as morphine and codeine should be used sparingly, as these drugs have active metabolites that are renally cleared and may cause delirium and myoclonus (148). To avoid unwanted adverse effects of many long-acting opioids, these drugs should be given in consultation with palliative care physicians. Hospice referral during hospital discharge has been shown to reduce the risk of readmission (90). Primary care physicians should consider referring patients for hospice and palliative care, where they can receive treatment by specially trained staff who are skilled in end-of-life communications with patients and family members and in providing spiritual and bereavement counseling and support (148).

Although comfort and relief of symptoms are more important goals than prolongation of life in patients with end-stage HF, neurohormonal blocking medication should not be discontinued, as these drugs also improve symptoms and reduce hospitalizations (149, 150). However, these drugs should be discontinued when necessary to treat specific side effects such as hypotension, bradycardia, worsening kidney function, hyperkalemia, or adverse gastrointestinal effects. Selective patients may benefit from intermittent inotropes or mechanical support. Shocks from ICDs at the end of life are generally undesirable, and patients should be offered the option for elective device deactivation.

DISCLOSURES

Ali Ahmed was in part supported by research grants from the National Institutes of Health (1RF1AG069121, 1R01HL156518, and 1R01AG073474) and the Department of Veterans Affairs (I01HX002422 and 1I01HX003552). The contents of this manuscript are solely the responsibility of the authors and do not necessarily reflect or represent the official views of the National Heart, Lung, and Blood Institute; the National Institutes of Health; the Washington DC Veterans Affairs Medical Center; the Department of Veterans Affairs; or the US government.

REFERENCES

1. Inouye SK, Studenski S, Tinetti ME, Kuchel GA. Geriatric syndromes: clinical, research, and policy implications of a core geriatric concept. *J Am Geriatr Soc* 2007;55:780–91.
2. Martin SS, Aday AW, Almarzooq ZI et al. 2024 Heart disease and stroke statistics: a report of US and global data from the American Heart Association. *Circulation* 2024;149:e347–e913.
3. Vasan RS, Enserro DM, Beiser AS, Xanthakis V. Lifetime risk of heart failure among participants in the Framingham study. *J Am Coll Cardiol* 2022;79:250–63.
4. Gottdiener JS, Arnold AM, Aurigemma GP et al. Predictors of congestive heart failure in the elderly: the cardiovascular health study. *J Am Coll Cardiol* 2000;35:1628–37.
5. Ekundayo OJ, Allman RM, Sanders PW et al. Isolated systolic hypertension and incident heart failure in older adults: a propensity-matched study. *Hypertension* 2009;53:458–65.
6. Guichard JL, Desai RV, Ahmed MI et al. Isolated diastolic hypotension and incident heart failure in older adults. *Hypertension* 2011;58:895–901.
7. Roy B, Pawar PP, Desai RV et al. A propensity-matched study of the association of diabetes mellitus with incident heart failure and mortality among community-dwelling older adults. *Am J Cardiol* 2011;108:1747–53.
8. Zile MR, Gaasch WH, Patel K, Aban IB, Ahmed A. Adverse left ventricular remodeling in community-dwelling older adults predicts incident heart failure and mortality. *JACC Heart Fail* 2014;2:512–22.
9. Bowling CB, Feller MA, Mujib M et al. Relationship between stage of kidney disease and incident heart failure in older adults. *Am J Nephrol* 2011;34:135–41.
10. Alagiakrishnan K, Patel K, Desai RV et al. Orthostatic hypotension and incident heart failure in community-dwelling older adults. *J Gerontol A Biol Sci Med Sci* 2014;69:223–30.
11. Bowling CB, Fonarow GC, Patel K et al. Impairment of activities of daily living and incident heart failure

in community-dwelling older adults. *Eur J Heart Fail* 2012;14:581–7.

12. Desai RV, Ahmed MI, Fonarow GC et al. Effect of serum insulin on the association between hyperuricemia and incident heart failure. *Am J Cardiol* 2010;106:1134–8.
13. Filippatos GS, Ahmed MI, Gladden JD et al. Hyperuricaemia, chronic kidney disease, and outcomes in heart failure: potential mechanistic insights from epidemiological data. *Eur Heart J* 2011;32:712–20.
14. Filippatos GS, Desai RV, Ahmed MI et al. Hypoalbuminaemia and incident heart failure in older adults. *Eur J Heart Fail* 2011;13:1078–86.
15. Ahmed AA, Patel K, Nyaku MA et al. Risk of heart failure and death after prolonged smoking cessation: role of amount and duration of prior smoking. *Circ Heart Fail* 2015;8:694–701.
16. Bryson CL, Mukamal KJ, Mittleman MA et al. The association of alcohol consumption and incident heart failure: the cardiovascular health study. *J Am Coll Cardiol* 2006;48:305–11.
17. Faselis C, Safren L, Allman RM et al. Income disparity and incident cardiovascular disease in older Americans. *Prog Cardiovasc Dis* 2022;71:92–9.
18. Patel K, Sui X, Zhang Y et al. Prevention of heart failure in older adults may require higher levels of physical activity than needed for other cardiovascular events. *Int J Cardiol* 2013;168:1905–9.
19. Kitzman DW, Gardin JM, Gottdiener JS et al. Importance of heart failure with preserved systolic function in patients > or = 65 years of age. CHS research group. Cardiovascular health study. *Am J Cardiol* 2001;87:413–9.
20. de Boer RA, Nayor M, deFilippi CR, et al. Association of cardiovascular biomarkers with incident heart failure with preserved and reduced ejection fraction. *JAMA Cardiology* 2018;3(3):215–224.
21. Fleg JL, Morrell CH, Bos AG et al. Accelerated longitudinal decline of aerobic capacity in healthy older adults. *Circulation* 2005;112:674–82.
22. Lakatta EG. Deficient neuroendocrine regulation of the cardiovascular system with advancing age in healthy humans. *Circulation* 1993;87:631–6.
23. Desai RV, Ahmed MI, Mujib M, Aban IB, Zile MR, Ahmed A. Natural history of concentric left ventricular geometry in community-dwelling older adults without heart failure during seven years of follow-up. *Am J Cardiol* 2011;107:321–4.
24. Fleg JL. Normative aging changes in cardiovascular structure and function. *Am J Geriatr Cardiol* 1996;5:7–15.
25. Fleg JL, Tzankoff SP, Lakatta EG. Age-related augmentation of plasma catecholamines during dynamic exercise in healthy males. *J Appl Physiol* 1985;59:1033–9.
26. Fleg JL, O'Connor F, Gerstenblith G et al. Impact of age on the cardiovascular response to dynamic upright exercise in healthy men and women. *J Appl Physiol* 1995;78:890–900.
27. Dutka DP, Olivotto I, Ward S, Oakley CM, Impallomeni M, Cleland JG. Effects of aging on neuroendocrine activation in subjects and patients in the presence and absence of heart failure with left ventricular systolic dysfunction. *Am J Cardiol* 1996;77:1197–201.
28. Ahmed A. Myocardial beta-1 adrenoceptor down-regulation in aging and heart failure: implications for beta-blocker use in older adults with heart failure. *Eur J Heart Fail* 2003;5:709–15.
29. Ahmed A. Chronic heart failure in older adults. *Med Clin North Am* 2011;95:439–61, ix.
30. Senni M, Tribouilloy CM, Rodeheffer RJ et al. Congestive heart failure in the community: a study of all incident cases in Olmsted County, Minnesota, in 1991. *Circulation* 1998;98:2282–9.
31. Ekundayo OJ, Howard VJ, Safford MM et al. Value of orthopnea, paroxysmal nocturnal dyspnea, and medications in prospective population studies of incident heart failure. *Am J Cardiol* 2009;104:259–64.
32. Maisel AS, Krishnaswamy P, Nowak RM et al. Rapid measurement of B-type natriuretic peptide in the emergency diagnosis of heart failure. *N Engl J Med* 2002;347:161–7.
33. Wright SP, Doughty RN, Pearl A et al. Plasma amino-terminal pro-brain natriuretic peptide and accuracy of heart-failure diagnosis in primary care: a randomized, controlled trial. *J Am Coll Cardiol* 2003;42:1793–800.
34. Pfisterer M, Buser P, Rickli H et al. BNP-guided vs symptom-guided heart failure therapy: the trial of intensified vs standard medical therapy in elderly patients with congestive heart failure (TIME-CHF) randomized trial. *JAMA* 2009;301:383–92.
35. Ahmed A. DEFEAT heart failure: clinical manifestations, diagnostic assessment, and etiology of geriatric heart failure. *Heart Fail Clin* 2007;3:389–402.
36. Feller MA, Mujib M, Zhang Y et al. Baseline characteristics, quality of care, and outcomes of younger and older Medicare beneficiaries hospitalized with heart failure: findings from the Alabama Heart Failure Project. *Int J Cardiol* 2012;162:39–44.
37. Bhatia V, Ahmed MI, Desai RV et al. Incidence and predictors of hospitalization due to heart failure among Medicare-eligible community-dwelling older adults with prevalent heart failure: insights from a prospective population study. *Circulation* 2010;122 (Supplement: Abstract):A20952.
38. Stein GY, Kremer A, Shochat T et al. The diversity of heart failure in a hospitalized population: the role of age. *J Card Fail* 2012;18:645–53.
39. Carson P, Anand I, O'Connor C et al. Mode of death in advanced heart failure: the comparison of medical, pacing, and defibrillation therapies in heart failure (COMPANION) trial. *J Am Coll Cardiol* 2005;46:2329–34.

40. Zile MR, Gaasch WH, Anand IS et al. Mode of death in patients with heart failure and a preserved ejection fraction: results from the Irbesartan in heart failure with preserved ejection fraction study (I-Preserve) trial. *Circulation* 2010;121:1393–405.
41. Wahle C, Adamopoulos C, Ekundayo OJ, Mujib M, Aronow WS, Ahmed A. A propensity-matched study of outcomes of chronic heart failure (HF) in younger and older adults. *Arch Gerontol Geriatr* 2009;49:165–71.
42. Ahmed MI, Mujib M, Desai RV et al. Outcomes in younger and older adults with chronic advanced systolic heart failure: a propensity-matched study. *Int J Cardiol* 2012;154:128–33.
43. Ahmed MI, Lainscak M, Mujib M et al. Gender-related dissociation in outcomes in chronic heart failure: reduced mortality but similar hospitalization in women. *Int J Cardiol* 2011;148:36–42.
44. Gambassi G, Agha SA, Sui X et al. Race and the natural history of chronic heart failure: a propensity-matched study. *J Card Fail* 2008;14:373–8.
45. Ahmed A. A propensity matched study of New York Heart Association class and natural history end points in heart failure. *Am J Cardiol* 2007;99:549–53.
46. Ahmed A, Aronow WS. A propensity-matched study of the association of physical function and outcomes in geriatric heart failure. *Arch Gerontol Geriatr* 2008;46:161–72.
47. Ahmed A, Aronow WS, Fleg JL. Higher New York Heart Association classes and increased mortality and hospitalization in patients with heart failure and preserved left ventricular function. *Am Heart J* 2006;151:444–50.
48. Ahmed A. Association of diastolic dysfunction and outcomes in ambulatory older adults with chronic heart failure. *J Gerontol A Biol Sci Med Sci* 2005;60:1339–44.
49. MAGGIC Investigators. The survival of patients with heart failure with preserved or reduced left ventricular ejection fraction: an individual patient data meta-analysis. Meta-analysis global group in chronic heart failure (MAGGIC). *Eur Heart J* 2012;33:1750–7.
50. Meyer P, Desai RV, Mujib M et al. Right ventricular ejection fraction <20% is an independent predictor of mortality but not of hospitalization in older systolic heart failure patients. *Int J Cardiol* 2012;155:120–5.
51. Ahmed A, Aban IB, Vaccarino V et al. A propensity-matched study of the effect of diabetes on the natural history of heart failure: variations by sex and age. *Heart* 2007;93:1584–90.
52. Ahmed MI, White M, Ekundayo OJ et al. A history of atrial fibrillation and outcomes in chronic advanced systolic heart failure: a propensity-matched study. *Eur Heart J* 2009;30:2029–37.
53. Patel SS, Raman VK, Zhang S et al. Identification and outcomes of KDIGO-defined chronic kidney disease in 1.4 million U.S. veterans with heart failure. *Eur J Heart Fail* 2024;26:1251–60.
54. Patel S, Raman VK, Faselis C et al. Outcomes of KDIGO-defined CKD in U.S. Veterans with HFpEF, HFmrEF, and HFrEF. *JACC Heart Fail* 2025;13:467–79.
55. Ahmed A, Zannad F, Love TE et al. A propensity-matched study of the association of low serum potassium levels and mortality in chronic heart failure. *Eur Heart J* 2007;28:1334–43.
56. Alper AB, Campbell RC, Anker SD et al. A propensity-matched study of low serum potassium and mortality in older adults with chronic heart failure. *Int J Cardiol* 2009;137:1–8.
57. Valentova M, Patel S, Lam PH et al. Hypokalaemia and outcomes in older patients hospitalized for heart failure. *ESC Heart Fail* 2020;7:794–803.
58. Ahmed MI, Ekundayo OJ, Mujib M et al. Mild hyperkalemia and outcomes in chronic heart failure: a propensity matched study. *Int J Cardiol* 2010;144:383–8.
59. Adamopoulos C, Pitt B, Sui X, Love TE, Zannad F, Ahmed A. Low serum magnesium and cardiovascular mortality in chronic heart failure: a propensity-matched study. *Int J Cardiol* 2009;136:270–7.
60. Pulignano G, Del Sindaco D, Di Lenarda A et al. Incremental value of gait speed in predicting prognosis of older adults with heart failure: insights from the IMAGE-HF study. *JACC Heart Fail* 2016;4:289–98.
61. Sims RV, Mujib M, McGwin G, Jr. et al. Heart failure is a risk factor for incident driving cessation among community-dwelling older adults: findings from a prospective population study. *J Card Fail* 2011;17:1035–40.
62. Lovasi GS, Richardson JM, Rodriguez CJ et al. Residential relocation by older adults in response to incident cardiovascular health events: a case-crossover analysis. *J Environ Public Health* 2014;2014:951971.
63. Gupta D, Georgiopoulou VV, Kalogeropoulos AP et al. Dietary sodium intake in heart failure. *Circulation* 2012;126:479–85.
64. Gheorghiade M, Abraham WT, Albert NM et al. Relationship between admission serum sodium concentration and clinical outcomes in patients hospitalized for heart failure: an analysis from the OPTIMIZE-HF registry. *Eur Heart J* 2007;28:980–8.
65. Kenchaiah S, Evans JC, Levy D et al. Obesity and the risk of heart failure. *N Engl J Med* 2002;347:305–13.
66. Wannamethee SG, Shaper AG, Whincup PH, Lennon L, Sattar N. Obesity and risk of incident heart failure in older men with and without pre-existing coronary heart disease: does leptin have a role? *J Am Coll Cardiol* 2011;58:1870–7.

67. Fonarow GC, Srikanthan P, Costanzo MR et al. An obesity paradox in acute heart failure: analysis of body mass index and inhospital mortality for 108,927 patients in the acute decompensated heart failure national registry. *Am Heart J* 2007;153:74–81.
68. Hu G, Jousilahti P, Antikainen R, Katzmarzyk PT, Tuomilehto J. Joint effects of physical activity, body mass index, waist circumference, and waist-to-hip ratio on the risk of heart failure. *Circulation* 2010;121:237–44.
69. Wang Y, Tuomilehto J, Jousilahti P et al. Occupational, commuting, and leisure-time physical activity in relation to heart failure among Finnish men and women. *J Am Coll Cardiol* 2010;56:1140–8.
70. Fleg JL. Exercise therapy for older heart failure patients. *Heart Fail Clin* 2017;13:607–17.
71. Austin J, Williams R, Ross L, Moseley L, Hutchison S. Randomised controlled trial of cardiac rehabilitation in elderly patients with heart failure. *Eur J Heart Fail* 2005;7:411–17.
72. O'Connor CM, Whellan DJ, Lee KL et al. Efficacy and safety of exercise training in patients with chronic heart failure: HF-ACTION randomized controlled trial. *JAMA* 2009;301:1439–50.
73. Flynn KE, Pina IL, Whellan DJ et al. Effects of exercise training on health status in patients with chronic heart failure: HF-ACTION randomized controlled trial. *JAMA* 2009;301:1451–9.
74. Blumenthal JA, Babyak MA, O'Connor C et al. Effects of exercise training on depressive symptoms in patients with chronic heart failure: the HF-ACTION randomized trial. *JAMA* 2012;308:465–74.
75. Pandey A, Segar MW, Singh S et al. Frailty status modifies the efficacy of exercise training among patients with chronic heart failure and reduced ejection fraction: an analysis from the HF-ACTION trial. *Circulation* 2022;146:80–90.
76. Takeda A, Martin N, Taylor RS, Taylor SJ. Disease management interventions for heart failure. *Cochrane Database Syst Rev* 2019;1:CD002752.
77. Lindenfeld J, Costanzo MR, Zile MR et al. Implantable hemodynamic monitors improve survival in patients with heart failure and reduced ejection fraction. *J Am Coll Cardiol* 2024;83:682–94.
78. Cohn JN, Goldstein SO, Greenberg BH et al. A dose-dependent increase in mortality with vesnarinone among patients with severe heart failure. Vesnarinone trial investigators. *N Engl J Med* 1998;339:1810–6.
79. Massie B, Bourassa M, DiBianco R et al. Long-term oral administration of amrinone for congestive heart failure: lack of efficacy in a multicenter controlled trial. *Circulation* 1985;71:963–71.
80. Curtiss C, Cohn JN, Vrobel T, Franciosa JA. Role of the renin-angiotensin system in the systemic vasoconstriction of chronic congestive heart failure. *Circulation* 1978;58:763–70.
81. Packer M. Role of the sympathetic nervous system in chronic heart failure. A historical and philosophical perspective. *Circulation* 1990;82:11–6.
82. The SOLVD Investigators. Effect of enalapril on survival in patients with reduced left ventricular ejection fractions and congestive heart failure. *N Engl J Med* 1991;325:293–302.
83. Granger CB, McMurray JJ, Yusuf S et al. Effects of candesartan in patients with chronic heart failure and reduced left-ventricular systolic function intolerant to angiotensin-converting-enzyme inhibitors: the CHARM-Alternative trial. *Lancet* 2003;362:772–6.
84. McMurray JJ, Packer M, Desai AS et al. Angiotensin-neprilysin inhibition versus enalapril in heart failure. *N Engl J Med* 2014;371:993–1004.
85. Packer M, Coats AJ, Fowler MB et al. Effect of carvedilol on survival in severe chronic heart failure. *N Engl J Med* 2001;344:1651–8.
86. The MERIT-HF Investigators. Effect of metoprolol CR/XL in chronic heart failure: metoprolol CR/XL randomised intervention trial in congestive heart failure (MERIT-HF). *Lancet* 1999;353:2001–7.
87. Pitt B, Zannad F, Remme WJ et al. The effect of spironolactone on morbidity and mortality in patients with severe heart failure. Randomized Aldactone Evaluation Study Investigators. *N Engl J Med* 1999;341:709–17.
88. Zannad F, McMurray JJ, Krum H et al. Eplerenone in patients with systolic heart failure and mild symptoms. *N Engl J Med* 2011;364:11–21.
89. Masoudi FA, Havranek EP, Wolfe P et al. Most hospitalized older persons do not meet the enrollment criteria for clinical trials in heart failure. *Am Heart J* 2003;146:250–7.
90. Heidenreich PA, Bozkurt B, Aguilar D et al. 2022 AHA/ACC/HFSA Guideline for the management of heart failure: a report of the American Cardiology/American Heart Association Joint Committee on Clinical Practice Guidelines. *J Am Coll Cardiol* 2022;79:e263–e421.
91. Faselis C, Arundel C, Patel S et al. Loop diuretic prescription and 30-day outcomes in older patients with heart failure. *J Am Coll Cardiol* 2020;76:669–79.
92. Faselis C, Lam PH, Patel S et al. Loop diuretic prescription and long-term outcomes in heart failure: association modification by congestion. *Am J Med* 2021;134:797–804.
93. Lopez B, Querejeta R, Gonzalez A, Sanchez E, Larman M, Diez J. Effects of loop diuretics on myocardial fibrosis and collagen type I turnover in chronic heart failure. *J Am Coll Cardiol* 2004;43:2028–35.
94. Mentz RJ, Anstrom KJ, Eisenstein EL et al. Effect of torsemide vs furosemide after discharge on all-cause mortality in patients hospitalized with heart failure: the TRANSFORM-HF randomized clinical trial. *JAMA* 2023;329:214–23.

95. Ekundayo OJ, Markland A, Lefante C et al. Association of diuretic use and overactive bladder syndrome in older adults: a propensity score analysis. *Arch Gerontol Geriatr* 2009;49:64–8.
96. Ahmed A, Fonarow GC, Zhang Y et al. Renin-angiotensin inhibition in systolic heart failure and chronic kidney disease. *Am J Med* 2012;125:399–410.
97. Sanam K, Bhatia V, Bajaj NS et al. Renin-angiotensin system inhibition and lower 30-day all-cause readmission in medicare beneficiaries with heart failure. *Am J Med* 2016;129:1067–73.
98. Sin MK, Allman RM, Faselis C et al. Lower risk of death and kidney failure associated with higher target (vs below-target) doses of RAS inhibitors in octogenarians withHFrEF. *Am J Med* 2025;138:639–649.e4.
99. Jhund PS, Fu M, Bayram E et al. Efficacy and safety of LCZ696 (sacubitril-valsartan) according to age: insights from PARADIGM-HF. *Eur Heart J* 2015;36:2576–84.
100. Deedwania PC, Gottlieb S, Ghali JK, Waagstein F, Wikstrand JC, Group M-HS. Efficacy, safety and tolerability of beta-adrenergic blockade with metoprolol CR/XL in elderly patients with heart failure. *Euro Heart J* 2004;25:1300–9.
101. Poole-Wilson PA, Swedberg K, Cleland JG et al. Comparison of carvedilol and metoprolol on clinical outcomes in patients with chronic heart failure in the Carvedilol Or Metoprolol European Trial (COMET): randomised controlled trial. *Lancet* 2003;362:7–13.
102. Ferreira JP, Rossello X, Eschalier R et al. MRAs in elderly hf patients: individual patient-data meta-analysis of RALES, EMPHASIS-HF, and TOPCAT. *JACC Heart Fail* 2019;7:1012–21.
103. Taylor AL, Ziesche S, Yancy C et al. Combination of isosorbide dinitrate and hydralazine in blacks with heart failure. *N Engl J Med* 2004;351:2049–57.
104. The Digitalis Investigation Group. The effect of digoxin on mortality and morbidity in patients with heart failure. *N Engl J Med* 1997;336:525–33.
105. Ahmed A, Rich MW, Love TE et al. Digoxin and reduction in mortality and hospitalization in heart failure: a comprehensive post hoc analysis of the DIG trial. *Eur Heart J* 2006;27:178–86.
106. Bourge RC, Fleg JL, Fonarow GC et al. Digoxin reduces 30-day all-cause hospital admission in older patients with chronic systolic heart failure. *Am J Med* 2013;126:701–8.
107. Ahmed A, Bourge RC, Fonarow GC et al. Digoxin use and lower 30-day all-cause readmission for Medicare beneficiaries hospitalized for heart failure. *Am J Med* 2014;127:61–70.
108. Sheriff HM, Thogaripally MR, Panjrath G et al. Digoxin and 30-day all-cause readmission in long-term care residents hospitalized for heart failure. *J Am Med Dir Assoc* 2017;18:761–5.
109. Ahmed A. Digoxin and reduction in mortality and hospitalization in geriatric heart failure: importance of low doses and low serum concentrations. *J Gerontol A Biol Sci Med Sci* 2007;62:323–9.
110. Malik A, Masson R, Singh S et al. Digoxin discontinuation and outcomes in patients with heart failure with reduced ejection fraction. *J Am Coll Cardiol* 2019;74:617–27.
111. Lam PH, Liu K, Ahmed AA et al. Digoxin discontinuation in patients with HFrEF on beta-blockers: implication for future 'knock-out trials' in heart failure. *Am J Med* 2024 Oct 17:S0002-9343(24)00638-7 doi: 101016/jamjmed202410015 2024.
112. Abraham WT, Adams KF, Fonarow GC et al. In-hospital mortality in patients with acute decompensated heart failure requiring intravenous vasoactive medications: an analysis from the Acute Decompensated Heart Failure National Registry (ADHERE). *J Am Coll Cardiol* 2005;46:57–64.
113. Slawsky MT, Colucci WS, Gottlieb SS et al. Acute hemodynamic and clinical effects of levosimendan in patients with severe heart failure. Study investigators. *Circulation* 2000;102:2222–7.
114. Mebazaa A, Nieminen MS, Packer M et al. Levosimendan vs dobutamine for patients with acute decompensated heart failure: the SURVIVE randomized trial. *JAMA* 2007;297:1883–91.
115. Rich MW, Imburgia M. Inotropic response to dobutamine in elderly patients with decompensated congestive heart failure. *Am J Cardiol* 1990;65:519–21.
116. McMurray JJV, Solomon SD, Inzucchi SE et al. Dapagliflozin in patients with heart failure and reduced ejection fraction. *N Engl J Med* 2019;381:1995–2008.
117. Packer M, Anker SD, Butler J et al. Cardiovascular and renal outcomes with empagliflozin in heart failure. *N Engl J Med* 2020;383:1413–24.
118. Zannad F, Ferreira JP, Pocock SJ et al. SGLT2 inhibitors in patients with heart failure with reduced ejection fraction: a meta-analysis of the EMPEROR-Reduced and DAPA-HF trials. *Lancet* 2020;396:819–29.
119. Rashid AM, Khan MS, Fudim M, DeWald TA, DeVore A, Butler J. Management of heart failure with reduced ejection fraction. *Curr Probl Cardiol* 2023;48:101596.
120. Armstrong PW, Pieske B, Anstrom KJ et al. Vericiguat in patients with heart failure and reduced ejection fraction. *N Engl J Med* 2020;382:1883–93.
121. Teerlink JR, Diaz R, Felker GM et al. Cardiac myosin activation with omecamtiv mecarbil in systolic heart failure. *N Engl J Med* 2021;384:105–16.
122. Swedberg K, Komajda M, Bohm M et al. Ivabradine and outcomes in chronic heart failure (SHIFT): a randomised placebo-controlled study. *Lancet* 2010;376:875–85.

123. Anand I, McMurray J, Cohn JN et al. Long-term effects of darusentan on left-ventricular remodelling and clinical outcomes in the EndothelinA receptor antagonist trial in heart failure (EARTH): randomised, double-blind, placebo-controlled trial. *Lancet* 2004;364:347–54.
124. Kalra PR, Cleland JGF, Petrie MC et al. Intravenous ferric derisomaltose in patients with heart failure and iron deficiency in the UK (IRONMAN): an investigator-initiated, prospective, randomised, open-label, blinded-endpoint trial. *Lancet* 2022;400:2199–209.
125. Abraham WT, Fisher WG, Smith AL et al. Cardiac resynchronization in chronic heart failure. *N Engl J Med* 2002;346:1845–53.
126. Bristow MR, Saxon LA, Boehmer J et al. Cardiac-resynchronization therapy with or without an implantable defibrillator in advanced chronic heart failure. *N Engl J Med* 2004;350:2140–50.
127. Zeitler EP, Dalgaard F, Abraham WT et al. Benefit of cardiac resynchronization therapy among older patients: a patient-level meta-analysis. *Am Heart J* 2024;267:81–90.
128. Moss AJ, Zareba W, Hall WJ et al. Prophylactic implantation of a defibrillator in patients with myocardial infarction and reduced ejection fraction. *N Engl J Med* 2002;346:877–83.
129. Bardy GH, Lee KL, Mark DB et al. Amiodarone or an implantable cardioverter-defibrillator for congestive heart failure. *N Engl J Med* 2005;352:225–37.
130. Mark DB, Anstrom KJ, Sun JL et al. Quality of life with defibrillator therapy or amiodarone in heart failure. *N Engl J Med* 2008;359:999–1008.
131. Kadish A, Dyer A, Daubert JP et al. Prophylactic defibrillator implantation in patients with nonischemic dilated cardiomyopathy. *N Engl J Med* 2004;350:2151–8.
132. Rose EA, Gelijns AC, Moskowitz AJ et al. Long-term use of a left ventricular assist device for end-stage heart failure. *N Engl J Med* 2001;345:1435–43.
133. Kim JH, Singh R, Pagani FD et al. Ventricular assist device therapy in older patients with heart failure: characteristics and outcomes. *J Card Fail* 2016;22:981–7.
134. Mehra MR, Uriel N, Naka Y et al. A fully magnetically levitated left ventricular assist device – final report. *N Engl J Med* 2019;380:1618–27.
135. Levinson JR, Akins CW, Buckley MJ et al. Octogenarians with aortic stenosis. Outcome after aortic valve replacement. *Circulation* 1989;80:I49–56.
136. Leon MB, Smith CR, Mack M et al. Transcatheter aortic-valve implantation for aortic stenosis in patients who cannot undergo surgery. *N Engl J Med* 2010;363:1597–607.
137. Siemieniuk RA, Agoritsas T, Manja V et al. Transcatheter versus surgical aortic valve replacement in patients with severe aortic stenosis at low and intermediate risk: systematic review and meta-analysis. BMJ 2016;354:i5130.
138. Smith CR, Leon MB, Mack MJ et al. Transcatheter versus surgical aortic-valve replacement in high-risk patients. *N Engl J Med* 2011;364:2187–98.
139. Stone GW, Lindenfeld J, Abraham WT et al. Transcatheter mitral-valve repair in patients with heart failure. *N Engl J Med* 2018;379:2307–18.
140. Velazquez EJ, Lee KL, Deja MA et al. Coronary-artery bypass surgery in patients with left ventricular dysfunction. *N Engl J Med* 2011;364:1607–16.
141. Velazquez EJ, Lee KL, Jones RH et al. Coronary-artery bypass surgery in patients with ischemic cardiomyopathy. *N Engl J Med* 2016;374:1511–20.
142. Sollie ZW, Kwon JH, Usry B et al. Changes in heart transplant outcomes of elderly patients in the new allocation era. *J Thorac Cardiovasc Surg* 2025;169:134–45 e1.
143. Bozkurt B, Ahmad T, Alexander K et al. HF STATS 2024: heart failure epidemiology and outcomes statistics an updated 2024 report from the heart failure society of America. *J Card Fail* 2025;31:66–116.
144. Felker GM, Lee, Bull DA et al. Diuretic strategies in patients with acute decompensated heart failure. *N Engl J Med* 2011;364:797–805.
145. Konstam MA, Gheorghiade M, Burnett JC, Jr. et al. Effects of oral tolvaptan in patients hospitalized for worsening heart failure: the EVEREST outcome trial. *JAMA* 2007;297:1319–31.
146. O'Connor CM, Starling RC, Hernandez AF et al. Effect of nesiritide in patients with acute decompensated heart failure. *N Engl J Med* 2011;365:32–43.
147. Metra M, Teerlink JR, Cotter G et al. Effects of serelaxin in patients with acute heart failure. *N Engl J Med* 2019;381:716–26.
148. Goodlin SJ. Palliative care in congestive heart failure. *J Am Coll Cardiol* 2009;54:386–96.
149. Tomasoni D, Vishram-Nielsen JKK, Pagnesi M et al. Advanced heart failure: guideline-directed medical therapy, diuretics, inotropes, and palliative care. *ESC Heart Fail* 2022;9:1507–23.
150. Chuzi S, Saylor MA, Allen LA et al. Integration of palliative care into heart failure care: consensus-based recommendations from the heart failure society of America. *J Card Fail* 2024;S1071-9164(24)00882-0. doi.org/10.1016/j.cardfail.2024.10.435.

20

Heart failure with preserved ejection fraction in older adults

BHARATHI UPADHYA, AKSHAY PENDYAL, AND PARAG GOYAL

Key points

- HFpEF is the most common form of heart failure in the community, particularly among older persons and women.
- Initially, HFpEF was viewed as a disorder due solely to abnormalities in LV diastolic function. However, our understanding has evolved to an appreciation that HFpEF is a systemic syndrome involving multiple organ systems influenced by aging, lifestyle factors, genetic predisposition, and multiple comorbidities.
- Treatment strategies include pharmacologic therapy, nonpharmacologic therapy, and management of multimorbidity.
- Pharmacologic therapy includes the use of loop diuretics, sodium-glucose cotransporter 2 inhibitors, and mineralocorticoid antagonists for most, and angiotensin receptor blockers/angiotensin receptor–neprilysin inhibitors and glucagon-like peptide 1 receptor agonists as add-on therapies for some.
- Nonpharmacologic therapy may include exercise training and caloric restriction.
- The concurrence of geriatric conditions should impact care and treatment priorities, with explicit integration of shared decision-making, multidisciplinary team use, and palliative care principles applicable across the disease spectrum starting as early as the diagnosis.

INTRODUCTION

Heart failure with preserved ejection fraction (HFpEF) is the most common form of heart failure in the community, particularly among older persons and women.[1] HFpEF is associated with high morbidity and mortality. After HF hospitalization (HFH), the 5-year survival of HFpEF is a dismal 35%, worse than many cancers.[2] During the last decade, our understanding of the pathophysiology (and our diagnostic approach) for HFpEF has markedly evolved. We now appreciate HFpEF as a systemic syndrome with pathogenesis involving multiple interacting pathways, including but not limited to aging processes, lifestyle factors, and genetic predisposition. HFpEF is a heterogeneous syndrome of multiple discrete phenotypes characterized by multiple intersecting cardiovascular (CV) and non-CV comorbidities.[3]

EPIDEMIOLOGY

HFpEF increases progressively with age; even within the older age range, and among older women, >80% of new cases of heart failure (HF) are HFpEF.[1] In the highest age decile (≥90 years old), nearly all patients with HF have HFpEF. The lifetime risk of HFpEF is nearly double that of HF with reduced ejection fraction (HFrEF) among women (10.7% vs. 5.8%), whereas the lifetime risk of

DOI: 10.1201/9781003568933-20

HFpEF and HFrEF are similar among men.[4] Although the incidence of HFpEF is similar among men and women, the prevalence of HFpEF is higher in women compared with men.[5] The overall incidence of HF in the United States appears to be stable or even decreasing, though the incidence of HFpEF continues to rise. Similarly, the prevalence of HFpEF is increasing and is expected to exceed that of HFrEF soon.[6]

In-hospital mortality in HFpEF ranges from 2.4% to 4.9%, with higher mortality rates at 30 days (5%) and 60–90 days (9.5%).[6–9] At 1 year, mortality in HFpEF varies from 20% to 29%.[2,8,10] By 5 years, at least half of patients with HFpEF have died.[2,10] The risk of death in patients with HFpEF increases with increasing comorbidity burden.[11] Even after adjustment of comorbid conditions, the mortality rates associated with HFpEF are higher compared with the general population of similar age.[12] While CV causes are a common cause of death, non-CV causes of death are very common and account for a significant proportion of deaths in HFpEF.[13] HFH is common in patients with HFpEF and frequently owing to non-CV causes.[14] In patients hospitalized with HFpEF, 20% are readmitted within 30 days of hospital discharge and >50% within 1 year.[15] Data from the National Inpatient Sample demonstrate that the number of HFpEF hospitalizations more than doubled from 189,260 in 2008 to 495,095 in 2018.[16] In addition, patients with HFpEF have poor quality of life (QOL), similar in severity to patients with HFrEF.[17]

DIAGNOSIS OF HFPEF AND CHALLENGES

Clinical manifestations of HFpEF are generally similar to those of HFrEF. HF is a clinical diagnosis made by routine history and physical examination. The cardinal manifestations of HF are exertional dyspnea and fatigue. In the chronic, stable state, even when relatively euvolemic and well compensated, patients with HFpEF may have severe exercise intolerance. Patients with HFpEF are at risk for acute exacerbations, marked by severe dyspnea, volume overload, peripheral edema, and pulmonary edema. Several precipitating factors can cause an episode of HFpEF decompensation (Table 20.1).[18] The most frequent are pneumonia and respiratory processes, arrhythmia, uncontrolled hypertension, and noncompliance with pharmacological treatment and diet. On clinical examination during acute decompensation, increased jugular venous pressure (JVP), peripheral edema, and pulmonary rales may be noted. An S4 gallop is caused by increased left ventricle (LV) stiffness and is often present in older adults with or without HF.

The most common symptom of HFpEF is exertional dyspnea. However, symptoms of reduced exercise tolerance are common in older adults and have been shown to reflect normal physiological changes related to aging or those due to noncardiac etiologies. Accordingly, exertional dyspnea poses a diagnostic challenge since multiple potential etiologies exist for such symptoms (pulmonary causes, anemia, or physical deconditioning). Similarly, elevated JVP is relatively specific but insensitive and often difficult to elicit, especially among those with obesity. Pulmonary rales are a hallmark of pulmonary edema but may also be caused by atelectasis or chronic lung disease in older patients. Lower extremity edema is another potential sign of HFpEF that may be caused by other conditions, such as medications (especially calcium channel blockers), venous insufficiency, lymphedema, kidney disease, or malnutrition in the geriatric population. Several other medical conditions can mimic HFpEF and create diagnostic uncertainty (Table 20.2).

Table 20.1 Common precipitating factors of HFpEF

- Dietary or medication nonadherence
- Excess fluid intake (including intravenous fluids-Iatrogenic)
- Alcohol or illicit drugs (especially cocaine, amphetamines)
- Infection (pneumonia, sepsis)
- Myocardial infarction/ischemia
- Poorly controlled hypertension
- Arrhythmias (especially atrial fibrillation/atrial flutter)
- Anemia
- Renal insufficiency
- Pulmonary embolism
- Valvular dysfunction
- Medication withdrawal (e.g., diuretics)
- Stress (e.g., major surgery, major life events)
- Chronic obstructive pulmonary disease exacerbation
- Drugs: steroids, TZDs, NSAIDs

Abbreviations: TZD, thiazolidinediones; NSAIDs, nonsteroidal anti-inflammatory drugs.

Basic laboratory evaluation for suspected HF includes a chest x-ray, 12-lead electrocardiogram, and selected blood tests such as renal and liver function panels and natriuretic peptides (NPs). The Heart Failure Society of America (HFSA) and Heart Failure Association of the European Society of Cardiology (HFA/ESC) guidelines recommend measuring NPs to support or exclude the diagnosis of HF.[19,20] This includes B-type NP (BNP) and N-terminal prohormone BNP (NT-proBNP). BNP accurately diagnoses HF in patients presenting to the emergency department with dyspnea, with a sensitivity of 90% and specificity of 76% at a 100 pg/ml cutoff value.[21,22] ESC guidelines recommend the following cutoff points for the exclusion of HF: 35 pg/mL for BNP, 125 pg/mL for NT-proBNP in the chronic setting; 100 pg/mL for BNP, 300 pg/mL for NT-proBNP in the acute setting.

Age and gender can affect NP levels, reducing their diagnostic value in older persons. Interpreting NP results requires additional information, especially in older

Table 20.2 Common comorbidities complicating the diagnosis of HFpEF and their management

Problem	Comments
Obesity	Alternative causes for breathlessness create diagnostic uncertainty. A hypocaloric diet can benefit highly selected patients. Data suggest symptomatic benefits from treating obesity using GLPIRAs.
COPD	Alternative causes for breathlessness create diagnostic uncertainty. Patients with HFpEF and COPD have a worse prognosis. Optimize therapy and smoking cessation.
SDB	Formal sleep assessment in patients with HFpEF suspected of SDB or excessive daytime sleepiness; routine screening is advised. Refer to a sleep study to confirm the diagnosis. Continuous positive airway pressure in patients with obstructive sleep apnea.
Atrial fibrillation (AF)	AF may cause HF and vice versa. Restoration and maintenance of sinus rhythm; control of heart rate in patients with permanent AF. Optimal ventricular rate control may be about 80 bpm at rest. Anticoagulation with DOAC is recommended over warfarin in eligible patients. Catheter ablation should be considered when there is an association between AF episodes and HFpEF decompensation.
Ischemic heart disease	Search for and treat symptomatic myocardial ischemia. Revascularize in appropriate patients with HFpEF and suitable coronary anatomy.
Hypertension	Most treatments for HFpEF reduce blood pressure. Blood pressure goal <130/80 mmHg.
Anemia	Often associated with iron deficiency. Consider intravenous iron replacement for symptom improvement. Consider transfusion in severe cases.
Diabetes mellitus	This indicates a worse prognosis. HbA1c goal of <7% for most adults, allowing for individualization based on patient characteristics and comorbid conditions. SGLT2 inhibitors for all patients with HFpEF and T2DM. SGLT2 inhibitors are contraindicated in patients with eGFR <30 mL/min/m^2. TZDs are contraindicated in patients with NYHA class III–IV HF.
Chronic kidney disease	Often due to preexisting renal damage and exacerbated by hypotension and low renal blood flow. Often limits the doses of medication that can be given. Can influence drug clearance. Adverse effects from drug treatment, including dehydration and electrolyte abnormalities. Optimize RAAS inhibitor therapy.
Stroke	They are related mainly to preexisting hypertension, atherosclerosis, and AF.
Dementia	Age often brings deterioration in cognitive as well as cardiac function. Dementia reduces the ability for self-care and adherence to advice and medication. Worsening HF may impair cognitive function.
Viral infection	Vaccination is encouraged.
Aortic stenosis	Diuretics may reduce congestion and symptoms. SAVR or TAVR for severe aortic stenosis.
Mitral regurgitation	Percutaneous correction of secondary mitral regurgitation should be considered if the patient fulfills the criteria for reducing HF hospitalizations.

Abbreviations: GLP1RAs, glucagon-like peptide 1 receptor agonists; HF, heart failure; HFpEF, HF with preserved ejection fraction; COPD, chronic obstructive lung disease; SDB, sleep disordered breathing; DOAC, direct oral anticoagulants; SGLT2, sodium-glucose cotransporter 2; T2DM, type 2 diabetes; eGFR, estimated glomerular filtration rate; TZD, thiazolidinediones; NYHA, New York Heart Association; RAAS, renin–angiotensin–aldosterone system; SAVR, surgical aortic valve replacement; TAVR, transcatheter aortic valve replacement.

adults, atrial fibrillation (AF), and renal dysfunction, where there is an increase in plasma NP concentrations.[22] This provides a rationale for age-stratified cutoff points for NT-proBNP (≥450 for ages <50 years, ≥900 for 50–75 years, and ≥1800 pg/mL for >75 years).[22,23] Female sex is an independent predictor of higher NP levels in older adults, even without cardiac dysfunction.[23] Importantly, NP levels are inversely related to body mass index (BMI), which is highly relevant since obesity is prevalent in HFpEF. This can create diagnostic challenges in patients with obesity, who may have normal levels of NP despite the diagnosis of HFpEF.[24,25] Other reasons for falsely low levels of NPs despite the presence of HFpEF include prior CV surgery, inflammation, hyperthyroidism, and prior use of angiotensin receptor–neprilysin inhibitors. Consequently, up to one third of ambulatory patients with HFpEF may have NPs below the typical diagnostic thresholds.[26] This highlights that NPs should be carefully evaluated within the context of all other clinical information on older patients with possible HFpEF.

A transthoracic echocardiogram (TTE) is important for all patients with suspected HF. Not only will a TTE assess left ventricular ejection fraction (LVEF), but it may also provide clues to other etiologies of a HFpEF syndrome, such as valvular disease, hypertrophic obstructive cardiomyopathy, and infiltrative cardiomyopathies such as cardiac amyloidosis. Patients presenting with HF with a preserved EF who have these diagnoses are not usually labeled as having HFpEF. Instead, they are considered distinct conditions with unique pathophysiologic mechanisms and therapeutic strategies despite being HF syndromes with normal or preserved EF. To definitively diagnose HFpEF, these conditions must be ruled out. In this way, HFpEF may be considered a diagnosis of exclusion, albeit a common one.

HFPEF SCORES TO PREDICT THE PROBABILITY OF HFPEF

Due to the lack of specific tests to definitively diagnose HFpEF, clinical scoring systems have been developed to diagnose suspected HFpEF. In 2018, the H_2FPEF algorithm was introduced to diagnose patients with HFpEF, a simple algorithm derived retrospectively from clinical characteristics and TTE measures.[27] The HFA/ESC has proposed utilizing different HFA–PEFF algorithms to diagnose HFpEF.[28] Both the H_2FPEF and HFA–PEFF scores can aid clinicians in diagnosing HFpEF. However, there are limitations. Each algorithm identified different HFpEF subgroups with different comorbid and imaging features, and there was little concordance between those.[29] Thus, using either the H_2FPEF or HFA–PEFF score must be undertaken with the expectation that further clinical evaluation will be needed (Table 20.3).

RISK FACTORS AND PATHOPHYSIOLOGY

Initially, HFpEF was viewed as a disorder due solely to abnormalities in LV diastolic function; however, our understanding has evolved now such that HFpEF is considered a systemic syndrome involving multiple organ systems, influenced by aging, lifestyle factors, genetic predisposition, and multiple comorbidities (Figure 20.1).[3,11] Normal aging is associated with extensive changes in the CV system that reduce CV reserve and predispose to the development of HFpEF (Table 20.4).[30,31] The new paradigm of HFpEF pathophysiology incorporates aging along with multiple comorbidities that may initiate chronic systemic inflammation that may affect myocardial remodeling and dysfunction in HFpEF through a signaling cascade, which may begin with coronary microvascular endothelial dysfunction.[11] The hemodynamic changes seen with adverse LV remodeling, along with this inflammatory response, activate the renin–angiotensin–aldosterone system (RAAS) and sympathetic nervous system. Their activation alters the phenotype of vascular and cardiac smooth muscle cells and produces proinflammatory cytokines, further damaging the myocardium and peripheral organ system, leading to clinical HF (Figure 20.1).[3,30,31]

MANAGEMENT OF HFPEF IN OLDER ADULTS

Effective management of HFpEF includes (1) pharmacologic therapy that includes symptomatic therapy with loop diuretics and disease-modifying therapy with sodium-glucose cotransporter 2 (SGLT2) inhibitors, mineralocorticoid antagonists (MRAs), glucagon-like peptide 1 receptor agonists (GLP-1RAs), angiotensin receptor blockers (ARBs), and ARB–neprilysin inhibitors (ARNIs); (2) nonpharmacologic therapy; (3) treatment of comorbid conditions that interact with the pathophysiology and the clinical course of HFpEF; and (4) patient education, self-management skills, care coordination across disciplines, and effective follow-up.

PHARMACOLOGIC THERAPY

Symptomatic treatment

Loop diuretics promote the excretion of sodium and chloride (along with potassium) by inhibiting the sodium potassium-chloride cotransporter of the ascending limb of the loop of Henle in the kidneys, resulting in significant diuresis.[32] Studies showed that loop diuretics, by lowering LV filling pressure, improved symptoms and reduced HFH, supporting the clinical benefit in HFpEF management.[33] Accordingly, they carry a class I indication in managing HFpEF in the HFA/ESC guidelines.[19,20] Loop diuretics are recommended in patients with volume overload. The goal is gentle diuresis to relieve symptoms, avoiding hypotension and its consequences. Overdiuresis should be avoided because patients may rely on high filling pressures to maintain cardiac output and may be preload dependent. Patients should weigh themselves regularly and know what steps to take if their weight exceeds the prespecified ranges by more than a few pounds. Recognizing that weight can fluctuate in older adults from other factors is important. In particular, many older adults may lose body mass over time, thus impacting their "dry weight"—such changes should be considered when using weight to guide diuresis to avoid causing

Table 20.3 H_2FPEF and HFA-PEFF scores

H_2FPEF score	Clinical variable	Value	Points
H_2	Heavy	BMI >30 kg/m^2	2
	Hypertensive	2 or more antihypertensives	1
F	Atrial Fibrillation	Paroxysmal or persistent	3
P	*Pulmonary hypertension	PASP >35 mmHg	1
E	Elder	>60 years	1
F	*Filling pressure	E/e′ >9	1
			Sum = 0–9
HFA-PEFF score			
	Major	Minor	
*Functional	Septal e′<7 cm/sec or Lateral e′<10 cm/sec or Average E/e′ ≥15 Or TR velocity >2.8 m/sec (PASP >35 mmHg)	Average E/e′: 9–14 or GLS <16%	
*Morphological	LAVi >34 ml/m^2 or LVMi ≥149/122 g/m^2 (M/F) RWT >0.42	LAVi 29–34 ml/m^2 or LVMi ≥115/95 g/m^2 (M/F) RWT >0.42 or LV wall thickness ≥12 mm	
Biomarker (SR)	NT-proBNP >220 pg/ml BNP >80 pg/ml	NT-proBNP 125–220 pg/ml BNP 35–80 pg/ml	
Biomarker (AF)	NT-proBNP >660 pg/ml BNP >240 pg/ml	NT-proBNP 365–660 pg/ml BNP 105–240 pg/ml	
Major criteria: 2 points			
Minor criteria: 1 point			
Probability of HFpEF	Low	Intermediate	High
H_2FPEF score	0–1	2–5	6–9
HFA-PEFF score	0–1	2–4	5–6

An H_2FPEF score ≥6 / HFA-PEFF ≥5 points: diagnostic of HFpEF.

An H_2FPEF score of 2–5 / HFA-PEFF of 2–4 points: the intermediate likelihood of HFpEF, wherein the authors propose invasive hemodynamic evaluation—preferably with exercise—or exercise echocardiography.

Abbreviations: BMI, body mass index; PASP, pulmonary artery systolic pressure; E, early diastolic transmitral inflow velocity; e′, early diastolic mitral annular velocities; GLS, global longitudinal strain; TR, tricuspid regurgitation; LAVi, left atrial volume index; LVMi, left ventricular mass index; M, male; F, female; RWT, relative wall thickness; LV, left ventricle; SR, sinus rhythm; AF, atrial fibrillation; BNP, B-type natriuretic peptide; NT-proBNP, N-terminal proBNP; HFpEF, heart failure with preserved ejection fraction.

*Assessed by echocardiography.

hypovolemia. Access to health care providers to address volume challenges before severe decompensation (periodic telephone calls, frequent follow-up appointments) is important to avoid hospitalizations. Serum electrolytes and renal function should be monitored frequently, and serum electrolytes should be repleted if necessary. Although metolazone can be added when the patient has a suboptimal response to a loop diuretic, extreme caution should be exercised to avoid an overexuberant response, which can cause hypovolemia, acute kidney injury, and electrolyte derangements, including hyponatremia and hypokalemia.

Disease-modifying therapy

SGLT2 INHIBITION

Initially, SGLT2 inhibitors were developed to improve glucose control in individuals with type 2 diabetes (T2DM); however, SGLT2 inhibitors have significant CV benefits in individuals with and without T2DM. Figure 20.2 shows

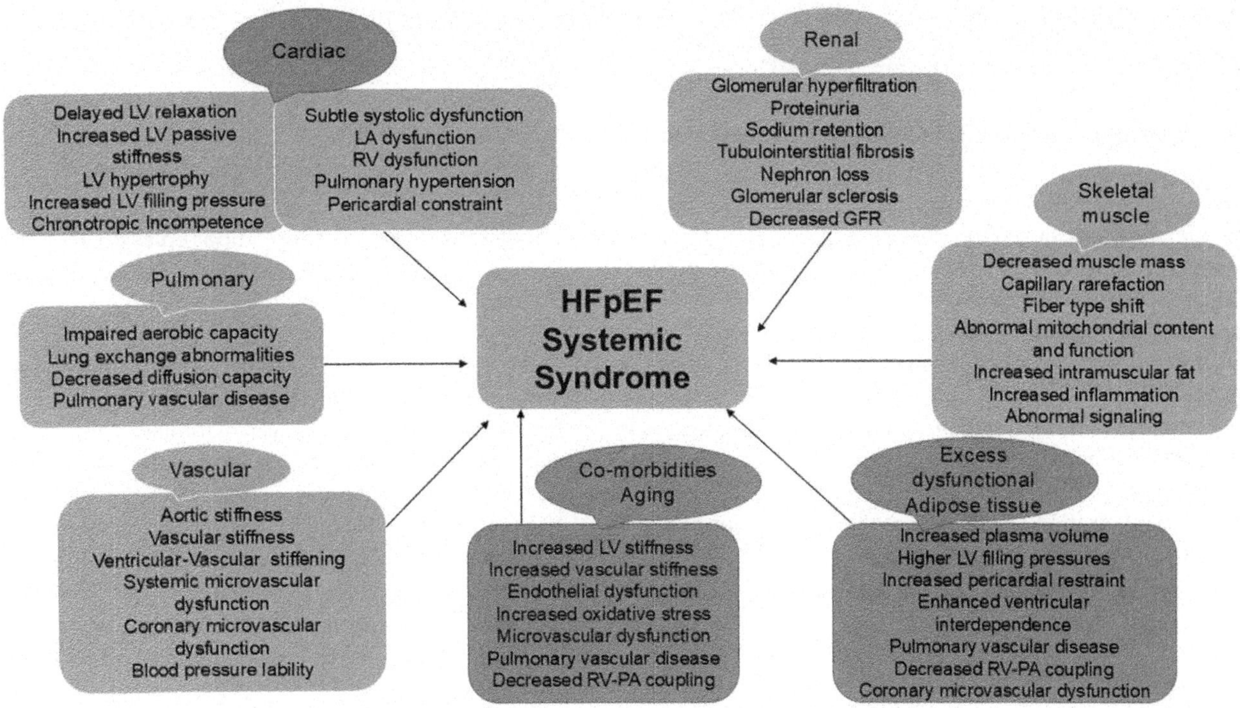

Figure 20.1 Heart failure with preserved ejection fraction (HFpEF) is a systemic syndrome. *Abbreviations*: LV, left ventricle; LA, left atrium; RV, right ventricle; GFR, glomerular filtration rate; PA, pulmonary artery.

the multiple mechanisms proposed for the pleiotropic effects of SGLT2 inhibitors in HFpEF. SGLT2 inhibitors, on top of other disease-modifying therapies, reduced the risk of HFH CV death, improved patient-reported symptoms, physical limitations, and exercise function in patients with LVEF ≥40% with or without T2DM.[34,35] SGLT2 inhibitors also improved health status, which had the most significant benefit for those with significant baseline impairment.[36] In patients with LVEF ≥40%, dapagliflozin improved QOL and 6-minute walk distance (6MWD).[37] The potential signal for a greater increase in 6MWD among patients with T2DM and higher BMI. 6MWD is more strongly tied to health status in older adults with HFpEF, providing insight into the origins of the improved QOL with SGLT2 inhibitors. This is supported by a meta-analysis that also showed a reduction in CV death and HFH among patients with LVEF ≥40% treated with SGLT2 inhibitors.[38] Of note, clinical trials of SGLT2 inhibitors included a substantial proportion of older adults, with over 40% aged ≥75 years. Post hoc analyses have demonstrated the efficacy of these agents across geriatric conditions, including frailty and polypharmacy, and showed a reduction in the composite endpoint of CV death and HFH and improvement in QOL measures.[37,39,40]

SGLT2-associated side effects such as volume depletion due to polyuria, genitourinary tract infections, leg amputation, and worsening urinary incontinence may be more common in older adults. Osmotic diuresis with SGLT2 inhibitors may lead to dehydration and orthostatic hypotension in older adults. Thus, a reduction in diuretic dose should be considered in patients vulnerable to volume depletion and dehydration who are on concomitant diuretic therapy. Genital mycotic infections are most common, occurring more frequently among women and uncircumcised men. Mild-to-moderate infections are responsive to topical antifungals, and occasionally oral fluconazole is required. Perineal necrotizing fasciitis (Fournier's gangrene) is a rare but severe and potentially disfiguring infection. Patient education and self-monitoring of genital/perineal symptoms are important. Another concern is acute kidney injury (AKI) or diabetic ketoacidosis (DKA), partially due to its effect on volume depletion. However, a recent meta-analysis showed no significant increase in AKI or DKA.[41] Early recognition and holding SGLT2 inhibitors in situations that could precipitate DKA are essential. Patients on dialysis should not be started on SGLT2 inhibitors.[19,20,42] The tolerability and safety appear to be preserved in older adults, with no notable rise in serious adverse events prompting medication discontinuation.[43,44] Older adults with T2DM are at an increased risk of CV complications irrespective of HF status and are consequently the group most likely to benefit most from SGLT2 inhibitors. Thus, we should not miss the opportunity to reduce the risks of adverse CV outcomes and avoid therapeutic inertia in this patient group when using SGLT2 inhibitors.

GLUCAGON-LIKE PEPTIDE 1 RECEPTOR AGONISM

GLP-1 is a hormone of the incretin family released from the gastrointestinal tract after food intake. Figure 20.3 shows the potential beneficial effect of GLP-1 receptor agonists (GLP-1RAs) in HFpEF with obesity. Among

Table 20.4 Major effects of normal aging on cardiovascular structure and function

Alteration	Impact
Vascular system	
Increased stiffness and decreased elasticity of large arteries	Increased impedance to LV ejection, gradual increase in SBP, ventricular aortic mismatch
Heart	
Collagen, amyloid, lipofuscin deposition Myocardium: Increased cardiomyocyte hypertrophy, increased fibrosis, increased myocardial stiffness and impaired LV relaxation, decreased microvascular density	Impaired diastolic function, impaired systolic reserve, increased LV filling pressure, and increased left atrial volume with predisposition to atrial fibrillation
Electrical system: Impaired responsiveness to beta-adrenergic stimulation	Declines in peak HR (220 – Age), peak contractility, and peripheral vasodilation
Decreased sinus node function and degenerative changes in the conduction system	Sick sinus syndrome, bradyarrhythmias, supraventricular and ventricular arrhythmias, conduction disturbances
Valves: Degeneration of the valves with calcium deposit	Valvular heart disease
Altered baroreceptor responsiveness	Predisposition to lightheadedness, falls, and syncope
Impaired endothelium-dependent vasodilation	
Microvascular dysfunction	Decline in peak coronary blood flow; predisposition to ischemia because of supply/demand mismatch Decreased peripheral blood flow
Skeletal muscles/body composition	
Decreased skeletal muscle mass and quality, muscle fat infiltration, changes in body composition predisposing sarcopenic obesity	Impaired peripheral oxygen utilization
Renal system	
Increased glomerulosclerosis, tubular atrophy, interstitial fibrosis	Decreased GFR further precipitates HF and complicates HF management
Respiratory system	
Increased alveolar dead space, decreased diffusion capacity, impaired chest compliance	Precipitates and complicates the diagnosis of HF
Brain	
Brain loss, decreased cerebral blood flow, amyloid deposition, increased senile plaques, and neurofibrillary tangles	Cognitive decline, memory loss, impaired coordination, missing outpatient visits, medications

Abbreviations: LV, left ventricle; SBP, systolic blood pressure; HR, heart rate; GFR, glomerular filtration rate.

patients with HFpEF and obesity (BMI ≥35 kg/m^2), treatment with semaglutide (a GLP-1RA) led to larger reductions in symptoms, greater improvements in exercise function, reduced inflammation, improved New York Heart Association (NYHA) functional class, and greater weight loss.[45,46] Recently, treatment with tirzepatide (a long-acting agonist of glucose-dependent insulinotropic polypeptide and GLP-1RA) led to a lower risk of a composite of death from CV causes or HFH and improved health status in patients with HFpEF and obesity.[47] However, clinical trials have not included large numbers of older adults, so specific data are unavailable for older adults. In addition, older adults have multiple other comorbidities and are on multiple medications, which puts them at high risk for adverse side effects. The gastrointestinal side effects of these medications can be worse in older adults, which can lead to dehydration or weakness and result in dizziness and falls. One potential concern of GLP-1RAs for older adults is related to the potential for exacerbating malnutrition and sarcopenia.[48] Data indicate that semaglutide reduces total energy intake by 24% compared to placebo while also inducing a significant loss of fat-free mass, including skeletal muscle. Given the prevalence of malnutrition and sarcopenia and their respective associations with adverse outcomes in patients with HFpEF, the safety of GLP-1RAs for older adults requires further investigation.

MINERALOCORTICOID RECEPTOR ANTAGONISM

Figure 20.4 shows the possible beneficial effects of MRA in HFpEF. A post hoc regional analysis from a large trial of the MRA spironolactone indicated that in the cohort from the Americas, which most closely matched characteristics observed in other randomized HFpEF trials, the rates of the primary composite outcome of CV death and HFH were significantly reduced.[49,50] MRAs significantly improve measures of diastolic function in individuals with HFpEF.[50,51] In a recent study, finerenone (a selective nonsteroidal MRA) reduced the composite risk of CV death and total HFH events in patients with HFpEF when

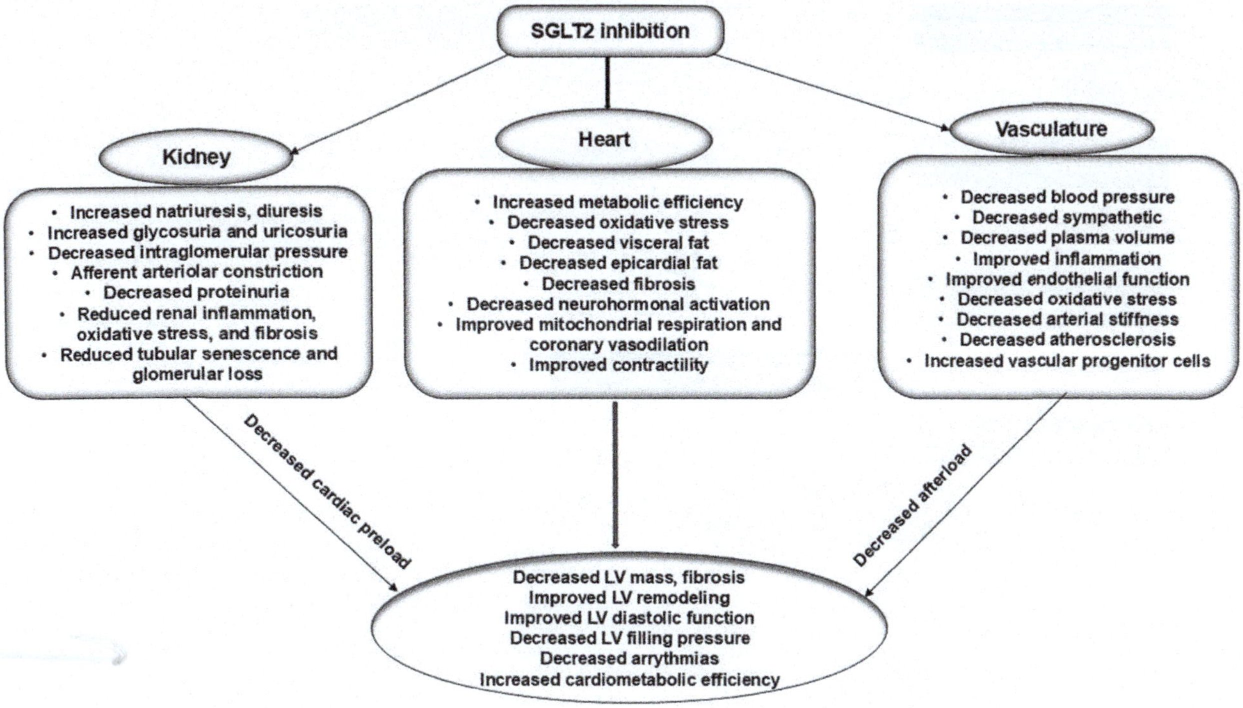

Figure 20.2 Beneficial effects of sodium-glucose cotransporter 2 (SGLT2) inhibitors. *Abbreviations*: LV, left ventricle. (Reproduced with permission from *Curr Hypertens Rep* 24, 1–20, 2022.)

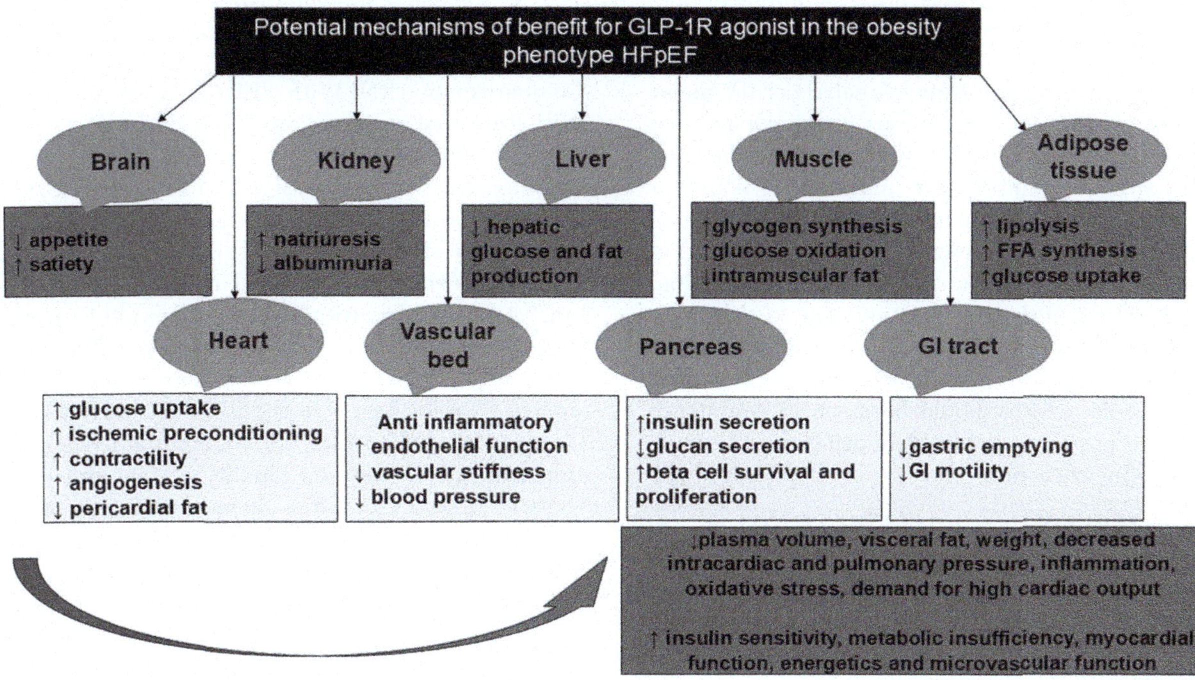

Figure 20.3 Potential mechanisms of benefit for GLP-1R agonist in the obesity phenotype HFpEF. *Abbreviations*: GLP-1R, glucagon-like peptide-1 receptor; HFpEF, heart failure with preserved ejection fraction; FFA, free fatty acid; GI, gastrointestinal.

added to background therapy.[52] The benefits of finerenone are consistent across all age groups, including patients aged ≥80 years.[53] MRA has a class IIb recommendation in the latest AHA/ACC/HFSA guidelines.[19,20]

Potential adverse effects of MRAs include hypotension, hyperkalemia, worsening renal function, and gynecomastia (for spironolactone, not eplerenone). MRAs are contraindicated if creatinine is >2.5 mg/dL or serum

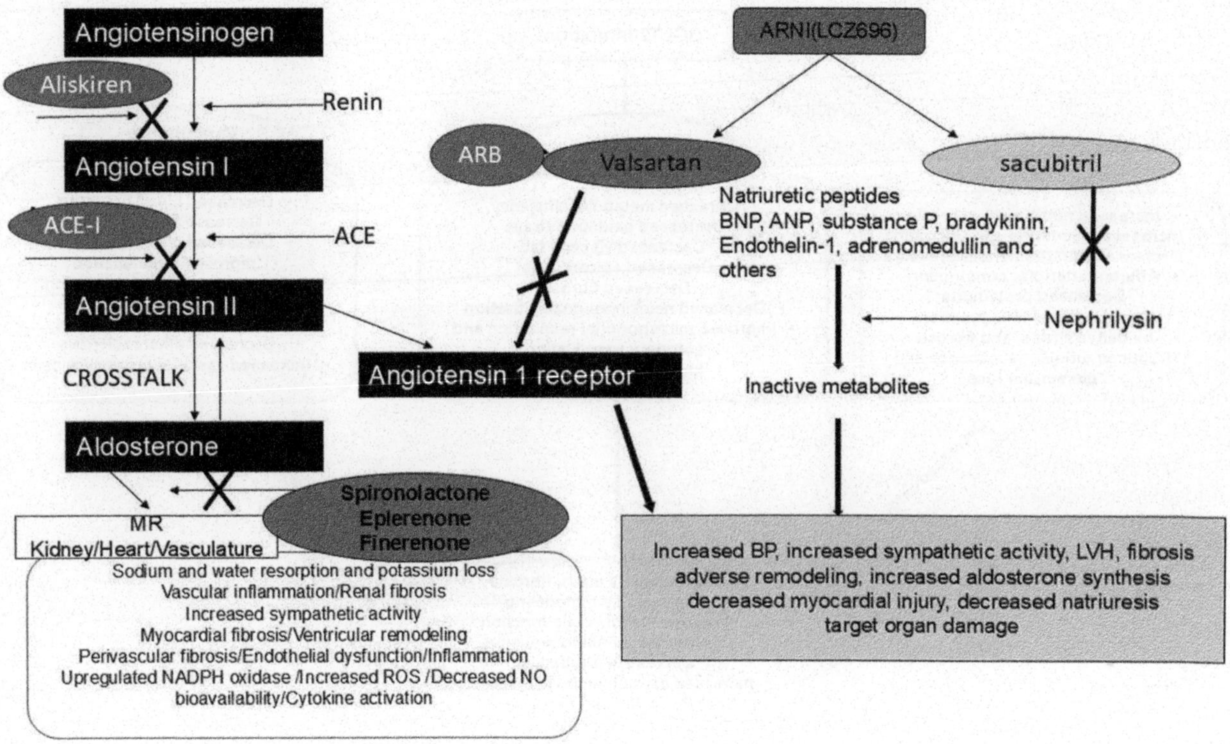

Figure 20.4 Beneficial effects of renin–angiotensin–aldosterone antagonism. *Abbreviations*: ACE, angiotensin converting enzyme; ACE-I, ACE inhibitor; ARB, angiotensin receptor blocker; MR, mineralocorticoid receptor; BNP, B-type natriuretic peptide; ANP, atrial natriuretic peptide; NADPH, nicotinamide adenine dinucleotide phosphate; ROS, reactive oxygen species; NO, nitric oxide; BP, blood pressure; LVH, left ventricular hypertrophy.

potassium is >5.0 mEq/L. A meta-analysis of the major MRA trials in older adults (≥75 years) demonstrated that MRA was equally beneficial in reducing morbidity and mortality in older adults.[54] It is important to note that hyperkalemia, AKI, hypotension, and hyponatremia may be more common among older adults compared to younger adults due to impairments in kidney function, increased chance of drug interactions due to polypharmacy and multimorbidity, and other geriatric syndromes such as frailty.[55] Since their beneficial effect is preserved in older people, efforts should be made to commence MRA where possible, closely monitoring serum potassium and kidney function.

RENIN–ANGIOTENSIN SYSTEM ANTAGONISTS (ANGIOTENSIN-CONVERTING ENZYME [ACE] INHIBITORS)/ANGIOTENSIN RECEPTOR BLOCKERS/ANGIOTENSIN RECEPTOR–NEPRILYSIN INHIBITORS)

Figure 20.4 shows the possible beneficial effects of ACE inhibitors, ARBs, and ARNIs in HFpEF. Of the three large randomized trials of ACE inhibitors/ARBs performed in HFpEF, only candesartan showed a nominal benefit in reducing HFH over 3 years of follow-up.[56] ARNI resulted in a lower level of NT-proBNP, a larger reduction in left atrial size, and greater improvement in the NYHA functional class than valsartan among the patients with HFpEF and LVEF ≥45%.[57] In the PARAGON-HF (Prospective Comparison of ARNI With ARB Global Outcomes in HF With Preserved Ejection Fraction) trial (LVEF ≥45%), the primary composite endpoint of total HFH and CV death was numerically lower with ARNI but was not statistically significant.[58] However, patients with recent HFH showed a substantially more significant reduction in risk from treatment with an ARNI compared with valsartan.[59] Analysis of prespecified subgroups of LVEF and sex showed a potential benefit in those with LVEF between 45% and 57%. There was a more significant benefit for women than for men.[60] In the PARALLAX (Prospective Comparison of ARNI vs. Comorbidity-Associated Conventional Therapy on Quality of Life and Exercise Capacity) trial (LVEF >40%, increased NPs), there was no salutary effect of ARNI on health status or submaximal exercise capacity compared with background medication–based individualized comparators.[61]

The average age of participants in the pivotal trials of ARBs and ARNIs in HFpEF ranged from 67 to 73 years. Importantly, data suggest their effectiveness is similar across age groups despite limited data in patients above 75 years. ACE inhibitors, ARBs, and ARNIs can also help manage hypertension, which is an important aspect of care for adults with HFpEF. ARNIs can be initiated in hospitalized patients with acute HF or outpatients to ensure the patient tolerates RAAS inhibition (starting dose: sacubitril/valsartan 24/26 mg and target dose 97/103 mg twice daily). If patients are already treated with an ACE inhibitor, a 36-hour washout is recommended before introducing the ARNI to reduce the risk of angioedema (a similar washout is not required with an ARB).

When using ACE inhibitors, ARBs, and ARNIs, it is important to monitor for hypotension, hyperkalemia, and AKI, which are more common in older adults due to age-related changes to the vascular system, kidneys, and known variations in pharmacodynamics and pharmacokinetics of drugs. In clinical trials, symptomatic hypotension was more common with ARNIs but was not associated with worsening kidney function. Angioedema was numerically higher but not statistically significantly different from ACE inhibitors. Careful attention should be given to initiation and titration for older patients to avoid hypotension. BP, potassium, and renal function should also be frequently monitored. Patients who are initiated on an ARNI and later find it cost-prohibitive or intolerant can be transitioned to an ARB. ACE inhibitors are not considered a reasonable alternative.

BETA-ADRENERGIC SIGNALING PATHWAYS

The drugs targeting beta-adrenergic signaling and heart rate modulation (beta-blockers [BBs], calcium channel blockers, and ivabradine) have shown no benefit in HFpEF. BBs can be used in patients with HFpEF who have specific indications, including myocardial infarction (for up to 3 years), angina, or AF requiring rate control. However, exercise tolerance should be monitored due to the potential for chronotropic incompetence, which can worsen exercise capacity.[62,63] There is emerging data about the potential benefits of withdrawing BBs, with a recent small study showing improvement in exercise tolerance.[64] An NIH-funded randomized controlled trial titled "DEPRESCRIBE-HFpEF" will examine the effects of BB withdrawal and hopefully address this question more definitively.

In conclusion, the first step is to ensure patients are adequately decongested using loop diuretics. SGLT2 inhibitors and MRAs are reasonable for all patients who can tolerate these agents and augment diuresis; MRAs can combat hypokalemia caused by loop diuretics.[19,20,42] SGLT2 inhibitors can prevent the progression of chronic kidney disease (CKD) and improve metabolic health. This combination may permit discontinuation or dosage reduction of loop diuretics in some patients. Coupling SGLT2 inhibitors with MRAs can mitigate the risk of hyperkalemia. When starting an MRA, it is important to check serum creatinine and potassium within 7 days, after 1 month, and then every 3–6 months. ARBs or ARNIs may be a beneficial agent for those with hypertension. Extra caution should be paid to those with orthostatic hypotension and/or a history of falls. Deprescribing BBs in the absence of a guideline-concordant indication is helpful. Among patients with HFrEF whose LVEF has improved to >45%, discontinuing BBs could lead to a relapse based on limited data about the withdrawal of guideline-directed medical therapy (GDMT) in this population.[65]

Nonpharmaceutical interventions

EXERCISE

Several clinical trials showed the beneficial effects of aerobic exercise training (ET) on exercise capacity, 6MWD, and QOL scores in older adults with HFpEF.[1] Moderate-intensity training appears equivalent to higher intensities.[1] The beneficial effects of ET appear mediated primarily by improvements in noncardiac factors.[1] In addition, clinical trials demonstrate a comparable or larger magnitude of improvement in exercise capacity from supervised ET in patients with chronic HFpEF compared to those with HFrEF.[66] However, the Centers for Medicaid and Medicare Services reimburse exercise-based cardiac rehabilitation coverage for only HFrEF after 4 weeks of stabilization from post-hospitalization;[67] and patients with HFpEF were explicitly excluded from Medicare coverage. Recently, a progressive, multidomain physical rehabilitation intervention started as early as possible following HFH among older patients with high comorbidity burden, severe physical dysfunction, and high rates of frailty showed it was feasible and safe, and resulted in improved physical function and reduced frailty, QOL, and depression.[68] Given that those with HFpEF had significantly greater impairments at baseline and derived greater benefit from the intervention,[69] the ongoing REHAB-HFPEF trial will definitively address whether such an intervention improves outcomes specifically in HFpEF and possibly pave the way for broad payer approval.

CALORIC RESTRICTION

Among older adults with obesity and HFpEF, weight loss via caloric restriction (CR) significantly improved exercise capacity to a degree similar to ET.[70] The combination of CR diet and ET produced a robust increase in exercise capacity. In addition, CR produced a moderate-sized improvement in QOL scores, greater than with ET.[70] It is well recognized that >80% of patients with HFpEF are overweight or obese.[71] Increased adipose tissue mass promotes systemic inflammation, insulin resistance, and diffuse endothelial dysfunction, impairing cardiac, arterial, and skeletal muscle function, all contributing to reduced exercise capacity in patients with HFpEF.[70,71] Similar to weight loss drugs, the potential risk for malnutrition will be important for understanding CR better. Combining CR and ET, including resistance exercise to minimize loss of muscle mass from CR, may be the ideal management for HFpEF and obesity.

Multimorbidity management

Older patients hospitalized with a primary diagnosis of HFpEF often have multiple cardiac and noncardiac comorbidities.[3] One recent study estimated that the average hospitalized patient with HFpEF had five other medical conditions.[72] A complex interplay between comorbidities influences the genesis of HFpEF and the outcomes of individuals with HFpEF. Life expectancy declines with the onset of each condition in patients with HFpEF.[73] Screening and effectively managing these comorbidities is essential to HFpEF management. Table 20.2 shows the appropriate management of HFpEF-associated comorbidities.[19,20,73,74] Pharmacologic agents that can concurrently treat multiple conditions are appealing strategies, well illustrated by SGLT2 inhibitors, which can concurrently treat HFpEF, T2DM, and CKD.[75] Due to its pleiotropic effects, exercise can positively impact multiple conditions and improve overall health.[1] We should also be aware that older patients with limited life expectancy from other comorbid conditions may not have the opportunity to derive as much lifetime benefit from pharmacotherapy.[76]

Embracing HFpEF as a true geriatric syndrome

Patients with HFpEF contend with impairments across multiple health domains, including the medical domain, mind/brain domain, physical function domain, and social environment. Multimorbidity, polypharmacy, cognitive impairment, depression, frailty, falls, and social isolation are highly prevalent in HFpEF.[73] These conditions have important implications for QOL, disability, hospitalization, and mortality in older adults.[73] Importantly, these conditions may be further exacerbated following a hospitalization. The "post-hospitalization syndrome" is an acquired, transient period of vulnerability.[77] The hospital environment (immobilization, fasting, sleep deprivation, and disorientation) is particularly problematic for physical frailty due to the risk of rapid, severe loss of muscle mass and function.[78] When deciding on therapeutic strategies for older adults with HFpEF, evaluating and integrating these conditions is essential since they likely impact the risk–benefit ratio of such therapeutic strategies.[48,73] Relatedly, eliciting patient priorities and health goals is important to ensure therapeutic decision-making is well aligned and remains patient-centric.[48,73]

PHYSICAL FUNCTION

HFpEF and frailty share common underlying mechanisms, often coexist, and represent each other's risk factors. It is important to consider routine assessment with well-validated tools and treat frailty in caring for older adults with HFpEF. Frailty is defined as a "multidimensional dynamic state, independent of age, that makes the individual with HF more vulnerable to the effect of stressors."[79] The prevalence of frailty in individuals with HFpEF ranges from 50% to 94% and is associated with a twofold increased risk for death, hospitalization, disability, nonadherence to medications, and lower QOL.[73,80–83] The pathophysiology of frailty and HFpEF is closely intertwined; both frailty and HFpEF are driven by a chronic inflammatory process associated with oxidative stress, neurohormonal derangement, sarcopenia, mitochondrial dysfunction, micronutrient deficiency, cellular senescence, and cellular necrosis.[80,83] Frail individuals with HF may present with significant disability that could be physical or mental, interfering with independent living, self-care, and overall health. Also, hospitalization leads to more hospitalization in frail older adults. In addition, older adults' degree of frailty often influences their care and treatment priorities.

Dietary counseling, along with nutritional and protein supplementation to increase muscle mass, potentially benefits frail patients with HFpEF. Physical exercise helps counter frailty and is strongly recommended for frail HF patients who can participate. Resistance and endurance exercise interventions have shown effectiveness in mitigating muscle loss and enhancing physical capacity in HF patients.[84,85] A recent study has shown that targeted interventions such as supervised ET and multidomain physical rehabilitation improved the QOL and physical function in frail older adults.[68] Thus, a comprehensive approach that targets multiple domains, including physical function and medical, cognitive, and social, is needed.

POLYPHARMACY

Aging is associated with altered pharmacokinetics and pharmacodynamics of most medications. Older patients are also more likely to have concomitant renal or liver disease that raises the risk of medication-related adverse events. Polypharmacy is generally described as taking five or more medications and is considered both a cause and consequence of geriatric syndromes.[86] Polypharmacy is common in patients with HFpEF due to coexisting multiple comorbidities. In an analysis of older adults aged ≥65 years who were hospitalized with HFpEF, 43% were on ten or more medications.[72] Polypharmacy can lead to adverse drug reactions that result in increased hospitalizations and more prescriptions to overcome the adverse effects, leading to prescription cascade, nonadherence, falls, disability, poor patient experience, and financial burden.[73,86] It is to be remembered that pharmacotherapy in older people requires an understanding not only of age-related physiological changes and pharmacokinetic changes but also of frailty-related physiological changes that predispose to adverse medication-related outcomes like orthostasis, risk of falls, worsening renal function, poor adherence, and need for emergency department visits.

Pharmacotherapy should be tailored to patients' needs rather than following a one-size-fits-all approach. For every patient encounter, medication lists should be thoroughly reviewed. Deprescribing should be done where there is a lack of evidence for medication or an adverse drug reaction, risks of medications outweigh their benefits, or where the time to benefit from treatment exceeds individual life expectancy. Simplifying complex regimens and the use of fixed-dose combination pills can increase adherence. Clinicians caring for older adults with HFpEF must consider goals of care, functional status, and new evidence-based therapies in order to optimize such polypharmacy for older adults.

GOALS OF CARE, PALLIATIVE CARE, AND ADVANCED CARE PLANNING

Discussions about the goals of care are important for older adults with HFpEF since HFpEF is a progressive, debilitating condition without a cure. Applying counseling skills that allow patients to raise issues such as death and identifying when a patient's condition is progressing with a paucity of additional therapeutic options and the need for palliative care is an integral part of an HF service. There is a misconception that palliative care is applicable only in the terminal phase of life when survival is no longer the goal; however, the goals of palliative care are applicable across the disease spectrum, starting as early as diagnosis. Prior work shows that palliative care services can improve HF symptoms, mental health, spiritual well-being, and social isolation.[87] In addition, opportunities should be taken to discuss disease trajectory and engage in advanced care planning in a timely fashion well ahead of the terminal stages of the disease.

DISCLOSURES

Parag Goyal received consulting fees from Agepha Pharma, Akros Pharma, Axon Therapies, Bayer HealthCare Pharmaceuticals, Pfizer, and Sensorum Health.

Bharathi Upadhya received support from Novartis and Corvia.

REFERENCES

1. Pandey A, Shah SJ, Butler J, Kellogg DL, Jr., Lewis GD, Forman DE, Mentz RJ, Borlaug BA, Simon MA, Chirinos JA, Fielding RA, Volpi E, Molina AJA, Haykowsky MJ, Sam F, Goodpaster BH, Bertoni AG, Justice JN, White JP, Ding J, Hummel SL, LeBrasseur NK, Taffet GE, Pipinos, II and Kitzman D. Exercise intolerance in older adults with heart failure with preserved ejection fraction: JACC state-of-the-art review. *J Am Coll Cardiol.* 2021;78:1166–87.
2. Owan TE, Hodge DO, Herges RM, Jacobsen SJ, Roger VL and Redfield MM. Trends in prevalence and outcome of heart failure with preserved ejection fraction. *N Engl J Med.* 2006;355:251–9.
3. Upadhya B, Pisani B and Kitzman DW. Evolution of a geriatric syndrome: pathophysiology and treatment of heart failure with preserved ejection fraction. *J Am Geriatr Soc.* 2017;65:2431–40.
4. Pandey A, Omar W, Ayers C, LaMonte M, Klein L, Allen NB, Kuller LH, Greenland P, Eaton CB, Gottdiener JS, Lloyd-Jones DM and Berry JD. Sex and race differences in lifetime risk of heart failure with preserved ejection fraction and heart failure with reduced ejection fraction. *Circulation.* 2018;137:1814–23.
5. Dunlay SM, Roger VL and Redfield MM. Epidemiology of heart failure with preserved ejection fraction. *Nat Rev Cardiol.* 2017;14:591–602.
6. Steinberg BA, Zhao X, Heidenreich PA, Peterson ED, Bhatt DL, Cannon CP, Hernandez AF and Fonarow GC. Trends in patients hospitalized with heart failure and preserved left ventricular ejection fraction: prevalence, therapies, and outcomes. *Circulation.* 2012;126:65–75.
7. Pérez de Isla L, Zamorano J, Hernández N, Contreras L, Rodrigo JL, Almería C, Aubele AL, Mataix L and Macaya C. Prognostic factors and predictors of in-hospital mortality of patients with heart failure with preserved left ventricular ejection fraction. *J Cardiovasc Med (Hagerstown).* 2008;9:1011–15.
8. Bhatia RS, Tu JV, Lee DS, Austin PC, Fang J, Haouzi A, Gong Y and Liu PP. Outcome of heart failure with preserved ejection fraction in a population-based study. *N Engl J Med.* 2006;355:260–9.
9. Fonarow GC, Stough WG, Abraham WT, Albert NM, Gheorghiade M, Greenberg BH, O'Connor CM, Sun JL, Yancy CW and Young JB. Characteristics, treatments, and outcomes of patients with preserved systolic function hospitalized for heart failure: a report from the OPTIMIZE-HF Registry. *J Am Coll Cardiol.* 2007;50:768–77.
10. Gerber Y, Weston SA, Redfield MM, Chamberlain AM, Manemann SM, Jiang R, Killian JM and Roger VL. A contemporary appraisal of the heart failure epidemic in Olmsted County, Minnesota, 2000 to 2010. *JAMA Intern Med.* 2015;175:996–1004.
11. Paulus WJ and Tschöpe C. A novel paradigm for heart failure with preserved ejection fraction: comorbidities drive myocardial dysfunction and remodeling through coronary microvascular endothelial inflammation. *J Am Coll Cardiol.* 2013;62:263–71.
12. Henkel DM, Redfield MM, Weston SA, Gerber Y and Roger VL. Death in heart failure: a community perspective. *Circ Heart Fail.* 2008;1:91–7.
13. Vaduganathan M, Patel RB, Michel A, Shah SJ, Senni M, Gheorghiade M and Butler J. Mode of death in heart failure with preserved ejection fraction. *J Am Coll Cardiol.* 2017;69:556–69.
14. Dunlay SM, Redfield MM, Weston SA, Therneau TM, Hall Long K, Shah ND and Roger VL. Hospitalizations after heart failure diagnosis a community perspective. *J Am Coll Cardiol.* 2009;54:1695–702.
15. Cheng RK, Cox M, Neely ML, Heidenreich PA, Bhatt DL, Eapen ZJ, Hernandez AF, Butler J, Yancy CW and Fonarow GC. Outcomes in patients with heart failure with preserved, borderline, and reduced ejection fraction in the Medicare population. *Am Heart J.* 2014;168:721–30.

16. Clark KAA, Reinhardt SW, Chouairi F, Miller PE, Kay B, Fuery M, Guha A, Ahmad T and Desai NR. Trends in heart failure hospitalizations in the US from 2008 to 2018. *J Card Fail.* 2022;28:171–80.
17. Hoekstra T, Lesman-Leegte I, van Veldhuisen DJ, Sanderman R and Jaarsma T. Quality of life is impaired similarly in heart failure patients with preserved and reduced ejection fraction. *Eur J Heart Fail.* 2011;13:1013–18.
18. Kapoor JR, Kapoor R, Ju C, Heidenreich PA, Eapen ZJ, Hernandez AF, Butler J, Yancy CW and Fonarow GC. Precipitating clinical factors, heart failure characterization, and outcomes in patients hospitalized with heart failure with reduced, borderline, and preserved ejection fraction. *JACC Heart Fail.* 2016;4:464–72.
19. Heidenreich PA, Bozkurt B, Aguilar D, Allen LA, Byun JJ, Colvin MM, Deswal A, Drazner MH, Dunlay SM, Evers LR, Fang JC, Fedson SE, Fonarow GC, Hayek SS, Hernandez AF, Khazanie P, Kittleson MM, Lee CS, Link MS, Milano CA, Nnacheta LC, Sandhu AT, Stevenson LW, Vardeny O, Vest AR and Yancy CW. 2022 AHA/ACC/HFSA guideline for the management of heart failure: executive summary: a report of the American College of Cardiology/American Heart Association Joint Committee on Clinical Practice Guidelines. *J Am Coll Cardiol.* 2022;79:1757–80.
20. McDonagh TA, Metra M, Adamo M, Gardner RS, Baumbach A, Böhm M, Burri H, Butler J, Čelutkienė J, Chioncel O, Cleland JGF, Coats AJS, Crespo-Leiro MG, Farmakis D, Gilard M, Heymans S, Hoes AW, Jaarsma T, Jankowska EA, Lainscak M, Lam CSP, Lyon AR, McMurray JJV, Mebazaa A, Mindham R, Muneretto C, Francesco Piepoli M, Price S, Rosano GMC, Ruschitzka F and Kathrine Skibelund A. 2021 ESC guidelines for the diagnosis and treatment of acute and chronic heart failure: developed by the task force for the diagnosis and treatment of acute and chronic heart failure of the European Society of Cardiology (ESC). With the special contribution of the Heart Failure Association (HFA) of the ESC. *Eur J Heart Fail.* 2022;24:4–131.
21. Maisel AS, Krishnaswamy P, Nowak RM, McCord J, Hollander JE, Duc P, Omland T, Storrow AB, Abraham WT, Wu AH, Clopton P, Steg PG, Westheim A, Knudsen CW, Perez A, Kazanegra R, Herrmann HC and McCullough PA. Rapid measurement of B-type natriuretic peptide in the emergency diagnosis of heart failure. *N Engl J Med.* 2002;347:161–7.
22. Chow SL, Maisel AS, Anand I, Bozkurt B, de Boer RA, Felker GM, Fonarow GC, Greenberg B, Januzzi JL, Jr., Kiernan MS, Liu PP, Wang TJ, Yancy CW and Zile MR. Role of biomarkers for the prevention, assessment, and management of heart failure: a scientific statement from the American Heart Association. *Circulation.* 2017;135:e1054–1.
23. Maisel AS, Clopton P, Krishnaswamy P, Nowak RM, McCord J, Hollander JE, Duc P, Omland T, Storrow AB, Abraham WT, Wu AH, Steg G, Westheim A, Knudsen CW, Perez A, Kazanegra R, Bhalla V, Herrmann HC, Aumont MC and McCullough PA. Impact of age, race, and sex on the ability of B-type natriuretic peptide to aid in the emergency diagnosis of heart failure: results from the Breathing Not Properly (BNP) multinational study. *Am Heart J.* 2004;147:1078–84.
24. Stavrakis S, Pakala A, Thomas J, Chaudhry MA and Thadani U. Obesity, brain natriuretic peptide levels and mortality in patients hospitalized with heart failure and preserved left ventricular systolic function. *Am J Med Sci.* 2013;345:211–7.
25. Obokata M, Reddy YNV, Pislaru SV, Melenovsky V and Borlaug BA. Evidence supporting the existence of a distinct obese phenotype of heart failure with preserved ejection fraction. *Circulation.* 2017;136:6–19.
26. Anjan VY, Loftus TM, Burke MA, Akhter N, Fonarow GC, Gheorghiade M and Shah SJ. Prevalence, clinical phenotype, and outcomes associated with normal B-type natriuretic peptide levels in heart failure with preserved ejection fraction. *Am J Cardiol.* 2012;110:870–6.
27. Reddy YNV, Carter RE, Obokata M, Redfield MM and Borlaug BA. A simple, evidence-based approach to help guide diagnosis of heart failure with preserved ejection fraction. *Circulation.* 2018;138:861–70.
28. Pieske B, Tschöpe C, de Boer RA, Fraser AG, Anker SD, Donal E, Edelmann F, Fu M, Guazzi M, Lam CSP, Lancellotti P, Melenovsky V, Morris DA, Nagel E, Pieske-Kraigher E, Ponikowski P, Solomon SD, Vasan RS, Rutten FH, Voors AA, Ruschitzka F, Paulus WJ, Seferovic P and Filippatos G. How to diagnose heart failure with preserved ejection fraction: the HFA-PEFF diagnostic algorithm: a consensus recommendation from the Heart Failure Association (HFA) of the European Society of Cardiology (ESC). *Eur Heart J.* 2019;40:3297–317.
29. Nikorowitsch J, Bei der Kellen R, Kirchhof P, Magnussen C, Jagodzinski A, Schnabel RB, Blankenberg S and Wenzel JP. Applying the ESC 2016, H(2) FPEF, and HFA-PEFF diagnostic algorithms for heart failure with preserved ejection fraction to the general population. *ESC Heart Fail.* 2021;8:3603–12.
30. Lakatta EG. So! What's aging? Is cardiovascular aging a disease? *J Mol Cell Cardiol.* 2015;83:1–13.
31. López-Otín C, Blasco MA, Partridge L, Serrano M and Kroemer G. The hallmarks of aging. *Cell.* 2013;153:1194–217.
32. Brater DC. Diuretic therapy. *N Engl J Med.* 1998;339:387–95.

33. Abraham WT, Adamson PB, Bourge RC, Aaron MF, Costanzo MR, Stevenson LW, Strickland W, Neelagaru S, Raval N, Krueger S, Weiner S, Shavelle D, Jeffries B and Yadav JS. Wireless pulmonary artery haemodynamic monitoring in chronic heart failure: a randomised controlled trial. *Lancet*. 2011;377:658–66.
34. Solomon SD, McMurray JJV, Claggett B, de Boer RA, DeMets D, Hernandez AF, Inzucchi SE, Kosiborod MN, Lam CSP, Martinez F, Shah SJ, Desai AS, Jhund PS, Belohlavek J, Chiang CE, Borleffs CJW, Comin-Colet J, Dobreanu D, Drozdz J, Fang JC, Alcocer-Gamba MA, Al Habeeb W, Han Y, Cabrera Honorio JW, Janssens SP, Katova T, Kitakaze M, Merkely B, O'Meara E, Saraiva JFK, Tereshchenko SN, Thierer J, Vaduganathan M, Vardeny O, Verma S, Pham VN, Wilderäng U, Zaozerska N, Bachus E, Lindholm D, Petersson M and Langkilde AM. Dapagliflozin in heart failure with mildly reduced or preserved ejection fraction. *N Engl J Med*. 2022;387:1089–98.
35. Anker SD, Butler J, Filippatos G, Ferreira JP, Bocchi E, Böhm M, Brunner-La Rocca HP, Choi DJ, Chopra V, Chuquiure-Valenzuela E, Giannetti N, Gomez-Mesa JE, Janssens S, Januzzi JL, Gonzalez-Juanatey JR, Merkely B, Nicholls SJ, Perrone SV, Piña IL, Ponikowski P, Senni M, Sim D, Spinar J, Squire I, Taddei S, Tsutsui H, Verma S, Vinereanu D, Zhang J, Carson P, Lam CSP, Marx N, Zeller C, Sattar N, Jamal W, Schnaidt S, Schnee JM, Brueckmann M, Pocock SJ, Zannad F and Packer M. Empagliflozin in heart failure with a preserved ejection fraction. *N Engl J Med*. 2021;385:1451–61.
36. Kosiborod MN, Bhatt AS, Claggett BL, Vaduganathan M, Kulac IJ, Lam CSP, Hernandez AF, Martinez FA, Inzucchi SE, Shah SJ, de Boer RA, Jhund PS, Desai AS, Fang JC, Han Y, Comin-Colet J, Vardeny O, Lindholm D, Wilderäng U, Bengtsson O, McMurray JJV and Solomon SD. Effect of dapagliflozin on health status in patients with preserved or mildly reduced ejection fraction. *J Am Coll Cardiol*. 2023;81:460–73.
37. Nassif ME, Windsor SL, Borlaug BA, Kitzman DW, Shah SJ, Tang F, Khariton Y, Malik AO, Khumri T, Umpierrez G, Lamba S, Sharma K, Khan SS, Chandra L, Gordon RA, Ryan JJ, Chaudhry SP, Joseph SM, Chow CH, Kanwar MK, Pursley M, Siraj ES, Lewis GD, Clemson BS, Fong M and Kosiborod MN. The SGLT2 inhibitor dapagliflozin in heart failure with preserved ejection fraction: a multicenter randomized trial. *Nat Med*. 2021;27:1954–60.
38. Vaduganathan M, Docherty KF, Claggett BL, Jhund PS, de Boer RA, Hernandez AF, Inzucchi SE, Kosiborod MN, Lam CSP, Martinez F, Shah SJ, Desai AS, McMurray JJV and Solomon SD. SGLT-2 inhibitors in patients with heart failure: a comprehensive meta-analysis of five randomised controlled trials. *Lancet*. 2022;400:757–67.
39. Butt JH, Jhund PS, Belohlávek J, de Boer RA, Chiang CE, Desai AS, Drożdż J, Hernandez AF, Inzucchi SE, Katova T, Kitakaze M, Kosiborod MN, Lam CSP, Maria Langkilde A, Lindholm D, Bachus E, Martinez F, Merkely B, Petersson M, Saraiva JFK, Shah SJ, Vaduganathan M, Vardeny O, Wilderäng U, Claggett BL, Solomon SD and McMurray JJV. Efficacy and safety of dapagliflozin according to frailty in patients with heart failure: a prespecified analysis of the DELIVER trial. *Circulation*. 2022;146:1210–24.
40. Peikert A, Goyal P, Vaduganathan M, Claggett BL, Kulac IJ, Miao ZM, Vardeny O, Kosiborod MN, Desai AS, Jhund PS, Lam CSP, Inzucchi SE, Martinez FA, de Boer RA, Hernandez AF, Shah SJ, Petersson M, Langkilde AM, McMurray JJV and Solomon SD. Dapagliflozin in heart failure with mildly reduced or preserved ejection fraction according to polypharmacy status. *JACC Heart Fail*. 2023;11:1380–93.
41. Aldafas R, Crabtree T, Alkharaiji M, Vinogradova Y and Idris I. Sodium-glucose cotransporter-2 inhibitors (SGLT2) in frail or older people with type 2 diabetes and heart failure: a systematic review and meta-analysis. *Age Ageing*. 2024;53;1.
42. Kittleson MM, Panjrath GS, Amancherla K, Davis LL, Deswal A, Dixon DL, Januzzi JL, Jr. and Yancy CW. 2023 ACC expert consensus decision pathway on management of heart failure with preserved ejection fraction: A Report of the American College of Cardiology Solution Set Oversight Committee. *J Am Coll Cardiol*. 2023;81:1835–78.
43. Goldman A, Fishman B, Twig G, Raschi E, Cukierman-Yaffe T, Moshkovits Y, Pomerantz A, Ben-Zvi I, Dankner R and Maor E. The real-world safety profile of sodium-glucose co-transporter-2 inhibitors among older adults (≥75 years): a retrospective, pharmacovigilance study. *Cardiovasc Diabetol*. 2023;22:16.
44. Evans M, Morgan AR, Davies S, Beba H and Strain WD. The role of sodium-glucose co-transporter-2 inhibitors in frail older adults with or without type 2 diabetes mellitus. *Age Ageing*. 2022;51(10).
45. Kosiborod MN, Abildstrøm SZ, Borlaug BA, Butler J, Rasmussen S, Davies M, Hovingh GK, Kitzman DW, Lindegaard ML, Møller DV, Shah SJ, Treppendahl MB, Verma S, Abhayaratna W, Ahmed FZ, Chopra V, Ezekowitz J, Fu M, Ito H, Lelonek M, Melenovsky V, Merkely B, Núñez J, Perna E, Schou M, Senni M, Sharma K, Van der Meer P, von Lewinski D, Wolf D and Petrie MC. Semaglutide in patients with heart failure with preserved ejection fraction and obesity. *N Engl J Med*. 2023;389:1069–84.
46. Schou M, Petrie MC, Borlaug BA, Butler J, Davies MJ, Kitzman DW, Shah SJ, Verma S, Patel S, Chinnakondepalli KM, Harring S, Abildstrøm SZ, Liisberg K and Kosiborod MN. Semaglutide and

NYHA functional class in obesity-related heart failure with preserved ejection fraction: the STEP-HFpEF program. *J Am Coll Cardiol.* 2024;84:247–57.
47. Packer M, Zile MR, Kramer CM, Baum SJ, Litwin SE, Menon V, Ge J, Weerakkody GJ, Ou Y, Bunck MC, Hurt KC, Murakami M and Borlaug BA. Tirzepatide for heart failure with preserved ejection fraction and obesity. *N Engl J Med.* 2024;392(5):427–37.
48. Hashemi A, Kwak MJ and Goyal P. Pharmacologic management of heart failure with preserved ejection fraction (HFpEF) in older adults. *Drugs Aging.* 2025;42(2):95–110.
49. Pfeffer MA, Claggett B, Assmann SF, Boineau R, Anand IS, Clausell N, Desai AS, Diaz R, Fleg JL, Gordeev I, Heitner JF, Lewis EF, O'Meara E, Rouleau JL, Probstfield JL, Shaburishvili T, Shah SJ, Solomon SD, Sweitzer NK, McKinlay SM and Pitt B. Regional variation in patients and outcomes in the treatment of preserved cardiac function heart failure with an aldosterone antagonist (TOPCAT) trial. *Circulation.* 2015;131:34–42.
50. Pitt B, Pfeffer MA, Assmann SF, Boineau R, Anand IS, Claggett B, Clausell N, Desai AS, Diaz R, Fleg JL, Gordeev I, Harty B, Heitner JF, Kenwood CT, Lewis EF, O'Meara E, Probstfield JL, Shaburishvili T, Shah SJ, Solomon SD, Sweitzer NK, Yang S and McKinlay SM. Spironolactone for heart failure with preserved ejection fraction. *N Engl J Med.* 2014;370:1383–92.
51. Edelmann F, Wachter R, Schmidt AG, Kraigher-Krainer E, Colantonio C, Kamke W, Duvinage A, Stahrenberg R, Durstewitz K, Löffler M, Düngen HD, Tschöpe C, Herrmann-Lingen C, Halle M, Hasenfuss G, Gelbrich G and Pieske B. Effect of spironolactone on diastolic function and exercise capacity in patients with heart failure with preserved ejection fraction: the Aldo-DHF randomized controlled trial. *Jama.* 2013;309:781–91.
52. Solomon SD, McMurray JJV, Vaduganathan M, Claggett B, Jhund PS, Desai AS, Henderson AD, Lam CSP, Pitt B, Senni M, Shah SJ, Voors AA, Zannad F, Abidin IZ, Alcocer-Gamba MA, Atherton JJ, Bauersachs J, Chang-Sheng M, Chiang CE, Chioncel O, Chopra V, Comin-Colet J, Filippatos G, Fonseca C, Gajos G, Goland S, Goncalvesova E, Kang S, Katova T, Kosiborod MN, Latkovskis G, Lee AP, Linssen GCM, Llamas-Esperón G, Mareev V, Martinez FA, Melenovský V, Merkely B, Nodari S, Petrie MC, Saldarriaga CI, Saraiva JFK, Sato N, Schou M, Sharma K, Troughton R, Udell JA, Ukkonen H, Vardeny O, Verma S, von Lewinski D, Voronkov L, Yilmaz MB, Zieroth S, Lay-Flurrie J, van Gameren I, Amarante F, Kolkhof P and Viswanathan P. Finerenone in heart failure with mildly reduced or preserved ejection fraction. *N Engl J Med.* 2024;391:1475–85.
53. Chimura M, Petrie MC, Schou M, Martinez FA, Henderson AD, Claggett BL, Desai AS, Kolkhof P, Viswanathan P, Lage A, Lam CSP, Senni M, Shah SJ, Rohwedder K, Mueller K, Voors AA, Zannad F, Pitt B, Vaduganathan M, Jhund PS, Solomon SD and McMurray JJV. Finerenone improves outcomes in patients with heart failure with mildly reduced or preserved ejection fraction irrespective of age: a prespecified analysis of FINEARTS-HF. *Circ Heart Fail.* 2024;17:e012437.
54. Ferreira JP, Rossello X, Eschalier R, McMurray JJV, Pocock S, Girerd N, Rossignol P, Pitt B and Zannad F. MRAs in elderly HF patients: individual patient-data meta-analysis of RALES, EMPHASIS-HF, and TOPCAT. *JACC Heart Fail.* 2019;7:1012–21.
55. Vardeny O, Claggett B, Vaduganathan M, Beldhuis I, Rouleau J, O'Meara E, Anand IS, Shah SJ, Sweitzer NK, Fang JC, Desai AS, Lewis EF, Pitt B, Pfeffer MA and Solomon SD. Influence of age on efficacy and safety of spironolactone in heart failure. *JACC Heart Fail.* 2019;7:1022–8.
56. Yusuf S, Pfeffer MA, Swedberg K, Granger CB, Held P, McMurray JJ, Michelson EL, Olofsson B and Ostergren J. Effects of candesartan in patients with chronic heart failure and preserved left-ventricular ejection fraction: the CHARM-preserved trial. *Lancet.* 2003;362:777–81.
57. Solomon SD, Zile M, Pieske B, Voors A, Shah A, Kraigher-Krainer E, Shi V, Bransford T, Takeuchi M, Gong J, Lefkowitz M, Packer M and McMurray JJ. The angiotensin receptor neprilysin inhibitor LCZ696 in heart failure with preserved ejection fraction: a phase 2 double-blind randomised controlled trial. *Lancet.* 2012;380:1387–95.
58. Solomon SD, McMurray JJV, Anand IS, Ge J, Lam CSP, Maggioni AP, Martinez F, Packer M, Pfeffer MA, Pieske B, Redfield MM, Rouleau JL, van Veldhuisen DJ, Zannad F, Zile MR, Desai AS, Claggett B, Jhund PS, Boytsov SA, Comin-Colet J, Cleland J, Düngen HD, Goncalvesova E, Katova T, Kerr Saraiva JF, Lelonek M, Merkely B, Senni M, Shah SJ, Zhou J, Rizkala AR, Gong J, Shi VC and Lefkowitz MP. Angiotensin-neprilysin inhibition in heart failure with preserved ejection fraction. *N Engl J Med.* 2019;381:1609–20.
59. Vaduganathan M, Claggett BL, Desai AS, Anker SD, Perrone SV, Janssens S, Milicic D, Arango JL, Packer M, Shi VC, Lefkowitz MP, McMurray JJV and Solomon SD. Prior heart failure hospitalization, clinical outcomes, and response to sacubitril/valsartan compared with valsartan in HFpEF. *J Am Coll Cardiol.* 2020;75:245–54.
60. McMurray JJV, Jackson AM, Lam CSP, Redfield MM, Anand IS, Ge J, Lefkowitz MP, Maggioni AP, Martinez F, Packer M, Pfeffer MA, Pieske B,

Rizkala AR, Sabarwal SV, Shah AM, Shah SJ, Shi VC, van Veldhuisen DJ, Zannad F, Zile MR, Cikes M, Goncalvesova E, Katova T, Kosztin A, Lelonek M, Sweitzer N, Vardeny O, Claggett B, Jhund PS and Solomon SD. Effects of sacubitril-valsartan versus valsartan in women compared with men with heart failure and preserved ejection fraction: insights from PARAGON-HF. *Circulation*. 2020;141:338–51.

61. Pieske B, Wachter R, Shah SJ, Baldridge A, Szeczoedy P, Ibram G, Shi V, Zhao Z and Cowie MR. Effect of sacubitril/valsartan vs standard medical therapies on Plasma NT-proBNP concentration and submaximal exercise capacity in patients with heart failure and preserved ejection fraction: the PARALLAX randomized clinical trial. *JAMA*. 2021;326:1919–29.
62. Heidenreich PA, Bozkurt B, Aguilar D, Allen LA, Byun JJ, Colvin MM, Deswal A, Drazner MH, Dunlay SM, Evers LR, Fang JC, Fedson SE, Fonarow GC, Hayek SS, Hernandez AF, Khazanie P, Kittleson MM, Lee CS, Link MS, Milano CA, Nnacheta LC, Sandhu AT, Stevenson LW, Vardeny O, Vest AR and Yancy CW. 2022 AHA/ACC/HFSA guideline for the management of heart failure: a report of the American College of Cardiology/American Heart Association Joint Committee on Clinical Practice Guidelines. *J Am Coll Cardiol*. 2022;79:e263–e421.
63. McDonagh TA, Metra M, Adamo M, Gardner RS, Baumbach A, Böhm M, Burri H, Butler J, Čelutkienė J, Chioncel O, Cleland JGF, Coats AJS, Crespo-Leiro MG, Farmakis D, Gilard M, Heymans S, Hoes AW, Jaarsma T, Jankowska EA, Lainscak M, Lam CSP, Lyon AR, McMurray JJV, Mebazaa A, Mindham R, Muneretto C, Piepoli MF, Price S, Rosano GMC, Ruschitzka F and Skibelund AK. [2023 Focused update of the 2021 ESC Guidelines for the diagnosis and treatment of acute and chronic heart failure]. *G Ital Cardiol (Rome)*. 2024;25:202–13.
64. Palau P, Seller J, Domínguez E, Gómez I, Ramón JM, Sastre C, de la Espriella R, Santas E, Miñana G, Chorro FJ, González-Juanatey JR and Núñez J. Beta-blockers withdrawal in patients with heart failure with preserved ejection fraction and chronotropic incompetence: effect on functional capacity rationale and study design of a prospective, randomized, controlled trial (The Preserve-HR trial). *Clin Cardiol*. 2020;43:423–29.
65. Halliday BP, Wassall R, Lota AS, Khalique Z, Gregson J, Newsome S, Jackson R, Rahneva T, Wage R, Smith G, Venneri L, Tayal U, Auger D, Midwinter W, Whiffin N, Rajani R, Dungu JN, Pantazis A, Cook SA, Ware JS, Baksi AJ, Pennell DJ, Rosen SD, Cowie MR, Cleland JGF and Prasad SK. Withdrawal of pharmacological treatment for heart failure in patients with recovered dilated cardiomyopathy (TRED-HF): an open-label, pilot, randomised trial. *Lancet*. 2019;393:61–73.
66. Sachdev V, Sharma K, Keteyian SJ, Alcain CF, Desvigne-Nickens P, Fleg JL, Florea VG, Franklin BA, Guglin M, Halle M, Leifer ES, Panjrath G, Tinsley EA, Wong RP and Kitzman DW. Supervised exercise training for chronic heart failure with preserved ejection fraction: a scientific statement from the American Heart Association and American College of Cardiology. *Circulation*. 2023;147:e699–e715.
67. Centers for Medicare & Medicaid Services. *Decision memo for cardiac rehabilitation (CR) programs—chronic heart failure (CAG-00437N)*. Medicare Coverage Database. U.S. Department of Health and Human Services; 2004.
68. Kitzman DW, Whellan DJ, Duncan P, Pastva AM, Mentz RJ, Reeves GR, Nelson MB, Chen H, Upadhya B, Reed SD, Espeland MA, Hewston L and O'Connor CM. Physical rehabilitation for older patients hospitalized for heart failure. *N Engl J Med*. 2021;385:203–16.
69. Mentz RJ, Whellan DJ, Reeves GR, Pastva AM, Duncan P, Upadhya B, Nelson MB, Chen H, Reed SD, Rosenberg PB, Bertoni AG, O'Connor CM and Kitzman DW. Rehabilitation intervention in older patients with acute heart failure with preserved versus reduced ejection fraction. *JACC Heart Fail*. 2021;9:747–57.
70. Kitzman DW, Brubaker P, Morgan T, Haykowsky M, Hundley G, Kraus WE, Eggebeen J and Nicklas BJ. Effect of caloric restriction or aerobic exercise training on peak oxygen consumption and quality of life in obese older patients with heart failure with preserved ejection fraction: a randomized clinical trial. *JAMA*. 2016;315:36–46.
71. Kitzman DW and Shah SJ. The HFpEF obesity phenotype: the elephant in the room. *J Am Coll Cardiol*. 2016;68:200–3.
72. Unlu O, Levitan EB, Reshetnyak E, Kneifati-Hayek J, Diaz I, Archambault A, Chen L, Hanlon JT, Maurer MS, Safford MM, Lachs MS and Goyal P. Polypharmacy in older adults hospitalized for heart failure. *Circ Heart Fail*. 2020;13:e006977.
73. Goyal P, Zainul O Bs MD, Marshall D and Kitzman DW. Geriatric domains in patients with heart failure with preserved ejection fraction. *Cardiol Clin*. 2022;40:517–32.
74. Baniak LM and Chasens ER. Sleep disordered breathing in older adults with heart failure with preserved ejection fraction. *Geriatr Nurs*. 2018;39:77–83.
75. Goyal P, Kneifati-Hayek J, Archambault A, Mehta K, Levitan EB, Chen L, Diaz I, Hollenberg J, Hanlon JT, Lachs MS, Maurer MS and Safford MM. Reply: toward improved understanding of potential harm in heart failure. *JACC Heart Fail*. 2020;8:247–8.

76. Goyal P, Sauer AJ and Rich MW. All-cause mortality as an end point for heart failure with preserved ejection fraction: underperformance or overambitious? *J Card Fail.* 2022;28:863–5.
77. Krumholz HM. Post-hospital syndrome--an acquired, transient condition of generalized risk. *N Engl J Med.* 2013;368:100–2.
78. Covinsky KE, Pierluissi E and Johnston CB. Hospitalization-associated disability: "She was probably able to ambulate, but I'm not sure." *JAMA.* 2011;306:1782–93.
79. Vitale C, Jankowska E, Hill L, Piepoli M, Doehner W, Anker SD, Lainscak M, Jaarsma T, Ponikowski P, Rosano GMC, Seferovic P and Coats AJ. Heart Failure Association/European Society of Cardiology position paper on frailty in patients with heart failure. *Eur J Heart Fail.* 2019;21:1299–305.
80. Pandey A, Kitzman D and Reeves G. Frailty is intertwined with heart failure: mechanisms, prevalence, prognosis, assessment, and management. *JACC Heart Fail.* 2019;7:1001–11.
81. Goyal P, Yum B, Navid P, Chen L, Kim DH, Roh J, Jaeger BC and Levitan EB. Frailty and post-hospitalization outcomes in patients with heart failure with preserved ejection fraction. *Am J Cardiol.* 2021;148:84–93.
82. Sanders NA, Supiano MA, Lewis EF, Liu J, Claggett B, Pfeffer MA, Desai AS, Sweitzer NK, Solomon SD and Fang JC. The frailty syndrome and outcomes in the TOPCAT trial. *Eur J Heart Fail.* 2018;20:1570–7.
83. Talha KM, Pandey A, Fudim M, Butler J, Anker SD and Khan MS. Frailty and heart failure: state-of-the-art review. *J Cachexia Sarcopenia Muscle.* 2023;14:1959–72.
84. Mudge AM, Pelecanos A and Adsett JA. Frailty implications for exercise participation and outcomes in patients with heart failure. *J Am Geriatr Soc.* 2021;69:2476–85.
85. Prokopidis K, Isanejad M, Akpan A, Stefil M, Tajik B, Giannos P, Venturelli M and Sankaranarayanan R. Exercise and nutritional interventions on sarcopenia and frailty in heart failure: a narrative review of systematic reviews and meta-analyses. *ESC Heart Fail.* 2022;9:2787–99.
86. Sukumar S, Orkaby AR, Schwartz JB, Marcum Z, Januzzi JL, Vaduganathan M and Warraich HJ. Polypharmacy in older heart failure patients: a multidisciplinary approach. *Curr Heart Fail Rep.* 2022;19:290–302.
87. Brännström M and Boman K. Effects of person-centred and integrated chronic heart failure and palliative home care. PREFER: a randomized controlled study. *Eur J Heart Fail.* 2014;16:1142–51.

21

Supraventricular tachyarrhythmias in older persons

SADE SOLOLA NUSSBAUM, SUBRAT K. DAS, SEI IWAI, WILBERT S. ARONOW, AND JASON T. JACOBSON

Key points

- Atrial fibrillation (AF), the most common cardiac arrhythmia, is associated with a higher incidence of mortality, stroke, and coronary events than is sinus rhythm.
- Indications for direct-current cardioversion, drug treatment of AF, and nonpharmacologic therapies are discussed.
- Patients with persistent or paroxysmal AF at high risk for stroke should be treated with long-term warfarin (with target international normalized ratio [INR] of 2.0 to 3.0) or with a direct oral anticoagulant (dabigatran, rivaroxaban, apixaban, or edoxaban).
- Patients with AF at low risk for stroke or with contraindications to anticoagulants can be treated with no antithrombotic therapy.
- Management of atrial flutter, paroxysmal supraventricular tachycardia, accelerated atrioventricular junctional rhythm, paroxysmal atrial tachycardia (PAT) with atrioventricular (AV) block, and multifocal atrial tachycardia is discussed.

ATRIAL FIBRILLATION

Atrial fibrillation (AF) is the most common cardiac arrhythmia, and manifests as irregular undulations on the baseline electrocardiogram (ECG) of varying amplitude, contour, and spacing known as fibrillatory waves, with the atrial rate between 350 and 600 beats per minute. These fibrillatory waves are seen best in leads V_1, II, III, and aVF. The fibrillatory waves may be large and coarse, or they may be fine with an almost flat ECG baseline. The ventricular rate in AF is irregular unless complete atrioventricular (AV) block is present. The morphology of the QRS complex in AF is normal unless there is prior bundle branch block, ventricular preexcitation, or other aberrant ventricular activation pattern.

If AF is associated with a slow and regular ventricular response, there is likely complete AV block with a junctional escape rhythm or idioventricular escape rhythm.

DOI: 10.1201/9781003568933-21

Myocardial infarction, degenerative changes in the conduction system, and drug toxicity, such as digitalis toxicity, are major causes of complete AV block. If AF is associated with a regular ventricular response between 60 and 130 beats per minute, this may be due to an accelerated junctional rhythm caused by an acute inferior myocardial infarction, digitalis toxicity, open heart surgery, or myocarditis. Regularization of the ventricular response in AF may also occur in patients with concomitant ventricular tachycardia (VT) or a ventricular paced rhythm.

Prevalence

The prevalence of AF increases with age (1–5) and thus is quite common in elderly patients. In the Framingham Heart Study, the prevalence of AF was 2%–5% in persons aged 60–69 years, 13%–14% in persons aged 70–90 years, and 22% in persons aged 91–103 years (1, 2). AF was present in 16% of 1160 men, mean age 80 years, and in 13% of 2464 women, mean age 81 years (3). In 5201 persons aged 65 years and older in the Cardiovascular Health Study, the prevalence of AF was 6% in men and 5% in women (4). In 1563 persons with a mean age 80 years, living in the community, the prevalence of AF was 9% (5). In the Cardiovascular Health Study, the incidence of AF was 19.2 per 1000 person-years (6).

AF is described as paroxysmal (PAF, with episodes lasting <7 days), persistent (PeAF, with episodes lasting 7-365 days; long-standing persistent [LSPAF] if >1 year), or permanent (patient and physician decide to stop further attempts at achieving sinus rhythm) (7).

Predisposing factors

AF is the result of electrophysiological abnormalities that are impulse-generating or structural abnormalities of cellular connections that facilitate rapid and nonuniform impulse conduction. AF often initiates as waves of electrical activity originating from ectopic action potentials generated in the pulmonary veins or left atrium, or in response to reentrant activity promoted by heterogeneous conduction due to interstitial fibrosis (7). There are multiple predisposing risk factors for AF such as age, genetics, lifestyle (smoking, obesity, alcohol), heart disease (CAD, CHF, valvular disease, congenital disease), or other medical conditions (obesity, OSA, thyroid disease) (7).

Studies conducted at Royal Adelaide Hospital in Australia assessed the impact of exercise and weight loss on symptomatic AF burden and rhythm control. The ACTIVE-AF trial randomized 120 patients into an exercise group versus control. Results showed freedom from AF in 24/60 (40%) patients in the exercise group and 12/60 (20%) patients in the control group (HR: 0.50; 95% CI: 0.33 to 0.78). There was a reduction of AF symptoms in the exercise group compared with the control group (mean difference −2.3; 95% CI: −4.3 to −0.2; P = 0.033). The LEGACY trial compared the AF burden and maintenance of sinus rhythm in 355 patients after 4 years of weight loss. Results showed a total weight loss ≥10% resulted in a decrease in AF burden and symptoms ($p <$ 0.001 for all) as well as a sixfold (95% confidence interval: 3.4 to 10.3; $p < 0.001$) greater probability of arrhythmia-free survival (8, 9). Treatment of predisposing factors can decrease the incidence of AF.

In a study of 30,000 patients who had coronary artery bypass surgery (CABS), preoperative AF was a predictor of postoperative complications, including death, and of a significant reduction in 3-year survival (10). Because of its anti-inflammatory effects, statin therapy might reduce the risk of postoperative AF (11). In addition, the anti-inflammatory drug colchicine has been shown to reduce inflammation-driven AF in the recovery period after catheter ablation (12).

The Framingham study demonstrated that low serum thyrotropin levels were independently associated with a 3.1 times increase in the development of new AF in older patients (13).

Associated risks

In the Framingham study, the incidence of death from cardiovascular causes was 2.7 times higher in women and 2.0 times higher in men with AF than in women and men with sinus rhythm (14). After adjustment for preexisting cardiovascular conditions, the odds ratio for mortality in persons with AF was 1.9 in women and 1.5 in men (15). In the Copenhagen City Heart Study, the effect of AF on the risk of cardiovascular death was significantly increased 4.4 times in women and 2.2 times in men (16).

AF was present in 22% of 106,780 persons aged ≥65 years with acute MI in the Cooperative Cardiovascular Project (17). Compared with sinus rhythm, patients with AF had a higher in-hospital mortality (25% vs. 16%), 30-day mortality (29% vs. 19%), and 1-year mortality (48% vs. 33%) (17).

In the Platelet Glycoprotein IIb/IIIa in Unstable Angina: Receptors Suppression Using Integrilin Therapy (PURSUIT) trial, AF developed in 6.4% of 9432 patients with acute coronary syndromes without ST-segment elevation (18). After adjustment for other variables, patients with AF had a higher 30-day mortality (hazard ratio = 4.0) and 6-month mortality (hazard ratio = 3.0) than patients without AF (18).

AF is also an independent risk factor for stroke, especially in elderly patients (1, 2). In the Framingham study, the relative risk of stroke in patients with nonvalvular AF compared with patients with sinus rhythm was increased 2.6 times in patients aged 60–69 years, 3.3 times in patients aged 70–79 years, and 4.5 times in patients aged 80–89 years (1). AF was an independent risk factor for thromboembolic (TE) stroke with a relative risk of 3.3 in 2101 persons, mean age 81 years (2). In addition, the 3-year incidence of TE stroke was 38% in older persons with AF and 11% in older persons with sinus rhythm, with a 5-year incidence of 72% in older persons with AF and 24% in older persons with sinus rhythm (2). At 37-month follow-up of 1476 patients who had 24-hour ambulatory ECGs (AECGs), the incidence of TE stroke was 43% for 201 patients with AF (relative risk = 3.3), 17% for 493 patients with paroxysmal supraventricular tachycardia, and 18% for 782 patients with sinus rhythm (19).

In the Copenhagen City Heart Study, the effect of AF on the risk of stroke was significantly increased 7.6 times in women and 1.7 times in men (16). AF is also a risk factor for impaired cognitive function (20).

In 2384 persons, mean age 81 years, AF was present in 17% of those with LV hypertrophy and in 8% of persons without LV hypertrophy. Both AF (risk ratio [RR] = 3.2) and LV hypertrophy (RR = 2.8) were independent risk factors for new TE stroke at 44-month follow-up (21). The higher prevalence of LV hypertrophy in older patients with AF contributes to the increased incidence of TE stroke in this population.

Both AF (RR = 3.3) and extracranial carotid arterial disease (ECAD) with 40%–100% occlusion (RR = 2.5) were independent risk factors for new TE stroke at 45-month follow-up of 1846 persons, mean age 81 years. Older persons with both AF and 40%–100% ECAD had a 6.9 times higher probability of developing new TE stroke than older persons with sinus rhythm and no significant ECAD (22).

AF predisposes to CHF in older patients. As much as 30%–40% of LV end-diastolic volume may be attributable to left atrial contraction in older persons. Absence of a coordinated left atrial contraction reduces late diastolic filling of the LV because of loss of the atrial kick. In addition, a fast ventricular rate in AF shortens the LV diastolic filling period, further reducing LV filling and stroke volume.

In 2708 patients with chronic advanced systolic heart failure, AF was associated with increased risk of hospitalization for CHF compared with patients without AF (hazard ratio of 1.28; 95% confidence interval [CI], 1.00–1.63; $p = 0.049$) (23).

A fast ventricular rate associated with persistent or paroxysmal AF may cause a tachycardia-related cardiomyopathy, which may be an unrecognized treatable cause of CHF (24). In six studies of 768 patients with CHF and AF treated with CRT, AV nodal ablation was performed in 339 patients (25). Compared with medical therapy to control ventricular rate, AV nodal ablation was associated with a significant 58% reduction in all-cause mortality, 56% reduction in cardiovascular mortality, and 48% improvement in New York Heart Association (NYHA) functional class (25).

Clinical symptoms

Patients with AF may be symptomatic or asymptomatic (with their arrhythmia diagnosed by physical examination or by ECG). Evaluation of a patient after a thromboembolic stroke may lead to the diagnosis of AF. Symptoms caused by AF may include palpitations, exercise intolerance, dyspnea or fatigue on exertion, cough, chest pain, dizziness, and/or syncope. A rapid ventricular rate and loss of atrial contraction decrease cardiac output and may lead to angina pectoris, CHF, hypotension, acute pulmonary edema, and syncope, especially in patients with significant valvular disease (especially aortic or mitral stenosis), diastolic or systolic dysfunction, or hypertrophic cardiomyopathy.

Diagnostic tests

When AF is suspected, a 12-lead ECG with a rhythm strip should be obtained to confirm the diagnosis. If paroxysmal AF is suspected, extended cardiac monitoring should be considered. This can include an event monitor, an extended Holter monitor, mobile cardiac outpatient telemetry, or an implantable loop recorder. Twenty-four-hour AECG is rarely sufficient. All patients with AF should have a transthoracic echocardiogram to determine the presence and severity of any cardiac abnormalities causing AF and to identify risk factors for stroke. Appropriate tests for noncardiac causes of AF should be obtained when clinically indicated. Thyroid function tests should be obtained, as AF or CHF may be the only clinical manifestations of apathetic hyperthyroidism in older patients.

Treatment of underlying causes

Management of AF should include therapy of the underlying disease (such as hyperthyroidism, pneumonia, or pulmonary embolism) when possible. Surgical candidates for mitral valve replacement should have mitral valve surgery (with surgical ablation of the AF) if it is clinically indicated. Precipitating factors such as CHF, infection, hypoglycemia, hypokalemia, hypovolemia, and hypoxia should be treated immediately. Alcohol, energy drinks, and drugs (especially sympathomimetics) that precipitate AF should be avoided. Patients with paroxysmal AF associated with the tachycardia–bradycardia (sick sinus syndrome) should be considered for treatment with permanent pacing in combination with drugs to decrease a rapid ventricular rate associated with AF or, in some cases, AF ablation (which may obviate the need for a pacemaker, especially if medications are exacerbating sinus node dysfunction).

Acute control of very rapid ventricular rate

Direct current (DC) cardioversion should be performed immediately in patients who have AF with a very fast ventricular rate associated with an acute MI, chest pain caused by myocardial ischemia, hypotension, severe CHF, syncope, or preexcitation syndromes. Intravenous β-blockers, diltiazem, or verapamil may be used to immediately reduce a very rapid ventricular rate associated with AF except in patients with preexcitation syndromes. In patients with ventricular dysfunction, diltiazem and verapamil should be used with extreme care, if at all, as they can precipitate cardiogenic shock in this population.

Control of rapid ventricular rate

Digoxin should be considered to decrease a rapid ventricular rate in AF unassociated with increased sympathetic tone, hypertrophic cardiomyopathy, or Wolff–Parkinson–White syndrome, especially if there is LV systolic dysfunction.

The usual initial dose of digoxin administered to patients with AF who are naïve to the drug is 0.5 mg orally. Depending on the clinical response, a second oral dose of 0.25 mg may be given in 6–8 hours, and a third oral dose of 0.25 mg may be given in another 6–8 hours to slow a rapid ventricular rate. The usual maintenance oral dose of digoxin given to patients with AF is 0.25–0.5 mg daily, with the dose reduced to 0.125–0.25 mg daily for older patients who are more susceptible to digitalis toxicity (26). Since digoxin is renally cleared, it should be avoided in patients with significant underlying renal disease.

Oral β-blockers, diltiazem, or verapamil should be added to the therapeutic regimen if a rapid ventricular rate in AF occurs at rest or during exercise. Of note, these drugs act synergistically with digoxin to depress conduction through the AV junction. In a study of atenolol 50 mg daily, digoxin 0.25 mg daily, diltiazem-CD 240 mg daily, digoxin 0.25 mg plus atenolol 50 mg daily, and digoxin 0.25 mg plus diltiazem-CD 240 mg daily, digoxin and diltiazem as single drugs were least effective and digoxin plus atenolol was most effective in controlling the ventricular rate in AF during daily activities (27). Oral β-blockers and the non-dihydropyridine calcium channel blockers should be considered first-line therapy, with digoxin being added if these drugs do not achieve the desired effect at maximally tolerated doses.

Amiodarone is the most effective drug for reducing a rapid ventricular rate in AF (28). The noncompetitive β-receptor inhibition and calcium channel blockade are powerful AV nodal conduction depressants. However, the adverse side effect profile of amiodarone limits its use in the treatment of AF. Daily oral doses of 200–400 mg of amiodarone may be given to selected patients with symptomatic life-threatening AF refractory to other drugs. It should be noted that amiodarone may also convert AF to sinus rhythm, therefore it should not be used for ventricular rate control if anticoagulation status is insufficient for cardioversion.

Dronedarone was found to be effective in treating patients with intermittent AF. However, in 3236 patients with permanent AF at risk for major vascular events, dronedarone was found to significantly increase rates of CHF (81%), stroke (232%), and cardiovascular death (211%), and should not be used in patients with permanent AF, class IV CHF, or unstable class II or III CHF (29).

Therapeutic concentrations of digoxin do not decrease the frequency of episodes of paroxysmal AF or the duration of episodes of paroxysmal AF diagnosed by 24-hour AECGs (30). In fact, digoxin has been shown to increase the duration of episodes of PAF, a result consistent with its action in reducing the atrial refractory period. Therapeutic concentrations of digoxin also do not prevent a fast ventricular rate from developing in patients with PAF (30). After a brief episode of AF, digoxin increases the shortening that occurs in atrial refractoriness and predisposes to the reinduction of AF (31). Therefore, digoxin should be avoided in patients with sinus rhythm with a history of PAF.

Nondrug therapies

Catheter ablation (CA) has become a mainstay therapy for patients with AF, especially those with AF refractory to antiarrhythmic drug (AAD) therapy. The cornerstone of CA is the electrical isolation of the pulmonary veins (PVs). For patients with paroxysmal AF, this often suffices as the sole ablation target. However, patients with persistent AF may need more extensive ablation. Other targets can include non-PV triggers (such as the superior vena cava), complex fractionated atrial electrograms (CFAEs), empiric linear lesions (LA roof, mitral isthmus, cavotricuspid isthmus) with or without posterior left atrial wall isolation, atrial scar, and rotors (32). That said, the STAR AF II trial found no benefit to either CFAE ablation or empiric linear lesions over PV isolation (PVI) alone (33). Evolving data, however, suggest that identification and ablation of scar areas, in addition to PVI, can increase success in both paroxysmal and persistent AF (34).

Ablation utilizing modern technology and techniques can afford freedom from AF significantly greater than that of AAD. Current technologies include open-irrigated ablation catheters that create deeper lesions and prevent char/thrombus on the catheter tip, contact-force sensing ablation catheters, and three-dimensional electroanatomic mapping systems (32). Initially, studies suggested that long-term success was dependent on the classification of AF; patients with PAF had the greatest success and patients with LSPAF the least. However, recent data suggest that a more prognostically accurate distinction lies in the presence or absence of atrial scarring. Those without scarring, despite designation as PAF or PeAF, have success rates of 70%–80% with PVI alone, while those with atrial scarring can achieve similar results when scar modification is added to PVI (35).

As worldwide experience with catheter ablation has grown, complication rates have fallen. While PV stenosis was more common at the dawn of PVI, this has become infrequent and usually of limited consequence if it does occur (36). TE risk periprocedure has also decreased dramatically in the era of uninterrupted anticoagulation (37). The most dreaded complications remain the most infrequent: atrio- and pericardio-esophageal fistula. The esophagus lies directly adjacent to the posterior LA and is usually in "the line of fire" at some point during ablation. Many techniques have been adopted to help prevent esophageal damage, but due to the rare occurrence, it is difficult to know their impact (38). Postprocedural cerebral magnetic resonance imaging showed new silent embolic lesions in 33 of 232 patients (14%), mean age 58 years, with paroxysmal or persistent AF who had radiofrequency left atrial catheter ablation (39). Most of these lesions resolve over time. This finding is not isolated to catheter ablation and has been seen in other left heart catheterization procedures, as well as cardiac surgery. The long-term significance of these transient lesions is unknown; however, since the first description, changes in ablation techniques have decreased their incidence (32). Regarding long-term stroke risk, it remains recommended to continue anticoagulation after ablation based on individual patient cerebrovascular accident (CVA) risk and not on the success of ablation (7, 32).

The first randomized study of ablation versus AAD as first-line therapy, the RAAFT-1 trial, was published in 2005 utilizing older ablation techniques and technology. Despite this, it demonstrated that circumferential pulmonary vein radiofrequency ablation was significantly more effective than antiarrhythmic drug therapy in preventing recurrence of symptomatic AF (13% vs. 63%) in 70 patients at 1 year (40).

The RAAFT-2 trial was published in 2014 and randomized 127 patients to ablation and AAD therapy (41). The ablation techniques and technology were more in line with current practice. The primary outcome was quite stringent: documented atrial tachyarrhythmia of more than 30 seconds (symptomatic or asymptomatic AF, atrial flutter, or atrial tachycardia) detected by either scheduled or unscheduled electrocardiogram, Holter, transtelephonic monitor, or rhythm strip. Of the AAD group, 72% experienced the primary outcome at 2 years versus 54% in the ablation group.

Many trials have been performed for ablation as second-line therapy in comparison to AAD. Those investigating PAF have largely focused on pulmonary vein isolation and show a success rate of 59%–89% at 1 year compared with 5%–23% success with AAD (32). For PeAF, 6–12 month success rates are 59%–80% with ablation, as opposed to 9%–58% with AAD (32). It is important to note that the ablation targets in these trials are heterogeneous; which ablation strategy is the most efficacious remains an area of intense debate.

Studies of AF ablation in the elderly have shown similar success and complication rates as in younger patients. Zado et al. (42) compared AF control (no AF on or off AADs or rare AF) and complication rates in patients <65, 65–74, and ≥75 years old. There was no significant difference in AF control (89% in group 1, 84% in group 2, and 86% in group 3, p = NS) during a mean follow-up of 27 months, or major complications (1.6% in group 1, 1.7% in group 2, 2.9% in group 3, p = NS). Corrado et al. found similar results in their cohort of septuagenarian patients (73% single procedure success at 20 months) (43), as did Tan et al. in their octogenarians (70% success at 18 months) (44).

The CASTLE AF study evaluated the efficacy of catheter ablation in improving death or progression of heart failure. The 363 patients with AF (median age of 64) with left ventricular ejection fraction ≤35% and NYHA class >2 HF were randomized 1:1 into catheter ablation or medical therapy (rate or rhythm control). The primary endpoint was death from any cause or worsening of HF with unplanned hospitalization. Results showed significantly fewer primary endpoints in the ablation group than in the medical-therapy group (51 patients [28.5%] vs. 82 patients [44.6%]; hazard ratio, 0.62; 95% confidence interval [CI], 0.43 to 0.87; P = 0.007). There were also significantly fewer deaths [(24 [13.4%] vs. 46 [25.0%]; hazard ratio, 0.53; 95% CI, 0.32 to 0.86; P = 0.01] and less heart failure [(37 [20.7%] vs. 66 [35.9%]; hazard ratio, 0.56; 95% CI, 0.37 to 0.83; P = 0.004)] in the ablation group (45).

Similarly, the CASTLE-HTx trial assessed the safety and efficacy of catheter ablation in patients with end-stage heart failure and symptomatic atrial fibrillation in patients referred for cardiac transplant or left ventricular assist device (LVAD). In the trial, 194 patients, mean age 65 years old, with symptomatic AF and NYHA class >2 HF were randomized 1:1 into a catheter ablation with guideline medical therapy and guideline medical therapy alone. The primary endpoint was a composite of death from any cause, implantation of an LVAD, or urgent heart transplantation. Results showed primary endpoint events occurred in 8 patients (8%) in the ablation group and in 29 patients (30%) in the medical-therapy group (hazard ratio, 0.24; 95% CI, 0.11 to 0.52; $P < 0.001$). Death from any cause occurred in 6 patients (6%) in the ablation group and in 19 patients (20%) in the medical-therapy group (hazard ratio, 0.29; 95% CI, 0.12 to 0.72) (46). This trial was stopped early due to the efficacy of catheter ablation.

The CABANA study, the largest AF ablation trial to date, evaluated the efficacy of catheter ablation therapy for AF compared to drug therapy in symptomatic patients with AF, NYHA class >2 HF, and risk of stroke. In this multicenter RCT, 2204 patients (mean age 67.5) were randomized to either catheter ablation (n = 1108) or drug therapy (n = 1096). Primary outcome was a composite of death, disabling stroke, serious bleeding, or cardiac arrest. Although there was no significant difference in this composite primary outcome endpoint (8.0% in the ablation group vs. 9.2% in the drug therapy group; HR 0.86; 95% CI 0.65–1.15; p = 0.30), there was significant crossover between groups, which likely diluted the actual treatment effect. However, there was a significant reduction in mortality or cardiovascular hospitalization (HR

0.83; 95% CI 0.74–0.93; $p = 0.001$). In addition, in a "per-protocol" analysis of the primary composite endpoint, at 12 months there was a significant benefit to catheter ablation (HR 0.73; 95% CI 0.54–0.99; $p = 0.46$). Recurrent AF was also decreased in the ablation group (HR 0.52; 95% CI 0.45–0.60; $p < 0.001$) (47).

In the Cryo-FIRST study, cryoballoon catheter ablation was compared to antiarrhythmic therapy undergoing first-line rhythm control treatment for symptomatic paroxysmal AF. In the trial, 218 patients with symptomatic PAF were randomized 1:1 to cryoballoon catheter ablation or antiarrhythmic therapy. The primary endpoint was ≥1 episode of recurrent atrial arrhythmia for >30 seconds, after a 90-day blanking period. Results showed freedom from atrial arrhythmia in the cryoballoon arm was 82.2% and 67.6% in the antiarrhythmic arm (HR = 0.48, $P = 0.01$) (48).

A newer ablation modality, pulse field ablation (PFA), uses high-amplitude electrical pulses to desiccate tissue by electroporation without heating tissue. A multicenter prospective study compared the safety and efficacy of PFA, cryoablation, and radiofrequency ablation specifically in elderly patients (>75 years old). Results showed no significant difference in complications or recurrence of atrial tachyarrhythmia at one year, with shorter procedure times associated with PFA. Thus, PFA appears safe and effective at PVI in the elderly population, without significant thermal injury risk (49).

Radiofrequency catheter modification of AV conduction has been promoted in patients with symptomatic AF in whom a rapid ventricular rate cannot be decreased by drugs (50) in the past, but has fallen into relative disfavor and is not utilized as often, especially given the improvements in safety seen with catheter ablation of AF. Complete AV block produced by radiofrequency catheter ablation followed by permanent pacemaker implantation is the procedure of choice in patients with AF who are refractory to, or not candidates for, a sinus rhythm maintenance strategy (51). In a randomized controlled study of 66 persons with CHF and persistent AF, AV junction ablation with implantation of a VVIR pacemaker was superior to drug treatment in controlling symptoms (52). In 44 patients, mean age 78 ± 5 years, radiofrequency catheter ablation followed by pacemaker implantation was successful in ablating the AV junction in 43 of 44 patients (98%) with AF and a rapid ventricular rate not controlled by drug therapy (53). Those with a low EF prior to ablation should be considered for a CRT device. When 77 patients, mean age 75.4 years, with persistent AF were randomized (1:1:1) to AF ablation with amiodarone (±DCCV), PPM with AVNA (+DCCV), or DCCV with amiodarone. Patients who underwent AF ablation with amiodarone had a lower 12-month AF burden compared to both DCCV with amiodarone and PPM and AVNA (without amiodarone) (17.0 ± 37.9% compared with 61.7 ± 48.6% and 76.4 ± 41.6%, respectively, $p < 0.0001$) (54).

Surgical techniques have been developed for use in patients with AF refractory to medical therapy (55). The MAZE procedure is a surgical dissection ("cut-and-sew") of the right and left atrium creating a maze through which the electrical activation is compartmentalized, preventing the formation and perpetuation of the multiple wavelets needed for maintenance of AF. This procedure is typically performed in association with mitral valve surgery or CABS. At 2- to 3-year follow-up, 74% of 39 patients and 90% of 100 patients undergoing the MAZE procedure remained in sinus rhythm (56). Another surgical technique for lesion formation is cryoablation, which restored sinus rhythm in 20 of 29 patients (69%) with persistent AF undergoing this procedure (57). In a trial of surgical ablation at the time of mitral valve surgery, those randomized to ablation had greater freedom from atrial arrhythmias than those in the control group at 6 and 12 months (63.2% vs. 29.4%, $p < 0.001$), with a higher rate of pacemaker implantation postoperatively (21.5 vs. 8.1 per 100 patient-years, $p = 0.01$) (56). Additionally, those in the ablation group randomized to PVI alone showed a similar success rate compared to those randomized to PVI plus additional atrial lesions (58).

Pacing

PAF associated with tachycardia–bradycardia (sick sinus) syndrome can be treated with a permanent pacemaker combined with drugs to slow a rapid ventricular rate associated with AF. AF ablation is also a consideration. Ventricular pacing is an independent risk factor for the development of chronic AF in patients with PAF associated with the tachycardia–bradycardia syndrome (59). Patients with PAF associated with the tachycardia–bradycardia syndrome and no signs of AV conduction abnormalities should be treated with atrial pacing or dual-chamber pacing with programming to minimize ventricular pacing because atrial pacing is associated with less AF and fewer TE complications, compared with ventricular pacing (60).

Many older patients are able to tolerate AF without the need for therapy because the ventricular rate is slow due to concomitant AV nodal disease. These patients should not be treated with drugs that depress AV conduction. A permanent pacemaker should be implanted in patients with AF who develop symptoms such as dizziness or syncope associated with ventricular pauses longer than 3 seconds that are not drug-induced, as documented by a 24-hour AECG or 5-second asymptomatic pauses (61). If patients with AF have drug-induced symptomatic bradycardia, and the causative drug cannot be discontinued, a permanent pacemaker should be implanted.

Percutaneous left atrial appendage transcatheter occlusion

Left atrial appendage occlusion or exclusion, either by percutaneous or surgical methods, is an alternative to anticoagulation in select patient populations. In the PROTECT-AF trial, 707 patients with AF (and a $CHADS_2$ score of at least 1) were randomized to percutaneous closure of the left atrial appendage with the Watchman 2.5 left atrial appendage occlusion device (463 patients) or to warfarin therapy to maintain an international normalized ratio (INR) between 2.0 and 3.0 (244 patients). The primary endpoint of stroke, cardiovascular death, and systemic embolism was not statistically different between the two groups. However, primary safety events were 69% higher in the intervention group than in the warfarin control group (62). The follow-up PREVAIL study narrowly missed the prespecified criteria for non-inferiority regarding the first efficacy endpoint (any stroke, systemic embolism, cardiovascular or unexplained death) but did meet the criteria for the second primary efficacy endpoint (ischemic stroke, systemic embolism 7 days or more post-randomization), and safety endpoints were significantly reduced compared with those in PROTECT-AF (63). Of note, the Watchman device has undergone design improvements and studies, including the PINNACLE FLX IDE study, and showed favorable performance with respect to meeting safety and efficacy endpoints (64).

The Amulet IDE trial evaluated the safety and effectiveness of the Amulet LAA occlusion device compared with the Watchman device. The Amulet device was noninferior to the Watchman device for the primary safety endpoint, which was a composite of procedure-related complications, all-cause death, or major bleeding at 12 months (14.5% vs. 14.7%; $p < 0.001$ for noninferiority), although procedure-related complications were higher for the Amulet (4.5% vs. 2.5%). The Amulet was also noninferior for the primary effectiveness endpoint, which was a composite of ischemic stroke or systemic embolism at 18 months (2.8% for both groups) (65). In a 3-year follow-up of these patients, the Amulet occlude showed continued safety and effectiveness with 96.2% free of oral anticoagulation usage, compared with 92.5% for Watchman ($p < 0.01$). Furthermore, clinical outcomes were comparable for the composite of ischemic stroke or systemic embolism (5.0% vs. 4.6%; $p = 0.69$) between the two devices (66).

The LARIAT device is a suture placed around the LAA via a percutaneous subxiphoid, and although it has 501K FDA clearance, there are no randomized trials for this device evaluating it for CVA prevention (67). The aMAZE trial is an RCT that evaluated the efficacy of percutaneous LAAO with LARIAT in adjunct to PVI in 404 patients with AF. Results showed no statistical superiority in efficacy for freedom from AF recurrence with adjuvant LAAO at time of PVI (68).

WOLFF–PARKINSON–WHITE SYNDROME

DC cardioversion should be performed if a rapid ventricular rate in patients with AF associated with Wolff–Parkinson–White (WPW) syndrome is life threatening or fails to respond to drug therapy. Drug treatment for PAF associated with WPW syndrome includes procainamide, disopyramide, quinidine (69), and ibutilide. Adenosine, β-blockers, digoxin, IV amiodarone, diltiazem, and verapamil are contraindicated to treat AF in patients with WPW syndrome because these drugs shorten (directly or indirectly) the refractory period of the accessory AV pathway, potentially resulting in more rapid conduction down the accessory pathway. This results in a marked increase in ventricular rate, potentially degenerating to ventricular fibrillation (VF). Radiofrequency catheter ablation of the accessory pathway is considered first-line therapy in patients with AF and rapid AV conduction over the accessory pathway (70). In 500 patients with an accessory pathway, radiofrequency catheter ablation of the accessory pathway was successful in 93% of patients (71).

Elective cardioversion

Elective DC cardioversion has a higher success rate than does medical cardioversion in converting AF to sinus rhythm (72). Table 21.1 shows favorable and unfavorable conditions for elective cardioversion of persistent AF.

The American College of Cardiology (ACC)/American Heart Association (AHA)/European Society for Cardiology (ESC) guidelines state that class I indications for cardioversion of AF to sinus rhythm include (i) hemodynamic instability due to AF and (ii) initial rhythm control or after unsuccessful chemical cardioversion in hemodynamically stable patients (7).

Elective cardioversion of AF, either by DC or by antiarrhythmic drugs, should not be performed in asymptomatic elderly patients with persistent AF. The EAST-AFNET 4 trial randomized 2789 patients, mean age of 70 years old, and atrial fibrillation into early rhythm (AAD or ablation) or rate-control strategies. The primary outcome was death from cardiovascular causes, stroke, hospitalization with worsening HF, or acute coronary syndrome, and follow-up was for a median of 5 years. Results showed a first primary-outcome event occurred in 249 of the patients assigned to early rhythm control (3.9 per 100 person-years) and in 316 patients assigned to usual care (5.0 per 100 person-years) (hazard ratio, 0.79; 96% confidence interval, 0.66 to 0.94; $P = 0.005$), indicating that a rhythm-control strategy is superior to rate control in the majority of cases in improving CV outcomes at 5 years among AF patients diagnosed within 1 year of AF (73).

Antiarrhythmic drugs that have been used to convert AF to sinus rhythm include amiodarone, disopyramide, dofetilide, flecainide, ibutilide, procainamide,

Table 21.1 Conditions favorable and unfavorable for cardioversion of atrial fibrillation

Favorable conditions	<1-year duration of AF No or minimal cardiomegaly Echocardiographic left atrial dimension <45 mm After treatment of a precipitating cause such as acute MI, cardiac or thoracic surgery, hyperthyroidism, pneumonia, or pericarditis After corrective valvular surgery Symptomatic AF with hemodynamic improvement and decrease in symptoms expected from sinus rhythm, especially in patients with valvular aortic stenosis or hypertrophic cardiomyopathy
Unfavorable conditions	Duration of atrial fibrillation >1 year Moderate to severe cardiomegaly Echocardiographic left atrial dimension >45 mm Digitalis toxicity (contraindicated) Slow ventricular rate Sick sinus syndrome Chronic obstructive lung disease Mitral valve disease Heart failure Recurrent AF despite antiarrhythmic drugs Inability to tolerate antiarrhythmic drugs

Abbreviations: AF, atrial fibrillation; MI, myocardial infarction.

propafenone, quinidine, and sotalol. None of these drugs is as successful as DC cardioversion, which has a success rate of at least 80%–90% in converting AF to sinus rhythm. All of these drugs are proarrhythmic and may aggravate or cause other cardiac arrhythmias.

Class IC drugs such as flecainide and propafenone should not be used in patients with prior MI and abnormal LV ejection fraction because these drugs may cause life-threatening ventricular tachyarrhythmias in these patients (74). Despite a lack of specific data, the results of the CAST trial are often generalized to patients with any structural heart disease or significant CAD. However, these drugs may be used carefully in these other populations under expert supervision (75).

Dofetilide and ibutilide are class III antiarrhythmic drugs that have been used for the conversion of AF to sinus rhythm. Eleven of 75 patients (15%) with AF treated with intravenous dofetilide converted to sinus rhythm (76). Torsade de pointes occurred in up to 3% of patients treated with intravenous dofetilide (76). After 1 month, 22 of 190 patients (11.6%) with AF and CHF had sinus rhythm restored with dofetilide compared to 3 of 201 patients (1.5%) treated with placebo (149). Torsade de pointes developed in 25 of 762 patients (3%) treated with dofetilide and in none of 756 patients (0%) treated with placebo (77). Twenty-three of 79 patients (29%) with AF treated with intravenous ibutilide converted to sinus rhythm (78). Polymorphic VT developed in 4% of patients who received intravenous ibutilide in this study (78). Baseline bradycardia with AF may predispose to ibutilide-induced polymorphic VT.

DC cardioversion of AF has a higher success rate in converting AF to sinus rhythm and a lower incidence of cardiac adverse effects than treatment with any antiarrhythmic drug. However, pretreatment with ibutilide has been found to facilitate DC cardioversion of AF (79).

Unless transesophageal echocardiography has demonstrated no thrombus in the LAA before cardioversion (80), therapeutic oral anticoagulants should be administered for at least 3 weeks before elective DC or drug conversion of patients with AF to sinus rhythm (81). Anticoagulant therapy should also be given at the time of cardioversion and continued until sinus rhythm has been maintained for at least 4 weeks (81). After DC or drug cardioversion of AF to sinus rhythm, the left atrium becomes stunned and can contract poorly for up to 3–4 weeks, predisposing to TE stroke unless the patient is maintained on oral warfarin (82) or one of the direct oral anticoagulants. The maintenance dose of oral warfarin should be titrated by serial prothrombin times so that the INR is 2.0–3.0 (82).

In a multicenter, randomized, prospective study, 1222 patients with AF of >2 days duration were randomized to either treatment guided by the findings on transesophageal echocardiography or to management with conventional therapy (83). The primary endpoint was CVA, transient ischemic attack, and peripheral embolism within 8 weeks. At 8 weeks, the incidence of embolic events was 0.8% in the transesophageal echocardiography treatment group and 0.5% in the conventional treatment group, and there were also no significant differences between the two groups in the rates of death, maintenance of sinus rhythm, or functional status (83). There was a higher rate of death from any cause in the transesophageal echocardiography treatment group (2.4%) than in the conventional treatment group (1.0%) ($p = 0.06$) (83).

It is important to maintain therapeutic anticoagulation in the period after cardioversion even if there is no transesophageal echocardiographic evidence of thrombus (82).

Use of antiarrhythmic drugs to maintain sinus rhythm

The efficacy and safety of antiarrhythmic drugs after cardioversion of AF to maintain sinus rhythm have been questioned. A meta-analysis of six double-blind, placebo-controlled studies of quinidine involving 808 patients who had DC cardioversion of persistent AF to sinus rhythm demonstrated that 50% of patients treated with quinidine and 25% of patients treated with placebo remained in sinus rhythm at 1-year follow-up (84). However, the mortality was significantly higher in patients treated with quinidine (2.9%) than in patients treated with placebo (0.8%) (84).

In another study, 85 patients were randomized to quinidine and 98 patients to sotalol after DC cardioversion of AF to sinus rhythm (85). At 6-month follow-up, 48% of quinidine-treated patients and 52% of sotalol-treated patients remained in sinus rhythm (85). At 1-year follow-up of 100 patients with AF cardioverted to sinus rhythm, 37% of 50 patients randomized to sotalol and 30% of 50 patients randomized to propafenone remained in sinus rhythm (86).

In a study of 403 patients with at least one episode of AF in the prior 6 months, 201 patients were treated with amiodarone and 202 patients were treated with sotalol or propafenone (87). At 16-month follow-up, AF recurred in 35% of patients treated with amiodarone and in 63% of patients treated with sotalol or propafenone (87). Adverse effects causing discontinuation of the drug occurred in 18% of patients treated with amiodarone and in 11% of patients treated with sotalol or propafenone (87).

After cardioversion of 394 patients with AF to sinus rhythm, 197 patients were randomized to metoprolol CR/XL and 197 patients to placebo (88). At 6-month follow-up, the percent of patients in sinus rhythm was significantly higher on metoprolol CR/XL (51%) than on placebo (40%) (88). The heart rate in patients who relapsed into AF was also significantly lower in patients treated with metoprolol CR/XL than in patients treated with placebo (88).

Of the 1330 patients in the Stroke Prevention in Atrial Fibrillation (SPAF) Study, 127 persons were taking quinidine, 57 procainamide, 34 flecainide, 20 encainide, 15 disopyramide, and 7 amiodarone (89). Patients who were taking an antiarrhythmic drug had a 2.7 times higher adjusted relative risk of cardiac mortality and a 2.3 times higher adjusted relative risk of arrhythmic death compared with patients not taking an antiarrhythmic drug (89). Patients with a history of CHF who were taking an antiarrhythmic drug had a 4.7 times increased risk of cardiac death and a 3.7 times increased risk of arrhythmic death than patients with a history of CHF not taking an antiarrhythmic drug (89).

A meta-analysis of 59 randomized, controlled trials comprising 23,229 patients that investigated the use of aprindine, disopyramide, encainide, flecainide, imipramine, lidocaine, mexiletine, moricizine, phenytoin, procainamide, quinidine, and tocainide after MI also demonstrated that mortality was significantly higher in patients receiving class I antiarrhythmic drugs (odds ratio = 1.14) than in patients not receiving an antiarrhythmic drug (90). None of the 59 studies showed a decrease in mortality by antiarrhythmic drugs (90).

Amiodarone is the antiarrhythmic drug with the highest success rate in maintenance of sinus rhythm after cardioversion of AF (87). However, in the Cardiac Arrest in Seattle: Conventional Versus Amiodarone Drug Evaluation Study, the incidence of pulmonary toxicity was 10% at 2 years in patients receiving amiodarone in a mean dose of 158 mg daily (91). The incidence of adverse effects from amiodarone also approaches 90% after 5 years of therapy (92).

Ventricular rate control

Because maintenance of sinus rhythm with antiarrhythmic drugs may require serial cardioversions; exposes patients to the risks of proarrhythmia, sudden cardiac death, and other adverse effects; and requires the use of anticoagulants in patients in sinus rhythm who have a high risk of recurrence of AF, some cardiologists prefer the management strategy of ventricular rate control plus use of anticoagulants in patients with AF, especially in elderly patients with AF who are not candidates for catheter ablation.

The Atrial Fibrillation Follow-Up Investigation of Rhythm Management (AFFIRM) Study was a randomized trial in AF patients over 65 or who had other risk factors for stroke to assess rate versus rhythm control treatment strategy using antiarrhythmic therapy. All-cause mortality at 5 years was numerically higher in the maintenance of sinus rhythm group compared to the ventricular rate control group, but this did not reach statistical significance (23.8% vs. 21.3%, respectively; HR 1.15; $p = 0.08$). TE stroke was also statistically insignificantly lower in the ventricular rate control group (5.5% vs. 7.1%; $p = 0.79$). Of note, the majority of the strokes in both groups occurred in patients who had stopped taking warfarin or whose INR was subtherapeutic at the time of the stroke. The RACE (Rate Control Versus Electrical Cardioversion for Persistent Atrial Fibrillation) and AF-CHF (Atrial Fibrillation and Congestive Heart Failure) trials also showed no difference in treatment strategies between rate versus pharmacologic rhythm control. Due to the results of the AFFIRM trial, many physicians had considered it appropriate to avoid a rhythm control strategy, due to the proarrhythmic or other significant side effects of antiarrhythmic medications (93).

However, more recently, multiple recent studies have demonstrated the positive effects of rhythm control in patients with high risk of cardiovascular disease regardless of symptoms. The most notable trial, EAST-AFNET 4, is an international multicenter RCT that showed a rhythm-control strategy is superior to rate control in the majority of cases in improving CV outcomes at 5 years among AF patients diagnosed within 1 year of AF (73).

It is important to recognize the benefits of sinus rhythm, and it should be discussed with the patient when AF is first diagnosed. Rhythm control is preferred in HF and most patients <70 years of age. However, the final

Table 21.2 Risk factors for stroke in patients with atrial fibrillation

Age (1, 21, 94)
Echocardiographic left ventricular dysfunction (95)
History of heart failure (95)
Hypertension (95)
Prior thromboembolic events (95)
Women older than 75 years of age (96)
Rheumatic mitral stenosis (94)
Mitral annular calcium (97)
Diabetes mellitus (94)
History of myocardial infarction (94, 95)
Echocardiographic left atrial enlargement (95)
Echocardiographic left ventricular hypertrophy (21, 22, 95)
Extracranial carotid arterial disease (22)
Hypercholesterolemia (94)
Low serum high-density lipoprotein cholesterol (94)

decision should be shared between the patient and physician after a discussion of the risks and benefits of rhythm and rate strategy.

Risk factors for thromboembolic stroke

Table 21.2 lists risk factors for TE stroke in patients with AF (1, 2, 21, 22). In the SPAF Study involving patients (mean age 67 years) with recent CHF (within 3 months), a history of hypertension, previous thromboembolism, echocardiographic left atrial enlargement, and echocardiographic LV systolic dysfunction were associated independently with the development of new TE events (95).

The CHA_2DS_2-VASc score has largely supplanted the previously used $CHADS_2$ criteria. In this newer system, along with the points in the $CHADS_2$ criteria, 1 point is given for age 65–74, 2 points for age 75 and up, 1 point for female sex, and 1 point for vascular disease (99). The addition of these factors better defines the low-risk population (100).

Antithrombotic therapy

Prospective, randomized trials (94, 101) and prospective, nonrandomized observational data from patients, mean age 83 years (96), have documented that warfarin is effective in decreasing the incidence of TE stroke in patients with nonvalvular AF (101). Analysis of pooled data from five randomized, placebo-controlled studies showed that warfarin significantly decreased the incidence of new TE stroke by 68% and was significantly more effective than aspirin in decreasing the incidence of new TE stroke (94).

Nonrandomized observational data from older patients with AF, mean age 83 years, found that 141 patients treated with oral warfarin to achieve an INR between 2.0 and 3.0 (mean INR was 2.4) had a 67% significant decrease in new TE stroke compared with 209 patients treated with oral aspirin (96). Compared with aspirin, warfarin caused a 40% significant decrease in new TE stroke in patients with prior stroke, a 31% significant decrease in new TE stroke in patients with no prior stroke, a 45% significant reduction in new TE stroke in patients with abnormal LV ejection fraction, and a 36% significant reduction in new TE stroke in patients with normal LV ejection fraction (96).

In the Second Copenhagen Atrial Fibrillation, Aspirin, Anticoagulation (AFASAK) study, low-dose warfarin plus aspirin was also less effective in reducing stroke or systemic TE events in patients with AF (7.2% after 1 year) than was adjusted-dose warfarin to achieve an INR between 2.0 and 3.0 (2.8% after 1 year). The incidence of major hemorrhage in older patients with chronic AF, mean age 83 years, was 4.3% (1.4% per year) in patients treated with warfarin to maintain an INR between 2.0 and 3.0 and 2.9% (1.0% per year) in patients treated with aspirin 325 mg daily (98).

Analysis of pooled data from five randomized controlled studies demonstrated that the annual incidence of major hemorrhage was 1.0% for the control group, 1.0% for the aspirin group, and 1.3% for the warfarin group (94). The incidence of major hemorrhage in patients, mean age 72 years, taking adjusted-dose warfarin to achieve an INR of 2.0 to 3.0 in the SPAF III Study was 2.1% (77). The incidence of major hemorrhage in older patients with chronic AF, mean age 83 years, was 4.3% (1.4% per year) in patients treated with warfarin to maintain an INR between 2.0 and 3.0 and 2.9% (1.0% per year) in patients treated with aspirin 325 mg daily (96).

In the SPAF III Study, 892 patients, mean age 67 years, at low risk for developing TE stroke were treated with oral aspirin 325 mg daily. The incidence of ischemic stroke or systemic embolism was 2.2% per year (102). The incidence of ischemic stroke or systemic embolism was 3.6% per year in patients with a history of hypertension and 1.1% per year in patients with no history of hypertension (102).

In a study of 13,559 patients with nonvalvular AF hospitalized with an outpatient stroke, compared to an INR of 2.0 or greater, an INR of <2.0 at hospital admission significantly increased the odds of a severe stroke by 1.9 times and the risk of death within 30 days by 3.4 times (103). The 30-day mortality was similar among patients who were taking aspirin or warfarin with an INR of <2.0 (103). Elderly patients taking warfarin should have an INR maintained between 2.0 and 3.0, not one <2.0 or >3.5 (104).

At 2.7-year follow-up of 973 patients, mean age 82 years, with AF randomized to warfarin to maintain an INR between 2.0 and 3.0 or aspirin 75 mg daily, warfarin significantly reduced fatal or disabling stroke, intracranial hemorrhage, or arterial embolism 52% ($p = 0.003$) (105). The yearly risk of extracranial hemorrhage was similar in both treatment groups (105).

Patients with AF and a left atrial thrombus diagnosed by transesophageal echocardiography should be treated with anticoagulant (if warfarin, aim to achieve an INR between 2.5 and 3.5) because they are at a high risk for new TE events (106). Of 399 patients with chronic kidney disease and AF (23% on hemodialysis and 33% with an estimated glomerular filtration rate <15 mL/min/1.73 m^2), 232 (58%) were treated with warfarin to maintain an INR between 2.0 and 3.0 (107). At 31-month follow-up of warfarin-treated patients and 23-month follow-up of patients not treated with warfarin, warfarin significantly reduced TE stroke by 72% (9% vs. 26%, $p < 0.001$) without significantly increasing major bleeding (14% vs. 9%) (107).

On the basis of the available data, patients with persistent or paroxysmal AF at high risk for developing TE stroke or with a history of hypertension and who have no contraindications to anticoagulation therapy should be treated with long-term oral anticoagulant (if warfarin, to achieve an INR between 2.0 and 3.0) (108).

Patients younger than age 60 years in Olmstead County, Minnesota, with lone AF (no heart disease) had a low risk of TE stroke at 15-year follow-up. At 30-year follow-up of this study, increased age and development of hypertension significantly increased the risk of TE events (109). Table 21.3 shows the ACC/AHA/Heart Rhythm Society (HRS) class I indications for antithrombotic therapy in the management of patients with AF (7).

Despite the data showing the efficacy of oral warfarin used in a dose to achieve an INR between 2.0 and 3.0 in reducing the incidence of new TE events in patients with paroxysmal or chronic AF, only about one third of patients with AF who should be taking warfarin receive it (110).

Elderly patients have a higher prevalence and incidence of AF than younger patients (1–6). Elderly patients with AF are at higher risk for developing TE stroke than are younger patients with AF (1, 19, 21, 94). However, physicians are more reluctant to treat elderly patients with AF with oral anticoagulant therapy. Hopefully, intensive physician education will help solve this important clinical problem.

In the Anticoagulation and Risk Factor in Atrial Fibrillation Study, women off warfarin had significantly higher annual rates of thromboembolism (3.5%) than men (1.8%) (111). Warfarin was associated with significantly lower adjusted TE rates for both women (60% reduction) and men (40% reduction) with similar annual rates of major bleeding (1.0% and 1.1%, respectively) (111).

Of 2580 patients, mean age 77 years, with hypertension and no history of AF in whom a pacemaker or defibrillator had been implanted, subclinical atrial tachyarrhythmias occurred in 10.1% by 3 months (112). Of 51 patients who had ischemic stroke or systemic embolism by 3 months, 11 (22%) had subclinical atrial tachyarrhythmias (112).

Multiple studies have been performed to assess the utility of OAC (edoxaban) for stroke prevention in patients with subclinical atrial fibrillation detected on implantable devices. The NOAH-AFNET 6 study compared the

Table 21.3 2023 American College of Cardiology/American Heart Association/Heart Rhythm Society class I indications for treating patients with atrial fibrillation with antithrombotic therapy

1. Antithrombotic therapy based on shared decision-making, discussion of risks of stroke and bleeding, and patient's preferences
2. Antithrombotic therapy to reduce the risk of stroke should be based on the risk of thromboembolism, regardless of AF pattern (pAF, perAF, LSPAF)
3. CHA_2DS_2-VASc score is recommended to assess annual risk of thromboembolic events, anticoagulation recommended for score >2 men, >3 women
4. DOAC recommended over warfarin if AF without history of moderate to severe rheumatic mitral stenosis or a mechanical heart valve
5. With prior stroke, TIA, or CHA_2DS_2-VASc score ≥2, oral anticoagulants recommended; options include warfarin, dabigatran, rivaroxaban, or apixaban
6. With warfarin, determine INR at least weekly during initiation of therapy and monthly when stable
7. Direct thrombin or factor Xa inhibitor recommended if unable to maintain therapeutic INR
8. Reevaluate the need for anticoagulation at periodic intervals
9. Surgical LAA exclusion with anticoagulation recommended if AF with CHA2DS2-VASc score ≥2 or equivalent stroke risk, undergoing cardiac surgery
10. If life-threatening bleeding on dabigatran, treat with idarucizumab; on warfarin, treat with PCC and vitamin K; on factor Xa inhibitor, treat with andexanet alfa or prothrombin complex concentrate
11. Bridging therapy with UFH or LMWH recommended with a mechanical heart valve if warfarin is interrupted. Bridging therapy should balance risks of stroke and bleeding
12. For patients without mechanical heart valves, bridging therapy decisions should balance stroke and bleeding risks against duration of time patient will not be anticoagulated
13. Evaluate renal function before initiation of direct thrombin or factor Xa inhibitors, and reevaluate when clinically indicated and at least annually
14. For atrial flutter, antithrombotic therapy is recommended as for AF

Abbreviations: INR, international normalized ratio; LMWH, low-molecular-weight heparin; UFH, unfractionated heparin.

efficacy and safety of OAC therapy to no anticoagulation in patients with atrial high-rate episodes detected on implantable devices. In 2536 patients, mean age 78 years old, with device-detected atrial high-rate episodes lasting ≥6 minutes and one stroke risk factor were randomized to edoxaban versus placebo. Results showed death from any cause or major bleeding occurred in 149 patients (5.9% per patient-year) in the edoxaban group and in 114 patients (4.5% per patient-year) in the placebo group (hazard ratio, 1.31; 95% CI 1.02 to 1.67; $P = 0.03$). Edoxaban leads to a significantly higher incidence of major bleeding when compared to placebo (113).

In the ARTESIA study, 4012 patients, mean age 78 years old, with subclinical AF detected on an implantable device with episodes lasting 6 minutes to 24 hours and mean CHA_2DS_2-VASc score >3 were randomized 1:1 to apixaban or aspirin. Results showed stroke or TE occurred in 55 patients in the apixaban group (0.78% per patient-year) and in 86 patients in the aspirin group (1.24% per patient-year) (hazard ratio, 0.63; 95% CI 0.45 to 0.88; $P = 0.007$). Major bleeding was 1.71% per patient-year in the apixaban group and 0.94% per patient-year in the aspirin group (hazard ratio, 1.80; 95% CI 1.26 to 2.57; $P = 0.001$). Thus, in patients with subclinical atrial fibrillation detected on an implantable device with high stroke risk, apixaban resulted in a lower risk of stroke or systemic embolism than aspirin but a higher risk of major bleeding (114).

Non-vitamin K-dependent oral anticoagulants (NOACs)

In the Randomized Evaluation of Long-Term Anticoagulation Therapy (RE-LY) study, 18,113 patients, mean age 72 years, with nonvalvular AF and a risk of stroke were randomized in a blinded fashion to the direct thrombin inhibitor dabigatran 150 mg twice daily, 110 mg twice daily, or (in an unblinded fashion) to warfarin to maintain an INR between 2.0 and 3.0 (115). Median follow-up was 2.0 years. The primary outcome was stroke or systemic embolism. Compared with warfarin, dabigatran 150 mg twice daily reduced the primary outcome by 34% ($p < 0.001$), reduced all-cause mortality from 4.13% per year to 3.64% per year ($p = 0.051$), and had a similar incidence of major bleeding (Table 21.4) (115). Compared with warfarin, dabigatran 110 mg twice daily had a similar incidence of the primary outcome and of all-cause mortality but reduced major bleeding per year from 3.36% to 2.71% ($p = 0.003$) (Table 21.4) (115). The US Food and Drug Administration (FDA) approved the 150 mg dose of dabigatran but not the 110 mg dose of dabigatran for treating AF because the 150 mg dose reduced TE events better than warfarin (116). The FDA approved a 75 mg dose twice daily of dabigatran in patients with an estimated glomerular filtration rate between 15 and 29 mg/mL/1.73 m², although patients with an estimated glomerular filtration rate <30 mg/mL/1.73 m² were excluded

Table 21.4 Effect of newer antithrombotic agents in treating patients with nonvalvular atrial fibrillation

Study	Results
Connolly et al. (115)	At 2-year follow-up, compared with warfarin, dabigatran 150 mg twice daily reduced stroke or systemic embolism from 1.69% per year to 1.11% per year ($p < 0.001$), reduced mortality from 4.13% per year to 3.64% per year ($p = 0.051$), and had a similar incidence of major bleeding (3.36% per year for warfarin and 3.11% per year for dabigatran). Compared with warfarin, dabigatran 110 mg twice daily had a similar incidence of stroke or systemic embolism and of mortality but reduced major bleeding per year from 3.36% to 2.71% ($p = 0.003$).
Patel et al. (118)	At 707-day follow-up, compared with warfarin, rivaroxaban 20 mg daily caused a similar incidence of stroke or systemic embolism and of major bleeding but less intracranial hemorrhage (0.5% vs. 0.7% per year, $p = 0.02$) and less fatal bleeding (0.2% vs. 0.5% per year, $p = 0.003$).
Connolly et al. (119)	Compared with aspirin, apixaban 5 mg twice daily reduced stroke or systemic embolism 55% from 3.7% per year to 1.6% per year ($p < 0.001$), reduced mortality 22% from 4.4% per year to 3.5% per year ($p = 0.07$), reduced first hospitalization for cardiovascular causes from 15.9% per year to 12.6% per year ($p < 0.001$), and did not increase major bleeding or intracranial hemorrhage.
Granger et al. (120) Giugliano et al. (121)	Compared with warfarin, apixaban reduced ischemic or hemorrhagic stroke by 21% from 1.60% per year to 1.27% per year ($p = 0.01$), all-cause mortality 11% from 3.94% per year to 3.52% per year ($p = 0.047$), major bleeding 31% from 3.09% per year to 2.13% per year ($p < 0.001$), and hemorrhagic stroke 49% from 0.47% per year to 0.24% per year ($p < 0.001$) (187). Compared with warfarin, high-dose edoxaban reduced stroke or systemic embolism by 21% from 1.50% per year to 1.18% per year ($p < 0.001$), cardiovascular mortality 14% from 3.17% per year to 2.74% per year ($p = 0.01$), major bleeding 20% from 3.43% per year to 2.75% per year ($p < 0.001$), and hemorrhagic stroke 46% from 0.47% per year to 0.26% per year ($p < 0.001$).

in the RE-LY trial (116). An antidote for dabigatran has recently been developed (117).

In the Rivaroxaban Once Daily Oral Direct Factor Xa Inhibition Compared with Vitamin K Antagonism for Prevention of Stroke and Embolism Trial in Atrial Fibrillation (ROCKET AF), 14,264 patients, mean age 73 years, with nonvalvular AF at increased risk for stroke were randomized to the direct factor Xa inhibitor rivaroxaban 20 mg daily or to warfarin to maintain an INR between 2.0 and 3.0. Median follow-up was 707 days. The primary outcome was stroke or systemic embolism. The primary endpoint and major bleeding were similar in both treatment groups. Significant reductions in intracranial hemorrhage (0.5% vs. 0.7% per year, $p = 0.02$) and in fatal bleeding (0.2% vs. 0.5%, $p = 0.003$) occurred in the rivaroxaban group (118).

In the Apixaban Versus Acetylsalicylic Acid (ASA) to Prevent Stroke in Atrial Fibrillation Patients Who Have Failed or Are Unsuitable for Vitamin K Antagonist Treatment (AVERROES) study, 5599 patients, mean age 70 years, with nonvalvular AF at increased risk for stroke for whom vitamin K antagonist therapy was unsuitable were randomized to the direct factor Xa inhibitor apixaban 5 mg twice daily or to aspirin 81–324 mg daily. Mean follow-up was 1.1 years. The primary outcome was stroke or systemic embolism. Compared with aspirin, apixaban reduced the primary outcome 55% from 3.7% per year to 1.6% per year ($p < 0.001$), reduced mortality 22% from 4.4% per year to 3.5% per year ($p = 0.07$), reduced first hospitalization for cardiovascular causes from 15.9% per year to 12.6% per year ($p < 0.001$), and did not increase major bleeding or intracranial hemorrhage (119).

In the Apixaban for Reduction in Stroke and Other Thromboembolic Events in Atrial Fibrillation (ARISTOTLE) trial, 18,201 patients, mean age 70 years, with nonvalvular AF and at least one additional risk factor for stroke were randomized to apixaban 5 mg twice daily or to warfarin to maintain an INR between 2.0 and 3.0 (120). Median follow-up was 1.8 years. The primary outcome was ischemic or hemorrhagic stroke or systemic embolism. Compared to warfarin, apixaban reduced ischemic or hemorrhagic stroke by 21% from 1.60% per year to 1.27% per year ($p = 0.01$), all-cause mortality 11% from 3.94% per year to 3.52% per year ($p = 0.047$), major bleeding 31% from 3.09% per year to 2.13% per year ($p < 0.001$), and hemorrhagic stroke 49% from 0.47% per year to 0.24% per year ($p < 0.001$) (120).

In the Edoxaban versus Warfarin in Patients with Atrial Fibrillation (ENGAGE AF-TIMI 48) trial, 21,105 patients, median age 72 years and $CHADS_2$ score of at least 2, were randomized to edoxaban 60 mg daily, 30 mg daily, or warfarin to maintain an INR between 2.0 and 3.0 (121). Moderate to severe mitral stenosis was an exclusion criterion. The primary efficacy endpoint was time to first stroke (ischemic or hemorrhagic) or systemic embolism. Compared with warfarin, high-dose edoxaban reduced stroke or systemic embolism by 21% from 1.50% per year to 1.18% per year ($p < 0.001$), cardiovascular mortality 14% from 3.17% per year to 2.74% per year ($p = 0.01$), major bleeding 20% from 3.43% per year to 2.75% per year ($p < 0.001$), and hemorrhagic stroke 46% from 0.47% per year to 0.26% per year ($p < 0.001$). For low-dose edoxaban, the primary endpoint was reached in 1.61%, which was noninferior to warfarin (hazard ratio, 1.07; 97.5% CI 0.87 to 1.31; $p = 0.005$ for noninferiority) (121).

An antidote for factor Xa inhibitors has been approved by the FDA after the ANNEXA-4 trial showed the use of a factor Xa inhibitor (andexanet alfa) in patients with major bleeding was associated with good or excellent hemostatic efficacy in 80% of the patients (122). Additionally, all the DOACs can be somewhat reversed with prothrombin complex concentrate (123), which has been utilized during ablation for AF under uninterrupted anticoagulation, to address bleeding complications.

Regarding initiation of anticoagulation in the setting of acute stroke, the OPTIMAS (Optimal Timing of Anticoagulation After Acute Ischemic Stroke) was a multicenter randomized control trial that assessed 3621 patients over the age of 78 years old with AF and acute stroke who were randomized into early (≤4 days within stroke onset) versus delayed (7–14 days) initiation of anticoagulation. Results showed a primary outcome occurred in 59 (3.3%) of 1814 participants in the early DOAC initiation group compared with 59 (3.3%) of 1807 participants in the delayed DOAC initiation group (adjusted risk difference [RD] 0.000, 95% CI −0.011 to 0.012). Early DOAC initiation within 4 days after ischemic stroke associated with atrial fibrillation was noninferior to delayed initiation for the composite outcome of ischemic stroke, intracranial hemorrhage, unclassifiable stroke, or systemic embolism at 90 days (124).

ATRIAL FLUTTER

Atrial flutter (AFL) may be paroxysmal or persistent. Episodes of AFL and AF may occur in the same patient. The AFL waves are usually best seen in leads II, III, aVF, and V_1. The atrial rate usually ranges from 250 to 350 beats per minute and is most commonly 300 beats per minute. Classically, there is no isoelectric interval between the AFL waves. In the absence of drug therapy, there is usually a 2:1 AV conduction response.

In the general population, the incidence of AFL increases with age and ranges from 5 per 100,000 persons younger than 50 years of age to 587 per 100,000 persons older than 80 years of age (125). At highest risk of developing AFL are the elderly, men, and patients with CHF or chronic obstructive lung disease (125). Documented structural heart disease or a predisposing condition such as a major surgical procedure or pneumonia was present in 178 of 181 patients (98%) with AFL (125).

The acute onset of AFL with a rapid ventricular rate reduces cardiac output and may lead to angina pectoris, CHF, hypotension, acute pulmonary edema, and syncope. Persistent AFL with a rapid ventricular rate can cause a tachycardia-mediated cardiomyopathy. Patients with AFL are also at increased risk for developing new TE stroke (126). LAA stunning occurs after cardioversion in patients with AFL, although to a lesser degree than in patients with AF (127).

Management

Management of AFL is similar to management of AF. DC cardioversion is the treatment of choice for acutely converting AFL to sinus rhythm (128). Of 78 patients with AFL, 38% treated with intravenous ibutilide converted to sinus rhythm (78), and 54% of 16 patients with AFL treated with intravenous dofetilide converted to sinus rhythm (77). Atrial pacing may also be used to try to convert AFL to sinus rhythm (129). This approach is only used in patients with cardiac implantable electronic devices that have a functioning atrial lead.

Intravenous verapamil, diltiazem, or β-blockers may be used to immediately slow a very rapid ventricular rate associated with AFL. Oral verapamil, diltiazem, or β-blockers (27) should be added to the therapeutic regimen if a rapid ventricular rate associated with AFL occurs at rest or during exercise. Amiodarone is the most effective drug for slowing a rapid ventricular rate associated with AFL (28), but it can also restore sinus rhythm, so care must be taken to confirm proper anticoagulation prior. Adenosine, intravenous amiodarone, β-blockers, digoxin, verapamil, and diltiazem are contraindicated in patients with AFL associated with WPW syndrome because these drugs shorten the refractory period of the accessory AV pathway, causing more rapid conduction down the accessory pathway. Class I antiarrhythmic drugs such as flecainide should never be used to treat patients with AFL who are not being treated with digoxin, a β-blocker, verapamil, or diltiazem as a 1:1 AV conduction response may develop.

Since patients with AFL are at increased risk for developing new TE stroke (130), anticoagulant therapy should be administered prior to DC cardioversion or drug cardioversion of AFL patients to sinus rhythm using the same guidelines as for converting AF (81). Patients with chronic AFL should be treated with oral warfarin with the INR maintained between 2.0 and 3.0 (81) or with dabigatran (115), rivaroxaban (118), apixaban (120), or edoxaban (121). Both $CHADS_2$ and CHA_2DS_2-VASc scores are useful for stroke risk stratification in patients with AFL (129).

Radiofrequency catheter ablation of AFL is a highly successful procedure, especially when the right atrial isthmus is incorporated in the AFL circuit (131, 132). Demonstration of bidirectional isthmus block after catheter ablation predicts a high long-term success rate (132). A second radiofrequency catheter ablation may be needed in up to one third of patients, especially in those with right atrial enlargement (131). Radiofrequency catheter ablation was successful in converting 63 of 70 patients (90%), mean age 78 ± 5 years, with AFL to sinus rhythm (53). It is important to note that up to 55% of patients will develop AF in long-term follow-up after successful AFL ablation (133), therefore lifelong anticoagulation should be considered in those at high risk for CVA.

PAROXYSMAL SUPRAVENTRICULAR TACHYCARDIA

Paroxysmal supraventricular tachycardia (PSVT) is a regular narrow complex tachycardia with a rate usually between 140 and 220 beats per minute. A wide QRS complex occurs in the presence of bundle branch block or aberrant ventricular conduction. If aberrant ventricular conduction is present, the QRS complex is usually <140 ms, and a right bundle branch block pattern is present 85% of the time.

PSVT is usually caused by reentry but may be caused by abnormal automaticity or by triggered activity. AV nodal reentrant tachycardia (AVNRT) accounts for 60% of episodes of PSVT (134). Discrete P waves are not seen on the 12-lead ECG in two thirds of these patients. Retrograde P waves (inverted in leads II, III, and aVF) following the QRS complex occur in approximately 30% of these patients. In approximately 10% of patients, the reentry circuit is reversed, with anterograde conduction over the fast pathway and retrograde conduction over the slow pathway (134). This type of PSVT is referred to as atypical AVNRT, and the RP interval is longer than the PR interval.

PSVT secondary to accessory pathway conduction occurs in approximately 30% of patients with sustained PSVT (135). Accessory pathway conduction can be overt, as in WPW syndrome, or concealed because accessory pathways are capable of either unidirectional or bidirectional conduction.

Paroxysmal atrial tachycardia (PAT) includes those forms of PSVT that do not involve the AV node as an obligate part of the tachycardia circuit (136). Atrial tachycardias can be reentrant, automatic, or triggered in origin (136).

The prevalence of short bursts of PSVT diagnosed by 24-hour ambulatory ECGs in 1476 elderly persons, mean age 81 years, with heart disease was 33% (19). At 43-month follow-up of 1476 persons, mean age 81 years, with heart disease, short bursts of PSVT were not associated with an increased incidence of new TE stroke (19).

Management

Sustained episodes of supraventricular tachycardia (SVT) should first be treated by increasing vagal tone by carotid sinus massage (in the absence of carotid disease/bruit), the Valsalva maneuver, and facial immersion in cold water (137). If vagal maneuvers are unsuccessful, intravenous adenosine is the drug of choice. Intravenous verapamil, diltiazem, or β-blockers may also be used. If these measures do not convert SVT to sinus rhythm, DC cardioversion should be considered.

Most patients with SVT do not require long-term therapy. If long-term treatment is required because of symptoms due to frequent episodes of SVT, digoxin, β-blockers, verapamil, or diltiazem may be administered. These are the initial drugs of choice for AVNRT and AV reciprocating tachycardia. For SVT associated with WPW syndrome, catheter ablation is considered first-line therapy. If medical therapy is preferred, flecainide or propafenone may be used if there is no associated heart disease (138). If heart disease is present, quinidine, procainamide, or disopyramide plus a β-blocker or verapamil should be used (138). Radiofrequency catheter ablation should be used to treat older persons with symptomatic, drug-resistant SVT and should be considered an early treatment option (139). Catheter ablation can be successfully performed in older patients with low complication rates. Some patients with baseline first-degree AV block can safely undergo ablation for AVNRT; however, extreme PR prolongation in older patients may identify a higher risk for complete AV block. Cardiac perforation risk is also increased in elderly women. For example, radiofrequency catheter ablation was successful in treating 60 of 66 patients with SVT (mean age 78 ± 5 years) (53).

Accelerated atrioventricular junctional rhythm

Accelerated AV junctional rhythm, also called nonparoxysmal AV junctional tachycardia, (NPJT) is a form of SVT caused by enhanced impulse formation within the AV junction rather than by reentry (140). This arrhythmia is usually due to recent aortic or mitral valve surgery, acute MI, or digitalis toxicity. The ventricular rate usually ranges between 70 and 130 beats per minute. Treatment of NPJT is directed toward correction of the underlying disorder. Hypokalemia, if present, should be treated with potassium. Digitalis should be stopped if digitalis toxicity is present. β-blockers may be given cautiously if this is warranted by clinical circumstances.

PAT with atrioventricular block

Digitalis toxicity causes 70% of cases of PAT with AV block. Digoxin and diuretics causing hypokalemia should be stopped in these patients. If the serum potassium is low or low-normal, potassium chloride is the treatment of choice. Intravenous propranolol will cause conversion to sinus rhythm in about 85% of patients with digitalis-induced PAT with AV block and in about 35% of patients with PAT with AV block not induced by digitalis (137). By increasing AV block, propranolol may also be beneficial in slowing a rapid ventricular rate in PAT with AV block (137).

Multifocal atrial tachycardia

Multifocal atrial tachycardia (MAT) is usually associated with acute illness, especially in older persons with pulmonary disease. MAT is best managed by treatment of the underlying disorder. Intravenous verapamil has been reported to be effective in controlling the ventricular rate in MAT, with occasional conversion to sinus rhythm (141). The tendency of intravenous verapamil to aggravate preexisting arterial hypoxemia also limits its use in the group of patients most likely to develop MAT (141).

CONCLUSION

The preponderance of supraventricular arrhythmias in the elderly is AF. Important management decisions revolve around stroke prevention, rate control, and rhythm control. AAD is often first-line therapy for rhythm control; however, catheter ablation has become an effective option. AFL is also commonly seen in this population, but even after successful ablation, AF frequently occurs. The same stroke risk stratification should be applied to patients with AFL. Other SVTs can be seen in the elderly as well, and their management echoes that of the general population.

REFERENCES

1. Wolf PA, Abbott RD, Kannel WB. Atrial fibrillation as an independent risk factor for stroke: The Framingham study. *Stroke* 1991; *22*: 983–988.
2. Aronow WS, Ahn C, Gutstein H. Prevalence of atrial fibrillation and association of atrial fibrillation with prior and new thromboembolic stroke in older patients. *J Am Geriatr Soc* 1996; *44*: 521–523.
3. Aronow WS, Ahn C, Gutstein H. Prevalence and incidence of cardiovascular disease in 1,160 older men and 2,464 older women in a long-term health care facility. *J Gerontol Med Sci* 2002; *57A*: M45–M46.
4. Furberg CD, Psaty BM, Manolio TA et al. Prevalence of atrial fibrillation in elderly subjects (the Cardiovascular Health Study). *Am J Cardiol* 1994; *74*: 236–241.
5. Mendelson G, Aronow WS. Underutilization of warfarin in older persons with chronic nonvalvular atrial fibrillation at high risk for developing stroke. *J Am Geriatr Soc* 1998; *46*: 1423–1424.
6. Psaty BM, Manolio TA, Kuller LH et al. Incidence of and risk factors for atrial fibrillation in older adults. *Circulation* 1997; *96*: 2455–2461.
7. Joglar JA, Chung MK, Armbruster AL, Benjamin EJ, Chyou JY, Cronin EM, Deswal A, Eckhardt LL, Goldberger ZD, Gopinathannair R, Gorenek B, Hess PL, Hlatky M, Hogan G, Ibeh C, Indik JH, Kido K, Kusumoto F, Link MS, Linta KT, Marcus GM, McCarthy PM, Patel N, Patton KK, Perez

MV, Piccini JP, Russo AM, Sanders P, Streur MM, Thomas KL, Times S, Tisdale JE, Valente AM, Van Wagoner DR; Peer Review Committee Members. 2023 ACC/AHA/ACCP/HRS guideline for the diagnosis and management of atrial fibrillation: a report of the American College of Cardiology/American Heart Association Joint Committee on Clinical Practice Guidelines. *Circulation* 2024 Jan 2; *149*(1): e1–e156.
8. Elliott AD, Verdicchio CV, Mahajan R, Middeldorp ME, Gallagher C, Mishima RS, Hendriks JML, Pathak RK, Thomas G, Lau DH, Sanders P. An exercise and physical activity program in patients with atrial fibrillation: The ACTIVE-AF randomized controlled trial. *JACC Clin Electrophysiol* 2023 Apr; *9*(4): 455–465.
9. Pathak RK, Middeldorp ME, Meredith M, Mehta AB, Mahajan R, Wong CX, Twomey D, Elliott AD, Kalman JM, Abhayaratna WP, Lau DH, Sanders P. Long-term effect of goal-directed weight management in an atrial fibrillation cohort: A long-term follow-up study (LEGACY). *J Am Coll Cardiol* 2015 May 26; *65*(20): 2159–2169.
10. Banach M, Goch A, Misztal M et al. Relation between postoperative mortality and atrial fibrillation before surgical revascularization – 3-year follow-up. *Thorac Cardiovasc Surg* 2008; *56*: 20–23.
11. Banach M, Ugurlucan M, Mariscalco G et al. Statins in the prevention of postoperative atrial fibrillation. Is there really no effect? *Am Heart J* 2008; *155*: e53.
12. Deftereos S, Giannopoulos G, Efremidis M et al. Colchicine for prevention of atrial fibrillation recurrence after pulmonary vein isolation: Mid-term efficacy and effect on quality of life. *Heart Rhythm* 2014; *11*: 620–628.
13. Sawin CT, Geller A, Wolf PA et al. Low serum thyrotropin concentration as a risk factor for atrial fibrillation in older persons. *N Engl J Med* 1994; *331*: 1249–1252.
14. Kannel WB, Abbott RD, Savage DD et al. Epidemiologic features of chronic atrial fibrillation: The Framingham study. *N Engl J Med* 1982; *306*: 1018–1022.
15. Benjamin EJ, Wolf PA, D'Agostino RB et al. Impact of atrial fibrillation on the risk of death. The Framingham heart study. *Circulation* 1998; *98*: 946–952.
16. Friberg J, Scharling H, Gadsboll N et al. Comparison of the impact of atrial fibrillation on the risk of stroke and cardiovascular death in women versus men (The Copenhagen City Heart Study). *Am J Cardiol* 2004; *94*: 889–894.
17. Rathore SS, Berger AK, Weinfurt KP et al. Acute myocardial infarction complicated by atrial fibrillation in the elderly: Prevalence and outcomes. *Circulation* 2000; *101*: 969–974.
18. Al-Khatib SM, Pieper KS, Lee KL et al. Atrial fibrillation and mortality among patients with acute coronary syndromes without ST-segment elevation: Results from the PURSUIT trial. *Am J Cardiol* 2001; *88*: 76–79.
19. Aronow WS, Ahn C, Mercando AD et al. Correlation of paroxysmal supraventricular tachycardia, atrial fibrillation, and sinus rhythm with incidences of new thromboembolic stroke in 1,476 old-old patients. *Aging Clin Experimental Res* 1996; *8*: 32–34.
20. Jozwiak A, Guzik P, Mathew A et al. Association of atrial fibrillation and focal neurologic deficits with impaired cognitive function in hospitalized patients ≥65 years of age. *Am J Cardiol* 2006; *98*: 1238–1241.
21. Aronow WS, Ahn C, Kronzon I et al. Association of left ventricular hypertrophy and chronic atrial fibrillation with the incidence of new thromboembolic stroke in 2,384 older persons. *Am J Cardiol* 1999; *84*: 468–469.
22. Aronow WS, Ahn C, Schoenfeld MR et al. Association of extracranial carotid arterial disease and chronic atrial fibrillation with the incidence of new thromboembolic stroke in 1,846 older persons. *Am J Cardiol* 1999; *83*: 1403–1403.
23. Ahmed MI, White M, Ekundayo OJ et al. A history of atrial fibrillation and outcomes in chronic advanced systolic heart failure: A propensity-matched study. *Eur Heart J* 2009; *30*: 2029–2037.
24. Schumacher B, Luderitz B. Rate issues in atrial fibrillation: Consequences of tachycardia and therapy for rate control. *Am J Cardiol* 1998; *82*: 29N–36N.
25. Ganesan AN, Brooks AG, Roberts-Thomson KC et al. Role of AV nodal ablation in cardiac resynchronization in patients with coexistent atrial fibrillation and heart failure. A systematic review. *J Am Coll Cardiol* 2012; *59*: 719–726.
26. Aronow WS. Digoxin or angiotensin converting enzyme inhibitors for congestive heart failure in geriatric patients: Which is the preferred treatment? *Drugs Aging* 1991; *1*: 98–103.
27. Farshi R, Kistner D, Sarma JSM et al. Ventricular rate control in chronic atrial fibrillation during daily activity and programmed exercise: A crossover open-label study of five drug regimens. *J Am Coll Cardiol* 1999; *33*: 304–310.
28. Chun SH, Sager PT, Stevenson WG et al. Long-term efficacy of amiodarone for the maintenance of normal sinus rhythm in patients with refractory atrial fibrillation or flutter. *Am J Cardiol* 1995; *76*: 47–50.
29. Connolly SJ, Camm AJ, Halperin JL et al. Dronedarone in high-risk permanent atrial fibrillation. *N Engl J Med* 2011; *365*: 2268–2276.
30. Murgatroyd FD, Gibson SM, Baiyan X et al. Double-blind placebo controlled trial of digoxin in symptomatic paroxysmal atrial fibrillation. *Circulation* 1999; *99*: 2765–2770.

31. Sticherling C, Oral H, Horrocks J et al. Effects of digoxin on acute, atrial fibrillation-induced changes in atrial refractoriness. *Circulation* 2000; *102*: 2503–2508.
32. Calkins H, Hindricks G, Cappato R et al. 2017 HRS/EHRA/ECAS/APHRS/SOLAECE expert consensus statement on catheter and surgical ablation of atrial fibrillation. *Heart Rhythm* 2017; *14*: e275–e444.
33. Verma A, Jiang CY, Betts TR et al. Approaches to catheter ablation for persistent atrial fibrillation. *N Engl J Med* 2015; *372*: 1812–1822.
34. Kottkamp H, Berg J, Bender R et al. Box isolation of fibrotic areas (BIFA): A patient-tailored substrate modification approach for ablation of atrial fibrillation. *J Cardiovasc Electrophysiol* 2016; *27*: 22–30.
35. Blandino A, Bianchi F, Grossi S et al. Left atrial substrate modification targeting low-voltage areas for catheter ablation of atrial fibrillation: A systematic review and meta-analysis. *Pacing Clin Electrophysiol* 2017; *40*: 199–212.
36. Rostamian A, Narayan SM, Thomson L et al. The incidence, diagnosis, and management of pulmonary vein stenosis as a complication of atrial fibrillation ablation. *J Interv Card Electrophysiol* 2014; *40*: 63–74.
37. Cardoso R, Knijnik L, Bhonsale A et al. An updated meta-analysis of novel oral anticoagulants versus vitamin K antagonists for uninterrupted anticoagulation in atrial fibrillation catheter ablation. *Heart Rhythm* 2018; *15*: 107–115.
38. Medeiros De Vasconcelos JT, Filho S, Atie J et al. Atrial-oesophageal fistula following percutaneous radiofrequency catheter ablation of atrial fibrillation: The risk still persists. *Europace* 2017; *19*: 250–258.
39. Gaita F, Caponi D, Pianelli M et al. Radiofrequency catheter ablation of atrial fibrillation: A cause of silent thromboembolism? Magnetic resonance imaging assessment of cerebral thromboembolism in patients undergoing ablation of atrial fibrillation. *Circulation* 2010; *122*: 1667–1673.
40. Wazni OM, Marrouche NF, Martin DO et al. Radiofrequency ablation vs antiarrhythmic drugs as first-line treatment of symptomatic atrial fibrillation. A randomized trial. *JAMA* 2005; *293*: 2634–2640.
41. Morillo CA, Verma A, Connolly SJ et al. Radiofrequency ablation vs antiarrhythmic drugs as first-line treatment of paroxysmal atrial fibrillation (RAAFT-2): A randomized trial. *JAMA* 2014; *311*: 692–700.
42. Zado E, Callans DJ, Riley M et al. Long-term clinical efficacy and risk of catheter ablation for atrial fibrillation in the elderly. *J Cardiovasc Electrophysiol* 2008; *19*: 621–626.
43. Corrado A, Patel D, Riedlbauchova L et al. Efficacy, safety, and outcome of atrial fibrillation ablation in septuagenarians. *J Cardiovasc Electrophysiol* 2008; *19*: 807–811.
44. Tan HW, Wang XH, Shi HF et al. Efficacy, safety and outcome of catheter ablation for atrial fibrillation in octogenarians. *Int J Cardiol* 2010; *145*: 147–148.
45. Marrouche NF, Brachmann J, Andresen D, Siebels J, Boersma L, Jordaens L, Merkely B, Pokushalov E, Sanders P, Proff J, Schunkert H, Christ H, Vogt J, Bänsch D; CASTLE-AF Investigators. Catheter ablation for atrial fibrillation with heart failure. *N Engl J Med* 2018 Feb 1; *378*(5): 417–427.
46. Sohns C, Fox H, Marrouche NF, Crijns HJGM, Costard-Jaeckle A, Bergau L, Hindricks G, Dagres N, Sossalla S, Schramm R, Fink T, El Hamriti M, Moersdorf M, Sciacca V, Konietschke F, Rudolph V, Gummert J, Tijssen JGP, Sommer P; CASTLE HTx Investigators. Catheter ablation in end-stage heart failure with atrial fibrillation. *N Engl J Med* 2023 Oct 12; *389*(15): 1380–1389.
47. Packer DL, Mark DB, Robb RA, Monahan KH, Bahnson TD, Poole JE, Noseworthy PA, Rosenberg YD, Jeffries N, Mitchell LB, Flaker GC, Pokushalov E, Romanov A, Bunch TJ, Noelker G, Ardashev A, Revishvili A, Wilber DJ, Cappato R, Kuck KH, Hindricks G, Davies DW, Kowey PR, Naccarelli GV, Reiffel JA, Piccini JP, Silverstein AP, Al-Khalidi HR, Lee KL; CABANA Investigators. Effect of catheter ablation vs antiarrhythmic drug therapy on mortality, stroke, bleeding, and cardiac arrest among patients with atrial fibrillation: The CABANA randomized clinical trial. *JAMA* 2019 Apr 2; *321*(13): 1261–1274.
48. Kuniss M, Pavlovic N, Velagic V, Hermida JS, Healey S, Arena G, Badenco N, Meyer C, Chen J, Iacopino S, Anselme F, Packer DL, Pitschner HF, Asmundis C, Willems S, Di Piazza F, Becker D, Chierchia GB; Cryo-FIRST Investigators. Cryoballoon ablation vs. antiarrhythmic drugs: First-line therapy for patients with paroxysmal atrial fibrillation. *Europace* 2021 Jul 18; *23*(7): 1033–1041.
49. Nakasone K, Della Rocca DG, Magnocavallo M, Betancur A, Vetta G, Pannone L, Sorgente A, Audiat C, Rodriguez J, Doundoulakis I, Nekic A, Velagić V, Polselli M, Mohanty S, Marcon L, Sieira J, Ströker E, Bala G, Bianchi S, Almorad A, Combes S, Tsiachris D, Sarkozy A, Natale A, Boveda S, Rossi P, de Asmundis C, Chierchia GB; HRMC Investigators. Pulsed field ablation in the elderly via a pentaspline multielectrode catheter: Safety, efficacy, and comparison with cryoballoon and radiofrequency devices. *Heart Rhythm* 2025 Jan 24: S1547–5271(25)00094-3.
50. Feld GK, Fleck P, Fujimura O et al. Control of rapid ventricular response by radiofrequency catheter modification of the atrioventricular node in patients with medically refractory atrial fibrillation. *Circulation* 1994; *90*: 2299–307.

51. Fitzpatrick AP, Kourouyan HD, Siu A et al. Quality of life and outcomes after radiofrequency His bundle catheter ablation and permanent pacemaker implantation: impact of treatment in paroxysmal and established atrial fibrillation. *Am Heart J* 1996; *131*: 499–507.
52. Brignole M, Menozzi C, Gianfranchi L et al. Assessment of atrioventricular junction ablation and VVIR pacemaker versus pharmacological treatment in patients with heart failure and chronic atrial fibrillation. A randomized, controlled study. *Circulation* 1998; *98*: 953–960.
53. Ozcan C, Jahangir A, Friedman PA et al. Long-term survival after ablation of the atrioventricular node and implantation of a permanent pacemaker in patients with atrial fibrillation. *N Engl J Med* 2001; *344*: 1043–1051.
54. Channamsetty V, Aronow WS, Sorbera C et al. Efficacy of radiofrequency catheter ablation in treatment of elderly patients with supraventricular tachyarrhythmias and ventricular tachycardia. *Am J Ther* 2006; *13*: 513–515.
55. Cox JL, Boineau JP, Schuessler RB et al. Successful surgical treatment of atrial fibrillation: Review and clinical update. *JAMA* 1991; *266*: 1976–1980.
56. Handa N, Scaff HV, Morris JJ et al. Outcome of valve repair and the Cox maze procedure for mitral regurgitation and associated atrial fibrillation. *J Thorac Cardiovasc Surg* 1999; *118*: 628–635.
57. Gaita F, Gallotti R, Calo L et al. Limited posterior left atrial cryoablation in patients with chronic atrial fibrillation undergoing valvular heart surgery. *J Am Coll Cardiol* 2000; *36*: 159–166.
58. Gillinov AM, Gelijns AC, Parides MK et al. Surgical ablation of atrial fibrillation during mitral-valve surgery. *N Engl J Med* 2015; *372*: 1399–1409.
59. Sgarbossa EB, Pinski SL, Maloney JD et al. Chronic atrial fibrillation and stroke in paced patients with sick sinus syndrome. Relevance of clinical characteristics and pacing modalities. *Circulation* 1993; *88*: 1045–1053.
60. Andersen HR, Thuesen L, Bagger JP et al. Prospective randomised trial of atrial versus ventricular pacing in sick-sinus syndrome. *Lancet* 1994; *344*: 1523–1528.
61. Epstein AE, DiMarco JP, Ellenbogen KA et al. ACC/AHA/HRS 2008 guidelines for device-based therapy of cardiac rhythm abnormalities: A report of the American College of Cardiology/American Heart Association Task Force on Practice Guidelines (writing committee to revise the ACC/AHA/NASPE 2002 guideline update for implantation of cardiac pacemakers and antiarrhythmia devices): developed in collaboration with the American Association for Thoracic Surgery and Society of Thoracic Surgeons. *Circulation* 2008; *117*: e350–e408.
62. Holmes DR, Reddy VY, Turi ZG et al. Percutaneous closure of the left atrial appendage versus warfarin therapy for prevention of stroke in patients with atrial fibrillation: A randomized non-inferiority trial. *Lancet* 2009; *374*: 534–542.
63. Holmes DR, Jr., Kar S, Price MJ et al. Prospective randomized evaluation of the Watchman left atrial appendage closure device in patients with atrial fibrillation versus long-term warfarin therapy: The PREVAIL trial. *J Am Coll Cardiol* 2014; *64*: 1–12.
64. Kar S, Doshi SK, Sadhu A, Horton R, Osorio J et al on behalf of the PINNACLE FLX Investigators. Primary outcome evaluation of the next-generation left atrial appendage closure device: Results from the PINNACLE FLX trial. *Circulation* 2021; *143*: 1754–1762.
65. Lakkireddy D, Thaler D, Ellis CR, Swarup V, Sondergaard L, Carroll J, Gold MR, Hermiller J, Diener HC, Schmidt B, MacDonald L, Mansour M, Maini B, O'Brien L, Windecker S. Amplatzer amulet left atrial appendage occluder versus watchman device for stroke prophylaxis (Amulet IDE): A randomized, controlled trial. *Circulation* 2021 Nov 9; *144*(19): 1543–1552.
66. Lakkireddy D, Thaler D, Ellis CR, Swarup V, Gambhir A et al. 3-year outcomes from the Amplatzer Amulet left atrial appendage occlude randomized controlled trial (Amulet IDE). *J Am Coll Cardiol Intv* 2023; *16*: 1902–1913.
67. Bartus K, Gafoor S, Tschopp D et al. Left atrial appendage ligation with the next generation LARIAT(+) suture delivery device: Early clinical experience. *Int J Cardiol* 2016; *215*: 244–7.
68. Lakkireddy DR, Wilber DJ, Mittal S et al. Pulmonary vein isolation with or without left atrial appendage ligation in atrial fibrillation: The aMAZE randomized clinical trial. *JAMA* 2024; *331*(13): 1099–1108.
69. Michelson EL. Clinical perspectives in management of Wolff–Parkinson–White syndrome. Part 2: Diagnostic evaluation and treatment strategies. *Mod Concepts Cardiovasc Dis* 1989; *58*: 49–54.
70. Jackman WM, Wang X, Friday KJ et al. Catheter ablation of accessory atrioventricular pathways (Wolff–Parkinson–White syndrome) by radiofrequency current. *N Engl J Med* 1991; *324*: 1605–1611.
71. Calkins H, Yong P, Miller JM et al. Catheter ablation of accessory pathways, atrioventricular nodal reentrant tachycardia, and the atrioventricular junction. Final results of a prospective, multicenter clinical trial. *Circulation* 1999; *99*: 262–270.
72. Morris JJ Jr, Peter RH, McIntosh HD. Electrical conversion of atrial fibrillation: Immediate and long-term results and selection of patients. *Ann Intern Med* 1966; *65*: 216–231.
73. Kirchhof P, Camm AJ, Goette A, Brandes A, Eckardt L, Elvan A, Fetsch T, van Gelder IC, Haase D,

Haegeli LM, Hamann F, Heidbüchel H, Hindricks G, Kautzner J, Kuck KH, Mont L, Ng GA, Rekosz J, Schoen N, Schotten U, Suling A, Taggeselle J, Themistoclakis S, Vettorazzi E, Vardas P, Wegscheider K, Willems S, Crijns HJGM, Breithardt G; EAST-AFNET 4 trial investigators. Early rhythm-control therapy in patients with atrial fibrillation. *N Engl J Med* 2020 Oct 1; *383*(14): 1305–1316.
74. Cardiac Arrhythmia Suppression Trial. Preliminary report: Effect of encainide and flecainide on mortality in a randomized trial of arrhythmia suppression after myocardial infarction. *N Engl J Med* 1989; *329*: 406–412.
75. Kiani S, Sayegh MN, Ibrahim R, Bhatia NK, Merchant FM, Shah AD, Westerman SB, De Lurgio DB, Patel AM, Thompkins CM, Leon AR, Lloyd MS, El-Chami MF. The feasibility and safety of flecainide use among patients with varying degrees of coronary disease. *JACC Clin Electrophysiol* 2023 Jul; 9(7 Pt 2): 1172–1180.
76. Falk RH, Pollak A, Singh SN et al. Intravenous dofetilide, a Class III antiarrhythmic agent, for the termination of sustained atrial fibrillation or flutter. *J Am Coll Cardiol* 1997; *29*: 385–390.
77. Torp-Pedersen C, Moller M, Bloch-Thomsen PE et al. Dofetilide in patients with congestive heart failure and left ventricular dysfunction. *N Engl J Med* 1999; *341*: 857–865.
78. Ellenbogen KA, Stambler BS, Wood MA et al. Efficacy of intravenous ibutilide for rapid termination of atrial fibrillation and atrial flutter: A dose-response study. *J Am Coll Cardiol* 1996; *28*: 130–136.
79. Oral H, Souza JJ, Michaud GF et al. Facilitating transthoracic cardioversion of atrial fibrillation with ibutilide pretreatment. *N Engl J Med* 1999; *340*: 1849–1854.
80. Manning WJ, Silverman DI, Keighley CS et al. Transesophageal echocardiographically facilitated early cardioversion from atrial fibrillation using short-term anticoagulation: Final results of a prospective 4.5-year study. *J Am Coll Cardiol* 1995; *25*: 1354–1361.
81. Laupacis A, Albers G, Dalen J et al. Antithrombotic therapy in atrial fibrillation. *Chest* 1998; *114*: 579S–589S.
82. Black IW, Fatkin D, Sagar KB et al. Exclusion of atrial thrombus by transesophageal echocardiography does not preclude embolism after cardioversion of atrial fibrillation: A multicenter study. *Circulation* 1994; *89*: 2509–2513.
83. Klein AL, Grimm RA, Murray RD et al. Use of transesophageal echocardiography to guide cardioversion in patients with atrial fibrillation. *N Engl J Med* 2001; *344*: 1411–1420.
84. Coplen SE, Antmann EM, Berlin JA et al. Efficacy and safety of quinidine therapy for maintenance of sinus rhythm after cardioversion: A meta-analysis of randomized control trials. *Circulation* 1990; *82*: 1106–1116.
85. Juul-Moller S, Edvardsson N, Rehnqvist-Ahlberg N. Sotalol versus quinidine for the maintenance of sinus rhythm after direct current conversion of atrial fibrillation. *Circulation* 1990; *82*: 1932–1939.
86. Reimold SC, Cantillon CO, Friedman PL et al. Propafenone versus sotalol for suppression of recurrent symptomatic atrial fibrillation. *Am J Cardiol* 1993; *71*: 558–563.
87. Roy D, Talajic M, Dorian P et al. Amiodarone to prevent recurrence of atrial fibrillation. *N Engl J Med* 2000; *342*: 913–920.
88. Kuhlkamp V, Schirdewan A, Stangl K et al. Use of metoprolol CR/XL to maintain sinus rhythm after conversion from persistent atrial fibrillation. A randomized, double-blind, placebo-controlled study. *J Am Coll Cardiol* 2000; *36*: 139–146.
89. Flaker GC, Blackshear JL, McBride R et al. Antiarrhythmic drug therapy and cardiac mortality in atrial fibrillation. *J Am Coll Cardiol* 1992; *20*: 527–532.
90. Teo KK, Yusuf S, Furberg CD. Effects of prophylactic antiarrhythmic drug therapy in acute myocardial infarction: An overview of results from randomized controlled trials. *JAMA* 1993; *270*: 1589–1595.
91. Greene HL, CASCADE Investigators. The CASCADE study: Randomized antiarrhythmic drug therapy in survivors of cardiac arrest in Seattle. *Am J Cardiol* 1993; *72*: 70F–74F.
92. Herre J, Sauve M, Malone P et al. Long-term results of amiodarone therapy in patients with recurrent sustained ventricular tachycardia or ventricular fibrillation. *J Am Coll Cardiol* 1989; *13*: 442–449.
93. The Atrial Fibrillation Follow-Up Investigation of Rhythm Management (AFFIRM) Investigators. A comparison of rate control and rhythm control in patients with atrial fibrillation. *N Engl J Med* 2002; *347*: 1825–1833.
94. Atrial Fibrillation Investigators. Risk factors for stroke and efficacy of antithrombotic therapy in atrial fibrillation. Analysis of pooled data from five randomized controlled trials. *Arch Intern Med* 1994; *154*: 1449–1457.
95. Stroke Prevention in Atrial Fibrillation Investigators. Predictors of thromboembolism in atrial fibrillation: II. Echocardiographic features of patients at risk. *Ann Intern Med* 1992; *116*: 6–12.
96. Aronow WS, Ahn C, Kronzon I et al. Effect of warfarin versus aspirin on the incidence of new thromboembolic stroke in older persons with chronic atrial fibrillation and abnormal and normal left ventricular ejection fraction. *Am J Cardiol* 2000; *85*: 1033–1035.
97. Aronow WS, Ahn C, Kronzon I et al. Association of mitral annular calcium with new thromboembolic

stroke at 44-month follow-up of 2,148 persons, mean age 81 years. *Am J Cardiol* 1998; *81*: 105–106.

98. Peterson P, Kastrup J, Helweg-Larsen S et al. Risk factors for thromboembolic complications in chronic atrial fibrillation. *Arch Intern Med* 1990; *150*: 819–821.
99. Lip GYH, Nieuwlaat R, Pisters R et al. Refining clinical risk stratification for predicting stroke and thromboembolism in atrial fibrillation using a novel risk factor-based approach. The Euro Heart Survey on Atrial Fibrillation. *Chest* 2010; *137*: 263–272.
100. Mason PK, Lake DE, DiMarco JP et al. Impact of the CHA2DS2-VASc score on anticoagulation recommendations for atrial fibrillation. *Am J Med* 2012; *125(6)*: 603.e1–603.e6.
101. Ezekowitz MD, Bridgers SL, James KE et al. Warfarin in the prevention of stroke associated with nonrheumatic atrial fibrillation. *N Engl J Med* 1992; *327*: 1406–1412.
102. The SPAF III Writing Committee for the Stroke Prevention in Atrial Fibrillation Investigators. Patients with nonvalvular atrial fibrillation at low risk of stroke during treatment with aspirin. Stroke prevention in atrial fibrillation III study. *JAMA* 1998; *279*: 1273–1277.
103. Hylek EM, Go AS, Chang Y et al. Effect of intensity of oral anticoagulation on stroke severity and mortality in atrial fibrillation. *N Engl J Med* 2003; *349*: 1019–1026.
104. Fang MC, Chang Y, Hylek EM et al. Advanced age, anticoagulation intensity, and risk for intracranial hemorrhage among patients taking warfarin for atrial fibrillation. *Ann Intern Med* 2004; *141*: 745–752.
105. Mant J, Hobbs R, Fletcher K et al. Warfarin versus aspirin for stroke prevention in an elderly community population with atrial fibrillation (the Birmingham Atrial Fibrillation Treatment of the Aged Study, BAFTA): A randomised controlled trial. *Lancet* 2007; *370*: 493–503.
106. Nair CK, Holmberg MJ, Aronow WS et al. Thromboembolism in patients with atrial fibrillation with and without left atrial thrombus documented by transesophageal echocardiography. *Am J Ther* 2009; *16*: 385–392.
107. Lai HM, Aronow WS, Kalen P et al. Incidence of thromboembolic stroke and of major bleeding in patients with atrial fibrillation and chronic kidney disease treated with and without warfarin. *Int J Nephrol Renovasc Dis* 2009; *2*: 33–37.
108. Fuster V, Ryden LE, Cannom DS et al. ACCF/AHA/HRS focused updates incorporated into the ACC/AHA/ESC 2006 guidelines for the management of patients with atrial fibrillation. A report of the American College of Cardiology Foundation/American Heart Association Task Force on Practice Guidelines and the European Society of Cardiology Committee for Practice Guidelines. Developed in partnership with the European Society of Cardiology and in collaboration with the European Heart Rhythm Association and the Heart Rhythm Society. *J Am Coll Cardiol* 2011; *57*: e101–e198.
109. Jahangir A, Lee V, Friedman PA et al. Long-term progression and outcomes with aging in patients with lone atrial fibrillation. A 30-year follow-up study. *Circulation* 2007; *115*: 3050–3056.
110. Gage BF, Boechler M, Doggette AL et al. Adverse outcomes and predictors of underuse of antithrombotic therapy in Medicare beneficiaries with chronic atrial fibrillation. *Stroke* 2000; *31*: 822–827.
111. Fang MC, Singer DE, Chang Y et al. Gender differences in the risk of ischemic stroke and peripheral embolism in atrial fibrillation. The Anticoagulation and Risk Factors in Atrial Fibrillation (ATRIA) study. *Circulation* 2005; *112*: 1687–1691.
112. Healey JS, Connolly SJ, Gold MR et al. Subclinical atrial fibrillation and the risk of stroke. *N Engl J Med* 2012; *366*: 120–129.
113. Kirchhof P, Toennis T, Goette A, Camm J, Diener HC, Becher N, Bertaglia E, Lundqvist CB, Borlich M, Brandes A, Cabanelas N, Calvert M, Chlouverakis G, Gheorghe-Andrei D, Groot J, Dichtl W, Kravchuk B, Lubiński A, Marijon E, Merkely B, Mont L, Ozga, Rajappan K, Sarkozy A, Scherr D, Sznajder R, Velchev V, Wichterle D, Sehner, Simantirakis E, Lip G, Vardas P, Schotten U, Zapf A. Anticoagulation with edoxaban in patients with atrial high-rate episodes. *N Engl J Med* 2023 Sept 28; *389*(13): 1167–1179.
114. Healey JS, Lopes RD, Granger CB, Alings M, Rivard L, McIntyre WF, Atar D, Birnie DH, Boriani G, Camm AJ, Conen D, Erath JW, Gold MR, Hohnloser SH, Ip J, Kautzner J, Kutyifa V, Linde C, Mabo P, Mairesse G, Benezet Mazuecos J, Cosedis Nielsen J, Philippon F, Proietti M, Sticherling C, Wong JA, Wright DJ, Zarraga IG, Coutts SB, Kaplan A, Pombo M, Ayala-Paredes F, Xu L, Simek K, Nevills S, Mian R, Connolly SJ; ARTESIA Investigators. Apixaban for stroke prevention in subclinical atrial fibrillation. *N Engl J Med* 2024 Jan 11; *390*(2): 107–117.
115. Connolly SJ, Ezekowitz MD, Yusuf S et al. Dabigatran versus warfarin in patients with atrial fibrillation. *N Engl J Med* 2009; *361*: 1139–1151.
116. Beasley BN, Unger EF, Temple R. Anticoagulant options-why the FDA approved a higher but not a lower dose of dabigatran. *N Engl J Med* 2011; *364*: 1788–1790.
117. Glund S, Moschetti V, Norris S et al. A randomised study in healthy volunteers to investigate the safety,

tolerability and pharmacokinetics of idarucizumab, a specific antidote to dabigatran. *Thromb Haemost* 2015; *113*: 943–951.
118. Patel MR, Mahaffey KW, Garg J et al. Rivaroxaban versus warfarin in nonvalvular atrial fibrillation. *N Engl J Med 2011*; *365*: 883–891.
119. Connolly SJ, Eikelboom J, Joyner C et al. Apixaban in patients with atrial fibrillation. *N Engl J Med* 2011; *364*: 806–817.
120. Granger CB, Alexander JH, McMurray JJV et al. Apixaban versus warfarin in patients with atrial fibrillation. *N Engl J Med* 2011; *365*: 981–992.
121. Giugliano RP, Ruff CT, Braunwald E et al. Edoxaban versus warfarin in patients with atrial fibrillation. *N Engl J Med* 2013; *369*: 2093–2104.
122. Milling TJ Jr, Middeldorp S, Xu L, Koch B, Demchuk A, Eikelboom JW, Verhamme P, Cohen AT, Beyer-Westendorf J, Gibson CM, Lopez-Sendon J, Crowther M, Shoamanesh A, Coppens M, Schmidt J, Albaladejo P, Connolly SJ; ANNEXA-4 Investigators. Final study report of andexanet alfa for major bleeding with factor Xa inhibitors. *Circulation* 2023 Mar 28; *147*(13): 1026–1038.
123. Grandhi R, Newman WC, Zhang X et al. Administration of 4-factor prothrombin complex concentrate as an antidote for intracranial bleeding in patients taking direct factor Xa inhibitors. *World Neurosurg* 2015; *84*: 1956–1961.
124. Best JG, Arram L, Ahmed N, Balogun M, Bennett K, Bordea E, Campos MG, Caverly E, Chau M, Cohen H, Dehbi HM, Doré CJ, Engelter ST, Fenner R, Freemantle N, Hunter R, James M, Lip GY, Murray ML, Norrving B, Sprigg N, Veltkamp R, Zaczyk I, Werring DJ; OPTIMAS investigators. Optimal timing of anticoagulation after acute ischemic stroke with atrial fibrillation (OPTIMAS): Protocol for a randomized controlled trial. *Int J Stroke* 2022 Jun; *17*(5): 583–589.
125. Granada J, Uribe W, Chyou P-H et al. Incidence and predictors of atrial flutter in the general population. *J Am Coll Cardiol* 2000; *36*: 2242–2246.
126. Grimm RA, Stewart WJ, Arheart KL et al. Left atrial appendage "stunning" after electrical cardioversion of atrial flutter: An attenuated response compared with atrial fibrillation as the mechanism for lower susceptibility to thromboembolic events. *J Am Coll Cardiol* 1997; *29*: 582–589.
127. Van Gelder IC, Tuinenburg AE, Schoonderwoerd BS et al. Pharmacologic versus direct-current electrical cardioversion of atrial flutter and fibrillation. *Am J Cardiol* 1999; *84*: 147R–151R.
128. Orlando J, Del Vicario M, Aronow WS. High reversion of atrial flutter to sinus rhythm after atrial pacing in patients with pulmonary disease. *Chest* 1977; *71*: 580–582.
129. Parikh MG, Aziz Z, Krishnan K et al. Usefulness of transesophageal echocardiography to confirm clinical utility of CHA_2DS_2-VASc and $CHADS_2$ scores in atrial flutter. *Am J Cardiol* 2012; *109*: 550–555.
130. Lanzarotti CJ, Olshansky B. Thromboembolism in chronic atrial flutter: Is the risk underestimated? *J Am Coll Cardiol* 1997; *30*: 1506–1511.
131. Saxon LA, Kalman JM, Olgin JE et al. Results of radiofrequency catheter ablation for atrial flutter. *Am J Cardiol* 1996; *77*: 1014–1016.
132. Poty H, Saoudi N, Aziz AA et al. Radiofrequency of catheter ablation of type 1 atrial flutter: Prediction of late success by electrophysiological criteria. *Circulation* 1995; *92*: 1389–1392.
133. Voight J, Akkaya M, Somasundaram P et al. Risk of new-onset atrial fibrillation and stroke after radiofrequency ablation of isolated, typical atrial flutter. *Heart Rhythm* 2014; *11*: 1884–1889.
134. Akhtar M, Jazayeri MR, Sra J et al. Atrioventricular nodal reentry: Clinical, electrophysiological, and therapeutic considerations. *Circulation* 1993; *88*: 282–295.
135. Josephson ME. Paroxysmal supraventricular tachycardia. An electrophysiologic approach. *Am J Cardiol* 1978; *41*: 1123–1126.
136. Stein KM, Mittal S, Slotwiner DJ et al. Atrial tachycardia: Update. *Cardiac Electrophysiol Rev* 2001; *5*: 290–293.
137. Aronow WS. Management of supraventricular tachyarrhythmias. *Compr Ther* 1989; *15*: 11–16.
138. Ganz LI, Friedman PL. Supraventricular tachycardia. *N Engl J Med* 1995; *332*: 162–173.
139. Epstein LM, Chiesa N, Wong MN et al. Radiofrequency catheter ablation in the treatment of supraventricular tachycardia in the elderly. *J Am Coll Cardiol* 1994; *23*: 1356–1362.
140. Rosen KM. Junctional tachycardia: Mechanisms, diagnosis, differential diagnosis, and management. *Circulation* 1973; *47*: 654–664.
141. Hazard PB, Burnett CR. Verapamil in multifocal atrial tachycardia. Hemodynamic and respiratory changes. *Chest* 1987; *91*: 68–70.

22

Ventricular arrhythmias in older persons

JASON T. JACOBSON, SEI IWAI, WILBERT S. ARONOW, AND MAHMOUD SAMY AHMED

Key points

- Effective risk stratification in patients with structural heart disease, such as ischemic or nonischemic cardiomyopathy, requires an integrated approach utilizing clinical assessment, imaging modalities, and electrophysiologic procedures to guide therapies such as ICD implantation and pharmacologic or interventional treatment.
- Beta-blockers remain the cornerstone therapy for reducing mortality and the burden of ventricular arrhythmias in patients with ICDs. Studies demonstrate that beta-blockers effectively decrease ICD shocks and improve survival compared to other antiarrhythmic drug therapies. The role of amiodarone and sotalol should be reserved for selected patients, with careful monitoring for potential side effects.
- GDMT is critical in managing patients with HFrEF and associated arrhythmic complications. ACE inhibitors, ARBs, ARNIs, SGLT2 inhibitors, and MRAs not only improve survival and reduce heart failure hospitalizations but also confer significant antiarrhythmic benefits. These agents improve cardiac remodeling, suppress neurohormonal activation, and may stabilize cardiac electrophysiology, reducing the risk of malignant ventricular arrhythmias and sudden cardiac death.
- Catheter ablation has evolved as an important treatment strategy for ventricular tachycardia in structurally abnormal hearts. Ablation of low-voltage areas and zones of slow conduction provides long-term success in arrhythmia control. This approach is most effective when integrated with comprehensive imaging, substrate mapping techniques, both endocardially and epicardially.

PREVALENCE OF COMPLEX VENTRICULAR ARRHYTHMIAS

The prevalence of nonsustained ventricular tachycardia (VT) detected by 24-hour ambulatory electrocardiograms (AECGs) was 4% in 98 older, disease-free persons in the Baltimore Longitudinal Study of Aging (1); 2% in 50 older persons without cardiovascular disease (3); 4% in 729 older women and 13% in 643 older men in the Cardiovascular Health Study (4); 3% in 135 older men and 2% in 297 older women without cardiovascular disease (5); 9% in 385 older men and 8% in 806 older women with hypertension, valvular disease, or cardiomyopathy (5); and 16% in 395 older men and 15% in 771 older women with coronary artery disease (CAD) (5). The prevalence of complex ventricular arrhythmia (VA) in older persons in these studies was 50% (1), 20% (3), 16% in women and 28% in men (4); 31% in older men and 30% in older

DOI: 10.1201/9781003568933-22

women without cardiovascular disease (5); 54% in older men and 55% in older women with hypertension, valvular disease, or cardiomyopathy (5); and 69% in older men and 68% in older women with CAD (5).

In older persons with cardiovascular disease, those with an abnormal left ventricular (LV) ejection fraction (6), with echocardiographic LV hypertrophy (7), or with asymptomatic myocardial ischemia (8) have a higher prevalence of VT and of complex VA than those with normal LV ejection fraction, normal LV mass, and no myocardial ischemia.

PROGNOSIS OF VENTRICULAR ARRHYTHMIAS

Idiopathic

Ventricular ectopy and tachycardia in the absence of structural heart disease are classified as idiopathic. For the most part, this type of VT is not associated with increased mortality. In the Baltimore Longitudinal Study of Aging, nonsustained VT or complex VA were not associated with an increased incidence of new coronary events at 10-year follow-up in 98 older subjects with no clinical evidence of heart disease (9). In addition, in this study, exercise-induced nonsustained VT was not associated with an increased incidence of new coronary events at 2-year follow-up in older persons with no clinical evidence of heart disease (10). And at 5.6-year follow-up in this study, exercise-induced frequent or repetitive ventricular premature complexes (VPCs) also were not associated with an increased incidence of new coronary events in older persons with no clinical evidence of heart disease (11).

Nonsustained VT or complex VA diagnosed by 24-hour AECGs were not associated with an increased incidence of new coronary events or primary ventricular fibrillation (VF)/sudden cardiac death in multiple studies involving older individuals without clinical evidence of heart disease. Specifically, no significant correlation was found in cohorts of 76 and 86 patients over a 2-year follow-up (12, 13), in 135 men over 45 months, and in 297 women over 47 months (5). These findings suggest that asymptomatic nonsustained VT or complex VA in elderly individuals without heart disease may not warrant antiarrhythmic treatment.

Because simple and complex VAs as well as nonsustained VT are not associated with an increased incidence of new coronary events in older persons with no evidence of structural heart disease, asymptomatic episodes in older patients without structural heart disease should not be treated with antiarrhythmic drugs (5, 9, 12, 13).

Treatment

Since idiopathic VAs are not associated with sudden cardiac death (SCD), pharmacologic management is often first-line therapy in those with symptoms or with (or at risk for) VA-induced cardiomyopathy. Given the mechanism of triggered activity for most idiopathic VA, the first option for medical therapy would be either beta-blockade (BB) or the use of a non-dihydropyridine calcium channel blocker (CCB). In a retrospective analysis of ventricular premature beat (VPB) management, Zhong et al. found that BB decreased VPB burden by 36% and CCB by 43% (14). Of interest, in a randomized placebo-controlled trial of 52 patients, both atenolol (50 mg if resting heart rate <70, 100 mg if >70) and placebo improved symptom frequency and quality of life, yet only atenolol decreased VPB frequency by an average of 33%, $P = 0.19$, while only 24% showed at least 80% decrease in VPB burden in the placebo group (15). In many patients, symptom control may be enough, however, a true reduction in VPB burden is required to reverse premature ventricular contraction-induced cardiomyopathy.

Antiarrhythmic drugs (AADs) that act directly on the ion channels subtending the cardiac action potential (Vaughan-Williams Class I and III) do offer superior control over BB and CCB; Zhong et al. found an 82% reduction in VPBs with these medications, compared with the lower rates with BB and CCB mentioned in the previous paragraph (14), specifically, Class III AAD (amiodarone 84%, sotalol 70%) and Class Ib (mexiletine 89%) and Ic (flecainide 83%, propafenone 73%). Stec and colleagues compared propafenone, verapamil, and metoprolol in an open-label prospective crossover study in 84 patients. Efficacy was defined as a ≥90% decrease in VPB burden on follow-up Holter compared with baseline. Patients were randomized as to the order in which the drugs were given, and each drug was given for a 2-week period at a stable dose with a washout period of 5 half-lives in between drug trials. Starting doses were 50 mg slow-release metoprolol daily, 120 mg slow-release verapamil daily, and 150 mg propafenone three times per day. Dosage was adjusted based on heart rate and tolerance. The mean daily dosages achieved were 67 ± 24 mg metoprolol, 171 ± 73 mg verapamil, and 704 ± 113 mg propafenone. Propafenone showed efficacy in 42%, verapamil in 15%, and metoprolol in 10% ($P < 0.01$) (16), and 51%, 24%, and 14%, respectively, achieved at least 80% decrease in burden. Proarrhythmia (>twofold increase in burden, development of nonsustained VT, sustained VT, or torsades de pointes) was seen in two patients on propafenone and one on metoprolol. Side effects causing drug discontinuation during the 2-week assessment period were seen in 21% of subjects on metoprolol, 17% on propafenone, and 15% on verapamil (16). This study suffers from a lack of a control group, which makes it difficult to rule out the natural variation in arrhythmia frequency over time that may occur. Additionally, all patients were offered ablation at the end of the study period, 60% of whom elected to take this path, so long-term efficacy is difficult to assess (although the short-term efficacy is modest at best).

Regarding VT, Gill et al. tested flecainide, sotalol, and verapamil in a serial drug study in 23 patients with sustained (10 patients) and nonsustained (13 patients) VT from the right ventricular outflow tract (RVOT) (17). Dosages were as follows: verapamil 120 mg TID, sotalol 120 mg BID (160 mg if patient weight >80 kg), and flecainide 100 mg BID (150 mg BID if weight >80 kg). Drugs were continued for a minimum of 5 half-lives for effect and then discontinued for 5 half-lives between drug trials. Efficacy was evaluated with a 24-hour Holter monitor, exercise testing, and programmed ventricular stimulation (PVS), and compared to drug-free results of these tests. While no statistically significant difference was found between these agents in efficacy, sotalol was the numerically superior drug. Episodes of VT (defined as ≥5 consecutive beats) on Holter decreased by >90% in 48% of subjects on flecainide and sotalol and 43% on verapamil. Compared with a baseline of 14 subjects inducible at exercise testing, flecainide decreased this number to 4 subjects, sotalol to 2, and verapamil to 5. With PVS, 17 subjects were inducible at baseline, while flecainide decreased this number to 4, sotalol to 2, and verapamil to 6. Some proarrhythmia was seen with all three drugs, defined as a 150% increase in hourly VT episodes (1 flecainide, 1 sotalol, 2 verapamil), VT on exercise testing when not seen at baseline (2 flecainide, 1 sotalol, 3 verapamil), and sustained VT with PVS when only nonsustained VT seen at baseline (2 flecainide, 1 sotalol, 3 verapamil) (17). Similar to the Stec study (16) discussed in the previous paragraph, this study suffers from both an absence of a control group and an inability to determine long-term efficacy. While the noninducibility rates at exercise testing and PVS are encouraging, the Holter results were modest at best.

Regarding fascicular VT, verapamil sensitivity has been a defining feature of this arrhythmia since its first description (18, 19). Verapamil exerts its effect on the Purkinje fibers of the slow conduction zone of the VT circuit and has a high success rate of acute termination (20). That said, the long-term recurrence with chronic oral CCB is 21%–28% (21). Other agents may be used when CCB fail, such as BB or Class I/III AAD, but little data exist for these drugs as applied to fascicular VT (22).

The dearth of trials evaluating medical therapy for idiopathic VA is an effect of the nonpharmacologic options for treating these arrhythmias, as well as the concern for side effects of chronic AAD, including proarrhythmia. Catheter ablation has proven quite successful in long-term prevention of recurrent idiopathic VPBs and VT, superior to that of medical therapy (14, 23).

STRUCTURAL HEART DISEASE

Numerous studies have documented that patients with VT or with complex VA associated with heart disease are at increased risk for developing new coronary events (24). Prospective studies in older persons, mean age 82 years, with heart disease also demonstrated that nonsustained VT and complex VA were significantly associated with an increased incidence of new coronary events and with an increased incidence of primary VF or sudden cardiac death (5, 9, 12, 13).

MEDICAL THERAPY

General measures

Underlying causes of complex VA should be treated, if possible. Guideline-directed medical therapy (GDMT) optimization for patients with congestive heart failure (CHF), reversal of digitalis toxicity, hypokalemia, hypomagnesemia, hypertension, myocardial ischemia by anti-ischemic drugs such as beta-blockers or by coronary revascularization, hypoxia, and other conditions may abolish or reduce complex VA. Smoking cessation and alcohol discontinuation as well as avoiding illicit drugs may improve complex VAs.

All older persons with CAD should be treated with aspirin or another antiplatelet agent (25), beta-blockers (25), and statins (25) unless there are contraindications to these drugs. The serum low-density lipoprotein (LDL) cholesterol level should be reduced to <70 mg/dl (25).

Age-related physiologic changes may affect the absorption, distribution, metabolism, and excretion of cardiovascular drugs. There are numerous physiologic changes with aging that affect pharmacodynamics with alterations in end-organ responsiveness to cardiovascular drugs. Drug interactions between antiarrhythmic drugs and other cardiovascular drugs are common, especially in older persons. There are also important drug-disease interactions that occur in older persons (26). Class Ic antiarrhythmic drugs have an unacceptable proarrhythmia rate in patients with ischemic heart disease and should be avoided. Class III antiarrhythmic drugs should also be used with caution in older patients with heart disease since multiple factors may increase the incidence of proarrhythmia. Except for beta-blockers, all antiarrhythmic drugs may cause torsades de pointes (VT with polymorphic appearance associated with prolonged QT interval).

Class I antiarrhythmic drugs

Class I antiarrhythmic drugs are sodium channel blockers. Class Ia antiarrhythmic drugs have intermediate channel kinetics and prolong repolarization. These drugs include quinidine, procainamide, and disopyramide. Class Ib antiarrhythmic drugs have rapid channel kinetics and slightly shorten repolarization. These drugs include lidocaine and mexiletine. Class Ic drugs have slow channel kinetics and have little effect on repolarization. Available Ic drugs include flecainide and propafenone. None of the Class I antiarrhythmic drugs has been demonstrated in controlled, clinical trials to reduce sudden cardiac death, total cardiac death, or total mortality.

The International Mexiletine and Placebo Antiarrhythmic Coronary Trial (IMPACT) was a prospective, double-blind, randomized study in survivors of myocardial infarction (MI), mean age 57 years, in whom 317 persons were randomized to mexiletine and 313 persons to placebo. Complex VA were present on 24-hour AECGs at study entry in 31% of persons randomized to mexiletine and in 38% of persons randomized to placebo. At 1-year follow-up, mortality was 7.6% for mexiletine-treated patients versus 4.8% for placebo-treated patients (27).

The Cardiac Arrhythmia Suppression Trial (CAST) I was a prospective, double-blind, randomized study in survivors of MI with asymptomatic or mildly symptomatic VA in which 730 patients were randomized to Class Ic agents encainide or flecainide and 725 patients to placebo (28). The prevalence of nonsustained VT was 21%. Mean LV ejection fraction (LVEF) was 40%. Thirty-eight percent of patients were 66–79 years of age. Adequate suppression of VA by encainide or flecainide was required before randomization. Despite adequate suppression of VA, at 10-month follow-up, encainide and flecainide significantly increased mortality from arrhythmia or cardiac arrest (relative risk = 3.6; 95% CI 1.7–8.5) and significantly increased total mortality (relative risk = 2.5; 95% CI 1.6–4.5) (28). Older age increased the likelihood of adverse events, including death, in patients receiving encainide and flecainide (29).

CAST II was a prospective, double-blind, randomized study in survivors of MI with asymptomatic or mildly symptomatic VA in which 581 patients were randomized to Ic agent moricizine and 574 patients to placebo (30). The prevalence of nonsustained VT was 30%. Mean LVEF was 33%. Thirty-eight percent of patients were 66–79 years of age. Adequate suppression of VA by moricizine was required before randomization. At 18-month follow-up, the mortality from arrhythmia or cardiac arrest was 8.4% for patients treated with moricizine and 7.3% for patients treated with placebo. The 2-year survival rate was 81.7% for patients treated with moricizine and 85.6% for patients treated with placebo. The investigators concluded that the use of moricizine in this study was "not only ineffective but also harmful" (30). Older age increased the likelihood of adverse events, including death, in patients receiving moricizine (29).

An analysis of the CAST I and II studies showed that older age was an independent predictor of adverse events (relative risk 1.30 per decade of age) (29). On the basis of the CAST I and CAST II data, use of Ic agents is avoided for the treatment of VT or complex VA in older or younger patients with heart disease, especially prior MI or unrevascularized CAD.

Aronow et al. studied the effect of quinidine or procainamide versus no antiarrhythmic drug on sudden cardiac death, total cardiac death, and total death in elderly patients with heart disease and complex VA, in a prospective study in 406 older persons, mean age 82 years, with heart disease (58% with prior MI) and asymptomatic complex VA diagnosed by 24-hour AECGs. The prevalence of nonsustained VT was 20%. The prevalence of an abnormal ejection fraction was 32%. The incidence of adverse effects causing cessation of drug was 48% for quinidine and 55% for procainamide. Of 406 older persons, 220 were treated with quinidine ($n = 213$) or procainamide ($n = 7$) and 186 with no antiarrhythmic drug. Follow-up 24-hour AECGs in 25 persons with nonsustained VT and in 104 persons with complex VA showed that quinidine or procainamide decreased nonsustained VT more than 90% in 84% of the persons and decreased the average number of VPCs/hour more than 70% in 84% of the persons (31). At 24-month follow-up, the incidences of sudden cardiac death, total cardiac death, and total death were not significantly different in persons treated with quinidine or procainamide or with no antiarrhythmic drug (31). The incidence of total mortality was 65% for persons treated with quinidine or procainamide and 63% for persons treated with no antiarrhythmic drug. Quinidine or procainamide did not decrease sudden cardiac death, total cardiac death, or total death in comparison with no antiarrhythmic drug in older patients with ischemic or nonischemic heart disease, abnormal or normal LVEF, and presence versus absence of VT (31).

Moosvi et al. (63) performed a retrospective analysis of the effect of empiric antiarrhythmic therapy in 209 resuscitated out-of-hospital cardiac arrest patients, mean age 62 years, with CAD. Of the 209 patients, 48 received quinidine, 45 received procainamide, and 116 received no antiarrhythmic drug. The 2-year sudden death survival was 69% for quinidine-treated patients, 69% for procainamide-treated patients, and 89% for patients treated with no antiarrhythmic drug ($p < 0.01$). The 2-year total survival was 61% for quinidine-treated patients, 57% for procainamide-treated patients, and 71% for patients treated with no antiarrhythmic drug ($p < 0.05$) (32).

Hallstrom et al. performed a retrospective analysis of the effect of antiarrhythmic drug use in 941 patients, mean age 62 years, resuscitated from prehospital cardiac arrest attributable to VF between 1970 and 1985. Quinidine was administered to 19% of the patients, procainamide to 18% of the patients, beta-blockers to 28% of the patients, and no antiarrhythmic drug to 39% of the patients. There was an increased incidence of death or recurrent cardiac arrest in patients treated with quinidine or procainamide versus no antiarrhythmic drug (adjusted relative risk = 1.17; 95% CI 0.98–1.41). Survival was significantly worse for patients treated with procainamide than for patients treated with quinidine (adjusted relative risk = 1.57; 95% CI 1.21–2.07) (33).

Morganroth and Goin performed a meta-analysis of four randomized, double-blind controlled trials lasting 2–12 weeks in which quinidine ($n = 502$) was compared with flecainide ($n = 141$), mexiletine ($n = 246$), tocainide ($n = 67$), and propafenone ($n = 53$) in the treatment of complex VA. There was an increased risk of mortality in patients treated with quinidine compared with patients treated with the other antiarrhythmic drugs (absolute risk increase = 1.6%; 95% CI 0–3.1%) (34).

Teo et al. analyzed 59 randomized controlled trials comprising 23,229 patients that investigated the use of Class I antiarrhythmic drugs after MI. The Class I drugs investigated included quinidine, procainamide, disopyramide, imipramine, moricizine, lidocaine, tocainide, phenytoin, mexiletine, aprindine, encainide, and flecainide. Mortality was significantly higher in patients receiving Class I antiarrhythmic drugs than in patients receiving no antiarrhythmic drugs (odds ratio = 1.14; 95% CI 1.01–1.28). None of the 59 studies demonstrated that the use of a Class I antiarrhythmic drug decreased mortality in postinfarction patients (35).

On the basis of the data from the studies discussed in this section, none of the Class I antiarrhythmic drugs should be used for the treatment of VT or complex VA in older or younger patients with heart disease in the absence of an implantable cardioverter-defibrillator (ICD).

Calcium channel blockers

Calcium channel blockers are not useful in the treatment of complex VA. Although verapamil and diltiazem can terminate a left septal fascicular VT, hemodynamic collapse can occur if intravenous verapamil is administered to patients with the more common forms of reentry VT. Teo et al. analyzed randomized controlled trials comprising 20,342 patients that investigated the use of calcium channel blockers after MI. Mortality was insignificantly higher in patients receiving calcium channel blockers than in patients receiving no antiarrhythmic drugs (odds ratio = 1.04; 95% CI 0.95–1.14) (35). On the basis of these data, none of the calcium channel blockers should be used in the treatment of VT or complex VA in older or younger patients with heart disease.

Beta-blockers

Teo et al. analyzed 55 randomized controlled trials comprising 53,268 patients that investigated the use of beta-blockers after MI. Mortality was significantly reduced in patients receiving beta-blockers compared with control patients (odds ratio = 0.81; 95% CI 0.75–0.87) (35).

Beta-blockers caused a greater reduction in mortality in older persons after MI than in younger persons after MI. The decrease in mortality after MI in persons treated with beta blockers was due to both a reduction in sudden cardiac death and recurrent MI (36–38).

The Beta-Blocker Heart Attack Trial was a double-blind, randomized study that included 3290 patients after MI. Thirty-three percent of the patients were 60–69 years of age. At 25-month follow-up, propranolol decreased sudden cardiac death by 28% in patients with complex VA and by 16% in patients without complex VA. Propranolol significantly reduced total mortality by 34% in patients aged 60–69 years (p = 0.01) and insignificantly reduced total mortality by 19% in patients aged 30–59 years (38, 39).

In the retrospective study by Hallstrom et al. in 941 patients, mean age 62 years, resuscitated from prehospital cardiac arrest attributed to VF, beta-blockers were administered to 28% of the patients and no antiarrhythmic drug to 39% of the patients. At 108-month follow-up, patients treated with beta-blockers had a significant decreased incidence of death or recurrent cardiac arrest compared to patients treated with no antiarrhythmic drug (adjusted relative risk = 0.62; 95% CI 0.50–0.77) (33).

In a retrospective analysis of the data from the CAST study, Kennedy et al. found that 30% of patients with a LVEF <40% were receiving beta-blockers. Forty percent of the patients were between 66 and 79 years of age. Patients on beta-blockers had a significant decrease in all-cause mortality of 43% at 30 days (p = 0.03), of 46% at 1 year (p = 0.001), and of 33% at 2 years (p < 0.001) (40). Patients receiving beta-blockers had a significant reduction in arrhythmic death or cardiac arrest of 66% at 30 days (p = 0.002), of 53% at 1 year (p = 0.001), and of 36% at 2 years (p = 0.001). Multivariate analysis showed that beta-blockers were an independent factor for decreasing arrhythmic death or cardiac arrest by 40% (95% CI 0.36–0.99), for reducing all-cause mortality by 33% (p = 0.05), and for decreasing the occurrence of new or worsened CHF by 32% (95% CI 0.49–0.94) (40).

A meta-analysis of ten randomized trials showed that the use of beta-blockers significantly reduced 2-year mortality in patients receiving ICD therapy (p < 0.01) (41).

CLASS III ANTIARRHYTHMIC DRUGS

Class III antiarrhythmic drugs are potassium channel blockers that prolong repolarization manifested by an increase in QT interval on the ECG. These drugs suppress VA by increasing the refractory period. However, prolonging cardiac repolarization and the refractory period can trigger after depolarizations and resultant torsade de pointes.

In the Survival With Oral d-Sotalol (SWORD) trial, 3121 survivors of MI, mean age 60 years, with a LVEF <40% were randomized to d-sotalol, a pure potassium channel blocker with no beta-blocking activity, or to a double-blind placebo (Table 22.1). At 148-day follow-up, mortality was 5.0% in patients treated with d-sotalol versus 3.1% in patients treated with placebo (relative risk = 1.65; 95% CI 1.15–2.36). Presumed arrhythmic deaths accounted for the increased mortality (relative risk = 1.77; 95% CI 1.15–2.74) (42).

In a study of 1486 patients with prior MI, compared with placebo, sotalol did not significantly reduce mortality in patients followed for 1 year (Table 22.1) (43).

In the Electrophysiologic Study versus Electrocardiographic Monitoring (ESVEM) study, 74% of 486 patients were >60 years of age (94). In this study, Holter monitor-guided therapy significantly predicted antiarrhythmic drug efficacy more often than did the electrophysiologic study in patients with sustained VT or survivors of

Table 22.1 Effect of Class III antiarrhythmic drugs on mortality in patients with heart disease and complex ventricular arrhythmias

Study	Results
Waldo et al. (42)	At 148-day follow-up, mortality was 5.0% for d-sotalol versus 3.1% for placebo (relative risk = 1.65; 95% CI 1.15–2.36).
Julian et al. (43)	At 1-year follow-up, compared with placebo, d,l-sotalol caused an insignificant reduction in mortality.
Singh et al. (44)	Compared with placebo, amiodarone significantly suppressed VT and complex VA ($p < 0.001$); 2-year survival was not significantly different for amiodarone (69.4%) versus placebo (70.8%).
Canadian Amiodarone Myocardial Infarction Arrhythmia Trial (45)	Amiodarone was very effective in suppressing VT and complex VA; at 1.8-year follow-up, compared with placebo, amiodarone caused an 18% insignificant reduction in mortality.
European Myocardial Infarct Amiodarone Trial (46)	At 21-month follow-up, mortality was similar for amiodarone (13.9%) versus placebo (13.7%).
Sudden Cardiac Death in Heart Failure Trial (47)	At 45.5-month follow-up, compared with placebo, amiodarone caused a 6% insignificant increase in mortality, and implantable cardioverter-defibrillator therapy reduced mortality by 23% ($p = 0.007$).

Abbreviations: VA, ventricular arrhythmia; VT, ventricular tachycardia.

cardiac arrest (77% vs. 45% of patients). However, there was no significant difference in the success of drug therapy selected by the two methods in preventing recurrences of ventricular tachyarrhythmias.

In the ESVEM study, d,l-sotalol was more effective than the other six antiarrhythmic drugs (imipramine, mexiletine, pirmenol, procainamide, propafenone, and quinidine) used in reducing recurrence of arrhythmia, death from arrhythmia, death from cardiac causes, and death from any cause. However, 7 of 10 episodes of torsade de pointes during this study occurred in patients receiving d,l-sotalol (48).

Amiodarone is very effective in suppressing VT and complex VA associated with heart disease (44, 45, 49). Unfortunately, the incidence of adverse effects from amiodarone approaches 90% after 5 years of therapy (50). In the Cardiac Arrest in Seattle: Conventional Versus Amiodarone Drug Evaluation (CASCADE) study, the incidence of pulmonary toxicity was 10% at 2 years in patients receiving an amiodarone dose of 158 mg/day (49). Amiodarone can also cause other adverse effects including hepatitis, hyperthyroidism, and hypothyroidism, and neurologic, dermatologic, and ophthalmologic adverse effects.

A double-blind study randomized 674 patients with CHF and complex VA to amiodarone or placebo. Compared with placebo, amiodarone significantly reduced the number of episodes of VT ($p < 0.001$) and the frequency of complex VA ($p < 0.001$). Twenty-seven percent of patients discontinued amiodarone in this study. At 2-year follow-up, survival was not significantly different in patients treated with amiodarone (69.4%) or placebo (70.8%) (Table 22.1) (44).

The Canadian Amiodarone Myocardial Infarction Arrhythmia Trial (CAMIAT) randomized 1202 survivors of MI with nonsustained VT or complex VA to amiodarone or placebo (Table 22.1). Amiodarone was very effective in suppressing VT and complex VA in this study. Early permanent discontinuation of amiodarone for reasons other than adverse events occurred in 36% of patients taking this drug. At 1.8-year follow-up, amiodarone caused an 18% insignificant reduction in mortality (45).

The European Myocardial Infarction Amiodarone Trial (EMIAT) randomized 1486 survivors of MI with a LVEF <40% to amiodarone or placebo (Table 22.1). Early permanent discontinuation of amiodarone occurred in 38.5% of patients taking this drug. At 21-month follow-up, mortality was similar in patients treated with amiodarone (13.9%) or with placebo (13.7%) (46).

In the Sudden Cardiac Death in Heart Failure Trial (SCD-HeFT), 2521 patients, mean age 60 years, with New York Heart Association (NYHA) Class II or III CHF due to ischemic or nonischemic heart disease, a LVEF of 35% or less, and a mean QRS duration on the resting ECG of 120 ms were randomized to placebo, amiodarone, or an ICD (Table 22.1). At 45.5-month median follow-up, compared with placebo, amiodarone insignificantly increased mortality by 6%. At 45.5-month median follow-up, compared with placebo, ICD therapy significantly reduced all-cause mortality by 23% ($p = 0.007$), with an absolute reduction in mortality of 7.2% after 5 years (47).

In a study of 965 patients, mean age 70 years, with ICDs, at 32-month mean follow-up, use of beta-blockers significantly reduced all-cause mortality by 46% ($p < 0.001$), whereas use of amiodarone or sotalol did not significantly affect mortality (51).

During 33-month mean follow-up of 1038 patients with ICDs, use of beta-blockers significantly reduced appropriate ICD shocks ($p < 0.001$). Use of amiodarone plus a beta-blocker was not more effective than beta-blocker therapy alone in reducing ICD shocks for any reason. In this study, use of sotalol did not decrease appropriate ICD shocks (52). These studies were not designed to compare the efficacy of AAD and beta-blockers for prevention of ICD therapies, and therefore should be interpreted with caution.

Sotalol has been shown to decrease ICD shocks or death from any cause by 44% compared to placebo in patients with ICD for secondary prevention (53). The OPTIC trial randomized patients receiving ICD shocks for VA to three AAD arms: Amiodarone plus beta-blockers, sotalol, and beta-blockers alone. At one year, the percentage of patients receiving ICD therapy for VA (antitachycardia pacing or shocks) was as follows: Amiodarone plus beta-blockers 13%, followed by sotalol 38.9%, and then beta-blockers alone 45% (54). Of note, the rate of drug discontinuation was 18.2% for amiodarone and 23.5% for sotalol (versus 5.3% for beta-blocker alone), due to side effects (54).

One other Class III AAD has been suggested to decrease ICD therapy for VA: dofetilide. In one brief observational report, 50% of patients had a decrease in ICD therapies after starting treatment with dofetilide (55). Additionally, Baquero et al. found a significant reduction in monthly VT/VF episodes (1.8 ± 4.5/month before vs. 1.0 ± 3.5/month on dofetilide, $p = 0.006$) in 30 patients with ICDs that had failed at least one other AAD (63% amiodarone) (56).

GUIDELINE-DIRECTED MEDICAL THERAPY FOR HEART FAILURE

Heart failure (HF) is highly prevalent among older adults, and its management requires a comprehensive approach using GDMT to improve survival and reduce arrhythmic complications. Older patients with heart failure with reduced ejection fraction (HFrEF) are particularly vulnerable to ventricular arrhythmias. While beta-blockers are Class II AADs and were discussed earlier in this chapter, this section will focus on the role of renin–angiotensin–aldosterone system (RAAS) inhibitors, sodium-glucose cotransporter-2 (SGLT2) inhibitors, and mineralocorticoid receptor antagonists (MRAs) in reducing ventricular arrhythmias in older HF patients. Numerous clinical trials have evaluated the effects of these GDMT agents on heart failure-related mortality, but their impact on ventricular arrhythmias and SCD is often underreported or analyzed in post hoc studies. Next, we review the available landmark trials and their findings regarding the antiarrhythmic benefits of angiotensin-converting enzyme (ACE) inhibitors, angiotensin II receptor blockers (ARBs), angiotensin receptor-neprilysin inhibitors (ARNIs), SGLT2 inhibitors, and MRAs in older adults with CHF.

ACE inhibitors, ARBs, and ARNIs

The CONSENSUS trial evaluated enalapril, an ACE inhibitor, in older patients with severe HF (NYHA class IV, mean age ~71 years). The trial demonstrated a 40% reduction in 12-month mortality compared to placebo, with a significant reduction in SCD. The survival benefit was primarily attributed to improved hemodynamics, neurohormonal modulation, and reduced electrical instability in the failing myocardium. These findings provided early evidence that ACE inhibitors lower the risk of fatal ventricular arrhythmias in severe HF (57).

The SOLVD trial included older patients (mean age ~63 years) with symptomatic and asymptomatic HFrEF and demonstrated that enalapril reduced total mortality by 16.5% ($p = 0.003$), primarily due to fewer SCDs and fatal ventricular arrhythmias. The trial highlighted that ACE inhibitors not only improve survival but also reduce ventricular arrhythmias, likely through favorable LV remodeling, sympathetic inhibition, and reduced myocardial fibrosis (58).

The Val-HeFT trial evaluated valsartan, an ARB, in CHF patients (mean age ~65 years) and demonstrated a post hoc reduction in SCD among patients not on beta-blockers. While all-cause mortality was not significantly reduced, valsartan led to a 13% decrease in HF hospitalizations ($p < 0.001$) and likely contributed to lower ventricular arrhythmic events by reducing myocardial fibrosis and RAAS activation (59).

The PARADIGM-HF (Prospective Comparison of ARNI with ACEI to Determine Impact on Global Mortality and Morbidity in Heart Failure) trial compared sacubitril/valsartan (ARNI) to enalapril in patients with HFrEF (mean age ~64 years) and demonstrated a 20% reduction in cardiovascular mortality and a 21% reduction in HF hospitalizations. Notably, SCD was reduced by 20% ($p < 0.001$), suggesting greater protection against ventricular arrhythmias than ACE inhibitors alone. The mechanisms of antiarrhythmic benefit might include enhanced natriuretic peptide activity, reduced myocardial fibrosis, and suppression of sympathetic drive, all of which stabilize cardiac electrophysiology (60).

SGLT2 inhibitors

The DAPA-HF (Dapagliflozin and Prevention of Adverse Outcomes in Heart Failure) trial investigated dapagliflozin in older CHF patients (mean age ~66 years) and showed significant reductions in cardiovascular death and HF hospitalizations (61). Importantly, post hoc analyses demonstrated that dapagliflozin significantly reduced serious ventricular arrhythmias, including VT, VF, and resuscitated cardiac arrest (62). This suggests that SGLT2 inhibitors may confer protective effects against malignant ventricular arrhythmias in HFrEF patients through mechanisms including reduced oxidative stress, decreased myocardial sodium retention, and improved cardiac metabolism.

The EMPEROR-Reduced (Empagliflozin Outcome Trial in Patients with Chronic Heart Failure and a Reduced Ejection Fraction) trial evaluated empagliflozin in older HFrEF patients (mean age ~67 years) and found significant reductions in cardiovascular death and HF hospitalizations. Although a trend toward reduced SCD was noted, it did not reach statistical significance. Nevertheless, empagliflozin has been associated with improved myocardial energetics, reduced sympathetic activation, and suppression of arrhythmogenic remodeling, which may contribute to reduced ventricular arrhythmia burden (63).

A meta-analysis encompassing multiple SGLT2 inhibitor trials found a significant reduction in SCD among heart failure patients receiving SGLT2 inhibitors. However, the effect on ventricular ectopy, nonsustained VT, and VT was less conclusive, suggesting the need for dedicated rhythm monitoring in future trials (64).

Mineralocorticoid receptor antagonists (MRAs)

The RALES (Randomized Aldactone Evaluation Study) assessed spironolactone in older CHF patients (mean age ~67 years, NYHA Class II–IV) and demonstrated a 30% reduction in all-cause mortality. Notably, SCD was significantly lower in the spironolactone group, suggesting a protective effect against ventricular arrhythmias. Potential mechanisms include reduced myocardial fibrosis, prevention of potassium and magnesium loss, and modulation of autonomic tone (65).

The EPHESUS (Eplerenone Post-Acute Myocardial Infarction Heart Failure Efficacy and Survival Study) evaluated eplerenone in older post-MI patients (mean age ~64 years) with LVEF ≤40% and found a 15% reduction in all-cause mortality and a 21% reduction in SCD. The antiarrhythmic benefits were attributed to decreased myocardial fibrosis, improved LV function, and reduced sympathetic activation (66).

GDMT, including ACE inhibitors, ARBs, ARNIs, SGLT2 inhibitors, and MRAs, has been shown to reduce the incidence of ventricular arrhythmias and SCD in older patients with CHF. These medications exert mostly indirect antiarrhythmic effects through multiple mechanisms, including improved cardiac remodeling, suppression of neurohormonal activation, and stabilization of cardiac electrophysiology. Given the high risk of malignant ventricular arrhythmias and sudden cardiac death in older CHF patients, optimizing GDMT remains essential for arrhythmic risk reduction.

INVASIVE INTERVENTION

If patients have life-threatening recurrent VT or VF resistant to antiarrhythmic drugs, invasive intervention should be performed. Patients with critical coronary artery stenosis and severe myocardial ischemia should undergo coronary revascularization (67). In the Coronary Artery Bypass Graft (CABG) Patch Trial, there was no evidence of improved survival among patients with CAD, LVEF <36%, and an abnormal signal-averaged ECG undergoing complete coronary revascularization, in whom an ICD was implanted prophylactically at the time of elective coronary artery bypass graft surgery (68).

Surgical ablation of the arrhythmogenic substrate in patients with life-threatening VT can be curative in selected patients with prior infarction. This technique is based on the early experience of surgical subendocardial resection of infarcted myocardium pioneered at the University of Pennsylvania (69, 70). This therapy includes aneurysmectomy or infarctectomy and subendocardial resection with or without adjunctive cryoablation based on activation mapping in the operating room, or endoaneurysmorrhaphy with a pericardial patch combined with mapping-guided subendocardial resection (71). However, the perioperative morbidity and mortality rates are high, therefore this approach has largely been abandoned, aside from empiric cryoablation of infarcted areas.

Catheter ablation offers a minimally invasive approach with less morbidity and has largely supplanted surgical resection. The most current ablation techniques consist of extensive ablation targeting all signals that display evidence of slow conduction in the hope of interrupting all possible VT circuits. The complete elimination of all these sites, both endocardially and epicardially, does show promise and does predict long-term success independent of non-inducibility of VT at the end of a procedure (72, 73).

A number of randomized trials of VT ablation in patients with ICM have been published. The SMASH-VT (Substrate Mapping and Ablation in Sinus Rhythm to Halt Ventricular Tachycardia) trial was a randomized controlled study that evaluated the role of prophylactic catheter ablation in reducing ICD therapies in 128 patients with prior MI and spontaneous VT or VF requiring ICD implantation for secondary prevention, or recent primary prevention ICD with recent therapy for VT/VF. Patients were randomized to ICD implantation alone (n = 64) or ICD implantation with adjunctive catheter ablation (n = 64). Ablation was performed using substrate-based mapping in sinus rhythm, and patients on Class I or III antiarrhythmic drugs were excluded. Over a mean follow-up of 22.5 months, catheter ablation significantly reduced the need for appropriate ICD therapy (antitachycardia pacing or shocks), occurring in 33% of the ICD-only group versus 12% in the ablation group (HR 0.35, P = 0.007). The incidence of ICD shocks specifically was also lower (31% vs. 9%, P = 0.003). Mortality did not significantly differ between groups (9% vs. 17%, P = 0.29), and there were no procedural deaths within 30 days. Ventricular function and functional class remained stable throughout follow-up. These findings demonstrated that substrate-based VT ablation significantly reduces ICD therapies, including shocks, without increasing mortality or worsening cardiac function, supporting its role in patients with prior MI undergoing ICD implantation for secondary prevention of sudden cardiac death (74).

The VTACH trial was a randomized controlled study conducted at 16 centers across four European countries to evaluate prophylactic VT ablation before ICD implantation in patients with prior MI, stable monomorphic VT, and LVEF ≤50%. A total of 110 patients were randomized to ICD alone (n = 56) or ICD with catheter ablation (n = 54). The ablation approach included activation mapping of the stable VT and substrate modification. Over 22.5 months of follow-up, the median time to VT/VF recurrence was significantly longer in the ablation group (18.6 vs. 5.9 months, HR 0.61, P = 0.045), with 47% versus 29% remaining arrhythmia-free at 2 years. Mortality did not differ significantly (5 vs. 4 deaths), and no procedural deaths occurred. Ablation-related complications were minimal (2 cases), while device-related interventions were fewer in the ablation group (4 vs. 9 cases). These findings support prophylactic VT ablation as an effective adjunct to ICD therapy in reducing arrhythmia burden in post-MI patients with reduced LVEF (75). A follow-up on treatment analysis (13% of the ablation group did not undergo the procedure, 19% of the control group were ablated) did show a greater effect of ablation when compared to the intention-to-treat analysis: relative risk reduction of VA, 49% versus 39%; and relative risk reduction in cardiac hospitalization, 52% versus 45% (76).

The CALYPSO trial was a pilot multicenter randomized controlled study designed to compare catheter ablation and AAD therapy in patients with ischemic heart disease and ICDs who had experienced at least one ICD shock or three antitachycardia pacing therapies for VT. Of 243 screened patients, only 27 were enrolled due to strict eligibility criteria, such as the exclusion of those already on AADs (41% of screen failures) and VT caused by reversible factors (11%). The median age of participants was 64 years (range: 43–83), with 85% having a history of heart failure and a median LVEF of 25%. Patients were randomized to receive either catheter ablation (n = 13) or AAD therapy (n = 14). Over a follow-up period of up to 6 months, VT recurrence rates were high in both groups (62% for ablation vs. 43% for AAD), and the median time to VT recurrence was 75 days for ablation versus 57 days for AAD. Mortality rates were similarly high, with 15% in the ablation group and 14% in the AAD group. These findings demonstrated the significant morbidity and mortality associated with recurrent VT in elderly patients and highlighted the challenges of identifying patients for earlier intervention. While CALYPSO underscored the importance of exploring earlier VT ablation, it lacked the power to assess survival benefits (77).

The PARTITA (Does Timing of Ventricular Tachycardia Ablation Affect Prognosis in Patients With an Implantable Cardioverter Defibrillator?) trial was a two-phase, prospective, multicenter, randomized controlled trial that assessed the impact of early catheter ablation after the first ICD shock in patients with ischemic or nonischemic cardiomyopathy. The study included 517 patients in an observational Phase A until their first appropriate ICD shock. Patients who experienced an ICD shock were reconsented and randomized (Phase B, n = 47) to either immediate catheter ablation within 2 months (n = 23) or standard medical therapy without ablation (n = 24). Over a median follow-up of 24.2 months, the primary composite endpoint (all-cause mortality or hospitalization for worsening heart failure) occurred in 4% of the ablation group versus 42% of the control group (HR 0.11, 95% CI 0.01–0.85, P = 0.034). All-cause mortality was significantly lower in the ablation group (0% vs. 33%, P = 0.004), and ICD shocks were reduced (9% vs. 42%, P = 0.039). Though heart failure hospitalizations were lower in the ablation group (4% vs. 17%), the difference was not statistically significant (P = 0.159) (78).

These findings suggest that early VT ablation following the first ICD shock significantly reduces mortality, hospitalizations for worsening heart failure, and ICD shocks compared to standard therapy. The trial supports considering early VT ablation as a proactive strategy in ICD patients to improve long-term outcomes. Despite its compelling findings, the PARTITA trial has several limitations, most notably its premature discontinuation, which limits the robustness of its conclusions. The trial was stopped early due to the strong observed benefit of catheter ablation, particularly in reducing all-cause mortality, which may have introduced potential overestimation of treatment effects due to truncated follow-up. Additionally, the small sample size in Phase B (only 47 randomized patients) significantly limits statistical power and generalizability. The exclusion of patients on amiodarone (except for atrial arrhythmias) may also have limited the applicability of the results to real-world clinical practice, where amiodarone is frequently used in patients with recurrent VT. It did not show a statistically significant reduction in heart failure hospitalizations, which is an important endpoint for quality of life and long-term prognosis (78).

While the majority of VT circuits in ICM can be ablated endocardially, some patients have extension of their substrate to the deeper myocardium and epicardium. The advent of a percutaneous subxiphoid approach to accessing the pericardial space for VT ablation has allowed for targeting of many VT previously inaccessible (79). The ability to identify and ablate mid-myocardial circuits remains a challenge. In refractory cases, selective intracoronary alcohol ablation can be effective but needs to be used cautiously (80). New ablation technologies able to deliver deeper lesions will hopefully address this issue in the near future.

Pulsed-field ablation (PFA) is an emerging nonthermal ablation modality that utilizes irreversible electroporation to selectively target myocardial cells while minimizing damage to surrounding structures. A systematic review of case reports and a case series demonstrated its high procedural success rate (87.5%) and absence of complications, suggesting its potential as a viable alternative for VT ablation (81). Compared to traditional radiofrequency and cryoablation, PFA offers benefits such as precise, uniform lesions; reduced collateral damage; and shorter procedural times (82). However, despite these promising results, PFA remains investigational and is not yet FDA-approved for the treatment of ventricular arrhythmias. The available evidence is still limited to small-scale studies, emphasizing the need for larger clinical trials to establish its long-term efficacy and safety (83).

Once considered an arrhythmia not amenable to ablation, techniques to address VF have been pioneered over the past few years. As SMASH-VT suggests, ablation of VT has the additional effect of decreasing ICD therapies for VF as well (74), likely explained by the fact that many VF episodes begin as VT, but also likely due to the extensive substrate ablation. Specifically, surviving Purkinje fibers located in areas of scarring can induce VF in ICM (84). These areas can be identified as displaying early signals that precede the QRS during sinus rhythm and during ectopic beats. Ablation of these areas can prevent further VF episodes, even if the exact site of ectopic beat origination is not identified (84).

Until recently, no randomized trials comparing ablation and AAD had been published. The Ventricular Tachycardia Ablation versus Escalation of Antiarrhythmic Drugs (VANISH) trial was designed to compare escalation of AAD therapy with VT ablation in patients with ICM and recurrent VT despite ongoing treatment with an AAD (85). All patients had a previously implanted ICD and had an episode of VT (either below the detection rate of the ICD or ICD-terminated episodes) during treatment with amiodarone or another Class I or III AAD within the previous 6 months. Patients were randomized (1:1) to either ablation or intensification of AAD therapy. For patients initially treated with another AAD, this was discontinued, and amiodarone was started (400 mg twice daily for 2 weeks, then 400 mg daily for 4 weeks, then 200 mg daily). For patients initially treated with amiodarone <300 mg daily, a loading of 400 mg twice for 2 weeks, followed by 400 mg daily for 1 week was followed by maintenance of 300 mg daily. Those patients who were taking at least 300 mg amiodarone daily had mexiletine 200 mg thrice daily added to their regimen. The primary endpoint was a composite of death or VT storm (at least three episodes in a 24-hour period) or appropriate ICD shocks (85).

Of 132 patients randomized to ablation, 129 underwent the procedure (2 died, 1 withdrew consent). All patients in the escalated-therapy group (127 patients) received the assigned treatment. The primary outcome rate was lower in the ablation group (HR 0.72; 95% CI 0.53–0.98; p = 0.04), which was mostly due to decreases in VT storm and appropriate ICD shocks (130). Of interest, in subgroup analysis, those patients who were on amiodarone prior to the start of the study, outcomes were superior in the ablation group (HR 0.55; 95% CI 0.38–0.80; p = 0.001). Of note, no mortality benefit was seen for ablation, even on subgroup analysis, although the study was not powered for this endpoint alone. While VANISH does not directly answer the question of superiority of ablation over AAD as first-line therapy, it does complement the data from OPTIC that amiodarone is superior to sotalol (the only other AAD used at baseline in the escalated-therapy arm) for the prevention of recurrent VA in this patient population. Additionally, it does aid in the decision for ablation, suggesting that those naïve to amiodarone may benefit from this drug (if not averse/susceptible to its toxicities), while those already on amiodarone would be less likely to benefit from increasing the dose or adding mexiletine (85).

While the VANISH trial established that catheter ablation is superior to AAD escalation in patients with ischemic cardiomyopathy and recurrent VT despite AAD therapy, it did not address whether catheter ablation should be used as first-line therapy instead of AADs in this population. To answer this question, the VANISH 2 trial was designed to compare first-line catheter ablation versus AAD therapy in patients with prior MI and clinically significant VT who had not yet failed AAD therapy (86).

The VANISH 2 trial was a multicenter, randomized controlled trial that enrolled 416 patients with ischemic cardiomyopathy, an ICD, and a recent VT event (defined as VT storm, appropriate ICD therapy, or sustained VT requiring intervention). Patients were randomized 1:1 to catheter ablation within 14 days (n = 203) or AAD therapy (sotalol or amiodarone, n = 213). Over a median follow-up of 4.3 years, the primary composite endpoint (death, VT storm, appropriate ICD shock, or treated sustained VT below ICD detection threshold) occurred in 50.7% of the ablation group versus 60.6% of the drug therapy group (HR 0.75; 95% CI 0.58–0.97; P = 0.03). ICD shocks and VT burden were significantly lower in the ablation group, though no significant mortality benefit was observed (22.2% vs. 25.4%, HR 0.84, P = 0.25) (86).

Subgroup analysis revealed that amiodarone was superior to sotalol in preventing primary outcome events, consistent with prior evidence favoring amiodarone use for VT. Patients eligible for amiodarone showed a significantly greater reduction in the primary composite endpoint compared to those eligible for sotalol (HR 0.64, 95% CI 0.43–0.94 vs. HR 0.86, 95% CI 0.61–1.22, respectively). This reinforces amiodarone's efficacy in patients with VT events but must be weighed against its high rates of noncardiac toxicities, observed in 21.6% of patients.

Although catheter ablation was associated with a higher rate of early procedural complications (1% mortality, 11.3% nonfatal adverse events), AAD therapy was also linked to significant toxicity, including pulmonary complications requiring treatment in 21.6% of patients. These findings suggest that first-line catheter ablation may be a preferable strategy in patients with ischemic cardiomyopathy and VT, reducing VT burden and ICD therapies compared to AADs. However, individualized decision-making is needed, given the procedural risks and lack of a mortality benefit (86).

Rademaker et al. (87) evaluated the outcomes of first-line catheter ablation in post-MI patients with tolerated VT and LVEF >35%, challenging the necessity of automatic ICD implantation in this population. This single-center, prospective observational study included 86 patients undergoing VT ablation between 2009 and 2022, of whom 51 patients with tolerated VT and LVEF >35% received ablation as first-line therapy without prior ICD implantation. Ablation was performed using a substrate-based approach, and post-procedural programmed electrical stimulation (PES) was used to assess VT inducibility, guiding ICD implantation decisions. Over a median follow-up of 40 months, patients rendered noninducible after ablation (n = 37, 73%) had no VT recurrence or SCD, with 86% discharged without an ICD. In contrast, patients with residual inducible VT (n = 14, 27%) had a 29% VT recurrence rate, and all were recommended for ICD implantation, though three declined. Overall, 27% of the total cohort died, but no SCD occurred in the noninducible subgroup. These findings suggest that first-line VT ablation may be an effective alternative to ICD implantation in select post-MI patients with tolerated VT and LVEF >35%, particularly when noninducibility is achieved. However, given the single-center design and observational nature of the study, further randomized trials are needed to determine whether this strategy can safely alter current ICD guidelines for secondary prevention (87).

The most recent ACC/AHA/HRS guidelines (88) provide clear recommendations for catheter ablation in patients with ischemic heart disease (IHD) and nonischemic cardiomyopathy (NICM) who experience recurrent VAs despite optimal medical therapy. In IHD patients with recurrent VA and significant symptoms or ICD shocks, catheter ablation is recommended (Class I) if they have failed or are intolerant of amiodarone or other antiarrhythmic drugs. Additionally, for patients with sustained monomorphic VT or VT storm, ablation may be considered as a first-line therapy (Class IIb) in those with hemodynamically stable arrhythmias. In NICM patients, catheter ablation is reasonable (Class IIa) for those with sustained VT who have failed or are intolerant of antiarrhythmic drugs. Notably, in both populations, beta-blockers, amiodarone, and sotalol remain first-line pharmacologic treatments, and ICD implantation is crucial for secondary prevention of SCD. These recommendations highlight the expanding role of catheter ablation in managing VT, particularly as an alternative to escalating antiarrhythmic therapy in select patients (88).

Despite the extensive body of literature on ablation and the expanding application to multiple VA substrates and areas of origin, a definitive mortality benefit has not been proven. For these reasons, at this writing, ablation of VA in structural heart disease is largely adjunctive to patients with an ICD that fails, and who do not tolerate or do not wish to take AAD.

IMPLANTABLE CARDIOVERTER-DEFIBRILLATOR

The ICD has been widely accepted as the most effective treatment for patients with life-threatening VT or VF. Tresch et al. (89, 90) showed in retrospective studies that the ICD was very effective in treating life-threatening VT in older as well as in younger patients.

Secondary prevention

In the Antiarrhythmics versus Implantable Defibrillators (AVID) trial, 1016 patients, mean age 65 years, were randomized to an ICD or Class III antiarrhythmic drug therapy (Table 22.2) (91). Forty-five percent of the patients had been resuscitated from near-fatal VF. The other 55% of the patients had sustained VT with syncope or sustained VT with a LVEF ≤40% and symptoms suggesting severe hemodynamic compromise due to the arrhythmia (near-syncope, CHF, and angina pectoris) (91).

Amiodarone was administered to 96% of patients randomized to medical therapy and to 2% of patients who had the ICD. Sotalol was administered to 3% of patients randomized to medical therapy and to 0.2% of patients who had the ICD. Beta-blockers were administered to 17% of patients randomized to medical therapy and to 42% of patients who had the ICD. The 1-year survival was 89.3% for patients who had the ICD versus 82.3% for patients treated with drug therapy (95% CI, 39 ± 20% decrease in mortality). The 2-year survival was 81.6% for patients who had the ICD versus 74.7% for patients treated with drug therapy (95% CI, 27 ± 21% reduction in mortality). The 3-year survival was 75.4% for patients who had the ICD versus 64.1% for patients treated with drug therapy (95% CI, 31 ± 21% decrease in mortality) (91).

The Canadian Implantable Defibrillator Study (CIDS) randomized 659 patients with VF, cardiac arrest, or hypotensive VT to an ICD or amiodarone therapy (Table 22.2) (92). Cardiac arrhythmic mortality was 4.5% per year in patients treated with amiodarone versus 3% per year in patients treated with an ICD (relative risk reduction = 33%; p = 0.094). Total mortality was 10.2% per year in patients treated with amiodarone versus 8.3% per year in patients treated with an ICD (relative risk reduction = 20%; p = 0.142) (92).

The Cardiac Arrest Study Hamburg (CASH) (93) was a prospective, multicenter, randomized trial comparing ICD therapy with antiarrhythmic drug therapy in 288 patients resuscitated from cardiac arrest due to documented sustained ventricular arrhythmias. Patients were initially randomized to ICD therapy, amiodarone, metoprolol, or propafenone, but the propafenone arm was discontinued in 1992 after interim analysis showed a 61% higher all-cause mortality in this group compared with

Table 22.2 Effect of the implantable cardioverter-defibrillator on mortality in patients with structural heart disease

Study	Results
Multicenter Automatic Defibrillator Implantation Trial (94)	At 27-month follow-up, the ICD caused a 54% significant reduction in mortality (95% CI 0.26–0.82).
Antiarrhythmics versus Implantable Defibrillators Trial (91)	One-year survival was 89.3% for ICD versus 82.3% for drug therapy (95% CI, 39 ± 20% decrease in mortality); 2-year survival was 81.6% for ICD versus 74.7% for drug therapy (95% CI, 27±21% decrease in mortality); 3-year survival was 75.4% for ICD versus 64.1% for drug therapy (95% CI, 31 ± 21% decrease in mortality).
Canadian Implantable Defibrillator Study (92)	Mortality was 10.2% per year for amiodarone and 8.3% per year for an ICD (risk reduction = 20%; p = 0.072).
Cardiac Arrest Study Hamburg (93)	Propafenone was discontinued at 11 months after interim analysis showed a 61% higher all-cause mortality in the propafenone group compared with the ICD group during a mean follow-up of 11.3 months. Crude death rate: 36.4% (ICD) versus 44.4% (amiodarone/metoprolol) over 57 months. ICD therapy significantly reduced sudden cardiac death: 13% (ICD) versus 33% (amiodarone/metoprolol), HR 0.42, *P* = 0.005.
Multicenter Unsustained Tachycardia Trial (95)	Compared with electrophysiologically guided antiarrhythmic drug therapy, the 5-year total mortality was reduced 20% by an ICD (95% CI 0.64–1.01), and the 5-year risk of cardiac arrest or death from an arrhythmia was reduced 76% by an ICD (95% CI 0.13–0.45).
Multicenter Automatic Defibrillator Implantation Trial II (96)	At 20-month follow-up, the ICD caused a 31% significant reduction in mortality (95% CI 0.51–0.93).
Multicenter Automatic Defibrillator Implantation Trial II (97)	At 8-year follow-up, the cumulative probability of all-cause mortality was 49% for patients treated with an ICD versus 62% for patients not treated with an ICD (*p* < 0.001).
Amiodarone or an Implantable Cardioverter–Defibrillator for Congestive Heart Failure (47)	At 45.5 month follow-up, ICD therapy was associated with a decreased risk of death of 23% (*p* = 0.007), while amiodarone was not.
Prophylactic Defibrillator Implantation in Patients with Nonischemic Dilated Cardiomyopathy (98)	Mortality rate at 2 years was 14.1% in the standard-therapy group and 7.9% in the ICD group (HR 0.65; 95% CI 0.40–1.06; *p* = 0.08). SCD from arrhythmia was lower in the ICD group, HR 0.20 (95% CI 0.06–0.71; *p* = 0.006).
Defibrillator Implantation in Patients with Nonischemic Systolic Heart Failure (99)	At 67.6 month follow-up, mortality was 21.6% in the ICD group and 23.4% in the control group (HR 0.87; 95% CI 0.68–1.12; *p* = 0.28). The HR for SCD was 0.50 (95% CI 0.31–0.82; *p* = 0.0005).

Abbreviations: ICD, implantable cardioverter-defibrillator; SCD, sudden cardiac death.

the ICD group during a mean follow-up of 11.3 months. Following this, randomization continued between ICD (n = 99), amiodarone (n = 92), and metoprolol (n = 97). Over a mean follow-up of 57 ± 34 months, the crude death rate was 36.4% in the ICD group compared with 44.4% in the amiodarone/metoprolol group, reflecting a nonsignificant 23% reduction in all-cause mortality (HR 0.77, P = 0.081). However, ICD therapy significantly reduced the rate of sudden cardiac death, with a 61% relative risk reduction (13% vs. 33%, HR 0.42, P = 0.005) (93).

Primary prevention

The Multicenter Automatic Defibrillator Implantation Trial (MADIT) randomized 196 patients, mean age 63 years, with a prior MI, an LVEF ≤35%, a documented episode of asymptomatic nonsustained VT, and inducible nonsuppressible ventricular tachyarrhythmia on electrophysiologic study to receive an ICD or conventional medical therapy (Table 22.2) (94). Amiodarone was given to 74% of patients receiving conventional medical therapy versus 2% of patients receiving an ICD. Beta-blockers were given to 8% of patients receiving conventional medical therapy versus 26% of patients receiving an ICD. At 27-month follow-up, patients receiving an ICD had a 54% significant reduction in mortality (95% CI 0.26–0.82) (94).

The Multicenter Unsustained Tachycardia Trial randomized 704 patients with ischemic cardiomyopathy, EF ≤40% and inducible, sustained ventricular tachyarrhythmias to three treatment groups (Table 22.2) (95).

Compared with electrophysiologically guided antiarrhythmic drug therapy, the 5-year total mortality was reduced 20% by an ICD (95% CI 0.64–1.01), and the 5-year risk of cardiac arrest or death from an arrhythmia was reduced 76% by an ICD (95% CI 0.13–0.45) (95). Neither the total mortality incidence nor the rate of cardiac arrest or death from arrhythmia was lower in patients randomized to electrophysiologically guided therapy and treated with antiarrhythmic drugs than in patients randomized to no antiarrhythmic treatment (95).

MADIT II randomized 1232 patients, mean age 64 years, with a prior MI and a LVEF of ≤30% to an ICD or to conventional medical therapy (Table 22.2) (96). Beta-blockers were given to 70% of ICD patients versus 70% of conventional medical therapy patients. ACE inhibitors were given to 68% of ICD patients versus 72% of conventional medical therapy patients. Amiodarone was given to 13% of ICD patients versus 10% of conventional medical therapy patients. At 20-month follow-up, compared with conventional medical therapy, the ICD reduced all-cause mortality from 19.8% to 14.2%, $p = 0.016$ (hazard ratio = 0.69; 95% CI 0.51–0.93). The effect of ICD therapy in improving survival was similar in patients stratified according to age, sex, LVEF, New York Heart Association Class, and QRS interval (96).

In MADIT-II, the reduction in sudden cardiac death in patients treated with an ICD was significantly reduced by 68% in 574 patients aged <65 years ($p = 0.02$), by 65% in 455 patients aged 65–74 years ($p = 0.005$), and by 68% in 204 patients aged >75 years ($p = 0.05$) (100). The median survival in 348 octogenarians treated with ICD therapy was >4 years (101).

At 8-year follow-up in MADIT II, the cumulative probability of all-cause mortality was 49% for patients treated with an ICD versus 62% for patients not treated with an ICD ($p < 0.001$). ICD treatment caused a 34% reduction in mortality during treatment years 1–4 ($p < 0.001$) and a 26% reduction in mortality during years 5–8 ($p = 0.02$) (97).

The Amiodarone or an Implantable Cardioverter–Defibrillator for Congestive Heart Failure Trial (SCD-HeFT) included 2521 patients with ischemic and nonischemic cardiomyopathy, EF ≤35% and NYHA Class II–III symptoms. Patients were randomized to three arms: conventional therapy, conventional therapy plus amiodarone, and conventional therapy plus prophylactic ICD implantation. The primary endpoint was all-cause mortality. This was the first trial that included NICM and found a mortality benefit from the ICD, but not from amiodarone. At 45.5 months follow-up, ICD therapy was associated with a decreased risk of death of 23% ($p = 0.007$) (47).

The Prophylactic Defibrillator Implantation in Patients with Nonischemic Dilated Cardiomyopathy (DEFINITE) trial (98) randomized 458 patients with NICM, EF <36%, history of symptomatic heart failure, and nonsustained VT or frequent VPCs on monitoring to standard medical therapy alone or with a single-chamber ICD. While this trial showed a significant decrease in SCD in the ICD arm (hazard ratio, 0.20; 95% CI 0.06–0.71; $P = 0.006$) at 2 years, overall mortality benefit did not reach statistical significance (hazard ratio, 0.65; 95% CI 0.40–1.06; $P = 0.08$) (98).

The Defibrillator Implantation in Patients with Nonischemic Systolic Heart Failure (DANISH) trial (99) was designed to evaluate prophylactic ICD use in NICM with the background of modern heart failure management, including CRT pacing in those who qualify. This trial enrolled 1116 patients between 2008 and 2014 with NICM, EF ≤35, NYHA Class II or III CHF, or Class IV CHF if CRT was planned, and elevated N-terminal pro-brain natriuretic peptide (>200 pg/ml). Patients were required to be on maximally tolerated stable doses of beta-blockers and ACEI/ARB. Patients were randomized to standard medical therapy (which could include CRT pacing) or ICD (with CRT if indicated). The primary outcome was all-cause mortality. While the primary outcome was similar between groups (HR 0.87; 95% CI 0.68–1.12; $p = 0.28$), there was a benefit for the prevention of SCD (HR 0.50; 95% CI 0.31–0.82; $p = 0.0005$). In subgroup analysis, patients younger than 68 years of age did show a significantly lower mortality (HR 0.64; 95% CI 0.45–0.90; $P = 0.01$). This trial would suggest that when considering an ICD in NICM patients, other factors such as age and comorbidities should be taken into account (99).

After ICD implantation, 35 patients were randomized to treatment with metoprolol and 35 patients to treatment with d,l-sotalol (102). VT recurrence was 17% at 1 year and 20% at 2 years for patients treated with metoprolol versus 43% at 1 year and 49% at 2 years for patients treated with d,l-sotalol ($p = 0.016$). At 26-month follow-up, survival was 91% for patients treated with metoprolol plus an ICD versus 83% for patients treated with d,l-sotalol plus an ICD ($p = 0.287$) (102). In MADIT-II, use of higher doses of beta-blockers in patients with ischemic heart disease and an ICD significantly reduced mortality by 56%–58% compared with non-use of beta-blockers ($p < 0.01$) (103). These data favor using a beta-blocker in patients with an ICD.

The American College of Cardiology (ACC)/American Heart Association (AHA) guidelines for ICD implantation in patients with VAs (88) are listed in Tables 22.3–22.7.

An ICD is also effective in preventing sudden death in patients with hypertrophic cardiomyopathy at high risk for sudden death (104) and in patients at high risk for sudden death because of a long QT interval or the Brugada syndrome (105).

ICDs were implanted in 378 men and 95 women, mean age 69 ± 12 years (106). At 3.6-year follow-up, survival was 76% in patients who had an ICD because of cardiac arrest due to VF or VT not due to a transient or reversible cause; 85% in patients who had an ICD because of spontaneous sustained VT in association with structural heart disease; 92% in patients who had an ICD because of

Table 22.3 Primary prevention ICD indications

Recommendation	Recommendation
In patients with LVEF of 35% or less that is due to ischemic heart disease who are at least 40 days post-MI and at least 90 days post-revascularization, and with NYHA class II or III HF despite GDMT, an ICD is recommended if meaningful survival of greater than 1 year is expected.	Class I
In patients with LVEF of 30% or less that is due to ischemic heart disease who are at least 40 days post-MI and at least 90 days post-revascularization, and with NYHA Class I HF despite GDMT, an ICD is recommended if meaningful survival of greater than 1 year is expected.	Class I
In patients with ischemic heart disease and unexplained syncope who have inducible sustained monomorphic VT on electrophysiological study, an ICD is recommended if meaningful survival of greater than 1 year is expected.	Class I
In patients with NSVT due to prior MI, LVEF of 40% or less and inducible sustained VT or VF at electrophysiological study, an ICD is recommended if meaningful survival of greater than 1 year is expected.	Class I
In patients with NICM, HF with NYHA Class II–III symptoms and an LVEF of 35% or less, despite GDMT, an ICD is recommended if meaningful survival of greater than 1 year is expected.	Class I
In patients with NICM, HF with NYHA Class I symptoms and an LVEF of 35% or less, despite GDMT, an ICD may be considered if meaningful survival of greater than 1 year is expected.	Class IIb
In patients with NICM who experience syncope presumed to be due to VA and who do not meet indications for a primary prevention ICD, an ICD or an electrophysiological study for risk stratification for SCD can be beneficial if meaningful survival greater than 1 year is expected.	Class IIa
In non-hospitalized patients with NYHA Class IV symptoms who are candidates for cardiac transplantation or an LVAD, an ICD is reasonable if meaningful survival of greater than 1 year is expected.	Class IIa
In patients with HFrEF who are awaiting heart transplant and who otherwise would not qualify for an ICD (e.g., NYHA Class IV and/or use of inotropes) with a plan to discharge home, an ICD is reasonable.	Class IIa

Abbreviations: ICD, implantable cardioverter-defibrillator; LVEF, left ventricular ejection fraction; MI, myocardial infarction; NYHA, New York Heart Association; GDMT, guideline-directed medical therapy; NSVT, nonsustained ventricular tachycardia; HF, heart failure; VA, ventricular arrhythmia; SCD, sudden cardiac death; CRT, cardiac resynchronization therapy; LVAD, left ventricular assist device.

Table 22.4 Secondary prevention ICD indications

Condition	Recommendation
In patients with ischemic or nonischemic heart disease, who either survive SCA due to VT/VF or experience hemodynamically unstable VT or stable sustained VT not due to reversible causes, an ICD is recommended if meaningful survival greater than 1 year is expected.	Class I
In patients with giant cell myocarditis with VF or hemodynamically unstable VT treated according to GDMT, an ICD and/or an antiarrhythmic medication may be considered if meaningful survival of greater than 1 year is expected.	Class IIb
Patients resuscitated from SCA due to coronary artery spasm for whom medical therapy is ineffective or not tolerated, an ICD is reasonable if meaningful survival of greater than 1 year is expected.	Class IIa
Patients resuscitated from SCA due to coronary artery spasm, an ICD in addition to medical therapy may be reasonable if meaningful survival of greater than 1 year is expected.	Class IIb

Abbreviations: ICD, implantable cardioverter-defibrillator; SCA, sudden cardiac arrest; VA, ventricular arrhythmias; VF, ventricular fibrillation; VT, ventricular tachycardia; GDMT, guideline-directed medical therapy.

Table 22.5 ICD indications in cardiomyopathies and infiltrative diseases

Recommendation
Class IIa
Class IIa
Class IIb
Class IIa
Class IIa
Class IIa
Class IIa
Class I
Class IIa

Abbreviations: ICD, implantable cardioverter-defibrillator; HCM, hypertrophic cardiomyopathy; SCD, sudden cardiac death; LVEF, left ventricular ejection fraction; NICM, nonischemic cardiomyopathy; PET, positron emission tomography; NSVT, nonsustained ventricular tachycardia; MRI, magnetic resonance imaging.

syncope of undetermined origin with clinically relevant, hemodynamically sustained VT or VF induced at electrophysiological study when drug therapy is ineffective, not tolerated, or not preferred; 84% in patients who had an ICD because of nonsustained VT with CAD, MI, LV dysfunction, and inducible VF or sustained VT at electrophysiological study that is not suppressible by a Class I antiarrhythmic drug; and 85% in all 473 patients (106).

ICDs are not effective in treating patients with LV dysfunction scheduled for elective CABG (107) or in patients who have had an acute MI within 40 days of the procedure (108). ICDs should also not be used to treat patients with NYHA Class IV CHF despite optimal medical management (unless they have an indication for CRT) or in patients with a life expectancy <1 year.

ICDs were implanted in 485 patients with ischemic cardiomyopathy and in 299 patients with nonischemic cardiomyopathy. At 33-month follow-up, appropriate ICD shocks occurred in 179 of 485 patients (37%) with ischemic cardiomyopathy and in 93 of 299 patients (31%) with nonischemic cardiomyopathy (p not significant). All-cause mortality occurred in 162 of 485 patients (33%) with ischemic cardiomyopathy and in 70 of 299 patients (23%) with nonischemic cardiomyopathy ($p = 0.002$) (109).

During implantation and during 38-month follow-up of 1060 patients who had ICDs, complications occurred in 60 patients (5.7%) (110). These complications consisted of fractured leads requiring lead revision in 36 patients (3.4%), lead infection requiring antibiotics in 5 patients (0.5%), device replacement because of malfunction in 5 patients (0.5%), repositioning of leads in 3 patients (0.3%), a hematoma at the time of implantation in 3 patients (0.3%), pneumothorax at the time of implantation in 2 patients (0.2%), repair of a defective generator in 1 patient (0.1%), replacement of the device because of atrophy of the skin over the device in 1 patient (0.1%), a transient ischemic attack because of atrial fibrillation developing during implantation in 1 patient (0.1%), device replacement because of a recall from Guidant in 1 patient (0.1%), pocket revision because of pain when lying on the side of the pacemaker in 1 patient (0.1%), and pacemaker infection in 1 patient (0.1%) (110). A downloadable algorithm has been developed to reduce inappropriate shocks caused by fractures of implantable ICD leads (111).

Table 22.6 ICD indications in cardiac channelopathies

Condition	Recommendation
In patients with catecholaminergic polymorphic ventricular tachycardia and recurrent sustained VT or syncope, while receiving adequate or maximally tolerated beta-blocker, treatment intensification with either combination medication therapy (e.g., beta-blocker, flecainide), left cardiac sympathetic denervation, and/or an ICD is recommended.	Class I
In patients with Brugada syndrome with spontaneous type 1 Brugada electrocardiographic pattern and cardiac arrest, sustained VA, or a recent history of syncope presumed due to VA, an ICD is recommended if meaningful survival of greater than 1 year is expected.	Class I
In high-risk patients with symptomatic long QT syndrome in whom a beta-blocker is ineffective or not tolerated, intensification of therapy with additional medications (guided by consideration of the particular long QT syndrome type), left cardiac sympathetic denervation, and/or an ICD is recommended.	Class I
In asymptomatic patients with long QT syndrome and a resting QTc greater than 500 ms while receiving a beta-blocker, intensification of therapy with medications (guided by consideration of the particular long QT syndrome type), left cardiac sympathetic denervation, or an ICD may be considered.	Class IIb
In patients with short QT syndrome who have a cardiac arrest or sustained VA, an ICD is recommended if meaningful survival greater than 1 year is expected.	Class I

Abbreviations: ICD, implantable cardioverter-defibrillator; VT, ventricular tachycardia; VA, ventricular arrhythmia.

Table 22.7 ICD indications in special populations

Condition	Recommendation
For older patients and those with significant comorbidities, who meet indications for a primary prevention ICD, an ICD is reasonable if meaningful survival of greater than 1 year is expected.	Class IIa
In patients with an LVAD and sustained VA, an ICD can be beneficial.	Class IIa
In patients with a heart transplant and severe allograft vasculopathy with LV dysfunction, an ICD may be reasonable if meaningful survival of greater than 1 year is expected.	Class IIb

Abbreviations: ICD, implantable cardioverter-defibrillator; NYHA, New York Heart Association; GDMT, guideline-directed medical therapy; EF, ejection fraction; SCD, sudden cardiac death.

Persistent atrial fibrillation is associated with appropriate shocks and with CHF in patients with LV dysfunction treated with an ICD (112). One or more inappropriate ICD shocks occurred in 83 of 719 MADIT II patients (11.5%) and comprised 31.2% of 590 shocks (113). Triggers for inappropriate shocks were atrial fibrillation (44%), supraventricular tachycardia (36%), and abnormal sensing (20%). Patients with inappropriate shocks had 2.3 times increase in mortality ($p = 0.025$) (113).

In 1193 patients with combined CRT-ICD therapy, atrial tachycardia/atrial fibrillation lasting longer than 10 minutes occurred in 361 patients (30%) (114). Device-detected atrial tachycardia/atrial fibrillation was associated with a 2.16 times increased mortality at 13 months median follow-up ($p = 0.032$) (114) .

Of 958 with an ICD, chronic kidney disease was a significant independent predictor of 1-year mortality ($p < 0.001$) (115). The 1-year mortality was 1.8%, 5.3%, 9.0%, 22%, and 38% for stages 1, 2, 3, 4, and 5, respectively, of renal function (115).

Successful radiofrequency ablation was performed in 22 of 84 patients with an ICD who had inappropriate shocks from atrial tachycardia, atrial flutter, or atrioventricular nodal reentrant tachycardia (116). Ninety-five percent of 22 patients who underwent successful radiofrequency ablation for supraventricular tachycardia had no inappropriate ICD shocks at 21-month follow-up compared to 63% of patients with inappropriate shocks for supraventricular tachycardia who did not have radiofrequency ablation ($p = 0.04$) (116).

In patients with ICDs, compared to patients treated with ventricular backup pacing at a rate of 40/minute, patients treated with dual-chamber rate-responsive pacing at a rate of 70/minute (DDDR-70) had an increase in mortality (117), worsening of LVEF (118), and an increase in new LV wall motion abnormality (118). One reason why DDDR-70 pacing may increase mortality and worsen LV systolic function is that ventricular electrical activation proceeds from the right ventricular apex instead of through the existing conduction system.

In patients with ICDs and no indication for pacing for bradycardia, 22 of 80 patients (28%) treated with right ventricular pacing died at 45-month follow-up, and 8 of 81 patients (10%) treated with biventricular pacing died at 53-month follow-up ($p < 0.01$) (119). At 23-month follow-up, the LVEF decreased from 36% to 30% in patients treated with right ventricular pacing and increased at 38-month follow-up from 35% to 40% in patients treated with biventricular pacing ($p < 0.001$). New LV wall motion abnormality developed at 23-month follow-up in 23 of 80 patients (29%) treated with right ventricular pacing and at 38-month follow-up in 7 of 81 patients (9%) treated with biventricular pacing ($p < 0.005$) (119). On the basis of the available data, patients with ICDs should be treated with biventricular pacing, not with DDDR-70 right ventricular pacing (119, 120). However, it is not recommended that patients without need for ventricular pacing due to AV block, or those with left bundle branch block and Class II-IV CHF, undergo biventricular pacing.

Autonomic modulation

Based on the known benefits of beta-adrenergic blockade previously discussed, and the success of left cardiac sympathetic denervation for long QT syndrome patients (121), invasive approaches to autonomic modulation have generated increasing interest for the treatment of VA in cardiomyopathy (CMP). The stellate ganglia provide direct sympathetic innervation to the heart. A number of case reports and series have investigated the surgical destruction of the lower third to half of the stellate ganglia for arrhythmia control (122, 123). In 41 patients refractory to AAD and ablation for VA, Vaseghi et al. found bilateral stellate ganglia destruction more effective than left-sided ganglion destruction alone (ICD shock-free survival 48% vs. 30%, $p = 0.04$) (123).

The development of renal artery denervation for the treatment of hypertension has generated much interest in the effects on arrhythmia prevention. A number of case reports and series have displayed potential benefit in cardiomyopathy patients with refractory VA (124–126). These data must be tempered by uncertain efficacy of renal denervation for the treatment of hypertension, as initial results from SYMPLICITY HTN-3 (127) showed no significant benefit, though long-term follow-up demonstrated sustained blood pressure reductions (128). Furthermore, the RADIANCE II trial recently confirmed the safety and efficacy of ultrasound renal denervation in lowering blood pressure in patients with mild to moderate hypertension, renewing interest in this therapy (129).

Lastly, direct spinal cord stimulation, which can help prevent angina by suppressing sympathetic effects on the heart, has been utilized in two patients with refractory VA with good effect (130). These invasive approaches to cardiac sympathetic blockade offer unique insights into arrhythmogenesis and offer potential future therapies, but have yet to be proven in large-scale trials.

EMERGING THERAPIES

Stereotactic body radiation therapy

Stereotactic body radiation therapy (SBRT) is an emerging noninvasive approach for VT ablation, offering a treatment option for patients who are poor candidates for catheter ablation or have refractory VT despite conventional therapies (131). Unlike catheter-based approaches, SBRT delivers focused high-dose radiation to arrhythmogenic substrates, inducing fibrosis and electrical inactivation over weeks to months. Early studies suggest that this approach may significantly reduce VT burden and ICD shocks while avoiding procedural risks associated with invasive ablation (131).

The feasibility of SBRT for VT was first demonstrated in a proof-of-concept study by Cuculich et al., published in the *New England Journal of Medicine*. In this study, five patients with drug-refractory VT despite prior catheter ablation underwent noninvasive radioablation guided by electrocardiographic imaging, receiving a single 25 Gy fraction of radiation. Over a median follow-up of 46 patient-months, VT burden was reduced by 99.9%, with VT episodes dropping from 6577 pre-treatment to just 4 post-ablation. There were no procedural complications, and LVEF remained stable. Imaging at 3 months showed mild inflammatory changes, which resolved by 1 year. This study provided initial evidence that SBRT can dramatically suppress VT noninvasively, offering an alternative to patients with refractory arrhythmias (132).

Subsequent studies have reinforced these findings. A study by Ninni et al. evaluated SBRT in electrical storm, enrolling 17 patients with recurrent VT despite optimal medical therapy and prior ablation. After a median follow-up of 12.5 months, VT burden was reduced by 91% beyond 6 weeks ($p < 0.0001$). However, in incessant VT, efficacy was observed within 1 to 7 weeks, while in non-incessant VT, early recurrences occurred in 7 of 12 patients during the first 6 weeks. Despite this delayed treatment effect, SBRT significantly reduced VT burden and ICD shocks, providing a potential life-saving intervention in electrical storm (133).

A review by Kim et al. highlighted the advantages and limitations of stereotactic arrhythmia radioablation (STAR). Unlike catheter ablation, which immediately interrupts reentrant circuits, SBRT induces delayed fibrosis and electrical inactivation, leading to gradual VT suppression. Early data suggested that SBRT reduces VT burden by >80% in most patients, particularly in those with intramural arrhythmogenic substrates not accessible to catheter ablation. However, concerns remain regarding long-term safety, radiation-induced fibrosis, and treatment durability, emphasizing the need for further studies (134).

The VT-ART Consortium, an ongoing multicenter observational study, is assessing the long-term efficacy and safety of SBRT for VT. This study compares patients undergoing 25 Gy SBRT to a matched cohort receiving standard VT therapy, evaluating overall cardiovascular survival, VT reduction, and hospitalizations. Preliminary results indicate that SBRT significantly reduces VT episodes, with an efficacy similar to catheter ablation. However, long-term data are still needed to define its role in routine clinical practice (135).

While SBRT remains an investigational therapy, early studies suggest it may provide a viable alternative for high-risk patients with refractory VT. The delayed treatment effect, potential for myocardial fibrosis, and lack of long-term randomized data remain key limitations. However, as ongoing trials continue to refine patient selection and dosing strategies, SBRT may emerge as an important tool in the management of VT, particularly for those ineligible for conventional ablation. The RADIATE-VT trial (NCT05765175), a multicenter randomized study, is currently evaluating the safety and efficacy of SBRT in patients with recurrent VT who have undergone prior catheter ablation, and its findings are anticipated to provide critical data to guide future practice (136).

REFERENCES

1. Fleg JL, Kennedy HL. Cardiac arrhythmias in a healthy elderly population. *Chest*. 1982;81(3):302–7.
2. Aronow WS, Mercando AD, Epstein S. Prevalence of arrhythmias detected by 24-hour ambulatory electrocardiography and value of antiarrhythmic therapy in elderly patients with unexplained syncope. *The American Journal of Cardiology*. 1992;70(3):408–10.
3. Kantelip J-P, Sage E, Duchene-Marullaz P. Findings on ambulatory electrocardiographic monitoring in subjects older than 80 years. *The American Journal of Cardiology*. 1986;57(6):398–401.
4. Manolio TA, Furberg CD, Rautaharju PM, Siscovick D, Newman AB, Borhani NO, et al. Cardiac arrhythmias on 24-h ambulatory electrocardiography in older women and men: the cardiovascular health study. *Journal of the American College of Cardiology*. 1994;23(4):916–25.
5. Aronow WS, Ahn C, Mercando AD, Epstein S, Kronzon I. Prevalence and association of ventricular tachycardia and complex ventricular arrhythmias with new coronary events in older men and women with and without cardiovascular disease. *The Journals of Gerontology Series A: Biological Sciences and Medical Sciences*. 2002;57(3):M178–M80.

6. Aronow WS, Epstein S, Schwartz KS, Koenigsberg M. Prevalence of arrhythmias detected by ambulatory electrocardiographic monitoring and of abnormal left ventricular ejection fraction in persons older than 62 years in a long-term health care facility. *The American Journal of Cardiology.* 1987;59(4):368–9.
7. Aronow WS, Epstein S, Schwartz KS, Koenigsberg M. Correlation of complex ventricular arrhythmias detected by ambulatory electrocardiographic monitoring with echocardiographic left ventricular hypertrophy in persons older than 62 years in a long-term health care facility. *The American Journal of Cardiology.* 1987;60(8):730–2.
8. Aronow WS, Epstein S. Usefulness of silent ischemia, ventricular tachycardia, and complex ventricular arrhythmias in predicting new coronary events in elderly patients with coronary artery disease or systemic hypertension. *The American Journal of Cardiology.* 1990;65(7):511–2.
9. Fleg JL, Kennedy HL. Long-term prognostic significance of ambulatory electrocardiographic findings in apparently healthy subjects ≥60 years of age. *The American Journal of Cardiology.* 1992;70(7):748–51.
10. Fleg JL, Lakatta EG. Prevalence and prognosis of exercise-induced nonsustained ventricular tachycardia in apparently healthy volunteers. *The American Journal of Cardiology.* 1984;54(7):762–4.
11. Janette Busby M, Shefrin EA, Fleg JL. Prevalence and long-term significance of exercise-induced frequent or repetitive ventricular ectopic beats in apparently healthy volunteers. *Journal of the American College of Cardiology.* 1989;14(7):1659–65.
12. Aronow WS, Epstein S, Koenigsberg M, Schwartz KS. Usefulness of echocardiographic abnormal left ventricular ejection fraction, paroxysmal ventricular tachycardia and complex ventricular arrhythmias in predicting new coronary events in patients over 62 years of age. *The American Journal of Cardiology.* 1988;61(15):1349–51.
13. Aronow WS, Epstein S, Koenigsberg M, Schwartz KS. Usefulness of echocardiographic left ventricular hypertrophy, ventricular tachycardia and complex ventricular arrhythmias in predicting ventricular fibrillation or sudden cardiac death in elderly patients. *The American Journal of Cardiology.* 1988;62(16):1124–5.
14. Zhong L, Lee Y-H, Huang X-M, Asirvatham SJ, Shen W-K, Friedman PA, et al. Relative efficacy of catheter ablation vs antiarrhythmic drugs in treating premature ventricular contractions: a single-center retrospective study. *Heart Rhythm.* 2014;11(2):187–93.
15. Krittayaphong R, Bhuripanyo K, Punlee K, Kangkagate C, Chaithiraphan S. Effect of atenolol on symptomatic ventricular arrhythmia without structural heart disease: a randomized placebo-controlled study. *American Heart Journal.* 2002;144(6):1–5.
16. Stec S, Sikorska A, Zaborska B, Kryński T, Szymot J, Kułakowski P. Benign symptomatic premature ventricular complexes: short- and long-term efficacy of antiarrhythmic drugs and radiofrequency ablation. *Kardiologia Polska* (Polish Heart Journal). 2012;70(4):351–58. (1897–4279 (Electronic)).
17. Gill JS, Mehta D, Ward DE, Camm AJ. Efficacy of flecainide, sotalol, and verapamil in the treatment of right ventricular tachycardia in patients without overt cardiac abnormality. *British Heart Journal.* 1992;68(4):392–7.
18. Belhassen B, Rotmensch HH, Laniado S. Response of recurrent sustained ventricular tachycardia to verapamil. *British Heart Journal.* 1981;46(6):679–82.
19. Belhassen B, Shapira I, Pelleg A, Copperman I, Kauli N, Laniodo S. Idiopathic recurrent sustained ventricular tachycardia responsive to verapamil: an ECG-electrophysiologic entity. *American Heart Journal.* 1984;108(4):1034–7.
20. Okumura K, Yamabe H, Tsuchiya T, Tabuchi T, Iwasa A, Yasue H. Characteristics of slow conduction zone demonstrated during entrainment of idiopathic ventricular tachycardia of left ventricular origin. *The American Journal of Cardiology.* 1996;77(5):379–83.
21. Collins KK, Schaffer MS, Liberman L, Saarel E, Knecht M, Tanel RE, et al. Fascicular and nonfascicular left ventricular tachycardias in the young: an international multicenter study. *Journal of Cardiovascular Electrophysiology.* 2013;24(6):640–8.
22. Morgera T, Hrovatin E, Mazzone C, Humar F, De Biasio M, Salvi A. Clinical spectrum of fascicular tachycardia. *Journal of Cardiovascular Medicine.* 2013;14(11):791–8.
23. Liu Y, Fang Z, Yang B, Kojodjojo P, Chen H, Ju W, et al. Catheter Ablation of fascicular ventricular tachycardia: long-term clinical outcomes and mechanisms of recurrence. *Circulation: Arrhythmia and Electrophysiology.* 2015;8(6):1443–51.
24. Kostis JB, Byington R, Friedman LM, Goldstein S, Furberg C. Prognostic significance of ventricular ectopic activity in survivors of acute myocardial infarction. *Journal of the American College of Cardiology.* 1987;10(2):231–42.
25. Virani SS, Newby LK, Arnold SV, Bittner V, Brewer LC, Demeter SH, et al. 2023 AHA/ACC/ACCP/ASPC/NLA/PCNA guideline for the management of patients with chronic coronary disease: a report of the American Heart Association/American College of Cardiology joint committee on clinical practice guidelines. *Circulation.* 2023;148(9):E9–E119. (1524–4539 (Electronic)).
26. Frishman WH, Aronow WS, Cheng-Lai A. *Cardiovascular Drug Therapy in the Elderly.* Fundamental and Clinical Cardiology Series: Informa Healthcare; 2008. p. 99–136.

27. International mexiletine and placebo antiarrhythmic coronary trial: I. Report on arrhythmia and other findings. Impact Research Group. *Journal of the American College of Cardiology*. 1984;4(6):1148–63. (0735–1097 (Print)).
28. Echt DS, Liebson PR, Mitchell LB, Peters RW, Obias-Manno D, Barker AH, Arensberg D, et al. Mortality and morbidity in patients receiving encainide, flecainide, or placebo: the Cardiac Arrhythmia Suppression Trial. *The New England Journal of Medicine*. 1991;324(12):781–8. (0028–4793 (Print)).
29. Akiyama T, Pawitan Y, Campbell WB, Papa L, Barker AH, Rubbert P, et al. Effects of advancing age on the efficacy and side effects of antiarrhythmic drugs in post-myocardial infarction patients with ventricular arrhythmias. *Journal of the American Geriatrics Society*. 1992;40(7):666–72.
30. Cardiac Arrhythmia Suppression Trial II Investigators. Effect of the antiarrhythmic agent moricizine on survival after myocardial infarction. *The New England Journal of Medicine*. 1992;327(4):227–33. (0028–4793 (Print)).
31. Aronow WS, Mercando AD, Epstein S, Kronzon I. Effect of quinidine or procainamide versus no antiarrhythmic drug on sudden cardiac death, total cardiac death, and total death in elderly patients with heart disease and complex ventricular arrhythmias. *The American Journal of Cardiology*. 1990;66(4):423–8.
32. Moosvi AR, Goldstein S, Medendorp SV, Landis JR, Wolfe RA, Leighton R, et al. Effect of empiric antiarrhythmic therapy in resuscitated out-of-hospital cardiac arrest victims with coronary artery disease. *The American Journal of Cardiology*. 1990;65(18):1192–7.
33. Hallstrom AP, Cobb LA, Yu BH, Weaver WD, Fahrenbruch CE. An antiarrhythmic drug experience in 941 patients resuscitated from an initial cardiac arrest between 1970 and 1985. *The American Journal of Cardiology*. 1991;68(10):1025–31.
34. Morganroth J, Goin JE. Quinidine-related mortality in the short-to-medium-term treatment of ventricular arrhythmias. A meta-analysis. *Circulation*. 1991;84(5):1977–83.
35. Teo KK. Effects of prophylactic antiarrhythmic drug therapy in acute myocardial infarction. *JAMA*. 1993;270(13):1589.
36. Hjalmarson Å, Herlitz J, Málek I, Rydén L, Vedin A, Waldenström A, et al. Effect on mortality of metoprolol in acute myocardial infarction. *The Lancet*. 1981;318(8251):823–7.
37. A randomized trial of propranolol in patients with acute myocardial infarction. *JAMA*. 1982;247(12):1707. doi: 10.1001/jama.1982.03320370021023.
38. Hawkins CM, Richardson DW, Vokonas PS. Effect of propranolol in reducing mortality in older myocardial infarction patients. The Beta-Blocker Heart Attack Trial experience. *Circulation*. 1983;67(6 Pt 2):I94–7. (0009–7322 (Print)).
39. A randomized trial of propranolol in patients with acute myocardial infarction. I. Mortality results. *JAMA*. 1982;247(12):1707. doi: 10.1001/jama.1982.03320370021023. (0098–7484 (Print)).
40. Kennedy HL, Brooks MM, Barker AH, Bergstrand R, Huther ML, Beanlands DS, et al. Beta-blocker therapy in the cardiac arrhythmia suppression trial. *The American Journal of Cardiology*. 1994;74(7):674–80.
41. Mäkikallio TH, Huikuri HV. Association between usage of beta-blocking medication and benefit from implantable cardioverter therapy. *The American Journal of Cardiology*. 2006;98(9):1245–7.
42. Waldo AL, Camm AJ, deRuyter H, Friedman PL, MacNeil DJ, Pauls JF, et al. Effect of d-sotalol on mortality in patients with left ventricular dysfunction after recent and remote myocardial infarction. *The Lancet*. 1996;348(9019):7–12.
43. Julian DG, Jackson FS, Prescott RJ, Szekely P. Controlled trial of sotalol for one year after myocardial infarction. *The Lancet*. 1982;319(8282):1142–7.
44. Singh SN, Fletcher RD, Fisher SG, Singh BN, Lewis HD, Deedwania PC, et al. Amiodarone in patients with congestive heart failure and asymptomatic ventricular arrhythmia. *New England Journal of Medicine*. 1995;333(2):77–82.
45. Cairns JA, Connolly SJ, Roberts R, Gent M. Randomised trial of outcome after myocardial infarction in patients with frequent or repetitive ventricular premature depolarisations: CAMIAT. *The Lancet*. 1997;349(9053):675–82.
46. Julian DG, Camm AJ, Frangin G, Janse MJ, Munoz A, Schwartz PJ, et al. Randomised trial of effect of amiodarone on mortality in patients with left-ventricular dysfunction after recent myocardial infarction: EMIAT. *The Lancet*. 1997;349(9053):667–74.
47. Bardy GH, Lee KL, Mark DB, Poole JE, Packer DL, Boineau R, et al. Amiodarone or an implantable cardioverter–defibrillator for congestive heart failure. *New England Journal of Medicine*. 2005;352(3):225–37.
48. Mason JW. A comparison of seven antiarrhythmic drugs in patients with ventricular tachyarrhythmias. *New England Journal of Medicine*. 1993;329(7):452–8.
49. Greene HL, The CI. The CASCADE study: randomized antiarrhythmic drug therapy in survivors of Cardiac Arrest in Seattle. *The American Journal of Cardiology*. 1993;72(16):F70-F4.
50. Herre JM, Sauve MJ, Malone P, Griffin JC, Helmy I, Langberg JJ, et al. Long-term results of amiodarone therapy in patients with recurrent sustained ventricular tachycardia or ventricular fibrillation. *Journal of the American College of Cardiology*. 1989;13(2):442–9.

51. Lai HM, Aronow WS, Kruger A, Desai H, Amin H, Frishman WH, et al. Effect of beta blockers, angiotensin-converting enzyme inhibitors or angiotensin receptor blockers, and statins on mortality in patients with implantable cardioverter-defibrillators. *The American Journal of Cardiology.* 2008;102(1):77–8.
52. Kruger A, Aronow WS, Lai H, Desai H, Singla A, Frishman WH, et al. Prevalence of appropriate cardioverter-defibrillator shocks in 1038 consecutive patients with implantable cardioverter-defibrillators. *American Journal of Therapeutics.* 2009;16(4):323–5.
53. Pacifico A, Hohnloser SH, Williams JH, Tao B, Saksena S, Henry PD, et al. Prevention of implantable-defibrillator shocks by treatment with sotalol. *New England Journal of Medicine.* 1999;340(24):1855–62.
54. Connolly SJ. Comparison of β-Blockers, Amiodarone Plus β-Blockers, or sotalol for prevention of shocks from implantable cardioverter defibrillators: the OPTIC study: a randomized trial. *JAMA.* 2006;295(2):165.
55. Pinter A, Akhtari S, O'Connell T, O'Donnell S, Mangat I, Korley V, et al. Efficacy and safety of dofetilide in the treatment of frequent ventricular tachyarrhythmias after amiodarone intolerance or failure. *Journal of the American College of Cardiology.* 2011;57(3):380–1.
56. Baquero GA, Banchs JE, Depalma S, Young SK, Penny-Peterson ED, Samii SM, et al. Dofetilide reduces the frequency of ventricular arrhythmias and implantable cardioverter defibrillator therapies. *Journal of Cardiovascular Electrophysiology.* 2011;23(3):296–301.
57. The CONSENSUS Trial Study Group. Effects of enalapril on mortality in severe congestive heart failure. Results of the Cooperative North Scandinavian Enalapril Survival Study (CONSENSUS). *New England Journal of Medicine.* 1987;316(23):1429–35. (0028–4793 (Print)).
58. Yusuf S, Pitt B, Davis CE, Hood WB, Cohn JN. Effect of enalapril on survival in patients with reduced left ventricular ejection fractions and congestive heart failure. *New England Journal of Medicine.* 1991;325(5):293–2. (0028–4793 (Print)).
59. Cohn JN, Tognoni G. A randomized trial of the angiotensin-receptor blocker valsartan in chronic heart failure. *New England Journal of Medicine.* 2001;345(23):1667–75. (0028–4793 (Print)).
60. McMurray JJ, Packer M, Desai AS, Gong J, Lefkowitz MP, Rizkala AR, Rouleau JL, et al. Angiotensin-neprilysin inhibition versus enalapril in heart failure. *New England Journal of Medicine.* 2014;371(11):993–1004. (1533–4406 (Electronic)).
61. McMurray JJV, Solomon SD, Inzucchi SE, Køber L, Kosiborod MN, Martinez FA, et al. Dapagliflozin in patients with heart failure and reduced ejection fraction. *New England Journal of Medicine.* 2019;381(21):1995–2008. (1533–4406 (Electronic)).
62. Curtain JA-O, Docherty KA-O, Jhund PA-O, Petrie MA-O, Inzucchi SE, Køber LA-O, et al. Effect of dapagliflozin on ventricular arrhythmias, resuscitated cardiac arrest, or sudden death in DAPA-HF. *Journal of the American College of Cardiology.* 2021;77(12):1460–1. (1522–9645 (Electronic)).
63. Packer MA-O, Anker SD, Butler J, Filippatos G, Pocock SJ, Carson P, et al. Cardiovascular and renal outcomes with empagliflozin in heart failure. *New England Journal of Medicine.* 2020;383(15):1413–24. (1533–4406 (Electronic)).
64. Vaduganathan M, Docherty KF, Claggett BL, Jhund PS, de Boer RA, Hernandez AF, et al. SGLT-2 inhibitors in patients with heart failure: a comprehensive meta-analysis of five randomised controlled trials. *Lancet.* 2022;400(10354):757–67. (1474–547X (Electronic)).
65. Pitt B, Zannad F, Remme WJ, Cody R, Castaigne A, Perez A, Palensky J, et al. The effect of spironolactone on morbidity and mortality in patients with severe heart failure. Randomized aldactone evaluation study investigators. *New England Journal of Medicine.* 1999;341(10):709–17. (0028–4793 (Print)).
66. Pitt B, Remme W, Zannad F, Neaton J, Martinez F, Roniker B, Bittman R, et al. Eplerenone, a selective aldosterone blocker, in patients with left ventricular dysfunction after myocardial infarction. *New England Journal of Medicine.* 2003;348(14):1309–21. (1533–4406 (Electronic)).
67. O'Rourke RA. Role of myocardial revascularization in sudden cardiac death. *Circulation.* 1992;85(1 Suppl):I112–7.
68. Bigger JT, Fleiss JL, Kleiger R, Miller JP, Rolnitzky LM. The relationships among ventricular arrhythmias, left ventricular dysfunction, and mortality in the 2 years after myocardial infarction. *Circulation.* 1984;69(2):250–8.
69. Josephson ME, Harken AH, Horowitz LN. Endocardial excision: a new surgical technique for the treatment of recurrent ventricular tachycardia. *Circulation.* 1979;60(7):1430–9.
70. Miller JM, Kienzle MG, Harken AH, Josephson ME. Subendocardial resection for ventricular tachycardia: predictors of surgical success. *Circulation.* 1984;70(4):624–31.
71. Rastegar H, Link MS, Foote CB, Wang PJ, Manolis AS, Estes NAM. Perioperative and long-term results with mapping-guided subendocardial resection and left ventricular endoaneurysmorrhaphy. *Circulation.* 1996;94(5):1041–8.
72. Jaïs P, Maury P, Khairy P, Sacher F, Nault I, Komatsu Y, et al. Elimination of local abnormal ventricular activities. *Circulation.* 2012;125(18):2184–96.

73. Di Biase L, Santangeli P, Burkhardt DJ, Bai R, Mohanty P, Carbucicchio C, et al. Endo-epicardial homogenization of the scar versus limited substrate ablation for the treatment of electrical storms in patients with ischemic cardiomyopathy. *Journal of the American College of Cardiology.* 2012;60(2):132–41.
74. Reddy VY, Reynolds MR, Neuzil P, Richardson AW, Taborsky M, Jongnarangsin K, et al. Prophylactic catheter ablation for the prevention of defibrillator therapy. *New England Journal of Medicine.* 2007;357(26):2657–65.
75. Kuck K-H, Schaumann A, Eckardt L, Willems S, Ventura R, Delacrétaz E, et al. Catheter ablation of stable ventricular tachycardia before defibrillator implantation in patients with coronary heart disease (VTACH): a multicentre randomised controlled trial. *The Lancet.* 2010;375(9708):31–40.
76. DelacrÉTaz E, Brenner R, Schaumann A, Eckardt L, Willems S, Pitschner HF, et al. Catheter ablation of stable ventricular tachycardia before defibrillator implantation in patients with coronary heart disease (VTACH): an on-treatment analysis. *Journal of Cardiovascular Electrophysiology.* 2013;24(5):525–9.
77. Al-Khatib SM, Daubert JP, Anstrom KJ, Daoud EG, Gonzalez M, Saba S, Jackson KP, et al. Catheter ablation for ventricular tachycardia in patients with an implantable cardioverter defibrillator (CALYPSO) pilot trial. *Journal of Cardiovascular Electrophysiology.* 2015 Feb;26(2):151–7. (1540–8167 (Electronic)).
78. Della Bella PA-O, Baratto F, Vergara P, Bertocchi P, Santamaria M, Notarstefano P, et al. Does timing of ventricular tachycardia ablation affect prognosis in patients with an implantable cardioverter defibrillator? results from the multicenter randomized PARTITA trial. *Circulation.* 2022 Jun 21;145(25):1829–38. (1524–4539 (Electronic)).
79. Sosa E, Scanavacca M, d'Avila A, Oliveira F, Ramires JAF. Nonsurgical transthoracic epicardial catheter ablation to treat recurrent ventricular tachycardia occurring late after myocardial infarction. *Journal of the American College of Cardiology.* 2000;35(6):1442–9.
80. Tokuda M, Sobieszczyk P, Eisenhauer AC, Kojodjojo P, Inada K, Koplan BA, et al. Transcoronary ethanol ablation for recurrent ventricular tachycardia after failed catheter ablation. *Circulation: Arrhythmia and Electrophysiology.* 2011;4(6):889–96.
81. Lozano-Granero C, Hirokami J, Franco E, Tohoku S, Matía-Francés R, Schmidt B, et al. Case series of ventricular tachycardia ablation with pulsed-field ablation: pushing technology further (Into the Ventricle). *JACC: Clinical Electrophysiology.* 2023;9(9):1990–4.
82. Weyand S, Löbig S, Seizer P. First in human focal pulsed field ablation to treat an epicardial VT focus with an endocardial approach in non-ischemic cardiomyopathy. *Journal of Interventional Cardiac Electrophysiology.* 2023;66(5):1057–8.
83. Adragão P, Matos D, Carmo P, Costa FM, Ramos S. Pulsed-field ablation vs radiofrequency ablation for ventricular tachycardia: first in-human case of histologic lesion analysis. *Heart Rhythm.* 2023;20(10):1395–8.
84. Marrouche NF, Verma A, Wazni O, Schweikert R, Martin DO, Saliba W, et al. Mode of initiation and ablation of ventricular fibrillation storms in patients with ischemic cardiomyopathy. *Journal of the American College of Cardiology.* 2004;43(9):1715–20.
85. Sapp JL, Wells GA, Parkash R, Stevenson WG, Blier L, Sarrazin J-F, et al. Ventricular tachycardia ablation versus escalation of antiarrhythmic drugs. *New England Journal of Medicine.* 2016;375(2):111–21.
86. Sapp JL, Tang ASL, Parkash R, Stevenson WG, Healey JS, Wells G. A randomized clinical trial of catheter ablation and antiarrhythmic drug therapy for suppression of ventricular tachycardia in ischemic cardiomyopathy: the VANISH2 trial. *American Heart Journal.* 2024;274:1–10.
87. Rademaker R, de Riva M, Piers SRD, Wijnmaalen AP, Zeppenfeld K. Excellent outcomes after first-line ablation in post-MI patients with tolerated VT and LVEF >35. *JACC: Clinical Electrophysiology.* 2024 Nov;10(11):2303–11. (2405–5018 (Electronic)).
88. Al-Khatib SM, Stevenson WG, Ackerman MJ, Bryant WJ, Callans DJ, Curtis AB, Deal BJ, et al. 2017 AHA/ACC/HRS guideline for management of patients with ventricular arrhythmias and the prevention of sudden cardiac death: executive summary: a report of the American College of Cardiology/American Heart Association Task Force on Clinical Practice Guidelines and the Heart Rhythm Society. *Circulation.* 2018;138(13):e210–e271. (1556–3871 (Electronic)).
89. Tresch DD, Platia EV, Guarnieri T, Reid PR, Griffith LSC. Refractory symptomatic ventricular tachycardia and ventricular fibrillation in elderly patients. *The American Journal of Medicine.* 1987;83(3):399–404.
90. Tresch DD, Troup PJ, Thakur RK, Veseth-Rogers J, Tucker V, Wetherbee JN, et al. Comparison of efficacy of automatic implantable cardioverter defibrillator in patients older and younger than 65 years of age. *The American Journal of Medicine.* 1991;90(1):717–24.
91. Moss AJ, Hall WJ, Cannom DS, Daubert JP, Higgins SL, Klein H, et al. Improved survival with an implanted defibrillator in patients with coronary disease at high risk for ventricular arrhythmia. *New England Journal of Medicine.* 1996;335(26):1933–40.
92. Connolly SJ, Gent M, Roberts RS, Dorian P, Roy D, Sheldon RS, et al. Canadian implantable defibrillator study (CIDS): a randomized trial of the implantable cardioverter defibrillator against amiodarone. *Circulation.* 2000;101(11):1297–302.

93. Kuck KH, Cappato R, Siebels J, Rüppel R. Randomized comparison of antiarrhythmic drug therapy with implantable defibrillators in patients resuscitated from cardiac arrest: the Cardiac Arrest Study Hamburg (CASH). *Circulation.* 2000;102(7):748–54.
94. Moss AJ, Hall WJ, Cannom DS, Daubert JP, Higgins SL, Klein H, et al. Improved survival with an implanted defibrillator in patients with coronary disease at high risk for ventricular arrhythmia. Multicenter automatic defibrillator implantation trial investigators. *New England Journal of Medicine.* 1996;335(26):1933–40.
95. Buxton AE, Lee KL, Fisher JD, Josephson ME, Prystowsky EN, Hafley G. A randomized study of the prevention of sudden death in patients with coronary artery disease. *New England Journal of Medicine.* 1999;341(25):1882–90.
96. Moss AJ, Zareba W, Hall WJ, Klein H, Wilber DJ, Cannom DS, et al. Prophylactic implantation of a defibrillator in patients with myocardial infarction and reduced ejection fraction. *New England Journal of Medicine.* 2002;346(12):877–83.
97. Goldenberg I, Gillespie J, Moss AJ, Hall WJ, Klein H, McNitt S, et al. Long-term benefit of primary prevention with an implantable cardioverter-defibrillator. *Circulation.* 2010;122(13):1265–71.
98. Kadish A, Dyer A, Daubert JP, Quigg R, Estes NAM, Anderson KP, et al. Prophylactic defibrillator implantation in patients with nonischemic dilated cardiomyopathy. *New England Journal of Medicine.* 2004;350(21):2151–8.
99. Køber L, Thune JJ, Nielsen JC, Haarbo J, Videbæk L, Korup E, et al. Defibrillator implantation in patients with nonischemic systolic heart failure. *New England Journal of Medicine.* 2016;375(13):1221–30.
100. Goldenberg I, Moss AJ. Treatment of arrhythmias and use of implantable cardioverter-defibrillators to improve survival in elderly patients with cardiac disease. *Clinics in Geriatric Medicine.* 2007;23(1):205–19.
101. Koplan BA, Epstein LM, Albert CM, Stevenson WG. Survival in octogenarians receiving implantable defibrillators. *American Heart Journal.* 2006;152(4):714–9.
102. Seidl K, Hauer B, Schwick NG, Zahn R, Senges J. Comparison of metoprolol and sotalol in preventing ventricular tachyarrhythmias after the implantation of a cardioverter/defibrillator. *The American Journal of Cardiology.* 1998;82(6):744–8.
103. Brodine WN, Tung RT, Lee JK, Hockstad ES, Moss AJ, Zareba W, et al. Effects of beta-blockers on implantable cardioverter defibrillator therapy and survival in the patients with ischemic cardiomyopathy (from the multicenter automatic defibrillator implantation Trial-II). *The American Journal of Cardiology.* 2005;96(5):691–5.
104. Maron BJ, Shen W-K, Link MS, Epstein AE, Almquist AK, Daubert JP, et al. Efficacy of implantable cardioverter–defibrillators for the prevention of sudden death in patients with hypertrophic cardiomyopathy. *New England Journal of Medicine.* 2000;342(6):365–73.
105. Brugada P, Brugada R, Brugada J, Geelen P. Use of the prophylactic implantable cardioverter defibrillator for patients with normal hearts. *The American Journal of Cardiology.* 1999;83(5):98–100.
106. Aronow WS, Sorbera C, Chagarlamudi A, Tabandeh H, Gupta S, Cohen M. Indications for and long-term survival in patients with automatic implantable cardioverter-defibrillators. *Cardiology in Review.* 2005;13(1):50–1.
107. Bigger JT. Prophylactic use of implanted cardiac defibrillators in patients at high risk for ventricular arrhythmias after coronary-artery bypass graft surgery. *New England Journal of Medicine.* 1997;337(22):1569–75.
108. Steinbeck G, Andresen D, Seidl K, Brachmann J, Hoffmann E, Wojciechowski D, et al. Defibrillator implantation early after myocardial infarction. *New England Journal of Medicine.* 2009;361(15):1427–36.
109. Gandhi K, Aronow WS, Desai H, Amin H, Lai HM, Frishman WH, et al. Incidence of appropriate cardioverter-defibrillator shocks and mortality in patients with implantable cardioverter-defibrillators with ischemic cardiomyopathy versus nonischemic cardiomyopathy at 33-month follow-up. *Archives of Medical Science.* 2010;6(6):900–3.
110. Tsai FS, Aronow WS, Devabhaktuni S, Desai H, Kruger A, Lai HM, et al. Prevalence of complications during implantation and during 38-month follow-up of 1060 consecutive patients with implantable cardioverter-defibrillators. *American Journal of Therapeutics.* 2010;17(1):e8–e10.
111. Swerdlow CD, Gunderson BD, Ousdigian KT, Abeyratne A, Stadler RW, Gillberg JM, et al. Downloadable algorithm to reduce inappropriate shocks caused by fractures of implantable cardioverter-defibrillator leads. *Circulation.* 2008;118(21):2122–9.
112. Rienstra M, Smit MD, Nieuwland W, Tan ES, Wiesfeld ACP, Anthonio RL, et al. Persistent atrial fibrillation is associated with appropriate shocks and heart failure in patients with left ventricular dysfunction treated with an implantable cardioverter defibrillator. *American Heart Journal.* 2007;153(1):120–6.
113. Daubert JP, Zareba W, Cannom DS, McNitt S, Rosero SZ, Wang P, et al. Inappropriate implantable cardioverter-defibrillator shocks in MADIT II. *Journal of the American College of Cardiology.* 2008;51(14):1357–65.
114. Santini M, Gasparini M, Landolina M, Lunati M, Proclemer A, Padeletti L, et al. Device-detected

atrial tachyarrhythmias predict adverse outcome in real-world patients with implantable biventricular defibrillators. *Journal of the American College of Cardiology*. 2011;57(2):167–72.
115. Hager CS, Jain S, Blackwell J, Culp B, Song J, Chiles CD. Effect of renal function on survival after implantable cardioverter defibrillator placement. *The American Journal of Cardiology*. 2010;106(9):1297–300.
116. Mainigi SK, Almuti K, Figueredo VM, Guttenplan NA, Aouthmany A, Smukler J, et al. Usefulness of radiofrequency ablation of supraventricular tachycardia to decrease inappropriate shocks from implantable cardioverter–defibrillators. *The American Journal of Cardiology*. 2012;109(2):231–7.
117. Wilkoff BL, Cook JR, Epstein AE, Greene HL, Hallstrom AP, Hsia H, et al. Dual-chamber pacing or ventricular backup pacing in patients with an implantable defibrillator: the Dual Chamber and VVI Implantable Defibrillator (DAVID) trial. *JAMA*. 2002;288(24):3115–23.
118. Sukhija R, Aronow WS, Sorbera C, Kakar P, Peterson SJ, Frishman WH, et al. Left ventricular ejection fraction and prevalence of new left ventricular wall motion abnormality at long-term follow-up in patients with automatic implantable cardioverter-defibrillators treated with dual-chamber rate-responsive pacing at a rate of 70/minute versus backup ventricular pacing at a rate of 40/minute. *The American Journal of Cardiology*. 2005;96(3):412–3.
119. Sukhija R, Aronow WS, Sorbera C, Peterson SJ, Frishman WH, Cohen M. Mortality, Left ventricular ejection fraction, and prevalence of new left ventricular wall motion abnormality at long-term follow-up in patients with implantable cardioverter defibrillators treated with biventricular pacing versus right ventricular pacing. *American Journal of Therapeutics*. 2007;14(4):328–30.
120. Sukhija R, Aronow WS, Sorbera C, Yalamanchili K, Cohen M. Patients, mean age 70 years, with automatic implantable cardioverter-defibrillators treated with dual-chamber rate responsive pacing (DDDR-70) have a higher mortality than patients with backup ventricular pacing (VVI-40) at 3.7-year follow-up. *The Journals of Gerontology Series A: Biological Sciences and Medical Sciences*. 2005;60(5):603–4.
121. Schwartz PJ, Locati EH, Moss AJ, Crampton RS, Trazzi R, Ruberti U. Left cardiac sympathetic denervation in the therapy of congenital long QT syndrome. A worldwide report. *Circulation*. 1991;84(2):503–11.
122. Hayase J, Patel J, Narayan SM, Krummen DE. Percutaneous stellate ganglion block suppressing VT and VF in a patient refractory to VT ablation. *Journal of Cardiovascular Electrophysiology*. 2013;24(8):926–8.
123. Vaseghi M, Gima J, Kanaan C, Ajijola OA, Marmureanu A, Mahajan A, et al. Cardiac sympathetic denervation in patients with refractory ventricular arrhythmias or electrical storm: intermediate and long-term follow-up. *Heart Rhythm*. 2014;11(3):360–6.
124. Ukena C, Bauer A, Mahfoud F, Schreieck J, Neuberger H-R, Eick C, et al. Renal sympathetic denervation for treatment of electrical storm: first-in-man experience. *Clinical Research in Cardiology*. 2011;101(1):63–7.
125. Hoffmann BA, Steven D, Willems S, Sydow K. Renal sympathetic denervation as an adjunct to catheter ablation for the treatment of ventricular electrical storm in the setting of acute myocardial infarction. *Journal of Cardiovascular Electrophysiology*. 2013;24(10):1175–8.
126. Remo BF, Preminger M, Bradfield J, Mittal S, Boyle N, Gupta A, et al. Safety and efficacy of renal denervation as a novel treatment of ventricular tachycardia storm in patients with cardiomyopathy. *Heart Rhythm*. 2014;11(4):541–6.
127. Bhatt DL, Kandzari DE, O'Neill WW, D'Agostino R, Flack JM, Katzen BT, et al. A controlled trial of renal denervation for resistant hypertension. *New England Journal of Medicine*. 2014;370(15):1393–401.
128. Bhatt DL, Vaduganathan M, Kandzari DE, Leon MB, Rocha-Singh K, Townsend RR, et al. Long-term outcomes after catheter-based renal artery denervation for resistant hypertension: final follow-up of the randomised SYMPLICITY HTN-3 trial. *Lancet*. 2022;400(10361):1405–16.
129. Azizi M, Saxena M, Wang Y, Jenkins JS, Devireddy C, Rader F, et al. Endovascular ultrasound renal denervation to treat hypertension: the RADIANCE II randomized clinical trial. *JAMA*. 2023;329(8):651–61.
130. Grimaldi R, de Luca A, Kornet L, Castagno D, Gaita F. Can spinal cord stimulation reduce ventricular arrhythmias? *Heart Rhythm*. 2012;9(11):1884–7.
131. Miszczyk M, Hoeksema WF, Kuna K, Blamek S, Cuculich PS, Grehn M, et al. Stereotactic arrhythmia radioablation (STAR)-A systematic review and meta-analysis of prospective trials on behalf of the STOPSTORM.eu consortium. *Europace*. 2023;25(1):1–10. (1556–3871 (Electronic)).
132. Cuculich PS, Schill MR, Kashani R, Mutic S, Lang A, Cooper D, et al. Noninvasive Cardiac Radiation for Ablation of Ventricular Tachycardia. *New England Journal of Medicine*. 2017;377(24):2325–36. (1533–4406 (Electronic)).
133. Ninni SA-O, Gallot-Lavallée TA-O, Klein C, Longère BA-O, Brigadeau F, Potelle C, et al. Stereotactic radioablation for ventricular tachycardia in the setting of electrical storm. *Circulation: Arrhythmia and*

Electrophysiology. 2022;15(9):e010955. (1941–3084 (Electronic)).

134. Kim EJ, Davogustto G, Stevenson WG, John RM. Non-invasive cardiac radiation for ablation of ventricular tachycardia: a new therapeutic paradigm in electrophysiology. *Arrhythmia & Electrophysiology Review.* 2018;7(1):8–10. (2050–3369 (Print)).
135. Cellini F, Narducci ML, Pavone C, Bencardino G, Perna F, Pinnacchio G, et al. Ventricular tachycardia ablation through radiation therapy (VT-ART) consortium: concept description of an observational multicentric trial via matched pair analysis. *Frontiers in Cardiovascular Medicine.* 2023;10:1020966. (2297–055X (Print)).
136. RADIATE-VT. *Randomized Study to Evaluate the Safety and Effectiveness of Stereotactic Body Radiation Therapy in Patients With Recurrent VT Post-Catheter Ablation.* U.S. National Library of Medicine; 2023. https://clinicaltrials.gov/ct2/show/NCT05765175.

23

Bradyarrhythmias and cardiac pacemakers in the elderly

MICHAEL LIU AND WIN-KUANG SHEN

Key points

- The incidence of bradyarrhythmias is high among older patients.
- Pacemakers have been proven to improve the quality of life and reduce symptoms of patients affected by sinus node dysfunction, AV block, and carotid sinus syndrome.
- Physiologic pacing reduces long-term adverse consequences from the conventional RV apical pacing. Many randomized clinical trials are ongoing, including those for the older population. It is anticipated that physiologic pacing will become the standard as techniques and technologies advance.
- Deactivation of pacemakers near the end of life should be discussed with older patients and their families.

INTRODUCTION

The aging population in North America has grown exponentially over the past several decades. The US Census Bureau 2020 estimated that 16.8% of the US population was older than 65, with a growth rate of 38.6%, the fastest of any decade from 1880 to 1890 and more than twice as fast as the previous decade [1]. The need for pacemaker implantation is highly prevalent among older adults, with a mean age at implant of 75 ± 12 years [2].

Sinus node dysfunction (SND) is the leading cause of bradyarrhythmias requiring pacing in the US, followed by atrioventricular (AV) conduction disorders and hypersensitivity of the carotid sinus [3]. The use of pacing for the treatment of neurocardiogenic syncope is still controversial, especially in younger patients (<40 years of age), and its indication is much less frequent.

SINUS NODE DYSFUNCTION

SND, also known as sick sinus syndrome (SSS), is a sinoatrial node disorder that generates an appropriate heart rate to meet one's physiologic needs. It is the most common cause of bradyarrhythmia requiring pacing, and it is predominant among elderly patients [4]. The average age of patients at the time of diagnosis of SND is 74 years, with equal distribution between men and women [5].

The most common cause of SND in older patients is idiopathic degeneration of the sinus node, with fibrotic infiltration on histology. The causes of SND are summarized in Table 23.1 [6–8].

DOI: 10.1201/9781003568933-23

Table 23.1 Causes of sinus node dysfunction (SND)

Intrinsic SND	Extrinsic SND
• Cardiomyopathy • Long-standing hypertension infiltrative disease (e.g., amyloidosis and sarcoidosis) • Inflammation o Collagen vascular disease o Rheumatic fever • Surgical trauma • Orthotropic cardiac transplantation with atrial–atrial anastomosis • Congenital heart disease (e.g., sinus venosus and secundum atrial septal defects) • Genetic defects o Musculoskeletal disorders (e.g., myotonic dystrophy and Friedreich ataxia) o Familial SSS (SCN5A gene, HCN4 gene, KCNQ1 gene, CJA5 gene, ANK2 gene, or EMD gene) • Infection o Viral myocarditis o Lyme disease • Pericardial disease (e.g., pericarditis or tumor)	• Drugs o Antiarrhythmic agents (Class IC, Class II, Class III, and Class IV) o Cardiac glycosides o Antihypertensive agents (e.g., clonidine, reserpine, and methyldopa) o Antipsychotic agents (e.g., lithium, phenothiazines, and amitriptyline) • Autonomically mediated, vagal stimulation, and hypervagotonia o Vasovagal syncope (cardioinhibitory) o Carotid sinus hypersensitivity o Valsalva maneuvers o Endotracheal intubation and suction o Vomiting o Trained athletes • Hypothyroidism • Intracranial hypertension (Cushing response) • Electrolytes imbalance (e.g., hyperkalemia) • Hypothermia • Hypoxia • Sleep apnea • Hypercapnia • Advanced liver disease • Infection (e.g., typhoid fever, brucellosis, and sepsis)

Electrocardiographic findings of sinus node dysfunction

A wide range of electrocardiographic findings can be seen in SND.

Sinus bradycardia is defined as a heart rate below 60 beats per minute (bpm). Modest sinus bradycardia, defined by heart rates of 40–59 bpm, can be seen in athletes and healthy nonathletic older adults due to a physiologic increase in vagal tone. However, a sinus rate below 40 bpm is most likely pathological [6].

Sinoatrial (SA) exit block is defined as the inability to propagate impulses generated in the sinus node to adjacent atrial tissue. In these situations, the sinus node impulse formation is appropriate, but the failure to conduct the impulse to atrial tissue results in various degrees of sinus pauses, including sinus arrest. SA exit block, similar to AV block, is classified into three types: first-degree, second-degree, and third-degree exit block. **First-degree SA exit block** can present as a simple slowing of conduction to the atria but with preserved 1:1 conduction. In other words, every impulse generated at the level of the sinus node will have a delayed conduction to atrial tissue with no real block. The conventional ECG cannot recognize this form of SA block because the heart rate is preserved. **Second-degree SA exit block** is characterized by intermittent failure of the sinus impulse to exit the sinus node. **The second-degree type I block** happens because of Wenckebach periodicity at the SA junction, leading to the progressive prolongation of conduction time from the sinus node to the atrial tissue and ultimately resulting in a conduction block. The SA conduction is then restored, repeating the same cycle of progressive prolongation of conduction time, as described before. The ECG representation of sinoatrial Wenckebach is repetitive group beating, characterized by progressive shortening of the PP interval, followed by a sinus pause (blocked SA impulse); the pauses in this type of block typically are less than twice the shortest sinus cycle (Figure 23.1a). With **second-degree type II block**, there is intermittent and abrupt failure of the impulse to exit the sinus node without incremental progression in the sinoatrial conduction time. This phenomenon can be intermittent, and it will manifest as episodic sinus pauses with a specific feature: the PP interval that encompasses the pause will be exactly twice as long or multiples (3×, 4×, etc.) of the PP interval during normal sinus rhythm (Figure 23.1b). **Third-degree or complete SA exit block** marks the absence of SA conduction, leading to sinus pause or atrial asystole. This ECG feature does not allow differentiation between complete SA exit block and primary failure of sinus node impulse formation.

Sinus arrest is seen because of cessation of impulse formation within the sinus node. The pause is not an exact multiple of the preceding PP interval.

Chronotropic incompetence is the inability of the heart rate (HR) to increase with increased activity or demand. The definition of chronotropic response is relatively ambiguous, but the inability to achieve ≥85% of age-predicted maximum HR during maximal exercise testing has been considered chronotropic incompetence

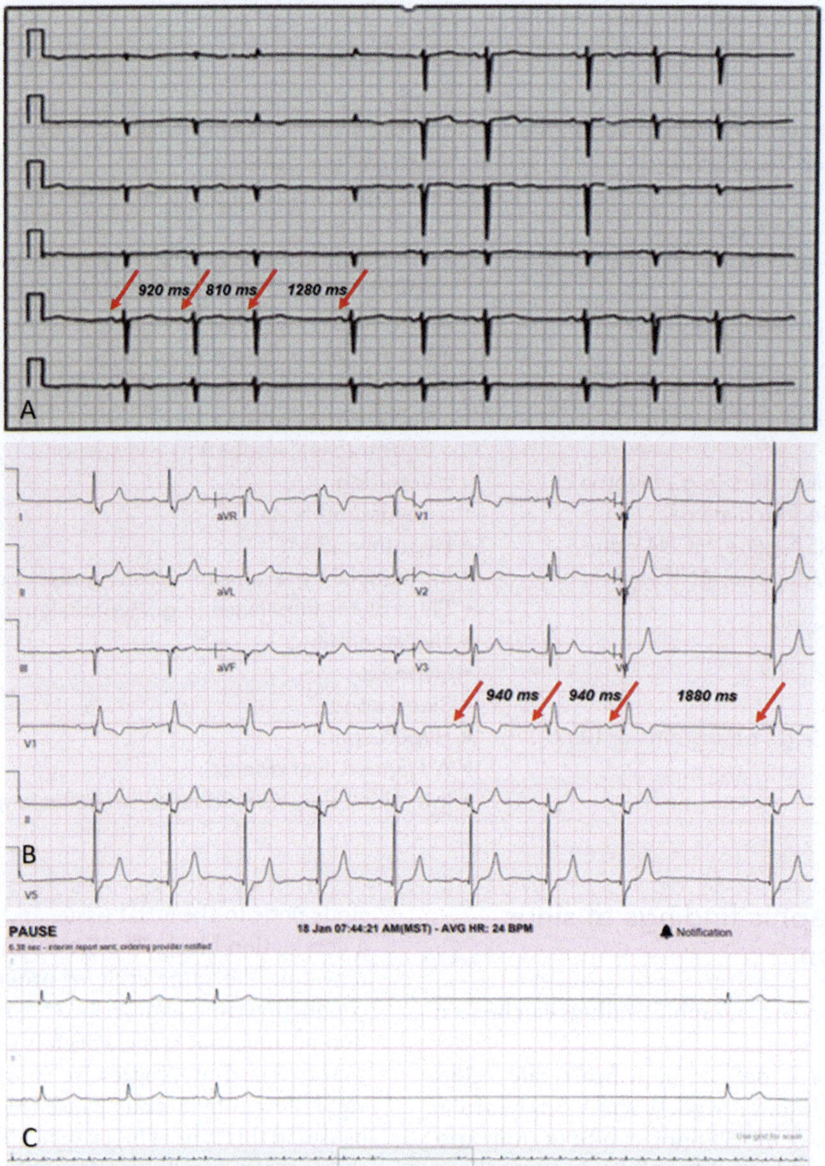

Figure 23.1 Second-degree SA exit block. (a) Type I block. Notice repetitive group beating, characterized by progressive shortening of the PP interval, followed by a sinus pause that is less than twice the sinus cycle length. (b) Type II block. Notice the pause is twice the sinus cycle length. (c) Sinus pause of 6 seconds.

[8]. Revised formulas for more precise determination of age-predicted maximal HR in healthy adults (208 – 0.7 × Age), in women (206 – 0.88 × Age), and in patients with coronary artery disease (CAD) (164 – 0.72 × Age) have been proposed. For patients taking beta-blockers, a value ≤62% of age-predicted maximal HR is significant. Since baseline functional capacity and resting HR have a bearing on chronotropic responses, an alternative approach to determine chronotropic incompetence has been proposed using the percent of heart rate reserve (HRR):

% HRR = [(HR achieved – HR rest) / (220 – Age – HR rest)] × 100

A proportional HR reserve of ≤80% has been used to define significant chronotropic incompetence [9, 10].

Because of the complexities of these assessments, individualized clinical evaluation is the best approach for this form of SND. In clinical practice, the inability to reach more than 70% of the maximum predicted rate during exertion or the inability to achieve HR above 90 bpm has been used as an indicator of chronotropic incompetence.

Tachycardia–bradycardia syndrome is characterized by periods of significant sinus or junctional bradycardia, alternating with episodes of atrial tachyarrhythmia, most commonly paroxysmal atrial fibrillation (AF) or atrial flutter. It is common to observe marked bradycardia immediately after termination of episodes of tachycardia, which can be associated with presyncope or syncope.

Atrial quiescence is a rare condition with no spontaneous atrial rhythm and should be differentiated from low-voltage P waves. This can sometimes occur after surgery, such as the MAZE procedure for atrial fibrillation.

Natural history of sinus node dysfunction

The natural history of SND is variable. It is frequently associated with the development of AV block and/or AF [11]. Development of AV block occurs at a rate of 1.7%/year among patients with SND and 8.5% over 5 years, with a significant increase to 35% in the same period if bundle branch block or bifascicular block was present at initial evaluation [12]. The prevalence of AF varies from 40% to 70% at the time of diagnosis of SND. For people without a history of AF at the initial presentation, 4%–22% will develop it during long-term follow-up [11]. SND does not significantly impact survival (see Figure 23.2) [13]. The incidence of sudden death is very low among patients with isolated SND [14]. A longitudinal study with 30 years of follow-up found that patients with pacemakers for SND had higher survival than AV block, which in turn had higher survival than atrial fibrillation [15]. Interestingly, that same study found a higher survival in women than men (Table 23.2).

Evaluation of sinus node dysfunction

The diagnosis of SND requires documentation of sinus bradycardia, sinus node pauses, or chronotropic incompetence during physical activity. ECG and Holter monitors are useful in documenting frequent or persistent episodes. Transient or reversible causes such as drug effects, especially beta-blockers, and electrolyte or endocrinologic abnormalities must be excluded. An ambulatory event recorder or implantable loop recorder can be considered when clinical episodes are intermittent or infrequent. A treadmill or cycle exercise test is helpful in evaluating the response of sinus rate to exercise in patients with chronotropic incompetence. Invasive electrophysiology study is no longer routinely recommended for diagnosis of SND due to its low sensitivity and specificity. The inability to correlate symptoms to sinus node abnormalities induced by programmed stimulation is another limitation of electrophysiologic studies for evaluating SND.

INDICATION FOR PACING

The AHA/ACC/HRS guidelines for pacing in patients with sinus node dysfunction were updated in 2018 [16]. The ESC guidelines were updated in 2021 [17]. The key indications for pacing in patients with sinus node dysfunction, AV block, and carotid sinus syndrome are summarized in Table 23.3. For SND, there is a Class I recommendation for pacing when there are symptoms directly attributable to SND or when there is symptomatic sinus bradycardia from required drug therapy for medical conditions. There is a Class IIa recommendation for pacing in tachycardia–bradycardia syndrome and symptomatic chronotropic incompetence. Without reversible causes, permanent pacemaker implantation is the only available treatment for SND. Several pacing modes are available for this condition, including single atrial lead or dual-chamber pacemaker. A single right atrial (RA) lead is a reasonable option if the AV conduction system is intact. However, elderly patients are likely to have some degree of conduction system disease, such as bundle branch block, or are at risk of developing AV block in the future, so most elderly patients are recommended to receive a dual-chamber pacemaker. Rate-adaptive pacing is available in most implantable devices and can be activated in cases of symptomatic chronotropic insufficiency.

ATRIOVENTRICULAR BLOCK

Atrioventricular (AV) block is a pathological conduction of an atrial impulse to the ventricles. The AV block can be defined based on the ECG characteristics into first-degree,

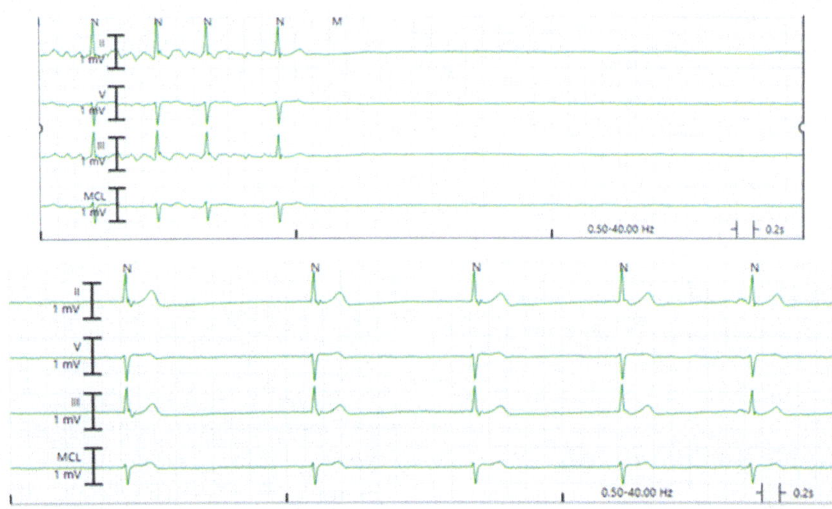

Figure 23.2 Tachycardia–bradycardia syndrome (from top to bottom). The telemetry strip shows the termination of atrial fibrillation, followed by post-conversion pauses. The continuous telemetry strip showed a junctional rhythm with a gradual return of sinus bradycardia.

Table 23.2 Survival rate after pacemaker implantation of patients with sick sinus syndrome compared to atrioventricular block and atrial fibrillation as well as male versus female gender

	5-year survival	10-year survival	15-year survival	20-year survival
Overall	65.5%	44.8%	30.8%	21.4%
SSS	73.5%	53.5%	38.9%	26.6%
AVB	62.0%	41.1%	28.1%	19.2%
AFIB	58.6%	38.3%	22.3%	14.9%
Male gender	61.4%	40.4%	26.8%	16.8%
Female gender	70.1%	49.5%	34.8%	25.5%

Source: Adapted from Brunner, M., et al., *Eur Heart J*, 25(1), 88–95, 2004.
Abbreviations: SSS, sick sinus syndrome; AVB, high-degree AV block; AFIB, bradycardic atrial fibrillation.

Table 23.3 AHA/ACC/HRS guidelines for device-based therapy of cardiac rhythm abnormalities

Class of recommendation	Sinus node dysfunction	Atrioventricular block	Carotid sinus syndrome
Class I	• Symptoms directly attributable to SND (Level of Evidence: C) • Symptomatic sinus bradycardia that results from required drug therapy for medical conditions (Level of Evidence: C)	• Second-degree Mobitz II AV block, high-grade AV block, or third-degree AV block not attributable to reversible of physiologic causes (Level of Evidence: B) • Permanent AF and symptomatic bradycardia (Level of Evidence: C) • Symptomatic AV block as a consequence of guideline-directed management (Level of Evidence: C)	• Recurrent syncope caused by spontaneously occurring carotid sinus stimulation and carotid sinus pressure that induces ventricular asystole of more than 3 seconds (Level of Evidence: C)
Class IIa	• Tachy-brady syndrome and symptoms related to bradycardia • Symptomatic chronotropic incompetence	• Patients with infiltrative cardiomyopathy and second-degree Mobitz II AV block, high-grade AV block, or third-degree AV block (Level of Evidence: B) • Patients with symptoms from marked first-degree or second-degree Mobitz I AV block (Level of Evidence: C)	• Syncope without clear, provocative events and with a hypersensitive cardioinhibitory response of 3 seconds or longer (Level of Evidence: C)
Class IIb indication: Permanent pacemaker implantation may be considered	• For patients with symptoms likely attributable to SND, a trial of oral theophylline may be considered to help determine the potential effects of permanent pacing	• Neuromuscular disease with PR >240 ms, QRS >120 ms, fascicular block (Level of Evidence: C)	• Significantly symptomatic neuro cardiogenic syncope associated with bradycardia documented spontaneously or at the time of tilt table testing (Level of Evidence: B)

second-degree, 2:1, high-grade, and complete AV block. A patient can exhibit different degrees of AV block at various times and under different pathophysiological conditions. Causes of AV block are summarized in Table 23.4 [6, 18, 19].

Electrocardiographic evaluation of atrioventricular block

First-degree AV block refers to a prolongation in AV conduction but with consistent conduction of atrial impulse to ventricles, excluding premature atrial beats. On the ECG, normal sinus P waves are followed by QRS complexes but with a PR interval that exceeds 0.20 seconds (Figure 23.3a). A narrow QRS usually indicates disease in the AV node, but a first-degree AV block with a widened QRS morphology usually suggests a conduction delay in the His–Purkinje system with or without a delay in the AV node (35). Normal QRS duration, very long PR interval (more than 0.3 seconds), and highly variable PR interval are features of AVN conduction delay.

Second-degree AV block is manifested by intermittent lack of conduction from the atria to the ventricles.

Table 23.4 Causes of AV block

1. Acquired
Drugs
• Digoxin
• Beta-blockers
• Calcium channel blockers
• Class I and III antiarrhythmic
Acute myocardial infarction
Chronic ischemic heart disease
Degenerative disease (e.g., Lev disease or Lenègre disease)
Calcific valve disease (aortic stenosis and mitral annulus calcification)
Rheumatic disease
Infiltrative disease (e.g., amyloidosis, sarcoidosis, and hemochromatosis)
Tumors (e.g., mesothelioma, rhabdomyoma, Hodgkin's lymphoma, and melanoma)
Neuromyopathies (Becker muscular dystrophy, peroneal muscular dystrophy, Kearns–Sayre syndrome, Erb dystrophy, and myotonic muscular dystrophy)
Infectious disease: Infective endocarditis and myocarditis of various viral, bacterial, and parasitic causes (including Lyme disease, rheumatic fever, Chagas disease, tuberculosis, measles, rickettsia, Aspergillus, and mumps)
Iatrogenic
• Cardiac surgery
• Intracardiac catheter manipulation
• Alcohol septal ablation
• Catheter ablation
• Radiation
Autonomically mediated, vagal stimulation, and hypervagotonia
• Vasovagal syncope (cardioinhibitory)
• Carotid sinus hypersensitivity
• Valsalva maneuvers
• Endotracheal intubation and suction
• Vomiting
• Trained athletes
Autoimmune disorder (e.g., ankylosing spondylitis HLA-B27, systemic sclerosis, Sjögren's syndrome, systemic lupus erythrocytosis, Wegener's granulomatosis, and Behçet's disease)
Metabolic (e.g., hyperkalemia, hypermagnesemia, and Addison's disease)
2. Congenital AV block
3. Genetic
(e.g., SCN5A, KCNJ2, TRPM4, GJA5, DES, PRKAG2, DMPK, BMP2 TBX5, NKX2-5, LMNA, and EMD)

Mobitz type I second-degree AV block (Wenckebach block) gradually prolongs PR intervals in successive beats until a P wave is blocked for one beat. Other features of typical Wenckebach AV block include lengthening of the PR interval at progressively decreasing increments, with the greatest increase in PR interval noted in the second beat of the cycle, resulting in progressively shorter RR intervals and a grouped beating pattern (Figure 23.3b). Mobitz type I block is usually considered benign and does not require permanent pacing unless symptoms are correlated to the bradycardia. **Mobitz type II second-degree AV block** usually involves disease below the AV node and produces a P wave with a dropped QRS without prior prolongation of the PR interval. Type II AV block usually occurs in the presence of a bundle branch block and is almost always caused by a block below the AV node. It requires permanent pacing due to the high risk of developing a complete heart block (Figure 23.3c).

A **2:1 atrioventricular block** is a form of second-degree AV block in which every other P wave does not produce a QRS, making it challenging to determine whether it is Mobitz I or Mobitz II (Figure 23.3d). The following features help in the differential diagnosis: (1) A 2:1 AV block pattern with normal QRS duration or a very long PR interval (more than 0.3 seconds) generally suggests the block in the AV node. (2) A short PR interval (less than 0.16 seconds) or the presence of bundle branch block favors block below the AV node. (3) Carotid sinus stimulation may worsen the degree of block in the AV node, whereas slowing the sinus rate may paradoxically improve the ratio of AV conduction and increase the ventricular rate if the block is located below the AV node. (4) Exercise or atropine can improve AV nodal conduction but may worsen AV conduction in patients with infranodal block (Figure 23.3d).

A **high-grade AV block** involves two or more consecutive P waves that fail to conduct to the ventricles. It may resemble a complete heart block, but the RR intervals are irregular due to intermittent AV conduction.

Third-degree or complete AV block (CHB) is characterized by total failure of all atrial impulses to conduct to the ventricles. The ECG during CHB usually exhibits four features: (1) nonconducted P waves, with continuously changing PR relationship, (2) AV dissociation, (3) a regular ventricular response produced by the escape rhythm, and (4) an atrial rate higher than the ventricular

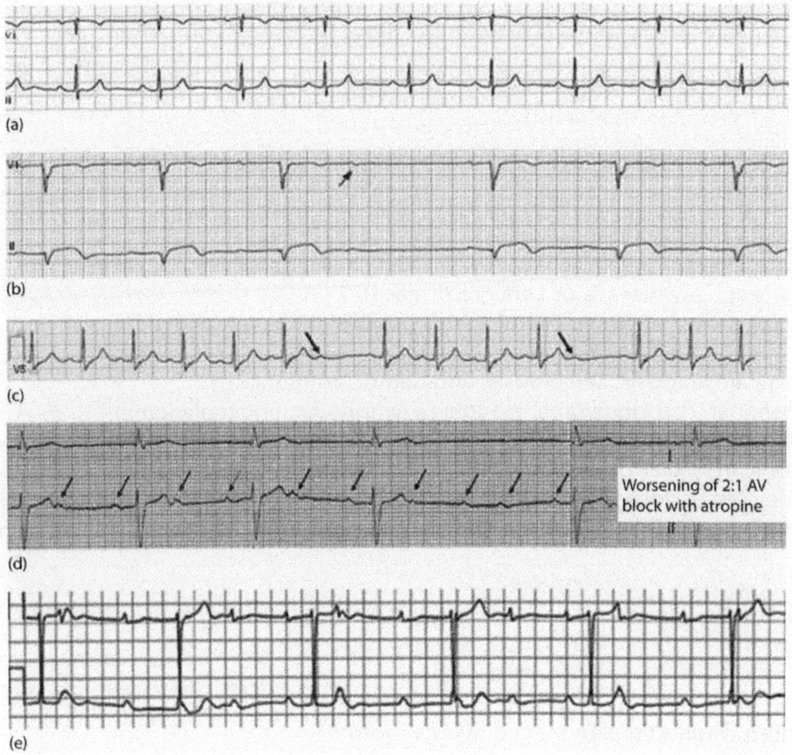

Figure 23.3 AV block examples. (a) First-degree AV block. Notice prolonged PR interval (more than 0.2 seconds but with 1:1 AV conduction). (b) Second-degree AV block, Mobitz I. Notice progressive prolongation of the PR interval followed by a blocked P wave (arrow). (c) Second-degree AV block, Mobitz II. The PR interval is constant if AV conduction is present with intermittent AV block (arrows). (d) 2:1 AV block. Notice the worsening of AV conduction with atropine, indicating His–Purkinje block. (e) Complete AV block. Complete dissociation between P waves and QRS complexes.

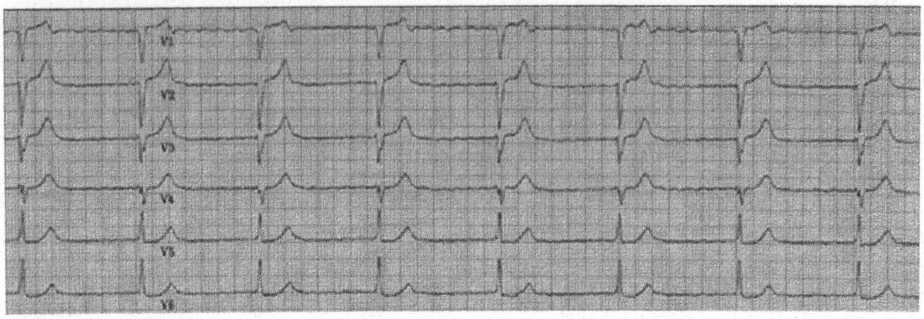

Figure 23.4 Atrial fibrillation with junctional rhythm.

rate and the P waves march through all phases of the ventricular cycle (Figure 23.3e). Regular RR intervals can identify a complete heart block in atrial fibrillation (Figure 23.4).

NATURAL HISTORY OF AV BLOCK

The natural history of AV block depends on the block type and whether the cause is reversible. First-degree AV block and Mobitz I second-degree AV block are considered benign and usually do not progress to higher degrees of block. Mobitz II second-degree AV block has a higher risk of progression to complete heart block. With a complete heart block that is not reversible, the risk of sudden cardiac death is 25% [20].

EVALUATION FOR AV BLOCK

Diagnosing an AV block requires ECG and/or cardiac monitoring, which shows documentation of Mobitz II second-degree AV block, third-degree AV block, or high-grade AV block. If there is Mobitz I second-degree AV block, there must be a correlation of symptoms to warrant pacemaker placement. Transient or reversible causes such as drug effects, especially beta-blockers, and electrolyte or endocrinologic abnormalities need to be excluded.

Current guidelines for pacing therapy in AV block

The ACC, AHA, and HRS jointly developed the current guidelines for pacemaker implantation [16, 21]. The recommendations for pacing in AV block are detailed in Table 23.3.

There is a Class I indication for pacing in second-degree Mobitz II AV block, high-grade AV block, or third-degree AV block without a reversible cause. There is a Class I indication for pacing in permanent atrial fibrillation and symptomatic bradycardia. There is a Class I indication for pacing in symptomatic AV block as a consequence of necessary guideline-directed medical therapy. There is a Class IIa recommendation for permanent pacing in patients with symptoms attributed to first-degree AV block and Mobitz I second-degree AV block.

CAROTID SINUS HYPERSENSITIVITY

Carotid sinus hypersensitivity (CSH) is an exacerbation of the carotid sinus reflex leading to vagal activation or sympathetic inhibition, with consequent bradycardia and/or hypotension. This condition is commonly seen in the elderly population. When CSH is associated with syncope or presyncope, it defines carotid sinus syndrome (CSS) [22]. This syndrome is responsible for up to 10%–25% of syncopal events in the elderly [23]. Syncope is a classic presentation of CSS. However, only a small proportion will have the classic presentation of symptoms during manipulation of the neck/carotid sinus region, representing less than 1% of all cases of syncope [24]. More commonly, patients will present with complaints of unexplained syncope without a clear trigger, and further tests will reveal the presence of CSH. Up to 37% of patients with CSS will present with dizziness and recurrent falls. These falls can be secondary to syncope, but some patients, especially at an advanced age, will not notice the loss of consciousness, either because it was too brief or because they do not recollect the symptoms preceding the event of the fall [25].

Evaluation and diagnosis of carotid sinus syndrome

Carotid sinus massage (CSM) can induce a physiologic response with bradycardia associated with mild hypotension, especially in people older than 40 years of age. The diagnostic criteria for CSH have been standardized as a pause of 3 seconds (cardioinhibitory response) and/or >50 mmHg drop in systolic blood pressure (vasodepressor response) in response to 3–5 seconds of CSM [26]. It is classified as a mixed response when both criteria are met. The CSM should be performed on both sides, along with beat-to-beat blood pressure and HR monitoring. If no abnormal response is detected while the patient is supine, the maneuver should be repeated upright (commonly done during a tilt table test, with the table inclined at 70 degrees). Up to 30% of patients will only have a positive CSM test in the upright position [18]. The CSM is considered positive only if the test reproduces the clinical symptoms. Up to 10% of the asymptomatic population can have a pronounced physiologic response to CSM, meeting the described criteria for CSH, without relevant clinical significance as in patients with CSS [25].

CSM is considered safe, even in elderly patients. The neurologic complication rate is between 0.28% and 0.45% [25]. This test, however, should not be performed in patients with carotid bruits, prior history of transient ischemic attack (TIA), stroke, or myocardial infarction in the past 3 months, except if carotid Doppler excludes significant stenosis [26].

Atropine can be used to differentiate mixed responses to CSM from hypotension secondary to prolonged bradycardia in cases of cardioinhibitory response. In a mixed response, atropine will prevent the induction of bradycardia during CSM when hypotension persists. In patients with cardioinhibitory response, hypotension subsides when bradycardia is prevented after atropine administration.

Carotid sinus syndrome treatment

Despite the high prevalence of CSS in the elderly population, there is limited data on ideal treatment for this condition. Medical therapy with anticholinergic drugs, fludrocortisone, beta-blockers, and serotonin reuptake inhibitors is potentially an option for the treatment of CSS, but the data are limited to small series and case reports.

Several randomized studies have shown that pacing reduces the rate of syncope, falls, and incidence of injury related to falls in patients with CSH [27–29]. However, it is essential to mention that most of these studies were small and unblinded. Up to 15% of patients will continue to present with recurrent syncope, and up to 50% will continue to report symptoms of dizziness and orthostatic hypotension after pacemaker implantation [25].

DDD pacing with rate-drop response was initially developed to treat patients with reflex syncope. Once a sudden drop in HR is detected, the pacemaker is programmed to intervene at a higher rate temporarily to increase cardiac output and compensate for possible hypotension associated with these events. The evidence of incremental benefit from the rate-drop response in patients with CSS is limited. McLeod et al. could not demonstrate the superiority of any pacing mode in elderly patients with CSS without other indications for pacing [23]. It is likely due to low event rates with infrequent episodes of CSH-mediated bradycardia in patients without other coexisting SND or AV conduction abnormalities.

Contemporary and advancing pacing methods and technology

LEADLESS PACEMAKERS

Leadless pacemaker systems were conceptualized several decades ago, and the first system, which contained a venous catheter implanted in leadless pacemakers in animals, was published in 1970 [30]. Leadless pacemakers can decrease lead- and pocket-related complications seen with conventional transvenous pacemakers. Leadless pacemakers are suitable for patients who meet indications for single-chamber right ventricular pacing, such as permanent AF with AV block or frequent pauses. Leadless dual-chamber pacemakers were recently approved for clinical use to preserve AV synchrony. These pacemakers are self-contained devices implanted by the femoral percutaneous approach. The reported successful implant rate is above 95%. The leadless ventricular pacemaker provides VVIR pacing mode, and long-term follow-up observations show good device performance with stable pacing threshold and impedance and no device-related complications [31–33]. The long-term follow-up experience from dual-chamber leadless pacemakers is limited.

The complication rate is comparable to conventional transvenous pacemakers; however, the nature of complications is not the same. Overall, based on indirect comparisons with historical cohorts, leadless pacemakers are associated with a reduced risk of pneumothorax, subclavian vein thrombosis or occlusion, lead-related complications such as dislodgement or fracture, and pocket hematoma. However, there is an increased risk of femoral vein complications and cardiac perforation. The risk of infection in the leadless pacemaker is exceedingly low [31–33].

Contemporary pacing methods

Dual-chamber pacemakers traditionally have involved a lead in the right atrium, specifically in the right atrial appendage, and the right ventricle, specifically at the apex. Procedural expertise in this method of pacemaker implantation leads to shorter procedural times, less use of fluoroscopy, and less use of intravenous contrast, which can be beneficial for elderly patients with comorbidities who may not tolerate more prolonged procedures or contrast exposure. However, the risks of RV apical pacing are well known. Chronic RV pacing can lead to pacing-induced cardiomyopathy, characterized by a decline in ejection fraction and heart failure symptoms when other causes of heart failure have been ruled out. The mechanism of pacing-induced cardiomyopathy has been attributed to mechanical and electrical dyssynchrony, as the right ventricle is activated first, with the left ventricle activated by myocyte-to-myocyte conduction rather than efficient activation through the conduction system [34].

The term "physiologic pacing" was clarified in the most recent HRS/APHRS/LAHRS guidelines (2023). Briefly, it is defined as pacing methods that restore or preserve ventricular synchrony (as opposed to conventional RV pacing). Physiologic methods include cardiac resynchronization therapy (CRT, or biventricular pacing) and conduction system pacing (CSP). CSP includes His bundle pacing (HBP) and left bundle branch area pacing (LBBAP). A summary of these contemporary pacing methodologies, clinical indications, and pros and cons will be provided. The guidelines apply to patients of all ages with established pacing indications, including the elderly patient population.

Biventricular pacing (cardiac resynchronization therapy)

Biventricular pacing is characterized by simultaneous or near-simultaneous pacing of both the left and right ventricles to avoid the problem of dyssynchrony with RV pacing. Biventricular pacing, or CRT, can be accomplished with a traditional RV lead (or a defibrillator lead) and a coronary sinus lead to pace the left ventricle. The indications of CRT are for patients with heart failure with reduced ejection fraction of ≤35% and wide QRS, particularly with left bundle branch block [35]. Selected patients may benefit from CRT if the expected pacing burden is expected to be high (20%–40%) with mildly to moderately reduced ejection fraction (EF 36%–50%) or if they have developed pacing-induced cardiomyopathy [35]. Achieving CRT involves locating an optimal branch of the coronary sinus, which is typically done under fluoroscopic guidance and utilization of intravenous contrast. This can lead to longer procedure times and more contrast exposure, which are considerations with older patients, especially if they have chronic kidney disease.

Conduction system pacing

Conduction system pacing seeks to avoid the risks of RV pacing with a single pacemaker lead that captures the His–Purkinje conduction system, which is more physiologic than pacing at the RV apex [36]. One solution is to pace the His bundle, but this pacing method is less frequently used currently for several reasons. Procedural times can be longer due to the technical challenges of locating and placing the lead at the bundle of His [37–39]. High capture thresholds can lead to early battery depletion [38, 40, 41]. The lead can be unstable and have a higher risk of lead dislodgment, requiring revision [41]. As the lead is located close to the atrium, atrial oversensing can occur [42].

Due to these disadvantages of His bundle pacing, the left bundle branching area pacing (LBBAP) is gaining acceptance to achieve physiologic pacing. A pacemaker lead is placed distal to the bundle of His and screwed into the ventricular septum until it captures the left bundle branch or in the area near the left bundle. There can be selective and nonselective capture of the left bundle depending on the location of the lead within the interventricular septum. These differences in capturing can be seen during threshold testing when the QRS duration and morphology change: at a higher output, there can be more nonselective as both LBB and surrounding myocardium are captured, and as the output decreases (LBBAP), the LBB is more selectively captured. Typically, the 12-lead ECG morphology of LBBAP should include a terminal R wave in the V1, signaling activation of the right bundle. The 12-lead ECG should also show a left ventricle activation time (LVAT) of less than 80 milliseconds, defined as the time from the pacing stimulus to the R wave in V5 or V6, which signals rapid activation of the lateral wall. A V6 to V1 interpeak interval greater than or equal to 45 milliseconds can confirm that the left bundle branch is captured, so there is sequential activation from LV to RV. If the criteria for LBBAP are not met, a short QRS duration of less than 120 milliseconds can indicate that the septum, rather than the left bundle area, is paced. This can still be beneficial as LV septal or deep septal pacing may also reduce the dyssynchrony in RV pacing [43]. An example of LBBAP is shown in Figure 23.5.

Observational studies of LBBAP have been promising, demonstrating favorable narrower pacing QRS duration, possibly lower atrial fibrillation occurrence, mitral regurgitation, pacing-induced cardiomyopathy, and hospital admissions for heart failure compared to conventional RV apical pacing. Many randomized clinical trials are currently under investigation in different pacing populations.

Smaller observational trials have suggested that LBBAP can benefit the elderly [44, 45]. Wang et al. compared LBBAP with RV pacing in patients aged 75 years and older, with 110 patients undergoing LBBAP and 157 patients undergoing RV pacing. There were longer procedural duration and fluoroscopy times in the LBBAP group but a lower composite endpoint of all-cause mortality, heart failure hospitalization, and upgrade to biventricular pacing [44]. While observational trials and limited clinical experience of LBBAP have been promising, there is a lack of long-term data and randomized controlled trials with LBBAP.

Specifically in the elderly, there may be some merit with RV apical pacing due to shorter procedural times, no routine need for intravenous contrast, and more clinical experience requiring less technical expertise. Especially if the ventricular pacing burden is expected to be low, an RV apical lead may still be desired in older patients.

PACEMAKER COMPLICATIONS

See Table 23.5 for a list of complications related to pacemaker implantation. Early complications include pneumothorax, bleeding, hematoma, infection, lead dislodgment, and cardiac perforation, which are complications related to the procedure itself. Late complications

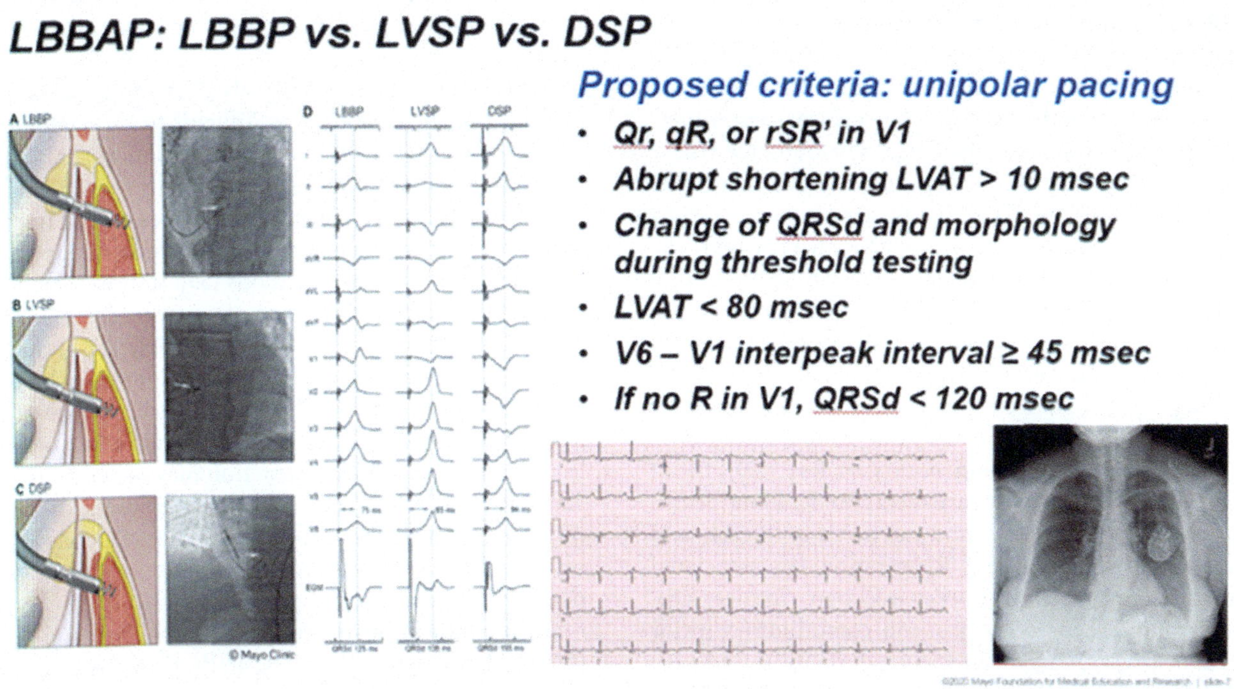

Figure 23.5 Left bundle branch area pacing (LBBAP), left ventricular septal pacing (LVSP), deep septal pacing (DSP). The left panel shows schematic and fluoroscopic views of LBBP, LVSP, and DSP. The 12-lead ECG shows LBBAP with characteristic QRS morphology. The CXR shows the AP view of a dual chamber PM with the ventricular lead in the LBB area. See details in the text.

Table 23.5 Pacemaker complications

Early complications	Late complications
Pneumothorax occurs in 1.1%–1.3% of cases due to accidental puncture of the lung while accessing the vasculature [46, 47]. Bleeding and hematoma occur in 2%–3% of cases, with a higher risk in patients on antithrombotic and antiplatelet medications [48–50]. Infection occurs in less than 1% of cases, with a higher risk in patients undergoing device replacements or revisions [51]. Lead dislodgment occurs in 1%–2% of cases [53]. Cardiac perforation occurs in less than 1% of cases [55–57].	Lead failure rates vary widely depending on the type of lead. Venous thrombosis can occur in 23%–45% of cases [60, 61]. Device-related infection can occur in the setting of any systemic infection.

include lead fracture, venous thrombosis, and device-related infection, which can occur regardless of procedural expertise.

Pneumothorax occurs in 1.1%–1.3% of cases due to accidental puncture of the lung while accessing the vasculature [46, 47]. Most commonly, the left subclavian vein is accessed with a needle (18–21 gauge) under fluoroscopic or ultrasound guidance. The apex of the lung is in close proximity to that area. A portable chest x-ray is commonly obtained immediately after the procedure is completed to evaluate for pneumothorax. If a pneumothorax is found, the management depends on the size of the pneumothorax. If large, a chest tube may be indicated. If small, supplemental oxygen is recommended. Serial chest x-rays are then obtained until resolution of the pneumothorax. Age greater than 80 years, female gender, Caucasian race, chronic obstructive pulmonary disease, and dual-chamber (versus single-chamber) device were associated with a higher risk of pneumothorax [46].

Bleeding and hematoma are common complications whose risk increases with use of antithrombotic and antiplatelet medications. Appropriate pocket closure and hemostasis during the procedure are critical to minimize the risk of pocket hematoma. One study found the risk of pocket hematoma to be 11% in patients on dual-antiplatelet therapy versus 3% in patients on aspirin monotherapy and 2% in patients without antiplatelet therapy [48]. The risk of hematoma in patients on warfarin or direct oral anticoagulants is 3.3%–3.5% [49, 50]. If significant bleeding or hematoma is deemed clinically significant, management typically consists of pocket evacuation. Minor bleeding can be managed conservatively without need for an additional procedure.

Device-related infection occurs in less than 1% of cases, with a higher risk in patients undergoing device replacements or revisions, and can occur both early and late after implantation [51]. Reoperation was associated with the highest risk of pocket infection. Younger age, more complex type of device, and comorbidities (prior valvular surgery, renal insufficiency, dermatitis) were also risk factors for device infection [52]. If there is evidence of device infection, extraction is indicated with reimplantation when deemed safe (usually 2–3 days after extraction if there is no systemic infection, and 2–4 weeks after extraction if there is bacteremia).

Lead dislodgment occurs in 1%–3% of cases [53]. It is important to restrict arm and shoulder movement on the side of device placement for 4–6 weeks after the procedure to minimize the risk of dislodgment. Independent risk factors include use of MRI-conditional leads, female sex, and higher body mass index [54]. If the lead is dislodged, lead revision is indicated.

Cardiac perforation occurs in less than 1% of cases [55–57]. Pacemaker leads can perforate through the myocardium and enter the pericardium causing cardiac tamponade, which can be fatal if not promptly addressed. Risk factors include older age, female sex, and active fixation leads [56, 57]. If perforation is suspected, immediate assessment of hemodynamic instability and echocardiography is indicated. If there is evidence of cardiac tamponade, pericardiocentesis, and sometimes a pericardial window, should be emergently performed. If there is a pericardial effusion without cardiac tamponade, the lead can be revised urgently rather than emergently, and pericardiocentesis can often be avoided.

Lead failure rates vary widely depending on the type of lead, but the incidence is difficult to ascertain. Lead failure can present as inappropriate shocks, inhibition of pacing, and lead alerts such as changes in impedance [58]. Defibrillator leads have higher rates of lead fracture compared to pacemaker leads. Lead fracture appears to be higher in younger populations [59]. If there is evidence of lead failure, then placement of a new lead is indicated. Extraction of the previous lead can be deferred at the discretion of the operator with considerations to include the total number of leads in the vasculature, the age of the leads, and operator expertise. If there are three or more leads in the vasculature, extraction may of benefit to prevent occlusion of the vein. The newer the leads, the easier it is the extract the leads. Lead extraction depends highly on operator and institutional expertise and should be performed at specialized centers.

Venous thrombosis can be quite common and occur in 23%–45% of cases [60, 61]. Usually, patients are asymptomatic, and thrombosis is found incidentally. Risk factors include the presence of multiple leads [61]. Management usually consists of therapeutic anticoagulation and reimaging with echocardiography or computed tomography after a period of time (usually 3 months). The pacemaker lead usually still functions normally and does not need to be revised.

PACEMAKERS IN VERY ELDERLY PATIENTS

The older population is rapidly growing in the US [62]. However, there is a paucity of data on outcomes in octogenarians or nonagenarians after pacemaker implantation. In a series of 149 pacemaker implants in a single center, Stevenson et al. reported that the rate of complications among very elderly patients (>80 years) was comparable with those previously reported in the literature, generally including younger patients (0.7% incidence of major complications in hospital, and 5.4% during 30-day follow-up) [63]. However, the 30-day all-cause mortality rate was higher among elderly patients when compared to historical data from other trials, including younger patients (cardiovascular mortality of 0.7% and all-cause mortality of 2% in 30 days). A short-term follow-up and modest number of patients limited this study. The investigators suggested that the higher mortality rate was inherent to the older population and unrelated to the procedure.

In another study, 481 octogenarians (86.2 ± 4.5 years) underwent pacemaker implantation for bradycardia in the Netherlands, and the rates of complications were similar (around 18%) over 5 years of follow-up when compared to patients <80 years old [64]. The survival rate was comparable to age- and sex-matched controls, suggesting that pacing for bradycardia can restore life expectancy to that expected in the general population.

Contrary to these previous studies, a meta-analysis of three major trials in bradycardia pacing (CTOPP, DANISH, and UKPACE) revealed modestly increased rates of acute complications in the elderly (>75 years), most commonly pneumothorax (1.6% vs. 0.8%) and lead dislodgement/loss of capture (2.0% vs. 1.1%). The risk of lead fracture, however, was lower among the elderly when compared to younger patients (2.7% vs. 3.6%, respectively) [65]. In patients greater than 80 years of age, comorbidities such as renal failure, active cancer, connective tissue disorder, cerebrovascular disease, and use of a single-lead device were associated with worse survival [66]. A study in 172 nonagenarian patients found 9 patients (5.2%) with short-term complications, 29 patients (16.8%) with post-procedure complications, including 4 patients (2.3%) with complications leading to death, and an 82.9% survival rate at 1 year [67]. In summary, despite some evidence of modestly increased mortality and procedural complications in older adults, the evidence does not preclude the recommendation of pacing therapy for these patients.

PACEMAKERS AND END OF LIFE

As previously discussed, the number of cardiac implantable electronic devices (CIEDs) continues to grow in the elderly. Despite these devices' proven efficacy in improving the quality of life or survival in selected patients, all patients will eventually reach the end of their lives. Once the patient becomes terminally ill, patients, family members, or health professionals should initiate a discussion about device deactivation. This discussion encompasses ethical, legal, and, oftentimes, religious issues, rendering the decision-making process complex and challenging.

A survey performed among internists about the cessation of pacing therapy or implantable cardioverter-defibrillator (ICD) deactivation in terminally ill patients showed that most internists were less comfortable discussing cessation of pacemaker and ICD therapy compared to other life-sustaining therapies, with only 34% of physicians reporting participation in this decision at some point in their practice [68]. Internists commonly reported a lack of experience with this practice. Some physicians erroneously classified the deactivation of the pacemaker in a pacemaker-dependent patient as assisted suicide (19%) or euthanasia (9%) [68].

Several key issues of patients nearing the end of life requesting withdrawal from therapy are summarized next [69, 70]:

1. Every patient with decision-making capacity has the right to refuse a new therapy or to choose the discontinuation of any medical treatment or intervention, even if its withdrawal will result in death. Patient autonomy is the fundamental principle in the decision-making process.
2. Patients can refuse any therapy and request the discontinuation of any intervention/therapy. CIEDs are no exception to this rule.
3. Ethically, CIED deactivation is neither physician-assisted suicide nor euthanasia. The deactivation of these devices will allow the patient to follow the natural course of their terminal condition.
4. In some cases, physicians may disagree with the deactivation of the device based on the physician's personal, moral, or religious values. In that case, another physician should proceed to reach a shared decision on the patient's wishes.
5. Advance directives are strongly recommended and ideally should be established as soon as the device is implanted.
6. Patients have the right to refuse any CIED therapy but do not have the right to demand removal of it, which would impose more risks and have the same effect as simply turning off the device.

REFERENCES

1. Caplan, Z. *U.S. Older population grew from 2010 to 2020 at fastest rate since 1880 to 1890.* 2023 [cited 2024 October 2]; Available from: https://www.census.gov/library/stories/2023/05/2020-census-united-states-older-population-grew.html#:~:text=The%20older%20population%20reached%2055.8,less%20than%201%20in%2020.

2. Kurtz, S.M., et al., Implantation trends and patient profiles for pacemakers and implantable cardioverter defibrillators in the United States: 1993–2006. *Pacing Clin Electrophysiol*, 2010. **33**(6): p. 705–11.
3. Gillis, A.M., et al., HRS/ACCF expert consensus statement on pacemaker device and mode selection. Developed in partnership between the Heart Rhythm Society (HRS) and the American College of Cardiology Foundation (ACCF) and in collaboration with the Society of Thoracic Surgeons. *Heart Rhythm*, 2012. **9**(8): p. 1344–65.
4. Menozzi, C., et al., The natural course of untreated sick sinus syndrome and identification of the variables predictive of unfavorable outcome. *Am J Cardiol*, 1998. **82**(10): p. 1205–9.
5. Lamas, G.A., et al., The mode selection trial (MOST) in sinus node dysfunction: design, rationale, and baseline characteristics of the first 1000 patients. *Am Heart J*, 2000. **140**(4): p. 541–51.
6. Vijayaraman, P. and K.A. Ellenbogen, Bradyarrhythmias, in V. Fuster, R.A. Harrington, J. Narula, and Z.J. Eapen, editors. *Hurst's the heart*. 14th ed. New York, NY: McGraw-Hill Education; 2017.
7. Sanders, P., D.H. Lau, and J.M. Kalman, Sinus node abnormalities, in D.P. Zipes, J. Jalife, and W.G. Stevenson, editors. *Cardiac electrophysiology: from cell to bedside*. 6th ed. Philadelphia, PA: Elsevier Saunders; 2014: p. 691–7.
8. Issa, Z.F., J.M. Miller, and D.P. Zipes, Chapter 8 - Sinus node dysfunction, in Z.F. Issa, J.M. Miller, and D.P. Zipes, editors. *Clinical arrhythmology and electrophysiology: a companion to Braunwald's heart disease*. 2nd ed. Philadelphia: W.B. Saunders; 2012: p. 164–74.
9. Fletcher, G.F., et al., Exercise standards for testing and training. *Circulation*, 2013. **128**(8): p. 873–934.
10. Lauer, M.S., et al., Impaired chronotropic response to exercise stress testing as a predictor of mortality. *JAMA*, 1999. **281**(6): p. 524–9.
11. Sutton, R. and R.A. Kenny, The natural history of sick sinus syndrome. *Pacing Clin Electrophysiol*, 1986. **9**(6): p. 1110–4.
12. Brandt, J., et al., Natural history of sinus node disease treated with atrial pacing in 213 patients: implications for selection of stimulation mode. *J Am Coll Cardiol*, 1992. **20**(3): p. 633–9.
13. Alt, E., et al., Survival and follow-up after pacemaker implantation: a comparison of patients with sick sinus syndrome, complete heart block, and atrial fibrillation. *Pacing Clin Electrophysiol*, 1985. **8**(6): p. 849–55.
14. Simon, A.B. and N. Janz, Symptomatic bradyarrhythmias in the adult: natural history following ventricular pacemaker implantation. *Pacing Clin Electrophysiol*, 1982. **5**(3): p. 372–83.
15. Brunner, M., et al., Long-term survival after pacemaker implantation. Prognostic importance of gender and baseline patient characteristics. *Eur Heart J*, 2004. **25**(1): p. 88–95.
16. Kusumoto, F.M., et al., 2018 ACC/AHA/HRS guideline on the evaluation and management of patients with bradycardia and cardiac conduction delay: a report of the American College of Cardiology/American Heart Association Task Force on Clinical Practice Guidelines and the *Heart Rhythm* Society. *J Am Coll Cardiol*, 2019. *74*(7): p. e51–e156.
17. Glikson, M., et al., 2021 ESC Guidelines on cardiac pacing and cardiac resynchronization therapy. *Eur Heart J*, 2021. **42**(35): p. 3427–520.
18. Zipes, D.P., J. Jalife, and W.G. Stevenson, *Cardiac electrophysiology: from cell to bedside*. 7th ed. Philadelphia, PA: Elsevier; 2018.
19. Issa, Z.F., J.M. Miller, and D.P. Zipes, *Clinical arrhythmology and electrophysiology: a companion to Braunwald's heart disease*. 4th ed. Philadelphia, PA: Elsevier; 2024.
20. Zehender, M., et al., Prevalence, circumstances, mechanisms, and risk stratification of sudden cardiac death in unipolar single-chamber ventricular pacing. *Circulation*, 1992. **85**(2): p. 596–605.
21. Epstein, A.E., et al., ACC/AHA/HRS 2008 Guidelines for device-based therapy of cardiac rhythm abnormalities: a report of the American College of Cardiology/American Heart Association Task Force on Practice Guidelines (writing committee to revise the ACC/AHA/NASPE 2002 guideline update for implantation of cardiac pacemakers and antiarrhythmia devices) developed in collaboration with the American Association for Thoracic Surgery and Society of Thoracic Surgeons. *J Am Coll Cardiol*, 2008. **51**(21): p. e1–62.
22. Moya, A., et al., Guidelines for the diagnosis and management of syncope (version 2009). *Eur Heart J*, 2009. **30**(21): p. 2631–71.
23. McLeod, C.J., et al., Method of pacing does not affect the recurrence of syncope in carotid sinus syndrome. *Pacing Clin Electrophysiol*, 2012. **35**(7): p. 827–33.
24. Brignole, M., et al., Guidelines on management (diagnosis and treatment) of syncope. *Eur Heart J*, 2001. **22**(15): p. 1256–306.
25. Healey, J., S.J. Connolly, and C.A. Morillo, The management of patients with carotid sinus syndrome: is pacing the answer? *Clin Auton Res*, 2004. **14** (Suppl 1): p. 80–6.
26. Shen, W.K., et al., 2017 ACC/AHA/HRS guideline for the evaluation and management of patients with syncope: a report of the American College of Cardiology/American Heart Association Task Force on Clinical Practice Guidelines and the Heart Rhythm Society. *Circulation*, 2017. **136**(5): p. e60–e122.

27. Huang, S.K., et al., Carotid sinus hypersensitivity in patients with unexplained syncope: clinical, electrophysiologic, and long-term follow-up observations. *Am Heart J*, 1988. **116**(4): p. 989–96.
28. Morley, C.A., et al., Carotid sinus syncope treated by pacing. Analysis of persistent symptoms and role of atrioventricular sequential pacing. *Br Heart J*, 1982. **47**(5): p. 411–8.
29. Kenny, R.A., et al., Carotid sinus syndrome: a modifiable risk factor for nonaccidental falls in older adults (SAFE PACE). *J Am Coll Cardiol*, 2001. **38**(5): p. 1491–6.
30. Spickler, J.W., et al., Totally self-contained intracardiac pacemaker. *J Electrocardiol*, 1970. **3**(3–4): p. 325–31.
31. Tjong, F.V. and V.Y. Reddy, Permanent leadless cardiac pacemaker therapy: a comprehensive review. *Circulation*, 2017. **135**(15): p. 1458–70.
32. Lee, J.Z., S.K. Mulpuru, and W.K. Shen, Leadless pacemaker: performance and complications. *Trends Cardiovasc Med*, 2018. **28**(2): p. 130–41.
33. Miller, M.A., et al., Leadless cardiac pacemakers: back to the future. *J Am Coll Cardiol*, 2015. **66**(10): p. 1179–89.
34. Ponnusamy, S.S., T. Syed, and P. Vijayaraman, Pacing induced cardiomyopathy: recognition and management. *Heart*, 2023. **109**(18): p. 1407–1415.
35. Heidenreich, P.A., et al., 2022 AHA/ACC/HFSA Guideline for the management of heart failure: a report of the American College of Cardiology/American Heart Association Joint Committee on Clinical Practice Guidelines. *J Am Coll Cardiol*, 2022. **79**(17): p. e263–e421.
36. Chung, M.K., et al., 2023 HRS/APHRS/LAHRS guideline on cardiac physiologic pacing for the avoidance and mitigation of heart failure. *Heart Rhythm*, 2023. **20**(9): p. e17–e91.
37. Zhang, S., X. Zhou, and M.R. Gold, Left bundle branch pacing: JACC review topic of the week. *J Am Coll Cardiol*, 2019. **74**(24): p. 3039–49.
38. Yuan, Z., L. Cheng, and Y. Wu, Meta-analysis comparing safety and efficacy of left bundle branch area pacing versus his bundle pacing. *Am J Cardiol*, 2022. **164**: p. 64–72.
39. Jastrzębski, M., et al., His-bundle pacing as a standard approach in patients with permanent atrial fibrillation and bradycardia. *Pacing Clin Electrophysiol*, 2018. **41**(11): p. 1508–12.
40. Cheng, L.T., et al., Recent approaches to His-Purkinje system pacing. *Chin Med J (Engl)*, 2019. **132**(2): p. 190–6.
41. Teigeler, T., et al., Intermediate-term performance and safety of his-bundle pacing leads: a single-center experience. *Heart Rhythm*, 2021. **18**(5): p. 743–9.
42. Lustgarten, D.L., P.S. Sharma, and P. Vijayaraman, Troubleshooting and programming considerations for His bundle pacing. *Heart Rhythm*, 2019. **16**(5): p. 654–62.
43. McBride, K.W., et al., Mitigation of pacing-induced cardiomyopathy with superficial right ventricular mid-septal pacing: a long-term retrospective comparison with apical pacing. *J Cardiovasc Electrophysiol*, 2025. **36**(1): p. 62–70.
44. Wang, Q., et al., Comparison of clinical and echocardiographic outcomes between left bundle branch area pacing and right ventricular pacing in older patients. *Pacing Clin Electrophysiol*, 2024. **47**(10): p. 1346–57.
45. Rijks, J.H.J., et al., Left bundle branch area pacing and atrioventricular node ablation in a single-procedure approach for elderly patients with symptomatic atrial fibrillation. *J Clin Med*, 2023. **12**(12): p. 4028.
46. Ogunbayo, G.O., et al., Incidence, predictors, and outcomes associated with pneumothorax during cardiac electronic device implantation: a 16-year review in over 3.7 million patients. *Heart Rhythm*, 2017. **14**(12): p. 1764–70.
47. Shepherd, E., et al., Extraction of select secure leads compared to conventional pacing leads in patients with congenital heart disease and congenital atrioventricular block. *Heart Rhythm*, 2015. **12**(6): p. 1227–32.
48. Said, S.M., et al., Influence of oral antiplatelet therapy on hemorrhagic complications of pacemaker implantation. *Clin Res Cardiol*, 2013. **102**(5): p. 345–9.
49. Birnie, D.H., et al., Pacemaker or defibrillator surgery without interruption of anticoagulation. *N Engl J Med*, 2013. **368**(22): p. 2084–93.
50. Martin, A.C., et al., Impact of peri-procedural management of direct oral anticoagulants on pocket haematoma after cardiac electronic device implantation: the StimAOD multicentre prospective study. *Europace*, 2023. **25**(5).
51. Johansen, J.B., et al., Infection after pacemaker implantation: infection rates and risk factors associated with infection in a population-based cohort study of 46299 consecutive patients. *Eur Heart J*, 2011. **32**(8): p. 991–8.
52. Olsen, T., et al., Risk factors for cardiac implantable electronic device infections: a nationwide Danish study. *Eur Heart J*, 2022. **43**(47): p. 4946–56.
53. Wang, Y., et al., Meta-analysis of the incidence of lead dislodgement with conventional and leadless pacemaker systems. *Pacing Clin Electrophysiol*, 2018. **41**(10): p. 1365–71.
54. Qin, D., et al., Short- and long-term risk of lead dislodgement events: real-world experience from product surveillance registry. *Circ Arrhythm Electrophysiol*, 2022. **15**(8): p. e011029.
55. Waddingham, P.H., et al., Iatrogenic cardiac perforation due to pacemaker and defibrillator leads:

a contemporary multicentre experience. *Europace*, 2022. **24**(11): p. 1824–33.

56. Cano, Ó., et al., Incidence and predictors of clinically relevant cardiac perforation associated with systematic implantation of active-fixation pacing and defibrillation leads: a single-centre experience with over 3800 implanted leads. *Europace*, 2017. **19**(1): p. 96–102.
57. Vamos, M., et al., Incidence of cardiac perforation with conventional and with leadless pacemaker systems: a systematic review and meta-analysis. *J Cardiovasc Electrophysiol*, 2017. **28**(3): p. 336–46.
58. Kusumoto, F.M., et al., 2017 HRS expert consensus statement on cardiovascular implantable electronic device lead management and extraction. *Heart Rhythm*, 2017. **14**(12): p. e503–e51.
59. Morrison, T.B., et al., Risk factors for implantable defibrillator lead fracture in a recalled and a nonrecalled lead. *J Cardiovasc Electrophysiol*, 2010. **21**(6): p. 671–7.
60. Spittell, P.C. and D.L. Hayes, Venous complications after insertion of a transvenous pacemaker. *Mayo Clin Proc*, 1992. **67**(3): p. 258–65.
61. van Rooden, C.J., et al., Incidence and risk factors of early venous thrombosis associated with permanent pacemaker leads. *J Cardiovasc Electrophysiol*, 2004. **15**(11): p. 1258–62.
62. Perls, T., Health and disease in people over 85. *BMJ*, 2009. **339**: p. b4715.
63. Stevenson, R.T., et al., Pacemaker implantation in the extreme elderly. *J Interv Card Electrophysiol*, 2012. **33**(1): p. 51–8.
64. Udo, E.O., et al., Long-term outcome of cardiac pacing in octogenarians and nonagenarians. *Europace*, 2012. **14**(4): p. 502–8.
65. Armaganijan, L.V., et al., Are elderly patients at increased risk of complications following pacemaker implantation? A meta-analysis of randomized trials. *Pacing Clin Electrophysiol*, 2012. **35**(2): p. 131–4.
66. Balla, C., et al., Prognosis after pacemaker implantation in extreme elderly. *Eur J Intern Med*, 2019. **65**: p. 37–43.
67. Dang, D., et al., Procedural safety and long-term follow-up after pacemaker implantation in nonagenarians. *Clin Cardiol*, 2018. **41**(10): p. 1315–21.
68. Kramer, D.B., et al., Ethical and legal views of physicians regarding deactivation of cardiac implantable electrical devices: a quantitative assessment. *Heart Rhythm*, 2010. **7**(11): p. 1537–42.
69. Lampert, R., et al., HRS expert consensus statement on the management of cardiovascular implantable electronic devices (CIEDs) in patients nearing end of life or requesting withdrawal of therapy. *Heart Rhythm*, 2010. **7**(7): p. 1008–26.
70. Padeletti, L., et al., EHRA Expert Consensus Statement on the management of cardiovascular implantable electronic devices in patients nearing end of life or requesting withdrawal of therapy. *Europace*, 2010. **12**(10): p. 1480–9.

24

Cerebrovascular disease in older adults

EMMA M. LOEBEL AND LAURA K. STEIN

Key points

- Stroke is highly prevalent and disproportionately affects older adults. With almost 800,000 strokes in the United States annually, approximately 75% occur in patients over 65 years of age and 20% in patients older than 85 years. Forecasting suggests the incidence of stroke among older adults will continue to increase.[1–3]
- Stroke is caused by the disruption of the circulation of blood to the brain and can be ischemic due to occlusion of an artery or hemorrhagic due to rupture of an artery. Ischemia accounts for ~85% of stroke, while hemorrhage accounts for ~15%.[3]
- Elucidating etiology of a stroke is critical for optimal management. Ischemic stroke etiology can be classified by the TOAST criteria, which includes cardioembolism, large artery atherosclerosis, small vessel disease, cryptogenic (includes embolic stroke of underdetermined source), and other (e.g., hypercoagulable state).[4]
- Stroke prevention is paramount. Over 80% of strokes can be prevented through management of modifiable risk factors.[5] High blood pressure is the most significant modifiable risk factor, and management of diabetes, high cholesterol, and healthy lifestyle factors are essential to stroke prevention.[6]
- Thrombolysis and mechanical thrombectomy are the cornerstone of hyperacute stroke therapy and have demonstrated benefit in the older adult population.[7,8]
- High-risk transient ischemic attacks and certain acute minor ischemic strokes may benefit from short-term dual antiplatelet therapy.[9–11]
- The direct oral anticoagulants are now widely prescribed and should be first-line for patients with nonvalvular atrial fibrillation and high thromboembolic risk or prior stroke, regardless of age.[5]

DEFINITION OF STROKE AND TIA

Stroke is highly prevalent and disproportionately affects older adults. With almost 800,000 strokes in the United States annually, approximately 75% occur in patients over 65 years and 20% in patients older than 85 years. Forecasting suggests the incidence of stroke among older adults will continue to increase.[1–3]

Stroke is defined as the sudden onset of a focal neurologic dysfunction caused by either a lack of blood flow

DOI: 10.1201/9781003568933-24

or rupture of a blood vessel. Ischemic stroke accounts for ~85% of all strokes and occurs when there is a blockage of blood flow through the arteries supplying the brain.[3] Hemorrhagic stroke includes both rupture of blood vessels in the brain parenchyma (intracerebral hemorrhage, ICH) and in the cerebrospinal fluid surrounding the surface of the brain (subarachnoid hemorrhage, SAH).

A transient ischemic attack (TIA) is a transient focal neurologic deficit caused by the temporary blockage of blood flow to the brain. TIAs are a warning sign of impending stroke and should be managed as a stroke.[12] Around 80% of strokes after TIA can be avoided by implementing timely, appropriate stroke prevention management.[12] Historically, the risk of stroke after TIA was estimated as high as 20% within 90 days, however, with proper management based on evidence-based guidelines,[13] that risk is estimated at closer to ~4%.[14] The risk remains highest within the first 2 days after the event.[15] The risk calculator, known as the ABCD2 score,[16] described later, can be useful in clinical practice for risk stratification and management.[15] The modern definition of TIA is imaging-based, as opposed to the formerly time-based, so while most may last a few minutes, if a patient presents with transient symptoms and has a correlating acute infarct on MRI diffusion weighted imaging (DWI), it is considered a stroke.[12,15] About one third of patients who present with transient stroke-like symptoms lasting less than 24 hours will have an infarct on MRI, confirming a stroke.[13,17]

ANATOMY AND PHYSIOLOGY OF THE CEREBRAL CIRCULATION

Blood flow to the brain is comprised of the anterior and posterior circulation, which form a network of vasculature called the circle of Willis at the base of the brain. The anterior circulation includes each internal carotid artery (ICA), which branches into the middle cerebral arteries (MCAs) over the lateral surfaces and the anterior cerebral arteries (ACAs) over the medial surface of the brain. The posterior circulation includes each vertebral artery, which joins to form the basilar artery to supply the brain stem and cerebellum. The basilar artery terminates in the posterior cerebral arteries (PCAs), feeding the posterior hemispheres and the thalamus. These major arteries of the circle of Willis are termed large vessels, and their blockage is referred to as a large vessel occlusion (LVO) in clinical practice.

Connections between the left and right anterior circulation exist between the two carotid arteries through the anterior communicating artery. The anterior and posterior circulation often connect through posterior communicating arteries, however, several anatomic variants exist. Collateral circulation to the brain can come from several sources, including the external carotid artery and anastomoses of meningeal branches of the external carotid artery and surface branches of the cerebral arteries. Because of this collateral circulation, at times the brain can tolerate complete occlusion of a carotid artery without injury or symptoms, and there are case reports of patients with bilateral carotid artery occlusion and unilateral vertebral artery occlusion whose only symptoms are nonspecific dizziness.[18]

Another protective mechanism for circulation to the brain is autoregulation, as blood flow is maintained at constant velocities without fluctuations due to pressure.[19] Blood flow fluctuates with the blood partial pressure of carbon dioxide (PCO_2), which ensures that there will be increased blood supply to metabolically active regions of the brain that are producing large amounts of carbon dioxide so that sufficient oxygen can be delivered.

PATHOPHYSIOLOGY OF ISCHEMIC STROKE AND TIA

Classifying stroke etiology is paramount to identifying risk factors and guiding appropriate therapy for secondary prevention. While multiple classifications systems exist, ischemic stroke etiology is commonly classified by one of five TOAST[4] classification subtypes: (1) large artery atherosclerosis, (2) cardioembolism, (3) small vessel disease (lacune), (4) stroke of other determined etiology, and (5) stroke of undetermined etiology (or cryptogenic). Stroke of undetermined etiology has been modified to include embolic strokes of undetermined source (ESUS)[20,21] (Figures 24.1 and 24.2).[22]

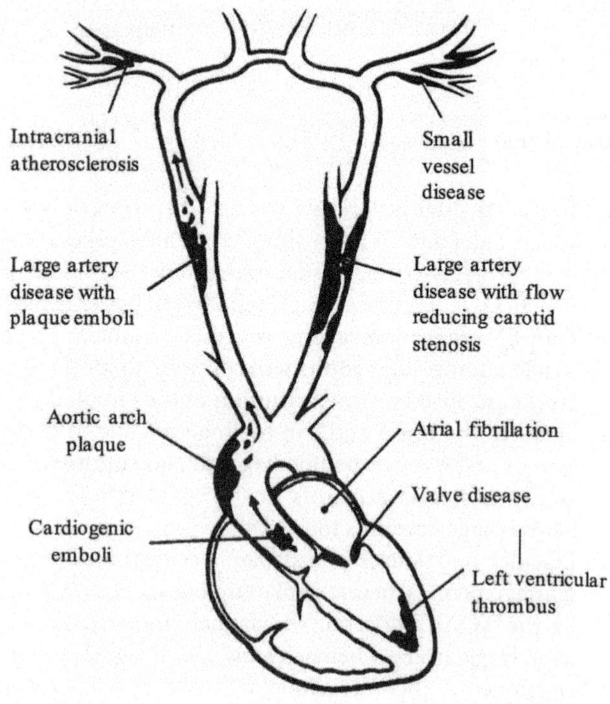

Figure 24.1 The anatomy of the cerebral circulation is diagrammed demonstrating potential etiologies of ischemic stroke. (Modified from Sherman DG et al., *Chest*, 108, 444S–456S, 1995. Copyright 1995 The American College of Chest Physicians.)

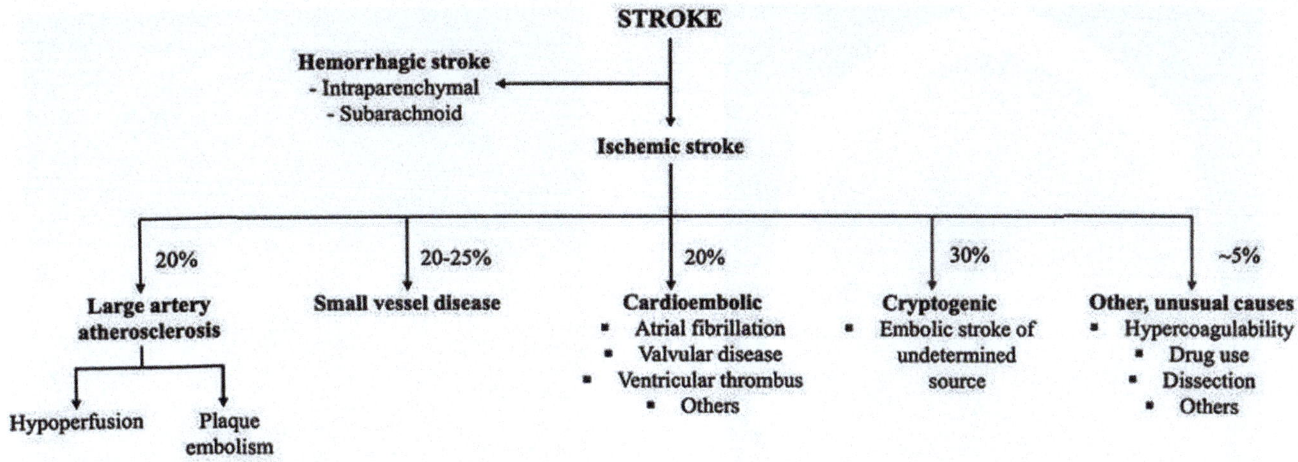

Figure 24.2 The estimated incidences of the various etiologies of ischemic stroke. (Modified from Sherman DG et al., *Chest*, 108, 444S–456S, 1995. Copyright 1995 The American College of Chest Physicians.)

Large artery atherosclerosis (LAA)

Large artery atherosclerotic disease accounts for ~20% of ischemic strokes, about equally split between involvement of the extracranial and intracranial arteries (known as intracranial atherosclerotic disease, or ICAD), and carries a higher risk of recurrent stroke[23,24] (Figure 24.3). Typical vascular risk factors can contribute to LAA, including high blood pressure, diabetes, high cholesterol, and more. Lipoprotein biomarkers can be useful to assess LAA severity and as therapeutic targets.[23] LAA can cause strokes through various mechanisms, including artery–artery embolization (e.g., embolization of thrombus or atherosclerotic debris from plaque), reduced perfusion (e.g., hypoperfusion event), or deep perforator disease. Due to collateral cerebral circulation, ischemic stroke more rarely occurs on a hemodynamic basis (e.g., due to a hypoperfusion event) unless there are significant blockages in the circle of Willis that prevent compensatory flow. Such infarcts may present in a watershed distribution, or areas supplied by the distal territories of two arterial trees (e.g., where the frontal lobe receives terminal branches from both the anterior and middle cerebral arteries). Watershed infarcts (Figure 24.4) may occur with hypoperfusion in settings of cardiac arrhythmia or arrest, fluid shifts during dialysis, or sepsis, for example. A solitary deep lesion in the territory of LAA may suggest perforator disease due to proximal atherosclerosis.

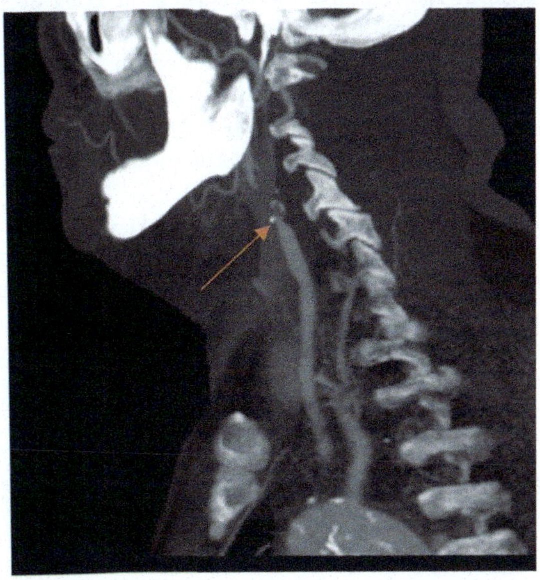

Figure 24.3 ICA occlusion. Sagittal CTA demonstrating stenosis and an occlusion of the left cervical carotid artery (arrow). *Abbreviations*: ICA, internal carotid artery; CTA, computed tomography angiography.

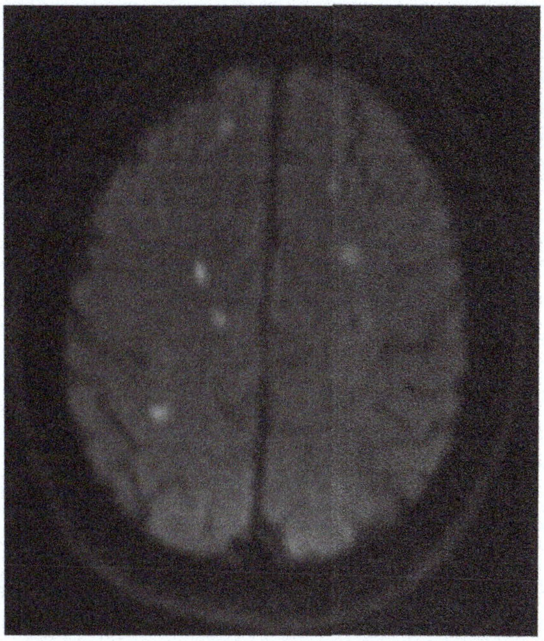

Figure 24.4 Multiple watershed infarcts. Diffusion-weighted image on MRI showing bilateral watershed acute infarcts in the ACA–MCA border zone areas *Abbreviations*: MRI, magnetic resonance imaging; ACA, anterior cerebral artery; MCA, middle cerebral artery.

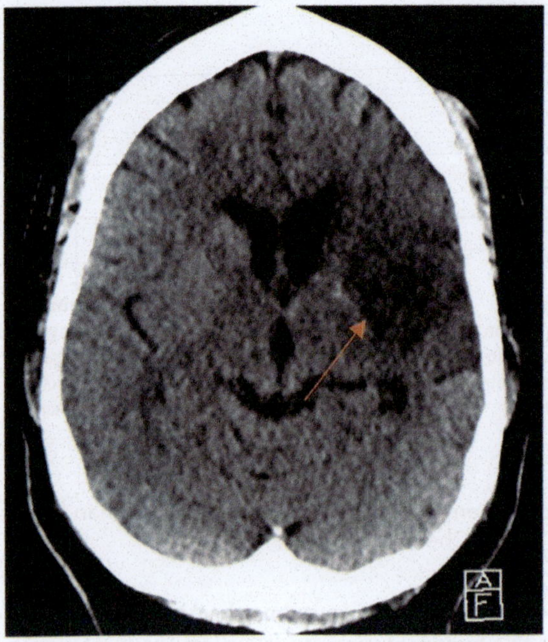

Figure 24.5 Left MCA territory stroke. Axial non-contrast CT scan at the level of the basal ganglia demonstrating a hypodensity in the left MCA territory involving the gray and white matter (arrow), indicating a subacute stroke (likely 3–5 days) due to distal MCA occlusion. *Abbreviations*: MCA, middle cerebral artery; CT, computed tomography.

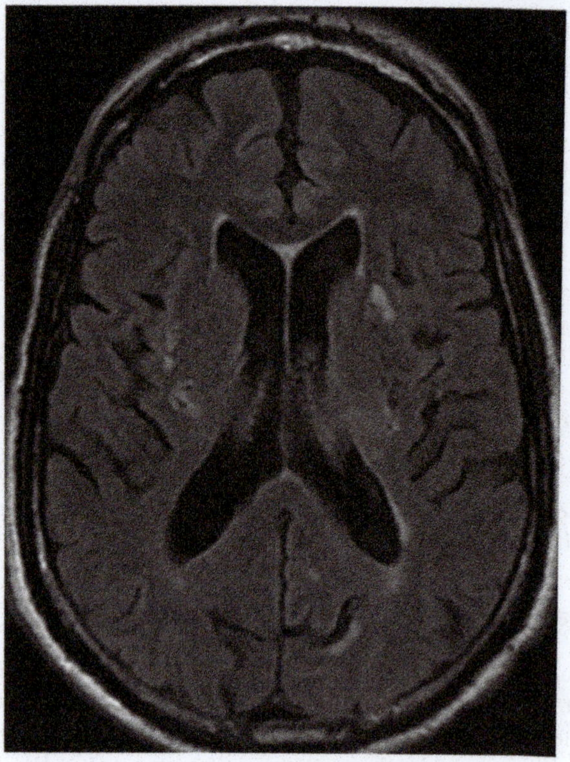

Figure 24.6 Multiple lacunar infarcts. Axial T2-weighted FLAIR MRI sequence demonstrating small bilateral areas of high signal intensity and areas of encephalomalacia in subcortical territory, indicating chronic lacunar infarcts. *Abbreviations*: FLAIR, fluid-attenuated inversion recovery; MRI, magnetic resonance imaging.

Cardioembolism

Cardioembolic sources account for ~20% of ischemic strokes through a variety of mechanisms including, most importantly, atrial fibrillation (AF).[24] AF is present in almost 10% of people over 80 years of age and contributes to a greater risk of stroke.[25] AF accounts for the greatest source of cardioembolism in patients >75 years and particularly women >80 years.[26] Other cardioembolic mechanisms that cause stroke include cardiomyopathy, valvular heart disease, recent myocardial infarction, patent foramen ovale (PFO), and aortic arch disease. Cardioembolic strokes usually occur by occluding major branches of the internal carotid artery, such as the middle cerebral artery or the more distal branches, causing cortical infarctions (Figure 24.5). Around half of cardioembolic strokes involve more than one vascular territory.[25]

Small vessel disease

Intracranial thrombosis of small penetrating vessels supplying the deep structures of the brain, such as the internal capsule and basal ganglia, account for ~20% of ischemic stroke.[24] These end arteries do not have collateral flow to the regions they supply. Thrombosis usually occurs because of proliferative thickening of arterial walls from fibrinoid necrosis or lipohyalinosis secondary to hypertension and diabetes, among other vascular and behavioral risk factors.[27] When these arteries occlude, they produce small holes in the deep white subcortical structures, known as lacunes (≤1.5 cm in size)[27] (Figure 24.6). While lacunes may be small, if they occur in significant white matter tracts, they may cause significant deficits of contralateral sensory and motor function.

Stroke of other determined etiology

Unusual causes of stroke, such as vasculitis, hypercoagulable state from anticardiolipin antibody or thrombophilia, arterial dissection, and hematologic disorders such as sickle cell disease, account for the vast minority of strokes and often occur in younger patients.[24,28]

Stroke of undetermined etiology (cryptogenic) and embolic stroke of undetermined source (ESUS)

Even with the advent of noninvasive imaging techniques to identify the nature and causes of ischemic stroke, in up to 30% of strokes the etiology cannot be identified, and these

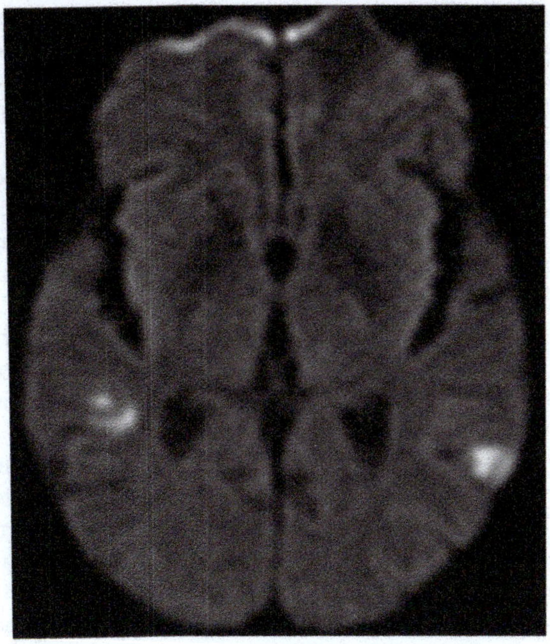

Figure 24.7 ESUS. Axial diffusion-weighted image on MRI showing bilateral temporal acute infarcts involving the cortex, suspicious of embolic etiology, with no known proximal embolic source. *Abbreviations*: ESUS, embolic stroke of undetermined source; MRI, magnetic resonance imaging.

are classified as cryptogenic strokes.[29,30] Approximately 17% of cryptogenic strokes are classified as ESUS, a new classification proposed in 2014 to identify nonlacunar strokes without proximal arterial stenosis, major cardioembolic risk source, or other identifiable stroke etiology after sufficient diagnostic workup, with suspected embolic origin.[31] While both the etiology of ESUS and cryptogenic strokes are unknown, ESUS is suspected to have an embolic origin based on the appearance (Figure 24.7).

Cancer may represent an important risk factor for ESUS, as data shows approximately 5%–10% of patients with ESUS have an active cancer, and stroke may even be the presenting sign. Rates of recurrent stroke classified as ESUS in patients with cancer at 1 year are about three times higher than those without cancer. While the mechanisms are likely heterogeneous, cancer-related hypercoagulability may be considered.[32]

Transient ischemic attack

A TIA is caused by a temporary blockage of blood flow, most often by a blood clot that may dissolve or dislodge. The ABCD2 score estimates the early risk of stroke after TIA and can be used in risk stratification and management decisions.[16] The result provides a score from 0 to 6 that correlates to the estimated risk of stroke after 2, 7, and 90 days, with a higher score estimating a higher risk of near-term stroke. This tool considers patient age, blood pressure at presentation, clinical features (unilateral weakness or speech impairment without weakness), duration of symptoms, and history of diabetes.[16]

PATHOPHYSIOLOGY OF HEMORRHAGIC STROKE

Spontaneous ICH is generally caused by arteriosclerosis, notably due to hypertension, or cerebral amyloid angiopathy (CAA), and both pathologies are prevalent in older adults.[33] Hypertensive hemorrhages typically occur in subcortical, deep structures of the brain, such as in the basal ganglia (Figure 24.8).

In older adults, lobar hemorrhages are most often due to CAA[34,35] (Figure 24.9). CAA is an age-related disease caused by the accumulation of cerebral amyloid-beta in the cerebral vessels, making them prone to rupture even in patients with normotension. CAA can clinically manifest with cognitive decline, focal neurologic deficits (due to stroke), and transient neurologic episodes, known as "amyloid spells," which can often mimic TIA. The recent Boston criteria 2.0 proposed in 2022 for CAA helps better diagnose possible or probable CAA in patients with

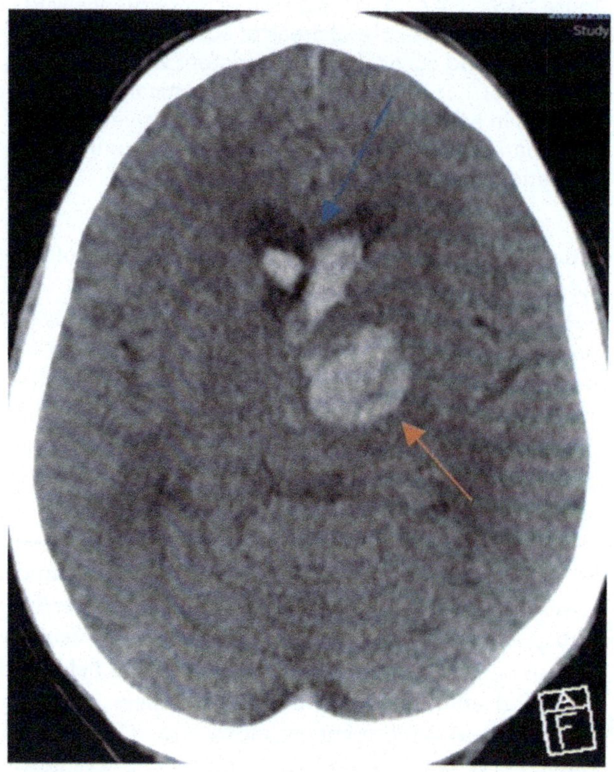

Figure 24.8 Subcortical deep hemorrhage. Axial noncontrast CT head at the level of the basal ganglia showing acute hypertensive hemorrhage in the left thalamus (orange arrow) with intraventricular extension into the lateral ventricles (blue arrow). There is rightward mass effect displacing the ventricles. *Abbreviations*: CT, computed tomography.

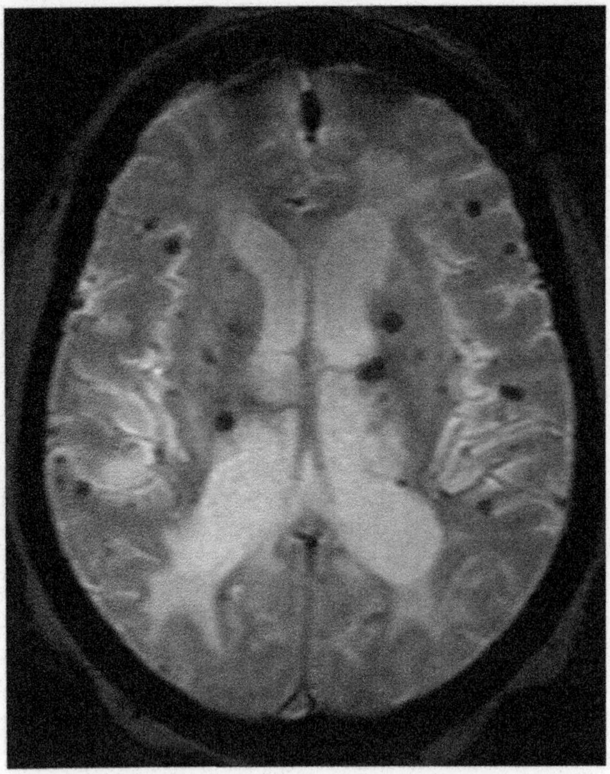

Figure 24.9 CAA. Axial gradient echo sequence MRI showing multiple bilateral areas of susceptibility in subcortical and cortical areas consistent with chronic microhemorrhages. The presence of cortical microhemorrhages in an older adult is highly suggestive of CAA. *Abbreviations*: CAA, cerebral amyloid angiopathy; MRI, magnetic resonance imaging.

clinical and radiographic features. The diagnosis of definite CAA requires postmortem pathology.[34]

Aneurysmal SAH can occur in older adults but is less common than in younger patients. Around 15%–20% of aneurysmal SAH occurs in patients >70 years, and these patients have higher morbidity and mortality than their younger counterparts.[36]

DIAGNOSIS OF STROKE AND TIA

The anatomic location of the stroke determines clinical signs and symptoms. Most strokes involve the cerebral hemispheres with contralateral hemiparesis or sensory loss, loss of vision in the contralateral visual field, and behavioral and speech disturbances. Strokes involving the brain stem can present with ipsilateral deficits of the cranial nerve function such as abnormality of eye movements and a contralateral hemiparesis. Dizziness is a common symptom in older adults, but dizziness alone rarely indicates stroke unless accompanied by signs of dysfunction in the cerebellum or brain stem.

One must establish stroke etiology by examining the patient's risk factors and brain imaging, often classified by the TOAST criteria,[4] to establish appropriate management. Clinical history, physical examination, imaging, and laboratory analysis help guide investigation of stroke risk factors.

Neurological examination helps determine if there is an extensive lesion caused by LVO or major hemorrhage, by determining if there is an alteration in level of consciousness, along with the focal deficits involved. The presence of cortical signs (i.e., focal neurologic deficits that localize to the cortex), including gaze palsy, visual field cut, neglect, or aphasia, increase suspicion of LVO. Small vessel lacunar strokes can be identified if typical syndromes of pure motor, pure sensory, dysarthria-clumsy hand, or ataxic hemiparesis are present in an alert patient.[27]

Computed tomography (CT) of the brain is absolutely necessary to differentiate between hemorrhagic and ischemic stroke. Many centers also perform CT angiography (CTA) of the head and neck as part of the acute stroke protocol to assess for LVO, as well as stenosis, dissection, or vascular malformation in the extracranial or intracranial circulation. CT perfusion of the brain can be used to identify hypoperfused tissue at risk of infarction that may benefit from revascularization. Signs of infarction are not always visualized on CT scan within the first 4–12 hours after ischemic stroke, but early ischemic changes are assessed using the Alberta Stroke Program Early CT Score (ASPECTS) and can aid in hyperacute revascularization decision-making for patients with LVO.[37] Diffusion-weighted magnetic resonance imaging (MRI) is more sensitive than CT scan for detecting early signs of infarction in the first 4–12 hours[38] (Figure 24.4 and Figure 24.7).

The appearance of the stroke on imaging, ideally MRI, is key to contributing to establishing stroke etiology. For example, a single small infarct ≤1.5 cm in a deep structure of the brain is generally sufficient to presume small vessel disease. An infarct in the territory distal to significant atherosclerosis of the proximal artery is reason to suspect atherosclerotic origin. In addition to CTA or MRA (MRI angiography), carotid duplex ultrasonography can be performed to further assess characteristics of known atherosclerosis in the cervical vessels. Transcranial Doppler (TCD) can identify occlusive disease of large intracranial arteries, however, CTA and MRA are typically sufficient for evaluation of the intracranial vessels, and TCD is frequently used to evaluate for microemboli.

While a cortical infarct in a patient with a known cardiogenic source such as AF is usually sufficient to diagnose cardioembolic stroke, transthoracic echocardiography helps identify a cardiogenic source for stroke. If the suspicion for cardioembolic stroke is high and no obvious source is identified, transesophageal echocardiography (TEE) is often indicated. TEE can confirm thrombus in the atrium, right-to-left shunts in the heart, such as PFO or atrial septal defect, and plaque in the arch of the aorta.[32] If no source is found, prolonged cardiac monitoring by Holter or loop recorder may be used to assess for occult arrhythmia.

Table 24.1 Stroke etiology, risk factors, and management

Stroke type	Etiology	Most common risk factors	Most common management
Ischemic stroke	Small vessel disease	Hypertension, diabetes, smoking, hyperlipidemia	Control of vascular risk factors, antithrombotic(s), statin, healthy lifestyle modifications
	Large artery atherosclerosis	Hyperlipidemia, hypertension, diabetes, smoking, metabolic syndrome	Control of vascular risk factors, antithrombotic(s), statin, healthy lifestyle modifications, surgical consideration for extracranial disease
	Cardioembolic	Atrial fibrillation, valvular disease, ventricular thrombus	Anticoagulation
Hemorrhagic stroke	Intracerebral	Hypertension, cerebral amyloid angiopathy	Control of hypertension, consideration of surgical evacuation
	Subarachnoid	Aneurysm, arteriovenous malformation, trauma	Control of hypertension, nimodipine, aneurysm clipping/coiling, management of delayed ischemia and vasospasm

PREVENTION OF CEREBROVASCULAR DISEASE

Management for primary and secondary prevention of ischemic stroke is summarized in Table 24.1. Despite significant advances in acute treatment for stroke, the major goal is prevention of stroke and cannot be overemphasized in older adults. Approximately one quarter of strokes annually are recurrent.[3] Stroke is a major contributor to cognitive impairment and can significantly impair quality of life, to the point that some older adults see severe stroke as worse than death.[5] Over 80% of strokes can be prevented[5] through management of modifiable risk factors such as hypertension, diabetes, high cholesterol, and lifestyle modifications, and it is never too late to implement prevention strategies. By some estimates, over a third of strokes globally could be due to patient lifestyle choices such as smoking, unhealthy diet, and minimal physical activity.[39] Given the disproportionate impact on older adults, a healthy 80-year-old patient carries a lifetime risk of stroke of about 20%.[5,40]

PRIMARY PREVENTION OF STROKE

Risk factor screening

The main components of preventative care for stroke are establishing a healthy lifestyle, screening for and managing common risk factors, and addressing social determinants of health.[6] Primary care physicians are at the forefront of stroke primary prevention and critical to patient education.

Hypertension is the most significant risk factor for stroke. All adults should be screened for high blood pressure. A normal blood pressure goal of <130/80 mmHg is recommended to reduce stroke risk.[6,41] Some guidelines suggest a higher threshold of 140/80 for hypertension in older adults age 65 and older and possibly even up to 150/80 in those 80 years and older.[42] Those with bilateral carotid artery stenosis and stiff arteries may need higher blood pressure goals as well.[5] Most adults with hypertension will need at least two hypertensive agents to attain proper blood pressure control.[6] Many classes of antihypertensive drugs are acceptable as first-line agents for hypertension.

Diabetes is a leading modifiable risk factor for stroke that can double the risk of ischemic stroke, independent of other factors, and contribute to worse stroke outcomes and a higher rate of complications.[43] The latest secondary stroke prevention guidelines recommend adding glucagon-like peptide-1(GLP-1) receptor agonist to first-line therapy in patients with diabetes to reduce stroke risk,[13] while the evidence for primary stroke prevention is still pending.[6] The benefit of GLP-1 in stroke risk reduction is likely multifactorial, although these agents may provide some neuroprotection and reduction in atherosclerosis.[43] Management of high cholesterol should follow the same guidelines as primary prevention of cardiovascular disease for primary stroke prevention.

Healthy lifestyle measures have a major impact on stroke risk, most notably a Mediterranean diet, physical activity, and tobacco cessation. Physical activity is integral to stroke prevention, and people should be encouraged to avoid long periods of sedentary behavior. Guidelines recommend engaging in at least 150 minutes of moderate intensity or 75 minutes of high intensity exercise per week to reduce risk of stroke.[6] Addressing obesity and weight loss are important to control the risk of stroke as a higher body mass index is associated with a higher risk of stroke. Some patients may benefit from bariatric surgery, and newer evidence suggests that certain groups may benefit from the new GLP-1 receptor agonists to control weight, cardiovascular, and stroke risk.[6]

Cigarette smoking is a significant risk factor for stroke. Cessation of smoking reduces the risk of stroke to a level similar to nonsmokers after 5–15 years of abstinence. Older adults should still be encouraged to stop smoking.[44] Guidelines support the use of pharmacologic agents such as nicotine replacement therapy, varenicline, or bupropion in addition to counseling for smoking cessation.[13]

Antiplatelet and anticoagulant use in primary prevention

Antiplatelet or anticoagulant therapy is only recommended for primary prevention of cerebrovascular disease in a few patient populations. Antiplatelet is recommended for those with systemic lupus erythematosus or antiphospholipid syndrome without any stroke or systemic clot history.[6] Even though older age is a vascular risk factor, studies have shown no stroke risk reduction and a higher risk of bleeding when initiating antiplatelet therapy in this population as primary prevention.[5,6,45] In the setting of incidentally found silent infarcts, controversy in the field exists on the use of antiplatelet agents in patients without any clinical stroke symptoms, and bleeding risk must be weighed.[6]

Patients with AF should be prescribed anticoagulation if their estimated annual risk of stroke or thromboembolic event is 2% or more, equaling a CHA2DS2-VASc ≥2 for men and ≥3 for women.[46] The major risk for cardioembolic stroke in older adults is nonvalvular AF,[26,47] and antiplatelets are not effective in this population.[5] The Framingham Study demonstrated an increasing incidence of AF and that 36.2% of strokes in patients ages 80–89 can be attributed to AF.[47] In patients >70 years, clinical trials for stroke prevention in AF have shown that aspirin is ineffective in preventing embolic stroke, and anticoagulation with warfarin had a significant protective effect.[48–51] In the Stroke Prevention in Atrial Fibrillation (SPAF) trial, the risk of hemorrhagic stroke and other hemorrhagic complications in those over 75 years equaled the risk reduction of cardioembolic stroke for warfarin compared with aspirin.[48]

Direct oral anticoagulants (DOACs), including the direct thrombin inhibitor dabigatran and the factor Xa inhibitors apixaban, rivaroxaban, and edoxaban, are the mainstream anticoagulants used in nonvalvular AF instead of warfarin given their advantages in dosing, drug interactions, and side effects. These should be considered as first-line at all ages.[52–57] Agents may require dose reduction based on age, renal function, or weight. A meta-analysis of randomized clinical trials of patients 75 years and older with AF showed no significant difference in stroke outcome between DOACs and warfarin. Additionally, DOACs overall carry about half the risk of intracerebral hemorrhage when compared with warfarin,[46] however, some evidence suggests a higher risk of bleeding with rivaroxaban.[57] For this reason, the American Geriatric Society 2023 guidelines recommend avoiding rivaroxaban in adults age 65 years and older with AF due to higher bleeding risk when compared with other DOACs, except for special circumstances such as the need for improved medication adherence with once daily dosing.[58] Some may want to avoid dabigatran in older adults, as it is the most renally excreted and can have large variations in blood levels.[5] Apixaban had a lower risk of stroke compared to warfarin as well as a lower rate of hemorrhagic complications,[52] and the American Geriatric Society favors apixaban as well based on safety profile.[58] At this time, DOACs have not been compared head-to-head in a randomized clinical trial, making the decision of which to use often dependent on clinician practice or insurance access. The efficacy and low rate of hemorrhagic complications have made apixaban a popular choice in the stroke neurology and geriatric community. To date, only warfarin is approved for use in valvular AF.[13]

At times there is a hesitancy to anticoagulate older adults because of a fear of intracerebral hemorrhage and risk of falls. One study has suggested that a patient would have to fall 295 times per year for the risk of traumatic subdural hematoma to outweigh the benefit of anticoagulation.[59] In the BAFTA trial, adults with AF ≥75 years randomized to warfarin had a lower relative risk of stroke, ICH, or systemic embolus than the aspirin group.[60] In light of the positive outcomes of the DOAC trials on stroke prevention and data indicating that certain DOACs may not have significantly higher major bleeding risk than aspirin,[61] DOACs are encouraged in older adults.[5] Studies have evaluated whether hypertensive or CAA-related hemorrhages are more common in patients on anticoagulation, and while results have varied, it is clear that control of blood pressure is key to reducing the risk of hemorrhage.[62] The HAS-BLED score was developed to help compare the risk of bleeding with anticoagulation to the risk of stroke with AF and can be used in treatment decision-making.[63,64] Two reversal agents are FDA approved for DOAC-related hemorrhage: idarucizumab for dabigatran and andexanet alfa for factor Xa inhibitors, although many centers continue rely on four-factor prothrombin complex concentrate due to availability, cost, and thrombotic risk with andexanet alfa.[65]

Cardioversion of patients with AF can be utilized to prevent cerebral emboli, although patients may still require anticoagulation. Additionally, certain patients with AF and contraindications to long-term anticoagulation may undergo left atrial appendage (LAA) closure. Placement of the device is designed to prevent embolization of LAA clot, but does require that the patient tolerate short-term periprocedural anticoagulation and long-term antiplatelet therapy.[46]

Anticoagulation with warfarin has also been beneficial in preventing stroke during the first 3 months after myocardial infarction[66] although aspirin is usually used for long-term prophylaxis. Patients with heart failure and dilated cardiomyopathy with enlarged left ventricle and have normal sinus rhythm are at risk for cardioembolic stroke. However, the large WARCEF trial showed no significant difference in a primary composite endpoint of ischemic stroke, ICH, and death comparing treatment with warfarin versus aspirin for patients with ejection fraction ≤35%.[67] Notably, in adults 60 years and older, the rate of ischemic stroke did not differ significantly between treatment groups, but there was a higher rate of ICH and death in the warfarin group.[68]

Atherosclerotic plaque in the ascending aorta and aortic arch has also been implicated as a potential, likely underrecognized, source of embolic stroke.[25] When these plaques are identified as an incidental finding with TEE performed for cardiac disease, then stroke prophylaxis may be indicated with aspirin therapy and cholesterol management, as well as overall consideration of atherosclerotic risk factor profile. Routine screening for carotid artery stenosis is not recommended in patients who are asymptomatic.[6]

SECONDARY PREVENTION OF STROKE

Secondary stroke prevention pertains to anyone who has had a stroke or TIA. Similar to primary prevention, control of blood pressure, diabetes, and high cholesterol is essential to preventing recurrent cerebrovascular events (Table 24.1). Once someone has had a stroke, pharmacologic treatment with antithrombotic therapy is indicated. In selected patients, surgical interventions such as carotid artery stenting or endarterectomy may prevent recurrent stroke.

Antiplatelet therapy is the mainstay of secondary prevention in patients with noncardioembolic stroke and TIA and should be implemented as soon as possible after the event. The International Stroke Trial, which included >60% of participants over age 70, demonstrated a beneficial effect of aspirin 300 mg at the time of onset of noncardioembolic ischemic stroke. A reduction in the outcomes of recurrent stroke and death or nonfatal recurrent stroke was seen at 14 days.[69] A 2014 Cochrane review analyzed eight trials of over 40,000 participants evaluating the initiation of immediate aspirin therapy (largely within 48 hours of the event) after acute ischemic stroke. This review suggested a significant reduction in recurrent ischemic stroke, significantly outweighing a small increase in intracranial hemorrhage, and a long-term decrease in death or dependency.[70] Guidelines currently recommend aspirin 81–325 mg within 24–48 hours of the stroke onset if no thrombolysis is given and once hemorrhage is ruled out.[71]

Both aspirin and clopidogrel have been shown to significantly reduce the risk of stroke, and the CAPRIE trial suggested that in patients with preexisting vascular risk factors, stroke occurred in similar numbers among patients taking aspirin versus clopidogrel.[72] In 2020, ticagrelor, a reversible, direct inhibitor of the P2Y12 adenosine diphosphate receptor, was demonstrated to have benefit in stroke patients.[73] A single antiplatelet is indicated for long-term secondary stroke prevention in patients without indication for anticoagulation for confirmed cardioembolic stroke or an alternative secondary prevention regimen. Since 2013, a few landmark trials support short-term dual antiplatelet (DAPT) in select patients with stroke and TIA.[9–11,74]

High-risk TIA and minor ischemic stroke

The following patient populations benefit from a course of DAPT: (1) acute minor stroke, (2) high-risk TIA, and (3) stroke due to symptomatic large artery atherosclerosis.

Early initiation of DAPT in patients with high-risk TIA and minor stroke has been studied in multiple randomized controlled trials. The first trial to support this practice was the CHANCE trial, published in 2013. In CHANCE, over 5000 Chinese patients of median age 62 treated with 21 days of aspirin and clopidogrel started within 24 hours of onset of a high-risk TIA or minor stroke had a lower rate of recurrent stroke than those treated with aspirin alone, without significant risk of bleeding.[9] The POINT[10] trial followed, published in 2018, redemonstrating the benefit of aspirin and clopidogrel for high-risk TIA and minor stroke. POINT included almost 5000 patients of median age 65 from an international population. The study assessed use of DAPT for 90 days initiated within 12 hours of symptom onset, and results revealed a lower risk of major ischemic events and a higher risk of major hemorrhage at 90 days.[10] Subsequent analysis of CHANCE and POINT suggested maximum benefit and safety of DAPT use within the first 21 days, and longer use may expose patients to excess risk without significant benefit.[75]

While both CHANCE and POINT had stringent inclusion criteria and defined high-risk TIA as ABCD2 score ≥4 and minor stroke as National Institutes of Health Stroke Scale (NIHSS) ≤3, significant variation in real-world practice exists. The READAPT study in 2023 explored real-world DAPT use for over 1000 stroke and TIA patients at multiple centers across Italy. Results showed ~30% of the ischemic stroke patients did not meet the trial criteria because of NIHSS >3, and ~7% with NIHSS >5. Almost 20% of the TIA patients did not meet trial criteria due to ABCD2 <4. Other common reasons that patients would not have met the trial criteria were DAPT initiation after 24 hours, undergoing revascularization procedures, and variations in the loading doses of aspirin and clopidogrel.[76] We encourage individualized decision-making in all patients with acute stroke and consideration of the suspected mechanism.

More recently, the international THALES trial evaluated the use of aspirin and ticagrelor for 30 days in mild-moderate stroke (NIHSS ≤5) or high-risk TIA (ABCD2 ≥6 or presence of symptomatic atherosclerosis) within 24 hours of stroke onset.[74] Results revealed a lower risk of stroke or death at 30 days in the DAPT group compared to aspirin monotherapy in over 11,000 patients with mean age 65.[74] This trial provides evidence that ticagrelor may be an alternative to clopidogrel in DAPT, which is important because up to ~60% of Asian patients and ~25% of

White patients may have a resistance to clopidogrel due to a loss-of-function genetic variant thus making the medication ineffective.[74] For this reason, the CHANCE-2 trial in 2021 investigated the use of ticagrelor versus clopidogrel in addition to aspirin in patients with the CYP2C19 loss-of-function variant. The trial involved DAPT for 21 days for minor stroke (NIHSS ≤3) or high-risk TIA (ABCD2 ≥4) within 24 hours of symptom onset. Risk of stroke at 90 days was lower with ticagrelor use compared to clopidogrel in this patient population, and risk of hemorrhage did not significantly differ.[77] Subsequent analysis of CHANCE-2 suggested patients 80 years and older had a higher risk of vascular events, disabling stroke, moderate to severe hemorrhage, and mortality within 90 days of DAPT use, and ticagrelor showed equal efficacy and safety to clopidogrel in this age group despite the genetic variant.[78]

Atherosclerotic disease and carotid revascularization

Secondary prevention guidelines recommend treating patients ≤75 years with stroke of presumed atherosclerotic origin with the highest intensity statin tolerated, regardless of LDL, with a goal of LDL <70. Patients >75 years who are not a candidate for high-intensity statin should be treated with moderate-intensity statin.[79] For those requiring additional agents to effectively reduce LDL, or not tolerating high-dose statin therapy, ezetimibe and proprotein convertase subtilisin–kexin type 9 (PCSK-9) inhibitors can be considered as adjunctive therapy.[5,80] Even in older adults, studies have demonstrated reduced major cardiovascular outcomes with lower LDL.[5]

Symptomatic atherosclerosis is typically treated with DAPT for 90 days. The SAMMPRIS trial investigated 451 patients of average age ~60 years with recent TIA or nondisabling stroke attributed to symptomatic ICAD (stenosis of 70%–99% of a proximal intracranial artery) treated with aggressive medical management versus intracranial stent. Aggressive medical management included 90 days of aspirin and clopidogrel with risk factor reduction measures, notably targeting normotensive blood pressure, an LDL cholesterol <70mg/dL, and a strict lifestyle modification program. Aggressive medical management was superior to surgical intervention, as the rate of stroke or death was significantly lower (5.8% medical management vs. 14.7% surgical intervention) at 30 days in the medical management group, and this trend continued at 1-year follow-up (12.2% medical management vs. 20% surgical intervention).[11]

The INSPIRES trial, published in 2023, provided further evidence for the use of DAPT for stroke due to intracranial or extracranial atherosclerosis. This trial included over 6000 patients of median age 65 in China enrolled within 72 hours of high-risk TIA (ABCD2 ≥4) or mild-moderate stroke (NIH ≤5) due to at least 50% atherosclerotic disease of a major intracranial or extracranial artery. Results demonstrated lower risk of stroke at 90 days (7.3% in DAPT vs. 9.2% aspirin only) but a higher risk of moderate-severe bleeding (0.9% in DAPT vs. 0.4% in aspirin only).[81] What constitutes the optimal antithrombotic regimen for symptomatic ICAD is currently under investigation in the CAPTIVA trial.[82]

Patients with cervical carotid artery disease may be eligible and benefit from a carotid revascularization procedure for stroke prevention, including carotid endarterectomy (CEA), carotid artery stenting (CAS), or, more recently, transcarotid revascularization (TCAR). Diagnosis of carotid artery disease is generally made through noninvasive imaging. Ultrasound, CTA, or MRA all have an accuracy of about ~90% in identifying stenosis >70% compared to gold-standard angiography.[83] When the results of the CTA/MRA agree, the accuracy is ~99%.[84] When the two studies do not agree, angiography is usually performed to determine if there is greater than 70% stenosis, or to be certain that there is not an inoperable complete occlusion of the internal carotid. Lately, advances in MRA vessel wall imaging have enhanced stroke etiology investigation by providing information about vessel wall properties in patients with vasculopathy.[85]

In patients with symptomatic carotid artery disease (i.e., ipsilateral TIA or stroke) with at least 50% stenosis, revascularization may be indicated to prevent stroke. Guidelines support early CEA in patients with at least 50% symptomatic carotid stenosis and low surgical risk. Data have suggested that the benefit of CEA is higher with severe (70%–99%) compared to moderate (50%–69%) stenosis, and improved outcomes in early revascularization within 2 weeks of nondisabling ischemic event. No benefit has been shown for carotid revascularization in patients with <50% carotid stenosis.[13]

Patients 70 years and older eligible for carotid revascularization should receive CEA over CAS to reduce periprocedural stroke risk.[13] In the landmark CREST Trial, the risk of ischemic stroke, myocardial infarction, or death in patients undergoing CEA and CAS for carotid stenosis was equivalent.[86] However, patients treated with CAS had a higher risk of stroke, and patients treated with CEA had a great risk of myocardial infarction.[86] A meta-analysis of four randomized controlled trials of almost 5000 patients with symptomatic carotid stenosis demonstrated that CEA was superior to CAS in patients aged 70–74 years and older.[87] Data showed that the periprocedural risk of stroke or death in CAS increased with older age, while age did not significantly impact periprocedural risk in CEA.[87] For older patients who are not surgical candidates, CAS can be considered. Initiating patients on DAPT prior to timely carotid surgery (generally within 1–2 weeks from the event) for symptomatic stenosis may improve neurologic outcomes without significantly increasing perioperative hemorrhagic complications.[88]

TCAR is another option that avoids manipulating the aortic arch as access goes directly into the common carotid artery. Assessment of outcomes with the more recent utilization of TCAR is limited so far.[13]

Surgical management of asymptomatic carotid stenosis remains controversial, and the asymptomatic carotid artery revascularization trials published decades ago do not reflect the current era of maximal medical therapy.[89] All patients with asymptomatic carotid stenosis should receive intensive medical management and counseling on healthy lifestyle measures, such as the importance of a healthy diet and exercise, and smoking cessation. Medical management generally includes an antiplatelet (most commonly aspirin), agents for high cholesterol to reach LDL <70, normotensive blood pressure, and hemoglobin A1c <7%.[90]

In the SPACE-2 trial, published in 2022, patients 50–85 years old with high-grade asymptomatic carotid artery stenosis ≥70% received intensive medical management and were randomized to CEA, CAS, or medical treatment alone.[91] While the sample size was insufficient, results did not show superiority of the revascularization procedures in addition to medical management over medical management alone on risk of any stroke or death within 30 days or ipsilateral stroke over the 5-year study period.[91] The ECST-2 trial randomized patients over 18 years with low to intermediate stroke risk with both symptomatic and asymptomatic carotid artery stenosis ≥50% to revascularization (mostly CEA) plus intensive medical management versus intensive medical management alone.[92] This trial also had a low, insufficient sample size, however, preliminary results indicate there was no significant difference in stroke outcomes between the two groups.[93] Both trials had insufficient power to produce conclusive results. Currently, the CREST-2 trial is attempting to answer the question of how maximal medical therapy compares to CEA and CAS plus maximal medical therapy for asymptomatic carotid artery stenosis.[94]

Overall, the incidence of stroke ipsilateral to carotid stenosis has declined over the past decades thanks to aggressive medical management and lifestyle modifications. There are certain patients with asymptomatic carotid stenosis who may benefit from revascularization, and the decision should be individualized. Important considerations include imaging features of the atherosclerosis that may increase the risk for ipsilateral stroke as well as a patient's surgical risk and life expectancy.[90]

Cardioembolic stroke

Unlike immediate implementation of antiplatelet therapy in noncardioembolic ischemic stroke, immediate anticoagulation after cardioembolic stroke can worsen the neurologic condition by contributing to hemorrhagic transformation of the infarct. This is particularly applicable to older patients, as the risk of major hemorrhagic transformation increases with age.[95,96] In several studies, the risk of re-embolization in patients with AF is about 2%, while the risk of major hemorrhagic transformation resulting in clinical deterioration is about 8% in the first 48 hours after stroke.[95,96] A small area of infarction on the initial CT scan does not indicate that it is safe to anticoagulate acutely because the full extent of the lesion may not be detected on CT initially. Diffusion weighted MRI is more sensitive in identifying the extent of early infarction, and when the region of infarcted brain is small, early anticoagulation can be instituted.

While there is no definitive guidance in the secondary stroke prevention guidelines, the 1–3–6–12 day rule can be adopted for patients with AF and acute stroke, referring to starting anticoagulation after 1 day for TIA, 3 days for minor (NIHSS <8), 6 days for moderate (NIHSS 8–15), and 12 days for severe stroke or with hemorrhagic transformation (NIHSS ≥16).[97] Often a CT scan is repeated prior to initiating anticoagulation to ensure hemorrhagic transformation has not occurred to make initiation of anticoagulation unsafe. The Early versus Later Anticoagulation for Stroke with Atrial Fibrillation (ELAN) trial in 2023 suggested that earlier anticoagulation with DOACs after acute ischemic stroke may be safe and effective.[98] Patients were randomly assigned to early anticoagulation (within 48 hours after minor or moderate stroke, or 6–7 days after major stroke) or later anticoagulation (3–4 days after minor stroke, 6–7 days after moderate stroke, 12–24 days after major stroke). Of note, the ELAN trial used imaging criteria to define the severity of stroke as opposed to NIHSS. The median age of over 2000 patients enrolled was 77 years. Results indicated that after 30 days, recurrent ischemic strokes occurred in 1.4% and 2.5% of the early anticoagulation and late anticoagulation group, respectively. Incidence of intracranial hemorrhage was about equal at 0.2% in both groups.[98] While no hypothesis was tested for superiority or noninferiority in this study, this large randomized clinical trial suggests that earlier initiation of DOACs in patients with acute ischemic stroke and AF is safe and may reduce adverse neurological outcomes.

Early anticoagulation is also necessary in patients with prosthetic cardiac valves who experience stroke because the risk of early re-embolization is greater, particularly when noninfectious vegetations are seen on the prosthesis with echocardiography. However, bacterial endocarditis must be ruled out in these instances prior to anticoagulation because mycotic aneurysms can form from infected emboli and can cause hemorrhage when the patient is anticoagulated.[99,100] In addition to AF, patients with stroke and heart failure with reduced ejection fraction <15% may benefit from anticoagulation to reduce stroke risk.[101]

Cryptogenic and embolic stroke of undetermined source

Patients with cryptogenic stroke, or ESUS, are typically treated with antiplatelet therapy. ESUS has been the subject of several studies to assess the hypothesis that treatment with anticoagulation is superior to antiplatelet, however, so far no clear evidence exists to support this approach.[13,30,80,102] In addition to the typical stroke workup, patients with cryptogenic stroke, and especially ESUS, typically undergo prolonged cardiac monitoring to assess for occult AF. Monitors are generally either a Holter monitor for 30 days or an implantable loop recorder (ILR) for up to 3 years. Studies have shown higher AF detection rates for patients with ischemic stroke with ILR. In randomized studies, detection of AF in patients with ILR was estimated at 30% after 3 years of monitoring post-stroke, while those who underwent a 30-day Holter monitor or usual care showed AF detection at 3% after 3 years.[46] AF detected at the time of stroke has the strongest association with risk of recurrent stroke. More research is needed to better understand the mechanistic significance of AF detected long after stroke, as well as the impact of short paroxysms of AF on stroke risk, although anticoagulation is often initiated for secondary prevention in such patients.[103]

PFO is a major cause of cryptogenic stroke and ESUS in the young, and trials have suggested that PFO closure may be beneficial in patients under 60 years.[104] The major PFO randomized trials did not sufficiently include patients over 60 years, so current data do not provide strong evidence for closure as part of secondary stroke prevention in this population. The RoPE score and PASCAL classification system are used to estimate the likelihood that a cryptogenic stroke is due to PFO.[105]

HYPERACUTE THERAPY FOR ISCHEMIC STROKE

Thrombolysis

In 1995, acute stroke care was revolutionized by the adoption of intravenous thrombolysis for hyperacute management. The National Institute of Neurological Disorders and Stroke (NINDS) rt-PA Stroke Study Group assessed intravenous alteplase (IV tPA) for acute ischemic stroke within 3 hours of onset (Table 24.2). Part 1 of the trial, which assessed neurologic outcome 24 hours after tPA, did not show a significant benefit in resolution or marked improvement of neurologic deficits. Part 2 of the trial, however, demonstrated that patients were >30% more likely to have minimal or no disability at 3 months compared to placebo.[8] Evidence suggests tPA can be administered safely to patients older than 80 years without a significant increase in the incidence of symptomatic cerebral hemorrhage.[106] In NINDS, 44 patients >80 years received tPA, and there was a consistent treatment effect by age.[8,107,108] Additionally, post hoc and pooled analyses have supported a consistent treatment effect by age.[107]

The ECASS III trial helped extend the treatment window to 4.5 hours after demonstrating that more patients had a favorable outcome when treated with alteplase administered between 3 and 4.5 hours from symptom onset (Table 24.2). The incidence of symptomatic intracranial hemorrhage was higher in the alteplase group, but there was no significant mortality difference. However, patients >80 years were not included in ECASS III, and no rigorous evidence for thrombolysis in the 3–4.5 hour time window exists for this age group.[109] Regardless, most clinicians do not exclude patients on the basis of age alone in the extended time window. A 2017 nationwide cohort study of thrombolysis in older adult stroke patients with and without dementia demonstrated that patients with dementia are less likely to receive tPA. This study included patients of median age 82 who received thrombolysis up to 4.5 hours from symptom onset. There was no significant difference in symptomatic ICH or death at 3 months in patients with or without dementia.[110]

Tenecteplase (TNK), a genetically modified form of alteplase, has pharmacologic and administrative advantages over tPA and is increasingly used instead of tPA for thrombolysis in acute ischemic stroke. TNK has higher fibrin specificity and resistance to plasminogen activator inhibitor-1, longer half-life, and easier administration as

Table 24.2 Thrombolysis trials comparison: NINDS versus ECASS III

Characteristic	NINDS	ECASS III
Hours from onset to thrombolysis	0–3	3–4.5
Number of patients	624	821
Location	United States	Europe
Age criteria (years)	18+	18–80
Age of intervention cohort*	Part 1: 67 ± 10 Part 2: 69 ± 12	64.9 ± 12.2
Male sex (%)	Part 1: 59 Part 2: 58	60
Primary outcome	Part 1: Early neurologic improvement (24 hours) Part 2: Sustained improvement (3 months)	Functional outcome at 90 days
Age subanalysis	Consistent treatment effect by age	Consistent treatment effect in <65 vs. ≥65

a single bolus as opposed to an infusion.[111] Multiple trials comparing TNK to tPA have supported its safety and efficacy, and TNK at a dose of 0.25mg/kg in a single IV bolus has become an accepted alternative to tPA in acute ischemic stroke.[71] Further analysis of the EXTEND-IA trial investigated the safety and efficacy of TNK in older patients aged over 80 years with LVO. Patients were randomized to receive TNK at two different doses versus tPA. Results showed that TNK at the accepted dose of 0.25 mg/kg had better functional outcome at 90 days compared to the higher dose of TNK 0.40 mg/kg and tPA 0.90mg/kg.[112]

Current guidelines support the use of IV thrombolysis in patients with disabling deficits from acute ischemic stroke within the appropriate time window, regardless of severity or NIHSS.[71] However, use of thrombolysis in patients with mild, nondisabling stroke is not supported by current evidence. The PRISMS trial in 2018 evaluated outcomes of tPA versus aspirin monotherapy within 3 hours of symptom onset in patients with nondisabling, mild symptoms (NIHSS ≤5). The study did not reach target recruitment, limiting conclusions, however, results indicated no significant difference in use of IV thrombolysis compared to aspirin in a favorable functional outcome at 90 days.[113] The ARAMIS trial, published in 2023, investigated the noninferiority of DAPT (aspirin and clopidogrel) versus IV thrombolysis for patients with acute minor nondisabling (NIHSS ≤5) ischemic stroke within 4.5 hours of symptom onset in China. Results suggested that DAPT was noninferior to IV alteplase with respect to a favorable functional outcome at 90 days.[114] Perceptions of what constitutes a disabling deficit can differ among patients and providers, and shared decision-making is crucial.

Care must be taken in selecting patients for administration of thrombolysis, and stroke centers have guidelines to avoid hemorrhagic complications. Administration of IV thrombolysis to patients more than 4.5 hours after ischemic stroke or to patients who have evidence of extensive infarction on CT scan leads to a greater risk of hemorrhagic complications and should be avoided.[109]

Mechanical thrombectomy

Acute stroke care underwent another revolution in 2015 with the establishment of mechanical thrombectomy (MT) as standard of care for eligible patients with LVO. Five landmark trials published in 2015 demonstrated the superiority of MT in addition to intravenous tPA for patients with confirmed LVO of the anterior circulation presenting within 6 hours of onset (Table 24.3).[115–121] The HERMES meta-analysis evaluated patient-level data from the five pivotal MT trials comparing standard care (including thrombolysis in eligible patients) to standard care plus MT.[121] The analysis included 1287 patients

Table 24.3 Landmark mechanical thrombectomy trials for anterior vessel occlusions[116–120]

	MR CLEAN	ESCAPE	REVASCAT	SWIFT PRIME	EXTEND IA
Hours from onset to thrombectomy	6	12	8	6	6
Number of patients	500	316	206	196	70
Location	Netherlands	International	Spain	United States and Europe	Australia and New Zealand
Age criteria (years)	18+	18+	18–85	18–80	18+
Age of intervention cohort*	65.8 (54.5–76.0)	71 (60–81)	65.7 ± 11.3	65.0 ± 12.5	68.6 ± 12.3
Male sex (%)	58	48	55	52	49
Thrombolysis use (%)	89	76	73	100	100
Primary outcome	Functional outcome at 90 days	Functional outcome at 90 days	Functional outcome at 90 days	Functional outcome at 90 days	Reperfusion at 24 hours and neurologic improvement on day 3
Age subanalysis	Consistent treatment effect in <80 vs. ≥80 years	Consistent treatment effect in <80 vs. ≥80 years	Consistent treatment effect in 70 vs. ≥70 years	Consistent treatment effect in 70 vs. ≥70 years	None

*Age reported in years as mean ± standard deviation or median (interquartile range).

with a median age of 68 years old, and 15% of the trial population was at least 80 years old. HERMES redemonstrated that those who underwent MT had lower levels of disability at 90 days compared to the control group. Subgroup analysis by age showed no difference in treatment effect.[121,122]

The evidentiary trials only included patients functionally independent at baseline, meaning the benefit of MT in patients with pre-stroke disability is not as clear.[7] A retrospective cohort study between 2015 and 2017 at two tertiary care centers aimed to evaluate this question and included 96 patients ≥80 years with baseline mild to moderate disability.[122] Successful MT occurred in almost 85% of the study population, with no difference between the two disability groups in return to independent or baseline functional status at 90 days, which occurred in about a third of the study population. Of note, mortality was significantly higher in patients with moderate baseline disability.[122] While a large international survey study in 2019 suggested that stroke experts consider age a key decision factor in pursuing MT,[123] this study had similar rates of good outcome in patients over 80 years with minimal disability as found in HERMES, supporting the notion that the level of disability should likely factor more into the decision to pursue MT than age.[122]

Subsequently, in 2018, trials were published extending the window for MT up to 24 hours in select patients with mismatch between the severity of the clinical deficit and the infarct volume, as determined by advanced perfusion imaging.[124,125] Recently, studies have explored the benefit of MT for the treatment of large ischemic strokes within 24 hours, with or without advanced perfusion imaging, and results suggest that patients with large infarcts still benefit from MT compared to standard care. However, age may play a role in functional outcomes, and those >80 years were underrepresented in trial populations.[126]

Hyperacute treatment of stroke with thrombolysis and MT has altered the landscape of stroke. Stroke is just as much of an emergency as a heart attack. Early recognition of stroke and emergency transport to a hospital capable of modern acute stroke care saves lives.

Nonpharmacological acute management and prevention of progression

Acute management of stroke requires careful monitoring, often in a stroke or telemetry unit. Blood pressure must be maintained at a level to ensure perfusion of the ischemic penumbra, or the region around the core infarct that is ischemic but not irreversibly damaged. Most stroke patients have an elevation of blood pressure for the first 48 hours, a response to the ischemic event, which improves without treatment.[127] In the acute setting, permissive hypertension is generally allowed for the first 24–48 hours, followed by a gradual reduction in blood pressure. Drastic reduction in blood pressure can cause worsening of the stroke.[71]

In patients who develop cerebral edema after LVO, mannitol or hypertonic saline may reduce cytotoxic edema, but steroids have no benefit.[128,129] In extreme cases, hemicraniectomy of the skull on the affected side relieves intracranial pressure and prevents herniation. After the HAMLET trial, DESTINY II provided evidence that hemicraniectomy offers some benefit in patients >60 years.[130,131] Patients age 61–82 with malignant middle cerebral artery who received hemicraniectomy had improved survival but were left requiring assistance with bodily needs.[130]

Patients who are immobilized from stroke should wear intermittent pneumatic compression stockings, and some may benefit from deep vein thromboprophylaxis. If there is a substantial risk of bleeding, low-dose anticoagulation for prophylaxis is held.[71] Physical and occupational, as well as speech therapy, if indicated, as soon as possible after a stroke can benefit recovery.[132]

Medical complications

The major medical complications associated with stroke are myocardial infarction, pulmonary emboli, aspiration pneumonia, airway obstruction, and reduction in the level of consciousness compromising respiration. An electrocardiogram is imperative to rule out concurrent myocardial infarction, and if there is any suggestive history of myocardial infarction, serial enzymes are obtained. Stroke units with monitored beds are useful in detecting and preventing complications of arrhythmia that could occur with concomitant myocardial infarction, or as the result of the stroke itself.

Post-stroke depression (PSD) occurs in approximately one third of stroke patients and can significantly impact recovery and quality of life.[133] History of psychiatric conditions may increase the risk of PSD, while older age may be protective against PSD. Interestingly, one large Medicare data study suggests that there is a >50% greater risk of developing depression after stroke compared to after myocardial infarction.[133] Timely diagnosis and management of PSD are crucial for optimizing recovery.

Post-stroke cognitive impairment is highly prevalent, occurring in approximately half of stroke patients. Severity of stroke likely plays a role, and over one third of patients with moderate-severe stroke may show signs of dementia after 1 year.[134]

Of note, older adults often have small infarcts or ischemic changes found on imaging without a known history of stroke or focal neurologic deficits, and these ischemic changes may contribute to cognitive decline.[135] When ischemia is identified as a contributor to the dementia, identification of stroke risk factors is essential, and appropriate vascular health management, including antithrombotic therapy, should be initiated when indicated. Adults with cognitive impairment on anti-amyloid antibody therapies for Alzheimer's disease should not receive thrombolysis due to risk of amyloid-related imaging abnormalities, including hemorrhage.[136]

MANAGEMENT OF HEMORRHAGIC STROKE

Appropriate blood pressure management is of the utmost importance in ICH management. The INTERACT-2 trial demonstrated that rapid lowering of systolic blood pressure to <140 mmHg within 1 hour resulted in lower death or major disability.[137] The ATACH2 trial demonstrated no difference in the risk of death or disability at 3 months in intensive management of SBP <140 but did demonstrate higher rates of adverse renal events.[138] Current guidelines recommend the goal of SBP 130–150 when patients present with SBP between 150 and 220 mmHg in the setting of spontaneous ICH. Drastic blood pressure fluctuations and SBP <130 can negatively impact outcomes.[33]

Unless emergent neurosurgical management is undertaken, the literature does not support the routine use of platelet transfusions in patients taking antiplatelet agents at the time of hemorrhage.[139] Patients on anticoagulation with spontaneous ICH should stop the agent immediately and receive reversal agents to improve survival outcomes.

Endotracheal intubation may be necessary for airway protection and for impending brain herniation with respiratory failure. Hyperventilation may be helpful to reduce increased intracranial pressure. Mannitol can reduce cerebral edema acutely in cases of impending herniation. Steroids do not provide any benefit in improving outcomes of patients with ICH and should not be incorporated in treatment even in cases of high ICP due to ICH.[33]

Surgical management of intracranial hemorrhage is employed in certain instances. Shunting of fluid and removal of blood from the ventricular system can reduce intracranial pressure and prevent hydrocephalus. In cerebellar hemorrhage, surgical drainage of the hematoma can be performed without inordinate risk to prevent compression of the brain stem and death.[33]

Currently, minimally invasive, stereotactic approaches to surgical management of ICH are being investigated. The recently published ENRICH study included adults up to 80 years to examine the effect of minimally invasive surgical intervention for anterior basal ganglia and lobar hemorrhages.[140] Surgical intervention led to improved functional outcomes at 6 months compared to medical management, given limitations in the study population and analysis, these results are most likely attributable to the lobar hemorrhage group.[140]

SUBARACHNOID HEMORRHAGE (SAH)

The major intracranial vessels are located in the subarachnoid space between the pia mater and dura mater. Aneurysms form at branch points from the vessels of the Circle of Willis at the base of the brain. Rupture of these aneurysms produces severe headache, photophobia, and stiff neck. The patient may become somnolent or comatose. A third nerve paralysis with ptosis, pupillary dilation, and ophthalmoplegia can result when a hematoma forms on the oculomotor nerve running just below the posterior communicating artery. Focal neurological disturbances such as hemiparesis can also occur acutely, and focality and obtundation portend a worse prognosis. Head CT can diagnose SAH in most cases, and within the first 6 hours a negative CT on a high-quality scanner read by a neuroradiologist is sufficient to reasonably exclude SAH given the high sensitivity of the image. After 6 hours of presentation, lumbar puncture may be necessary when the CT scan is negative and there is a high clinical suspicion of SAH. The gold standard to identify the aneurysm is cerebral angiography.[141]

Optimal care for aneurysmal SAH involves prevention of rebleeding and management of delayed cerebral ischemia (DCI). Most importantly, patients should receive timely intervention either by surgical clipping or coiling of the aneurysm, ideally within the first 24 hours.[141,142] For patients >70 years, no clear evidence suggests that coiling or clipping is superior.[141] Older age is not a reason to necessarily forgo surgical intervention; consideration of intervention should be individualized and involve shared decision-making.[141]

Vasospasm is the most common and serious complication in SAH, as it can contribute to DCI and lead to worsening neurologic deficits and death. Spasm can be detected by measurement of increased flow velocities with TCD. The calcium channel blocker nimodipine should be initiated early after SAH to prevent DCI and improve functional outcomes. When vasospasm occurs postoperatively, the blood pressure can be elevated to increase cerebral perfusion. When vasospasm is severe, intra-arterial vasodilators and angioplasty can be considered.[141]

Arteriovenous malformation (AVM) of the brain, in which arteries feed directly into the venous system without going through a capillary bed, can also cause SAH. Surgical extirpation can eliminate the source of the bleeding, but often the AVM can recur or too much brain parenchyma is at risk for resection to be feasible.[143] Embolization of colloidal particles or endovascular insertion of coils can be employed to thrombose the AVM. It is unusual to be able to eliminate the AVM by these methods, but the size can be reduced so that it becomes amenable to surgical removal. Radiosurgery with gamma knife technology can also eliminate or reduce the volume of the AVM.[144] In 2013, enrollment for the ARUBA trial was stopped when medical management of unruptured AVMs was found to be superior to interventional therapy with neurosurgery, embolization, or stereotactic radiotherapy alone or in combination.[145]

CONCLUSION

New treatments for stroke have dramatically improved outcomes. While prevention is still paramount to stroke management, the use of dual antiplatelet regimens, DOACs, IV thrombolysis, and MT for a wide range of patients has changed the concept of stroke from hopeless to a highly treatable condition. Stroke should be treated as an acute emergency, or brain attack, to optimize patient outcomes regardless of age.

REFERENCES

1. Mozaffarian D, Benjamin EJ, Go AS, et al. Heart disease and stroke statistics-2016 update: a report from the American Heart Association. *Circulation* 2016;133(4):e38–360. (In Eng). DOI: 10.1161/cir.0000000000000350.
2. Howard G, Goff DC. Population shifts and the future of stroke: forecasts of the future burden of stroke. *Ann N Y Acad Sci* 2012;1268:14–20. DOI: 10.1111/j.1749-6632.2012.06665.x.
3. Martin SS, Aday AW, Almarzooq ZI, et al. 2024 Heart disease and stroke statistics: a report of US and global data from the American Heart Association. *Circulation* 2024;149(8):e347–e913. DOI: 10.1161/CIR.0000000000001209.
4. Adams HP, Jr., Bendixen BH, Kappelle LJ, et al. Classification of subtype of acute ischemic stroke. Definitions for use in a multicenter clinical trial. TOAST. Trial of Org 10172 in acute stroke treatment. *Stroke* 1993;24(1):35–41. (In Eng). DOI: 10.1161/01.str.24.1.35.
5. Spence JD, Azarpazhooh MR, Larsson SC, Bogiatzi C, Hankey GJ. Stroke prevention in older adults. *Stroke* 2020;51(12):3770–77. DOI: 10.1161/STROKEAHA.120.031707.
6. Bushnell C, Kernan WN, Sharrief AZ, et al. 2024 Guideline for the primary prevention of stroke: a guideline from the American Heart Association/American Stroke Association. *Stroke* 2024;55(12):e344–e424. DOI: 10.1161/STR.0000000000000475.
7. Creutzfeldt CJ, Levitt MR, Leslie-Mazwi TM. Is endovascular thrombectomy for the very elderly? *Stroke* 2022;53(7):2227–9. DOI: 10.1161/STROKEAHA.122.039340.
8. Tissue plasminogen activator for acute ischemic stroke. *N Engl J Med* 1995;333(24):1581–7. (In Eng). DOI: 10.1056/nejm199512143332401.
9. Wang Y, Wang Y, Zhao X, et al. Clopidogrel with aspirin in acute minor stroke or transient ischemic attack. *N Engl J Med* 2013;369(1):11–9. (In Eng). DOI: 10.1056/NEJMoa1215340.
10. Johnston SC, Easton JD, Farrant M, et al. Clopidogrel and Aspirin in acute ischemic stroke and high-risk TIA. *N Engl J Med* 2018;379(3):215–25. DOI: 10.1056/NEJMoa1800410.
11. Chimowitz MI, Lynn MJ, Derdeyn CP, et al. Stenting versus aggressive medical therapy for intracranial arterial stenosis. *N Engl J Med* 2011;365(11):993–1003. DOI: 10.1056/NEJMoa1105335.
12. Coutts SB. Diagnosis and management of transient ischemic attack. *Continuum (Minneap Minn)* 2017;23(1, Cerebrovascular Disease):82–92. (In Eng). DOI: 10.1212/con.0000000000000424.
13. Kleindorfer DO, Towfighi A, Chaturvedi S, et al. 2021 Guideline for the prevention of stroke in patients with stroke and transient ischemic attack: a guideline from the American Heart Association/American Stroke Association. *Stroke* 2021;52(7):e364–e467. DOI: 10.1161/STR.0000000000000375.
14. Amarenco P, Lavallee PC, Labreuche J, et al. One-year risk of stroke after transient ischemic attack or minor stroke. *N Engl J Med* 2016;374(16):1533–42. DOI: 10.1056/NEJMoa1412981.
15. Amin HP, Madsen TE, Bravata DM, et al. Diagnosis, workup, risk reduction of transient ischemic attack in the emergency department setting: a scientific statement from the American Heart Association. *Stroke* 2023;54(3):e109–e121. DOI: 10.1161/STR.0000000000000418.
16. Johnston SC, Rothwell PM, Nguyen-Huynh MN, et al. Validation and refinement of scores to predict very early stroke risk after transient ischaemic attack. *Lancet* 2007;369(9558):283–92. DOI: 10.1016/S0140-6736(07)60150-0.
17. Brazzelli M, Chappell FM, Miranda H, et al. Diffusion-weighted imaging and diagnosis of transient ischemic attack. *Ann Neurol* 2014;75(1):67–76. (In Eng). DOI: 10.1002/ana.24026.
18. Doniger DE. Bilateral complete carotid and basilar artery occlusion in a patient with minimal deficit. case report and discussion of diagnostic and therapeutic implications. *Neurology* 1963;13:673–8. (In Eng). DOI: 10.1212/wnl.13.8.673.
19. Obrist WD, Thompson HK, Jr., Wang HS, Wilkinson WE. Regional cerebral blood flow estimated by 133-xenon inhalation. *Stroke* 1975;6(3):245–56. (In Eng). DOI: 10.1161/01.str.6.3.245.
20. Hart RG, Diener HC, Coutts SB, et al. Embolic strokes of undetermined source: the case for a new clinical construct. *Lancet Neurol* 2014;13(4):429–38. (In Eng). DOI: 10.1016/s1474-4422(13)70310-7.
21. Hart RG, Catanese L, Perera KS, Ntaios G, Connolly SJ. Embolic stroke of undetermined source: a systematic review and clinical update. *Stroke* 2017;48(4):867–72. (In Eng). DOI: 10.1161/strokeaha.116.016414.
22. Sherman DG, Dyken ML, Jr., Gent M, Harrison JG, Hart RG, Mohr JP. Antithrombotic therapy for cerebrovascular disorders. An update. *Chest* 1995;108(4 Suppl):444s–456s. (In Eng). DOI: 10.1378/chest.108.4_supplement.444s.
23. Yaghi S, Prabhakaran S, Khatri P, Liebeskind DS. Intracranial atherosclerotic disease. *Stroke* 2019;50(5):1286–93. DOI: 10.1161/STROKEAHA.118.024147.

24. Ornello R, Degan D, Tiseo C, et al. Distribution and temporal trends from 1993 to 2015 of ischemic stroke subtypes. *Stroke* 2018;49(4):814–19. DOI: 10.1161/STROKEAHA.117.020031.
25. Kamel H, Healey JS. Cardioembolic stroke. *Circ Res* 2017;120(3):514–26. DOI: 10.1161/CIRCRESAHA.116.308407.
26. Wolf PA, Dawber TR, Thomas HE, Jr., Kannel WB. Epidemiologic assessment of chronic atrial fibrillation and risk of stroke: the Framingham study. *Neurology* 1978;28(10):973–7. (In Eng). DOI: 10.1212/wnl.28.10.973.
27. Fisher CM. Lacunes: small, deep cerebral infarcts. *Neurology* 1965;15:774–84. (In Eng). DOI: 10.1212/wnl.15.8.774.
28. Kim H, Kim J-T, Lee JS, et al. Stroke of other determined etiology: results from the nationwide multicenter stroke registry. *Stroke* 2022;53(8):2597–606. DOI: 10.1161/STROKEAHA.121.037582.
29. Li L, Yiin GS, Geraghty OC, et al. Incidence, outcome, risk factors, and long-term prognosis of cryptogenic transient ischaemic attack and ischaemic stroke: a population-based study. *Lancet Neurol* 2015;14(9):903–13. (In Eng). DOI: 10.1016/s1474-4422(15)00132-5.
30. Diener H-C, Sacco RL, Easton JD, et al. Dabigatran for prevention of stroke after embolic stroke of undetermined source. *N Engl J Med* 2019;380(20):1906–17. DOI: 10.1056/NEJMoa1813959.
31. Hart RG, Diener HC, Coutts SB, et al. Embolic strokes of undetermined source: the case for a new clinical construct. *Lancet Neurol* 2014;13(4):429–38. DOI: 10.1016/S1474-4422(13)70310-7.
32. Navi BB, Kasner SE, Elkind MSV, Cushman M, Bang OY, DeAngelis LM. Cancer and embolic stroke of undetermined source. *Stroke* 2021;52(3):1121–30. DOI: 10.1161/STROKEAHA.120.032002.
33. Greenberg SM, Ziai WC, Cordonnier C, et al. 2022 Guideline for the management of patients with spontaneous intracerebral hemorrhage: a guideline from the American Heart Association/American Stroke Association. *Stroke* 2022;53(7):e282–e361. DOI: 10.1161/STR.0000000000000407.
34. Charidimou A, Boulouis G, Frosch MP, et al. The Boston criteria version 2.0 for cerebral amyloid angiopathy: a multicentre, retrospective, MRI-neuropathology diagnostic accuracy study. *Lancet Neurol* 2022;21(8):714–25. (In Eng). DOI: 10.1016/s1474-4422(22)00208-3.
35. Viswanathan A, Greenberg SM. Cerebral amyloid angiopathy in the elderly. *Ann Neurol* 2011;70(6):871–80. DOI: 10.1002/ana.22516.
36. Fehnel CR, Gormley WB, Dasenbrock H, et al. Advanced age and post-acute care outcomes after subarachnoid hemorrhage. *J Am Heart Assoc* 6(10):e006696. DOI: 10.1161/JAHA.117.006696.
37. Barber PA, Demchuk AM, Zhang J, Buchan AM. Validity and reliability of a quantitative computed tomography score in predicting outcome of hyperacute stroke before thrombolytic therapy. ASPECTS study group. Alberta stroke programme early CT score. *Lancet* 2000;355(9216):1670–4. (In Eng). DOI: 10.1016/s0140-6736(00)02237-6.
38. Warach S, Gaa J, Siewert B, Wielopolski P, Edelman RR. Acute human stroke studied by whole brain echo planar diffusion-weighted magnetic resonance imaging. *Ann Neurol* 1995;37(2):231–41. (In Eng). DOI: 10.1002/ana.410370214.
39. Feigin VL, Abate MD, Abate YH, et al. Global, regional, and national burden of stroke and its risk factors, 1990–2021: a systematic analysis for the Global Burden of Disease Study 2021. *The Lancet Neurology* 2024;23(10):973–1003. DOI: 10.1016/S1474-4422(24)00369-7.
40. Seshadri S, Wolf PA. Lifetime risk of stroke and dementia: current concepts, and estimates from the Framingham study. *The Lancet Neurology* 2007;6(12):1106–14. DOI: 10.1016/S1474-4422(07)70291-0.
41. Whelton PK, Carey RM, Aronow WS, et al. 2017 ACC/AHA/AAPA/ABC/ACPM/AGS/APhA/ASH/ASPC/NMA/PCNA guideline for the prevention, detection, evaluation, and management of high blood pressure in adults: a report of the American College of Cardiology/American Heart Association Task Force on Clinical Practice Guidelines. *Hypertension* 2018;71(6):e13–e115. DOI: 10.1161/HYP.0000000000000065.
42. Williams B, Mancia G, Spiering W, et al. 2018 ESC/ESH guidelines for the management of arterial hypertension: the task force for the management of arterial hypertension of the European Society of Cardiology (ESC) and the European Society of Hypertension (ESH). *Eur Heart J* 2018;39(33):3021–104. DOI: 10.1093/eurheartj/ehy339.
43. Goldenberg RM, Cheng AYY, Fitzpatrick T, Gilbert JD, Verma S, Hopyan JJ. Benefits of GLP-1 (glucagon-like peptide 1) receptor agonists for stroke reduction in type 2 diabetes: a call to action for neurologists. *Stroke* 2022;53(5):1813–22. DOI: 10.1161/STROKEAHA.121.038151.
44. Wu J, Sin DD. Improved patient outcome with smoking cessation: when is it too late? *Int J Chron Obstruct Pulmon Dis* 2011;6:259–67. (In Eng). DOI: 10.2147/copd.S10771.
45. McNeil JJ, Nelson MR, Woods RL, et al. Effect of Aspirin on all-cause mortality in the healthy elderly. *N Engl J Med* 2018;379(16):1519–28. DOI: 10.1056/NEJMoa1803955.
46. Ko D, Chung MK, Evans PT, Benjamin EJ, Helm RH. Atrial fibrillation: a review. *JAMA* 2024. DOI: 10.1001/jama.2024.22451.

47. Wolf PA, Abbott RD, Kannel WB. Atrial fibrillation: a major contributor to stroke in the elderly. The Framingham study. *Arch Intern Med* 1987;147(9):1561–4. (In Eng).
48. Warfarin versus aspirin for prevention of thromboembolism in atrial fibrillation: stroke prevention in atrial fibrillation II study. *Lancet* 1994;343(8899):687–91. (In Eng).
49. Petersen P, Boysen G, Godtfredsen J, Andersen ED, Andersen B. Placebo-controlled, randomised trial of warfarin and aspirin for prevention of thromboembolic complications in chronic atrial fibrillation. The Copenhagen AFASAK study. *Lancet* 1989;1(8631):175–9. (In Eng). DOI: 10.1016/s0140-6736(89)91200-2.
50. Singer DE, Hughes RA, Gress DR, et al. The effect of low-dose warfarin on the risk of stroke in patients with nonrheumatic atrial fibrillation. *N Engl J Med* 1990;323(22):1505–11. (In Eng). DOI: 10.1056/nejm199011293232201.
51. Ezekowitz MD, Bridgers SL, James KE, et al. Warfarin in the prevention of stroke associated with nonrheumatic atrial fibrillation. Veterans Affairs Stroke prevention in Nonrheumatic Atrial Fibrillation Investigators. *N Engl J Med* 1992;327(20):1406–12. (In Eng). DOI: 10.1056/nejm199211123272002.
52. Granger CB, Alexander JH, McMurray JJ, et al. Apixaban versus warfarin in patients with atrial fibrillation. *N Engl J Med* 2011;365(11):981–92. (In Eng). DOI: 10.1056/NEJMoa1107039.
53. Connolly SJ, Ezekowitz MD, Yusuf S, et al. Dabigatran versus warfarin in patients with atrial fibrillation. *N Engl J Med* 2009;361(12):1139–51. (In Eng). DOI: 10.1056/NEJMoa0905561.
54. Patel MR, Mahaffey KW, Garg J, et al. Rivaroxaban versus warfarin in nonvalvular atrial fibrillation. *N Engl J Med* 2011;365(10):883–91. (In Eng). DOI: 10.1056/NEJMoa1009638.
55. Giugliano RP, Ruff CT, Braunwald E, et al. Edoxaban versus warfarin in patients with atrial fibrillation. *N Engl J Med* 2013;369(22):2093–104. (In Eng). DOI: 10.1056/NEJMoa1310907.
56. Ng KH, Hart RG, Eikelboom JW. Anticoagulation in patients aged ≥75 years with atrial fibrillation: role of novel oral anticoagulants. *Cardiol Ther* 2013;2(2):135–49. (In Eng). DOI: 10.1007/s40119-013-0019-y.
57. Lin DSH, Lo HY, Huang KC, Lin TT, Lee JK. Efficacy and safety of direct oral anticoagulants for stroke prevention in older patients with atrial fibrillation: a network meta-analysis of randomized controlled trials. *J Am Heart Assoc* 2023;12(23):e030380. DOI: 10.1161/JAHA.123.030380.
58. American Geriatrics Society 2023 updated AGS Beers Criteria® for potentially inappropriate medication use in older adults. *J Am Geriatr Soc* 2023;71(7):2052–81. (In eng). DOI: 10.1111/jgs.18372.
59. Man-Son-Hing M, Nichol G, Lau A, Laupacis A. Choosing antithrombotic therapy for elderly patients with atrial fibrillation who are at risk for falls. *Arch Intern Med* 1999;159(7):677–85. (In Eng). DOI: 10.1001/archinte.159.7.677.
60. Mant J, Hobbs FD, Fletcher K, et al. Warfarin versus aspirin for stroke prevention in an elderly community population with atrial fibrillation (the Birmingham Atrial Fibrillation Treatment of the Aged Study, BAFTA): a randomised controlled trial. *Lancet* 2007;370(9586):493–503. (In Eng). DOI: 10.1016/s0140-6736(07)61233-1.
61. Connolly SJ, Eikelboom J, Joyner C, et al. Apixaban in patients with atrial fibrillation. *N Engl J Med* 2011;364(9):806–17. DOI: 10.1056/NEJMoa1007432.
62. Wilson M, Incontri D, Vu S, et al. Association of anticoagulant use with hemorrhage location and etiology in incident spontaneous intracerebral hemorrhage. *Stroke* 2024;55(11):2677–84. DOI: 10.1161/STROKEAHA.124.048243.
63. Pisters R, Lane DA, Nieuwlaat R, de Vos CB, Crijns HJ, Lip GY. A novel user-friendly score (HAS-BLED) to assess 1-year risk of major bleeding in patients with atrial fibrillation: the Euro Heart Survey. *Chest* 2010;138(5):1093–100. (In Eng). DOI: 10.1378/chest.10-0134.
64. Lip GY, Frison L, Halperin JL, Lane DA. Comparative validation of a novel risk score for predicting bleeding risk in anticoagulated patients with atrial fibrillation: the HAS-BLED (Hypertension, Abnormal Renal/Liver Function, Stroke, Bleeding History or Predisposition, Labile INR, Elderly, Drugs/Alcohol Concomitantly) score. *J Am Coll Cardiol* 2011;57(2):173–80. (In Eng). DOI: 10.1016/j.jacc.2010.09.024.
65. Chaudhary R, Singh A, Chaudhary R, et al. Evaluation of direct oral anticoagulant reversal agents in intracranial hemorrhage: a systematic review and meta-analysis. *Jama Netw Open* 2022;5(11):e2240145–e2240145. DOI: 10.1001/jamanetworkopen.2022.40145.
66. Smith P, Arnesen H, Holme I. The effect of warfarin on mortality and reinfarction after myocardial infarction. *N Engl J Med* 1990;323(3):147–52. (In Eng). DOI: 10.1056/nejm199007193230302.
67. Homma S, Thompson JL, Pullicino PM, et al. Warfarin and aspirin in patients with heart failure and sinus rhythm. *N Engl J Med* 2012;366(20):1859–69. (In Eng). DOI: 10.1056/NEJMoa1202299.
68. Homma S, Thompson JLP, Sanford AR, et al. Benefit of warfarin compared with aspirin in patients with heart failure in sinus rhythm. *Circ Heart Fail* 2013;6(5):988–97. DOI: 10.1161/CIRCHEARTFAILURE.113.000372.
69. The International Stroke Trial (IST): a randomised trial of aspirin, subcutaneous heparin, both, or neither among 19435 patients with acute ischaemic

stroke. International Stroke trial collaborative group. *Lancet* 1997;349(9065):1569–81. (In Eng).

70. Sandercock PA, Counsell C, Tseng MC, Cecconi E. Oral antiplatelet therapy for acute ischaemic stroke. *Cochrane Database Syst Rev* 2014;2014(3):Cd000029. (In eng). DOI: 10.1002/14651858.CD000029.pub3.
71. Powers WJ, Rabinstein AA, Ackerson T, et al. Guidelines for the early management of patients with acute ischemic Stroke: 2019 update to the 2018 guidelines for the early management of acute ischemic Stroke: a guideline for healthcare professionals from the American Heart Association/American Stroke Association. *Stroke* 2019;50(12):e344–e418. DOI: 10.1161/STR.0000000000000211.
72. A randomised, blinded, trial of clopidogrel versus aspirin in patients at risk of ischaemic events (CAPRIE). CAPRIE steering committee. *Lancet* 1996;348(9038):1329–39. (In Eng). DOI: 10.1016/s0140-6736(96)09457-3.
73. Wallentin L, Becker RC, Budaj A, et al. Ticagrelor versus clopidogrel in patients with acute coronary syndromes. *N Engl J Med* 2009;361(11):1045–57. (In Eng). DOI: 10.1056/NEJMoa0904327.
74. Johnston SC, Amarenco P, Denison H, et al. Ticagrelor and Aspirin or Aspirin alone in acute ischemic stroke or TIA. *N Engl J Med* 2020;383(3):207–17. DOI: 10.1056/NEJMoa1916870.
75. Pan Y, Elm JJ, Li H, et al. Outcomes associated with clopidogrel-aspirin use in minor stroke or transient ischemic attack: a pooled analysis of clopidogrel in high-risk patients with acute non-disabling cerebrovascular events (CHANCE) and platelet-oriented inhibition in new TIA and minor ischemic stroke (POINT) Trials. *JAMA Neurology* 2019;76(12):1466–73. DOI: 10.1001/jamaneurol.2019.2531.
76. De Matteis E, De Santis F, Ornello R, et al. Divergence between clinical trial evidence and actual practice in use of dual antiplatelet therapy after transient ischemic attack and minor stroke. *Stroke* 2023;54(5):1172–81. DOI: 10.1161/STROKEAHA.122.041660.
77. Wang Y, Meng X, Wang A, et al. Ticagrelor versus clopidogrel in CYP2C19 loss-of-function carriers with stroke or TIA. *N Engl J Med* 2021;385(27):2520–30. DOI: 10.1056/NEJMoa2111749.
78. Zhang X, Jing J, Wang A, et al. Efficacy and safety of dual antiplatelet therapy in the elderly for stroke prevention: a subgroup analysis of the CHANCE-2 trial. *Stroke Vasc Neurol* 2024;9(5):541–50. (In Eng). DOI: 10.1136/svn-2023-002450.
79. Stone NJ, Robinson JG, Lichtenstein AH, et al. 2013 ACC/AHA guideline on the treatment of blood cholesterol to reduce atherosclerotic cardiovascular risk in adults: a report of the American College of Cardiology/American Heart Association Task Force on Practice Guidelines. *Circulation* 2014;129(25 Suppl 2):S1-45. (In Eng). DOI: 10.1161/01.cir.0000437738.63853.7a.
80. Kamel H, Longstreth WT, Jr, Tirschwell DL, et al. Apixaban to prevent recurrence after cryptogenic stroke in patients with atrial cardiopathy: the ARCADIA randomized clinical trial. *JAMA* 2024;331(7):573–81. DOI: 10.1001/jama.2023.27188.
81. Gao Y, Chen W, Pan Y, et al. Dual antiplatelet treatment up to 72 hours after ischemic stroke. *N Engl J Med* 2023;389(26):2413–24. DOI: 10.1056/NEJMoa2309137.
82. ISC 2023 Session: "Intracranial Atherosclerotic Disease After SAMMPRIS: looking to the Future After a 'Lost Decade'".
83. Faught E, Trader SD, Hanna GR. Cerebral complications of angiography for transient ischemia and stroke: prediction of risk. *Neurology* 1979;29(1):4–15. (In Eng). DOI: 10.1212/wnl.29.1.4.
84. Ringleb PA, Allenberg J, Brückmann H, et al. 30 day results from the SPACE trial of stent-protected angioplasty versus carotid endarterectomy in symptomatic patients: a randomised non-inferiority trial. *Lancet* 2006;368(9543):1239–47. (In Eng). DOI: 10.1016/s0140-6736(06)69122-8.
85. Demchuk AM, Menon BK, Goyal M. Comparing vessel imaging. *Stroke* 2016;47(1):273–81. DOI: 10.1161/STROKEAHA.115.009171.
86. Brott TG, Hobson RW, 2nd, Howard G, et al. Stenting versus endarterectomy for treatment of carotid-artery stenosis. *N Engl J Med* 2010;363(1):11–23. (In Eng). DOI: 10.1056/NEJMoa0912321.
87. Howard G, Roubin GS, Jansen O, et al. Association between age and risk of stroke or death from carotid endarterectomy and carotid stenting: a meta-analysis of pooled patient data from four randomised trials. *Lancet* 2016;387(10025):1305–11. (In Eng). DOI: 10.1016/s0140-6736(15)01309-4.
88. Batchelder A, Hunter J, Cairns V, Sandford R, Munshi A, Naylor AR. Dual antiplatelet therapy prior to expedited carotid surgery reduces recurrent events prior to surgery without significantly increasing peri-operative bleeding complications. *Eur J Vasc Endovasc Surg* 2015;50(4):412–19. DOI: 10.1016/j.ejvs.2015.07.019.
89. Brott TG, Roubin GS, Moore WS, Meschia JF. Carotid artery disease: then and now. Stroke: vascular and interventional *Neurology* 2024;4(2):e001076. DOI: 10.1161/SVIN.123.001076.
90. Hackam DG. Optimal medical management of asymptomatic carotid stenosis. *Stroke* 2021;52(6):2191–8. DOI: 10.1161/STROKEAHA.120.033994.
91. Reiff T, Eckstein HH, Mansmann U, et al. Carotid endarterectomy or stenting or best medical treatment alone for moderate-to-severe asymptomatic carotid artery stenosis: 5-year results of a multicentre, randomised controlled trial. *Lancet*

Neurol 2022;21(10):877–88. (In eng). DOI: 10.1016/s1474-4422(22)00290-3.

92. Cheng SF, van Velzen TJ, Gregson J, et al. The 2nd European Carotid Surgery Trial (ECST-2): rationale and protocol for a randomised clinical trial comparing immediate revascularisation versus optimised medical therapy alone in patients with symptomatic and asymptomatic carotid stenosis at low to intermediate risk of stroke. *Trials* 2022;23(1):606. (In eng). DOI: 10.1186/s13063-022-06429-z.
93. Interim data find "no evidence of benefit" for carotid revascularisation additional to optimised medical therapy. May 26, 2023. https://vascularnews.com/interim-data-find-no-evidence-of-benefit-for-carotid-revascularisation-additional-to-optimised-medical-therapy/#:~:text=From%20this%20interim%20analysis%20of,addition%20to%20optimised%20medical%20therapy.
94. Meschia JF, Edwards L, Roubin G, Brott TG, Lal BK. CREST-2 Commitment to rigorous assessment of carotid stenting for primary prevention of stroke. Stroke: vascular and interventional *Neurology* 2024;4(3):e001227. DOI: 10.1161/SVIN.123.001227.
95. Koller RL. Recurrent embolic cerebral infarction and anticoagulation. *Neurology* 1982;32(3):283–5. (In Eng).
96. Immediate anticoagulation of embolic stroke: a randomized trial. Cerebral embolism study group. *Stroke* 1983;14(5):668–76. (In eng). DOI: 10.1161/01.str.14.5.668.
97. Kirchhof P, Benussi S, Kotecha D, et al. 2016 ESC Guidelines for the management of atrial fibrillation developed in collaboration with EACTS. *Eur Heart J* 2016;37(38):2893–962. DOI: 10.1093/eurheartj/ehw210.
98. Fischer U, Koga M, Strbian D, et al. Early versus later anticoagulation for stroke with atrial fibrillation. *N Engl J Med* 2023;388(26):2411–21. DOI: 10.1056/NEJMoa2303048.
99. Pessin MS, Estol CJ, Lafranchise F, Caplan LR. Safety of anticoagulation after hemorrhagic infarction. *Neurology* 1993;43(7):1298–303. (In Eng). DOI: 10.1212/wnl.43.7.1298.
100. Pruitt AA, Rubin RH, Karchmer AW, Duncan GW. Neurologic complications of bacterial endocarditis. *Medicine (Baltimore)* 1978;57(4):329–43. (In Eng). DOI: 10.1097/00005792-197807000-00004.
101. Pullicino PM, Qian M, Sacco RL, et al. Recurrent stroke in the warfarin versus aspirin in reduced cardiac ejection fraction (WARCEF) trial. *Cerebrovasc Dis* 2014;38(3):176–81. DOI: 10.1159/000365502.
102. Hart RG, Sharma M, Mundl H, et al. Rivaroxaban for stroke prevention after embolic stroke of undetermined source. *N Engl J Med* 2018;378(23):2191–201. DOI: 10.1056/NEJMoa1802686.
103. Sposato LA, Chaturvedi S, Hsieh C-Y, Morillo CA, Kamel H. Atrial fibrillation detected after stroke and transient ischemic attack: a novel clinical concept challenging current views. *Stroke* 2022;53(3):e94–e103. DOI: 10.1161/STROKEAHA.121.034777.
104. Mas JL, Derumeaux G, Guillon B, et al. Patent foramen ovale closure or anticoagulation vs. Antiplatelets after stroke. *N Engl J Med* 2017;377(11):1011–21. (In Eng). DOI: 10.1056/NEJMoa1705915.
105. Sposato LA, Albin CSW, Elkind MSV, et al. Patent foramen ovale management for secondary stroke prevention: state-of-the-art appraisal of current evidence. *Stroke* 2024;55(1):236–47. DOI: 10.1161/STROKEAHA.123.040546.
106. Berrouschot J, Röther J, Glahn J, Kucinski T, Fiehler J, Thomalla G. Outcome and severe hemorrhagic complications of intravenous thrombolysis with tissue plasminogen activator in very old (> or = 80 years) stroke patients. *Stroke* 2005;36(11):2421–5. (In Eng). DOI: 10.1161/01.STR.0000185696.73938.e0.
107. Bluhmki E, Danays T, Biegert G, Hacke W, Lees KR. Alteplase for acute ischemic stroke in patients aged >80 years. *Stroke* 2020;51(8):2322–31. DOI: 10.1161/STROKEAHA.119.028396.
108. Generalized efficacy of t-PA for acute stroke. *Stroke* 1997;28(11):2119–25. DOI: 10.1161/01.STR.28.11.2119.
109. Hacke W, Kaste M, Bluhmki E, et al. Thrombolysis with alteplase 3 to 4.5 hours after acute ischemic stroke. *N Engl J Med* 2008;359(13):1317–29. (In eng). DOI: 10.1056/NEJMoa0804656.
110. Zupanic E, von Euler M, Kåreholt I, et al. Thrombolysis in acute ischemic stroke in patients with dementia: a Swedish registry study. *Neurology* 2017;89(18):1860–68. (In Eng). DOI: 10.1212/wnl.0000000000004598.
111. Rodriguez M, Sidebottom C, Wells DA, et al. A systematic review of the efficacy and safety of tenecteplase versus alteplase in acute ischemic stroke: a time to pass the torch. Stroke: vascular and interventional *Neurology* 2024;4(4):e001110. DOI: 10.1161/SVIN.123.001110.
112. Yogendrakumar V, Churilov L, Mitchell PJ, et al. Safety and efficacy of tenecteplase in older patients with large vessel occlusion. *Neurology* 2022;98(12):e1292–e301. DOI: 10.1212/WNL.0000000000013302.
113. Khatri P, Kleindorfer DO, Devlin T, et al. Effect of alteplase vs Aspirin on functional outcome for patients with acute ischemic stroke and minor nondisabling neurologic deficits: the PRISMS randomized clinical trial. *JAMA* 2018;320(2):156–66. DOI: 10.1001/jama.2018.8496.
114. Chen H-S, Cui Y, Zhou Z-H, et al. Dual antiplatelet therapy vs alteplase for patients with minor nondisabling acute ischemic stroke: the ARAMIS randomized clinical trial. *JAMA* 2023;329(24):2135–44. DOI: 10.1001/jama.2023.7827.

115. Bluhmki E, Chamorro Á, Dávalos A, et al. Stroke treatment with alteplase given 3·0–4·5 h after onset of acute ischaemic stroke (ECASS III): additional outcomes and subgroup analysis of a randomised controlled trial. The *Lancet Neurology* 2009;8(12):1095–102. DOI: https://doi.org/10.1016/S1474-4422(09)70264-9.
116. Berkhemer OA, Fransen PS, Beumer D, et al. A randomized trial of intraarterial treatment for acute ischemic stroke. *N Engl J Med* 2015;372(1):11–20. (In Eng). DOI: 10.1056/NEJMoa1411587.
117. Goyal M, Demchuk AM, Menon BK, et al. Randomized assessment of rapid endovascular treatment of ischemic stroke. *N Engl J Med* 2015;372(11):1019–30. (In Eng). DOI: 10.1056/NEJMoa1414905.
118. Saver JL, Goyal M, Bonafe A, et al. Stent-retriever thrombectomy after intravenous t-PA vs. t-PA alone in stroke. *N Engl J Med* 2015;372(24):2285–95. (In Eng). DOI: 10.1056/NEJMoa1415061.
119. Campbell BC, Mitchell PJ, Kleinig TJ, et al. Endovascular therapy for ischemic stroke with perfusion-imaging selection. *N Engl J Med* 2015;372(11):1009–18. (In Eng). DOI: 10.1056/NEJMoa1414792.
120. Jovin TG, Chamorro A, Cobo E, et al. Thrombectomy within 8 hours after symptom onset in ischemic stroke. *N Engl J Med* 2015;372(24):2296–306. (In Eng). DOI: 10.1056/NEJMoa1503780.
121. Goyal M, Menon BK, van Zwam WH, et al. Endovascular thrombectomy after large-vessel ischaemic stroke: a meta-analysis of individual patient data from five randomised trials. *Lancet* 2016;387(10029):1723–31. (In eng). DOI: 10.1016/s0140-6736(16)00163-x.
122. Slawski DE, Salahuddin H, Shawver J, et al. Mechanical thrombectomy in elderly stroke patients with mild-to-moderate baseline disability. *Interv Neurol* 2018;7(5):246–55. (In Eng). DOI: 10.1159/000487333.
123. Saposnik G, Menon BK, Kashani N, et al. Factors associated with the decision-making on endovascular thrombectomy for the management of acute ischemic stroke. *Stroke* 2019;50(9):2441–47. DOI: 10.1161/STROKEAHA.119.025631.
124. Nogueira RG, Jadhav AP, Haussen DC, et al. Thrombectomy 6 to 24 hours after stroke with a mismatch between deficit and infarct. *N Engl J Med* 2018;378(1):11–21. (In Eng). DOI: 10.1056/NEJMoa1706442.
125. Albers GW, Marks MP, Kemp S, et al. Thrombectomy for stroke at 6 to 16 hours with selection by perfusion imaging. *N Engl J Med* 2018;378(8):708–18. DOI: 10.1056/NEJMoa1713973.
126. Tsivgoulis G, Campbell BC. Endovascular thrombectomy for large core ischemic stroke—age matters. *Jama Netw Open* 2024;7(8):e2425958–e2425958. DOI: 10.1001/jamanetworkopen.2024.25958.
127. Wallace JD, Levy LL. Blood pressure after stroke. *JAMA* 1981;246(19):2177–80. (In Eng).
128. Mulley G, Wilcox RG, Mitchell JR. Dexamethasone in acute stroke. *Br Med J* 1978;2(6143):994–6. (In Eng). DOI: 10.1136/bmj.2.6143.994.
129. Candelise L, Colombo A, Spinnler H. Therapy against brain swelling in stroke patients. A retrospective clinical study on 227 patients. *Stroke* 1975;6(4):353–6. (In Eng). DOI: 10.1161/01.str.6.4.353.
130. Jüttler E, Unterberg A, Woitzik J, et al. Hemicraniectomy in older patients with extensive middle-cerebral-artery stroke. *N Engl J Med* 2014;370(12):1091–100. (In Eng). DOI: 10.1056/NEJMoa1311367.
131. Hofmeijer J, Kappelle LJ, Algra A, Amelink GJ, van Gijn J, van der Worp HB. Surgical decompression for space-occupying cerebral infarction (the Hemicraniectomy after middle cerebral artery infarction with life-threatening edema trial [HAMLET]): a multicentre, open, randomised trial. *Lancet Neurol* 2009;8(4):326–33. (In eng). DOI: 10.1016/s1474-4422(09)70047-x.
132. Winstein CJ, Stein J, Arena R, et al. Guidelines for adult stroke rehabilitation and recovery: a guideline for healthcare professionals from the American Heart Association/American Stroke Association. *Stroke* 2016;47(6):e98–e169. DOI: 10.1161/STR.0000000000000098.
133. Mayman N, Stein LK, Erdman J, et al. Risk and predictors of depression following acute ischemic stroke in the elderly. *Neurology* 2021;96(17):e2184–e91. DOI: 10.1212/WNL.0000000000011828.
134. Joundi RA, Fang J, Austin PC, et al. Magnitude and time-course of dementia risk in stroke survivors. *Neurology* 2025;104(1):e210131. DOI: 10.1212/WNL.0000000000210131.
135. Prins ND, van Dijk EJ, den Heijer T, et al. Cerebral white matter lesions and the risk of dementia. *Archives of Neurology* 2004;61(10):1531–4. DOI: 10.1001/archneur.61.10.1531.
136. Ryan D, Zwischenberger BA, Liu AJ. Pearls and Oy-sters:apatientonlecanemabnewlydiagnosedwith atrial fibrillation. *Neurology* 2024;103(12):e210125. DOI: 10.1212/WNL.0000000000210125.
137. Anderson CS, Heeley E, Huang Y, et al. Rapid blood-pressure lowering in patients with acute intracerebral hemorrhage. *N Engl J Med* 2013;368(25):2355–65. (In Eng). DOI: 10.1056/NEJMoa1214609.
138. Qureshi AI, Palesch YY, Barsan WG, et al. Intensive blood-pressure lowering in patients with acute cerebral hemorrhage. *N Engl J Med* 2016;375(11):1033–43. (In Eng). DOI: 10.1056/NEJMoa1603460.

139. Baharoglu MI, Cordonnier C, Al-Shahi Salman R, et al. Platelet transfusion versus standard care after acute stroke due to spontaneous cerebral haemorrhage associated with antiplatelet therapy (PATCH): a randomised, open-label, phase 3 trial. *Lancet* 2016;387(10038):2605–13. (In Eng). DOI: 10.1016/s0140-6736(16)30392-0.
140. Pradilla G, Ratcliff JJ, Hall AJ, et al. Trial of early minimally invasive removal of intracerebral hemorrhage. *N Engl J Med* 2024;390(14):1277–89. DOI: 10.1056/NEJMoa2308440.
141. Hoh BL, Ko NU, Amin-Hanjani S, et al. 2023 Guideline for the management of patients with aneurysmal subarachnoid hemorrhage: a guideline from the American Heart Association/American Stroke Association. *Stroke* 2023;54(7):e314–e70. DOI: 10.1161/STR.0000000000000436.
142. Molyneux AJ, Kerr RS, Yu LM, et al. International subarachnoid aneurysm trial (ISAT) of neurosurgical clipping versus endovascular coiling in 2143 patients with ruptured intracranial aneurysms: a randomised comparison of effects on survival, dependency, seizures, rebleeding, subgroups, and aneurysm occlusion. *Lancet* 2005;366(9488):809–17. (In Eng). DOI: 10.1016/s0140-6736(05)67214-5.
143. Spetzler RF, Zabramski JM. Grading and staged resection of cerebral arteriovenous malformations. *Clin Neurosurg* 1990;36:318–37. (In Eng).
144. Dawson RC, 3rd, Tarr RW, Hecht ST, et al. Treatment of arteriovenous malformations of the brain with combined embolization and stereotactic radiosurgery: results after 1 and 2 years. *AJNR Am J Neuroradiol* 1990;11(5):857–64. (In Eng).
145. Mohr JP, Parides MK, Stapf C, et al. Medical management with or without interventional therapy for unruptured brain arteriovenous malformations (ARUBA): a multicentre, non-blinded, randomised trial. *Lancet* 2014;383(9917):614–21. (In Eng). DOI: 10.1016/s0140-6736(13)62302-8.

25

Evaluation and management of syncope and related disorders in older adults

ANDREA UNGAR, MARTINA RAFANELLI, AND GIULIA MATTEUCCI

Key points

- Syncope is a transient loss of consciousness due to transient global cerebral hypoperfusion.
- Prevalence increases with age, particularly in individuals over 65 years.
- Older patients often present with atypical symptoms, making diagnosis challenging.
- Syncope is caused by decreased cerebral perfusion due to systemic blood pressure drops.
- Age-related physiological changes (e.g., reduced baroreceptor sensitivity, altered blood volume control) increase susceptibility.
- Noncardiac syncope includes reflex syncope (vasovagal, situational, carotid sinus syndrome) and orthostatic hypotension (OH).
- Cardiac syncope includes arrhythmic causes (bradycardia, tachycardia) and structural heart disease (valvular, myocardial, and congenital anomalies).
- A standardized approach can diagnose over 90% of cases and reduce healthcare costs.
- Initial evaluation includes clinical history, physical examination, active standing test, and ECG.
- Additional tests (tilt testing, carotid sinus massage, prolonged ECG monitoring) improve diagnostic accuracy.
- Risk stratification allows identification of high-risk patients requiring hospitalization and further cardiac evaluation.
- Various scoring systems (EGSYS, Canadian Syncope Arrhythmia Risk Score, OESIL, ROSE) help predict adverse outcomes.
- Treatment is based on the underlying cause of syncope.
- Nonpharmacological measures include lifestyle modifications, education, and physical counterpressure maneuvers.
- Pharmacological treatments include midodrine, fludrocortisone, or droxidopa for orthostatic hypotension.
- Cardiac pacing is considered for severe cardioinhibitory responses, especially in older adults.
- Syncope is often misdiagnosed as unexplained falls. A comprehensive evaluation can differentiate between the two and improve patient outcomes.
- Older adults with cognitive impairment are at higher risk of syncope-related falls.

DOI: 10.1201/9781003568933-25

- A systematic diagnostic approach helps identify treatable causes of syncope in older adults.

INTRODUCTION

Syncope is a transient loss of consciousness due to a transient global cerebral hypoperfusion, characterized by a rapid onset, short duration, and spontaneous and complete recovery (1). This condition is extremely frequent in the general population (2), but the estimation of the true incidence is challenging because different definitions have been used in the existing epidemiological studies, and the incidence derived from specific clinical settings probably underestimates the true value because most syncopal patients do not seek medical assistance. In the latest report of the Framingham Offspring Study, 10% of the 7814 participants (mean age 51, range 20–96 years) reported at least one syncope. The first-time incidence of syncope by age is bimodal; the prevalence is very high in patients between the age of 10 and 30 years, uncommon in adults with an average age of 40 years, and peaks again above the age of 65 years (3). From the age of 70 onward, its incidence increases rapidly, up to 81.2 per 1000 patient years ≥80 years of age (4).

The prevalence of the causes of syncope differs depending on the age: reflex syncope is the most frequent cause at all ages (5); cardiac syncope is the second most common cause (6); orthostatic hypotension (OH) is a frequent cause of syncope in very old patients. In the elderly, multiple causes are often present (7) and the diagnosis within this population can be complex due to atypical presentations, amnesia for events, absence of witnesses, and the overlap with other clinical presentations such as unexplained falls.

PATHOPHYSIOLOGY

Global cerebral hypoperfusion is responsible for an inadequate supply of oxygen and metabolic substrates to the brain (8) and is what differentiates syncope from other transient loss of consciousness (TLoC) without underlying cerebral hypoperfusion (1).

Cerebral autoregulation maintains a constant blood flow within a wide range of systolic blood pressure (SBP) between 60 and 190 mmHg. When SBP decreases below this threshold, the brain perfusion decreases slowly and progressively and, if this hemodynamic status lasts for 8–15 seconds, ischemia and ultimately loss of consciousness will follow (9). Therefore, the main mechanism is a fall in systemic blood pressure (BP), which may depend on a reduction of vascular total peripheral resistance (TPR) and/or cardiac output (CO) (1).

Advanced age might predispose to pathophysiological changes: a reduced left ventricular compliance increases the dependence of CO on preload and atrial contraction; an altered control of blood volume; and a decreased sensitivity of the baroreceptors may lead to cerebral hypoperfusion. Blood pressure adjustments on assuming the upright position rely primarily on an increase in TPR (10) in older patients, thus explaining the susceptibility to vasoactive drugs as precipitating factors for syncope (11). Age-related physiologic impairments of HR, BP, and cerebral blood flow, in combination with comorbid conditions, concurrent medications, and neurohumoral adjustments, contribute to the increased susceptibility of older adults to syncope.

CLASSIFICATION OF SYNCOPE

The principal causes of syncope are listed in Table 25.1.

NONCARDIAC SYNCOPE

Reflex or neurally mediated syncope

Vasovagal syncope (VVS) is induced by triggers, such as fear, pain, and instrumentation, or due to orthostatic stress or hot environment. In the elderly, the presentation is often atypical; the event can occur with uncertain stimuli or even without apparent triggers. Prodromal symptoms may be short and loss of consciousness may start abruptly, leading to falls and injuries (12). Nausea, blurred vision, and diaphoresis are the most common prodromal symptoms in VVS, whereas dyspnea is more predictive of cardiac syncope (13). Myoclonic movements have rarely been observed in older subjects, especially older than 74 years, as the occurrence of an asystolic response is less frequent in this age group, and there is often a slower reduction in BP. Even during recovery, the frequency of autonomic symptoms is lower in older subjects. Thus, in the elderly, the clinical features of VVS are very similar to those of cardiac syncope (14).

A vasovagal syncope, which occurs in the upright position, may lead to a fall, rendering the clinical finding of these two conditions very similar. In this context, retrograde amnesia has been demonstrated in patients with syncope induced on tilt testing (TT). Indeed, about 25% of patients fail to recall their prodromes and TLoC during tilt-induced syncope (15).

CAROTID SINUS SYNCOPE

Exerting pressure at the site of the neck where the common carotid artery bifurcates produces a slowing in HR and a fall in BP. In some individuals, the reflex, initiated by carotid sinus massage (CSM), elicits an exaggerated response which is defined as carotid sinus hypersensitivity (CSH), that can manifest as cardioinhibitory (CI-CSH; asystole ≥3 seconds during CSM), vasodepressor (VD-CSH; a fall in SBP ≥50 mmHg during CSM), or mixed (M-CSH) (1). CSH may have a role in predisposing to unexplained falls; in this condition, syncope has to be considered even if the clear dynamic of the event could not be recalled due to retrograde amnesia.

Table 25.1 Classification of syncope

NONCARDIAC SYNCOPE
Reflex (neurally mediated) syncope
Vasovagal (VVS)
• Orthostatic VVS: standing, or less commonly sitting
• Emotional: fear, pain, instrumentation, blood phobia
• Pain triggers: peripheral or visceral
Situational
• Micturition
• Gastrointestinal stimulation (swallow, defecation)
• Cough, sneeze
• Others (e.g., laughing, brass instrument playing, weight lifting, post-exercise)
Carotid sinus syncope
Syncope due to orthostatic hypotension
Drug-induced orthostatic hypotension (e.g., vasodilators, diuretics, phenothiazine, antidepressants)
Volume depletion (e.g., hemorrhage, diarrhea, vomiting, etc.)
Primary autonomic failure (pure autonomic failure, multiple system atrophy, Parkinson's disease, dementia with Lewy bodies)
Secondary autonomic failure (diabetes, amyloidosis, spinal cord injuries, autoimmune autonomic neuropathy, paraneoplastic autonomic neuropathy, kidney failure)
CARDIAC SYNCOPE
Arrhythmia as primary cause
• Bradycardia
• Sinus node dysfunction (including bradycardia/tachycardia syndrome)
• Atrioventricular conduction system disease
• Implanted device malfunction
• Tachycardia
• Supraventricular
• Ventricular (idiopathic, secondary to structural heart disease or to channelopathies)
Structural disease
Cardiac: cardiac valvular disease, acute myocardial infarction/ischemia, hypertrophic cardiomyopathy, cardiac masses (atrial myxoma, tumors, etc.), pericardial disease/tamponade, congenital anomalies of coronary arteries, prosthetic valves dysfunction
Pulmonary embolus, acute aortic dissection, pulmonary hypertension

Source: Moya A et al., *Eur Heart J*, 30, 2631–2671, 2009.

Maggi et al. (16) have shown that CI-CSH in patients with a clinical diagnosis of suspected neurally mediated syncope has been related to a long asystolic reflex detected by an implantable loop recorder (ILR) at the time of the spontaneous syncope. When CSH occurs in a patient who has previously had syncope with reproduction of symptoms, it is defined as carotid sinus syndrome (CSS) (1).

CSH is common in older males without a history of syncope, especially when affected by cardiovascular diseases (17). The prevalence of CSS has been estimated to range from <4% in patients <40 years to 41% in those >80 years attending a specialized syncope facility. The related syncope often has little or no prodrome, with a consequent increased risk of traumatic fall. Syncope recurrence is common and is reported to be 50% in 2 years (18).

Given the high rate of positive responses to CSM, even in subjects without a history of syncope, the 3-second cutoff for asystole has been considered too sensitive (17); in addition, clinical data suggest that asystole lasting less than 6 seconds is frequently asymptomatic (19). Indeed, the mean pause required to elicit symptoms during CSM is 7.9 seconds (20), and the mean asystole duration during spontaneous syncope is 9 seconds (16). A new 6-second cutoff has thus been proposed to define CSH (21). Moreover, several studies have demonstrated that an isolated cardioinhibitory response does not exist since vasodepression is found in nearly all patients, with variable intensity (18). Therefore, a revision of conventional CSS classification has been proposed, considering CSS as a continuum between cardioinhibition and vasodepression and including "predominant cardioinhibitory," "predominant vasodepressor," and "mixed" CSS (22). This new interpretation can influence referral for treatment since cardiac pacing is less effective in the presence of a significant vasodepressor response, which may be responsible for syncopal recurrence.

Syncope due to orthostatic hypotension

Orthostatic hypotension (OH) is defined as a fall in SBP from a baseline value ≥20 mmHg or diastolic BP (DBP) ≥10 mmHg or a sustained decrease in SBP to an absolute value <90 mmHg within 3 minutes of standing (1). Since the magnitude of BP drop also depends on baseline values, it was suggested that a drop of 30 mmHg may be a more appropriate criterion for OH in patients with supine hypertension (23).

OH increases with age, reaching 24% in the eighth decade and 31% in the ninth decade (24), and has a prevalence of 24% in patients older than 65 years consecutively referred to an emergency department (ED) for a TLoC (25).

The circulatory autonomic causes of orthostatic intolerance include initial OH (IOH), classical OH (COH), and delayed OH (DOH) (1). Initial OH is represented by a BP decrease of >40 mmHg for SBP and/or >20 mmHg for DBP within 15 seconds of standing, with quick and spontaneous recovery, which is detectable by beat-to-beat BP monitoring (1). IOH may have implications in older adults, particularly when on cardiovascular medications (26); approximately 15% of long-term care residents fall after rising to standing (27), and initial OH could potentially exacerbate this falling risk.

Classical OH is detected on active standing or passive standing on tilt of at least 60 degrees, within 3 minutes of standing.

Delayed OH is defined as OH occurring beyond 3 minutes of active standing or passive standing on tilt and is characterized by a slow and progressive decrease of SBP. Hypotension can manifest clinically up to 30 minutes after the achievement of the upright position, and passive TT is needed for the diagnosis (1). DOH is common in the elderly, due to impairment of compensatory reflexes and stiffer hearts more sensitive to a decrease in preload (28). It may also represent a mild form of COH, especially if associated with parkinsonism or diabetes (29).

Pharmacotherapy is the primary cause of OH in the older patient. A drug regimen based on alpha-receptor blockers, nitrates, or benzodiazepines was found to be a predictor of OH in this age group (24). Other causes of OH are represented by primary autonomic failure (e.g., idiopathic Parkinson's disease and multiple system atrophy), secondary autonomic failure (e.g., diabetic and alcoholic autonomic neuropathy), and dehydration. Occasionally, OH may be the first manifestation of malignancy or anemia, which should be excluded, particularly in the older population (30).

Mechanism-based classification of noncardiac syncope: Hypotensive and bradycardic phenotype

Due to advances in the understanding of the pathophysiology, a new classification of noncardiac syncope has recently been proposed.

Different phenotypes according to the predominant underlying hemodynamic mechanism, i.e., hypotension (vasodepression) or bradycardia, have been identified (Table 25.2).

Table 25.2 Classification of noncardiac syncope by mechanism

Intermittent bradycardia
Asystole
• Sinus arrest
• Sinus bradycardia plus atrioventricular block
Progressive sinus bradycardia
Intermittent tachycardia
Progressive sinus tachycardia
Intermittent hypotension
Supine hypotension
Orthostatic hypotension
• Early/classical or delayed

Source: Rivasi G et al., *Eur Heart J Suppl*, 23(Suppl B), B6–B16, 2021.

The *hypotensive phenotype* is caused by low blood pressure (vasodepression) and is more common in patients with a predisposition to hypotension, whether constitutional, drug-induced, or secondary to specific medical conditions. It is often associated with reduced cardiac filling and impaired vascular tone. Tilt testing, carotid sinus massage, and 24-hour ambulatory blood pressure monitoring (ABPM) are essential for identifying this phenotype. Treatment typically involves counteracting the hypotensive tendency through lifestyle modifications, optimizing medications, and, in selected cases, the use of drugs like midodrine or fludrocortisone to stabilize the blood pressure.

The *bradycardic phenotype* is characterized by an overactive cardioinhibitory response, leading to bradycardia or even asystole. Patients often experience sinus arrest or atrioventricular block triggered by reflex mechanisms, rather than structural cardiac abnormalities. Diagnosis is achieved through TT, CSM, or prolonged ECG monitoring. Management of this phenotype frequently involves cardiac pacing, especially in patients over 40 years old who suffer from severe and recurrent episodes without warning symptoms, which carry a high risk of injury.

Some patients may manifest both hypotensive and bradycardic phenotypes (*mixed phenotype*). In those cases, a comprehensive approach is required to address both mechanisms. For example, a patient with significant vasodepression might still benefit from cardiac pacing if cardioinhibitory episodes are also present.

This new classification highlights the importance of tailoring syncope management to the specific hemodynamic mechanism underlying each case. By focusing on these mechanisms, clinicians can provide more effective strategies to prevent syncope recurrence, improving both patient safety and quality of life (31).

CARDIAC SYNCOPE

Cardiac causes of syncope are highly prevalent in the older population (32). In the Framingham study, cardiac syncope doubled the risk of death from any cause and increased the risk of nonfatal and fatal cardiovascular events, compared to those without syncope (3).

Short-lived syncope of abrupt onset and recovery, occurring while supine, during (rather than after) exercise, or associated with palpitations or chest pain, should be considered cardiac until proven otherwise. A history of heart disease is an independent predictor of cardiac syncope with a sensitivity of 95% and specificity of 45% (33). In particular, cardiac syncope should be suspected in patients with known or suspected left ventricular systolic dysfunction, valvular disease, left ventricular outflow tract obstruction, an abnormal surface electrocardiogram (ECG), and where the clinical context and concomitant investigations suggest pulmonary embolism. A neurally mediated cause of symptoms cannot be assumed in any patient with these clinical and diagnostic features until a cardiac cause has been effectively ruled out.

Bradyarrhythmia and tachyarrhythmia are the most common cardiac causes of cardiac syncope. Guidelines (1) and clinical scoring systems (33–35) for identifying high-risk patients include arrhythmias as a predictor of death and adverse events.

Multifactorial causes

Elderly patients often have multiple coexisting potential causes of syncope, and a definite diagnosis is not always found. In 873 consecutive patients older than 65 years, the rate of "complex diagnoses," namely, the presence of more than one diagnosis on active standing test, TT, and CSM, was 23%; the most frequent association was between OH and VVS on TT in 15.8% of cases (23).

A high number of possible contributing causes of syncope was recently confirmed in a sample of very old patients evaluated in a syncope and falls clinic. The most common contributing causes of syncope in the elderly were orthostatic/postprandial hypotension, followed by cardiac disorders; reflex syncope was less common (36). It is therefore useful to run a comprehensive evaluation in every subject, without stopping at the first apparent etiological diagnosis.

INITIAL DIAGNOSTIC EVALUATION

The diagnostic protocol proposed by the European Society of Cardiology (ESC) guidelines on syncope (Figure 25.1) (1) is well enforceable at any age; when applied, the rate of unexplained syncope decreases to around 10% (7). The first-line evaluation relies on clinical history, physical examination, active standing test, and 12-lead ECG (1). The clinical history should include the collection of systemic diseases, physical frailty, and locomotor disabilities. Details of cognitive status, social circumstances, injuries, impact of the event on confidence, and ability to carry out basal/instrumental activities of daily living independently should also be recorded. The clinical history regarding the syncope should be pursued by a witness's account for the relevant presence of retrograde amnesia in the elderly. Particular attention should be paid to the time of the day, season, relationship with meals, nocturnal micturition, supine or upright position, drugs, duration of treatment, and time relationship between drug consumption and appearance of adverse effects (1).

Precise details of the drug regimen should be collected, as alpha-receptor blockers, nitrates, and benzodiazepines are predictors of OH. Therefore, attention should be paid to reappraisal of the drug regimen in the presence of OH in order to reduce syncope recurrence (23). Since the medical history has a limited value in the differential diagnosis between cardiac and neurally mediated causes of syncope in older patients (13), TT and CSM become essential in the diagnostic pathway.

A comprehensive cardiovascular and neurological assessment, searching for Parkinson's disease or other neurodegenerative conditions related to autonomic dysfunction, coupled with a careful observation of gait and standing balance for the evaluation of the locomotor

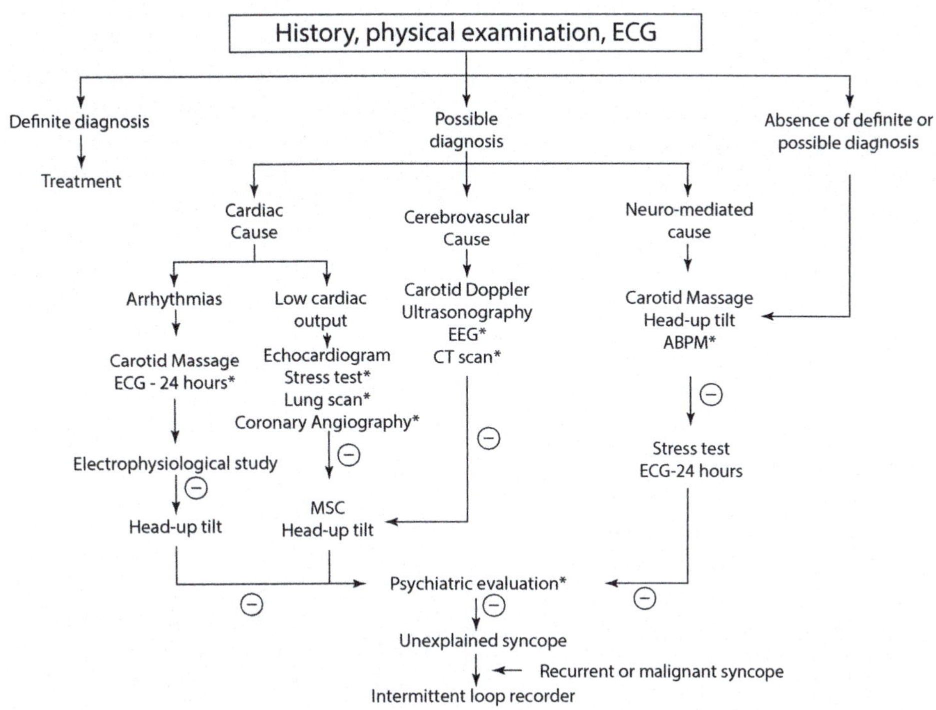

Figure 25.1 Standardized algorithm for the diagnosis of transient loss of consciousness. *Abbreviations*: ABPM, ambulatory blood pressure monitoring; ECG, electrocardiogram; EEG, electroencephalogram; CT scan, computed tomography scan. (Adapted from Moya A et al., *Eur Heart J*, 30, 2631–2671, 2009.)

system and the consequent risk of falling, are mandatory steps of the physical examination of the older patient with syncope.

The active standing test consists of measuring BP in the supine position and then immediately after changing from the supine to the upright position and after 1 and 3 minutes of standing. Given the age-related increase in OH, standing BP measurements are mandatory in the elderly and should be repeated, preferably in the morning and/or "promptly" after the syncope, as the standing fall in BP is not always reproducible, especially when related to drugs or predisposing conditions (1).

The 12-lead ECG can be considered diagnostic, requiring no further evaluation before institution of treatment in the following cases:

- Persistent sinus bradycardia <40 bpm in awake or repetitive sinus-atrial block or sinus pauses >3 seconds.
- Mobitz II second- or third-degree atrioventricular block, alternating left and right bundle branch block.
- Ventricular tachycardia (VT) or rapid paroxysmal supraventricular tachycardia.
- Nonsustained episodes of polymorphic VT and long or short QT interval.
- Acute ischemia with or without myocardial infarction (1).

However, studies have shown that an ECG will determine the cause of syncope in only ~5% of patients (37).

Given the high prevalence of CSS as a cause of syncope and unexplained falls in the elderly, the ESC guidelines on syncope (1) propose the execution of CSM during the initial evaluation. The test is performed under continuous HR and beat-to-beat BP monitoring for 10 seconds bilaterally, first in the supine and then in the upright position on TT at an angle of 60 degrees. The added diagnostic value of repeating CSM in the upright position has been well documented (38). In order to assess the contribution of the vasodepressive component, CSM may be repeated after intravenous administration of 0.02 mg/kg of atropine, which eliminates vagally induced asystole, thereby unmasking the vasodepression (39). This quantification of the vasodepressive component is clinically relevant, because it has been shown that pacemaker therapy is less effective when the vasodepressive effect is large, compared with predominant cardioinhibition (40). Transient ischemic attack or stroke during the prior 3 months or critical carotid artery stenosis on Doppler ultrasound performed in the presence of carotid bruits represent relative contraindications to CSM (41). In these situations, a careful risk–benefit assessment must be undertaken.

ADDITIONAL TESTS

Blood tests, head computed tomography (CT), echocardiogram, and carotid ultrasonography should be guided by history and physical examination (42). Routine blood tests typically only confirm clinical suspicion in syncope, as they only uncover an etiology in 2% of patients (37). Specifically, cardiac enzymes are of little value if drawn routinely from elderly patients who are admitted with syncope. Cardiac enzymes should only be drawn if the patient has other signs or symptoms suggestive of myocardial ischemia by history, such as chest pain, dyspnea, a concerning ECG, or an ECG that is uninterpretable for ischemia (43). Additional studies, such as electroencephalography and cardiac stress testing, have a low diagnostic benefit and should not be performed routinely (44). Telemetry can help determine the etiology of syncope in 3%–5% of patients, most commonly from causes such as AF or bradycardia (45).

If a new murmur is heard on examination, an echocardiogram should be obtained. However, if patients do not have a history of a murmur or have an audible murmur on examination, they are unlikely to have a valvular etiology for their syncope (46). An echocardiogram may give a diagnosis 2%–22% of the time, and most often it is aortic stenosis (45).

Head CT scans should be limited to patients presenting to the ED with syncope and either neurologic deficit, neurologic complaints, or concomitant signs of head trauma (47, 48). It is important to note that the elderly may have intracranial bleeds without evidence of trauma, emphasizing the importance of a neurologic assessment and evaluating for changes in a patient's baseline mental status. It is unlikely that a cerebral vascular event alone will cause syncope. However, neurologic complaints may be due to head trauma that occurred during the syncopal event. Grossman et al. (42) suggest that patients presenting with syncope without head trauma have a low likelihood of having abnormal findings on head CT and do not require a scan.

In addition to these tests, device interrogation is performed almost universally in patients with implantable cardiac defibrillators or pacemakers to assess for malfunctioning or new arrhythmias, despite little evidence to suggest its efficacy in the absence of concerning history, physical, or ECG findings (49). Choosing tests based on history and examination and prioritizing less expensive and higher yield tests may enable a more informed and cost-effective approach to evaluating syncope in the elderly.

RISK STRATIFICATION

When the cause of syncope remains uncertain after the initial evaluation, the next step is to assess the risk of major cardiovascular events or sudden cardiac death (1). Patients at low risk do not require further evaluation and can be discharged from the ED. Patients at moderate risk should undergo clinical and instrumental monitoring in observation units inside the ED. Patients at high risk should be monitored and treated properly in case of worsening (50).

Several risk stratification tools have been validated in the ED setting. The EGSYS score is a diagnostic score to identify cardiac syncope. Abnormal ECG and/or heart disease, palpitations before syncope, syncope during effort or in supine position, absence of autonomic prodromes, and absence of predisposing and/or precipitating factors were found to be predictors of cardiac syncope. To each variable, a score from +4 to −1 was assigned according to the magnitude of the regression coefficient. A score >3 identified cardiac syncope with a sensitivity of 95%/92% and a specificity of 61%/69% in the derivation and validation cohorts, respectively (33).

Recently, the Canadian Syncope Arrhythmia Risk Score was developed to predict the 30-day risk of arrhythmia or death after ED disposition among patients presenting with syncope. Abnormal ECG (QRS duration >130 ms and QTc interval >480 ms), heart disease, and absence of precipitating factors were associated with arrhythmia or death. A score of ≤0 was associated with <1% risk, scores of 1–3 were associated with 1.9%–7.5% risk, and scores of 4–8 were associated with 14.3%–22.2% risk of arrhythmia or death within 30 days of ED disposition (51).

Several additional studies have identified prognostic factors in patients with syncope. In the Short-Term Prognosis of Syncope (STePS) study, abnormal ECG, concomitant trauma, absence of prodrome, and male gender were associated with short-term unfavorable outcomes (52). Sun et al. (53) have identified age greater than 90 years, history of arrhythmia, triage SBP greater than 160 mmHg, abnormal ECG, and abnormal troponin I as predictors of 30-day serious events in older adults with syncope. The authors suggest inpatient evaluation for the high-risk individual (e.g., those with a syncope risk score of at least 3 points, when 1 point was given for each factor). In the San Francisco Syncope Rule study (35), abnormal ECG, complaint of shortness of breath, hematocrit <30%, SBP <90 mmHg, and history of congestive heart failure predicted 7-day serious outcomes. In the Risk Stratification of Syncope in the Emergency Department (ROSE) study (54), a serious outcome or all-cause mortality at 1 month were related to a brain natriuretic peptide concentration greater than or equal to 300 pg/mL, a positive fecal occult blood, hemoglobin ≤90 g/L, oxygen saturation ≤94%, and Q wave on the presenting ECG.

The Boston Syncope Criteria is an alternative method to identify ED patients at risk for adverse outcomes at 30 days. It is an eight-component decision tool, including signs and symptoms of acute coronary syndrome, worrisome cardiac history, family history of sudden cardiac death, valvular disease, signs of cardiac conduction disease, volume depletion, persistently abnormal vital signs for greater than 15 minutes, and primary neurological event (46). This tool has subsequently been validated and proved to safely reduce hospital admission by 11% (55).

Another simple risk classification system for patients presenting with syncope to the ED aimed at identifying independent predictors of 12-month total mortality after initial evaluation is the OESIL (Osservatorio Epidemiologico sulla Sincope nel Lazio) score, which considers age >65 years, history of cardiovascular disease, syncope without prodromes, and abnormal ECG (34). Nonetheless, these and others risk-stratification tools perform no better than clinician judgment at predicting short-term serious outcomes (56).

SECOND-LEVEL EVALUATION

When the cause of syncope remains uncertain after the initial evaluation, TT and/or prolonged ECG monitoring have been shown to yield a high diagnostic value in most severe cases.

Tilt testing

Tilt testing (TT) is the most validated test for the clinical assessment of neurally mediated reflexes, particularly for the diagnosis of VVS of undetermined origin after the initial evaluation. The *Traditional Italian Protocol*, which uses 300 μg of sublingual nitroglycerine, has long been the standard approach. It has been validated in older adults and shown to be well tolerated, with a positivity rate and specificity comparable to those observed in younger patients (57). Furthermore, a multicenter study (58) demonstrated that TT is safe and effective even in octogenarians, without major complications, confirming that the test can be safely performed at any age.

TT should be performed in the morning, in the fasting state, in a quiet and dimly lit room. Traditionally, TT involves 20 minutes of passive orthostatic positioning at an angle of 60 degrees, followed by the administration of 300 μg of nitroglycerine if syncope does not occur, and an additional 15 minutes of observation at the same angle. The test is considered positive if symptoms reproducing those reported by the patient during spontaneous syncope are associated with hypotension, bradycardia, or both (1).

More recently, the *"Fast Italian Protocol"* has been proposed as a time-efficient alternative. This newer approach reduces the total test duration from 40 to 25 minutes while maintaining diagnostic accuracy. The fast protocol consists of a 10-minute passive phase at 70 degrees, followed by a 10-minute active phase potentiated with 300 μg of sublingual nitroglycerin, if the passive phase is negative. Studies comparing the two protocols have shown similar positivity rates (~60%) and a comparable distribution of hemodynamic responses, including vasodepressor, cardioinhibitory, and mixed forms. Importantly, the shorter duration makes it more practical for widespread clinical use, reducing resource utilization and improving patient compliance without compromising safety or diagnostic yield.

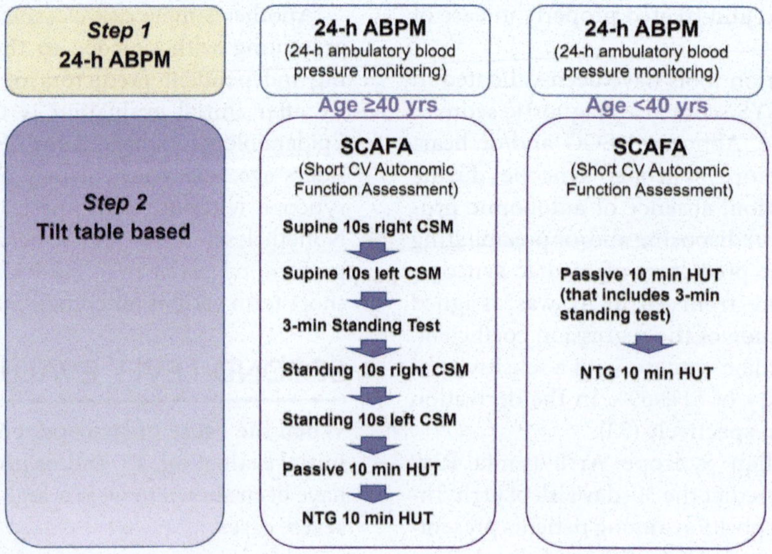

Figure 25.2 2STEPS assessment of noncardiac syncope.

Both protocols play critical roles in the evaluation of syncope, with the choice depending on clinical context and available resources. While the traditional protocol continues to be widely utilized, the fast protocol offers a promising alternative for streamlining diagnostic workflows (59).

The Fast Italian Protocol, while offering a faster and efficient alternative to traditional tilt testing, plays a central role in the recently introduced *2STEPS protocol* (Figure 25.2). This new diagnostic approach has been developed to provide a comprehensive evaluation of autonomic syncope by integrating two key steps that work together to identify the predominant hemodynamic mechanism behind the condition.

It consists of two complementary steps:

1. *Twenty-four-hour ambulatory blood pressure monitoring (ABPM)*, which helps detect persistent or episodic hypotension. This is particularly useful in uncovering cases of hypotensive susceptibility, where blood pressure drops might not be evident during routine clinical evaluations.
2. *Short cardiovascular autonomic function assessment (SCAFA)*, which includes carotid sinus massage (CSM), a 3-minute passive standing test, and tilt testing using the Fast Italian Protocol. These tests are conducted in a single session with continuous beat-to-beat hemodynamic monitoring, allowing for a detailed analysis of autonomic responses (60).

The 2STEPS protocol has shown high diagnostic efficacy, achieving positive results in 89% of cases. It has been particularly effective in classifying patients into the main three hemodynamic phenotypes:

- Hypotensive phenotype (68%)
- Bradycardic phenotype (6%)
- Mixed phenotype (15%) (59–61)

One of the major advantages of the 2STEPS protocol is its efficiency. The SCAFA session typically lasts only about 25 minutes, significantly reducing the time and resources needed for diagnostic evaluation while maintaining a high level of accuracy. This approach is particularly valuable for patients with recurrent or unexplained syncope, offering a structured framework to identify the underlying mechanisms and tailor treatment accordingly.

By incorporating the Fast Italian Protocol, the 2STEPS method bridges the gap between traditional diagnostic pathways and the need for faster, more precise evaluations. It also serves as an intermediate step before considering more invasive methods, such as implantable loop recorders, ensuring that patients receive a personalized and cost-effective diagnostic approach (61).

TT is also valuable for distinguishing syncope from other conditions, such as unexplained falls and epilepsy. The similar positivity rates of TT and CSM in these cases highlights the importance of routine neuroautonomic evaluation with these methods, especially in older patients with unexplained falls (64).

Syncope is a common cause of misdiagnosed epilepsy (65–68). Syncope and epilepsy can also coexist, either coincidentally or due to shared pathophysiologic mechanisms (69–71).

A standardized evaluation protocol, including TT, is crucial for differential diagnosis in such cases. This was confirmed in a study of patients with recurrent (TLoC of unknown cause. Among those referred to syncope units, isolated syncope was diagnosed in 42% of cases, most frequently in patients with possible epilepsy (~70%). Syncope and epilepsy coexisted in ~40% of patients. During follow-up, TLoC recurrence was ~50%. In patients previously treated with antiepileptic drugs, ~50% discontinued them, resuming only after confirmation of an epilepsy diagnosis (72).

Ambulatory blood pressure monitoring (ABPM)

ABPM is a reliable tool to detect and monitor hypotensive susceptibility in clinical practice.

The importance of optimizing blood pressure control in reflex syncope has been highlighted by recent evidence from the *synABPM1* and *synABPM2* studies. The synABPM1 study revealed that patients with reflex syncope frequently exhibit significant daytime SBP drops during ABPM, with one or more episodes of SBP <90 mmHg, or two or more episodes of SBP <100 mmHg, serving as highly specific markers of vasodepressor mechanisms (73).

Building on these findings, the synABPM2 study explored how ABPM can guide personalized treatment strategies for older adults with recurrent syncope. In this multicenter trial, patients were divided into two groups:

- Deprescription group: Discontinuing or reducing hypotensive medications resulted in an average SBP increase of +8.8 mmHg and a 64% reduction in episodes of SBP <90 mmHg, while also reducing syncope recurrence.
- BP-raising group: Introducing BP-raising drugs, such as fludrocortisone or midodrine, achieved an average SBP increase of +6.3 mmHg, with a 62% reduction in symptomatic hypotension episodes ().

These studies underline the value of ABPM not only as a diagnostic tool but also as a guide for individualized therapeutic approaches. By enabling precise identification of hypotensive susceptibility, ABPM supports targeted interventions that stabilize blood pressure, reduce symptom recurrence, and improve outcomes in patients with vasodepressor reflex syncope.

Prolonged electrocardiographic monitoring

ECG monitoring is aimed at diagnosing intermittent bradyarrhythmias and tachyarrhythmias and is indicated when there is a high pretest probability of identifying an arrhythmia associated with syncope (1).

- *In-hospital monitoring* is indicated when the patient is at high risk of life-threatening arrhythmia, and although the diagnostic yield varies from 1.9% to 16%, it is justified by the need to avoid immediate risk to the patient (45, 75).
- *Holter ECG monitoring* in syncope is of more value if symptoms are very frequent, as daily episodes might increase the potential for a correlation between symptoms and ECG. However, since symptoms do not relapse in most patients during the monitoring period, the true yield of Holter ECG in syncope may be as low as 1%–2% (76).
- *Loop recorders, external* (*ELR*) or *internal* (*ILR*), have a loop memory that continuously records and deletes ECG, including a manual function, through which the patient can activate ECG storage during symptoms and an automatic feature that allows the capture of arrhythmic events without relying on the patient's compliance or perception of symptoms. When activated by the patient, typically after a symptom has occurred, several seconds to minutes of preactivation ECG is stored and can be retrieved for analysis.

ELR can be useful in patients with relatively frequent syncope when used early after the last episode (1). A recent international multicenter registry showed a 24.5% diagnostic yield in patients with syncope (77). An ILR is implanted subcutaneously under local anesthesia, has a battery life of more than 36 months, and is indicated in patients with less frequent syncopal episodes. It appears to provide an ECG-syncope correlation in about 35% of patients during the lifetime of the device. Of these, 56% of patients had asystole or severe bradycardia. Similar findings were observed when an ILR was inserted in patients with suspected neurally mediated syncope early after the initial evaluation or in unexplained syncope at the end of the conventional workup (78). The newest devices are so small that they can be injected with a minimally invasive procedure and are able to send wireless transmissions automatically to a central server, allowing continuous patient monitoring.

Krahn et al. (79) have previously shown that age was the only independent variable that predicted bradyarrhythmic syncope and the need for pacing, as recently confirmed (80). Older patients are more likely to receive an ILR implantation than younger patients because of the need for a precise diagnosis in case of structural heart disease or bundle branch block, which are almost exclusively present in patients ≥65 years, because of the limited value of the clinical history in determining the causes of syncope, and because in the elderly the onset of syncope is often sudden with little or no prodrome and a consequent higher risk of trauma. These factors justify the need for ILR to detect the underlying mechanism and facilitate a precise treatment (81).

ILR has a high diagnostic value also in those conditions in which an initial diagnosis is only suspected, and the demonstration of an arrhythmic mechanism could definitively guide therapy. In a population of highly selected patients, with mean age 71 years and an initial diagnosis of either likely epilepsy or unexplained fall, the ILR device documented a relapse of their index attack; in about a quarter of patients, the final diagnosis was arrhythmic syncope. Moreover, when the arrhythmia was not documented at the time of a spontaneous attack, ILR monitoring definitely excluded an arrhythmic cause

(82). These observations have been recently confirmed in a single-center, prospective, observational cohort study of older recurrent fallers attending the ED, in whom an ILR was used to detect arrhythmia. Of older patients with unexplained falls who attend the ED, 71% had a cardiac arrhythmia that was not apparent at the time of presentation, but detected within 9 months of continuous monitoring using ILR. In 20% of these patients, events were directly attributable to a modifiable cardiac arrhythmia (83).

Treatment

The treatment of patients with syncope is based on risk stratification and identification of specific mechanisms leading to global cerebral hypoperfusion (1).

Therapeutic options in neurally mediated syncope

Physical counterpressure maneuvers such as leg crossing, hand grip, or arm tensing can induce a significant BP increase during impending reflex syncope, but given the frequent absence of prodromes in older adults, these maneuvers are difficult to apply in this age group. Education and reassurance and avoidance of triggering situations are cornerstones of behavioral strategies.

Particular consideration should be given to the reappraisal of hypotensive drugs regimens. In a recent randomized, parallel, prospective trial in older patients with vasodepressor reflex syncope (84), the recurrence of syncope and presyncope was safely reduced by discontinuing/reducing vasoactive therapy, without increasing the risk of cardiovascular and neurological events, and applying careful BP control, aimed at achieving average SBP values around 140 mmHg, or at least below 150 mmHg, as per current guideline recommendations in older adults (85).

Disappointing results have been obtained by the use of various drugs in the context of neurally mediated syncope (86). Recently, the multicenter POST 2 (Prevention of Syncope Trial 2), a randomized, placebo-controlled, double-blind trial, that assessed the effects of fludrocortisone in vasovagal syncope over a 1-year treatment period, did not meet its primary objective of demonstrating that fludrocortisone reduced the likelihood of VVS (87).

Cardiac pacing should be considered in patients with dominant cardioinhibitory CSS (1). The efficacy of pacing in patients with neurally mediated syncope has been controversial, until the results of the ISSUE 3 study were published, showing that pacing was effective in reducing the recurrence of syncope in patients ≥40 years with severe asystolic neurally mediated syncope, previously documented by an ILR (62). Nevertheless, 25% of the patients had syncope recurrence after 2 years despite pacemaker therapy. The benefit of pacemaker therapy was not substantial in patients with a positive TT, suggesting a hypotensive mechanism that cannot be prevented by cardiac pacing (63).

In a pragmatic study of patients aged >40 years affected by severe unpredictable recurrent reflex syncope, a guidelines-based diagnostic algorithm was proposed and the efficacy of cardiac pacing was assessed (88). Patients underwent CSM, followed by TT if CSM was negative, followed by implantation of an ILR, if TT was negative. Those who had an asystolic response to one of these tests received a dual-chamber pacemaker. The recurrence rate of syncope was highly reduced in the year following implantation compared to the prior year and was similar in CSM+, TT+, and ILR+ patients. The recurrence rate was also significantly lower than that observed in the group of patients with a nondiagnostic test who had received an ILR instead of a pacemaker. This guidelines-based diagnostic algorithm proved clinically useful for selection of candidates for cardiac pacing in everyday clinical practice. Follow-up data from this study showed that the effectiveness of this algorithm and the benefit of cardiac pacing were maintained up to 3 years (89). The benefit of pacing was irrespective of the index diagnostic test, but was influenced by the results of TT: in patients with negative TT, the syncope recurrence rate was very low; in those with a positive TT, the probability of recurrence of syncope within 3 years was 23% in patients with an asystolic TT response and 27% in patients with mixed or vasodepressor TT response.

Closed-loop stimulation pacemaker, a pacing program designed to detect and stop the abnormal heart rhythms that precede syncope, has shown promising results in preventing the recurrence of VVS in patients with a cardioinhibitory response to TT compared with conventional pacing. A possible explanation is its quick reaction in high-rate pacing delivered in the early phase of vasovagal reflex, which increase the CO and BP, preventing loss of consciousness (90).

Therapeutic options in orthostatic hypotension and orthostatic intolerance syndromes

The principal treatment strategies for OH involve elimination of hypotensive drugs and expansion of extracellular volume and salt and water intake in the absence of hypertension. Elevation of the head of the bed ameliorates nocturnal hypertension, maintains a more favorable distribution of body fluids, and prevents nocturnal polyuria. Gravitational venous pooling in older patients can be treated with abdominal binders or compression stockings (1).

If nonpharmacological measures do not attenuate symptoms sufficiently, pharmacological interventions may become necessary. Nevertheless, supine hypertension has to be considered in pharmacological treatment.

Volume expansion may be achieved with fludrocortisone, a synthetic mineralocorticoid that increases plasma volume by renal sodium retention. Unless peripheral vascular resistance (PVR) declines sufficiently, fludrocortisone treatment may result in dose-dependent supine hypertension.

The alpha-agonist midodrine has been used to treat OH by vasoconstriction of peripheral arteries; its major limitation is a short half-life, which requires frequent dosing and limits long-term compliance. Furthermore, it may have adverse effects on urinary outflow, which requires special caution in older men (91). Pyridostigmine, a cholinesterase inhibitor, improves ganglionic transmission and vascular adrenergic tone in the upright position, mediating a slight increase in DBP during standing without worsening supine hypertension (92). Droxidopa is an orally administered artificial amino acid converted both peripherally and centrally into norepinephrine. The enzyme responsible for the conversion, aromatic amino acid decarboxylase, is widely expressed; thus, administration of droxidopa increases norepinephrine even if postganglionic sympathetic neurons are not intact. The drug has received accelerated Food and Drug Administration (FDA) approval for the treatment of symptomatic OH. It has been recently demonstrated that droxidopa improved symptoms and their impact on daily activities, with an associated increase in standing SBP in patients with symptomatic OH due to different orthostatic intolerance syndromes, without worsening supine hypertension (93).

SPECIAL CONSIDERATIONS IN THE ELDERLY

Overlap between syncope and falls in the older patient

The clinical relevance of syncope in the older patient could be underestimated due to the overlap with other presentations such as falls. The incidence of syncope in older patients is thus likely to be considerably higher than current estimates, with attendant cost implications.

Between 1999 and 2000, falls accounted for 647,721 visits to United Kingdom accident and emergency departments, and 204,424 hospital admissions in people aged 60 years and over, with costs approaching 1 billion pounds, the majority of which was related to inpatient admissions (94). Falling is another major geriatric syndrome (95), affecting mortality, morbidity, and institutionalization (96). Thirty-four percent of community-dwelling patients older than 65 years and 50% of octogenarians fall at least once a year (97).

Ten percent of hospital admissions are due to fall-related trauma (98); 5%–10% of older patients who fall experience fractures or concussions (99), and in about 1% a hip fracture occurs, with a 20%–30% 1-year mortality and substantial loss of functional capacity (100). In 30%–70% of fallers, a depressive syndrome develops due to the fear of falling and consequent disability (101).

Falls that are not accidental, not related to a clear medical condition, or drug-induced are defined as "unexplained" (102) and represent a relevant cause of hospital admission and increased health care costs (95). Especially in older adults in whom the circumstances of a fall event cannot be established because of the lack of witnesses and amnesia for the episode, a misdiagnosed syncope may underlie an unexplained fall. About 20% of cardiovascular syncope in patients older than 70 years presents as a fall, especially in patients with CSS and OH; more than 20% of the older patients with CSS complain of falls as well as syncope (103). In a study of patients older than 60 years admitted to the hospital because of a fall or syncope, fallers who had CSS during CSM, showed retrograde amnesia for the loss of consciousness more frequently than patients with syncope (104). Furthermore, over one third of the falls in patients in orthopedic wards are unexplained, particularly in those with depressive symptoms and syncopal spells (105), underscoring the importance of a comprehensive history and assessment at the beginning of the medical evaluation.

Unexplained falls not initially thought due to syncope but in which a final diagnosis of syncope is confirmed after a diagnostic workup have been recently defined as "syncopal falls" (106); in a recent study (107), such falls accounted for 43% of the initially unexplained falls, which received a final diagnosis of syncope after a standardized and guidelines-based approach. Thus, a careful syncope workup may be useful in patients with unexplained falls.

Postural BP decreases could cause a falling event. It has been suggested that 2%–10% of falls in older adults may occur secondary to impaired orthostatic hemodynamic responses, and loss of consciousness is estimated to result in as many as 10% of falls (108). In many cases, loss of consciousness may not occur, but increased fall susceptibility remains through presyncope and associated physiological impairments (8). Results from the Irish Longitudinal Study on Ageing (109) proved that, with the exception of initial OH, beat-to-beat measures of impaired orthostatic BP recovery or sustained OH are independent risk factors for future falls, unexplained falls, and injurious falls. Finally, the presence of comorbidities could worsen the prognosis, as older adults with Parkinson's disease or diabetes mellitus and OH have poorer balance scores in comparison to those without OH (110, 111). Poor balance is a known risk factor for falls, and may increase this risk threefold (97).

Syncope in the older patient with dementia

BP impairments including OH and hypertension, as well as acute and chronic cerebral hypoperfusion are associated with impaired cognitive performance in older adults

(112, 113). This association has been confirmed in a large sample of the general population, in which patients with OH showed worse cognitive performance in the domains of memory, attention, and executive functions (114).

Frewen et al. (115) have shown an independent association between early OH and cognitive decline in patients with supine hypertension. A possible explanation is that high long-term BP levels, which are per se related to cognitive impairment, could be associated with OH, which in turn aggravates the cognitive deficit. The latter is also a risk factor for falls. Multivariable analyses suggest cognitive deficits increase falling risk threefold. Therefore, cognitive functioning could serve as an intermediary mechanism between BP impairments and falling risk in older adults (108). The risk of falling is eight times as high in elderly adults with dementia as in their cognitively intact counterparts and is frequently related to syncope (116).

Although neuroautonomic evaluation (TT, CSM, supine and upright BP measurement) is a reliable diagnostic tool in elderly adults with unexplained falls and syncope (64), individuals with dementia are a clinical subset in which suspected syncope is less likely to be fully investigated because of several factors, ranging from difficulty in collecting information on falls, to an ageist attitude that tends to underestimate the relevance of falls and syncope in older persons, particularly those with cognitive impairment.

Recently, a prospective, observational, multicenter study (117) was conducted to define the etiology of syncope and unexplained falls in elderly adults with dementia, using a simplified guidelines-based protocol. An initially suspected diagnosis of syncope was confirmed in 87% of the patients, and syncope was identified as the cause of the event in the 45% of those referred for unexplained falls. Orthostatic hypotension was the cause of the event in the 48% of the participants with a final diagnosis of syncope. The study proved that a guidelines-based diagnostic protocol can be used even in older patients with dementia referred for suspected syncope or unexplained falls. Unexplained falls may mask a diagnosis of syncope or pseudo-syncope in almost 50% of cases. Given the high prevalence of orthostatic syncope in participants (~50%), a systematic reappraisal of drugs potentially responsible for OH should be performed. Indeed, the prevalence of orthostatic syncope differs by setting: 10% in all patients admitted in the ED (EGSYS-2 study) (30), 30% in geriatric patients older than 75 years (GIS study) (6), and 50% in frail elderly patients affected by dementia (117) (Figure 25.3).

A recent analysis from the Syncope & Dementia registry (107) identified the presence of precipitant factors in the clinical history (mainly postural changes and neck movements) and better cognitive function as independent predictors of syncopal falls in patients with cognitive impairment. Conversely, subjects with nonsyncopal falls were more often treated with insulin and benzodiazepines

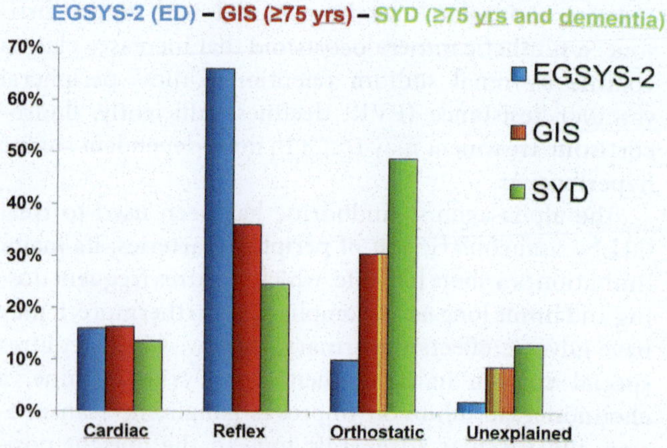

Figure 25.3 Prevalence of orthostatic syncope in different populations. *Abbreviations*: EGSYS, Evaluation of Guidelines in Syncope Study; GIS, Gruppo Italiano Sincope of Italian Geriatric Society; SYD, Syncope and Dementia study. (From Brignole M et al., *Eur Heart J*, 27, 76–82, 2006; Ungar A et al., *J Am Geriatr Soc*, 54, 1531–1536, 2006; Ungar A et al., *J Am Geriatr Soc*, 64, 1567–1573, 2016.)

and less often reported prodromes (especially neurovegetative symptoms) compared with those with syncopal falls. The identification of the causes of falls and of individuals with syncope-related falls may have important clinical and therapeutic implications that, in turn, may reduce the burden of falls-related morbidity and mortality in this subset of frequent fallers.

REFERENCES

1. Moya A, Sutton R, Ammirati F et al. Guidelines for the diagnosis and management of syncope (version 2009): The task force for the diagnosis and management of syncope of the European Society of Cardiology (ESC). *Eur Heart J* 2009; *30*: 2631–2671.
2. Soteriades ES, Evans JC, Larson MG et al. Incidence and prognosis of syncope. *N Engl J Med* 2002; *347*: 878–885.
3. Ruwald MH, Hansen ML, Lamberts M et al. The relation between age, sex, comorbidity, and pharmacotherapy and the risk of syncope: A Danish nationwide study. *Europace* 2012; *14*: 1506–1514.
4. Olde Nordkamp LAR, van Dijk N, Ganzeboom KS et al. Syncope prevalence in the ED compared to that in the general practice and population: A strong selection process. *Am J Emerg Med* 2009; *27*: 271–279.
5. Del Rosso A, Alboni P, Brignole M et al. Relation of clinical presentation of syncope to the age of patients. *Am J Cardiol* 2005; *96*: 1431–1435.
6. Ungar A, Mussi C, Del Rosso A et al. Diagnosis and characteristics of syncope in older patients referred to geriatric departments. *J Am Geriatr Soc* 2006; *54*: 1531–1536.

7. Van Lieshout JJ, Wieling W, Karemaker JM et al. Syncope, cerebral perfusion, and oxygenation. *J Appl Physiol* 2003; *94*: 833–848.
8. Wieling W, Thijs RD, van Dijk N et al. Symptoms and signs of syncope: A review of the link between physiology and clinical clues. *Brain* 2009; *132*: 2630–2642.
9. Serrador JM, Sorond FA, Vyas M et al. Cerebral pressure-flow relations in hypertensive elderly humans: Transfer gain in different frequency domains. *J Appl Physiol* 2005; *98*: 151–159.
10. Kenny RA. Syncope in the elderly: Diagnosis, evaluation, and treatment. *J Cardiovasc Electrophysiol* 2003; *14*: S74–S77.
11. Van Wijnen VK, Finucane C, Harms MPM et al. Noninvasive beat-to-beat finger arterial pressure monitoring during orthostasis: A comprehensive review of normal and abnormal responses at different ages. *J Intern Med* 2017; *282*: 468–483.
12. Galizia G, Abete P, Mussi C et al. Role of early symptoms in assessment of syncope in elderly people: Results from the Italian group for the study of syncope in the elderly. *J Am Geriatric Soc* 2009; *57*: 18–23.
13. Tan MP, Parry SW. Vasovagal syncope in the older patient. *J Am Coll Cardiol* 2008; *51*: 599–606.
14. O'Dwyer C, Bennett K, Langan Y et al. Amnesia for loss of consciousness is common in vasovagal syncope. *Europace* 2011; *13*: 1040–1045.
15. Maggi R, Menozzi C, Brignole M et al. Cardioinhibitory carotid sinus hypersensitivity predicts an asystolic mechanism of spontaneous neurally mediated syncope. *Europace* 2007; *9*: 563–567.
16. Kerr SR, Pearce MS, Brayne C et al. Carotid sinus hypersensitivity in asymptomatic older persons: Implications for diagnosis of syncope and falls. *Arch Intern Med* 2006; *166*: 515–520.
17. Sutton R. Carotid sinus syndrome: Progress in understanding and management. *Glob Cardiol Sci Pract* 2014 Jun 18; *2014*(2): 1–8. doi: 10.5339/gcsp.2014.18.
18. Menozzi C, Brignole M, Lolli G et al. Follow-up of asystolic episodes in patients with cardioinhibitory, neurally mediated syncope and VVI pacemaker. *Am J Cardiol* 1993; *72*: 1152–1155.
19. Puggioni E, Guiducci V, Brignole M et al. Results and complications of the carotid sinus massage performed according to the 'method of symptoms'. *Am J Cardiol* 2002; *89*: 599–601.
20. Krediet CT, Parry SW, Jardine DL et al. The history of diagnosing carotid sinus hypersensitivity: Why are the current criteria too sensitive? *Europace* 2011; *13*: 14–22.
21. Wieling W, Krediet CT, Solari D et al. At the heart of the arterial baroreflex: A physiological basis for a new classification of carotid sinus hypersensitivity. *J Intern Med* 2013; *273*: 345–358.
22. Freeman R, Wieling W, Axelrod FB et al. Consensus statement on the definition of orthostatic hypotension, neurally mediated syncope and the postural tachycardia syndrome. *Clin Auton Res* 2011; *21*: 69–72.
23. Rafanelli M, Morrione A, Landi A et al. Neuroautonomic evaluation of patients with unexplained syncope: Incidence of complex neurally mediated diagnoses in the elderly. *Clin Interv Aging* 2014; *9*: 333–338.
24. Mussi C, Ungar A, Salvioli G et al. Evaluation of Guidelines in Syncope Study 2 Group. Orthostatic hypotension as cause of syncope in patients older than 65 years admitted to emergency departments for transient loss of consciousness. *J Gerontol A Biol Sci Med Sci* 2009; *64*: 801–806.
25. Wieling W, Krediet CT, van Dijk N et al. Initial orthostatic hypotension: Review of a forgotten condition. *Clin Sci* 2007; *112*: 157–165.
26. Robinovitch SN, Feldman F, Yang Y et al. Video capture of the circumstances of falls in elderly people residing in long-term care: An observational study. *Lancet* 2013; *381*: 47–54.
27. Ricci F, De Caterina R, Fedorowski A. Orthostatic hypotension: Epidemiology, prognosis, and treatment. *J Am Coll Cardiol* 2015; *66*: 848–860.
28. Gibbons CH, Freeman R. Clinical implications of delayed orthostatic hypotension: A 10-year follow-up study. *Neurology* 2015; *85*: 1362–1367.
29. Marrison VK, Fletcher A, Parry SW. The older patient with syncope: Practicalities and controversies. *Int J Cardiol* 2012; *155*: 9–13.
30. Brignole M, Menozzi C, Bartoletti A et al. A new management of syncope: Prospective systematic guideline-based evaluation of patients referred urgently to general hospitals. *Eur Heart J* 2006; *27*: 76–82.
31. Rivasi G, Ungar A. Syncope: New solutions for an old problem. *Eur Heart J Suppl* 2021; *23*(Suppl B): B6–B16.
32. Alboni P, Brignole M, Menozzi C et al. Diagnostic value of history in patients with syncope with or without heart disease. *J Am Coll Cardiol* 2001; *37*: 1921–1928.
33. Del Rosso A, Ungar A, Maggi R et al. Clinical predictors of cardiac syncope at initial evaluation in patients referred urgently to general hospital: The EGSYS score. *Heart* 2008; *94*: 1620–1626.
34. Colivicchi F, Ammirati F, Melina D et al. OESIL (Osservatorio Epidemiologico sulla Sincope nel Lazio) study investigators. Development and prospective validation of a risk stratification system for patients with syncope in the emergency department: The OESIL risk score. *Eur Heart J* 2003; *24*: 811–819.
35. Quinn J, McDermott D, Stiell I et al. Prospective validation of the San Francisco syncope rule to

predict patients with serious outcomes. *Ann Emerg Med* 2006; *47*: 448–454.
36. de Ruiter SC, Wold JFH, Germans T et al. Multiple causes of syncope in the elderly: Diagnostic outcomes of a Dutch multidisciplinary syncope pathway. *Europace* 2018; *20*: 867–872.
37. Linzer M, Yang EH, Estes NA 3rd et al. Diagnosing syncope. Part 1: Value of history, physical examination, and electrocardiography. Clinical Efficacy Assessment Project of the American College of Physicians. *Ann Intern Med* 1997; *126*: 989.
38. Parry SW, Richardson DA, O'Shea D et al. Diagnosis of carotid sinus hypersensitivity in older adults: Carotid sinus massage in the upright position is essential. *Heart* 2000; *83*: 22–23.
39. Solari D, Maggi R, Oddone D et al. Assessment of the vasodepressor reflex in carotid sinus syndrome. *Circ Arrhythm Electrophysiol* 2014; *7*: 505–510.
40. Lopes R, Gonçalves A, Campos J et al. The role of pacemaker in hypersensitive carotid sinus syndrome. *Europace* 2011; *13*: 572–575.
41. Davies AG, Kenny RA. Neurological complication following carotid sinus massage. *Am J Cardiol* 1998; *81*: 1256–1257.
42. Grossman SA. Testing in syncope. *Intern Emerg Med* 2006; *1*: 135–136.
43. Grossman SA, Van Epp S, Arnold R et al. The value of cardiac enzymes in elderly patients presenting to the emergency department with syncope. *J Gerontol A Biol Sci Med Sci* 2003; *58*: 1055–1059.
44. Sun BC, Costantino G, Barbic F et al. Priorities for emergency department syncope research. *Ann Emerg Med* 2014; *64*: 649–655.
45. Chiu DT, Shapiro NI, Sun BC et al. Are echocardiography, telemetry, ambulatory electrocardiography monitoring and cardiac enzymes in emergency department patients presenting with syncope useful tests? A preliminary investigation. *J Emerg Med* 2014; *47*: 113–118.
46. Grossman SA, Fischer C, Lipsitz L et al. Predicting adverse outcomes in syncope. *J Emerg Med* 2007; *33*: 233–239.
47. Goyal N, Donnino MW, Vachhani R et al. The utility of head computed tomography in the emergency department evaluation of syncope. *Intern Emerg Med* 2006; *1*: 148–150.
48. Grossman SA, Fischer C, Bar JL et al. The yield of head CT in syncope: A pilot study. *Intern Emerg Med* 2007; *2*: 46–49.
49. D'Angelo RN, Pickett CC. Diagnostic yield of device interrogation in the evaluation of syncope in an elderly population. *Int J Cardiol* 2017; *236*: 164–167.
50. Casagranda I, Brignole M, Cencetti S et al. Management of transient loss of consciousness of suspected syncopal cause, after the initial evaluation in the Emergency Department. *Emerg Care J* 2016; *12*: 6046.
51. Thiruganasambandamoorthy V, Stiell IG, Sivilotti MLA, Rowe BH, Mukarram M, Arcot K, Kwong K, McRae AD, Wells GA, Taljaard M. Predicting short-term risk of arrhythmia among patients with syncope: the Canadian syncope arrhythmia risk score. *Acad Emerg Med.* 2017 Nov; *24*(11): 1315–1326. doi: 10.1111/acem.13275.
52. Costantino G, Perego F, Dipaola F et al. Short- and long-term prognosis of syncope, risk factors, and role of hospital admission: Results from the STePS (Short-term prognosis of syncope) study. *J Am Coll Cardiol* 2008; *51*: 276–283.
53. Sun BC, Derose SF, Liang LJ et al. Predictors of 30-day serious events in older patients with syncope. *Ann Emerg Med* 2009; *54*: 769–778; e1–e5.
54. Reed MJ, Newby DE, Coull AJ et al. The ROSE (risk stratification of syncope in the emergency department) study. *J Am Coll Cardiol* 2010; *55*: 713–721.
55. Grossman SA, Bar J, Fischer C et al. Reducing admissions utilizing the Boston Syncope Criteria. *J Emerg Med* 2012; *42*: 345–352.
56. Costantino G, Casazza G, Reed M et al. Syncope risk stratification tools vs. clinical judgment: An individual patient data meta-analysis. *Am J Med* 2014; *127*: *1126*.e13–25.
57. Del Rosso A, Bartoletti A, Bartoli P et al. Methodology of head-up tilt testing with sublingual nitroglycerin in unexplained syncope. *Am J Cardiol* 2000; *85*: 1007–1011.
58. Ungar A, Rivasi G, Rafanelli M et al. Safety and tolerability of tilt testing and carotid sinus massage in the octogenarians. *Age Ageing* 2016; *45*: 242–248.
59. Russo V, Parente F et al. Short-duration head-up tilt test potentiated with sublingual nitroglycerin in suspected vasovagal syncope: The fast Italian protocol. *European Heart Journal.* 2023. doi:10.1093/eurheartj/ehad123
60. Moya A, Sutton R, Ammirati F et al. Guidelines for the diagnosis and management of syncope (version 2009). *Eur Heart J.* 2009; *30*(21): 2631–2671.
61. Groppelli A, Russo V, Parente E, Comune A, de Lange FJ, Rivasi G, Rafanelli M, Deharo JC, Francisco-Pascual J, Maggi R, Fedorowski A, Ungar A, Parati G, Brignole M. Mechanism of syncope: Role of ambulatory blood pressure monitoring and cardiovascular autonomic function assessment. *Eur Heart J.* 2024 Dec 30: ehae907. doi: 10.1093/eurheartj/ehae907.
62. Brignole M, Menozzi C, Moya A et al. Pacemaker therapy in patients with neurally-mediated syncope and documented asystole. Third international study on syncope of unknown etiology (ISSUE-3): A randomized trial. *Circulation* 2012; *125*: 2566–2571.
63. Brignole M, Donateo P, Tomaino M et al. Benefit of pacemaker therapy in patients with presumed neurally-mediated syncope and documented asystole is greater when tilt test is negative. An analysis

from the Third International Study on Syncope of Uncertain Etiology (ISSUE-3). *Circ Arrhythm Electrophysiol* 2014; *7*: 10–16.
64. Rafanelli M, Ruffolo E, Chisciotti VM et al. Clinical aspects and diagnostic relevance of neuroautonomic evaluation in patients with unexplained falls. *Aging Clin Exp Res* 2014; *26*: 33–37.
65. Chowdhury FA, Nashef L, Elwes RD. Misdiagnosis in epilepsy: A review and recognition of diagnostic uncertainty. *Eur J Neurol* 2008; *15*: 1034–1042.
66. Angus-Leppan H. Diagnosing epilepsy in neurology clinics: A prospective study. *Seizure* 2008; *17*: 431–436.
67. Lempert T, Bauer M, Schmidt D. Syncope: A videometric analysis of 56 episodes of transient cerebral hypoxia. *Ann Neurol* 1994; *36*: 233–237.
68. Sander JW, O'Donoghue MF. Epilepsy: Getting the diagnosis right. *BMJ* 1997; *314*: 158–159.
69. Zaidi A, Clough P, Cooper P et al. Misdiagnosis of epilepsy: Many seizure-like attacks have a cardiovascular cause. *J Am Coll Cardiol* 2000; *36*: 181–184.
70. Rodrigues Tda R, Sternick EB, Moreira Mda C. Epilepsy or syncope? An analysis of 55 consecutive patients with loss of consciousness, convulsion, falls, and no EEG abnormalities. *PACE* 2010; *33*: 804–811.
71. Rangel I, Freitas J, Correia AS et al. The usefulness of the head-up tilt test in patients with suspected epilepsy. *Seizure* 2014; *23(5)*: 367–370.
72. Ungar A, Ceccofiglio A, Pescini F et al. Syncope and epilepsy coexist in 'possible' and 'drug-resistant' epilepsy (Overlap between Epilepsy and Syncope Study OESYS). *BMC Neurol* 2017; *17*: *45*. doi:10.1186/s12883-017-0822-5.
73. Sharad B, Rivasi G, Hamrefors V, Johansson M, Ungar A, Sutton R, Brignole M, Parati G, Fedorowski A. Twenty-four-hour ambulatory blood pressure profile in patients with reflex syncope and matched controls. *J Am Heart Assoc.* 2023 Apr 18; *12*(8): e028704. doi: 10.1161/JAHA.122.028704.
74. Groppelli A, Russo V, Parente E, Comune A, de Lange FJ, Rivasi G, Rafanelli M, Deharo JC, Francisco-Pascual J, Maggi R, Fedorowski A, Ungar A, Parati G, Brignole M. Mechanism of syncope: Role of ambulatory blood pressure monitoring and cardiovascular autonomic function assessment. *Eur Heart J.* 2024 Dec 30: ehae907. doi: 10.1093/eurheartj/ehae907.
75. Benezet-Mazuecos J, Ibanez B, Rubio JM et al. Utility of in-hospital cardiac remote telemetry in patients with unexplained syncope. *Europace* 2007; 9: 1196–1201.
76. Bass EB, Curtiss EI, Arena VC et al. The duration of Holter monitoring in patients with syncope. Is 24 hours enough? *Arch Intern Med* 1990; *150*: 1073–1078.
77. Locati ET, Moya A, Oliveira M et al. External prolonged electrocardiogram monitoring in unexplained syncope and palpitations: Results of the SYNARR-Flash study. *Europace* 2016; *18*: 1265–1272.
78. Brignole M, Vardas P, Hoffman E et al. Indications for the use of diagnostic implantable and external ECG loop recorders. *Europace* 2009; *11*: 671–687.
79. Krahn AD, Klein GJ, Fitzpatrick A et al. Predicting the outcome of patients with unexplained syncope undergoing prolonged monitoring. *Pacing Clin Electrophysiol* 2002; *25*: 37–41.
80. Palmisano P, Accogli M, Zaccaria M et al. Predictive factors for pacemaker implantation in patients receiving an implantable loop recorder for syncope remained unexplained after an extensive cardiac and neurological workup. *Int J Cardiol* 2013; *168*: 3450–3457.
81. Brignole M, Menozzi C, Maggi R et al. The usage and diagnostic yield of implantable loop-recorder in detection of the mechanism of syncope and in guiding effective antiarrhythmic therapy in older people. *Europace* 2005; *7*: 273–279.
82. Maggi R, Rafanelli M, Ceccofiglio A et al. Additional diagnostic value of implantable loop recorder in patients with initial diagnosis of real or apparent transient loss of consciousness of uncertain origin. *Europace* 2014; *16*: 1226–1230.
83. Bhangu J, McMahon CG, Hall P et al. Long-term cardiac monitoring in older adults with unexplained falls and syncope. *Heart* 2016; *102*: 681–686.
84. Solari D, Tesi F, Unterhuber M et al. Stop vasodepressor drugs in reflex syncope: A randomised controlled trial. *Heart* 2017; *103*: 449–455.
85. Mancia G, Fagard R, Narkiewicz K et al. ESH/ESC Guidelines for the management of arterial hypertension. *Eur Heart J* 2013; *34*: 2159–2219.
86. Sheldon RS, Grubb BP, Olshansky B et al. 2015 Heart rhythm society expert consensus statement on the diagnosis and treatment of postural tachycardia syndrome, inappropriate sinus tachycardia, and vasovagal syncope. *Heart Rhythm* 2015; *12*: e41–e63.
87. Sheldon R, Raj SR, Rose SM et al. Fludrocortisone for the prevention of vasovagal syncope: A randomized, placebo-controlled trial. *J Am Coll Cardiol* 2016; *68*: 1–9.
88. Brignole M, Ammirati F, Arabia F et al. Assessment of a standardized algorithm for cardiac pacing in older patients affected by severe unpredictable reflex syncopes. *Eur Heart J* 2015; *36*: 1529–1535.
89. Brignole M, Arabia F, Ammirati F et al. Standardized algorithm for cardiac pacing in older patients affected by severe unpredictable reflex syncope: 3-year insights from the Syncope Unit Project 2 (SUP 2) study. *Europace* 2016; *18*: 1427–1433.
90. Palmisano P, Dell'Era G, Russo V et al. Effects of closed-loop stimulation vs. DDD pacing on

haemodynamic variations and occurrence of syncope induced by head-up tilt test in older patients with refractory cardioinhibitory vasovagal syncope: The Tilt test-induced response in closed-loop stimulation multicentre, prospective, single blind, randomized study. *Europace* 2018; *20*: 859–866.
91. Metzler M, Duerr S, Granata R et al. Neurogenic orthostatic hypotension: Pathophysiology, evaluation and management. *J Neurol* 2013; *260*: 2212–2219.
92. Singer W, Sandroni P, Opfer-Gehrking TL et al. Pyridostigmine treatment trial in neurogenic orthostatic hypotension. *Arch Neurol* 2006; *63*: 513–518.
93. Kaufmann H, Freeman R, Biaggioni I et al. Droxidopa for neurogenic orthostatic hypotension A randomized, placebo-controlled, phase 3 trial. *Neurology* 2014; *83*: 328–335.
94. Scuffham P, Chaplin S, Legood R. Incidence and costs of unintentional falls in older people in the United Kingdom. *J Epidemiol Community Health* 2003; *57*: 740–744.
95. Malasana G, Brignole M, Daccarett M et al. The prevalence and cost of the faint and fall problem in the state of Utah. *PACE* 2011; *34*: 278–283.
96. Kenny RA, O'Shea D. Falls and syncope in elderly patients. *Clin Geriatr Med* 2002; *18*: XIII–XIV.
97. Rubenstein LZ, Josephson KR. The epidemiology of falls and syncope. *Clin Geriatr Med* 2002; *18*: 141–158.
98. Tinetti ME. Preventing falls in elderly persons. *N Engl J Med* 2003; *348*: 41–49.
99. Tinetti ME, Williams CS. Falls, injuries due to falls, and the risk of admission to a nursing home. *N Engl J Med* 1997; *337*: 1279–1284.
100. Marottoli RA, Berkman LF, Cooney LM. Decline in physical function following hip fracture. *J Am Geriatr Soc* 1992; *40*: 861–866.
101. Jørstad EC, Hauer K, Becker C et al. Measuring the psychological outcomes of falling: A systematic review. *J Am Geriatr Soc* 2005; *53*: 501–510.
102. Masud T, Morris RO. Epidemiology of falls. *Age Ageing* 2001; *30*: 3–7.
103. Carey BJ, Potter JF. Cardiovascular causes of falls. *Age Ageing* 2001; *30*: 19–24.
104. Kenny RA, Richardson DA, Steen N et al. Carotid sinus syndrome: A modifiable risk factor for non accidental falls in older adults (SAFE PACE). *J Am Coll Cardiol* 2001; *38*: 1491–1496.
105. Chiara M, Gianluigi G, Pasquale A et al. Unexplained falls are frequent in patients with fall-related injury admitted to orthopaedic wards: The UFO Study (Unexplained Falls in Older Patients). *Curr Gerontol Geriatr Res* 2013. doi:10.1155/2013/928603.
106. Alboni P, Coppola P, Stucci N et al. Differential diagnosis between 'unexplained' fall and syncopal fall: A difficult or impossible task. *J Cardiovasc Med (Hagerstown)* 2015; *16*: 82–89.
107. Mossello E, Ceccofiglio A, Rafanelli M et al. Differential diagnosis of unexplained falls in dementia: Results of "Syncope & Dementia" registry. *Eur J Intern Med* 2018; *50*: 41–46.
108. Shaw BH, Claydon VE. The relationship between orthostatic hypotension and falling in older adults. *Clin Auton Res* 2014; *24*: 3–13.
109. Finucane C, O'Connell MDL, Donoghue O et al. Impaired orthostatic blood pressure recovery is associated with unexplained and injurious falls. *J Am Geriatr Soc* 2017; *65*: 474–482.
110. Hohler AD, Zuzuarregui JR, Katz DI et al. Differences in motor and cognitive function in patients with Parkinson's disease with and without orthostatic hypotension. *Int J Neurosci* 2012; *122*: 233–236.
111. Cordeiro RC, Jardim JR, Perracini MR et al. Factors associated with functional balance and mobility among elderly diabetic outpatients. *Arq Bras Endocrinol Metabol* 2009; *53*: 834–843.
112. Kennelly SP, Lawlor BA, Kenny RA. Blood pressure and the risk for dementia: A double edged sword. *Ageing Res Rev* 2009; *8*: 61–70.
113. Mehrabian S, Duron E, Labouree F et al. Relationship between orthostatic hypotension and cognitive impairment in the elderly. *J Neurol Sci* 2010; *299*: 45–48.
114. Frewen J, Savva GM, Boyle G et al. Cognitive performance in orthostatic hypotension: Findings from a nationally representative sample. *J Am Geriatr Soc* 2014; *62*: 117–122.
115. Frewen J, Finucane C, Savva GM et al. Orthostatic hypotension is associated with lower cognitive performance in adults aged 50 plus with supine hypertension. *J Gerontol A Biol Sci Med Sci* 2014; *69*: 878–885.
116. Allan LM, Ballard CG, Rowan EN et al. Incidence and prediction of falls in dementia: A prospective study in older people. *PLoS One* 2009; *4*: e5521.
117. Ungar A, Mussi C, Ceccofiglio A et al. Etiology of syncope and unexplained falls in elderly adults with dementia: Syncope and Dementia (SYD) study. *J Am Geriatr Soc* 2016; *64*: 1567–1573.

26

Venous thromboembolic disease in older adults

WILBERT S. ARONOW

Key points

- Older patients with DVT require lower doses of warfarin than younger patients because of potential drug interactions and increased bleeding risk.
- Newer direct oral anticoagulants such as apixaban and rivaroxaban are preferred for older patients with DVT as they may require less monitoring compared with warfarin.
- Wearing compression stockings can help reduce swelling and improve lower extremity blood flow, which is especially important for older patients with reduced mobility.

It is important to treat underlying medical conditions that could contribute to DVT.

Venous thromboembolic (VTE) disease, comprising deep venous thrombosis (DVT) and pulmonary embolism (PE), is a common and potentially fatal cardiovascular condition, which reoccurs in one quarter of patients. Pulmonary hypertension and post-thrombotic syndrome (PTS) may result. The risk of VTE increases with age, cancer, male gender, and hypercoagulability, as well as other conditions, and is particularly prevalent in hospitalized patients, where VTE prophylaxis with mechanical and/or anticoagulant methods should be considered. Anticoagulant treatment with direct oral anticoagulants (DOACs), low-molecular-weight heparins (LMWHs), and warfarin for 3 months is recommended. Extended or indefinite therapy should be considered for patients at high risk for recurrent VTE, including those with unprovoked or recurrent VTE, thrombophilia, and in males, among others. Risk stratification for recurrence with use of compression ultrasonography (CUS) and D-dimer testing is recommended when considering extended therapy.

CLINICAL PRESENTATION

Epidemiology

Venous thromboembolism (VTE), a disease comprising deep vein thrombosis (DVT), most commonly of the leg or pelvis, and pulmonary embolism (PE), is a common cardiovascular disorder. VTE occurs in 700 per 100,000

DOI: 10.1201/9781003568933-26

(1)—somewhat less frequently than that of acute coronary syndromes and stroke; however, it is attributed as the etiology of 3.2% (>43,000) of cardiovascular deaths in the United States yearly (2, 3). The incidence of VTE is higher in African Americans and lower in Asians, as compared with Caucasians, somewhat higher in men than women, and increases 10- to 16-fold with age (4).

The costs of care of hospitalized patients who have a VTE are 2.5 times greater ($62,838 vs. $24,464) than in those patients who do not (5). In addition to causing sudden death, VTE is a chronic disease, recurring in 23% of patients in community populations more than a year later (6), although the rate of recurrence varies depending on the underlying cause and risk. Despite identifiable underlying conditions that predispose older adults to VTE, about 26%–45% of cases have no identifiable cause (7). Efforts at prevention, heightened clinical suspicion, understanding of diagnostic testing, and ultimately improved treatment and secondary prevention of VTE in older adults will result in improved outcomes of this disease.

Pathophysiology

Virchow's triad describes the pathophysiology of VTE, postulating that venous stasis, vascular injury, and hypercoagulability lead to thrombosis. Pulmonary emboli result from a portion of thrombus breaking away and flowing through the vasculature to lodge in the pulmonary arteries. Venous thrombi are often referred to as "red clots," rich in fibrin and trapped red cells (8).

Venous stasis results from obstructed flow. Most thrombi develop in areas with the slowest blood flow such as venous sinuses and bifurcations in the lower extremities. Venous stasis may result from an abrupt decline in mobility such as limb paralysis, following an orthopedic procedure or fracture, stroke, or an acute illness causing an individual to become bedfast. VTE is more frequently associated with acute rather than gradual development of immobility. Chronic medical conditions, such as heart failure, ischemic heart disease, chronic pulmonary disease, osteoarthritis, varicose veins, and other debilitating diseases can impact mobility and venous stasis, increasing VTE risk.

Vascular injury may result directly from trauma, producing endothelial disruption, or indirectly, from burns, endotoxin exposure, and increased release of inflammatory cytokines accompanying many medical and surgical conditions. Endothelial damage produces expression of tissue factor, directly from endothelial cells or from monocytes attracted to the site of damage, inducing factor VII activation and coagulation. Endothelial damage also results in subendothelial exposure of collagen and von Willebrand factor, which in turn lead to platelet adhesion and aggregation, resulting in local hypercoagulability at the site of injury.

Hypercoagulability due to congenital genetic abnormalities causing VTE usually presents prior to older age. The most frequent inherited (primary) hypercoagulable states are the factor V Leiden mutation and the prothrombin gene mutation, together accounting for 50%–60% of cases, followed by defects in protein S, protein C, and antithrombin III, and the antiphospholipid syndrome. In older adults, testing for genetic hypercoagulability rarely changes the overall management.

Acquired hypercoagulable states predominate in older adults in conjunction with malignancy, trauma, surgery, and systemic infections. Hypercoagulability associated with cancer may be produced by several mechanisms. Malignant cells may produce a procoagulant protein that stimulates factor X, accelerating conversion of prothrombin to thrombin. Tissue trauma during surgery increases thromboplastin, increasing levels of procoagulants and thrombosis (9). Cancer cells can also activate platelets, further promoting thrombosis. Blood concentration due to dehydration, blood loss, and transfusion, or associated with hematologic conditions such as polycythemia, hypergammaglobulinemia, dysproteinemia, or cryoglobulinemia, also promotes venous stasis and thrombosis.

Deep venous thrombosis

Although 22% of DVTs are asymptomatic at diagnosis, leg pain (83%) and swelling of an extremity (73%) are the most common signs and symptoms in clinical presentations, followed by calf tenderness, erythema, and/or skin discoloration (6). Other clinical features include venous distension, a palpable cord from a thrombosed vessel, and the prominence of superficial veins or cyanosis. There is no correlation between the intensity of signs or symptoms and the extent of thrombosis. The differential diagnosis for a lower extremity DVT includes muscle strain or tear, twisting injury, lymphangitis or lymphatic obstruction, venous reflux, popliteal cyst, cellulitis, chronic venous stasis, or post-thrombotic syndrome. In older adults, chronic medical conditions such as heart failure, kidney disease, peripheral vascular disease with venous stasis, and swelling of a paralyzed limb may also be considered in the differential diagnosis. As a result, the diagnosis of DVT requires confirmatory testing.

In about half of DVT patients, the clot recanalizes over time without further signs or symptoms. *Post-thrombotic syndrome* (PTS) is a chronic condition that develops in 20%–50%. It is defined by edema, skin changes, varicosities, leg ulcers, pain, and heaviness, often resulting in a negative impact on quality of life (10). The skin discoloration is described as "brawny" due to iron staining from red cell stasis. Tenderness of the medial lower leg is labeled as "lipodermatosclerosis." Venous stasis ulcers may develop, which heal slowly and often recur. PTS is a clinical diagnosis that can be confused with recurrent thrombosis. Elastic compression stockings are often applied to reduce edema and treat the symptoms of an acute DVT, however, they have not reduced the incidence of the PTS (11).

Pulmonary embolism

PE is underrecognized in older adults. It is estimated that 6.9% of PEs are asymptomatic (6), but the true prevalence may be much higher. Clinical signs and symptoms include dyspnea, tachypnea, pleuritic chest pain, cough, tachycardia, and hemoptysis. Cardiovascular collapse, hypotension, syncope, and coma can be associated with a massive PE. Other findings include unexplained arrhythmias, fever, wheezing, anxiety, and confusion. Electrocardiographic (ECG) findings including new-onset atrial fibrillation, right bundle branch block, or signs of right heart strain with an $S_1Q_3T_3$ pattern may be detected (12). The differential diagnosis of PE includes cardiopulmonary diseases such as pneumonia, myocardial infarction, heart failure, and cardiac tamponade. Absent the classic features of PE, physicians and older patients may attribute symptoms to exacerbations of chronic underlying cardiopulmonary conditions.

Older adults present more commonly with tachycardia and syncope, and less often with chest or pleuritic pain or abnormalities in vital signs, as compared with younger patients. Of a series of older patients (mean age 76) who presented with syncope, 17% were found to have a PE. After eliminating those with a low pretest probability for PE and a negative D-dimer test, 42% were ultimately diagnosed with a PE (13). Older adults develop acute pulmonary hypertension more often, perhaps accounting for the increase in syncope (14). PE causes about 10% of hospital deaths, disproportionately in older adults, which has led to standardized consideration of VTE prophylaxis in hospitalized patients.

Older and younger adults with DVT have a similar incidence of associated PE. However, older adults require hospitalization (74% vs. 65%) and have elevated troponin and B-type natriuretic protein (BNP) markers more often (15). Massive PE occurs in 5%–6% of older PE patients, but they undergo thrombectomy or thrombolytic therapy less often due to a perceived increased risk of bleeding and comorbidities.

Thromboembolic pulmonary hypertension (CTEPH) develops in 2%–4% of PE patients, particularly those with recurrent PEs due to persistent macrovascular obstruction and right ventricular failure. CTEPH is defined by a mean pulmonary artery pressure greater than 25 mmHg persisting 6 months following the diagnosis of a PE (3). Death may occur from right heart failure.

PRIMARY PREVENTION/ THROMBOPROPHYLAXIS

Risk assessment

The advent of safe and effective physical and pharmacologic methods to reduce the risk of VTE has enabled the identification of appropriate patients for prophylaxis. The public reporting of hospital quality measures, including VTE prophylaxis rates in medical (Centers for Medicare & Medicaid Services [CMS]) and surgical patients (Surgical Care Improvement Project [SCIP-VTE-2]), has enforced the use of either individualized risk assessment tools or screening by population and use of prophylaxis guidelines. Prophylaxis is generally not recommended for community-based populations as a group, but an individualized approach to risk assessment and prophylaxis is appropriate.

In the hospital setting, individualized risk assessment tools can be used, such as the Padua Prediction Score (16) (medical patients), Caprini Risk Assessment Method (17) (surgical patients), or Khorana or Ottawa Scores (18) (cancer patients), to identify appropriate candidates for prophylaxis. For example, the Padua Prediction Score stratifies patients into high or low VTE risk by assigning points to the presence of 11 possible clinical factors: 3 points each for active cancer, prior VTE, reduced mobility, or prior thrombophilic condition; 2 points for recent trauma or surgery; 1 point each for age ≥70, heart or respiratory failure, acute myocardial infarction or ischemic stroke, acute infection and/or rheumatologic disorder, obesity (body mass index [BMI] ≥30), or ongoing hormonal treatment. Patients with <4 points have a very low incidence of VTE (0.3%) not requiring prophylaxis, whereas patients with ≥4 points have higher risk (11%) (16). For surgical patients, a *Caprini score* of 7–8 is associated with a 4% VTE risk, whereas a score of >8 has a 10.7% risk (19). These scoring systems require that individual risk data be obtained by the clinical staff (or automated from electronic medical record data, if available). Once risk levels are established, guidelines and prophylaxis order sets can be implemented.

The American College of Chest Physicians (ACCP) (20) uses an alternative approach to individualized risk assessment by estimating risk by the site and type of care. Their guidelines focus on the following groups: community-dwelling patients, hospitalized medical patients, critical care patients, and surgical patients (including orthopedics), with risk modification for the presence of cancer and other known high-risk conditions such as a prior VTE.

Although use of standardized order sets achieves higher rates of adherence to prophylaxis recommendations, this has not proven to decrease hospital rates of VTE. A study of inpatients with cancer in whom VTE prophylaxis rates increased from 66% to 83% did not result in a reduction in the rate of new VTE diagnoses or death attributable to VTE, perhaps due to a baseline low prevalence of cases (0.41%–0.57%) (21).

Physical methods

Mechanical methods to prevent lower extremity thrombosis include graduated compression stockings (GCS), foot pumps, and intermittent pneumatic compression devices (IPCDs). *GCS* exerts constant pressure on the limb in order to compress the venous system and decrease stasis. Thigh-high stockings have been compared with a placebo in immobilized stroke patients and found not to reduce the incidence of VTE and were associated with an increase in skin breaks (5% vs. 1%) (22). When thigh-high stockings were compared with knee-high stockings there was a modest 2.5% absolute risk reduction in DVT (31% odds ratio) (23).

IPCDs consist of single-chamber or multichamber cuffs wrapped around the limb that apply constant or sequential pressure in slow or rapid inflation cycles by an electric pump to decrease venous stasis and induce fibrinolysis. In an immobilized stroke population, IPCDs demonstrated a 3.6% absolute risk reduction in DVT (24). A meta-analysis of high-risk surgical patients—largely total joint replacement patients—found IPCD use comparable to anticoagulant prophylaxis for VTE prevention, with a lower risk of bleeding. IPCD use with anticoagulants versus anticoagulants alone was comparable for VTE prophylaxis (25). Adherence to IPCDs use is challenging and requires nursing vigilance.

Anticoagulants

Anticoagulants employed for primary prevention of VTE have evolved as new agents have been developed. Effective pharmacologic agents include low-dose unfractionated heparin (UFH), low-molecular-weight heparins (LMWHs), fondaparinux, warfarin, and direct oral anticoagulants (DOACs). Aspirin has also been used for thromboprophylaxis, although with less supporting data (26). The site of activity of anticoagulants is depicted in Figure 26.1 and the pharmacology of DOACs is presented in Table 26.1. The use of these agents for prevention of VTE in several high-risk populations of older adults will be discussed—orthopedic surgical patients, other surgical patients, hospitalized medical patients, cancer patients and patients treated in post-acute care settings. Dosing recommendations are presented in Table 26.2.

OLDER ORTHOPEDIC SURGERY PATIENTS

Major orthopedic surgery, including hip fracture surgery and elective total knee replacement (TKR) and total hip replacement (THR), is commonly performed in older adults, and is associated with a very high risk (50%–60%) for the development of VTE due to a combination of procedure-associated and patient-specific risk factors (27, 28). National guidelines by the ACCP (2012) (29) and the American Academy of Orthopaedic Surgeons (AAOS) (2011) (30) have endorsed the use of anticoagulants and/or physical methods for VTE prophylaxis as the standard of care. Since publication of these guidelines, further clinical trials and comparative effectiveness data regarding existing as well as new anticoagulant agents have emerged, including a 2017 review of comparative effectiveness by the Agency for Healthcare Research and Quality (AHRQ) (31). A limited discussion of these trials of new agents follows.

The most recent ACCP guidelines (29) recommended LMWH with the addition of an IPCD during the hospital stay (Grade 2C) for VTE prophylaxis in patients undergoing THR and TKR surgery, as there had been more experience with these therapies. However, recent data regarding other anticoagulants now support their use for prophylaxis in orthopedic joint replacement surgery as well. Fondaparinux, dabigatran, apixaban, and rivaroxaban may be used effectively for THR or TKR, although data do not yet support their use in hip fracture surgery. In addition, UFH, adjusted-dose warfarin, aspirin (all Grade 1B), or IPCD use (Grade 1C) for a minimum of 10–14 days have demonstrated efficacy for this indication. Extending thromboprophylaxis for up to 35 days (Grade 2B) is also recommended, as VTE can occur days to weeks after surgery. In contrast to ACCP, the 2011 AAOS guideline does not advocate for a particular prophylactic agent or duration of therapy.

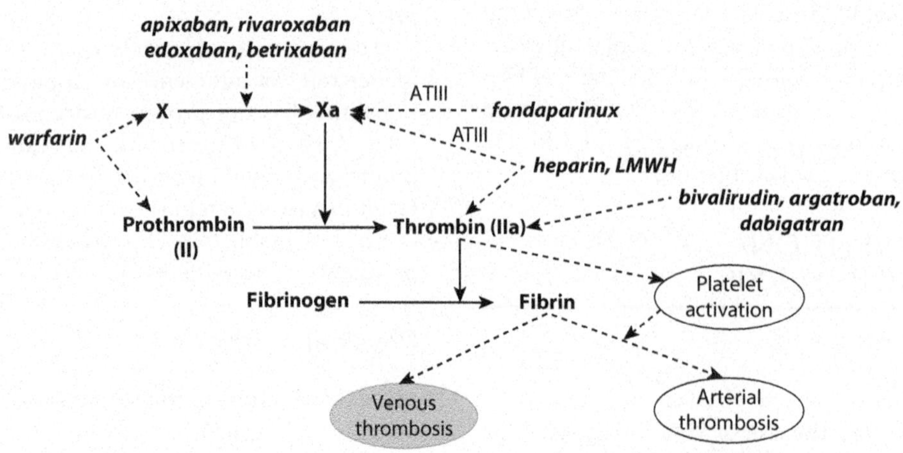

Figure 26.1 Anticoagulant sites of activity.

Table 26.1 Pharmacology of direct oral anticoagulants

	Apixaban	Betrixaban	Dabigatran	Edoxaban	Rivaroxaban
Target	Factor Xa	Factor Xa	Factor IIa	Factor Xa	Factor Xa
Half-life (hours)	9–14	19–27	12–17	10–14	5–9
Renal excretion	~25%	11%	80%	~50%	~36%
Interaction pathways	3A4/P-gp	P-gp	P-gp	3A4/P-gp	3A4/P-gp

Sources: Pradaxa® (package insert), Boehringer Ingelheim Pharmaceuticals, Ridgefield, CT, 2017; Xarelto® (package insert), Janssen Pharmaceuticals, Titusville, NJ, 2011; Eliquis® (package insert), Bristol-Myers Squibb Company and Pfizer, Princeton, NJ, 2016; http://www.bevyxxa.com/docs/Bevyxxa-Full-Prescribing-Information.pdf; SAVAYSA® (package insert), Daiichi Sankyo, Parsippany, NJ, 2017.

Table 26.2 VTE prophylaxis in various inpatient populations

Class	Drug	Dose	Medical	Orthopedic surgery	Nonorthopedic surgery
Heparin	UFH	5000 units SQ bid or tid	✓	✓	✓
LMWHs	Enoxaparin	40 mg SQ daily	✓	✓[a]	✓
		30 mg SQ bid		✓[b]	
	Dalteparin	5000 units SQ daily[c]	✓	✓	✓
Factor X inhibitor	Fondaparinux	2.5 mg SQ daily[d]	✓	✓	✓
DOACs	Apixaban	2.5 mg bid		✓[e]	
	Betrixaban	160 mg on day 1, then 80 mg daily	✓[f]		
	Dabigatran	110 mg 1–4 hours after surgery, then 220 mg daily		✓[g]	
	Rivaroxaban	10 mg daily		✓	

Abbreviations: DOACs, direct oral anticoagulants; LMWHs, low-molecular-weight heparins; SQ, subcutaneous; UFH, unfractionated heparin; VTE, venous thromboembolism.

Sources: Kearon C et al., *Chest*, 141, e419S–94S, 2012; Falck-Ytter Y et al., *Chest*, 141, e278S–e325S, 2012; Pradaxa® (package insert), Boehringer Ingelheim Pharmaceuticals, Ridgefield, CT, 2017; Xarelto® (package insert), Janssen Pharmaceuticals, Titusville, NJ, 2011; Eliquis® (package insert), Bristol-Myers Squibb Company and Pfizer, Princeton, NJ, 2016; Lovenox® (package insert), Sanofi-Aventis US, LLC, Bridgewater, NJ, 2013; Arixtra® (package insert), GlaxoSmithKline, Research Triangle Park, NC, 2010; Gould MK et al., *Chest*, 141, e227S–e277S, 2012; Kahn SR et al., *Chest*, 141, e195S–e226S, 2012; Cohen AT et al., *N Engl J Med*, 375, 534–544, 2016.

[a] Enoxaparin 40 mg SQ daily starting 9–15 hours before surgery, indicated for hip replacement only.
[b] Enoxaparin 30 mg SQ bid starting 12–24 hours after surgery, indicated for both hip and knee replacement.
[c] Dalteparin maintenance regimen; first dose and time vary by indication. See prescribing information.
[d] Fondaparinux is indicated for VTE prophylaxis only for adults weighing ≥50 kg.
[e] Apixaban may be started 12–24 hours after orthopedic surgery.
[f] Betrixaban duration for VTE prophylaxis is 35–42 days.
[g] Dabigatran is indicated for hip replacement only.

Direct oral anticoagulants

DOACs provide the opportunity for oral therapy without the requirements of complex monitoring and dosage adjustment. Despite emerging data regarding DOACs, it should be noted that safety and efficacy data for the use of DOACs after hip fracture surgery or traumatic lower extremity injuries are limited.

DOACs fall into two major groups: direct inhibitors of thrombin (factor II), of which dabigatran is the only US Food and Drug Administration (FDA)-approved agent in the United States; and factor Xa inhibitors, including rivaroxaban, apixaban, edoxaban, and betrixaban. Although all are approved for use in the United States, betrixaban does not have approval for prophylactic use in major orthopedic surgery. These agents are not interchangeable as they have significant pharmacokinetic differences that impact drug selection. In addition, dabigatran can be effectively reversed by idarucizumab, a monoclonal antibody fragment that binds with high affinity to dabigatran. In the RE-VERSE AD clinical trial (32) of patients with active bleeding, it reversed the anticoagulant effect in lab testing within minutes and hemostasis improved without significant thrombosis, although patient outcomes were unclear. Another agent, andexanet alfa (33), acts as a decoy to target and sequester factor Xa inhibitors and thereby reverse the anticoagulant activity of both oral direct Xa inhibitors (apixaban, edoxaban, and rivaroxaban) and injectable indirect Xa inhibitors (enoxaparin and fondaparinux). Andexanet alfa has been evaluated and approved by the FDA.

All of the major clinical trials of DOACs for thromboprophylaxis in major orthopedic surgery have used enoxaparin 40 mg daily or 30 mg twice daily as an active comparator. It is important to note that enoxaparin 30 mg twice daily is the preferred dosing regimen in North America; in contrast, enoxaparin 40 mg once daily is preferred in Europe. The timing of prophylaxis initiation also varies. Europeans administer prophylaxis prior to surgery, whereas in North America, prophylaxis is typically initiated postoperatively after hemostasis is established.

Dabigatran is the only *direct thrombin inhibitor* available Bivalirudin and argatroban are direct thrombin inhibitors that are administered intravenously. Dabigatran has been evaluated for VTE prophylaxis in THR patients in the RE-NOVATE trials. RE-NOVATE, a 3-month, phase 3, randomized, noninferiority study, compared the efficacy and safety of two doses of dabigatran. Noninferiority was achieved for both doses for the primary composite endpoint of total VTE (venographically detected or symptomatic VTE) and all-cause mortality (34). The RE-NOVATE II trial examined whether extended prophylaxis (28–35 days) with dabigatran 220 mg was as effective as enoxaparin 40 mg daily after primary THR. The primary outcome occurred in 7.7% of the dabigatran group and in 8.8% of the enoxaparin group, indicating noninferiority (35). Both studies found no significant difference in the rates of bleeding among groups.

In the RE-MODEL trial (36) of patients undergoing TKR, dabigatran 150 mg and 220 mg were found to be noninferior to enoxaparin 40 mg once daily administered for 6–10 days for the composite of symptomatic and venographic VTE and all-cause death, without a significant difference in bleeding events. When dabigatran was compared to the North American regimen in patients undergoing TKR, it was found to be inferior to the enoxaparin 30 mg twice daily regimen (RE-MOBILIZE trial) (37), attributed to several factors including the delayed starting time, mean duration of therapy, and the difference in dosing regimens. As a result, dabigatran is not currently approved for VTE prophylaxis after TKR in the United States, although it has gained approval elsewhere (38).

Factor Xa inhibitors currently available in the United States include rivaroxaban, apixaban, edoxaban, and betrixaban. Rivaroxaban has received FDA approval for VTE prophylaxis in patients undergoing either THR or TKR (39). The RECORD1 study compared rivaroxaban 10 mg once daily with enoxaparin 40 mg once daily for the prevention of VTE in THR patients. Rivaroxaban was initiated 6–8 hours after wound closure; enoxaparin 40 mg once daily was started 12 hours before surgery and restarted 6–8 hours after wound closure, for a duration of 35 days. Rivaroxaban was associated with a lower composite rate of DVT (symptomatic or venographic), nonfatal PE, and death, as compared to enoxaparin (1.1% vs. 3.7%, $p < 0.0001$), with a lower rate of major VTE (0.2% vs. 2.0%, $p < 0.0001$) without an increase in the rate of major bleeding (40). The RECORD2 study compared the same dosing regimens with rivaroxaban treatment for an extended duration (31–39 days) as compared with enoxaparin for the standard 10–14 days, and demonstrated a reduction in the rate of the composite endpoint (VTE, nonfatal PE, death) at 36 days (2% vs. 9.3%, $p < 0.0001$) (41). The mean age of patients across the two studies was 63 ± 12 years; about half were 65 years or older (39).

Although RECORD3 (42) and RECORD4 (43) found that rivaroxaban was superior to enoxaparin in reducing the primary composite endpoint for thromboprophylaxis after TKR, the rates of major VTE and symptomatic VTE and major bleeding were not statistically different. In a pooled analysis of the RECORD1–4 trials, the incidence of major and nonmajor clinically relevant bleeding occurred more commonly in the rivaroxaban group (44). This modest increase in bleeding observed with rivaroxaban, given the long-term safety data with the use of LMWH, is cited as the reason why enoxaparin is preferred for thromboprophylaxis (29) by the ACCP.

Apixaban is approved for the prophylaxis of DVT following THR and TKR based on the ADVANCE-1 (45) and ADVANCE-2 (46) studies, which compared apixaban 2.5 mg twice daily for 10–14 days with enoxaparin 30 mg twice daily and 40 mg once daily, respectively, for thromboprophylaxis after THR. The primary endpoint of both studies was a composite of symptomatic and asymptomatic DVT, nonfatal PE, and death. ADVANCE-2 demonstrated the superiority of apixaban to reduce the risk of the primary outcome as compared with enoxaparin 40 mg once daily (risk ratio [RR] 0.62, 95% confidence interval [CI] 0.51–0.74, $p < 0.0001$), without an increased risk of bleeding.

The ADVANCE-3 (47) study examined extended prophylaxis with apixaban for patients undergoing elective THR and demonstrated superiority as compared to enoxaparin for reduction in the composite of total VTE, nonfatal PE, and death without an increase in bleeding events. Across all three studies, 16% or 1866 patients aged 75 years or older were enrolled (48). The number of older adults included in the ADVANCE studies coupled with apixaban's lower dependence on renal function for elimination as compared to other DOACs may make apixaban an attractive option for thromboprophylaxis after orthopedic surgery in this population.

Edoxaban does not currently have an indication for VTE prophylaxis after orthopedic surgery in the United States, although a growing body of literature is emerging that should make this agent another viable option in the future (49). Betrixaban does not have an indication for thromboprophylaxis in orthopedic surgery patients.

Comparative effectiveness

The AHRQ conducted the most recent comparative effectiveness review of 127 randomized clinical trials and 15 nonrandomized clinical studies regarding VTE prophylaxis in major orthopedic surgery (31). They concluded that there are trade-offs between VTE risk reduction and bleeding risk between agents. Many studies used a composite outcome of "total DVT" that may not be as relevant as symptomatic VTE (to include PEs) as well as death. There are also trade-offs for patients and providers between oral and parenteral or subcutaneously administered thromboprophylaxis. For THR, the AHRQ concluded that LMWH prophylaxis provided the lowest risk for VTE and bleeding together, further commenting that aspirin has similar efficacy in reducing the risks of total PE, symptomatic DVT, as well as the risk for major bleeding, and that the DOAC group of direct thrombin inhibitors demonstrated lower VTE risk but not bleeding. LMWHs had a reduced rate of bleeding as compared with warfarin, and warfarin had a superior reduction in VTE, as compared with mechanical devices. For TKR patients, again LMWH has the greatest benefit for VTE risk with the lowest rate of bleeding. For hip fracture surgery, again, LMWH has a lower total DVT risk than factor Xa DOACs. Future prospective studies are needed to evaluate the safety and efficacy of DOACs as compared to other anticoagulants for thromboprophylaxis after orthopedic surgery.

With routine use of effective VTE prophylaxis, the rate of symptomatic VTE has been reduced to less than 2% in patients undergoing major orthopedic surgery (29). Further study of these and new agents is ongoing. With the abundance of data and contrasting recommendations from leading professional organizations, the choice and duration of VTE prophylaxis after orthopedic surgery, especially in older adults, should be made based on guidelines, a combination of the clinician's risk–benefit analysis, and patient preference.

HOSPITALIZED OLDER SURGICAL PATIENTS

As increasing numbers of older adults undergo elective or urgent major surgery, prevention of perioperative VTE is a major concern. Perioperative VTE risk depends on procedural features, patient-related individual risk factors, and bleeding risk. Examples of procedural risk factors include the degree of invasiveness, type and duration of anesthesia, and requirement for immobilization. Patient-related risk factors include, but are not limited to, increasing age, history of prior DVT, presence of malignancy, obesity, thrombophilia, or one or more significant medical conditions such as heart disease, infection, or recent stroke.

The risk for bleeding with anticoagulant thromboprophylaxis, although low, may be quite important in certain types or locations of surgery, such as neurosurgery or ophthalmic surgery, or related to the selection of the method for delivering postoperative analgesia. For example, pharmacologic VTE prophylaxis in patients with indwelling epidural catheters used for regional pain control are at risk for spinal hematomas and sequelae such as irreversible paralysis. The highest risk of complications is at the time of catheter insertion and removal.

Subcutaneous UFH is the only pharmacologic agent considered to be a safe option for VTE prophylaxis in patients with indwelling epidural catheters, according to the American Society of Regional Anesthesia (ASRA) (50). ASRA recommends subcutaneous UFH be held for a minimum of 8–10 hours prior to insertion of epidural catheters to allow the drug to wash out, and a minimum of 2 hours after insertion or removal before resuming UFH. Additionally, ASRA supports the use of twice daily UFH in this setting; the increased risk of bleeding and lack of safety data preclude thrice daily administration. Enoxaparin and fondaparinux should not be used with epidural analgesia. A minimum of 24 hours must elapse after catheter removal before considering initiation of either drug (51, 52).

The ACCP recommendations for VTE prophylaxis depend on the type of surgery and the presence of individual risk factors for VTE and for bleeding. Surgical patients can be stratified into low, moderate, and high risk for VTE, as previously discussed. Regardless of initial VTE risk, early patient ambulation as tolerated is recommended. In general, mechanical prophylaxis is recommended for those patients who are considered to be at high risk for bleeding or for whom the consequences of bleeding could cause significant harm until it is deemed safe for the use of pharmacologic prophylaxis (53).

General, abdominal–pelvic, or thoracic surgery patients who are considered to be at moderate or high risk for VTE and do not have significant bleeding concerns should receive LMWH or UFH. The addition of mechanical prophylaxis—IPC or compression stockings—is recommended for high-risk patients. Alternatives for pharmacologic prophylaxis in the setting of contraindications to UFH or LMWH include low-dose aspirin or fondaparinux. Anticoagulant prophylaxis should be continued at least until patients are fully ambulatory. The ACCP makes a strong recommendation that general or abdominal–pelvic surgery patients undergoing procedures for cancer preferentially receive LMWH and that the duration of therapy be extended to 4 weeks of prophylaxis (53).

Cardiac surgery patients are generally categorized as moderate risk for VTE and high risk for major bleeding complications. As a result, ACCP guidelines suggest mechanical over pharmacologic prophylaxis for patients with uncomplicated postoperative courses. For patients who have nonbleeding complications prolonging hospitalization after cardiac surgery, LMWH or UFH should be considered for VTE prophylaxis, as longer hospital courses are generally associated with prolonged immobility, whereas the bleeding risk typically subsides with time following the procedure (53). An individualized risk-benefit analysis should be performed to determine the need and optimal type of prophylaxis. Of note, one study showed that age greater than 65 years was independently associated with VTE after coronary artery bypass graft surgery, suggesting that older adults have a greater risk of VTE as compared with the general population (54).

Guideline recommendations for VTE prophylaxis after neurosurgery by the ACCP (52) and the Neurocritical Care Society (NCS) (55) depend on the type of procedure performed. After elective craniotomy, the ACCP recommends mechanical over pharmacologic prophylaxis except for very high-risk patients (e.g., craniotomy for tumor resection) (53). In contrast, the NCS recommends a combination of mechanical and pharmacologic prophylaxis with LMWH or UFH within 24 hours after craniotomy (55). Adequate hemostasis must be achieved postoperatively, often confirmed via neuroimaging, prior to the initiation of anticoagulant prophylaxis.

Options for VTE prophylaxis after major trauma include UFH, LMWH, and/or mechanical prophylaxis. The patient's specific injuries may guide the approach to VTE prophylaxis. For example, patients with acute spinal cord injury, spinal surgery for trauma, traumatic brain injury, or orthopedic fractures, particularly of long bones (e.g., femur), should receive a combination of mechanical and pharmacologic measures as long as the injuries do not preclude placement of IPCDs (53). Some trial data suggest that LMWH may be superior to UFH for prevention of VTE after major trauma, particularly data examining a more aggressive dosing regimen of enoxaparin 30 mg subcutaneously twice daily (56). Studies have suggested that even "standard" dosing of enoxaparin of 30 mg twice daily in trauma patients, however, may result in low anti-factor Xa levels. The optimal LMWH dosing for trauma remains unclear (57). In practice, the choice of agent and dose depends on injury type, bleeding risk, renal function, and the need for and timing of any future surgical interventions.

HOSPITALIZED OLDER MEDICAL PATIENTS

Hospitalized acutely ill medical patients also have an increased incidence of VTE as compared with community-dwelling adults and younger patients (3). Medical risk factors for VTE include active cancer, stroke, acute infectious process, myocardial infarction, acute respiratory illnesses, prolonged immobilization, heart failure, prior history of VTE, inflammatory disorders, age >70 years, and obesity (58). One large study indicated that prior VTE, bed rest, peripherally inserted central venous catheters, and cancer were the risk factors most predictive of a VTE among hospitalized medical patients (59).

For hospitalized cancer patients, VTE risk is associated with the type and location of cancer, stage and histology, and time from diagnosis. Malignant brain tumors; adenocarcinomas of the lung, ovary, pancreas, colon, stomach, prostate, and kidney; and hematologic malignancies are associated with higher risk. A variety of cancer biomarkers, hormonal therapy, angiogenesis inhibitors such as thalidomide or lenalidomide, radiation, transfusions, use of intravenous catheters for chemotherapy, as well as surgery increase the risk for VTE. Clinical decision-making regarding VTE prophylaxis must also consider prognosis and the goals of care. Patients with prolonged immobilization, such as older acute stroke patients, have an increased VTE risk.

Acutely ill older medical inpatients are at particularly high risk of developing VTE as compared with younger patients; however, there is a tendency to underprescribe VTE prophylaxis due to the fear of bleeding. Risk factors for bleeding in acutely ill medical inpatients identified at admission were derived from the International Medical Prevention Registry on Venous Thromboembolism (IMPROVE) (15,156 patients). Active gastroduodenal ulcer, prior bleeding, and low platelet count were the strongest independent risk factors at admission and a 3.2% cumulative 14-day incidence of major and nonmajor bleeding was identified (60).

UFH, a parenteral anticoagulant, remains one of the agents recommended for the prevention of VTE, particularly in patients with severe renal insufficiency. A major debate regarding the optimal frequency of dosing surrounds its use. No "head-to-head" randomized clinical trials compare twice with thrice daily administration regimens. A meta-analysis of 16 trials suggested that there is no significant difference in the rates of VTE or major bleeding between these different regimens (61). The choice of dosing interval (every 8 versus 12 hours) should be based on the patient's risk factors for developing thrombosis, cost, body weight, and risk of bleeding.

LMWHs (e.g., enoxaparin, dalteparin) are parenteral agents derived from UFH by chemical or enzymatic degradation. Their more predictable pharmacokinetics often makes them the preferred agents over UFH. None of the LMWHs has proven superiority over other LMWHs. Dosing for VTE prophylaxis depends on the patient population (see Table 26.2). LMWHs are eliminated primarily by the kidneys and more slowly than UFH, necessitating caution even when prescribed at prophylactic doses in patients with impaired renal function. Subgroup analyses of the PREVENT and MEDENOX trials in patients 75 years or older suggest a greater reduction of VTE with enoxaparin as compared with placebo (58, 62) with no increase in bleeding (62).

In randomized trials, pharmacologic prophylaxis with UFH, LMWH, or fondaparinux has been found to be superior to placebo in reducing the incidence of VTE in medical inpatients without increasing the risk of bleeding. A meta-analysis designed to evaluate other clinically important outcomes noted a statistically significant reduction in fatal PEs without affecting all-cause mortality or bleeding (63). While all of these agents have demonstrated superiority over placebo in clinical trials, a major criticism has been the lack of a comparator arm with the standard of care. Several meta-analyses have demonstrated a marginal superiority of LMWH as compared to low-dose UFH with respect to bleeding in medical patients; however, the heterogeneity of the study populations and their failure to distinguish symptomatic from asymptomatic VTE limits their applicability (64). No randomized controlled trials at present compare fondaparinux to either UFH or LMWH for VTE prevention in medical patients. Hence, the selection of an anticoagulant agent depends on patient characteristics, adverse effects, patient preference, compliance, and acquisition cost. If there is a contraindication to anticoagulant prophylaxis, mechanical prophylaxis with GCS or IPC devices should be used.

Betrixaban is approved for VTE prophylaxis in medical patients. Therapy is recommended for 35–42 days (65). Apixaban is also approved for VTE prophylaxis. Therapy is recommended for 6 months with a dose of 5mg twice daily. In a study of over 7000 hospitalized medically ill patients, the composite outcome of asymptomatic and symptomatic VTE plus VTE-related death was reduced in patients taking betrixaban as compared with enoxaparin, without an increase in bleeding. Rivaroxaban has also been studied in acutely ill general medical patients (66). In the MAGELLAN trial (67), rivaroxaban was demonstrated to be noninferior to enoxaparin for standard duration thromboprophylaxis and superior for extended duration prophylaxis, but at the cost of higher risk of bleeding. Thus, rivaroxaban is not recommended in this patient population.

Chemoprophylaxis with subcutaneous LMWH, UFH (twice or thrice daily), or fondaparinux continued until full mobility is restored or until hospital discharge, whichever comes first, is recommended by the ACCP guidelines for the prevention of VTE in general medical inpatients in whom the benefits of prophylaxis seem to outweigh the bleeding risks (64). Warfarin is not currently recommended. Betrixaban, approved for this indication subsequent to the 2012 guidelines, is prescribed for a longer duration as discussed.

OLDER ADULTS WITH CANCER

Patients with cancer are at significant risk for VTE for reasons stated earlier. The use of anticoagulants in this population, however, may also be associated with a higher risk for bleeding due to, for example, frequent procedures, thrombocytopenia related to bone marrow disease or other consequences of the malignancy, coagulopathy due to liver disease, coincident use of other drugs that increase bleeding risk, tumor growth, and vascularity. Patients with active cancer residing in the community generally do not require chemoprophylaxis. One exception is patients with multiple myeloma receiving angiogenesis agents with chemotherapy and/or dexamethasone, or thalidomide or lenalidomide in addition to chemotherapy or dexamethasone, who should receive prophylaxis with either LMWH or low-dose aspirin to prevent VTE (68).

The 2014 American Society of Clinical Oncology (ASCO) guidelines (68) address VTE prophylaxis in patients with active cancer and suggest that patients admitted for minor procedures or chemotherapy infusions do not require thromboprophylaxis. Most older adults with active cancer who are hospitalized either in a medical or surgical setting require thromboprophylaxis due to the risk of VTE associated with malignancy as well as other risk factors associated with admission. If major cancer surgery is contemplated, prophylaxis should be initiated before surgery and continue for at least 7–10 days, with extended prophylaxis considered for up to 4 weeks in those who undergo major abdominal or pelvic surgery with high-risk features. DOACs are not currently recommended for patients with malignancy and VTE until further data are available. ASCO comments that patients with cancer should be periodically assessed for VTE risk; however, anticoagulation should not be used to extend the survival of patients with cancer in the absence of other indications.

OLDER ADULTS IN COMMUNITY AND POST-ACUTE CARE SETTINGS

Primary prevention of VTE in community-dwelling individuals, including patients with cancer (except certain patients with multiple myeloma as discussed earlier) (68), is not recommended as the baseline risk is low and therefore the benefit is also low.

Patients in post-acute care settings may have a risk for VTE similar to hospitalized patients based on individual risk assessment and/or have continued high risk due to prior medical admission or surgical procedures. Patients who have not yet completed the recommended standard duration of therapy (7–10 days), and patients for whom extended prophylaxis is recommended (up to 35 days)—THR, TKR, and abdomino-pelvic surgery for cancer—should complete the course of thromboprophylaxis. Unfortunately, adequate studies of VTE risk and clinical trials of prophylaxis have not been undertaken in the post-acute care setting, and both risk and efficacy of thromboprophylaxis for individualized patients must be extrapolated from other data.

The selection of an anticoagulant and/or the use of mechanical methods of prophylaxis is dependent on the setting, patient population, and clinical status and indication.

DIAGNOSIS

Clinical decision rules

The clinical diagnosis of DVT and PE is challenging due to variable presentations and nonspecific symptoms. Objective testing is usually required. To avoid unnecessary testing and improve test utility, clinical decision rules are useful tools to assess the pretest probability of DVT or PE. These rules weigh signs, symptoms, and other risk factors which increase or decrease the likelihood of a diagnosis of DVT or PE. Validated instruments include the modified Wells score (69) for DVT, and the simplified Wells score (70) and the revised Geneva score (71) for PE.

The *modified Wells score* for DVT is a point system, with 1 point assigned for each of eight clinical characteristics: cancer, prior DVT, lower extremity immobilization, prior surgery (<4 weeks), bedridden (>3 days), leg edema, localized tenderness, and the presence of collaterals. If another diagnosis is more likely, 2 points are subtracted. A DVT is "likely" if the score is >2; "unlikely" if ≤1.

The *simplified Wells score* (70) for suspected PE is based on seven clinical parameters with 1 point each for clinical signs and symptoms of DVT (leg swelling, pain with palpation), tachycardia (>100 beats/min), immobilization (bedrest for 3 consecutive days) or surgery in prior 4 weeks, prior DVT or PE, hemoptysis, malignancy, or if "PE as likely as or more likely than an alternative diagnosis." A score of ≤1 signifies that a PE is unlikely.

The *revised Geneva score* (71), an alternative validated clinical decision rule for the diagnosis of PE, considers the patient's age, scoring 1 point each for age >65 years, prior history of DVT, active malignancy, surgery or fracture within a month, unilateral limb pain, hemoptysis, pain on deep vein palpation of lower limb and unilateral edema, or a heart rate 75–94 beats per minute (2 points if >94). A score of >2 suggests that a PE is likely. The *Pulmonary Embolism Rule-out Criteria* (PERC) is a validated tool to identify outpatients presenting with chest pain who are at low risk for PE so that further diagnostic testing can be avoided (72).

D-dimer testing

The D-dimer is a degradation product of cross-linked fibrin after plasmin undergoes proteolysis that can be detected in the blood by various assays. The quantitative enzyme-linked immunosorbent assay (ELISA) is most commonly used. A level >500 ng/mL is considered abnormal. D-dimer assays demonstrate good sensitivity (97% for PE) and negative predictive value, but poor specificity and positive predictive value (normal in only 40%–68% of patients without PE). Specificity decreases further with age. Age-specific cutoffs (Age × 10 μg/L in patients aged >50 years) for PE diagnosis increase specificity without compromising sensitivity (above 97% in all age categories); however, an age-adjusted cut-off value has reduced specificity (35%) in patients aged >80 years (73, 74).

Clinical prediction rules assist in determining whether to obtain further testing, as they alone cannot exclude or verify the diagnosis of DVT or PE. D-dimer testing is recommended for patients with "low pretest probability" as a low (negative) result has a high negative predictive value, essentially excluding the diagnosis of VTE without further testing. In patients with high pretest probability, D-dimer testing is not recommended as a stand-alone test. When pretest clinical probability is not low, or the D-dimer levels are increased, further diagnostic testing, usually imaging, is required.

Imaging

Although a number of noninvasive and invasive imaging modalities can be used to diagnose DVT, proximal compression ultrasonography (CUS) is the modality of choice as it is highly accurate when performed by an experienced technician, reproducible, and less costly than others. The diagnosis of DVT is established by abnormal compressibility of the vein, which has a high sensitivity (97%) and specificity (98%) for proximal thromboses, but reduced sensitivity (73%) for distal clots (75). CUS does not detect thrombi in the iliac vein. In patients with a high pretest probability and a positive proximal CUS, treatment is recommended. In patients with a high pretest probability but a negative proximal CUS, additional testing is warranted. Repeating CUS in 1 week along with a highly sensitive D-dimer is one approach. Computed tomography (CT) or magnetic resonance imaging (MRI) may be obtained in order to image the pelvis. Magnetic resonance venography (MRV) is noninvasive but more expensive. Changes in the signal from the clot over time may allow estimation of the age of the thrombus.

Although signs and symptoms may raise the suspicion of a PE, confirmatory tests are also necessary to establish an accurate diagnosis, as the prevalence of other diseases as an alternative diagnosis is significant. Clinical prediction rules and pretest assessment of the probability of PE are critical but not sufficient. However, the diagnostic imaging test of choice, computed tomographic pulmonary angiography (CTPA), requires a significant iodinated contrast load and radiation exposure. In the case of a low or moderate pretest probability of PE, D-dimer testing is recommended. If negative, the diagnosis of PE is unlikely (76). If a D-dimer test is positive, multidetector CTPA is the preferred imaging test as it is relatively safe and provides a rapid diagnosis of PE with a sensitivity of 100% and specificity of 89% by direct visualization of the pulmonary arterial circulation. Diagnostic criteria include a lack of opacification of the vascular lumen due to a central filling defect or a partial filling defect surrounded by contrast material on a cross-sectional image, contrast material between the central filling defect and the artery wall on a longitudinal image, or a peripheral intraluminal defect that forms an acute angle with the artery. PEs not identified by this diagnostic test tend to be more peripheral in the lung and smaller.

The ventilation/perfusion (V/Q) lung scan was extensively studied for the diagnosis of PE in the landmark PIOPED study (77). In patients with a high pretest probability who have significant renal dysfunction, the V/Q scan offers a reasonable alternative as long as the patient

(1) is able to participate in the ventilation portion and (2) does not have other pulmonary disease. For patients with an intermediate probability of PE, the diagnostic accuracy of the V/Q scan is less and additional testing may be required. In contrast to CTPA, PEs missed by a V/Q scan tend to be clinically more important central PEs. Although pulmonary angiography was once the gold standard, the invasiveness and morbidity generally preclude its use.

Echocardiography is not recommended for diagnosis of PE, but may be useful as it can identify patients with PE who are at risk for severe morbidity or mortality and who may benefit from more aggressive initial treatment, such as thrombolysis or thrombectomy. It is estimated that 30%–40% of patients with an acute PE have echocardiographic abnormalities, assisting in diagnosing hemodynamically significant PE, particularly those requiring thrombolytic therapy.

TREATMENT/SECONDARY PREVENTION

The intent of treatment is to reduce acute and chronic symptoms and pathology that result from VTE, as well as reduce the risk for VTE recurrence (secondary prevention). Accepted treatment of VTE necessitates the use of anticoagulants. Consideration of the risks and benefits of these agents in the context of the care plan is important for all patients, but particularly for older adults in whom the benefits but also the risks associated with bleeding are greater.

Acute symptom management

Venous distension and pressure from the thrombus obstructing venous flow can cause pain and swelling, which may be aggravated by upright posture. Local inflammation commonly produces erythema and induration. The application of heat to the site of pain and inflammation may palliate these initial symptoms. Although nonsteroidal anti-inflammatory drugs (NSAIDs) are often prescribed for pain and inflammation, they are generally contraindicated in the treatment of DVT, as their use increases the risk of bleeding. Acetaminophen may be prescribed, but its efficacy is limited.

Although there is limited data regarding early ambulation in patients with a DVT, studies indicate that ambulation is not associated with an increased risk for embolization. It is recommended that therapeutic anticoagulation be achieved when ambulation is initiated (78). Recent studies of leg compression using GCS indicate that the acute pain associated with DVT is not reduced, nor does GCS prevent PTS, although it does not appear to increase the risk of recurrent VTE (78).

Patients with an acute PE may present with hemodynamic instability and dyspnea that can progress to cardiovascular collapse, respiratory failure, and death. Management of patients presenting with hypotension parallels that of other critically ill patients who require hemodynamic support with fluids and vasopressors. Supplemental oxygen should be provided for hypoxemia, and intubation with mechanical ventilation is indicated for severe hypoxemia and impending respiratory failure.

Bleeding risk assessment

An individualized assessment of the risk for bleeding in VTE patients is an essential first step prior to initiating anticoagulant therapy. For some, the burden of anticoagulant therapy (drug administration, monitoring, cost, risk for bleeding) may outweigh the potential benefits. A clear understanding of the goals of care is essential prior to consideration of anticoagulant therapy. Clinical decision-making requires weighing potential risks for bleeding against potential benefits of therapy (i.e., reduced risk of death, pulmonary hypertension with VTE). Patients treated for VTE with anticoagulation have a case-fatality rate of 11.3% prior to anticoagulation, and 3.6% after anticoagulation (79), with a 0.2% rate of major bleeding events during the first 3 months of therapy. A study comparing treatment with warfarin versus DOACs found comparable case rates for fatality and recurrence with a lower rate of major bleeding for DOACs (0.58 vs. 1.6 per 100 patient-years), and the composite of fatal events was also less (incidence rate ratio [IRR] 0.40, 95% CI 0.14–1.0, $p = 0.03$) (80).

Anticoagulant therapy is often urgently initiated prior to laboratory testing when a VTE is suspected based on the medical history and physical examination. Required history includes prior bleeding episodes, questions about easy bruising, and inquiry about the use of medications and herbals that can influence platelet function, such as aspirin, P2Y12 inhibitors (ticagrelor, prasugrel, clopidogrel), NSAIDs, selective serotonin reuptake inhibitors (SSRIs), vitamin E, and ginkgo biloba, among others, which increase the risk for bleeding, sometimes substantially. Laboratory testing should include a complete blood count and coagulation parameters. The finding of anemia and/or coagulopathy should be explained and treated if possible.

Common sites for bleeding are the gastrointestinal and genitourinary tracts and soft tissues, but intracranial bleeding is associated with the greatest morbidity. Age is associated with an increased risk for bleeding in general, and for intracranial hemorrhage in particular. DOACs have been found to be associated with a somewhat lower rate of bleeding in patients with atrial fibrillation. Recent hemorrhage, concomitant medical conditions, particularly renal and liver disease, uncontrolled hypertension, stroke, and cancer increase bleeding risk. Although physicians often cite falls as a relative contraindication for anticoagulation, the risk of falling (30% yearly in older adults) and sustaining further injury that causes bleeding is generally much less than the morbidity of VTE during the initial 3 months of therapy.

The risk for bleeding can be estimated using the HAS-BLED score (81). This instrument assigns 1 point for the following risk factors: hypertension (systolic blood pressure >160), abnormal renal function, abnormal liver function, stroke, bleeding history or predisposition (anemia), labile INR (time in therapeutic range [TTR] <60%), age >65, and drugs or alcohol use concomitantly. Also, it was validated in patients with atrial fibrillation. A HAS-BLED score of 0 is associated with 1.13 bleeds per 100 patient-years; a score of 1 with 1.02 bleeds per 100 patient-years, 2 with 1.88 bleeds, 3 with 3.74 bleeds, 4 with 8.70 bleeds, and 5 with 12.50 bleeds. Assessment of gait and cognitive function is also recommended in the evaluation of bleeding risk in older adults.

Setting for initial therapy

The initial patient assessment should inform the decision whether to initiate therapy for VTE as an inpatient or outpatient. With patient selection criteria, outpatient treatment has achieved comparable outcomes to inpatient (82). Factors considered in selecting patients for inpatient therapy include a history of thrombotic and bleeding risk factors, unstable vital signs and physical examination, and diagnostic testing abnormalities. Because older patients exhibit instability in vital signs, ECG, and pulse oxygenation more often than younger patients, they are less likely to be suitable candidates for outpatient therapy. Contraindications include active bleeding or a notable bleeding history, significant alterations in blood pressure or respiration, significant anemia, thrombocytopenia, a history of heparin-induced thrombocytopenia (HIT) or heparin (or LMWH) allergy, severe renal insufficiency (creatinine clearance <30 mL/min), or the inability to obtain or administer the drug reliably. Signs of right ventricular failure, dyspnea, hypoxemia, elevated cardiac markers, and other clinical signs and symptoms of PE may necessitate hospital admission.

The cognitive ability to adhere to recommended therapy for VTE is critical. LMWH injections can be administered in the office, by self-injection, or by a home care nurse or other caregiver. Costs for the drug and its administration and monitoring are considerations. Although DOACs are oral, produce stable drug levels obviating monitoring, and have far fewer food and drug interactions, the initial clinical assessment is important as the patient's ability to adhere to scheduled dosing of DOACs is essential due to their relatively short half-life as compared with warfarin.

Inferior vena cava filters

Inferior vena cava (IVC) filters are often placed in DVT patients who may or may not be receiving anticoagulation, without strong data supporting this practice. A case series evaluating the use of filters in patients with and without anticoagulation failed to show any difference in outcomes (83). A landmark study (84) of IVC filters placed in anticoagulated DVT patients showed that at 8 years, use of IVC filters decreased subsequent PE but increased the incidence of DVT. The PREPIC trial (85) found that IVC filters with anticoagulation decreased PE, increased DVT, and did not affect VTE-related mortality. PREPIC2 (86) studied removable filter use for 3 months with anticoagulation, which did not reduce recurrent PE. Placement of an IVC filter is recommended only for patients in whom anticoagulation is contraindicated due to active or a very high risk of bleeding. If and when the bleeding risk is mitigated, anticoagulation should be initiated (87). Removable filter placement with an active filter tracking program to ensure prompt removal (<6 months) is preferred.

Operative thrombectomy and thrombolysis

Operative thrombectomy, catheter-directed thrombolysis (CDT) with or without mechanical thrombus fragmentation, and systemic thrombolytic therapy are interventions aimed at dissolving or removing proximal DVT or PE. It should be noted that in the absence of contraindications to anticoagulant therapy, the utilization of any of these interventional techniques does not preclude the use of anticoagulation, and the same intensity and duration of systemic anticoagulation should be prescribed (20).

Thrombus removal via *operative thrombectomy* is not currently recommended by the ACCP guidelines; standard systemic anticoagulation is recommended as the first-line approach. Less invasive catheter-directed thrombus removal is preferred over operative thrombectomy if an interventional technique is to be employed. If operative thrombectomy is considered, the following criteria must be met: acute iliofemoral DVT (symptoms <7 days), good functional status, life expectancy of at least 1 year, and treatment at an institution with the experience, resources, and expertise necessary to perform these procedures (20).

CDT is a method of delivering a thrombolytic agent via a catheter directly to the site of the thrombus. CDT may or may not involve methods of thrombus fragmentation (e.g., ultrasound-assisted CDT) to help break down the clot and enhance the permeability of the thrombolytic agent. Theoretical advantages of CDT include accelerated clot destruction and the potential to reduce the dose of locally administered thrombolytics as compared with systemic thrombolytic therapy (88, 89).

The role of CDT in the treatment of acute proximal DVT in the leg remains controversial. The CaVenT study is the largest randomized controlled trial of 209 patients randomized to CDT plus anticoagulation or anticoagulation alone for treatment of acute iliofemoral DVT (symptoms <21 days). The addition of CDT was associated with a significantly lower risk of PTS at 24 months and a greater incidence of iliofemoral patency after 6 months. Twenty patients in the CDT group had bleeding complications, however, as compared with none of those in the control group. There were no differences in VTE recurrence between groups (90). Based on this study, a cost-effectiveness analysis was undertaken that demonstrated that the quality-of-life impact, measured in quality-adjusted life years (QALYs), was similar with CDT or standard anticoagulation (91); however, patients older than 75 years were excluded (3, 4). Furthermore, large observational studies and systematic reviews of CDT for acute proximal lower extremity DVT have yielded conflicting results (85, 92, 93). As a result, the ACCP's 2016 guidelines continue to recommend anticoagulation alone over CDT for acute proximal DVT in the leg (20).

For acute PE, both *systemic thrombolysis* and CDT have been evaluated as initial treatment options. Systemic thrombolysis leads to more rapid clot resolution but is associated with an increased bleeding risk, particularly concerning for intracranial hemorrhage. The ACCP guidelines continue to recommend that systemic thrombolysis for acute PE should be limited to patients who present with hypotension (systolic blood pressure <90 mmHg) (20). Several studies have demonstrated that ultrasound-assisted CDT for intermediate or high-risk PE is associated with a significant reduction in right-to-left ventricular diameter ratio (94–96). A meta-analysis of 35 studies with 1253 patients who underwent all types of CDT for acute PE confirmed that CDT improved mean pulmonary artery pressure and right ventricular function regardless of whether patients presented with hemodynamic instability (97). Current ACCP guidelines, however, recommend that acute PE patients who are treated with thrombolytic therapy receive systemic thrombolysis rather than CDT, as the studies to date have small sample sizes and a low quality of evidence (20). More recently, a large propensity-matched study of PE using the National Readmission Database revealed that CDT was associated with significantly lower rates of in-hospital mortality, 30-day readmissions, and a composite of in-hospital mortality plus gastrointestinal or intracranial bleeding as compared to systemic thrombolysis (98). In addition, emerging data from the OPTALYSE PE study suggest that even lower doses and shorter-duration ultrasound-assisted CDT may be effective (99). CDT may play a larger role in the future management of acute PE.

Anticoagulant therapy

Anticoagulants are the cornerstone of therapy for treatment of VTE in patients of all age groups. Anticoagulant treatment, except for thrombolytic therapy, does not dissolve the clot; rather, it prevents clot extension, embolization, and recurrence (secondary prevention), and perhaps mitigates the PTS. Anticoagulant therapy should be initiated when there is a strong clinical suspicion of a DVT or PE while diagnostic testing is pursued, as the risk of thrombus extension or embolization generally outweighs the potential short-term harm unless there is evidence of acute bleeding. For patients with a low probability of VTE, diagnostic testing can be pursued without initiating anticoagulation as long as results are obtained in a timely manner. If the thrombosis is isolated to the distal veins of the lower extremity, and symptoms are mild, the risk of progression is low. Serial duplex ultrasound diagnostic images can be obtained over 2 weeks and a decision regarding anticoagulation made on the basis of progression. If a distal DVT is more symptomatic, anticoagulation is recommended for 3 months (78).

Special consideration regarding drug selection, dosing, and duration of anticoagulant therapy must be applied in prescribing for older adults who pose a greater risk for anticoagulant-associated bleeding. The use of thrombotic and bleeding risk models may help the clinician evaluate the net benefit of anticoagulation for an individual patient. Current evidence for anticoagulant use in older adults for the acute treatment and secondary prevention of VTE is presented herein with a focus on newer agents and recent data. A comprehensive discussion of conventional agents in the treatment of VTE is available elsewhere (100).

Traditionally, initial VTE treatment consisted of either parenteral UFH, LMWHs, or fondaparinux, alone or overlapped with an oral vitamin K antagonist (VKA) (warfarin). For most patients, the parenteral anticoagulant is administered for at least 5 days coincident with warfarin and is stopped when the target INR has reached 2 to 3. When choosing a lead-in parenteral agent, LMWH or fondaparinux is recommended over UFH due to more predictable pharmacokinetics and improved safety and efficacy (20). For patients with active cancer, the ASCO recommends LMWH for the initial 5–10 days of treatment of both DVT and PE, as well as for long-term secondary prophylaxis for at least 6 months. DOACs, specifically rivaroxaban and apixaban, are now an option for treatment of acute VTE based on the EINSTEIN and AMPLIFY trials, which supported the use of an all-oral approach without parenteral lead-in therapy (101–103). It should be noted that these trials required higher initial doses of the oral regimen for the first few weeks, followed by a dose reduction to address the issue of recurrence, as the risk is highest in the first month after diagnosis. In contrast, the studies evaluating use of dabigatran or edoxaban in patients with acute VTE—RE-COVER and Hokusai-VTE—were designed with a parenteral anticoagulant lead-in for a minimum of 5 days prior to DOAC initiation (104, 105).

The major limitation of UFH is the need to achieve rapid and consistent therapeutic anticoagulation, indicated by a prothrombin time (PTT) 1.5–2.5 times greater than the control value. This equates to a serum heparin level by protamine titration of 0.2–0.4 units/mL or an anti-Xa level of 0.3–0.7 units/mL (20). Due to the unpredictable binding of UFH to plasma proteins and cells, dosing is challenging, and although weight-based nomograms

(106) can assist, the PTT must be closely monitored with frequent adjustments in dose. Some data support the use of an unmonitored, weight-based subcutaneous UFH for the treatment of DVT (20, 107). If therapeutic levels of UFH are not achieved within 24 hours, the risk of recurrence is increased significantly (108). Additionally, UFH carries a risk, although low, of causing heparin-induced thrombocytopenia. Although UFH has largely been replaced by LMWHs and DOACs, UFH is still the preferred agent for initial anticoagulation in older adults with severe renal impairment, since it is not dependent on the kidneys for elimination, or with severe obesity (20). It may also be preferred for older adults with high bleeding risk or plans for a surgical procedure in the near future due to its short half-life, rapid onset and offset, and the ability to fully reverse its effects with protamine sulfate.

LMWHs are preferred to UFH for VTE treatment due to more predictable pharmacokinetics, which eliminates the need for routine monitoring, although different LMWHs have varying risks of accumulation in renal impairment (109). They also have a lower risk for bleeding, thrombocytopenia, VTE recurrence, and death (20). LMWHs are administered by subcutaneous injection, potentially limiting their long-term use due to patient preference.

Fondaparinux is a synthetic indirect factor Xa inhibitor that can be administered subcutaneously once daily for treatment of VTE owing to its long half-life (~17 hours). In the Matisse trials for treatment of DVT and PE, fondaparinux was shown to have similar efficacy and safety to initial treatment with LMWHs or UFH followed by warfarin (110, 111). It is contraindicated in patients with a creatinine clearance <30 mL/min; fondaparinux should be administered with caution to frail older adults or those with borderline renal function due to the risk of accumulation. No antidote is currently available, although andexanet alfa (33) is being evaluated as a reversal agent in the event that bleeding should occur on fondaparinux.

Until recently, the VKA warfarin was the only oral anticoagulant available for the treatment of VTE. Despite demonstrated efficacy in preventing recurrent thrombosis, the practical challenges associated with warfarin prescribing are well known, including delayed onset of action, multiple drug and dietary interactions, need for therapeutic drug monitoring, and the risk of INR variability due to genetic polymorphisms predisposing patients to both underanticoagulation and overanticoagulation. These issues predispose older adults to a higher risk for major hemorrhage, consistent with a report that warfarin is the most commonly implicated medication in emergency department visits for adverse drug events among older adults (112).

Four DOACs have been approved in the United States for the treatment of VTE: the direct thrombin inhibitor dabigatran, and direct factor Xa inhibitors rivaroxaban, apixaban, and edoxaban. When compared with warfarin, DOACs have been demonstrated to be noninferior with regard to efficacy with similar (dabigatran and rivaroxaban) or lower rates of major bleeding (apixaban or edoxaban) (101–105). A subgroup analysis of DOACs in older patients and the pooled results from large phase III trials have been described in two meta-analyses (113, 114), which indicated that DOACs are at least as efficacious as warfarin and possibly have a safer profile with respect to major bleeding in patients aged >75 years, as seen in Table 26.3. Apixaban or rivaroxaban appeared to have a greater safety benefit in older patients as compared with VKAs than dabigatran or edoxaban (113). The convenience of fixed-dose oral medications that do not need routine laboratory monitoring has made DOACs the preferred agents in the ACCP guidelines (20). The applicability of these results to older adults with VTE is less certain, as the total number of patients aged >75 years was considerably lower (12%–15%) in VTE trials as compared with those enrolled in atrial fibrillation (>40%) trials (114). Among all DOACs, apixaban appears to have the greatest safety with regard to bleeding and an overall reduction in medical expenditure as a result (115). The decision to choose a particular DOAC should be based on the pharmacokinetic profile of the drug (e.g., renal excretion), adverse effects, individual patient characteristics, affordability, and drug interactions, as no head-to-head DOAC trials are available to guide decision-making.

The most recent ACCP guidelines for VTE treatment (2016) recommend a DOAC over warfarin or LMWH due to the predictable pharmacokinetics, reduced associated bleeding, and greater convenience for patients and health care providers in patients who do not have cancer (87). When faced with the choice of prescribing a DOAC or warfarin, it is important to consider whether the patient is likely to achieve tight control of their anticoagulation on warfarin from a safety and efficacy viewpoint as assessed by the time that the INR falls in the TTR. Several cost-effectiveness studies suggest that DOAC use was not cost-effective as compared to patients on warfarin with excellent INR control (116). While TTR >65%–70% is considered ideal, even in the setting of controlled clinical trials, the mean TTR was observed to be approximately 60%. A population-based study identified a TTR of only 40%, supporting the recommendation that DOACs may be a superior alternative. The longer half-life of warfarin, however, is advantageous if a dose is accidentally omitted. Despite this, there are certain clinical situations where DOACs are not suitable anticoagulants because data regarding efficacy and safety are insufficient. Examples include thromboembolism associated with antiphospholipid syndrome, cancer, and pregnancy, which were not well represented in trials. In summary, treatment decisions should be individualized, taking into account the potential risks and benefits of therapy.

Table 26.3 Efficacy and safety of direct oral anticoagulants for acute VTE treatment in the elderly

		AMPLIFY (103)		RE-COVER I-II (135)		HOKUSAI (105)		EINSTEIN DVT-PE (101, 102)	
		Apixaban	Warfarin	Dabigatran	Warfarin	Edoxaban	Warfarin	Rivaroxaban	Warfarin
N		5395		5107		8292		8281	
Age ≥75 years, n (%)		768 (14%)		259 (12%)		1104 (13%)		1283 (15%)	
TTR (%) on warfarin		61		57–60		63.5		62	
Recurrent VTE[a]	Age (years)								
	≥75, n/N (%)	7/389 (1.85)	13/360 (3.6%)	3/253 (1.2%)	5/276 (1.8%)	14/560 (2.5%)	27/544 (5%)	15/656 (2.3%)	23/627 (3.7%)
	< 75, *n/N* (%)	52/2220 (2.3%)	58/2275 (2.5%)	57/2300 (2.5%)	50/2278 (2.2)	116/3558 (3.3%)	119/3578 (3.3%)	71/3494 (2%)	72/3504 (2.1%)
Major bleeding	≥75 *n/N* (%)	4/398 (1.0%)	16/370 (4.3)	8/231 (3.5%)	10/262 (3.8%)	70/560^ (12.5%)	82/544^ (15.1%)	8/655 (1.2%)	28/624 (4.5%)
P-value[b]		0.009		0.83		0.12		<0.001	
	<75, *n/N* (%)	11/2278 (0.5%)	33/2319 (1.4%)	16/2225 (0.7%)	30/2200 (1.4%)	279/3558^ (7.8%)	341/3578^ (9.5%)	32/3475 (0.9%)	44/3492 (1.3%)
P-value[b]		0.002		0.038		0.53		0.17	

Abbreviations: TTR, time in therapeutic range; VTE, venous thromboembolism.
[a] P-value not significant except HOSUSAI trial ≥75 years of age.
[b] Tested for noninferiority.
^ Includes major and clinically relevant nonmajor bleeding.

Duration of therapy

Following landmark clinical trials of VTE treatment for varying durations, 3 months of anticoagulant treatment is currently recommended (20) for most patients. Extended or indefinite therapy is considered for patients in whom the clinical risk for recurrence outweighs that of serious bleeding. Trials of extended therapy seem to indicate that longer durations seem only to delay a spike in recurrence rate that follows anticoagulant discontinuation, although the yearly risk appears to decline over time if no recurrent thromboses are observed (117, 118). Recurrence rates after 3–6 months of anticoagulation vary from 5% to 15% in the year following discontinuation. This then declines to 2%–4% yearly, with a 45% cumulative 8-year risk. DVT and PE have similar rates of recurrence, but PE patients are more likely to have a PE with recurrence. Bleeding rates on anticoagulants also decline over time (2% per year) (119).

Extended therapy beyond 3 months is suggested for patients with unprovoked VTE if the benefit of continued anticoagulation outweighs the risk of bleeding. Extended therapy implies that anticoagulation therapy will be continued beyond 3 months, but is not necessarily synonymous with lifelong treatment. Periodic reevaluation (e.g., annually) of the continued risks and benefits of anticoagulation therapy for VTE should be undertaken, particularly in older adults whose medical problems and pharmacotherapy may change frequently. The rationale for longer treatment for these patients is that they suffer from a higher rate of VTE recurrence following cessation of anticoagulation.

The challenge is to identify which patients have a high risk for recurrence and may be candidates for extended therapy, while considering patient preferences (to discontinue anticoagulants) and goals of care. Transient (provoked) risk factors, such as surgery, air travel (>8 hours), and hormone use are associated with a lower risk of recurrence than unprovoked VTE, although this difference declines over time as well. A large meta-analysis found that the rate of VTE recurrence at 24 months for those with a transient risk factor (surgical, 0.7%; nonsurgical, 4.2%) is 3.3% per patient-year, while that for patients with unprovoked VTE is 7.4% (120). Only about half of patients, however, have an identified major provoking risk factor (121). Independent risk factors associated with recurrence include male gender, age, active cancer, limb paralysis, obesity, genetic prothrombotic conditions, unprovoked VTE, proximal (vs. distal) DVT, and prior VTE (4, 20, 78, 119).

Extended or indefinite therapy is recommended for patients with high VTE recurrence risk (e.g., those with active cancer, hereditary or acquired thrombophilias, persistent residual vein thrombosis (RVT, defined as incompressibility ≥4 mm in the common femoral and/or the popliteal vein after 3 months), persistent positive D-dimer, many male patients), and those with an unprovoked VTE as long as the bleeding risk is low to moderate (20).

A CUS reassessment at 3 months helps define further low- or high-recurrence risk and establishes a baseline for high-risk individuals to help differentiate a recurrence from PTS in the future. RVT has been associated with increased risk, and one study identified RVT in almost half of DVT patients, particularly males and those with prior VTE or extensive thrombosis. Recurrent VTE developed in 20% of patients with RVT versus 10% (hazard ratio 2.03) in those without RVT during the 3-year follow-up (122).

An elevated plasma D-dimer obtained at 3 months after discontinuation of therapy has been used to identify the risk of recurrence as well. If the D-dimer result at 3 months is low (negative), the annual risk for recurrence is estimated to be 3.5%. A positive D-dimer (elevated) has been associated with an 8.9% annual risk for recurrence (123). A positive D-dimer after discontinuation of anticoagulation connotes a 2.6 increase in the risk of recurrence, regardless of the patient's age and timing of post-anticoagulant testing (124). The D-dimer is used in an algorithm with CUS after 3 months of therapy to determine risk for a first proximal DVT (124). In patients with no residual vein thrombosis and a negative D-dimer, anticoagulation was stopped. The D-dimer was repeated at 1 and 3 months, and was positive in 14% in whom anticoagulation was restarted. The rate of recurrence for those with negative results was 3.6% annually, 4.1% in those with an unprovoked DVT, and 2.2% for others, with a 7.7% total rate over the 3 years. In males with unprovoked VTE, however, 7.3% had recurrence in the first year. Thus, it is reasonable to use CUS and D-dimer to establish which patients should be considered for extended therapy.

Recently a study was undertaken to identify patients in whom a clinical decision rule could be used to identify patients at low risk of recurrent VTE who could discontinue anticoagulants (125). Only subgroups of women were identified as being at low risk. The HERDOO2 decision rule incorporates the following criteria: (1) *h*yperpigmentation, edema, or *r*edness in either leg; (2) *D*-dimer level ≥250 μg/L during treatment; (3) *o*besity with BMI ≥30 kg/M^2; and (4) *o*lder age ≥65 years. Women with one or none of these criteria are considered to be at low risk for recurrent VTE; 51% of patients (653/1213) were classified as low risk. In those who discontinued oral anticoagulant treatment, 3.0% (17/591) per year developed recurrent VTE. In the high-risk group, 8.1% (25/323) of those who discontinued anticoagulants had recurrent VTE as compared to 1.6% (28/1802) of those who continued anticoagulants (126).

Extended therapy

Controversy exists regarding optimal candidates for extended VTE therapy and the appropriate agent of choice after initial therapy is completed. Historically, the only viable oral anticoagulant option was warfarin therapy; extended treatment at full dosage is recommended over reduced intensity of anticoagulation (127, 128). DOACs have recently been approved as alternatives to warfarin for secondary prevention of VTE. For rivaroxaban and dabigatran, the full treatment dose is continued for extended therapy, while apixaban is approved at a reduced dosage (101, 129, 130). The treatment duration for the majority of the extension trials ranged from 6 to 12 months, with the exception of the REMEDY trial, which extended treatment to 36 months. Most of these studies compared a DOAC with a placebo, as definitive guidance on extended anticoagulation was not available at the time of patient enrollment. Dabigatran is the only DOAC that has been compared with warfarin for extended secondary prevention of VTE (129). All three DOACS demonstrated superiority at lowering the risk of VTE recurrence versus placebo. Additionally, there was no significant difference in major bleeding as compared to placebo with rivaroxaban and apixaban; however, the risk of major bleeding did increase with dabigatran versus placebo. In the second extension study comparing dabigatran with warfarin, there was no significant difference in VTE recurrence risk or major bleeding. Separate subgroup analyses in older adults have not been performed since only 10%–15% of the patients enrolled in each study were older than 75 years of age.

Lifelong treatment is recommended for most patients with a second unprovoked DVT or PE. In patients who have recurrent VTE on an oral anticoagulant and are adherent to therapy, guidelines suggest switching to treatment with LMWH for at least 1 month (20). If the recurrent VTE developed on LMWH, then the guidelines recommend increasing the dose of LMWH by approximately one quarter to one third of the previous dose (20). In general, for extended therapy, the same anticoagulant prescribed in the prior 3 months is continued unless treatment experience with that agent has identified bleeding or adherence issues, for example, due to cost or cognition.

A more recent study comparing rivaroxaban with aspirin for extended therapy found 1.2%–1.5% recurrent VTE with rivaroxaban (20 or 10 mg) versus 4.4% with aspirin (100 mg). Rates of major bleeding were comparable (0.4%–0.5% for rivaroxaban; 0.3% for aspirin) (131). Anticoagulant therapy, rather than aspirin, is recommended, but aspirin may be considered if a decision to discontinue anticoagulants is made for other reasons.

For patients refusing or stopping anticoagulant therapy, daily aspirin therapy has been shown to reduce the rate of VTE recurrence as compared with placebo, without increasing the risk of major bleeding (20). Clinicians must keep in mind, however, that aspirin only reduces the VTE recurrence rate by 30%–35% in comparison to an 80% reduction in recurrent VTE observed with oral anticoagulants (132–135).

CURRENT MANAGEMENT OF ACUTE PE

Treatment of acute PE includes cardiopulmonary support, anticoagulation to prevent extension and recurrence, and reperfusion of the pulmonary artery (136). Cardiopulmonary support begins with supplemental oxygen and inotropic agents. If the right ventricle does not respond to inotropes, surgery or extracorporeal membrane oxygenation may be needed. More than 70% of patients with massive PE receive advanced treatments for reperfusion of the PA including systemic thrombolysis, CDT, and surgical pulmonary embolectomy. Massive PE is associated with a 20% to 50% mortality rate with guideline-directed therapy. Overall mortality was 6.2% in 32 patients with massive PE treated with surgical embolectomy and 14.9% in 27 patients with massive PE treated with extracorporeal membrane oxygenation (137). Adverse outcomes were more closely associated with preoperative cardiopulmonary resuscitation than with treatment modality (137). Indications for surgical pulmonary embolectomy in older patients include massive or submassive PE with any of the following: contraindications to thrombolytic therapy, failed thrombolytic therapy, patent foramen ovale, right heart failure or cardiogenic shock, and thrombus-in-transit within the right heart chambers (138).

MANAGEMENT OF LOWER EXTREMITY VTE DISEASE

High-risk features of distal DVT include severe symptoms, extensive thrombosis (>5cm in length, involving multiple veins, >7 mm in diameter), thrombosis near the proximal veins, no reversible precipitating factor, active cancer, history of VTE, >3 days of immobility, and COVID-19 infection (139–141). These patients should be treated with anticoagulation for at least 3 months because they are at higher risk of progression to proximal DVT and PE (139, 141).

Risk factors for major bleeding on anticoagulation include age older than 75 years, recent major bleeding, severe liver dysfunction, severe renal impairment, severe thrombocytopenia, cancer, acute hemorrhagic stroke or cerebral lesions at high risk for bleeding, and severe uncontrolled hypertension (139, 141). Apixaban, rivaroxaban, or edoxaban are recommended for patients with active cancer with no gastrointestinal or genitourinary involvement, and apixaban for patients with gastrointestinal or genitourinary involvement (139, 141). Apixaban, rivaroxaban, or edoxaban is recommended for patients with a creatinine clearance rate of 30 to 50 mL/min (139, 141). Direct oral anticoagulants should be avoided in patients with an increased prothrombin time or a creatinine clearance rate <30 mL/min, and dabigatran should be avoided in patients with a recent acute coronary syndrome (139, 141). Low-molecular-weight heparins are recommended for active cancer patients and can be used in patients with an increased prothrombin time (139, 141). Fondaparinux is recommended for patients with high-risk superficial vein thrombosis (139, 141).

Warfarin is recommended for patients with antiphospholipid syndrome and can be used in patients with an increased prothrombin time and can be used in patients with a creatinine clearance rate <30 mL/min (139, 141). Older patients with DVT require lower doses of warfarin than younger patients because of potential drug interactions and increased bleeding risk. Newer direct oral anticoagulants such as apixaban and rivaroxaban are preferred for older patients with DVT as they may require less monitoring compared to warfarin.

In 1000,000 patients with DVT in the RIETE registry, patients aged 70 years and older (48%) with VTE were more frequently women (58% versus 44%), more likely to have unprovoked VTE (51% versus 45%), and were more likely to present with severe renal failure (10% versus 1%) and acute PE versus DVT (54% versus 45%) (142). Patients aged 70 years and older were less likely to receive advanced therapies. They had a 36% increased 30-day all-cause mortality, a 2.1 times increased incidence of major bleeding, but a 38% lower risk of 30-day VTE recurrences (142).

In the RIETE registry, 3262 patients with VTE were aged 90 years and older (143). Most of these patients (99.6%) were receiving anticoagulant treatment. These patients were more likely to have immobility, chronic heart failure, anemia, renal insufficiency, or dementia than younger patients with VTE. During the first 3 months, 564 died, 26 developed recurrent VTE, and 116 had major bleeding (143).

In a prospective, multicenter cohort study of 1106 patients with COVID-19-associated VTE, mean age 62.3 years, followed up for 12.5 months after stopping anticoagulant therapy, there were 38 recurrences (3.5%) (144). No patient died of recurrent PE.

Of 8261 patients with unprovoked VTE in the RIETE study, 48.6% of patients had isolated DVT, and 51.4% of patients had a PE (145). At median follow-up of 318 days after discontinuing anticoagulant therapy, 543 patients had recurrent DVTs, 540 patients had recurrent PEs, 71 patients had major bleeding episodes, and 447 patients died (145).

REFERENCES

1. Winter MP, Schernthaner GH, Lang IM. Chronic complications of venous thromboembolism. *J Thromb Haemo* 2017; *15*: 1531–1540.
2. Mozaffarian D, Benjamin EJ, Go AS et al. American Heart Association Statistics Committee and Stroke Statistics Subcommittee. Heart disease and stroke statistics—2015 update: A report from the American Heart Association. *Circulation* 2015; *131*(4): e29–e322.
3. Goldhaber SZ. Venous thromboembolism: Epidemiology and magnitude of the problem. *Best Pract Res Cl Ha* 2012; *25*: 235–242.
4. Heit JA, Spencer FA, White RH. The epidemiology of venous thromboembolism. *J Thromb Thrombolysis* 2016; *41*: 3–14.
5. Cohoon KP, Leibson CL, Ransom JE et al. Costs of venous thromboembolism associated with hospitalization for medical illness. *Am J Manag Care* 2015; *21*(4): e255–e263.
6. Cohen AT, Gitt AK, Bauersachs R et al. The management of acute venous thromboembolism in clinical practice. Results from the European PREFER in VTE Registry. *Thromb Haemost* 2017; *117*: 1326–1337.
7. Kroegel C, Reissig A. Principle mechanisms underlying venous thromboembolism: Epidemiology, risk factors, pathophysiology and pathogenesis. *Respiration* 2003; *70*: 7–30.
8. Mackman N. Triggers, targets and treatments for thrombosis. *Nature* 2008; *451*: 914–918.
9. Behranwala KA, Williamson RC. Cancer-associated venous thrombosis in the surgical setting. *Ann Surg* 2009; *249*: 366–375.
10. Kahn SR, Comerota AJ, Cushman M et al. The post-thrombotic syndrome: Evidence-based prevention, diagnosis, and treatment strategies: A scientific statement from the American Heart Association. *Circulation* 2014; *130*: 1636–1661.
11. Kahn SR, Shapiro S, Wells PS et al. SOX trial investigators. Compression stockings to prevent post-thrombotic syndrome: A randomised placebo-controlled trial. *Lancet* 2014; *383*: 880–888.
12. Wells PS, Anderson DR, Rodger M. Excluding pulmonary embolism at the bedside without diagnostic imaging: Management of patients with suspected pulmonary embolism presenting to the emergency department by using a simple clinical model and D-dimer. *Ann Intern Med* 2001; *135*: 98–107.
13. Prandoni P, Lensing AWA, Prins MA et al. Prevalence of pulmonary embolism among patients hospitalized for syncope. *N Engl J Med* 2016; *375*: 1524–1531.
14. Goldhaber S, Visani L, De Rosa M. Acute pulmonary embolism: Clinical outcomes in the international cooperative pulmonary embolism registry. *Lancet* 1999; *352*: 1386–1389.
15. Jimenez D, Aujesky D, Moores L et al. Simplification of the pulmonary embolism severity index for prognostication in patients with acute symptomatic pulmonary embolism. *Arch Intern Med* 2010; *170*: 1383–1389.
16. Barbar S, Noventa F, Rossetto V et al. A risk assessment model for the identification of hospitalized medical patients at risk for venous thromboembolism: The Padua prediction score. *J Thromb Haemost* 2010; *8*: 2450–2457.

17. Caprini JA. Risk assessment as a guide for the prevention of the many faces of venous thromboembolism. *Am J Surg* 2010; *199*; S3–S10.
18. Angelini D, Khorana AA. Risk assessment scores for cancer-associated venous thromboembolic disease. *Semin Thromb Hemost* 2017; *43*(5): 469–478.
19. Pannucci CJ, Swistun L, MacDonald JK et al. Individualized venous thromboembolism risk stratification using the 2005 Caprini Score to identify the benefits and harms of chemoprophylaxis in surgical patients. A meta-analysis. *Ann Surg* 2017 *265*(6): 1094–1103.
20. Kearon C, Akl EA, Comerota AJ et al. Antithrombotic therapy for VTE disease: Antithrombotic therapy and prevention of thrombosis, 9th ed: American College of Chest Physicians evidence based clinical practice guidelines. *Chest* 2012; *141*: e419S–94S.
21. Kukar M, Asaro J, Aquino A et al. Incidence of venous thromboembolic events in mandated risk assessment versus optional DVT prophylaxis era at a large tertiary cancer center. *Am Surg* 2015; *81*(9): 893–898.
22. The CLOTS Trials Collaboration. Effectiveness of thigh-length graduated compression stockings to reduce the risk of deep vein thrombosis after stroke (CLOTS trial 1): A multicentre, randomised controlled trial. *Lancet* 2009; *373*: 1958–1965.
23. CLOTS Trial Collaboration. Thigh-length versus below-knee stockings for deep venous thrombosis prophylaxis after stroke: A randomized trial. *Ann Intern Med* 2010; *153*: 553–562.
24. CLOTS (Clots in Legs Or sTockings after Stroke) Trials Collaboration. Effectiveness of intermittent pneumatic compression in reduction of risk of deep vein thrombosis in patients who have had a stroke (CLOTS 3): A multicentre randomized controlled trial. *Lancet* 2013, *382*: 516–524.
25. Pavon JM, Adam SS, Razouki ZA. Effectiveness of intermittent pneumatic compression devices for venous thromboembolism prophylaxis in high-risk surgical patients: A systematic review. *J Arthroplasty* 2016; *31*: 524–532.
26. Stewart DW, Freshour JE. Aspirin for the prophylaxis of venous thromboembolic events in orthopedic surgery patients: A comparison of the AAOS and ACCP guidelines with review of the evidence. *Ann Pharmacother* 2013; *47*(1): 63–74.
27. Warwick D, Rosencher N. The "critical thrombosis period" in major orthopedic surgery: When to start and when to stop prophylaxis. *Clin Appl Thromb Hemost* 2010; *16*(4): 394–405.
28. Arcelus JI, Kudrna JC, Caprini JA. Venous thromboembolism following major orthopedic surgery: What is the risk after discharge? *Orthopedics* 2006; *29*(6): 506–516.
29. Falck-Ytter Y, Francis CW, Johanson NA et al. Prevention of VTE in orthopedic surgery patients. Antithrombotic therapy and prevention of thrombosis 9th ed: American college of chest physicians evidence-based clinical practice guidelines. *Chest* 2012; *141*(2)(Suppl): e278S–e325S.
30. Jacobs JJ, Mont MA, Bozic KJ et al. American Academy of Orthopaedic Surgeons: preventing venous thromboembolic disease in patients undergoing elective hip and knee arthroplasty: An evidence-based guideline and evidence report. https://www.aaos.org/uploadedFiles/PreProduction/Quality/Guidelines_and_Reviews/VTE_full_guideline_10.31.16.pdf (Accessed October 29, 2017.)
31. Brown Evidence-based Practice Center. Venous thromboembolism prophylaxis in major orthopedic surgery: systematic review update. Comparative Effectiveness Review number 191. AHRQ Publication No. 17-EHC021-EF June 2017 https://effectivehealthcare.ahrq.gov/sites/default/files/pdf/thromboembolism-update_research-2017.pdf (Accessed November 21, 2017).
32. Pollack CV, Reilly PA, Eikelboom J et al. Idarucizumab for dabigatran reversal. *N Engl J Med* 2015; *373*(6): 511–520.
33. Siegal DM, Curnutte JT, Connolly SJ et al. Andexanet alfa for the reversal of factor Xa inhibitor activity. *N Engl J Med* 2015; *373*(25): 2413–2424.
34. Eriksson BI, Dahl OE, Rosencher N et al. Dabigatran etexilate versus enoxaparin for prevention of venous thromboembolism after total hip replacement: a randomized, double-blind, non-inferiority trial. *Lancet* 2007; *370*: 949–956.
35. Eriksson BI, Dahl OE, Huo MH et al. Oral dabigatran versus enoxaparin for thromboprophylaxis after primary total hip arthroplasty (RE-NOVATE II). *Thromb Haemost* 2011; *105*(4): 721–729.
36. Eriksson BI, Dahl OE, Rosencher N et al. Oral dabigatran etexilate vs. subcutaneous enoxaparin for the prevention of venous thromboembolism after total knee replacement: The RE-MODEL randomized trial. *Thromb Haemost* 2007; *5*(11): 2178–2185.
37. Ginsberg JS, Davidson BL, Comp PC et al. Oral thrombin inhibitor dabigatran etexilate vs North American enoxaparin regimen for prevention of venous thromboembolism after knee arthroplasty surgery. *J Arthroplasty* 2009; *24*(1): 1–9.
38. Pradaxa® [package insert]. Ridgefield, CT: Boehringer Ingelheim Pharmaceuticals; 2017.
39. Xarelto® [package insert]. Titusville, NJ: Janssen Pharmaceuticals; 2011.
40. Eriksson BI, Borris LC, Friedman RJ et al. Rivaroxaban versus enoxaparin for thromboprophylaxis after hip arthroplasty. *N Engl J Med* 2008; *358*(26): 2765–2775.
41. Kakkar AK, Brenner B, Dahl OE et al. Extended duration rivaroxaban versus short-term enoxaparin for the prevention of venous thromboembolism

after total hip arthroplasty: A double blind, randomised controlled trial. *Lancet* 2008; *372*: 31–39.
42. Lassen MR, Ageno W, Borris LC et al. RECORD3 Investigators. Rivaroxaban versus enoxaparin for thromboprophylaxis after total knee arthroplasty. *N Engl J Med* 2008; *358*: 2776–2786.
43. Turpie AG, Lassen MR, Davidson BL et al. RECORD4 Investigators. Rivaroxaban versus enoxaparin for thromboprophylaxis after total knee arthroplasty (RECORD4): A randomised trial. *Lancet* 2009; *373*: 1673–1680.
44. Turpie AG, Lassen MR, Eriksson BI et al. Rivaroxaban for the prevention of venous thromboembolism after hip or knee arthroplasty. Pooled analysis of four studies. *Thromb Haemost* 2011; *105*: 444–453.
45. Lassen MR, Raskob GE, Gallus A et al. Apixaban or enoxaparin for thromboprophylaxis after knee surgery. *N Engl J Med* 2009; *361*(6): 594–604.
46. Lassen MR, Raskob GE, Gallus A et al. Apixaban versus enoxaparin for thromboprophylaxis after knee replacement (ADVANCE-2): A randomised double-blind trial. *Lancet* 2010; *375*: 807–815.
47. Lassen MR, Gallus A, Raskob GE et al. Apixaban versus enoxaparin for thromboprophylaxis after hip replacement. *N Engl J Med* 2010; *363*(26): 2487–2498.
48. Eliquis® [package insert]. Princeton, NJ: Bristol-Myers Squibb Company and Pfizer; 2016.
49. AlHajri L, Jabbari S, AlEmad H et al. The efficacy and safety of edoxaban for VTE prophylaxis post-orthopedic surgery: A systematic review. *J Cardiovasc Pharmacol Ther* 2017; *22*(3): 230–238.
50. Narouze S, Benzon HT, Provenzano DA et al. Interventional spine and pain procedures in patients on antiplatelet and anticoagulant medications. Guidelines from the American society of regional anesthesia and pain therapy, the American academy of pain medicine, the international neuromodulation society, the North American neuromodulation society and the world institute of pain. *Reg Anesth Pain Med* 2015; *40*: 182–212.
51. Lovenox® [package insert]. Bridgewater, NJ: Sanofi-Aventis US, LLC; 2013.
52. Arixtra® [package insert]. Research Triangle Park, NC: GlaxoSmithKline; 2010.
53. Gould MK, Garcia DA, Wren SM et al. Prevention of VTE in nonorthopedic surgical patients. Antithrombotic therapy and prevention of thrombosis, 9th ed: American College of Chest Physicians evidence-based clinical practice guidelines. *Chest* 2012; *141*(2)(Suppl): e227S–e277S.
54. Ambrosetti M, Salerno M, Zambelli M et al. Deep vein thrombosis among patients entering cardiac rehabilitation after coronary artery bypass surgery. *Chest* 2004; *125*(1): 191–196.
55. Nyquist P, Bautista C, Jichici D et al. Prophylaxis of venous thromboembolism in neurocritical care patients: An evidence-based guideline: A statement for healthcare professionals from the neurocritical care society. *Neurocritical Care* 2016; *24*: 47–60.
56. Geerts WH, Jay RM, Code KI et al. A comparison of low-dose heparin with low-molecular-weight heparin as prophylaxis against venous thromboembolism after major trauma. *N Engl J Med* 1996; *335*(10): 701–707.
57. Malinoski D, Jafari F, Ewing T et al. Standard prophylactic enoxaparin dosing leads to inadequate anti-Xa levels and increase deep vein thrombosis rates in critically ill trauma and surgical patients. *J Trauma* 2010; *69*(4): 874–880.
58. Lacut K, Le Gal G, Mottier D. Primary prevention of venous thromboembolism in elderly medical patients. *Clin Interv Aging* 2008; *3*: 399–411.
59. Woller SC, Stevens SM, Jones JP et al. Derivation and validation of a simple model to identify venous thromboembolism risk in medical patients. *Am J Med* 2011; *124*: 947–954.
60. Decousus H, Tapson VF, Bergmann J-F et al. Factors at admission associated with bleeding risk in medical patients. Findings from the IMPROVE investigators. *Chest* 2011; *139*(1): 69–79.
61. Phung OJ, Kahn SR, Cook DJ et al. Dosing frequency of unfractionated heparin thromboprophylaxis: A meta-analysis. *Chest* 2011; *140*: 374–381.
62. Kucher N 1, Leizorovicz A, Vaitkus PT et al. Efficacy and safety of fixed low-dose dalteparin in preventing venous thromboembolism among obese or elderly hospitalized patients: A subgroup analysis of the PREVENT trial. *Arch Intern Med* 2005; *165*: 341–345.
63. Dentali F, Douketis JD, Gianni M et al. Meta-analysis: Anticoagulant prophylaxis to prevent symptomatic venous thromboembolism in hospitalized medical patients. *Ann Intern Med* 2007; *146*: 278–288.
64. Kahn SR, Lim W, Dunn AS et al. Prevention of VTE in nonsurgical patients: Antithrombotic therapy and prevention of thrombosis, 9th ed: American College of Chest Physicians evidence-based clinical practice guidelines. *Chest* 2012; *141*(2 Suppl): e195S–e226S.
65. http://www.bevyxxa.com/docs/Bevyxxa-Full-Prescribing-Information.pdf
66. Cohen AT, Harrington RA, Goldhaber SZ et al. Extended thromboprophylaxis with betrixaban in acutely ill medical patients. *N Engl J Med* 2016; *375*: 534–544.
67. Cohen AT, Spiro TE, Büller HR et al. MAGELLAN investigators. Rivaroxaban for Thromboprophylaxis in acutely Ill medical patients. *N Engl J Med* 2013; *368*: 513–523.
68. Lyman GH, Bohlke K, Khorana AA et al. Venous thromboembolism prophylaxis and treatment in patients with cancer: American Society of Clinical

Oncology clinical practice guideline update 2014. *J Clin Oncol* 2015; *33*: 654–656.

69. Wells PS, Anderson DR, Bormanis J et al. Value of assessment of pretest probability of deep-vein thrombosis in clinical management. *Lancet* 1997; *350*: 1795–1798.
70. Gibson NS, Sohne M, Kruip MJ et al. Further validation and simplification of the Wells clinical decision rule in pulmonary embolism. *Thromb Haemost* 2008; *99*(1): 229–234.
71. Le Gal G, Righini M, Roy PM et al. Prediction of pulmonary embolism in the emergency department: The revised Geneva score. *Ann Intern Med* 2006; *144*(3): 165–171.
72. Singh B, Mommer SK, Erwin PJ et al. Pulmonary embolism rule-out criteria (PERC) in pulmonary embolism-revisited: A systematic review and meta-analysis. *Emerg Med J* 2013; *30*(9): 701–706.
73. Schouten HJ, Geersing GJ, Koek HL et al. Diagnostic accuracy of conventional or age adjusted D-dimer cut-off values in older patients with suspected venous thromboembolism: Systematic review and meta-analysis. *Br Med J* 2013; *346*: f2492.
74. van Es N, van der Hulle T, van Es J et al. Rule and d-dimer testing to rule out pulmonary embolism: A systematic review and individual-patient data meta-analysis. *Ann Intern Med* 2016; *165*: 253–261.
75. Birdwell BG, Raskob GE, Whitsett TL et al. Predictive value of compression ultrasonography for deep vein thrombosis in symptomatic outpatients: Clinical implications of the site of vein noncompressibility. *Arch Intern Med* 2000; *160*: 309–313.
76. Le Gal G, Righini M, Wells PS. Computed tomographic pulmonary angiography for pulmonary embolism. *JAMA* 2015; *314*(1): 74–75.
77. The PIOPED Investigators. Value of the ventilation/perfusion scan in acute pulmonary embolism. Results of the prospective investigation of pulmonary embolism diagnosis (PIOPED). *JAMA* 1990; *263*(20): 2753–2759.
78. Streiff MB, Agnelli G, Connors JM et al. Guidance for the treatment of deep vein thrombosis and pulmonary embolism. *J Thromb Thrombolysis* 2016; *41*: 32–67.
79. Carrier M, Le Gal G, Wells PS et al. Systematic review: Case-fatality rates of recurrent venous thromboembolism and major bleeding events among patients treated for venous thromboembolism. *Ann Intern Med* 2010; *152*: 578–589.
80. Wu C, Alotaibi GS, Alsaleh K et al. Case-fatality of recurrent venous thromboembolism and major bleeding associated with aspirin, warfarin, and direct oral anticoagulants for secondary prevention. *Thromb Res* 2015; *135*: 243–248.
81. Pisters R, Lane DA, Nieuwlaat R et al. A novel user-friendly score (HAS-BLED) to assess 1-year risk of major bleeding in patients with atrial fibrillation: The Euro Heart Survey. *Chest* 2010; *138*: 1093–1100.
82. Otero R, Uresandi F, Jiménez D et al. Home treatment in pulmonary embolism. *Thromb Res* 2010; *126*(1): e1–e5.
83. Billett HH, Jacobs LG, Madsen EM et al. Efficacy of inferior vena cava filters in anticoagulated patients. *J Thromb Haemost* 2007; *5*: 1–6.
84. Decousus H, Leizorovicz A, Parent F et al. A clinical trial of vena caval filters in the prevention of pulmonary embolism in patients with proximal deep-vein thrombosis. Prévention du Risque d'Embolie Pulmonaire par interruption cave study group. *N Engl J Med* 1998; *338*: 409–415.
85. PREPIC Study Group. Eight-year follow-up of patients with permanent vena cava filters in the prevention of pulmonary embolism: The PREPIC (Prevention du Risque d'Embolie Pulmonaire par Interruption Cave) randomized study. *Circulation* 2005; *112*(3): 416–422.
86. Mismetti P, Laporte S, Pellerin O. Effect of a retrievable inferior vena cava filter plus anticoagulation vs anticoagulation alone on risk of recurrent pulmonary embolism. A randomized clinical trial. *JAMA* 2015; *313*(16): 1627–1635.
87. Kearon C, Akl EZ, Ornelas J et al. Antithrombotic therapy for VTE disease: CHEST guideline and expert panel report. *Chest* 2016; *149*: 315–352.
88. Grommes J, Strijkers R, Greiner A et al. Safety and feasibility of ultrasound-accelerated catheter-directed thrombolysis in deep vein thrombosis. *Eur J Vasc Endovasc Surg* 2011; *41*: 526–532.
89. Haig Y, Enden T, Slagsvold CE et al. Determinants of early and long-term efficacy of catheter-directed thrombolysis in proximal deep vein thrombosis. *J Vasc Interv Radiol* 2013; *24*: 17–24.
90. Enden T, Haig Y, Klow NE et al. Long-term outcome after additional catheter-directed thrombolysis versus standard treatment for acute iliofemoral deep vein thrombosis (the CaVenT study): A randomized controlled trial. *Lancet* 2012; *379*: 31–38.
91. Enden T, Resch S, White C et al. Cost-effectiveness of additional catheter-directed thrombolysis for deep vein thrombosis. *J Thromb Haemost* 2013; *11*: 1032–1042.
92. Guo-Cheng D, Zhang MC, Zhao JC. Catheter-directed thrombolysis plus anticoagulation versus anticoagulation alone in the treatment of proximal deep vein thrombosis—A meta analysis. *Vasa* 2015; *44*: 195–202.
93. Bashir R, Zack CJ, Zhao H et al. Comparative outcomes of catheter-directed thrombolysis plus anticoagulation vs anticoagulation alone to treat lower-extremity proximal deep vein thrombosis. *JAMA Intern Med* 2014; *174*(9): 1494–1501.
94. Kucher N, Boekstegers P, Muller OJ et al. Randomized, controlled trial of ultrasound-assisted

catheter-directed thrombolysis for acute intermediate-risk pulmonary embolism. *Circulation* 2014; *129*: 479–486.
95. Piazza G, Hohlfelder B, Jaff MR et al. A prospective, single-arm, multicenter trial of ultrasound-facilitated, catheter-directed, low-dose fibrinolysis for acute massive and submassive pulmonary embolism: The SEATTLE II study. *JACC Cardiovasc Interv* 2015; *8*: 1382–1392.
96. Kaymaz C, Ozturk S, Akbal O et al. Ultrasound-assisted catheter-directed thrombolysis in high-risk and intermediate-high-risk pulmonary embolism: Results from a single-center cohort. *Angiology* 2017; *68*(5): 433–440.
97. Bajaj NS, Kalra R, Arora P et al. Catheter-directed treatment for acute pulmonary embolism: Systematic review and single-arm meta analysis. *Int J Cardiol* 2016; *225*: 128–139.
98. Arora S, Panaich SS, Ainani N et al. Comparison of in-hospital outcomes and readmission rates in acute pulmonary embolism between systemic and catheter-directed thrombolysis (from the National Readmission Database). *Am J Cardiol* 2017; *120*: 1653–1661.
99. Tapson VF, Piazza G, Goldhaber SZ et al. Optimum duration and dose of R-Tpa with the acoustic pulse thrombolysis procedure for intermediate-risk (submassive) pulmonary embolism: OPTALYSE PE [Abstract]. *Am J Respir Crit Care Med* 2017; *195*: A2835.
100. Spyropoulos AC, Merli G. Management of venous thromboembolism in the elderly. *Drugs Aging* 2006; *23*: 651–671.
101. EINSTEIN Investigators. Oral rivaroxaban for symptomatic venous thromboembolism. *N Engl J Med* 2010; *363*: 2499–2510.
102. EINSTEIN-PE Investigators. Oral rivaroxaban for the treatment of symptomatic pulmonary embolism. *New Engl J Med* 2012; *366*: 1287–1297.
103. Agnelli G, Buller HR, Cohen A et al. Oral apixaban for the treatment of acute venous thromboembolism. *N Engl J Med* 2013; *369*: 799–808.
104. Schulman S, Kearon C, Kakkar AK et al. Dabigatran versus warfarin in the treatment of acute venous thromboembolism. *N Engl J Med* 2009; *361*: 2342–2352.
105. Hokusai-VTE Investigators, Büller HR, Décousus H et al. Edoxaban versus warfarin for the treatment of symptomatic venous thromboembolism. *N Engl J Med* 2013; *369*: 1406–1415.
106. Raschke R, Reilly BM, Srinivas S et al. The weight-based heparin dosing nomogram compared with a "standard care" nomogram: A randomized controlled trial. *Ann Intern Med* 1993; *119*: 874–881.
107. Kearon C, Ginsberg JS, Julian JA et al. Fixed-dose heparin (FIDO) Investigators. Comparison of fixed-dose weight-adjusted unfractionated heparin and low-molecular-weight heparin for acute treatment of venous thromboembolism. *JAMA* 2006; *296*: 935–942.
108. Hull RD, Raskob GE, Brant RF et al. Relation between the time to achieve the lower limit of the APTT therapeutic range and recurrent venous thromboembolism during heparin treatment for deep vein thrombosis. *Arch Intern Med* 1997; *157*: 2562–2568.
109. Tincani E, Crowther MA, Turrini F et al. Prevention and treatment of venous thromboembolism in the elderly patient. *Clin Interv Aging* 2007; *2*: 237–246.
110. The Matisse Investigators. Subcutaneous fondaparinux versus intravenous unfractionated heparin in the initial treatment of pulmonary embolism. *N Engl J Med* 2003; *349*: 1695–1702.
111. The Matisse Investigators. Fondaparinux or enoxaparin for the initial treatment of symptomatic deep venous thrombosis: A randomized trial. *Ann Intern Med* 2004; *140*: 867–873.
112. Shehab N, Lovegrove MC, Geller AI et al. Emergency department visits for outpatient adverse drug events, 2013–2014. *JAMA* 2016; *316*: 2115–2125.
113. Geldhof V, Vandenbriele C, Verhamme P et al. Venous thromboembolism in the elderly: Efficacy and safety of non-VKA oral anticoagulants. *Thromb J* 2014; *13*: 12–21.
114. Barco S, Cheung YW, Eikelboom JW et al. New oral anticoagulants in elderly patients. *Best Pract Res Clin Haematol* 2013; *26*: 215–224.
115. Amin A. Choosing non-Vitamin K antagonist oral anticoagulants: Practical considerations we need to know. *Ochsner J* 2016; *16*: 531–541.
116. Voukalis C, Lip G, Shantsila E. Non-vitamin K oral anticoagulants versus vitamin K antagonists in the treatment of venous thromboembolic disease. *Expert Opin Pharmacother* 2016; *17*: 2033–2047.
117. Agnelli G, Prandoni P, Becattini C et al. Warfarin optimal duration Italian trial investigators. Extended oral anticoagulant therapy after a first episode of pulmonary embolism. *Ann Intern Med* 2003; *139*: 19–25.
118. Couturaud F, Sanchez O, Pernod G et al. PADIS-PE Investigators. Six months vs extended oral anticoagulation after a first episode of pulmonary embolism: The PADIS-PE randomized clinical trial. *JAMA* 2015; *314*: 31–40.
119. Rodger M, Carrier M, Gandara E et al. Unprovoked venous thromboembolism: Short term or indefinite anticoagulation? Balancing long-term risk and benefit. *Blood Rev* 2010; *24*: 171–178.
120. Iorio A, Kearon C, Filippucci E et al. Risk of recurrence after first episode of symptomatic venous thromboembolism provoked by a transient risk factor: A systematic review. *Arch Intern Med* 2010; *170*(19): 1710–1716.

121. White RH. The epidemiology of venous thromboembolism. *Circulation* 2003; *107*(Suppl *1*): I4–I8.
122. Prandoni P, Lensing AWA, Prins MH. The impact of residual thrombosis on the long-term outcomes of patients with deep venous thrombosis treated with conventional anticoagulation. *Semin Thromb Hemost* 2015; *41*(2): 133–140.
123. Verhovsek M, Douketis JD, Yi Q et al. Systematic review: D-dimer to predict recurrent disease after stopping anticoagulant therapy for unprovoked venous thromboembolism. *Ann Intern Med* 2008; *149*: 481–490.
124. Douketis J, Tosetto A, Marcucci M et al. Patient-level meta-analysis: Effect of measurement timing, threshold, and patient age on ability of D-dimer testing to assess recurrence risk after unprovoked venous thromboembolism. *Ann Intern Med* 2010; *153*: 523–531.
125. Rodger MA, Kahn SR, Wells PS et al. Identifying unprovoked thromboembolism patients at low risk for recurrence who can discontinue anticoagulant therapy. *CMAJ* 2008; *179*: 417–426.
126. Rodger MA, Le Gal G, Anderson DR et al. Validating the HERDOO2 rule to guide treatment duration for women with unprovoked venous thrombosis: Multinational prospective cohort management study. *BMJ* 2017; *356*: j1065.
127. Ridker PM, Goldhaber SZ, Danielson E et al. Long-term, low-intensity warfarin therapy for the prevention of recurrent venous thromboembolism. *N Engl J Med* 2003; *348*: 1425–1434.
128. Kearon C, Ginsberg JS, Kovacs MJ et al. Comparison of low-intensity warfarin therapy with conventional-intensity warfarin therapy for long-term prevention of recurrent venous thromboembolism. *N Engl J Med* 2003; *349*: 631–639.
129. Schulman S, Kearon C, Kakkar AK et al. RE-MEDY and the RE-SONATE trials investigators. Extended use of dabigatran, warfarin, or placebo in venous thromboembolism. *N Engl J Med* 2013; *368*: 709–718.
130. Agnelli G, Buller HR, Cohen A et al. AMPLIFY-EXT Investigators. Apixaban for extended treatment of venous thromboembolism. *N Engl J Med* 2013; *368*: 699–708.
131. Weitz JI, Lensing AWA, Prins MH et al. Einstein choice investigators. Rivaroxaban or aspirin for extended treatment of venous thromboembolism. *N Engl J Med* 2017; *376*(13): 1211–1222.
132. Shapiro NL, Bhatt SH. Critical review and update on the treatment of acute and chronic pulmonary embolism. *J Pharm Pract* 2016; *29*: 35–45.
133. Becattini C, Agnelli G, Schenone A et al. WARFASA Investigators. Aspirin for preventing the recurrence of venous thromboembolism. *N Engl J Med* 2012; *366*: 1959–1967.
134. SAVAYSA® [package insert], Parsippany, NJ: Daiichi Sankyo; 2017.
135. Feuring M, Schulman S, Eriksson H et al. Net clinical benefit of dabigatran vs. warfarin in venous thromboembolism: Analyses from RE-COVER®, RE-COVER™ II, and RE-MEDY™. *J Thromb Thrombolysis* 2017; *43*(4): 484–489.
136. Licha CRM, McCurdy CM, Maldonado SM et al. Current management of acute pulmonary embolism. *Ann Thorac Carduiovasc Surg* 2019; *26*: 65–71.
137. Goldberg JB, Spevack DM, Ahsan S et al. Comparison of surgical embolectomy and venoarterial extracorporeal oxygenation for massive pulmonary embolism. *Semin Thorac Cardiovasc Surg* 2022; *34*: 934–942.
138. Konstantinides SV, Meyer G, Becattini C et al. 2019 ESC guidelines for the diagnosis and management of acute pulmonary embolism developed in collaboration with the European Respiratory Society (ERS): The task force for the diagnosis and management of acute pulmonary embolism of the European society of Cardiology (ESC). *Eur Resp J* 2019; *54*: 1901647.
139. Stevens SM Woller SC, Kreuziger LB et al. Antithrombotic therapy for VTE disease: second update of the chest guideline and expert panel report. *Chest* 2021; *160*: e545–e608.
140. Sartori M, Favaretto E, Cosmi B. Relevance of immobility as a risk factor for symptomatic proximal and isolated distal deep vein thrombosis in acutely ill medical patients. *Vasc Med* 2021; *26*: 542–548.
141. Ziyadeh F, Mauer Y. Management of lower-extremity venous thromboembolism: an updated review. *Cleve Clin J Med* 2024; *91*: 229–235.
142. Ortega AG, Jimenez D, Pedro-Tudela A et al. Age-related differences in the presentation, management, and clinical outcomes of 100,000 patients with venous thromboembolism in the RIETE registry. *Arch Bronchoneumol* 2024: 143–152.
143. Lafaie L, Poenou G, Hanon O et al. Anticoagulation and venous thromboembolism in patients aged 90 years and older: Data from the RIETE registry. *J Am Geriatr Soc* 2024; *72*: 113–125.
144. Jaro-Palomares L, Bikdeli B, Jiminez D et al. Risk of recurrence after discontinuing anticoagulation in patients with COVID-19-associated venous thromboembolism: a prospective multicentre cohort study. *E Clinical Medicine* 2024; *73*: 102659.
145. Gabara C,Aibar J, Nishimoto Y et al. Clinical outcomes after discontinuing anticoagulant therapy in patients with first unprovoked venous thromboembolism. *J Thromb Haemost* 2024; *22*: 2234–2246.

27

Management of peripheral arterial disease in older persons

WILBERT S. ARONOW

Key points

- Behavioral therapy, nicotine replacement therapy, and drug therapy with varenicline or bupropion should be considered for smoking cessation.
- Blood pressure should be reduced to less than 130 mm Hg.
- Serum LDL cholesterol should be reduced to less than 55 mg/dL.
- Diabetics should be treated with SGLT-2 inhibitors or glucagon-like peptide 1 receptor agonists as first-line hypoglycemic agents.
- Single antiplatelet therapy with either aspirin or clopidogrel, especially clopidogrel, should be administered in patients at high risk for bleeding.
- Rivaroxaban 2.5 mg twice daily plus aspirin 80 to 100 mg daily should be given to patients with lower extremity PAD at high risk for ischemic events and at low bleeding risk.
- Walking is the preferred form of exercise in exercise programs.
- Annual influenza vaccination and vaccination against COVID-19 are recommended.

INTRODUCTION

Peripheral arterial disease (PAD) is chronic arterial occlusive disease of the lower extremities caused by atherosclerosis. PAD may cause intermittent claudication, which is pain or weakness with walking that is relieved with rest. The muscle pain or weakness after exercise occurs distal to the arterial obstruction. Since the superficial femoral and popliteal arteries are most commonly affected by atherosclerosis, the pain of intermittent claudication is most commonly localized to the calf. Atherosclerotic obstruction of the distal aorta and its bifurcation into the two iliac arteries may cause pain in the buttocks, hips, thighs, or the inferior back muscles as well as the calves.

The Rutherford classification of PAD includes seven stages (1). PAD is classified as stage 0 if the person is asymptomatic, stage 1 if mild intermittent claudication is present, stage 2 if moderate intermittent claudication is present, stage 3 if severe intermittent claudication is present, stage 4 if ischemic rest pain is present, stage 5 if the person has minor tissue loss, and stage 6 if the person has ulceration or gangrene (1).

DOI: 10.1201/9781003568933-27

Only half of elderly persons with documented PAD are symptomatic. Persons with PAD may not walk far or fast enough to induce muscle ischemic symptoms because of comorbidities such as pulmonary disease or arthritis, may have atypical symptoms unrecognized as intermittent claudication, may fail to mention their symptoms to their physician, or may have sufficient collateral arterial channels to tolerate their arterial obstruction. Women with PAD have a higher prevalence of leg pain on exertion and at rest, poorer functioning, and greater walking impairment from leg symptoms than men with PAD (2). Poorer leg strength in women contributes to poorer lower extremity functioning in women with PAD than in men with PAD (2). Women with PAD develop a faster functional decline than men with PAD. More sedentary hours and slower outdoor walking speed are associated with faster decreases in functioning and adverse calf muscle changes in PAD. Increased physical activity levels during daily life are associated with less functional decline in patients with PAD (3).

Upper extremity PAD will cause unequal blood pressure measurements in each arm. PAD patients also have a higher prevalence of cognitive impairment and erectile dysfunction.

If the arterial flow to the lower extremities cannot meet the needs of resting tissue metabolism, critical lower extremity ischemia occurs with pain at rest or tissue loss. Critical ischemia causes rest pain in the toes or feet with progression to ulceration or gangrene. Chronic arterial insufficiency ulcers commonly develop at the ankle, heel, or leg. Mummified, dry, black toes or devitalized soft tissue covered by a crust is gangrene caused by ischemic infarction. Suppuration often develops with time, and dry gangrene changes to wet gangrene.

The vascular physical examination includes (1) measurement of the blood pressure in both arms; (2) palpation of the carotid pulses and listening for carotid bruits; (3) auscultation of the abdomen and flank for bruits; (4) palpation of the abdomen and notation of the presence of the aortic pulsation and its maximal diameter; (5) palpation of pulses at the brachial, radial, ulnar, femoral, popliteal, dorsalis pedis, and posterior tibial sites; and (6) auscultation of both femoral arteries for femoral bruits. The shoes and socks should be removed and the feet inspected. The color, temperature, and integrity of the skin should be evaluated, and the presence of distal hair loss, trophic skin changes, hypertrophic nails, and ulcerations noted (4). Persons with PAD of the lower extremities have reduced or absent arterial pulses.

NONINVASIVE DIAGNOSIS

Noninvasive tests used to assess lower extremity arterial blood flow include measurement of ankle and brachial artery systolic blood pressures, characterization of velocity waveform, and duplex ultrasonography. Measurement of ankle and brachial artery systolic blood pressures using a Doppler stethoscope and blood pressure cuffs allows calculation of the ankle–brachial index (ABI), which is normally 0.9–1.2. An ABI of less than 0.90 is 95% sensitive and 99% specific for the diagnosis of PAD (5). The lower the ABI, the more severe the restriction of arterial blood flow and the more serious the ischemia. ABIs of 0.6–0.9 usually correlate with mild to moderate intermittent claudication. ABIs of 0.4–0.6 usually correlate with severe intermittent claudication. With ABIs between 0.25 and 0.4, rest pain and tissue loss are often found. Patients with calcified arteries from diabetes mellitus or renal failure occasionally have relatively noncompressible arteries, leading to falsely elevated ABI values in the normal range. Patients with an ABI of 1.4 or higher also have an increased incidence of cardiovascular events (6) and lower quality of life (7).

In addition to measuring arterial pressure in nonpalpable arteries, Doppler ultrasound methods allow characterization of the flow versus time velocity waveform. Finding biphasic flow at the groin or monophasic flow more distally is evidence of arterial obstruction, even when ABI measurements are falsely increased to normal levels because of calcification.

Duplex ultrasonography combines Doppler frequency measurements with two-dimensional images of blood vessels. The severity of flow restriction caused by an arterial stenosis can be accurately assessed by this most comprehensive noninvasive method (8).

Duplex ultrasonography, computed tomographic angiography, and magnetic resonance angiography are useful in assessing the anatomic location and severity of PAD and in selecting suitable candidates for endovascular or surgical revascularization (4).

Treadmill exercise testing, with and without pre-exercise and post-exercise ABIs, helps differentiate claudication from pseudoclaudication in patients with exertional leg symptoms (4). Treadmill exercise testing may be useful to diagnose PAD with a normal resting ABI but a reduced post-exercise ABI (4). Treadmill exercise testing may objectively document the magnitude of symptom limitation in patients with claudication (4). The post-exercise ABI is a powerful independent predictor of all-cause mortality and provides more risk stratification than the resting ABI (9). The treadmill is a better functional test than the 6-minute walk test.

PREVALENCE

The prevalence of PAD increases with age (Table 27.1).

RISK FACTORS

Risk factors that predispose to PAD include cigarette smoking (10, 13, 17, 19, 20), diabetes mellitus (10, 13, 17, 20), hypertension (10, 13, 17, 19–21), dyslipidemia (10, 13, 17, 19, 20, 22–24), increased plasma homocysteine levels (25), reduced glomerular filtration rate (26–28),

Table 27.1 Prevalence of peripheral arterial disease

Study	Prevalence
360 men aged 60 years (10)	16%
306 women aged 60 years (10)	13%
158 persons aged 38–59 years (11)	5.6%
161 persons aged 60–69 years (11)	15.9%
294 persons aged 70–82 years (11)	33.8%
2214 women aged ≥65 years (12)	13.9%
2870 women aged ≥65 years (12)	11.4%
467 men, mean age 80 years (13)	20%[a]
1444 women, mean age 81 years (13)	13%[a]
2589 men aged ≥55 years (14)	16.9%
3861 women aged ≥55 years (14)	20.5%
1160 men, mean age 80 years (15)	32%[a]
2464 women, mean age 81 years (15)	26%[a]
268 Blacks, mean age 81 years (16)	29%[a]
71 Hispanics, mean age 81 years (16)	24%[a]
1310 Whites, mean age 82 years (17)	23%[a]
386 men, mean age 72 years (17)	26.7%[a]
620 women, mean age 72 years (17)	17.1%
6979 men and women, mean age 69 years (18)	29%

[a] Symptomatic peripheral arterial disease.

microalbuminuria (28), metabolic syndrome in women (29), inflammation (29), and a family history of PAD (30). Obesity is associated with a high ABI (31). Women are more likely than men to present with PAD at an older age, are often asymptomatic, and have poorer outcomes with revascularization than men (32).

Table 27.2 shows the significant independent risk factors for PAD in 467 men, mean age 80 years, and in 1444 women, mean age 81 years, living in the community and seen in an academic geriatrics practice.

In 147 men and women with PAD and 373 men and women without PAD, mean age 81 years, plasma homocysteine was a significant independent risk factor for PAD with an odds ratio of 1.13 for each 1 μmol/L increase (25). In 249 men and women, mean age 79 years, the prevalence of PAD was significantly higher in persons with subclinical hypothyroidism (14 of 18 persons or 78%) than in persons with euthyroidism (40 of 231 persons or 17%) (33).

COEXISTENCE OF OTHER ATHEROSCLEROTIC DISORDERS

PAD coexists with other atherosclerotic disorders (Table 27.3).

Patients with PAD and CAD have more extensive and calcified coronary atherosclerosis, constrictive arterial remodeling, and greater disease progression (40). Patients with PAD also have a higher prevalence of left ventricular systolic dysfunction than patients without PAD (41).

CARDIOVASCULAR MORTALITY AND MORBIDITY

Persons with PAD are at increased risk for all-cause mortality, cardiovascular mortality, and cardiovascular events (6, 30, 42–49). At 10-year follow-up of 565 men and women, mean age 66 years, PAD significantly increased the risk of all-cause mortality (relative risk = 3.1), of mortality from cardiovascular disease (relative risk = 5.9), and of mortality from CAD (relative risk = 6.6) (42). At 4-year follow-up of 1492 women, mean age 71 years, an ABI of 0.9 or less was associated with a relative risk of 3.1 for all-cause mortality after adjustment for age, smoking, and other risk factors (43).

In a prospective study of 291 men and women, mean age 82 years, with PAD, CAD was present in 160 persons (55%) (44). Silent myocardial ischemia detected by 24-hour ambulatory electrocardiography was present in 60 of 160 persons (38%) with PAD and CAD, and in 26 of 131 persons (20%) with PAD and no clinically evident CAD (44). At 43-month follow-up, new coronary events developed in 54 of 60 persons (90%) with PAD, CAD, and silent myocardial ischemia, and in 59 of 100 persons (59%) with PAD, CAD, and no silent myocardial ischemia (44). New coronary events also developed in 18 of 26 persons (69%) with PAD, no CAD, and silent myocardial ischemia, and in 34 of 105 persons (32%) with PAD, no CAD, and no silent myocardial ischemia (44).

Table 27.2 Significant independent risk factors for symptomatic peripheral arterial disease in 467 men, mean age 80 years, and in 1444 women, mean age 81 years

	Odds ratio	
Risk factor	Men	Women
Age (each 1-year increase)	1.05	1.03
Current cigarette smoking	2.6	4.6
Systolic or diastolic hypertension	2.2	2.8
Diabetes mellitus	6.1	3.6
High-density lipoprotein cholesterol	0.95 for 1 mg/dL increase	0.97 for 1 mg/dL increase
Low-density lipoprotein cholesterol	1.02 for 1 mg/dL increase	1.02 for 1 mg/dL increase

Table 27.3 Coexistence of peripheral arterial disease with other atherosclerotic disorders in older persons

Study	Result
1886 persons, mean age 81 years (34)	If PAD was present, 58% had coexistent CAD and 34% had prior ischemic stroke.
1802 persons, mean 80 years (35)	If PAD was present, 68% had coexistent CAD and 42% had prior ischemic stroke.
924 men, mean age 80 years (36)	PAD was 1.5 times higher in men with mitral annular calcium than in men without mitral annular calcium.
1881 women, mean age 81 years (36)	PAD was 1.6 times higher in women with mitral annular calcium than in women without mitral annular calcium.
989 men, mean age 80 years (37)	PAD was 1.6 times higher in men with aortic stenosis than in men without aortic stenosis.
1998 women, mean age 81 years (37)	PAD was 1.7 times higher in women with aortic stenosis than in women without aortic stenosis.
279 persons with PAD, mean age 71 years, undergoing coronary angiography for suspected CAD (20)	Obstructive CAD was present in 98% of persons, left main CAD in 18% of persons, and three- or four-vessel CAD in 63% of persons.
218 persons without PAD, mean age 70 years, undergoing coronary angiography for suspected CAD (20)	Obstructive CAD was present in 82% of persons, left main CAD in <1% of persons, and three- or four-vessel CAD in 11% of persons.
1006 persons, mean age 72 years (17)	If PAD was present, 63% had coexistent CAD, and 43% had prior ischemic stroke.
336 patients, mean age 73 years (38)	CAD was present in 75% of patients with a decreased ABI and in 29% of age- and gender-matched patients with a normal ABI.
273 patients, mean age 71 years, with CAD (39)	The lower the ABI, the higher the prevalence of three- or four-vessel CAD.

Abbreviations: ABI, ankle–brachial index; CAD, coronary artery disease; PAD, peripheral arterial disease.

A pooled analysis of mortality in eight large randomized percutaneous coronary intervention (PCI) trials of 19,867 patients showed that the presence of PAD was associated with higher rates of post-PCI death and myocardial infarction (50). PAD was an independent predictor of short-term and long-term mortality (45).

At 7.5-year follow-up of persons in the Cardiovascular Health study in a propensity-matched study of community-dwelling older adults, matched hazard ratios for PAD for all-cause mortality, incident heart failure, and symptomatic PAD were 1.57, 1.32, and 3.92, respectively (46). In a well-balanced propensity-matched population of 2689 patients with advanced chronic systolic heart failure, during 4.1 years of follow-up, PAD was significantly associated with increased mortality and hospitalization (47).

At 33-month follow-up of 414 patients with PAD and at 48-month follow-up of 89 patients without PAD followed in a vascular surgery clinic, the incidence of death, new stroke/transient ischemic attack, new myocardial infarction, new coronary revascularization, new carotid endarterectomy, or new PAD revascularization was significantly higher in patients with PAD (63%) than in patients without PAD (24%) (48). PAD was a significant independent risk factor for all-cause mortality with a hazard ratio of 2.2 (48). In 879 patients, mean age 67 years, with PAD (456 with coexistent CAD), despite a higher adherence to medical therapy in patients with concomitant CAD, the presence of CAD was an independent risk factor for 5-year all-cause mortality by 35% (49).

Of 710 patients, mean age 61 years, with CAD, 446 had no PAD, 83 had clinical PAD, and 181 had subclinical PAD diagnosed by an ABI ≤0.90 or >1.40 (50). At 7.2-year median follow-up, clinical PAD increased all-cause mortality 2.11 times, and subclinical PAD increased all-cause mortality 1.65 times (50).

Dipyridamole thallium scintigraphy also has prognostic value in the preoperative assessment of patients with PAD undergoing vascular surgery (51).

RISK FACTOR MODIFICATION

Continuing smoking increases the risk of amputation in patients with intermittent claudication (52). Patency in lower extremity bypass grafts is also worse in smokers than in nonsmokers. Smoking cessation reduces the progression of PAD to critical leg ischemia and reduces the risk of myocardial infarction and death from vascular causes (53). Smoking cessation programs should be strongly encouraged in persons with PAD (Table 27.4).

Table 27.4 Medical management of peripheral arterial disease

1. Smoking cessation program
2. Treatment of hypertension with blood pressure reduced to <130/80 mmHg
3. Control diabetes mellitus with the hemoglobin A1C level reduced to <7%
4. Treat dyslipidemia with high-dose statins and reduce serum low-density lipoprotein cholesterol to <70 mg/dL
5. Antiplatelet drug therapy with aspirin or preferably clopidogrel
6. Treatment with an angiotensin-converting enzyme inhibitor
7. Treatment with beta blockers in patients with coronary artery disease in the absence of contraindications to these drugs
8. Use of statins
9. Treatment with cilostazol in patients with intermittent claudication
10. Exercise rehabilitation program
11. Foot care
12. Annual influenza vaccination

Patients should be assisted with counseling and developing a plan for quitting that may include pharmacotherapy and/or referral to a smoking cessation program (54).

Approaches to smoking cessation include use of nicotine patches or nicotine polacrilex gum, which are available over the counter (55). If this therapy is unsuccessful, nicotine nasal spray or treatment with the antidepressant bupropion should be considered (55). A nicotine inhaler may also be used (56). The dosage and duration of treatment of each of these pharmacotherapies are discussed in detail elsewhere (56). Concomitant behavioral therapy may also be needed (57). Repeated physician advice is very important in the treatment of smoking addiction. Patients with PAD should also avoid passive smoking (4).

Hypertension should be adequately controlled to decrease cardiovascular mortality and morbidity in persons with PAD (21, 58, 59) (Table 27.4). Blood pressure should be reduced to <130/80 mmHg (59).

Among persons with PAD in the Appropriate Blood Pressure Control in Diabetes trial, the incidence of cardiovascular events in persons treated with antihypertensive drug therapy with enalapril or nisoldipine was 13.6% if the mean blood pressure was reduced to 128/75 mmHg versus 38.7% if the mean blood pressure was reduced to 137/81 mmHg (58).

Older persons with diabetes mellitus and PAD and no CAD have a 1.5 times higher incidence of new coronary events than elderly nondiabetics with PAD and prior myocardial infarction (60). The higher the hemoglobin A1C levels in patients with diabetes mellitus and PAD, the higher the prevalence of severe PAD (61). Diabetes mellitus should be treated with the hemoglobin A1C level decreased to less than 7% to decrease the incidence of myocardial infarction (62). The blood pressure should be reduced to less than 130/80 mmHg in elderly persons with PAD and diabetes mellitus (59). Elderly diabetics with PAD should also be treated with high-dose statins (4, 63, 64) and the serum LDL cholesterol reduced to <70 mg/dL (64).

Treatment of dyslipidemia with statins has been documented to reduce the incidence of mortality, cardiovascular events, and stroke in persons with PAD with and without CAD (23, 24, 63–73). At 5-year follow-up of 4444 men and women with CAD and hypercholesterolemia in the Scandinavian Simvastatin Survival Study, compared with placebo, simvastatin significantly decreased the incidence of intermittent claudication by 38% (65).

In a study of 264 men and 396 women, mean age 80 years, with symptomatic PAD and a serum LDL cholesterol of 125 mg/dL or higher, 318 of 660 persons (48%) were treated with a statin and 342 of 660 persons (52%) with no lipid-lowering drug (70). At 39-month follow-up, treatment with statins caused a significant independent reduction in the incidence of new coronary events of 58%, of 52% in persons with prior myocardial infarction, and of 59% in persons with no prior myocardial infarction (70).

In the Heart Protection Study, 6748 of the 20,536 persons (33%) had PAD (66). At 5-year follow-up, treatment with simvastatin 40 mg daily caused a significant 19% relative reduction and a 6.3% absolute reduction in major cardiovascular events independent of age, gender, or serum lipid levels (66). These data favor the administration of statins to elderly persons with PAD regardless of serum lipid levels.

On the basis of the available data, older persons with PAD and hypercholesterolemia should be treated with statins to reduce cardiovascular mortality and morbidity and progression of PAD (4, 23, 24, 63–70) and to improve exercise time until intermittent claudication (71–73) (Table 27.4). Statins also reduce perioperative myocardial infarction and mortality (74) and 2-year mortality (74) in patients undergoing noncardiac vascular surgery.

Since lipid-lowering therapy is underutilized in persons with PAD (75, 76), intensive educational programs are needed to educate physicians to use lipid-lowering therapy in elderly persons with cardiovascular disease and dyslipidemia (76–78). On the basis of data from the Heart Protection Study, persons with PAD should be treated with statins regardless of age, gender, or initial serum lipid levels (66).

Hypothyroidism is a risk factor for PAD (33). Older persons with clinical or subclinical hypothyroidism should be treated with l-thyroxine to decrease the development of CAD (79) and possibly of PAD (33). There is no evidence showing that treatment with l-thyroxine will reduce the development of PAD or improve symptoms.

ANTIPLATELET DRUGS

Antiplatelet drugs that have been shown to decrease the incidence of vascular death, nonfatal myocardial infarction, and nonfatal stroke in persons with PAD are aspirin, ticlopidine, clopidogrel, and ticagrelor (80–82). Aspirin plus dipyridamole has not been shown to be more efficacious than aspirin alone in the treatment of persons with PAD (80). Oral platelet glycoprotein IIb/IIIa inhibitors have been shown to increase mortality in the treatment of persons with CAD and have not been investigated in the treatment of persons with PAD (83). Ticagrelor and clopidogrel are equally effective in reducing cardiovascular events and cause a similar incidence of major bleeding (82).

Thromboxane A_2 induces platelet aggregation and vasoconstriction. Aspirin decreases the aggregation of platelets exposed to thrombogenic stimuli by inhibiting the cyclooxygenase enzyme reaction within the platelet and thereby blocking the conversion of arachidonic acid to thromboxane A_2 (84). Clopidogrel is a thienopyridine derivative that inhibits platelet aggregation by inhibiting the binding of adenosine 5′-diphosphate to its platelet receptor (85). Ticagrelor is a P2Y12 inhibitor (81, 82).

Vorapaxar is a novel antagonist of protease-activated receptor-1 (86). Vorapaxar has been approved by the US Food and Drug Administration to reduce the risk of myocardial infarction, stroke, cardiovascular death, and coronary revascularization in patients with a history of myocardial infarction or lower extremity PAD. Because of its increased risk of bleeding, vorapaxar should not be used in patients who have had a stroke, a transient ischemic attack, or bleeding in the head.

The Antithrombotic Trialists' Collaboration Group (ATCG) reported a meta-analysis of 26 randomized studies of 6263 persons with intermittent claudication due to PAD (80). At follow-up, the incidence of vascular death, nonfatal myocardial infarction, and nonfatal stroke was 6.4% in patients randomized to antiplatelet drugs versus 7.9% in the control group, a significant reduction of 23% caused by antiplatelet therapy. The reductions are significant for all subgroups.

The ATCG reported a meta-analysis of 12 randomized studies of 2497 persons with PAD undergoing peripheral arterial grafting (80). At follow-up, the incidence of vascular death, nonfatal myocardial infarction, and nonfatal stroke was 5.4% in persons randomized to antiplatelet drugs versus 6.5% in the control group, a significant reduction of 22% caused by antiplatelet therapy.

The ATCG also reported a meta-analysis of four randomized studies of 946 persons with PAD undergoing peripheral angioplasty (80). At follow-up, the incidence of vascular death, nonfatal myocardial infarction, and nonfatal stroke was 2.5% in patients randomized to antiplatelet drugs versus 3.6% in the control group, a significant reduction of 29% caused by antiplatelet therapy.

If one combines the 42 randomized studies of 9706 patients with intermittent claudication, peripheral arterial grafting, or peripheral angioplasty, the incidence of vascular death, nonfatal myocardial infarction, and nonfatal stroke at follow-up was significantly decreased 23% by antiplatelet drugs, with similar benefits among patients with intermittent claudication, those having peripheral arterial grafting, and those having peripheral angioplasty (120). These data favor the use of aspirin in men and women with PAD (80) (Table 27.4).

Antiplatelet therapy with aspirin alone or with clopidogrel alone is recommended by the 2016 American College of Cardiology (ACC)/American Heart Association (AHA) PAD guidelines to reduce myocardial infarction, stroke, and vascular death in patients with symptomatic PAD (4). These guidelines also recommend that this antiplatelet therapy is reasonable to reduce myocardial infarction, stroke, and vascular death in patients with asymptomatic PAD (4).

Aspirin

Table 27.5 shows the efficacy of different doses of aspirin in reducing the incidence of vascular death, nonfatal myocardial infarction, and nonfatal stroke in high-risk persons (80). Since aspirin doses greater than 150 mg daily do not reduce vascular death, nonfatal myocardial infarction, and nonfatal stroke more than does a dose of 75–150 mg daily and cause more gastrointestinal bleeding than the lower doses, this author prefers an aspirin dose of 81 mg daily in treating older persons with atherosclerotic vascular disease.

Clopidogrel

In the Clopidogrel versus Aspirin in Patients at Risk for Ischaemic Events (CAPRIE) trial, 5795 persons with PAD were randomized to clopidogrel 75 mg daily and 5797 persons with PAD were randomized to aspirin 325 mg daily (87). At 1.9-year follow-up, the annual incidence of vascular death, nonfatal myocardial infarction, and

Table 27.5 Efficacy of aspirin doses in decreasing vascular death, nonfatal myocardial infarction, and nonfatal stroke in high-risk patients

Aspirin dose	Decrease in vascular death, myocardial infarction, or stroke
500–1500 mg (34 trials)	19%
160–325 mg (19 trials)	26%
75–150 mg (12 trials)	32%
<75 mg (3 trials)	13%

Source: Antithrombotic Trialists' Collaboration, *BMJ*, 324, 71–86, 2002.

nonfatal stroke was 3.7% in persons randomized to clopidogrel versus 4.9% in persons randomized to aspirin, a 24% significant decrease with the use of clopidogrel (87).

On the basis of these data, it is reasonable to conclude that clopidogrel is superior to aspirin in the management of patients with PAD. On the basis of these data, the author also recommends the use of clopidogrel 75 mg daily in the treatment of patients with PAD (Table 27.4). In a vascular surgery clinic, 501 of 506 persons (83%) with PAD were treated with aspirin or clopidogrel (88). Aspirin 75–325 mg daily or clopidogrel 75 mg daily are recommended by the 2016 ACC/AHA guidelines to reduce the risk of myocardial infarction, stroke, or vascular death in patients with PAD (4).

ORAL ANTICOAGULANTS

In the Dutch Bypass Oral Anticoagulants or Aspirin Study, 2690 persons were randomized after infrainguinal bypass surgery to aspirin 80 mg daily or to oral anticoagulation with phenprocoumon or acenocoumarol to maintain an international normalized ratio (INR) of 3.0–4.5 (89). At 21-month follow-up, there was no significant difference between the two treatments in the primary outcome of infrainguinal graft occlusion (89). There was no significant difference between the two treatments in the secondary outcomes of myocardial infarction, stroke, amputation, or vascular death (89). However, persons treated with oral anticoagulant therapy had 1.96 times more major bleeding episodes than persons treated with oral aspirin (89). The ACC/AHA guidelines state that oral anticoagulant therapy with warfarin should not be given to reduce the risk of adverse cardiovascular ischemic events in persons with atherosclerotic lower extremity PAD (4).

ANGIOTENSIN-CONVERTING ENZYME INHIBITORS

The ACC/AHA guidelines recommend treating persons with PAD with ACE inhibitors unless there are contraindications to the use of these drugs to reduce cardiovascular mortality and morbidity (90) (Table 27.4). A randomized, double-blind, placebo-controlled trial of 212 patients, mean age 66 years, with intermittent claudication due to PAD also showed at 6-month follow-up that 10 mg daily of ramipril increased pain-free walking time 75 seconds and maximum walking time 255 seconds (91). This study also showed that ramipril increased the SF-36 median Physical Component Summary score by 8.2 (91).

BETA-BLOCKERS

A meta-analysis of 11 randomized controlled studies found that beta-blockers do not adversely affect walking capacity or the symptoms of intermittent claudication in persons with mild to moderate PAD (92).

An observational study was performed in 575 men and women, mean age 80 years, with symptomatic PAD and prior myocardial infarction (93). Of the 575 persons, 85 persons (15%) had contraindications to the use of beta-blockers. Of the 490 persons without contraindications to the use of beta-blockers, 257 persons (52%) were treated with beta-blockers. Adverse effects causing cessation of beta-blockers occurred in 31 of the 257 persons (12%). At 32-month follow-up, use of beta-blockers caused a 53% significant independent decrease in the incidence of new coronary events in elderly persons with PAD and prior myocardial infarction (93). In a vascular surgery clinic, 301 of 364 persons (83%) with PAD and CAD were treated with beta-blockers (88). Beta-blockers should be used to treat CAD in patients with PAD in the absence of contraindications to these drugs (Table 27.4).

STATINS

On the basis of data from the Heart Protection Study, persons with PAD should be treated with statins regardless of age, gender, or initial serum lipid levels (66) (Table 27.4). Three double-blind, randomized, placebo-controlled studies have also demonstrated that statins improve walking performance in persons with PAD (Table 27.6) (71–73).

Table 27.6 Effects of statins on walking performance in patients with intermittent claudication

Study	Results
69 persons, mean age 75 years, with intermittent claudication and hypercholesterolemia (71)	Compared with placebo, simvastatin 40 mg daily significantly increased treadmill exercise time until the onset of intermittent claudication by 24% at 6 months and by 42% at 1 year.
354 persons, mean age 68 years, with intermittent claudication and hypercholesterolemia (72)	At 1-year follow-up, compared with placebo, atorvastatin 80 mg daily significantly increased pain-free treadmill walking distance by 40% and community-based physical activity.
86 persons, mean age 67 years, with intermittent claudication and hypercholesterolemia (73)	At 6-month follow-up, compared with placebo, simvastatin 40 mg daily significantly increased pain-free walking distance and total walking distance on a treadmill, the mean ankle–brachial index at rest and after exercise, and symptoms of claudication.

Statin use is also associated with superior leg functioning independent of cholesterol levels and other potential confounders (94). The data suggest that non-cholesterol-lowering properties of statins may favorably influence functioning in persons with and without PAD (94).

Despite the data recommending use of statins, aspirin, and ACE inhibitors or angiotensin receptor blockers for secondary prevention in patients with PAD, millions of adults in the United States with PAD are not receiving these drugs (95). Use of these drugs in patients with PAD and no other cardiovascular disease was associated with a 65% significant reduction in all-cause mortality (95).

DRUGS TO INCREASE WALKING DISTANCE

Chelation therapy has been demonstrated to be ineffective in the therapy of PAD (4). Numerous drugs have been shown to be ineffective in improving walking distance in persons with intermittent claudication (96).

Two drugs, pentoxifylline and cilostazol, have been approved by the Food and Drug Administration for symptomatic treatment of intermittent claudication. However, many studies have found no consistent improvement with pentoxifylline in patients with intermittent claudication in comparison with placebo (97). The 2016 ACC/AHA PAD guidelines recommend the use of cilostazol but not of pentoxifylline to improve symptoms and increase walking distance in patients with claudication (4).

Cilostazol inhibits phosphodiesterase type 3, increasing intracellular concentration of cyclic adenosine monophosphate. Cilostazol suppresses platelet aggregation and also acts as a direct arterial vasodilator. Cilostazol has been documented in numerous trials to improve exercise capacity in patients with intermittent claudication (98–101), and at a dose of 100 mg twice daily, was shown to be superior to both placebo and pentoxifylline (100).

Cilostazol should be administered to patients with PAD to increase walking distance (Table 27.4) but should not be given to persons with PAD who also have heart failure. Other contraindications to the use of cilostazol include a creatinine clearance <25 mL/min, a known predisposition for bleeding, or coadministration of CYP3A4 or CYP2C19 inhibitors such as cimetidine, diltiazem, erythromycin, ketoconazole, lansoprazole, omeprazole, and HIV-1 protease inhibitors.

EXERCISE REHABILITATION

Exercise rehabilitation programs have been demonstrated to increase walking distance in persons with intermittent claudication through improvements in peripheral circulation, walking economy, and cardiopulmonary function (102). The optimal exercise program for improving claudication pain distance in persons with PAD uses intermittent walking to near-maximal pain during a program of at least 6 months (103). The 2016 ACC/AHA PAD guidelines recommend a supervised exercise program for patients with intermittent claudication (49) (Table 27.4).

Supervised exercise training is recommended for a minimum of 30–45 minutes in sessions performed at least 3 times per week for a minimum of 12 weeks and preferably for 6 months or longer (103). Among persons with PAD, self-directed walking exercise performed at least 3 times weekly is associated with significantly less functional decline during the subsequent year (104). However, patients with PAD with and without claudication symptoms who are unable or unwilling to participate in supervised exercise programs will benefit from a home-based walking exercise intervention program (105).

FOOT CARE

Persons with PVD must have proper foot care (4, 106) (Table 27.4). They must wear properly fitted shoes. Careless nail clipping or injury from walking barefoot must be avoided. Feet should be washed daily and the skin kept moist with topical emollients to prevent cracks and fissures, which may have portals for bacterial infection. Fungal infection of the feet must be treated. Socks should be wool or other thick fabrics, and padding or shoe inserts may be used to prevent pressure sores. When a wound of the foot develops, specialized foot gear, including casts, boots, and ankle foot orthoses, may be helpful in unweighting the affected area (106). Patients with PAD should also have an annual influenza vaccination to reduce all-cause mortality (4, 90).

LOWER EXTREMITY ANGIOPLASTY AND BYPASS SURGERY

Table 27.7 states that the indications for lower extremity percutaneous transluminal angioplasty or bypass surgery are (1) incapacitating claudication in persons interfering with work or lifestyle; (2) limb salvage in persons with limb-threatening ischemia as manifested by rest pain, nonhealing ulcers, and/or infection or gangrene; and (3) vasculogenic impotence (107). Percutaneous transluminal angioplasty can be performed if there is a skilled vascular interventionalist and the arterial disease is localized to a vessel segment less than 10 cm in length (107). Compared

Table 27.7 Indications for angioplasty or bypass surgery in lower extremities

1. Incapacitating intermittent claudication in persons interfering with work or lifestyle
2. Limb salvage in persons with limb-threatening ischemia as manifested by rest pain, nonhealing ulcers, and/or infection or gangrene
3. Vasculogenic impotence

Source: Weitz JI et al., *Circulation*, 94, 3026–3049, 1996.

to percutaneous transluminal angioplasty alone, stenting improves 3-year patency by 26% (108). After infrainguinal bypass surgery, oral anticoagulant therapy is preferable in persons with venous grafts, whereas aspirin is preferable in persons with nonvenous grafts (89).

Percutaneous balloon angioplasty and/or stenting is indicated for short-segment stenoses, whereas multisegment disease and occlusions are most effectively treated with surgical revascularization (109). Revascularization of PAD is discussed extensively elsewhere (4, 106). In patients presenting with severe limb ischemia caused by infrainguinal disease and who are suitable for either surgery or angioplasty, bypass surgery and balloon angioplasty are associated with similar outcomes in terms of amputation-free survival (110). Patients with intermittent claudication should be considered for revascularization to improve symptoms only in the absence of other diseases that would limit exercise improvement such as angina pectoris, heart failure, chronic pulmonary disease, or orthopedic limitations (4).

However, 6-month outcomes from 111 patients with claudication due to aortoiliac PAD randomized to optimal medical therapy, optimal medical therapy plus supervised exercise, or optimal medical therapy plus stent revascularization showed that the greatest increase in treadmill walking performance occurred in the patients randomized to optimal medical therapy plus supervised exercise (111).

An invasive treatment strategy improved health-related quality of life and intermittent claudication distance after 1 year in 158 patients, mean age 68 years, with stable lifestyle-limiting claudication receiving current medical treatment (112). In a study of 883 patients, mean age 67 years, undergoing peripheral endovascular interventions and 975 patients, mean age 67 years, undergoing lower extremity bypass surgery for treatment of symptomatic PAD, 30-day procedural complications were higher with bypass surgery (37.1% vs. 11.9%), revascularization rates were higher at 1 year and at 3 years with endovascular interventions, and there was no difference in subsequent amputations (113).

In a randomized trial of 212 patients, mean age 65 years, with intermittent claudication, at 1-year follow-up, a combination therapy of endovascular revascularization followed by supervised exercise caused greater improvement in walking distances and in health-related quality-of-life scores compared with supervised exercise alone (114). Research is needed to see if home-based exercise will improve walking performance when added to endovascular therapy for PAD (115). Despite a lack of clinical trial data supporting the use of dual antiplatelet therapy with aspirin plus clopidogrel after peripheral revascularization for lower extremity PAD, many operators treat these patients with a variable course of aspirin plus clopidogrel after peripheral revascularization (116). The 2016 ACC/AHA PAD guidelines state that endovascular procedures should not be performed in patients with PAD solely to prevent progression to critical limb ischemia (4).

AMPUTATION

Nonrandomized studies have demonstrated that both immediate and long-term survival are higher in patients having revascularization rather than amputation for limb-threatening ischemia (117). However, amputation of lower extremities should be performed if tissue loss has progressed beyond the point of salvage, if surgery is too risky, if life expectancy is very low, or if functional limitations diminish the benefit of limb salvage (106).

ABDOMINAL AORTIC ANEURYSM

The prevalence of abdominal aortic aneurysm (AAA) increases with advancing age, smoking, hypercholesterolemia, hypertension, male gender, and family history (4, 118, 119). The prevalence of an AAA varies from 1.3% for men aged 45–54 years to 12.5% for men aged 75–84 years (4). The prevalence of an AAA varies from 0% for women aged 45–54 years to 5.2% for women aged 75–84 years (4). Most patients with an AAA are asymptomatic, with their AAA noted on studies performed for other reasons rather than on physical examination. Of 110 men with an AAA, 71% had CAD, 46% had lower extremity PAD, and 27% had cerebrovascular disease (120). The prognosis of an AAA in women is worse than in men (121).

In patients who have evidence of back, abdominal, or groin pain in the presence of a pulsatile abdominal mass, the aorta needs to be evaluated immediately, preferably with computed tomographic scanning. In one study, the mortality rates were 35% for ruptured AAAs, 26% for symptomatic AAAs, and 5% for asymptomatic AAAs undergoing repair (122). In another study, treatment of 96 high-risk patients, mean age 72 years, with an AAA with an endovascular stent-graft prosthesis was associated with a 100% survival at 90-day follow-up (123).

The ACC/AHA PAD guidelines recommend that patients with infrarenal or juxtarenal AAAs measuring 5.5 cm or larger undergo repair to eliminate the risk of rupture (7, 8). Patients with infrarenal or juxtarenal AAAs measuring 4.0–5.4 cm in diameter should be monitored by ultrasound or computed tomographic scans every 6–12 months to detect expansion (4).

Patients with AAA should undergo intensive risk factor modification. In one study, use of ACE inhibitors was associated with a reduced risk of ruptured AAA (124). Of 130 patients with AAAs not treated surgically, patients treated with statins (58% of the group) had a significantly lower mortality at 45-month follow-up (5% for statin-treated patients versus 16% for patients not treated with statins) (125). The size of the AAA was 4.6 cm at baseline versus 4.5 cm at 23-month follow-up in patients treated with statins versus 4.5 cm at baseline and 5.3 cm at 24-month follow-up in patients not treated with statins (125). Use of statins also reduced perioperative and 2-year mortality in patients undergoing surgical AAA repair (74). In addition, long-term statin use was associated with decreased all-cause mortality and cardiovascular mortality after successful AAA surgery irrespective of clinical risk factors and use of beta-blockers (126).

In 400 patients ineligible for open repair of an AAA randomized to no repair or endovascular repair, at 8-year follow-up, endovascular repair was associated with a significant 47% reduction in aneurysm-related mortality but was not associated with a reduction in all-cause mortality (127). A study compared 39,966 matched pairs of Medicare patients, mean age 76 years, with an AAA who underwent open repair or endovascular repair (128). The perioperative mortality was 1.6% with endovascular repair versus 5.4% with open repair. Late survival was similar in both groups after 3 years. Through 8 years of follow-up, aneurysm rupture was more common with endovascular repair (5.4%) than with open repair (1.4%). Through 8 years, interventions related to management of the AAA or its complications were higher with endovascular repair, whereas interventions for complications related to laparotomy were higher with open repair (128).

CANADIAN CARDIOVASCULAR SOCIETY 2022 PAD GUIDELINES 129

Smoking cessation can prevent PAD and decrease major adverse cardiovascular events and evolution to limb-threatening ischemia or limb loss (MALE) in patients with symptomatic PAD (129). Behavioral therapy (130), nicotine replacement therapy (131), and drug therapy with varenicline (132) or bupropion (133) should be considered. Diabetics with PAD should be treated with a sodium-glucose cotransporter 2 (SGLT-2) inhibitor to reduce mortality, major adverse cardiovascular events, and MALE (134). Patients with PAD should be treated with a maximally tolerated dose of statin therapy (135, 136). Statin add-on treatments with ezetimibe and/or a PCSK9 inhibitor should be added if the serum LDL cholesterol is 55 mg/dL or higher to further reduce major adverse cardiovascular events and MALE (135, 136). Diet, exercise, weight management, alcohol reduction, stress management, and self-monitoring of blood pressure are important in managing blood pressure (59, 129). The blood pressure should be reduced to less than 130 mm Hg (59, 129). Most patients with PAD will require more than one antihypertensive drug to control hypertension. The Canadian guidelines recommend that the first antihypertensive drug be an ACE inhibitor or angiotensin receptor blocker (129, 137). Rivaroxaban 2.5 mg twice daily plus aspirin 80 to 100 mg daily should be administered to patients with symptomatic lower extremity PAD at high risk for ischemic events and low bleeding risk (129, 138, 139). Single antiplatelet treatment with either aspirin 75 to 325 mg or clopidogrel 75 mg daily should be considered for patients with symptomatic lower extremity PAD at high risk for bleeding who are eligible for antithrombotic treatment with clopidogrel being the preferred drug (129).

A subanalysis of the COMPASS trial included 4129 patients (71% men) with symptomatic lower extremity PAD, mean age 66.8 years, who were randomized to rivaroxaban 2.5 mg twice daily plus aspirin 100 mg once daily, rivaroxaban 5 mg twice daily plus aspirin 100 mg once daily, or to aspirin 100 mg once daily (140). The 30-month Kaplan–Meier incidence risk of major adverse cardiovascular events or MALE in patients with either high-risk limb presentations or high-risk comorbidities showed a 4.2% absolute reduction in patients treated with rivaroxaban plus aspirin compared with aspirin alone with a net clinical benefit after major bleeding of 3.2% (140).

The Canadian Cardiovascular Society 2022 PAD guidelines recommend treatment with rivaroxaban 2.5 mg twice daily plus aspirin 80 to 100 mg once daily with or without short-term treatment with clopidogrel 75 mg daily after elective endovascular revascularization of lower extremity PAD (129, 141). These guidelines recommend treatment with rivaroxaban 2.5 mg twice daily plus aspirin 80 to 100 mg once daily after elective open revascularization of lower extremity PAD (129). Treatment with rivaroxaban 2.5 mg twice daily plus aspirin 80 to 100 mg once daily plus short-term use (maximum of 30 days) of clopidogrel 75 mg daily can be considered in patients who have complex endovascular stenting of lower extremity PAD (129). Dual antiplatelet therapy with clopidogrel 75 mg daily plus aspirin 75 to 325 mg daily for at least 1 month should be used in patients with lower extremity PAD after elective endovascular revascularization who are unable to receive low-dose rivaroxaban (129).

The European Atherosclerosis Society/European Society of Vascular Medicine guidelines recommend the use of either clopidogrel 75 mg daily or aspirin 100 mg daily plus rivaroxaban 2.5 mg twice daily to reduce cardiovascular events in patients with lower extremity PAD (136). Dual antiplatelet therapy with aspirin plus clopidogrel should be given for at least 1 month after drug-coated balloon angioplasty, and for 3 months after either drug-eluting or covered stent implantation (136). Aspirin 100 mg daily plus rivaroxaban 2.5 mg twice daily should be considered for dual antiplatelet therapy post-intervention (136).

The Canadian Cardiovascular Society 2022 PAD guidelines recommend that for patients with intermittent claudication due to lower extremity PAD, a supervised exercise program, a home exercise program, or a community-based exercise therapy is efficacious in improving total walking time or distance, claudication, need for revascularization, and quality of life (129). Walking is the preferred form of exercise in exercise programs for intermittent claudication (129). The STARDUST randomized clinical trial showed that liraglutide increased peripheral perfusion in persons with type 2 diabetes and lower extremity PAD detected by peripheral transcutaneous oxygen pressure during 6 months of treatment (142).

2024 EUROPEAN SOCIETY FOR VASCULAR SURGERY GUIDELINES FOR INTERMITTENT CLAUDICATION

The 2024 European Society for Vascular Surgery Guidelines for intermittent claudication recommend both behavioral therapy and pharmacotherapy for smoking cessation for all patients with lower extremity PAD who smoke. Varenicline alone or in combination with nicotine replacement therapy is recommended as the first pharmacological smoking cessation treatment (143). Patients with intermittent claudication due to lower extremity PAD should be screened for obesity, diabetes, metabolic syndrome, and cardiovascular risk factors with subsequent optimal medical management (143). High-intensity statin treatment is recommended (143). The serum LDL cholesterol should be reduced to less than 55 mg/dL by high-dose statins plus ezetimibe if needed, plus a PCSK-9 inhibitor if needed (136, 143, 144). Blood pressure should be reduced to 120 to 129/80 mm Hg or lower in patients younger than 70 years and to 130 to 139/80 mm Hg in patients 70 years and older with intermittent claudication (143, 145). Diabetics with lower extremity PAD should have a hemoglobin A1c value of 7.0% and lower (143, 146). In type 2 diabetics with lower extremity PAD, both SGLT-2 inhibitors and glucagon-like peptide 1 receptor agonists are recommended as first-line hypoglycemic agents to decrease the risk of major cardiovascular and renal events (143, 146). Annual influenza vaccination and vaccination against COVID-19 are recommended for patients with lower extremity PAD (143). For all patients with lower extremity PAD, moderate intensity exercise for at least 150 to 300 minutes a week or vigorous intensity aerobic exercise for at least 75 to 150 minutes per week is recommended to decrease all-cause cardiovascular events and cardiovascular mortality (143, 147).

2024 ACC/AHA PAD GUIDELINES

In patients with symptomatic PAD, single antiplatelet therapy with clopidogrel 75 mg daily preferably or aspirin 75 mg to 325 mg daily is recommended to reduce the risk of MACE. In patients with symptomatic PAD, rivaroxaban 2.5 mg twice daily plus low-dose aspirin is recommended to reduce the risk of MACE and MALE. After endovascular or surgical revascularization for PAD, rivaroxaban 2.5 mg twice daily plus low-dose aspirin is recommended to reduce the risk of MACE and MALE. In patients with asymptomatic PAD, single antiplatelet therapy is reasonable to reduce the risk of MACE (148).

Patients with PAD should be treated with atorvastatin 40–80 mg daily or rosuvastatin 20–40 mg daily to achieve a decrease in serum LDL-C of 50% or more. If the serum LDL-C on maximally tolerated statin therapy is 70 mg/dL or higher, it is reasonable to add ezetimibe or a PCSK-9 inhibitor. Blood pressure should be treated to a level of <130/80 mm Hg. An ACE inhibitor or ARB is recommended in patients with PAD and hypertension to reduce the risk of MACE. Patients who smoke should be referred to a smoking cessation program and should avoid exposure to secondhand smoke. Diabetics with PAD should be treated with liraglutide or semaglutide or with an SGLT-2 inhibitor to reduce the risk of MACE. Exercise therapy is recommended to improve walking performance. Patients with PAD should have an annual influenza vaccination and be vaccinated to prevent COVID-19, including the boosters.

In patients with functionally limiting claudication and an inadequate response to guideline-directed medical treatment, including a structured exercise program, revascularization is a reasonable treatment to improve walking function and quality of life. Revascularization is also indicated in patients with acute limb ischemia and a salvageable limb to prevent irreversible tissue damage and major amputation.

REFERENCES

1. Dormandy JA, Rutherford RB, for the TASC Working Group. TransAtlantic Inter-Society Consensus (TASC). Management of peripheral arterial disease (PAD). *J Vasc Surg* 2000; *31*: S1–S296.
2. McDermott MM, Greenland P, Liu K et al. Sex differences in peripheral arterial disease: leg symptoms and physical functioning. *J Am Geriatr Soc* 2003; *51*: 222–228.
3. Garg PK, Liu K, Tian L et al. Physical activity during daily life and functional decline in peripheral arterial disease. *Circulation* 2009; *119*: 251–260.
4. Gerhard-Herman MD, Gornik HL, Barrett C et al. 2016 AHA/ACC guideline on the management of patients with lower extremity peripheral artery disease: executive summary. A report of the American College of Cardiology/American Heart Association Task Force on Clinical Practice Guidelines. *J Am Coll Cardiol* 2017; *69*: 1465–1508.
5. McDermott MM, Greenland P, Liu K et al. The ankle brachial index is associated with leg function and physical activity: the walking and leg circulation study. *Ann Intern Med* 2002; *136*: 873–883.
6. Criqui MH, McClelland RL, McDermott MM et al. The ankle-brachial index and incident cardiovascular events in the MESA (Multi-Ethnic Study of Atherosclerosis). *J Am Coll Cardiol* 2010; *56*: 1506–1512.
7. Allison MA, Hiatt WR, Hirsch AT et al. A high ankle-brachial index is associated with increased cardiovascular morbidity and lower quality of life. *J Am Coll Cardiol* 2008; *51*: 1292–1298.

8. Kohler TR, Nance DR, Cramer MM et al. Duplex scanning for diagnosis of aortoiliac and femoropopliteal disease: a prospective study. *Circulation* 1987; *76*: 1074–1080.
9. Sheikh MA, Bhatt DL, Li J et al. Usefulness of postexercise ankle-brachial index to predict all-cause mortality. *Am J Cardiol* 2011; *107*: 778–782.
10. Schroll M, Munck O. Estimation of peripheral arteriosclerotic disease by ankle blood pressure measurements in a population of 60-year-old men and women. *J Chron Dis* 1981; *34*: 261–269.
11. Criqui MH, Fronek A, Barrett-Connor E et al. The prevalence of peripheral arterial disease in a defined population. *Circulation* 1985; *71*: 510–515.
12. Newman A, Siscovick DS, Manolio TA et al. Ankle-arm index as a marker of atherosclerosis in the cardiovascular health study. *Circulation* 1993; *88*: 837–845.
13. Ness J, Aronow WS, Ahn C. Risk factors for peripheral arterial disease in an academic hospital-based geriatrics practice. *J Am Geriatr Soc* 2000; *48*: 312–314.
14. Meijer WT, Hoes AW, Rutgers D et al. Peripheral arterial disease in the elderly. The Rotterdam study. *Arterioscler Thromb Vasc Biol* 1998; *18*: 185–192.
15. Aronow WS, Ahn C, Gutstein H. Prevalence and incidence of cardiovascular disease in 1160 older men and 2464 older women in a long-term health care facility. *J Gerontol Med Sci* 2002; *57A*: M45–M46.
16. Aronow WS. Prevalence of atherothrombotic brain infarction, coronary artery disease and peripheral arterial disease in elderly blacks, Hispanics and whites. *Am J Cardiol* 1992; *70*: 1212–1213.
17. Ness J, Aronow WS, Newkirk E et al. Prevalence of symptomatic peripheral arterial disease, modifiable risk factors, and appropriate use of drugs in the treatment of peripheral arterial disease in older persons seen in a university general medicine clinic. *J Gerontol Med Sci* 2005; *60A*: M255–M257.
18. Hirsch AT, Criqui MH, Treat-Jacobson D et al. Peripheral arterial disease detection, awareness, and treatment in primary care. *JAMA* 2001; *286*: 1317–1324
19. Aronow WS, Sales FF, Etienne F et al. Prevalence of peripheral arterial disease and its correlation with risk factors for peripheral arterial disease in elderly patients in a long-term health care facility. *Am J Cardiol* 1988; *62*: 644–646.
20. Sukhija R, Yalamanchili K, Aronow WS. Prevalence of left main coronary artery disease, of 3-vessel or 4-vessel coronary artery disease, and of obstructive coronary artery disease in patients with and without peripheral arterial disease undergoing coronary angiography for suspected coronary artery disease. *Am J Cardiol* 2003; *92*: 304–305.
21. Aronow WS, Fleg JL, Pepine CJ et al. ACCF/AHA 2011 expert consensus document on hypertension in the elderly. A report of the American College of Cardiology Foundation Task Force on Clinical Expert Consensus Documents. Developed in collaboration with the American Academy of Neurology, American Geriatrics Society, American Society for Preventive Cardiology, American Society for Hypertension, American Society of Nephrology, Association of Black Cardiologists, and European Society of Hypertension. *J Am Coll Cardiol* 2011; *57*: 2037–2114.
22. Aronow WS, Ahn C. Correlation of serum lipids with the presence or absence of atherothrombotic brain infarction and peripheral arterial disease in 1,834 men and women aged ≥62 years. *Am J Cardiol* 1994; *73*: 995–997.
23. Aronow WS. Treatment of older persons with hypercholesterolemia with and without cardiovascular disease. *J Gerontol Med Sci* 2001; *56A*: M138–M145.
24. Aronow WS. Should hypercholesterolemia in older persons be treated to reduce cardiovascular events? *J Gerontol Med Sci* 2002; *57A*: M411–M413.
25. Aronow WS, Ahn C. Association between plasma homocysteine and peripheral arterial disease in older persons. *Coronary Artery Dis* 1998; *9*: 49–50.
26. Joseph J, Koka M, Aronow WS. Prevalence of moderate and severe renal insufficiency in older persons with hypertension, diabetes mellitus, coronary artery disease, peripheral arterial disease, ischemic stroke, or congestive heart failure in an academic nursing home. *J Am Dir Assoc* 2008; *9*: 257–259.
27. Duncan K, Aronow WS, Babu S. Prevalence of moderate or severe chronic kidney disease in patients with severe peripheral arterial disease versus mild or moderate peripheral arterial disease. *Med Sci Monit* 2010; *16*: CR584–CR587.
28. Baber U, Mann D, Shimbo D et al. Combined role of reduced estimated glomerular filtration rate and microalbuminuria on the prevalence of peripheral arterial disease. *Am J Cardiol* 2009; *104*: 1446–1451.
29. Conen D, Rexrode KM, Creager MA et al. Metabolic syndrome, inflammation, and risk of symptomatic peripheral arterial disease in women. A prospective study. *Circulation* 2009; *120*: 1041–1047.
30. Khaleghi M, Isseh IN, Bailey KR et al. Family history as a risk factor for peripheral arterial disease. *Am J Cardiol* 2014; *114*: 928–932.
31. Tison GH, Ndumele CE, Gerstenblith G et al. Usefulness of baseline obesity to predict development of a high ankle brachial index from the multi-ethnic study of atherosclerosis. *Am J Cardiol* 2011; *107*: 1386–1391.
32. Paul N, Vuddanda V, Mujib M et al. Advances in our understanding of the influence of gender on patient outcomes with peripheral arterial

disease co-occurring with diabetes. *Expert Rev of Endocrinol Metab* 2016; *11*: 271–279.
33. Mya MM, Aronow WS. Increased prevalence of peripheral arterial disease in older men and women with subclinical hypothyroidism. *J Gerontol Med Sci* 2003; *58A*: M68–M69.
34. Aronow WS, Ahn C. Prevalence of coexistence of coronary artery disease, peripheral arterial disease, and atherothrombotic brain infarction in men and women ≥62 years of age. *Am J Cardiol* 1994; *74*: 64–65.
35. Ness J, Aronow WS. Prevalence of coexistence of coronary artery disease, ischemic stroke, and peripheral arterial disease in older persons, mean age 80 years, in an academic hospital-based geriatrics practice. *J Am Geriatr Soc* 1999; *47*: 1255–1256.
36. Aronow WS, Ahn C, Kronzon I. Association of mitral annular calcium with symptomatic peripheral arterial disease in older persons. *Am J Cardiol* 2001; *88*: 333–334.
37. Aronow WS, Ahn C, Kronzon I. Association of valvular aortic stenosis with symptomatic peripheral arterial disease in older persons. *Am J Cardiol* 2001; *88*: 1046–1047.
38. Park H, Das M, Aronow WS et al. Relation of decreased ankle-brachial index to prevalence of atherosclerotic risk factors, coronary artery disease, aortic valve calcium, and mitral annular calcium. *Am J Cardiol* 2005; *95*: 1005–1006.
39. Sukhija R, Aronow WS, Yalamanchili K et al. Association of ankle-brachial index with severity of angiographic coronary artery disease in patients with peripheral arterial disease and coronary artery disease. *Cardiology* 2005; *103*: 158–160.
40. Hussein AA, Uno K, Wolski K et al. Peripheral arterial disease and progression of coronary atherosclerosis. *J Am Coll Cardiol* 2011; *57*: 1220–1225.
41. Ward RP, Goonewardena SN, Lammertin G et al. Comparison of the frequency of abnormal cardiac findings by echocardiography in patients with and without peripheral arterial disease. *Am J Cardiol* 2007; *99*: 499–503.
42. Criqui MH, Langer RD, Fronek A et al. Mortality over a period of 10 years in patients with peripheral arterial disease. *N Engl J Med.* 1992; *326*: 381–386.
43. Vogt MT, Cauley JA, Newman AB et al. Decreased ankle/arm blood pressure index and mortality in elderly women. *JAMA* 1993; *270*: 465–469
44. Aronow WS, Ahn C, Mercando AD et al. Prognostic significance of silent ischemia in elderly patients with peripheral arterial disease with and without previous myocardial infarction. *Am J Cardiol* 1992; *69*: 137–139.
45. Saw J, Bhatt DL, Moliterno DJ et al. The influence of peripheral arterial disease on outcomes. A pooled analysis of mortality in eight large randomized percutaneous coronary intervention trials. *J Am Coll Cardiol* 2006; *48*: 1567–1572.
46. Aronow WS, Ahmed MI, Ekundayo OJ et al. A propensity-matched study of the association of peripheral arterial disease with cardiovascular outcomes in community-dwelling older adults. *Am J Cardiol* 2009; *103*: 130–135.
47. Ahmed MI, Aronow WS, Criqui MH et al. Effect of peripheral arterial disease on outcomes in advanced chronic systolic heart failure. A propensity-matched study. *Circ Heart Fail* 2010; *3*: 118–124.
48. Chhabra A, Aronow WS, Ahn C et al. Incidence of new cardiovascular events in patients with and without peripheral arterial disease seen in a vascular surgery clinic. *Med Sci Monit* 2012; *18*: CR131–CR134.
49. Chen DC, Singh GD, Armstrong EJ et al. Long-term comparative outcomes of patients with peripheral artery disease with and without concomitant coronary artery disease. *Am J Cardiol* 2017; 119: 1146-1152.
50. Bouisset F, Bongard V, Ruidavets J-B et al. Prognostic usefulness of clinical and subclinical peripheral arterial disease in men with stable coronary heart disease. *Am J Cardiol* 2012; *110*: 197–202.
51. Hendel RC, Whitfield SS, Villegas BJ et al. Prediction of late cardiac events by dipyridamole thallium imaging in patients undergoing elective vascular surgery. *Am J Cardiol* 1992; *70*: 1243–1249.
52. Juergens IL, Barker NW, Hines EA. Arteriosclerosis of veterans: a review of 520 cases with special reference to pathogenic and prognostic factors. *Circulation* 1960; *21*: 188–199
53. Myers KA, King RB, Scott DF et al. The effect of smoking on the late patency of arterial reconstructions in the legs. *Br J Surg* 1978; *65*: 267–271.
54. Quick CRG, Cotton LT. The measured effect of stopping smoking on intermittent claudication. *Br J Surg* 1982; *69*(Suppl): S24–S26.
55. Creager MA, Belkin M, Bluth EI et al. 2012 ACCF/AHA/ACRSCAI/SIR/STS/SVM/SVN/SVS key data elements and definitions for peripheral atherosclerotic vascular disease. A report of the American College of Cardiology Foundation/American Heart Association Task Force on Clinical Data Standards (Writing committee to develop clinical data standards for peripheral atherosclerotic vascular disease). Developed in collaboration with the American Association of Cardiovascular and Pulmonary Rehabilitation, American Academy of Neurology, American Association of Neurological surgeons, American Diabetes Association, Society of Atherosclerosis Imaging and Prevention, Society of Cardiovascular Computed Tomography, Society for Cardiovascular Magnetic Resonance, and Vascular Disease Foundation. *J Am Coll Cardiol* 2012; *59*: 294–357.

56. Benowitz NL. Treating tobacco addiction: Nicotine or no nicotine. *N Engl J Med* 1997; *337*: 1230–1231.
57. Frishman WH, Ky T, Ismail A. Tobacco smoking, nicotine, and non-nicotine replacement therapies. *Heart Dis* 2001; *3*: 365–377.
58. Mehler PS, Coll JR, Estacio R et al. Intensive blood pressure control reduces the risk of cardiovascular events in patients with peripheral arterial disease and type 2 diabetes. *Circulation* 2003; *107*: 753–756.
59. Whelton PK, Carey RM, Aronow WS et al. 2017 ACC/AHA/AAPA/ABC/ACPM/AGS/APhA/ASH/ASPC/NMA/ PCNA Guideline for the prevention, detection, evaluation and management of high blood pressure in adults. A report of the American College of Cardiology/American Heart Association Task Force on Clinical Practice Guidelines. *J Am Coll Cardiol* 2018; *71*: e127–e248.
60. Aronow WS, Ahn C. Elderly diabetics with peripheral arterial disease and no coronary artery disease have a higher incidence of new coronary events than elderly nondiabetics with peripheral arterial disease and prior myocardial infarction treated with statins and with no lipid-lowering drug. *J Gerontol A Biol Sci Med Sci* 2003; *58*: M573–M575.
61. Aronow WS, Ahn C, Weiss MB et al. Relation of increased hemoglobin A_{1c} levels to severity of peripheral arterial disease in patients with diabetes mellitus. *Am J Cardiol* 2007; *99*: 1468–1469.
62. Stratton IM, Adler AI, Neil HAW et al. Association of glycaemia with macrovascular and microvascular complications of type 2 diabetes (UKPDS 35): prospective observational study. *Br Med J* 2000; *321*: 405–412.
63. Aronow WS, Ahn C, Gutstein H. Reduction of new coronary events and of new atherothrombotic brain infarction in older persons with diabetes mellitus, prior myocardial infarction, and serum low-density lipoprotein cholesterol ≥125 mg/dL treated with statins. *J Gerontol Med Sci* 2002; *57A*: M747–M750.
64. Stone NJ, Robinson J, Lichtenstein AH et al. 2013 ACC/AHA guideline on the treatment of blood cholesterol to reduce atherosclerotic cardiovascular risk in adults: a report on the American College of Cardiology/American Heart Association Task Force on Practice Guidelines. *J Am Coll Cardiol* 2014; *63*: 2889–2934.
65. Pedersen TR, Kjekshus J, Pyorala K et al. Effect of simvastatin on ischemic signs and symptoms in the Scandinavian Simvastatin Survival Study (4S). *Am J Cardiol* 1998; *81*: 333–336.
66. Heart Protection Study Collaborative Group. MRC/BHF Heart Protection Study of cholesterol lowering with simvastatin in 20,536 high-risk individuals: a randomised placebo-controlled trial. *Lancet* 2002; *360*: 7–22.
67. Aronow WS, Ahn C. Incidence of new coronary events in older persons with prior myocardial infarction and serum low-density lipoprotein cholesterol ≥125 mg/dL treated with statins versus no lipid-lowering drug. *Am J Cardiol* 2002; *89*: 67–69.
68. Aronow WS, Ahn C, Gutstein H. Incidence of new atherothrombotic brain infarction in older persons with prior myocardial infarction and serum low-density lipoprotein cholesterol ≥125 mg/dL treated with statins versus no lipid-lowering drug. *J Gerontol Med Sci* 2002; *57A*: M333–M335
69. Aronow WS, Ahn C. Frequency of congestive heart failure in older persons with prior myocardial infarction and serum low-density lipoprotein cholesterol ≥125 mg/dl treated with statins versus no lipid-lowering drug. *Am J Cardiol* 2002; *90*: 147–149.
70. Aronow WS, Ahn C. Frequency of new coronary events in older persons with peripheral arterial disease and serum low-density lipoprotein cholesterol ≥125 mg/dl treated with statins versus no lipid-lowering drug. *Am J Cardiol* 2002; *90*: 789–791.
71. Aronow WS, Nayak D, Woodworth S et al. Effect of simvastatin versus placebo on treadmill exercise time until the onset of intermittent claudication in older patients with peripheral arterial disease at 6 months and at 1 year after treatment. *Am J Cardiol* 2003: *92*: 711–712.
72. Mohler ER III, Hiatt WR, Creager MA for the Study Investigators. Cholesterol reduction with atorvastatin improves walking distance in patients with peripheral arterial disease. *Circulation* 2003; *108*: 1481–1486.
73. Mondillo S, Ballo P, Barbati R et al. Effects of simvastatin on walking performance and symptoms of intermittent claudication in hypercholesterolemic patients wit peripheral vascular disease. *Am J Med* 2003; *114*:359–364
74. Desai H, Aronow WS, Ahn C et al. Incidence of perioperative myocardial infarction and of 2-year mortality in 577 elderly patients undergoing noncardiac vascular surgery treated with and without statins. *Arch Gerontol Geriatr* 2010; *51*: 149–151.
75. Ghosh S, Ziesmer V, Aronow WS. Underutilization of aspirin, beta blockers, angiotensin-converting enzyme inhibitors, and lipid-lowering drugs and overutilization of calcium channel blockers in older persons with coronary artery disease in an academic nursing home. *J Gerontol Med Sci* 2002; *57A*: M398–M400.
76. Ghosh S, Aronow WS. Utilization of lipid-lowering drugs in elderly persons with increased serum low-density lipoprotein cholesterol associated with coronary artery disease, symptomatic peripheral arterial disease, prior stroke, or diabetes mellitus before and after an educational program to treat dyslipidemia. *J Gerontol Med Sci* 2003; *58A*: M432–M435.
77. Sanal S, Aronow WS. Effect of an educational program on the prevalence of use of antiplatelet drugs, beta blockers, angiotensin-converting enzyme

inhibitors, lipid-lowering drugs, and calcium channel blockers prescribed during hospitalization and at hospital discharge in patients with coronary artery disease. *J Gerontol Med Sci* 2003; *58A*: M1046–M1048.
78. Nayak D, Aronow WS. Effect of an ongoing educational program on the use of antiplatelet drugs, beta blockers, angiotensin-converting enzyme inhibitors, and lipid-lowering drugs in patients with coronary artery disease seen in an academic cardiology clinic. *Cardiol Rev* 2005; *13*: 95–97.
79. Mya MM, Aronow WS. Subclinical hypothyroidism is associated with coronary artery disease in older persons. *J Gerontol Med Sci* 2002; *57A*: M658–M659.
80. Antithrombotic Trialists' Collaboration. Collaborative meta-analysis of randomised trials of antiplatelet therapy for prevention of death, myocardial infarction, and stroke in high risk patients. *BMJ* 2002; *324*: 71–86.
81. Bonaca MP, Bhatt DL, Storey RF et al. Ticagrelor for prevention of ischemic events after myocardial infarction in patients with peripheral artery disease. *J Am Coll Cardiol* 2016; *67*: 2719–2728.
82. Hiatt WR, Fowkes FGR, Heizer G et al. Ticagrelor versus clopidogrel in symptomatic peripheral artery disease. *N Engl J Med* 2017; *376*: 32–40.
83. Chew DP, Bhatt DL, Sapp S et al. Increased mortality with oral platelet glycoprotein IIb/IIIa antagonists. A meta-analysis of phase III multicenter randomized trials. *Circulation* 2001; *103*: 201–206.
84. Roth GJ, Majerus PW. The mechanism of the effect of aspirin on human platelets: I. Acetylation of a particulate fraction protein. *J Clin Invest* 1975; *56*: 624–632.
85. Mills DC, Puri R, Hu CJ et al. Clopidogrel inhibits the binding of ADP analogues to the receptor mediating inhibition of platelet adenylate cyclase. *Arterioscler Thromb* 1992, *12*, 430–436.
86. Bonaca MP, Gutierrez JA, Creager MA et al. Acute limb ischemia and outcomes with vorapaxar in patients with peripheral artery disease. Results from the trial to assess the effects of vorapaxar in preventing heart attack and stroke in patients with atherosclerosis-thrombolysis in myocardial infarction 50 (TRA2°P-TIMI 50). *Circulation* 2016; *133*: 997–1005.
87. CAPRIE Steering Committee. A randomised, blinded, trial of clopidogrel versus aspirin in patients at risk of ischaemic events (CAPRIE). *Lancet* 1996; *348*: 1329–1339.
88. Sukhija R, Yalamanchili K, Aronow WS et al. Clinical characteristics, risk factors, and medical treatment of 561 patients with peripheral arterial disease followed in an academic vascular surgery clinic. *Cardiol Rev* 2005; *13*: 108–110.
89. Dutch Bypass Oral Anticoagulants or Aspirin (BOA) Study Group. Efficacy of oral anticoagulants compared with aspirin after infrainguinal bypass surgery (The Dutch Bypass Oral Anticoagulants or Aspirin Study): a randomized trial. *Lancet* 2000; *355*: 346–351.
90. Smith SC Jr, Blair SN, Bonow RO et al. A statement for healthcare professionals from the American Heart Association and the American College of Cardiology. *J Am Coll Cardiol* 2001; *38*: 1581–1583.
91. Ahimastos AA, Walker PJ, Askew C et al. Effect of ramipril on walking times and quality of life among patients with peripheral artery disease and intermittent claudication. A randomized controlled trial. *JAMA* 2013; *309*: 453–460.
92. Radack K, Deck C. Beta-adrenergic blocker therapy does not worsen intermittent claudication in subjects with peripheral arterial disease: meta-analysis of randomized controlled trials. *Arch Intern Med* 1991; *151*: 1769–1776.
93. Aronow WS, Ahn C. Effect of beta blockers on incidence of new coronary events in older persons with prior myocardial infarction and symptomatic peripheral arterial disease. *Am J Cardiol* 2001; *87*: 1284–1286.
94. McDermott MM, Guralnik JM, Greenland P et al. Statin use and leg functioning in patients with and without lower-extremity peripheral arterial disease. *Circulation* 2003; *107*: 757–761.
95. Pande RL, Perlstein TS, Beckman JA et al. Secondary prevention and mortality in peripheral artery disease. National Health and Nutrition Examination Study, 1999 to 2004. *Circulation* 2011; *96*: 1031–1033.
96. Hiatt WR. Medical treatment of peripheral arterial disease and claudication. *N Engl J Med* 2001; *344*: 1608–16
97. Eberhardt RT, Coffman JD. Drug treatment of peripheral vascular disease. In: Frishman WH, Sonnenblick EH, Sica DA, eds. *Cardiovascular Pharmacotherapeutics*, 2nd ed. New York: McGraw-Hill, 2003: pp. 919–934.
98. Dawson DL, Cutler BS, Meissner MH et al. Cilostazol has beneficial effects in treatment of intermittent claudication. Results from a multicenter, randomized, prospective, double-blind trial. *Circulation* 1998; *98*: 678–686.
99. Thompson PD, Zimet R, Forbes WP et al. Meta-analysis of results from eight randomized, placebo-controlled trials on the effect of cilostazol on patients with intermittent claudication. *Am J Cardiol* 2002; *90*: 1314–1319.
100. Dawson DL, Cutler BS, Hiatt WR et al. A comparison of cilostazol and pentoxifylline for treating intermittent claudication. *Am J Med* 2000; *109*: 523–530.
101. Money SR, Herd JA, Isaacsohn JL et al. Effect of cilostazol on walking distances in patients with intermittent claudication caused by peripheral vascular disease. *J Vasc Surg* 1998; *27*: 267–274.

102. Hamburg NM, Balady GJ. Exercise rehabilitation in peripheral artery disease. Functional impact and mechanisms of benefit. *Circulation* 2011; *123*: 87–97.
103. Gardner AW, Poehlman ET. Exercise rehabilitation programs for the treatment of claudication pain. A meta-analysis. *JAMA* 1995; *274*: 975–980.
104. McDermott MM, Liu K, Ferrucci L et al. Physical performance in peripheral arterial disease: a slower rate of decline in patients who walk more. *Ann Intern Med* 2006; *144*: 10–20.
105. McDermott MM, Polonsky TS. Home-based exercise. A therapeutic option for peripheral arterial disease. *Circulation* 2016; *134*: 1127–1129.
106. Fujitani RM, Gordon IL, Perera GB et al. Peripheral vascular disease in the elderly. In: Aronow WS, Fleg JL, eds. *Cardiovascular Disease in the Elderly Patient*, 3rd ed. New York: Marcel Dekker, 2003: pp. 707–763.
107. Weitz JI, Byrne J, Clagett GP et al. Diagnosis and treatment of chronic arterial insufficiency of the lower extremities: a critical review. *Circulation* 1996; *94*: 3026–3049.
108. Palmaz JC, Garcia OJ, Schatz RA et al. Placement of balloon-expandable intraluminal stents in iliac arteries. First 171 procedures. *Radiology* 1990; *174*: 969.
109. Comerota AJ. Endovascular and surgical revascularization for patients with intermittent claudication. *Am J Cardiol* 2001; *87* (Suppl): 34D–43D.
110. BASIL trial participants. Bypass versus angioplasty in severe ischaemia of the leg (BASIL): Multicentre, randomised controlled trial. *Lancet* 2005; *366*: 1925–1934.
111. Murphy TP, Cutlip DE, Regensteiner JG et al. Supervised exercise versus primary stenting for claudication resulting from aortoiliac peripheral artery disease. Six-month outcomes from the Claudication: exercise Versus Endoluminal Revascularization (CLEVER) study. *Circulation* 2012; *125*: 130–139.
112. Nordanstig J, Taft C, Hensater M et al. Improved quality of life after 1 year with an invasive versus a noninvasive treatment strategy in claudicants. One-year results of the Invasive Revascularization or Not in Intermittent Claudication (IRONIC) trial. *Circulation* 2014; *130*: 939–947.
113. Tsai TT, Rehring TF, Rogers RK et al. The contemporary safety and effectiveness of lower extremity bypass surgery and peripheral endovascular interventions in the treatment of symptomatic peripheral arterial disease. *Circulation* 2015; *132*: 1999–2011.
114. Fakhry F, Spronk S, van der Laan L et al. Endovascular revascularization and supervised exercise for peripheral arterial disease and intermittent claudication. A randomized clinical trial. *JAMA* 2015; *314*: 1936–1944.
115. McDermott MM, Kibbe MR. Improving lower extremity functioning in peripheral artery disease. Exercise, endovascular revascularization, or both? *JAMA* 2017; *317*: 689–690.
116. Hess CN, Norgren L, Ansel GM et al. A structured review of antithrombotic therapy in peripheral artery disease with a focus on revascularization. A TASC (Intersociety Consensus for the Management of Peripheral Artery Disease) initiative. *Circulation* 2017; *135*: 2534–2555.
117. DeFrang RD, Taylor LM Jr, Porter JM. Basic data related to amputations. *Ann Vasc Surg* 1991; *5*: 202–207.
118. Sule S, Aronow WS, Babu S. Prevalence of risk factors and of coronary artery disease, ischemic stroke, carotid arterial disease and lower extremity peripheral arterial disease in 96 patients undergoing elective surgery for an abdominal aneurysm. *Int J Angiol* 2008; *17*: 141–142.
119. Forsdahl SH, Singh K, Solberg S et al. Risk factors for abdominal aortic aneurysms. A 7-year prospective study: the Tromsø study, 1994–2001. *Circulation* 2009; *119*: 2202–2208.
120. Sukhija R, Aronow WS, Yalamanchili K et al. Prevalence of coronary artery disease, lower extremity peripheral arterial disease, and cerebrovascular disease in 110 men with an abdominal aortic aneurysm. *Am J Cardiol* 2004; *94*: 1358–1359.
121. Norman PE, Powell JT. Abdominal aortic aneurysm. The prognosis in women is worse. *Circulation* 2007; *115*: 2865–2869.
122. Sullivan CA, Rohrer MJ, Cutler BS. Clinical management of the symptomatic but unruptured abdominal aortic aneurysm. *J Vasc Surg* 1990; *11*: 799–803.
123. Sukhija R, Aronow WS, Mathew J et al. Treatment of abdominal aortic aneurysms with an endovascular stent-graft prosthesis in 96 high-risk patients. *Cardiol Rev* 2005; *13*: 165–166.
124. Hackam DG, Thiruchelvam D, Redelmeier DA. Angiotensin-converting enzyme inhibitors and aortic rupture: a population-based case-control study. *Lancet* 2006; *368*: 659–665.
125. Sukhija R, Aronow WS, Sandhu R et al. Mortality and size of abdominal aortic aneurysm at long-term follow-up of patients not treated surgically and treated with and without statins. *Am J Cardiol* 2006; *97*: 279–280.
126. Kertai MD, Boersma E, Westerhout CM et al. Association between long-term statin use and mortality after successful abdominal aortic aneurysm surgery. *Am J Med* 2004; *116*: 96–103.
127. The United Kingdom EVAR Trial investigators. Endovascular repair of aortic aneurysm in patients physically ineligible for open repair. *N Engl J Med* 2010; *362*: 1872–1880.
128. Schermerhorn ML, Buck DB, O'Malley AJ et al. Long-term outcomes of abdominal aortic aneurysm

in the Medicare population. *N Engl J Med* 2015; *373*: 328–338.

129. Abramson BL, Al-Omran M, Anand SS et al. Canadian Cardiovascular Society 2022 Guidelines for peripheral arterial disease. *Can J Cardiol* 2022; *38*: 560–587.
130. Hartmann-Boyce J, Livingstone-Banks J, Ordonez-Mena JM et al. Behavioural interventions for smoking cessation: an overview and network meta-analysis. *Cochrane Database Syst Rev* 2021; *1*: CD013229.
131. Hartmann-Boyce J, McRobbie H, LindsonN et al. Electronic cigarettes for smoking cessation. *Cochrane Database Syst Rev* 2021; *4*: CD010216.
132. Howes S, Hartmann-Boyce J, Livingstone Banks J et al. Antidepressants for smoking cessation. *Cochrane Database Syst Rev* 2020; *4*: CD.000031
133. Shang XEF, Guo K, Yang C et al. Effectiveness and safety of varenicline for smoking cessation: an overview and meta-analysis. *J Addict Med* 2023; *17*:P 536–543.
134. Bonaca MP, Wiviott SD, ZelnikerTA et al. Dapagliflozin and cardiac, kidney, and limb outcomes in patients with and without peripheral artery disease in DECLARE TIMI 58. *Circulation* 2020; *142*: 734–747.
135. Pearson GJ, Thanassoulis G, Anderson DJ et al. Canadian Cardiovascular Society guidelines for the management of dyslipidemia for the prevention of cardiovascular disease in adults. *Can J Cardiol* 2021; *37*: 1129–1150
136. Belch JJF, Brodmann M, Baumgartner I et al. Lipid-lowering and anti-thrombotic therapy in patients with peripheral arterial disease: European Atherosclerosis Society/European Society of Vascular Medicine joint statement. *Atherosclerosis* 2021; *338*: 55–63.
137. Armstrong FJ, Chen DC, Singh GD et al. Angiotensin-converting enzyme inhibitor or angiotensin receptor blocker use is associated with reduced major adverse cardiovascular events among patients with critical limb ischemia. *Vasc Med* 2015; *20*: 237–244.
138. Hess CN, Debus ES, Nehler MR et al. Reduction in acute limb ischemia with rivaroxaban versus placebo in peripheral artery disease after lower extremity revascularization: insights from VOYAGER PAD. *Circulation* 2021; *144*: 1831–1841.
139. Anand SS, Bosch J, Eikelboom JW et al. Rivaroxaban with or without aspirin in patients with stable peripheral or carotid artery disease: an international, randomized, double-blind, placebo-controlled trial. *Lancet* 2018; *391*: 219–229.
140. Kaplovitch E, Eikelboom JW, Dyal L et al. Rivaroxaban and aspirin in patients with symptomatic lower extremity peripheral artery disease: a subanalysis of the COMPASS randomized clinical trial. *JAMA Cardiology* 2021; *6*: 21–29.
141. Hiatt WR, Bonaca MP, Patel MR et al. Rivaroxaban and aspirin in peripheral artery disease revascularization: impact of concomitant clopidogrel on efficacy and safety. *Circulation* 2020; *142*: 2219–2230.
142. Caruso B, Maiorino MI, Longo M et al. Liraglutide for lower limb perfusion in people with type 2 diabetes and peripheral artery disease: the STARDUST randomized clinical trial. *JAMA Network Open* 2024; *7*: e241545.
143. Nordanstig J, Behrendt CA, Baumgartner I et al. European Society for Vascular Surgery (ESVS) 2024 clinical practice guidelines on the management of asymptomatic peripheral artery disease and intermittent claudication. *Eur J Vasc Endovasc Surg* 2024; *67*: 9–96.
144. Mach F, Baigent C, Catapano AL et al. 2019 ESC/EAS guidelines for the management of dyslipidaemias: lipid modification to reduce cardiovascular risk. *Eur Heart J* 2020; *44*: 111–118.
145. Visseren FLJ, Mach F, Smulders YM et al. 2021 ESC guidelines on cardiovascular disease prevention in clinical practice. *Eur Heart J* 2021; *42*: 3227–3337.
146. American Diabetes Association. Pharmacologic approaches to glycemic treatment: standards of medical care in diabetes–2021. *Diabetes Care* 2021; *44*: S111–S124.
147. Kraus WE, Powell KE, Haskell WL et al. Physical activity, all-cause and cardiovascular mortality, and cardiovascular disease. *Med Sci Sports Exerc* 2019; *51*: 1270–1281.
148. Gornik HL, Aronow HD, Goodney PP et al. 2024 ACC/AHA/ AACVPR/APMA/ABC/SCAI/SVM/SVN/SVS/SIR/VESS guideline for the management of lower extremity peripheral artery disease. *J Amer Coll Card* 2024; *83*: 2497–2604.

28

Perioperative cardiovascular evaluation and treatment of older adults undergoing noncardiac surgery

JEANNA D. BLITZ

Key points

- The preoperative evaluation of older adults has expanded beyond a limited risk assessment.
- The impact of preoperative interventions on long-term health outcomes should be considered.
- A broader approach to preoperative evaluation is now recommended. The identification and management of additional conditions (e.g., CIEDs, frailty, anemia, atrial fibrillation, and valvular heart disease) that increase perioperative risk are emphasized. These have not been well captured in historic surgical risk calculators.
- An estimation of functional capacity using a standardized tool such as the Duke Activity Status Index (DASI) is preferred over subjective assessment.
- Overtesting without clear opportunities for risk modification should be avoided.
- Multiple validated risk scoring tools exist; the most commonly used are the Revised Cardiac Risk Index (RCRI), the Gupta MICA score, and the American College of Surgeons NSQIP score.
- Perioperative measurement of biomarkers, including brain natriuretic peptide (BNP) or N-terminal fragment of pro-BNP (NT-proBNP), is recommended in patients at increased risk of MACE undergoing elevated risk surgery to improve risk prediction.
- Postoperative surveillance for myocardial injury after noncardiac surgery (MINS) should be considered in patients at elevated risk of MACE.
- The approach to the anesthetic care of the older surgical patient should be individualized based upon both patient- and surgery-specific factors.

DOI: 10.1201/9781003568933-28

INTRODUCTION

Over 5 million patients over the age of 65 years undergo noncardiac surgery annually in the United States.[3] The health care costs associated with adverse cardiac outcomes have been estimated to exceed $10 billion annually in the United States;[7] the costs of caring for frail patients after surgery are estimated to be 1.5 times greater.[1,5] With the shifting demographics of the US population, there is an increased need to identify those at highest risk of perioperative events and apply strategies to reduce their risk. However, preoperative risk-reduction interventions are often time and resource intensive and are only effective when applied to patients with significant, modifiable vulnerability and timed far enough in advance of surgery to make a clinically relevant impact.[6,7]

The preoperative evaluation and preparation of the older adult patient undergoing noncardiac surgery represent a unique challenge for the multidisciplinary care team. Undergoing surgery and anesthesia can result in significant morbidity in older adults, including postoperative cognitive decline, non-home discharge, decreased functional capacity, loss of the ability to independently perform activities of daily living, and lack of autonomy.[11] Global risk prediction models have become far more accurate for individual patients than prior risk scales and scores; however, no risk prediction model accounts for all factors that impact perioperative outcomes, including health behaviors and social drivers of health.[7] The decision to pursue cardiac testing preoperatively should be based upon the likelihood that the test result will necessitate a change in the perioperative management plan versus the likelihood that the test may cause harm or unnecessary costs and delays in surgery.[2] As a population, older adults are not well represented in current clinical trial data, making the extrapolation of study results to clinical decision-making in real-world clinical scenarios for older adults challenging. It is important not to perform testing unless the results will affect perioperative management and to consider alternative or palliative options when reasonable.[5] As the older adult surgical population grows, a deeper and more nuanced appreciation for what matters most to older adults has emerged: maintenance of independence, avoidance of physical and cognitive disability, and quality of life are cited as more important than length of life in many older adults.[6] A critical component of a thorough preoperative evaluation and consultation is discussion with the patient about how they define quality of life and their long-term health goals.

For many patients, the preoperative evaluation may be their first comprehensive health assessment in a long time, if ever.[12] Therefore, strategies to assess and modify perioperative cardiac risk may also have an important impact on the patient's long term health outcomes. We will highlight the factors associated with greatest perioperative risk in older adults and present perioperative interventions that may modify that risk.

Risk of major adverse cardiac events (MACE), including cardiac mortality, remains a focus of the preoperative evaluation of patients undergoing noncardiac surgery. This is especially relevant in older adults, who are more likely to have established cardiovascular disease and increased risk for MACE compared to younger patients without risk factors for cardiovascular disease.

There are several important physiologic cardiovascular changes that occur with aging that should be considered for the management of older surgical patients. Left ventricular (LV) wall thickness increases due to an increase in the size of cardiac myocytes. There is also an increased incidence of diastolic dysfunction and elevated left atrial pressures. Intimal thickening and stiffness may increase in the vasculature. These changes result in decreased resilience by the cardiovascular system in response to perioperative stress such as hemodynamic instability.[4] The presence of heart failure, even with preserved ejection fraction, increases the risk of perioperative mortality.[2]

Brain natriuretic peptide (BNP) is a hormone released from the ventricles in the presence of stretch.[10] Obtaining a preoperative BNP or N-terminal pro–B-type natriuretic peptide (NT-proBNP) is a low-cost, accessible way to enhance risk prediction in older adults with signs and symptoms of heart failure and poor functional capacity.[2,10–13] Baseline levels of serum BNP may be elevated in older adults compared to younger adults; however, an increase greater than 200–300 ng/mL has been recommended as associated with increased risk of MACE.[2,12]

ASSESSMENT OF THE PATIENT BEFORE NONCARDIAC SURGERY

History taking

MACE remains a leading cause of perioperative morbidity and mortality in older adults. Over time, the adverse events included within the composite outcome described as MACE have expanded to include death, cardiac arrest, myocardial infarction, stroke, malignant arrhythmia, hospitalization, heart failure, and myocardial injury after non-cardiac surgery (MINS).[14,15] Therefore, a key component of the preoperative consultation is a review of the patient's cardiovascular risk factors and symptoms of active cardiac conditions (Table 28.1). Patients with active cardiac conditions (unstable coronary syndromes, decompensated heart failure [HF], significant arrhythmias, severe valvular disease) should generally have these conditions corrected before proceeding with elective noncardiac surgery.[2] Appropriate use criteria and existing guidelines and practice parameters from the non-perioperative arena may be applied. The results of this risk assessment and evaluation process will drive recommendations for further testing or preoperative interventions to reduce perioperative risk and inform the shared decision-making discussion about whether the proposed

Table 28.1 Clinical predictors of increased perioperative cardiovascular risk (MI, CHF, death)

Active cardiac conditions
Unstable coronary syndromes
• Unstable or severe angina[a] (CCS class III or IV)[b]
• Recent MI[c]
Decompensated HF (NYHA functional class IV; worsening or new-onset HF)
Significant arrhythmias
• High-grade atrioventricular block
• Mobitz II atrioventricular block
• Third-degree atrioventricular heart block
• Symptomatic ventricular arrhythmias
• Supraventricular arrhythmias (including AF) with uncontrolled ventricular rate
• HR >100/min at rest
• Symptomatic bradycardia
• Newly recognized VT
Severe valvular disease
• Severe aortic stenosis (mean pressure gradient >40 mmHg, aortic valve area <1.0 cm^2, or symptomatic)
• Symptomatic mitral stenosis (progressive dyspnea on exertion, exertional presyncope, or heart failure)
Clinical predictors of risk in RCRI
History of ischemic heart disease
History of compensated or prior HF
History of cerebrovascular disease
Diabetes mellitus
Renal insufficiency

Abbreviations: AF, atrial fibrillation; CCS, Canadian Cardiovascular Society; CHF, congestive heart failure; ECG, electrocardiogram; HF, heart failure; HR, heart rate; MI, myocardial infarction; NYHA, New York Heart Association; RCRI, Revised Cardiac Risk Index; VT, ventricular tachycardia.

Source: Fleisher LA et al., *Circulation*, 120, e169–e276, 2009.

[a] May include "stable" angina in patients who are unusually sedentary.

[b] Campeau L, *Circulation*, 54, 522–523, 1976.

[c] The American College of Cardiology National Database Library defines recent MI as >7 days but <30 days.

surgery is aligned with the individual patient's longer-term goals.[2]

Several cardiac risk scores and models are widely available to estimate perioperative cardiac risk in patients before noncardiac surgery. Historically, the most widely used risk score has been the revised cardiac risk index (RCRI).[2,16] This risk index is based on six independent predictors of complications, including patient factors (e.g., renal failure, diabetes, age) and surgery-specific factors (emergency, severity of surgery).[16] Risk prediction models such as the Gupta MICA score[14] and the American College of Surgeons global NSQIP score[17] have become more widely accessible and have increased in use as part of a perioperative risk assessment process in recent years. Risk prediction models are discussed in more detail later.

Exercise tolerance is one of the most important determinants of perioperative risk.[17] A high level of exercise tolerance is associated with a low risk of adverse perioperative cardiac events. Estimated energy requirements for various activities can be defined by metabolic equivalent (MET) levels, where 1 MET equals resting energy expenditure of approximately 3.5 mL oxygen/kg/min. Perioperative cardiac risk is increased in patients unable to achieve 4 METs during normal daily activities.[18] Estimation of MET capacity can be done accurately by using simple questionnaires that have been developed for this purpose, such as the Duke Activity Status Index (DASI)[19,20] and MET-REPAIR.[21] The DASI is a 13-question survey with a maximum of 58.2 points.[19] A DASI score of <34 points is associated with an increased risk of adverse cardiac events.[22] While responses to the MET-REPAIR Questionnaire correlate well with METs measured by cardiopulmonary exercise testing (CPET), self-reported physical exertion correlate poorly with objectively measured METs.[21]

Disease-specific approach

CORONARY ARTERY DISEASE

Symptoms suggestive of cardiovascular disease, such as chest pain and dyspnea on exertion, should be carefully elicited. In patients with symptomatic coronary artery disease (CAD), the preoperative evaluation may identify an increase in the frequency or pattern of anginal symptoms. It is important to realize that certain populations of patients, such as older adults, women, and people with diabetes mellitus (DM), may present with more atypical symptoms of angina pectoris. Often, the presence of other comorbidities may obscure the detection of angina, such as concomitant dyspnea from pulmonary disease or physical deconditioning and limited activity/mobility. The mortality of acute myocardial infarction (MI) increases dramatically with age. If unstable angina is present, there is associated high perioperative risk of MI.[23] Stable angina is also associated with increased perioperative risk of MACE; patients with significant functional limitations may require additional preoperative cardiovascular testing or perioperative monitoring, depending on the clinical scenario.

Clinicians should conduct a thorough patient history and review of prior medical and surgical cardiac interventions in patients who report symptoms suggestive of CAD. Key questions include: (1) What is the exercise threshold that produces ischemia? (2) What is the patient's LV function? (3) Is the patient on an optimal guideline-directed medical therapy (GDMT) regimen? Current guidelines do not recommend coronary revascularization before noncardiac surgery, unless the patient is a candidate for coronary revascularization independent of the need for surgery. This guidance is based upon evidence from a clinical trial that failed to demonstrate a reduction in MACE via preoperative revascularization in patients with CAD.[24] For patients with known CAD and/or poor functional capacity undergoing elevated risk surgery, coronary computed tomography angiography (CCTA) may be considered to detect high-risk coronary anatomy; however, CCTA is known to overestimate the risk of MACE.[2] Testing, particularly cardiopulmonary exercise testing, may also be indicated to assess risk as part of the decision regarding the indication for surgery as opposed to nonsurgical treatment or palliative care.

The risk of perioperative events increases after an MI. Although early studies demonstrated an increased incidence of reinfarction if surgery was performed within 6 months of an MI, this time interval has evolved in the current era of thrombolytics, endovascular stenting, and aggressive medical management.[25–27] Timing of planned noncardiac surgery (NCS) in patients post-MI should be decided based upon consensus of the multidisciplinary team using shared decision-making.[2] Elective NCS should be scheduled for at least 14 days after balloon angioplasty without stent placement. Ideally, elective NCS should be delayed for 1 year after ACS with coronary stent placement if antiplatelet agents will require interruption.

HYPERTENSION

Hypertension (HTN) is a common condition in older adults. Although mild to moderate HTN is not an independent predictor of postoperative cardiac complications, extreme blood pressure elevation in the postoperative period, defined as a diastolic blood pressure greater than 120 mmHg with clinical evidence of impending or actual end-organ damage, poses a risk of MI and cerebrovascular accident. If the preoperative evaluation establishes HTN as mild or moderate, antihypertensive medications should be continued perioperatively, and blood pressure should be maintained near preoperative levels to reduce the risk of myocardial ischemia. In patients unable to take oral medications, parenteral β-blockers and transdermal clonidine may be used. In patients with more severe HTN, such as diastolic blood pressure higher than 110 mmHg, the potential benefits of delaying surgery to optimize antihypertensive medications should be weighed against the risk of delaying the surgical procedure.[2] A randomized trial of treated hypertensive patients without known CAD who presented the morning of surgery with an elevated diastolic blood pressure was unable to demonstrate any difference in outcome between those who were actively treated with intranasal nifedipine versus those in whom surgery was delayed.[28]

VALVULAR HEART DISEASE

Valvular heart disease is frequently encountered in older patients undergoing surgical procedures. The ACC/AHA guidelines indicate that severe valvular disease is a major clinical predictor of increased perioperative cardiovascular risk.[2] Patients with suspected valvular disease should undergo echocardiography to quantify the severity of valvular dysfunction. Those with known valvular disease of moderate severity or greater should undergo preoperative echocardiography if there is no recent echocardiogram in the past year or if there is a change in clinical status since the last evaluation. In addition to the hemodynamic considerations, the management of anticoagulation in the perioperative period in patients with prosthetic heart valves is an important consideration.[2]

AORTIC STENOSIS

Aortic stenosis is more common in men, with increased prevalence in older adults, and usually results from degenerative calcific aortic valve disease in this population. A substantially higher rate of perioperative complications has been reported in patients with severe aortic stenosis, compared with patients with moderate aortic stenosis—31% (5/16) versus 11% (10/92).[29] If the aortic stenosis is symptomatic, elective noncardiac surgery should generally be postponed until an intervention is performed to address the stenosis. An open surgical aortic valve replacement (AVR) or a transcatheter AVR (TAVR) might be indicated before non-time-sensitive noncardiac surgery. If a patient is not a candidate for AVR, percutaneous balloon aortic valvuloplasty may be reasonable as a bridge to surgery in hemodynamically unstable adult patients with aortic stenosis who require urgent noncardiac surgery.[2] The 2024 ACC/AHA guidelines provide a class 2b recommendation for proceeding with elective low-risk surgery in asymptomatic patients with moderate or severe aortic stenosis and normal LV systolic function as assessed by echocardiography within the past year.[2]

In patients with asymptomatic, severe aortic stenosis, including older adults, who undergo noncardiac surgery, intraoperative hypotension should be recognized promptly and treated aggressively with vasopressors, such as phenylephrine. Adequate preload should be maintained throughout the perioperative period. Maintenance of sinus rhythm is important since the atrial contraction contributes significantly to ventricular filling in patients with severe aortic stenosis.

General anesthesia may be preferable to spinal anesthesia in patients with aortic stenosis because the vasodilation and reduction in afterload associated with the onset of sympathetic blockade from spinal anesthesia may be undesirable. Patients with severe aortic stenosis may also benefit from close postoperative hemodynamic monitoring in an intensive care unit.[30]

MITRAL STENOSIS

Patients with severe mitral stenosis are at increased risk for complications from noncardiac surgery and should be managed similarly to patients with aortic stenosis. The major concerns in the patient with mitral stenosis undergoing noncardiac surgery are (1) maintaining hemodynamic stability and (2) decreasing the incidence of perioperative arrhythmia such as atrial fibrillation (AF). Increases in heart rate reduce LV filling across the stenotic mitral valve and increase the transmitral pressure gradient. Patients with mitral stenosis can become symptomatic with tachycardia, which frequently manifests during the perioperative period. β-Blockers may be used to reduce heart rate in an attempt to optimize hemodynamic conditions. Antiarrhythmic agents may be considered to prevent the development of AF since this arrhythmia is particularly likely in these patients.

PROSTHETIC HEART VALVES

The management of chronic anticoagulation in the perioperative period is of major importance in patients with mechanical prosthetic heart valves. The risk of temporarily discontinuing anticoagulation must be weighed against the benefit of a reduced risk of perioperative bleeding for all patients on chronic anticoagulation, especially those with prosthetic heart valves. In general, the incidence of thromboembolism in patients with valvular heart disease depends on the position of the valve involved, the type of prosthetic heart valve, the existence of concomitant heart disease, the presence of left atrial enlargement, and whether AF is present.

In patients at low risk of thrombosis, defined as those with a bileaflet mechanical AVR with no high-risk factors (AF, previous thromboembolism, LV dysfunction, hypercoagulable conditions, older-generation thrombogenic valves, mechanical tricuspid valves, or more than one mechanical valve), it is recommended that warfarin be stopped 5 days before the procedure and restarted the day after the procedure. A heparin bridge is rarely indicated. In patients at high risk of thrombosis, defined as those with any mechanical mitral valve replacement or a mechanical AVR with any high-risk factor, parenteral heparin should be started when the INR falls below the desired therapeutic range (typically 72 hours before surgery), stopped before the procedure, restarted as early after surgery as bleeding stability allows, and continued until the INR is again therapeutic with warfarin therapy.[2]

The use of low-molecular-weight heparins (LMWHs) in preoperative warfarin anticoagulation bridging was investigated in a multicenter, single-arm cohort study[31] of high-risk patients (prosthetic valves, AF, and a major risk factor). Warfarin was held for 5 days; LMWHs were given 3 days preoperatively and at least 4 days postoperatively. The overall rate of thromboembolism was 3.6%, and the overall rate of cardioembolism was 0.9%. Major bleeding was seen in 6.7% of subjects, although only 8 of 15 episodes occurred during LMWH administration. Regardless of the form of bridging therapy, it is recommended that warfarin be restarted as soon as possible following surgery, and that LMWH be resumed and continued until oral anticoagulation is in the therapeutic range.[2]

CONGESTIVE HEART FAILURE

The presence of HF preoperatively is associated with an increased incidence of perioperative cardiac morbidity.[2,16,32] Optimization of symptoms of pulmonary congestion and volume overload is prudent prior to elective surgery. Diastolic filling abnormalities are particularly common in older patients and may increase the risk of developing symptomatic HF or AF in the perioperative period.

DIASTOLIC DYSFUNCTION

Chronic hypertension results in concentric left ventricular hypertrophy (LVH), normal or above-normal systolic function, and diastolic dysfunction. In the older adult patient with marked concentric LVH and small end-systolic chamber sizes, diastolic dysfunction can lead to pulmonary congestion. The pathophysiology of this condition lies in impaired relaxation and increased LV diastolic stiffness. Increases in LV diastolic stiffness will mandate higher left atrial pressures to maintain filling and thus promote elevated pulmonary venous pressures and pulmonary congestion when left atrial pressures are elevated or promote reduced cardiac output when left atrial pressures are not elevated.

This population may be particularly sensitive to factors that affect diastolic filling of the LV, such as increased heart rate, AF, or volume depletion. Identifying patients with chronically elevated blood pressure and diastolic dysfunction via echocardiography may guide optimal perioperative fluid and blood pressure management.

Increased sympathetic nervous system activity may produce increases in blood pressure and heart rate as the patient emerges from anesthesia. This response may compromise diastolic filling, so it is critical to assess volume status at this time and may warrant continuous invasive hemodynamic monitoring in certain clinical scenarios.

ARRHYTHMIAS

Cardiac arrhythmias and conduction disturbances are common in the perioperative period, particularly in the geriatric patient population. High-grade atrioventricular block, symptomatic ventricular arrhythmias in the presence of underlying heart disease, and supraventricular arrhythmias with an uncontrolled ventricular response are considered major clinical predictors of increased perioperative risk.[2] The management of perioperative ventricular arrhythmias is not well studied. Reversible causes such as electrolyte disturbances, acid-base abnormalities, or decompensated HF should be corrected. A search for underlying cardiac or pulmonary disease or for potential drug toxicity is essential. More recent detailed studies using continuous electrocardiogram (ECG) monitoring found that asymptomatic ventricular arrhythmias, including couplets and nonsustained ventricular tachycardia, were not associated with an increase in cardiac complications after noncardiac surgery.[33] Nonsustained ventricular arrhythmias, whether single premature ventricular contractions, complex ventricular ectopy, or ventricular tachycardia, usually do not require therapy unless they result in hemodynamic compromise. No studies support the suppression of preoperative arrhythmias with antiarrhythmic drugs to reduce surgical morbidity and mortality.[33]

ATRIAL FIBRILLATION

The incidence of chronic AF doubles with each decade beginning at the age of 60 years; by the age of 80–89 years, the incidence of AF is estimated to be 8%–10%. The median age of patients with AF in the United States is about 75 years, with approximately 70% of such patients with AF between the ages of 65 and 85 years. The incidence of postoperative AF ranges from 0.37% to 30%. It usually occurs within the first 2 days postoperatively. Risk factors include older age, male sex, and preoperative tachycardia.[4] In patients undergoing vascular surgery, new-onset AF in the immediate perioperative period is associated with a more than sixfold increase in cardiovascular death, MI, unstable angina, and stroke in the first 30 days, and a fourfold increase in these endpoints over the next 12 months.

The main goal of treatment is to control the ventricular rate with nodal blocking agents, including β-blockers and calcium channel blockers (diltiazem, verapamil). Use of digoxin is reserved for patients who are refractory to these medications and in some cases of systolic HF. Caution should be exercised in using β-blockers and diltiazem in patients with systolic HF, as they can impair inotropy and result in worsening systolic function. Amiodarone can also be used in the acute postoperative setting for rate or rhythm control. The indication for electric cardioversion remains the same as for the general management of AF: when hemodynamic instability is present. The risks of cardioversion causing an embolic event should be weighed against the benefits of rhythm control.[2,34]

Management of anticoagulation for stroke prophylaxis is addressed on a case-by-case basis based on the ischemic event benefit and individual bleeding risk. In previous decades, warfarin, a vitamin K antagonist, was the most common anticoagulant used for stroke prophylaxis in patients with AF or mechanical heart valves, and for treatment of thromboembolism. However, there is increasing use of oral anticoagulants, including rivaroxaban, apixaban, and dabigatran, for stroke prophylaxis in AF and for treatment of thromboembolism. Specific novel oral anticoagulants are readily reversible with the administration of andexanet alfa or idarucizumab, respectively.[2]

The decision of whether and when to hold anticoagulation preoperatively depends upon the type of surgery being performed and associated bleeding risk, the thrombotic risk of being off anticoagulation, renal function, and planned use of neuraxial anesthesia. The PAUSE trial demonstrated that in older adult patients, not bridging with parenteral anticoagulation was noninferior to bridging for prevention of embolic events and superior to bridging in preventing bleeding events.[35] It is rare that the novel anticoagulants require bridging with parenteral anticoagulation, though unique situations may exist. Higher-risk procedures require team-based decision-making involving the proceduralist, the cardiologist and/or physician prescribing the anticoagulation, and the anesthesiologist. Patients scheduled to undergo neuraxial anesthesia should be counseled to hold oral anticoagulation for 72 hours prior to surgery. For other clinical scenarios of high-risk bleeding and normal renal function, novel oral anticoagulants may be held for 48 hours prior to the procedure.[2,36]

STROKE AND TRANSIENT ISCHEMIC ATTACK

Patients with a history of stroke or transient ischemic attack are at risk of recurrent stroke or worsening of neurological deficits perioperatively. Ideally, noncardiac surgery should be delayed for 3 months after the most recent cerebrovascular event to reduce the incidence of recurrent stroke and MACE.[37] While this risk decreases over time as inflammation subsides and cerebral autoregulation is reestablished, perioperative risk after stroke never returns to baseline. Patients with a history of stroke have a 12% recurrence rate over the subsequent 5 years.[2]

FRAILTY

Frailty represents a state of diminished reserves and increased vulnerability to stressors in the perioperative period.[38] Patients with frailty syndrome or who lack reserve in domains such as physical function, nutritional status, cognitive function, or social support are at increased risk of postoperative complications and require higher resource utilization for their perioperative care. Although frailty is not solely a geriatric syndrome, frailty is a common finding in older adults. All patients over age 65 years who are planning to undergo elevated-risk NCS should be screened for frailty preoperatively using a validated frailty screening tool.[2] Early preoperative identification of frailty may lead to better perioperative outcomes via the application of patient-specific interventions designed to improve functional capacity, nutrition, and psychological state, known as prehabilitation.[39] A recent systematic review and meta-analysis of the impact of prehabilitation for patients (mean age 64 years) undergoing orthopedic surgery revealed improvements in preoperative function, muscle strength, pain, and health-related quality of life, as well as improvements in postoperative function at 6 weeks and 6 months after surgery in patients who participated in prehabilitation compared to patients who received standard of care.[40]

ELEMENTS OF PHYSICAL EXAMINATION

Blood pressure and heart rate measurements in both the supine and standing positions are useful to assess intravascular volume status or autonomic dysfunction, which may be present in older adults. Careful cardiac auscultation may detect clinically important cardiac findings, including the presence of an S_3 gallop suggestive of HF and murmurs suggestive of significant valvular disease, particularly aortic stenosis. The pulmonary exam and evaluation of the jugular venous pulsations and lower extremity edema can also help determine intravascular volume status and the presence of HF. Peripheral arterial pulses that are diminished or bruits may suggest peripheral vascular disease or the presence of occult atherosclerotic disease.

APPROACH TO THE PATIENT

The decision to undertake further testing depends on the interaction of the clinical risk factors, surgery-specific risk, and functional capacity.

The identification of perioperative cardiac risk has been studied for three decades, and much of the work has focused on the development of clinical risk indices. The guidelines present a multitude of options including the RCRI, the Gupta MICA score, and the ACS NSQIP risk prediction model.

More recently, the American College of Surgeons created the National Surgery Quality Improvement Program Perioperative MI and Cardiac Arrest (NSQIP MICA) risk calculator, more commonly known as the Gupta risk model.[14] Based on multivariate logistic regression analysis, five predictors of perioperative MI or cardiac arrest were identified: type of surgery, dependent functional status, abnormal creatinine, American Society of Anesthesiologists Physical Status classification, and increasing age. The risk model was subsequently validated on multiple data sets and compared to the RCRI. Its predictive performance surpasses that of the RCRI.[14,41]

Another risk calculator was also created by the American College of Surgeons known as the NSQIP Surgical Risk Calculator.[17] Unlike the two aforementioned risk calculators that are specific to cardiovascular events, this calculator assesses the risk of numerous other types of adverse events (15 total). It incorporates 20 preoperative risk factors and therefore has more discriminative ability than the MICA-specific risk calculator. However, the amount of data required to calculate risk also makes it more time consuming and requires a web-based-only calculator.

DIAGNOSTIC TESTING

Resting electrocardiography

A routine ECG before noncardiac surgery based solely on age is no longer recommended.[2,42] Therefore, the clinical history and surgical risk of the patient should be utilized to determine the need for an immediate preoperative ECG. A preoperative resting ECG is recommended for patients with known coronary heart disease, peripheral arterial disease, or cerebrovascular disease who are undergoing intermediate-risk surgical procedures. A preoperative resting ECG should also be performed in any patient with at least one clinical risk factor who is undergoing vascular surgical procedures, and it is reasonable for an ECG to be performed in patients without clinical indicators undergoing vascular surgery.

It has been estimated that up to 30% of MIs are silent and only detected on routine ECG by the presence of Q waves, especially in patients with DM and HTN.[43] The baseline ECG has limited applicability in the assessment of myocardial ischemia but may be useful to detect significant conduction disturbances and arrhythmias. ECG abnormalities may not always lead to delay of a noncardiac surgical procedure.

High-grade atrioventricular block, symptomatic ventricular arrhythmias in the presence of underlying heart disease, and supraventricular arrhythmias with uncontrolled ventricular rate are considered high-risk clinical predictors by the ACC/AHA guidelines.[2] Pathological Q waves are considered intermediate-risk clinical predictors. The presence of LVH, left bundle branch block, ST-segment abnormalities, and rhythm other than sinus is considered a minor risk predictor. Despite the absence of evidence to suggest that a 12-lead ECG is required in all patients immediately prior to noncardiac surgery and is considered a class III recommendation in asymptomatic patients undergoing a low-risk surgery, the availability of an old ECG may be useful for comparison.[2]

Biomarkers

Preoperative measurement of BNP or NT-proBNP is recommended for risk stratification in higher-risk patients by multiple society guidelines.[2,12,13] The addition of postoperative measurement of BNP or NT-proBNP has been demonstrated to enhance risk prediction of MACE within 180 days of surgery.[2,13,44] Routine postoperative troponin screening is also recommended in the Canadian Cardiovascular Society, European Society of Cardiology, and the European Society of Anaesthesiologists and Intensive Care guidelines due to the increased ability to detect postoperative myocardial injury after noncardiac surgery (MINS).[12,13,45] The results of the MANAGE trial suggest an improvement in major vascular outcomes without an increase in major bleeding by treatment with 110 mg dabigatran twice daily in patients who develop MINS.[46]

Assessment of left ventricular function

In general, an assessment of baseline LV function should be reserved for those patients with unexplained cardiopulmonary symptoms. This can be accomplished using echocardiography, radionuclide angiography, and/or contrast ventriculography. Most commonly, however, echocardiography is used when assessment of LV function is thought to be warranted. LV ejection fraction has been correlated with short- and long-term prognosis in multiple studies in patients undergoing noncardiac surgery; in general, the lower the ejection fraction, the greater the perioperative risk. Importantly, preoperative echocardiographic information has not been demonstrated to improve risk stratification when added to clinical risk factors.[47] In open vascular surgery, both asymptomatic systolic and isolated diastolic LV dysfunction were associated with 30-day cardiovascular events and long-term cardiovascular mortality. In endovascular surgery, only symptomatic HF was associated with 30-day cardiovascular events and long-term cardiovascular mortality.[48]

The ACC/AHA task force guidelines recommend that preoperative assessment of LV systolic function prior to noncardiac surgery should be limited to patients with current or poorly controlled HF, but not used as a routine test in patients without prior HF.[2] Among patients without a history of HF and with dyspnea of unknown etiology, the indications are less clear. It is important to note that the 2024 ACC/AHA/ASE/ASNC/HFSA/HRS/SCAI /SCCT/SCMR/STS 2024 Appropriate Use Criteria for Multimodality Imaging in Cardiovascular Evaluation of Patients Undergoing Nonemergent, Noncardiac Surgery guidelines state it is rarely reasonable to assess ventricular function in patients without signs or symptoms of cardiovascular disease in the preoperative setting.[49]

Noninvasive cardiac stress testing

Preoperative stress testing has been deemphasized in the most recent 2024 version of the ACC/AHA guidelines.[2] In a patient with a negative stress test for myocardial ischemia, the risk of a perioperative cardiac event is relatively low. However, because the positive predictive values of stress tests are low, the perioperative risk for a patient with evidence of stress-induced myocardial ischemia is less clear.[50]

The risk of MACE in patients undergoing low-risk surgery is sufficiently low that it generally does not require an assessment of CAD to further stratify risk. Likewise, patients who have reasonably good functional status (i.e., those who can perform 4 METs of activity) may proceed with surgery at an acceptable risk without the need for preoperative noninvasive stress testing. Stress testing should only be considered in patients with poor or unknown functional status and clinical risk factors who are undergoing elevated-risk operations or when the results of the stress test will change the decision to proceed with surgery or the approach to the patient.[2]

CORONARY ANGIOGRAPHY AND REVASCULARIZATION BEFORE NONCARDIAC SURGERY

Coronary angiography

The present indications for coronary angiography in the preoperative evaluation before noncardiac surgery are adapted from the ACC/AHA guidelines for coronary angiography in the general population.[51] Coronary angiography should be considered in patients with unstable symptoms of angina pectoris, recent MI, or large areas of myocardium at risk on noninvasive stress tests if coronary revascularization would be considered outside of the surgical context. An abnormal stress test should not prompt coronary angiography or revascularization unless the test shows high-risk findings.

Coronary revascularization

The Coronary Artery Revascularization Prophylaxis (CARP) trial showed that coronary artery revascularization before elective vascular surgery did not significantly alter long-term outcomes.[24] In this trial, 510 patients at increased risk for perioperative cardiac complications were randomized to undergo either coronary artery revascularization or no revascularization before elective major vascular surgery. The average age was 65.6 years in the revascularization arm and 67.2 years in the no-revascularization arm. There was no difference between groups in either postoperative MI or in mortality at 2.7 years after randomization. When patients who underwent coronary angiography in both the randomized and non-randomized portions of the CARP trial were examined, only the subset of patients with unprotected left main disease showed a benefit with preoperative coronary artery revascularization.[2]

Percutaneous coronary intervention

Cardiac complications are less frequent in patients with stable and/or asymptomatic coronary stenosis, and percutaneous coronary intervention (PCI) may actually destabilize coronary plaques that manifest in the days or weeks after noncardiac surgery. PCI using coronary stenting poses several special issues including (1) the risk of stent thrombosis, especially if dual antiplatelet therapy (DAPT) needs to be interrupted; (2) the consequence of delaying the desired surgical procedure, which is especially important in time-sensitive situations such as malignancy; and (3) increased risk of intra- and periprocedural bleeding and the consequence of such bleeding if DAPT is continued.

Older observational studies found the risk of stent-related thrombotic complications to remain high for at least 1 year after drug-eluting stent (DES) placement; thus, DAPT was not to be interrupted for at least 1 year. However, newer-generation DES requires a shorter minimum duration of DAPT due to the lower risk of stent thrombosis.[52]

The 2024 AHA/ACC guidelines provide a class I recommendation that elective noncardiac surgery in patients treated with DES for an acute coronary syndrome be delayed 1 year if one or more antiplatelet agents will require interruption. Patients who undergo DES for chronic coronary disease are recommended to wait 6 months post-PCI to proceed with surgery if antiplatelet agents are to be interrupted. Aspirin should be continued perioperatively whenever possible in patients with cardiac stents who are undergoing surgery.[2] If a P2Y12 inhibitor is held before a surgical procedure, it is recommended to be restarted as soon as it is safe from a surgical perspective. Given the complexity of these decisions and considerations, a team-based approach involving the surgeon, anesthesiologist, cardiologist, and patient is recommended.

PERIOPERATIVE INTERVENTIONS TO REDUCE RISK

β-Blockers

In the POISE trial, 8351 high-risk patients (average age 69 years) undergoing noncardiac surgery were randomized to metoprolol succinate 200 mg daily or a matching placebo.[53] Active treatment with a β-blocker reduced the composite of cardiovascular death, nonfatal MI, and nonfatal cardiac arrest at 30 days after randomization by 1.1% but was associated with higher total mortality by 0.8% and stroke by 0.5%. Two possible explanations for the mildly increased mortality and stroke rate are (1) timing of medication administration and (2) lack of titration of the medication. Perioperative β-blockade administered according to the Perioperative Cardiac Risk Reduction protocol was associated with a reduction in 30-day and 1-year mortality. Conversely, perioperative withdrawal of β-blockers was associated with increased mortality.[54,55]

The 2024 update to the ACC/AHA guidelines on perioperative cardiovascular management for noncardiac surgery recommends the following: continuation of β-blockers in patients undergoing surgery who are on stable doses of β-blockers remains a class I recommendation; when indicated, preoperative initiation of β-blockade should occur at least 7 days prior to surgery; and it remains a class III recommendation (harmful) to start β-blockers on the day of surgery. Ideally, β-blocker therapy should be titrated to a heart rate of less than 70 beats per minute, and longer-acting agents such as atenolol or bisoprolol should be used.

Angiotensin-converting enzyme inhibitors, angiotensin receptor blockers, and aldosterone antagonists

The prevalence of HF in the surgical patient population has increased over time. Many older adults undergoing noncardiac surgery will be taking angiotensin receptor blockers (ARBs), angiotensin-converting enzyme inhibitors (ACEIs), or aldosterone antagonists (AAs) for treatment of HF or HTN. A large randomized controlled trial found that continuation of ACEIs was associated with higher rates of intraoperative hypotension but no effect on any other outcomes.[56] Another meta-analysis found that of those taking ACEIs, 50% experienced hypotension on the day of surgery without altering other important outcomes including perioperative cardiac events or death.[57] The 2024 guidelines recommend continuation of ACEIs and ARBs perioperatively in patients with a history of HF as a class IIa indication and to consider holding them for 24 hours prior to elevated-risk surgery in patients with controlled blood pressure to limit intraoperative hypotension.[2]

Statins

In addition to their cholesterol-lowering effects, statins have anti-inflammatory and plaque-stabilizing properties. A significant reduction in cardiovascular complications was demonstrated with the initiation of a statin 30 days prior to vascular surgery.[58] A meta-analysis on the overall effect of preoperative statin therapy on postoperative outcomes revealed a 59% reduction in the risk of mortality after vascular surgery.[59] When including all noncardiac surgery, a 44% reduction in mortality was observed. Statins should be continued perioperatively to reduce the risk of MACE (class I recommendation). Furthermore, statins should be initiated in statin-naïve patients who meet criteria to reduce long-term adverse cardiovascular outcomes.[2]

α-2-Adrenergic agonists

Clonidine stimulates central α-2-adrenergic receptors and thereby decreases sympathetic nervous outflow to the vasculature, producing vasodilation and lowering blood pressure. In POISE-2, one of the largest clinical trials looking at major cardiovascular outcomes after noncardiac surgery. Devereaux et al.[60] examined the efficacy of clonidine 0.2 mg versus placebo in 10,010 patients (mean age 68 years) across 23 countries with risk factors or evidence of cardiovascular disease. They found that low-dose clonidine compared with placebo did not improve the primary outcome of mortality and nonfatal MI at 30 days. In fact, the clonidine arm had a nonsignificant increase in rates of MI and clinically significant hypotension.[60] Thus, initiation of clonidine in the perioperative period to reduce cardiovascular risks is not recommended (class III).[2]

PERIOPERATIVE ANEMIA MANAGEMENT

Anemia of any degree is associated with increased perioperative morbidity and mortality and serves as a risk multiplier when it exists in the presence of other comorbidities.[61] Perioperative anemia has also been associated with an increased incidence of perioperative myocardial ischemia. A liberal transfusion strategy, as compared with a restrictive strategy, did not reduce rates of death or inability to walk independently on 60-day follow-up or reduce in-hospital morbidity in older adult patients at high cardiovascular risk. In patients undergoing elevated-risk NCS where significant blood loss is anticipated, it is reasonable to administer tranexamic acid. Patients with a diagnosis of iron deficiency anemia should undergo preoperative iron repletion with either intravenous or oral iron supplementation to increase their hemoglobin level and reduce the risk of perioperative blood transfusion.[2]

Prehabilitation

There is no doubt that surgery in the presence of high-risk factors can lead to worse short- and long-term recovery and outcomes, especially in the older adult population. There have been efforts made to optimize the intraoperative and postoperative periods to improve recovery, including early mobilization and rehabilitation pathways. However, the most opportune time to affect clinical recovery might be in the preoperative period with "prehabilitation," a method of improving a patient's functional status in anticipation of surgery. This includes structured exercise programs as well as nutritional counseling and supplementation. Several methods of intensification of exercise can be implemented, including gradually increasing target heart rate goals or gradually increasing the intensity of the workout based on the widely used Borg Rating of Perceived Exertion Scale. The goal of a prehabilitation program should be not only to improve functionality but also empower patients with the tools and motivation to continue their efforts after surgery and beyond to lead a healthy lifestyle.[39,62]

There is data to suggest that patients with good versus poor performance on cardiopulmonary exercise testing have better outcomes, making it a useful risk stratification tool. A meta-analysis of 17 randomized controlled trials looking at the effects of prehabilitation on function, pain, and quality of life postoperatively found that prehabilitation of varying duration did not correlate with improved quality of life or pain indices.[63] However, a prehabilitation program consisting of more than 500 minutes correlated with a decreased need for postoperative rehabilitation.[63] Although many studies have shown that preoperative exercise programs may not improve hard outcomes such as readmissions and postoperative placement in rehabilitation programs, improvements in patient satisfaction and improvement in physiology are not negligible. Ongoing randomized trials are further investigating the feasibility and effects of prehabilitation.

Cardiac devices

MANAGEMENT OF PERMANENT PACEMAKERS AND IMPLANTABLE CARDIOVERTER-DEFIBRILLATORS

Pacemakers and implantable cardioverter-defibrillators (ICDs) are collectively referred to as cardiovascular implantable electronic devices (CIEDs). To assist clinicians with the perioperative evaluation and management of patients with CIEDs, the AHA developed a multidisciplinary expert scientific statement published in July 2024.[64] The 2024 ACC/AHA guidelines for perioperative cardiovascular management also contain recommendations for the perioperative management of CIEDs.[2] The recommended team-based approach to management of CIEDs involves communication by the surgical team regarding the nature of the procedure and the plan for the type of electrocautery to be used. The perioperative management plan for CIEDs must be individualized for each patient depending on the type of device, degree of pacemaker dependence, current device settings, and types of therapies programmed. Patients who are pacemaker dependent should have their device set to an asynchronous mode either via magnet or reprogramming before having surgery above the umbilicus. Patients with leadless pacemakers will require reprogramming. Patients who are pacemaker dependent will require reprogramming of the CIED prior to surgery above the umbilicus to ensure the device is set to an asynchronous mode and tachytherapies have been inhibited. A magnet may be used to inhibit tachytherapy in patients with CIEDs who are non-pacemaker dependent. Preoperative device settings should be restored within the postoperative period. Major CIED manufacturers are often able to provide perioperative technical support for their particular devices.

INTRAOPERATIVE CONSIDERATIONS

Anesthetic agents

There are many different approaches to the anesthetic care and intraoperative monitoring of the older surgical patient, depending on the integration of patient- and surgery-specific factors. The type of anesthesia used is not an independent predictor of 30-day mortality, ambulation, length of hospitalization, or postoperative delirium in older patients undergoing repair of a hip fracture.[65]

GENERAL ANESTHESIA

General anesthesia can best be defined as a state of unconsciousness, during which the patient experiences amnesia, analgesia, immobility, and attenuation of autonomic responses to noxious stimulation. General anesthesia can be achieved with or without an endotracheal tube. Traditionally, laryngoscopy and intubation were thought to be the time of greatest stress and risk for myocardial ischemia, but there is newer evidence to suggest that extubation is the time of greatest risk.[66]

Three commonly used inhalational anesthetic agents are available in the United States, all of which have reversible myocardial depressant effects and decrease myocardial oxygen demand (Table 28.2). Overall, there appears to be no one best inhalation anesthetic for older adult patients with CAD.

Isoflurane is a potent vasodilator and has minimal effects on baroreceptor function. Despite initial concerns, several large-scale studies of isoflurane in patients undergoing CABG have not demonstrated any increased incidence of myocardial ischemia or infarction.[67]

Two other inhalation agents, desflurane and sevoflurane, are available. Desflurane has the fastest onset of inhaled anesthetics and is commonly used in the outpatient setting, although it has been shown to be associated with airway irritability leading to tachycardia. In a large-scale study comparing a narcotic-based anesthetic with desflurane, the desflurane group had a significantly higher incidence of myocardial ischemia.[68] By including narcotics with desflurane, tachycardia may be mitigated. Sevoflurane is the newest approved agent for use in the United States.

There are theoretical advantages to the use of inhalational anesthetics in patients with CAD. Several investigative groups have demonstrated in vitro and in animal models that these agents possess protective effects on the myocardium similar to ischemic preconditioning. This favorable effect on myocardial oxygen demand would serve to offset the theoretical effects of coronary steal in patients with chronic coronary occlusion.

High-dose narcotics are an alternative form of anesthesia and offer an advantage of hemodynamic stability and lack of myocardial depression. The disadvantage is the risk of postoperative respiratory depression and associated complications, especially in older adults who may be more sensitive to the effects of opioid analgesics. An ultra-short-acting narcotic may be considered in certain clinical scenarios to reduce the risk of respiratory suppression and prolonged ventilation. There has been no difference in survival or major morbidity between a high-dose narcotic technique and inhalation-based technique. Therefore, use of a "balanced" technique using lower doses of narcotics with an inhalational agent is common.[69] Intravenous propofol, an alkyl phenol that can be used for both induction and maintenance of general anesthesia, has gained popularity due to rapid clearance with few residual effects on awakening.

Table 28.2 Clinical qualities of inhaled anesthetics

Agent	Advantages	Disadvantages
Nitrous oxide	Rapid uptake and elimination Minimal respiratory depression Minimal circulatory depression Odorless, nonpungent	Supports combustion Expansion of closed air spaces Inactivates vitamin B12 Lack of anesthetic potency Suggestion of increased cardiac morbidity
Isoflurane	Decreases cerebral metabolic rate	Tachycardia at greater concentration
Desflurane	Cardiac output maintained Rapid uptake and elimination	Airway irritation Tachycardia with rapid increase in inspired concentration Requires specialized vaporizer for administration Expensive unless low flows are used
Sevoflurane	Rapid uptake and elimination Nonpungent Less depression of myocardial contractility Stable heart rate	Reacts with CO_2 absorbents Inorganic fluoride release Expensive unless low flows are used

REGIONAL ANESTHESIA

Regional anesthesia includes the techniques of spinal and epidural anesthesia, as well as peripheral nerve blocks. Peripheral techniques offer the advantage of being associated with minimal or no hemodynamic effects. In contrast, spinal or epidural techniques are associated with sympathetic blockade, which can lead to reduction in blood pressure, reflex sympathetic activation above the level of the blockade, and slowing of heart rate.

The associated autonomic effects of spinal anesthesia occur sooner than the same anesthetic agent administered through an epidural. Since a catheter is usually left in place for epidural anesthesia, it can be more easily titrated. Improved outcomes have been demonstrated with a combined regional and general anesthetic for patients with CAD, particularly in those undergoing vascular surgery.[70]

Maintenance of body temperature

Hypothermia has also been associated with an increased incidence of myocardial ischemia in vascular surgery patients. In a randomized trial involving patients either undergoing vascular surgery or with known risk factors for CAD, use of forced air warming to maintain normothermia was associated with a significant reduction in cardiac morbidity and myocardial ischemia for the first 24 postoperative hours.[71] Therefore, maintenance of normothermia should be a goal of perioperative management.

Surveillance for perioperative myocardial infarction

The optimal and most cost-effective strategy for monitoring high-risk patients for major cardiac morbidity after noncardiac surgery is unknown. Postoperative myocardial ischemia or infarction is often clinically silent, most likely due to the confounding effects of analgesics.[72] Myocardium-specific enzymes such as cardiac troponins (I or T) are quite sensitive in the detection of perioperative MI. Troponin I has a reported a specificity of 99%.

Traditionally, perioperative MI was associated with a 30%–50% short-term mortality. With greater perioperative surveillance, more asymptomatic MIs and myocardial injury after noncardiac surgery (MINS) are being detected. More recent series have reported that perioperative MI is associated with a short-term mortality of up to 20%.[72] The VISION trial determined the relationship between the peak fourth-generation troponin T (TnT) measurement in the first 3 days after noncardiac surgery and 30-day mortality in a total of 15,133 patients, 25% of whom were 75 years of age or older.[73] Peak TnT values of at least 0.02 ng/mL were associated with higher 30-day mortality compared to the reference group. The 2024 ACC/AHA guidelines recommend the use of cardiac biomarkers for patients at high risk and those with clinical, ECG, or hemodynamic evidence of cardiovascular dysfunction.[2]

REFERENCES

1. McGinn R, Agung Y, Grudzinski AL, Talarico R, Hallet J, McIsaac DI. Attributable perioperative cost of frailty after major, elective noncardiac surgery: a population-based cohort study. *Anesthesiology.* 2023;139(2):143–152.
2. Thompson A, Fleischmann KE, Smilowitz NR, Sr. ea, Peer Review Committee M. 2024 AHA/ACC/ACS/ASNC/HRS/SCA/SCCT/SCMR/SVM guideline for perioperative cardiovascular management for noncardiac surgery: a report of the American College of Cardiology/American Heart Association Joint Committee on Clinical Practice Guidelines. *Circulation.* 2024;150(19):e351–e442.
3. Becher RD, Vander Wyk B, Leo-Summers L, Desai MM, Gill TM. The incidence and cumulative risk of major surgery in older persons in the United States. *Ann Surg.* 2023;277(1):87–92.
4. Colloca G, Santoro M, Gambassi G. Age-related physiologic changes and perioperative management of elderly patients. *Surg Oncol.* 2010;19(3):124–130.
5. Daza JF, Wijeysundera HC, Diep C, et al. Healthcare costs of new functional impairment in the year after noncardiac surgery. *Anesthesiology.* 2023;139(6):902–904.
6. Goldenberg E, Saffary R, Schmiesing C. New Role for the anesthesia preoperative clinic: helping to ensure that surgery is the right choice for patients with serious illness. *Anesth Analg.* 2019;129(1):311–315.
7. Blitz JD. Preoperative evaluation in the 21st century. *Anesthesiology.* 2023;139(1):91–103.
8. Cooper L, Abbett SK, Feng A, et al. Launching a geriatric surgery center: recommendations from the Society for Perioperative Assessment and Quality Improvement. *J Am Geriatr Soc.* 2020;68(9):1941–1946.
9. Fleisher LA, Fleischmann KE, Auerbach AD, et al. 2014 ACC/AHA guideline on perioperative cardiovascular evaluation and management of patients undergoing noncardiac surgery: executive summary: a report of the American College of Cardiology/American Heart Association Task Force on Practice Guidelines. *Circulation.* 2014;130(24):2215–2245.
10. Rehn M, Chew MS, Kalliomaki M, Olkkola KT, Sigurethsson MI, Moller MH. ESAIC focused guideline for the use of cardiac biomarkers in perioperative risk evaluation: endorsement by the Scandinavian Society of Anaesthesiology and Intensive Care Medicine. *Acta Anaesthesiol Scand.* 2024;68(9):1179–1181.

11. Zhao BC, Lei SH, Zhuang PP, et al. Preoperative N-terminal pro-B-type natriuretic peptide and high-sensitivity cardiac troponin T and outcomes after major noncardiac surgery: a prospective cohort study. *Anesthesiology.* 2024;141(3):475–488.
12. Duceppe E, Parlow J, MacDonald P, et al. Canadian cardiovascular society guidelines on perioperative cardiac risk assessment and management for patients who undergo noncardiac surgery. *Can J Cardiol.* 2017;33(1):17–32.
13. Halvorsen S, Mehilli J, Cassese S, et al. 2022 ESC Guidelines on cardiovascular assessment and management of patients undergoing non-cardiac surgery. *Eur Heart J.* 2022;43(39):3826–3924.
14. Gupta PK, Gupta H, Sundaram A, et al. Development and validation of a risk calculator for prediction of cardiac risk after surgery. *Circulation.* 2011;124(4):381–387.
15. Liu JB, Liu Y, Cohen ME, Ko CY, Sweitzer BJ. Defining the intrinsic cardiac risks of operations to improve preoperative cardiac risk assessments. *Anesthesiology.* 2018;128(2):283–292.
16. Lee TH, Marcantonio ER, Mangione CM, et al. Derivation and prospective validation of a simple index for prediction of cardiac risk of major noncardiac surgery. *Circulation.* 1999;100(10):1043–1049.
17. Bilimoria KY, Liu Y, Paruch JL, et al. Development and evaluation of the universal ACS NSQIP surgical risk calculator: a decision aid and informed consent tool for patients and surgeons. *J Am Coll Surg.* 2013;217(5):833–842.
18. Reilly DF, McNeely MJ, Doerner D, et al. Self-reported exercise tolerance and the risk of serious perioperative complications. *Arch Intern Med.* 1999;159(18):2185–2192.
19. Hlatky MA, Boineau RE, Higginbotham MB, et al. A brief self-administered questionnaire to determine functional capacity (the Duke Activity Status Index). *Am J Cardiol.* 1989;64(10):651–654.
20. Wijeysundera DN, Pearse RM, Shulman MA, et al. Assessment of functional capacity before major non-cardiac surgery: an international, prospective cohort study. *Lancet.* 2018;391(10140):2631–2640.
21. Jaeger C, Burkard T, Kamber F, et al. Quantification of metabolic equivalents (METs) by the MET-REPAIR questionnaire: a validation study in patients with a high cardiovascular burden. *J Clin Anesth.* 2022;76:110559.
22. Wijeysundera DN, Beattie WS, Hillis GS, et al. Integration of the Duke Activity Status Index into preoperative risk evaluation: a multicentre prospective cohort study. *Br J Anaesth.* 2020;124(3):261–270.
23. Shah KB, Kleinman BS, Rao TL, Jacobs HK, Mestan K, Schaafsma M. Angina and other risk factors in patients with cardiac diseases undergoing noncardiac operations. *Anesth Analg.* 1990;70(3):240–247.
24. McFalls EO, Ward HB, Moritz TE, et al. Coronary-artery revascularization before elective major vascular surgery. *N Engl J Med.* 2004;351(27):2795–2804.
25. Rao TL, Jacobs KH, El-Etr AA. Reinfarction following anesthesia in patients with myocardial infarction. *Anesthesiology.* 1983;59(6):499–505.
26. Shah KB, Kleinman BS, Sami H, Patel J, Rao TL. Reevaluation of perioperative myocardial infarction in patients with prior myocardial infarction undergoing noncardiac operations. *Anesth Analg.* 1990;71(3):231–235.
27. Tarhan S, Moffitt EA, Taylor WF, Giuliani ER. Myocardial infarction after general anesthesia. *JAMA.* 1972;220(11):1451–1454.
28. Weksler N, Klein M, Szendro G, et al. The dilemma of immediate preoperative hypertension: to treat and operate, or to postpone surgery? *J Clin Anesth.* 2003;15(3):179–183.
29. Kertai MD, Bountioukos M, Boersma E, et al. Aortic stenosis: an underestimated risk factor for perioperative complications in patients undergoing noncardiac surgery. *Am J Med.* 2004;116(1):8–13.
30. Calleja AM, Dommaraju S, Gaddam R, Cha S, Khandheria BK, Chaliki HP. Cardiac risk in patients aged >75 years with asymptomatic, severe aortic stenosis undergoing noncardiac surgery. *Am J Cardiol.* 2010;105(8):1159–1163.
31. Kovacs MJ, Wells PS, Anderson DR, et al. Postoperative low molecular weight heparin bridging treatment for patients at high risk of arterial thromboembolism (PERIOP2): double blind randomised controlled trial. *BMJ.* 2021;373:n1205.
32. Goldman L, Caldera DL, Nussbaum SR, et al. Multifactorial index of cardiac risk in noncardiac surgical procedures. *N Engl J Med.* 1977;297(16):845–850.
33. O'Kelly B, Browner WS, Massie B, Tubau J, Ngo L, Mangano DT. Ventricular arrhythmias in patients undergoing noncardiac surgery. The Study of Perioperative Ischemia Research Group. *JAMA.* 1992;268(2):217–221.
34. Joglar JA, Chung MK, Armbruster AL, et al. 2023 ACC/AHA/ACCP/HRS guideline for the diagnosis and management of atrial fibrillation: a report of the American College of Cardiology/American Heart Association Joint Committee on Clinical Practice Guidelines. *Circulation.* 2024;149(1):e1–e156.
35. Douketis JD, Spyropoulos AC, Anderson JM, et al. The Perioperative Anticoagulant Use for Surgery Evaluation (PAUSE) study for patients on a direct oral anticoagulant who need an elective surgery or procedure: design and rationale. *Thromb Haemost.* 2017;117(12):2415–2424.
36. Kopp SL, Vandermeulen E, McBane RD, Perlas A, Leffert L, Horlocker T. Regional anesthesia in the patient receiving antithrombotic or thrombolytic therapy: American Society of Regional Anesthesia

and Pain Medicine evidence-based guidelines (fifth edition). *Reg Anesth Pain Med.* 2025.

37. Benesch C, Glance LG, Derdeyn CP, et al. Perioperative neurological evaluation and management to lower the risk of acute stroke in patients undergoing noncardiac, nonneurological surgery: a scientific statement from the American Heart Association/American Stroke Association. *Circulation.* 2021;143(19):e923–e946.
38. McIsaac DI, MacDonald DB, Aucoin SD. Frailty for perioperative clinicians: a narrative review. *Anesth Analg.* 2020;130(6):1450–1460.
39. Gillis C, Ljungqvist O, Carli F. Prehabilitation, enhanced recovery after surgery, or both? A narrative review. *Br J Anaesth.* 2022;128(3):434–448.
40. Punnoose A, Claydon-Mueller LS, Weiss O, Zhang J, Rushton A, Khanduja V. Prehabilitation for patients undergoing orthopedic surgery: a systematic review and meta-analysis. *JAMA Netw Open.* 2023;6(4):e238050.
41. Glance LG, Faden E, Dutton RP, et al. Impact of the choice of risk model for identifying low-risk patients using the 2014 American College of Cardiology/American Heart Association perioperative guidelines. *Anesthesiology.* 2018;129(5):889–900.
42. Committee on S, Practice P, Apfelbaum JL, et al. Practice advisory for preanesthesia evaluation: an updated report by the American Society of Anesthesiologists Task Force on Preanesthesia Evaluation. *Anesthesiology.* 2012;116(3):522–538.
43. Kannel WB, Cupples LA, Gagnon DR. Incidence, precursors and prognosis of unrecognized myocardial infarction. *Adv Cardiol.* 1990;37:202–214.
44. Rodseth RN, Biccard BM, Le Manach Y, et al. The prognostic value of pre-operative and post-operative B-type natriuretic peptides in patients undergoing noncardiac surgery: B-type natriuretic peptide and N-terminal fragment of pro-B-type natriuretic peptide: a systematic review and individual patient data meta-analysis. *J Am Coll Cardiol.* 2014;63(2):170–180.
45. Lurati Buse G, Bollen Pinto B, Abelha F, et al. ESAIC focused guideline for the use of cardiac biomarkers in perioperative risk evaluation. *Eur J Anaesthesiol.* 2023;40(12):888–927.
46. Devereaux PJ, Duceppe E, Guyatt G, et al. Dabigatran in patients with myocardial injury after non-cardiac surgery (MANAGE): an international, randomised, placebo-controlled trial. *Lancet.* 2018;391(10137):2325–2334.
47. Halm EA, Browner WS, Tubau JF, Tateo IM, Mangano DT. Echocardiography for assessing cardiac risk in patients having noncardiac surgery. Study of Perioperative Ischemia Research Group. *Ann Intern Med.* 1996;125(6):433–441.
48. Flu WJ, van Kuijk JP, Hoeks SE, et al. Prognostic implications of asymptomatic left ventricular dysfunction in patients undergoing vascular surgery. *Anesthesiology.* 2010;112(6):1316–1324.
49. Writing Group M, Doherty JU, Daugherty SL, et al. ACC/AHA/ASE/ASNC/HFSA/HRS/SCAI/SCCT/SCMR/STS 2024 appropriate use criteria for multimodality imaging in cardiovascular evaluation of patients undergoing nonemergent, noncardiac surgery. *J Am Coll Cardiol.* 2024;84(15):1455–1491.
50. Arora V, Velanovich V, Alarcon W. Preoperative assessment of cardiac risk and perioperative cardiac management in noncardiac surgery. *Int J Surg.* 2011;9(1):23–28.
51. Lawton JS, Tamis-Holland JE, Bangalore S, et al. 2021 ACC/AHA/SCAI guideline for coronary artery revascularization: a report of the American College of Cardiology/American Heart Association Joint Committee on Clinical Practice Guidelines. *Circulation.* 2022;145(3):e18–e114.
52. Feres F, Costa RA, Abizaid A, et al. Three vs twelve months of dual antiplatelet therapy after zotarolimus-eluting stents: the OPTIMIZE randomized trial. *JAMA.* 2013;310(23):2510–2522.
53. Group PS, Devereaux PJ, Yang H, et al. Effects of extended-release metoprolol succinate in patients undergoing non-cardiac surgery (POISE trial): a randomised controlled trial. *Lancet.* 2008;371(9627):1839–1847.
54. Wallace AW, Au S, Cason BA. Perioperative beta-blockade: atenolol is associated with reduced mortality when compared to metoprolol. *Anesthesiology.* 2011;114(4):824–836.
55. Wallace AW, Au S, Cason BA. Association of the pattern of use of perioperative beta-blockade and postoperative mortality. *Anesthesiology.* 2010;113(4):794–805.
56. Turan A, You J, Shiba A, Kurz A, Saager L, Sessler DI. Angiotensin converting enzyme inhibitors are not associated with respiratory complications or mortality after noncardiac surgery. *Anesth Analg.* 2012;114(3):552–560.
57. Roshanov PS, Rochwerg B, Patel A, et al. Withholding versus continuing angiotensin-converting enzyme inhibitors or angiotensin II receptor blockers before noncardiac surgery: an analysis of the vascular events in noncardiac surgery patients cohort evaluation prospective cohort. *Anesthesiology.* 2017;126(1):16–27.
58. Durazzo AE, Machado FS, Ikeoka DT, et al. Reduction in cardiovascular events after vascular surgery with atorvastatin: a randomized trial. *J Vasc Surg.* 2004;39(5):967–975; discussion 975–966.
59. Hindler K, Shaw AD, Samuels J, Fulton S, Collard CD, Riedel B. Improved postoperative outcomes associated with preoperative statin therapy. *Anesthesiology.* 2006;105(6):1260–1272; quiz 1289–1290.

60. Devereaux PJ, Sessler DI, Leslie K, et al. Clonidine in patients undergoing noncardiac surgery. *N Engl J Med.* 2014;370(16):1504–1513.
61. Musallam KM, Tamim HM, Richards T, et al. Preoperative anaemia and postoperative outcomes in non-cardiac surgery: a retrospective cohort study. *Lancet.* 2011;378(9800):1396–1407.
62. Carli F, Ferreira V. Prehabilitation: a new area of integration between geriatricians, anesthesiologists, and exercise therapists. *Aging Clin Exp Res.* 2018;30(3):241–244.
63. Cabilan CJ, Hines S, Munday J. The effectiveness of prehabilitation or preoperative exercise for surgical patients: a systematic review. *JBI Database System Rev Implement Rep.* 2015;13(1):146–187.
64. Wan EY, Rogers AJ, Lavelle M, et al. Periprocedural management and multidisciplinary care pathways for patients with cardiac implantable electronic devices: a scientific statement from the American Heart Association. *Circulation.* 2024;150(8):e183–e196.
65. Neuman MD, Feng R, Carson JL, et al. Spinal anesthesia or general anesthesia for hip surgery in older adults. *N Engl J Med.* 2021;385(22):2025–2035.
66. Zambouri A. Preoperative evaluation and preparation for anesthesia and surgery. *Hippokratia.* 2007;11(1):13–21.
67. Leung JM, Goehner P, O'Kelly BF, et al. Isoflurane anesthesia and myocardial ischemia: comparative risk versus sufentanil anesthesia in patients undergoing coronary artery bypass graft surgery. The SPI (Study of Perioperative Ischemia) Research Group. *Anesthesiology.* 1991;74(5):838–847.
68. Helman JD, Leung JM, Bellows WH, et al. The risk of myocardial ischemia in patients receiving desflurane versus sufentanil anesthesia for coronary artery bypass graft surgery. The S.P.I. Research Group. *Anesthesiology.* 1992;77(1):47–62.
69. Alwardt CM, Redford D, Larson DF. General anesthesia in cardiac surgery: a review of drugs and practices. *J Extra Corpor Technol.* 2005;37(2):227–235.
70. Salata K, Abdallah FW, Hussain MA, et al. Short-term outcomes of combined neuraxial and general anaesthesia versus general anaesthesia alone for elective open abdominal aortic aneurysm repair: retrospective population-based cohort study. *Br J Anaesth.* 2020;124(5):544–552.
71. Frank SM, Fleisher LA, Breslow MJ, et al. Perioperative maintenance of normothermia reduces the incidence of morbid cardiac events. A randomized clinical trial. *JAMA.* 1997;277(14):1127–1134.
72. Botto F, Alonso-Coello P, Chan MT, et al. Myocardial injury after noncardiac surgery: a large, international, prospective cohort study establishing diagnostic criteria, characteristics, predictors, and 30-day outcomes. *Anesthesiology.* 2014;120(3):564–578.
73. Devereaux PJ, Szczeklik W. Myocardial injury after non-cardiac surgery: diagnosis and management. *Eur Heart J.* 2020;41(32):3083–3091.

29

Ethical decisions and end-of-life care in older patients with cardiovascular disease

ESTHER S. PAK

Key points

- Despite numerous advancements in pharmacological and technological therapies, older adults with cardiovascular disease suffer high morbidity and mortality, especially at the end of life.
- Frequent discussions with patients about their prognosis, potential risks and benefits of treatment options, and their preferences and goals are required to ensure optimal goal-concordant care.
- In patients with compromised decision-making capacity, surrogate decision-makers must be effectively engaged.
- The nuances of managing complex medication regimens, implantable cardiac devices, and mechanical circulatory support can raise ethical issues at the end of life.
- Meeting the complex needs of older patients with cardiovascular disease at the end of life requires a multidisciplinary team approach that often includes palliative care.

INTRODUCTION

Cardiovascular disease (CVD) has an enormous impact on patients, their families, and healthcare systems worldwide. CVD, particularly in the advanced stages of disease, disproportionately affects older patients. Technologies such as cardiac resynchronization therapy (CRT) and implantable cardioverter-defibrillators (ICDs), transcatheter valvular procedures, and mechanical circulatory support (MCS) aim to improve symptoms, quality of life, and survival. However, management of these cardiac devices at the end of life raises complex ethical issues. Despite the availability of treatment options, older patients with CVD suffer high morbidity and mortality. In particular, older adults suffer high symptom burden and disability associated with CVD that may worsen toward the end of life. Older patients are usually more vulnerable to potential complications associated with CVD and its treatment. Comorbidities such as frailty, cognitive impairment, and chronic kidney disease further complicate CVD management. The variety of treatment options, potential

DOI: 10.1201/9781003568933-29

associated risks, and the presence of comorbidities have increased the complexity of decision-making processes and ethical issues for patients living with and dying from CVD.

Prognostication is difficult in CVD as death may be sudden or follow extended periods of decline. This uncertainty may cause providers to hesitate in initiating discussions regarding treatment preferences and goals of care. In light of this uncertainty, early and iterative conversations ensure thorough elicitation and implementation of patient preferences and goals.

This chapter discusses ethical issues commonly encountered in caring for older patients with CVD, including impaired decision-making capacity, surrogate decision-making, advance directives, and issues surrounding cardiopulmonary resuscitation (CPR). End-of-life issues in patients with CVD, device management at the end of life, and hospice care are also addressed. The chapter concludes with a discussion of coronary artery bypass grafting (CABG) and surgical and catheter-based treatment options for aortic stenosis in older patients. Concerns regarding distributive justice, disparities, cost, and appropriateness of treatment are important issues but are beyond the scope of this chapter.

DECISION-MAKING CAPACITY

Central to autonomy is the ability of patients to articulate preferences, values, and goals and to understand diagnosis, prognosis, and risks and benefits of treatments associated with their health. The assessment of decision-making capacity constitutes an essential skill for clinicians who aim to engage in shared decision-making, to educate patients regarding their illness and treatment options, and to obtain informed consent for treatments and procedures. As goal-directed CVD care can entail multiple decisions about treatments and procedures throughout a patient's disease course, assessment of decision-making capacity may be necessary at multiple time points. In clinical scenarios such as dementia or delirium, the patient's ability to make decisions may be impaired to varying degrees. Cognitive impairment is underrecognized in patients with CVD (1). Older patients have a higher prevalence of conditions such as dementia and challenges in communication due to visual and hearing impairment, which negatively impact decision-making capacity.

This section discusses assessment of the capacity to make treatment decisions and consent to treatment. This is only one domain of capacity (2), but it is the most relevant to ethical decision-making for inpatient care.

Determination of decision-making capacity

An informed patient understands the diagnosis, prognosis, nature of proposed treatments and procedures, the risks and benefits of treatments and procedures, and alternatives (3). Applebaum et al. (4) have described the fundamental components of capacity to make treatment decisions as the abilities to communicate a choice, to understand the relevant information, to appreciate the medical consequences of the situation, and to reason about treatment choices. These are further outlined in Table 29.1 with questions clinicians might use to assess each component. Decision-making capacity can be

Table 29.1 Criteria for decision-making capacity and questions for assessment

Criterion	Questions for assessment	Comments
Ability to communicate a choice	Which treatment do you prefer?	Frequent reversals of choice due to neurologic or psychiatric illness may be indicative of lack of capacity.
Ability to understand relevant information	What have you been told about: The current problem with your health? What treatment has been recommended? The possible risks or benefits of the treatment? The alternatives to this treatment? What would happen if you got no treatment?	Ask patient to answer these questions in his/her own words. Patient need not use medical terminology to demonstrate understanding.
Ability to appreciate the situation and its consequences	What do you know about your health? Tell me about the illness and the treatments you could choose. What is this treatment likely to do for you? What do you believe will happen if you do not get treatment?	Patients who do not acknowledge their illness cannot make valid treatment decisions. Choosing no treatment is acceptable as long as the explanation of the decision process is rational.
Ability to reason about treatment options	How did you make your decision? Why is the option you chose better than the alternative option?	This is to assess the *process* not content of the decision. Patients have the right to make poor choices

Source: Adapted from Appelbaum PS, *N Engl J Med*, 357, 1834–1840, 2007.

assessed by any provider caring for a patient. Patients may designate surrogate decision-makers or delegate certain kinds of decisions to others.

In cases involving mental illness, substance use, and delirium, psychiatric consultants may be helpful in determining decision-making capacity. When there is conflict between providers or between the provider and patient and/or family, an ethics consultant may provide valuable input. It should be noted that patients and their families are permitted to make decisions contrary to medical recommendations. Furthermore, patients may meet criteria for demonstrating capacity regardless of their compliance with medical recommendations, and they may have the capacity to make some decisions but not others (often depending on the complexity of the decision).

Formal assessment tools

Several tools have been developed to formally assess decision-making capacity (5). The best validated among these is the MacArthur Competence Assessment Tool for Treatment. This instrument involves a 15–20 minute semistructured interview that generates quantitative scores for each of the four criteria of decision-making capacity, including understanding of treatment options, understanding of the medical disorder, thinking rationally about treatment, and expressing a choice. Though this instrument can be a helpful guide (and can provide standardized data in the case of legal proceedings), the scores must be integrated with other available data when determining the decision-making capacity of the patient.

SHARED DECISION-MAKING

As patients age and technologies advance, the complexities of patients' comorbidities and of treatment options present challenges in determining outcomes and potential complications. Shared decision-making is the process through which providers and patients share information and reach decisions together (Table 29.2). In the process of shared decision-making, the roles of the provider include eliciting the values and preferences of patients and integrating those values and preferences with medically reasonable options. Both patients/families and clinicians are providing important information to guide the decision-making process. Patients and providers must consider outcomes relevant to each individual patient, including those associated with survival, functional capacity, quality of life, and costs. Shared decision-making recognizes that there are complex trade-offs regarding costs and burdens, survival, and quality of life (6). Ideally, this process occurs early and iteratively throughout a patient's disease course. As it incorporates outcomes meaningful to patients, shared decision-making ensures patient-centered care, as mandated by the Patient Protection and Affordable Care Act (7).

Table 29.2 Components of shared decision-making

Role of patient	Role of provider
Articulation of preferences, goals, values	Selection of appropriate diagnostic workup Selection of appropriate treatment options

Source: Allen LA et al., *Circulation*, 125, 1928–1952, 2012.

SURROGACY AND ADVANCE DIRECTIVES

When it is determined that an individual lacks the ability to make his or her own medical decisions, medical providers must turn to advanced directives and/or surrogates.

Ideally, the patient will have left specific instructions for medical providers and appointed surrogates to follow in the event of the loss of capacity, and such instructions would be clearly applicable to the patient's current condition. However, this ideal set of circumstances is rarely present. Furthermore, it is often difficult to predict which of many potential decisions any given patient will face in end-of-life situations.

The process of advance care planning (ACP) encompasses designating a surrogate decision-maker and defining preferences for surrogate decision-making. At a minimum, it is important to identify a surrogate who can act in the patient's best interest, even if they lack knowledge of the patient's preferences about specific circumstances. Most often a close family member such as a spouse or adult child is the natural surrogate, but this is not always the case. In the United States, all states have specific laws governing the hierarchy of surrogates for medical decision-making. Several European countries have similar laws, though there is more variability throughout Europe than within the United States (8). ACP also includes elucidating values related to survival and quality of life. These discussions may guide the formation of specific goals regarding medical treatments such as dialysis or invasive procedures. Knowledge of a person and their values and goals can help considerably in determining what a patient would have wanted. When choosing a surrogate, patients should be encouraged to discuss values and goals with that person. Documentation of these goals can serve as an advance directive (9).

Advance directives

Advance directives serve to formally designate surrogate decision-makers and to document preferences for future medical care. However, few patients complete such directives. Lack of timely advance care planning has been associated with poor patient quality of life, caregiver distress, hospitalizations, physician burnout, and higher costs (9).

Even when completed, advance directives have limited impact on end-of-life care (10), and patients can receive care discordant with their stated preferences. Reasons for failure of advance directives include overly vague or overly specific instructions that are inapplicable to clinical care and complex health decisions (11). Fortunately, there are emerging models of advance care planning that may overcome some of the failings of traditional advance directives. Respecting Choices is a community-wide advance planning system originally developed in La Crosse, Wisconsin. This program involves community-wide education of health care providers and patients, training of advance care planning facilitators, integration of advance care planning into clinical care, and written protocols allowing emergency personnel access to physician orders that reflect patient preferences (12). This program has been shown to increase the use of advance directives and the adherence to treatment preferences defined in advance directives; in addition, participants are less likely to die in the hospital. The Respecting Choices program is being implemented in communities and organizations in the United States, Canada, and Australia.

Another approach to end-of-life planning is the Physician Orders for Life-Sustaining Treatment (POLST) program. This model, originally developed in Oregon but now available in many states, is designed to be used with individuals who are frail or suffering from advanced illnesses. The main feature is a brightly colored physician order form that is completed following discussion between the physician and the patient and/or surrogates. This form orders the level of aggressiveness in medical care and serves to direct nurses in community-based settings and emergency personnel. The document accompanies the patient across care settings to ensure that orders directing resuscitation and transfer to the hospital accompany the patient. The POLST form has been shown to represent patient treatment preferences and to match actual treatment at the end of life (13). Additionally, use of the form reduces unwanted CPR, intensive care, and ventilator support (14). A national task force for implementation of the POLST paradigm was established in 2004. Rather than a stand-alone system, the POLST paradigm is complementary to other advance directive systems and its use is strongly encouraged within the Respecting Choices program (15). Another model, Five Wishes (https://agingwithdignity.org), is a legal advance directive in a growing number of states that can be used to guide decisions by surrogates even where it is not a formal advance directive (16). Five Wishes walks people through documentation of their end-of-life wishes, covering the following:

1. The person I want to make care decisions for me when I can't
2. The kind of medical treatment I want or don't want
3. How comfortable I want to be
4. How I want people to treat me
5. What I want my loved ones to know

It is important to note that the completion of an advance directive is one part of advance care planning, but a conversation about values and goals with surrogates and medical providers should accompany the execution of the directive. Existing advance directives often do not specifically address cardiac devices such as pacing, tachytherapies, and left ventricular assist devices. As such, advance care planning discussions are paramount between patients with CVD and their cardiologists. Future advance directives and programs will need to include cardiac devices.

CARDIOPULMONARY RESUSCITATION

History and outcomes of cardiopulmonary resuscitation

In the 1960s, multiple advanced life-support techniques were combined to form a new lifesaving intervention known as cardiopulmonary resuscitation (CPR). In its infancy, CPR was restricted to intraoperative use and cardiac arrest due to ventricular arrhythmias. Before long, however, CPR began to be applied more broadly both in and outside of health care facilities. In 1974, the American Medical Association recommended that "code status" be documented in the medical record. Hospital policies regarding do-not-resuscitate (DNR) orders first appeared in 1976, ushering in an era, extending to the present day, in which CPR became the default medical treatment after cardiopulmonary arrest in the absence of a DNR order (17). Patients undergoing in-hospital CPR have a rate of return of spontaneous circulation of 30%–45% but only between 10% and 18% survive to hospital discharge (18). Though older adults as a group have a lower rate of survival to discharge following CPR, there are conflicting data as to whether age predicts poorer outcome independent of illness burden (19). Cardiopulmonary arrest from cardiac disease may be more responsive to CPR than other disease states, especially in the case of cardioversion for witnessed ventricular fibrillation (20).

The ethics of cardiopulmonary resuscitation and do-not-resuscitate orders

Given the relatively poor outcomes of CPR described earlier and even poorer outcomes in those with advanced illnesses, there has been vigorous debate over the ethics of offering or withholding CPR. In recent decades, the rising prominence of autonomy as a driving force in medical care and medical ethics has steered away from unilateral decision-making on the part of providers to withhold CPR (21). Multiple professional societies now recommend routine discussions of resuscitation preferences with all patients suffering from chronic or advanced illness. However, there is evidence that physicians do not conduct these discussions as frequently as recommended

(22). Discussing resuscitation preferences can be seen as an informed consent discussion. Such conversations can begin by asking what patients have told other clinicians or their families that they would prefer when the time comes that their "breathing or heart stops." The choice should be presented as between allowing natural death versus having someone try to revive them. As patients may overestimate their prognosis, clinicians should be prepared to share available data and estimates of outcomes of CPR in the context of the patients' medical problems. Additionally, physicians should provide support for patients' choice to allow natural death and be prepared to make a recommendation based on the patients' goals, values, and medical condition. Most patients want their physician to initiate discussions of resuscitation preferences. This is true even in situations where patients find the topic upsetting (23). Table 29.3 describes the recommended content of resuscitation discussions as well as sample statements and questions that can be used in such discussions. To best support patient autonomy, these discussions should be ongoing rather than a single event. There is evidence that resuscitation preferences of older adults and those with advanced illness are not static and frequently change with changes in medical condition or other life circumstances (24). Additionally, many patients may not want to make their own health care decisions, and these patients should be asked to identify surrogates (25).

It is generally agreed that the wishes of the patient or their surrogate regarding resuscitation preferences should be followed. However, physicians are not required to provide interventions that are "futile," that may not benefit, or that may be deemed potentially harmful. Ethicists disagree on how such futility should be defined and even whether futility should ever be used as a reason not to initiate CPR outside of extreme circumstances (e.g., decapitation, rigor mortis, decomposition) (26, 27). There is also debate about the use of the term "futility" itself, with some experts recommending that the term "medically inappropriate" be used instead (28). Regardless of which term is used, clinicians should conduct empathetic explorations of patients' goals, values, and preferences, as well as educate patients about their illness and expected outcomes of potential resuscitation attempts. If a patient and/or surrogate continues to insist on resuscitation in a case in which it is believed to be medically futile/medically

Table 29.3 Discussing resuscitation preferences

General guidelines

- Eliminate distractions, sit at patient level, and be ready to listen
- Ask if the patient would like any family/loved ones present
- Name and validate emotions that arise
- Validate difficulty of discussing these issues
- Stress importance of discussion in order to provide care that is consistent with patient's goals/values

Step	Example of language to use
Setting context/normalizing discussion	"I talk with all of my patients about what to do when the time comes that their heart or breathing stops." "Given the change in your condition, we need to review what to do when the time comes that your heart or breathing stops."
Describe alternatives and use "when" rather than "if"	"When the time comes that your heart stops or you stop breathing, do you want us to try to revive you or allow you to die naturally?"
Probe for understanding of the patient's reasoning	"Help me understand how you think about this issue." "Have you or your family had experiences with being revived or resuscitated?"
Identify undesired states, describe broadly	"Are there states of health that you would never want to be kept alive in?" "Unable to communicate with family/friends?" "Unable to make decisions for yourself?" "Unable to live independently?"
Discuss preferences for level/location of care	"How would you feel about being cared for in the hospital, an intensive care unit, or a nursing home if your condition worsened?"
Closing the conversation Provide a professional recommendation Clarify the difference between do not resuscitate/ongoing treatment, state commitment to continue care Set expectation for ongoing discussions	"Given what you describe [restate details], I recommend that we enter a do-not-resuscitate order." "We will continue to treat your illnesses and try to improve your length and quality of life." "We will revisit these issues with you and/or your family if your condition changes or if you want to discuss this again."

Sources: Adapted from Tanner CE et al., *Congest Heart Fail*, 17, 235–240, 2011; Goodlin SJ et al., *J Card Fail*, 14, 106–113, 2008.

inappropriate, all attempts should be made to obtain consensus. In the absence of such consensus, involvement of ethics consultation is usually appropriate.

One concerning finding from multiple studies that may complicate the discussion of resuscitation preferences is that the presence of a DNR order affects physician decision-making and aggressiveness of care separate from resuscitation (29, 30). It has been stated by some authors that a "do-not-resuscitate" order may be interpreted as a "do-not-treat" order. It is not ethically justifiable to restrict non-resuscitation treatments based solely on the presence of a DNR order. It may be possible to avoid this problem by using explicit language in DNR orders clarifying that all other treatments should be continued or through educational initiatives targeted at medical and nursing staff.

ETHICAL DECISIONS IN THE MANAGEMENT OF HEART FAILURE

The treatment of heart failure (HF) presents many complex ethical issues (31). The epidemiology, impact, and treatment of HF in older adults are discussed in Chapters 19 and 20. A multitude of advances in the management of HF have improved both survival and quality of life. These advances include pharmaceutical approaches, chronic disease management, and therapy with devices, all of which may complicate end-of-life care. Despite these advances, HF is still a life-limiting illness and progressively results in high symptom burden and loss of function. There is also a high caregiver burden. This section addresses advance care or preparedness planning in HF patients in general, in the setting of inotropic support, and in the setting of treatment with implanted devices.

Advance care planning in heart failure

The variable trajectory of HF makes it difficult for clinicians to predict outcomes for individual patients and complicates advance care planning (30). Such discussions, however, are critical to supporting patient autonomy and allowing patients to avoid undue harm, unwanted interventions, and potential consequences of treatments and interventions. Unfortunately, such planning is often initiated in the last stages of HF (32). All patients should be given the opportunity to discuss the expected disease trajectory, prognosis, and the uncertainties associated with a HF diagnosis. Ideally, discussions of preparedness planning would be initiated at or near the time of the HF diagnosis. These discussions should focus on integrating the patient's beliefs, values, goals, and preferences considering the life-limiting nature of HF and the uncertainty in prognostication. Validated tools such as the Seattle Heart Failure Model (https://depts.washington.edu/shfm) can be applied to help in general prognostication (33). The American Heart Association proposed the "Annual Heart Failure Review" as a potential platform for these discussions that promote shared decision-making in an iterative manner (7, 34).

Treatment with inotropic agents

Inotropic agents such as milrinone and dobutamine may help relieve refractory symptoms, improve quality of life, and reduce hospitalizations for some patients with reduced ejection fraction. Inotropes may also be used with "palliative intent" for symptom relief in patients with end-stage HF who are not candidates for other advanced therapies. Inotropic agents may be associated with increased risk of arrhythmias (35). The risks may be further increased by renal dysfunction (36). Other complications are related to those associated with intravenous access and infection. As a result, though inotropes are used with the intent to relieve symptoms, the increased risk of arrhythmias may result in ICD shocks that may increase anxiety and pain at the end of life. Best practices regarding palliative inotropic agents have not been elucidated, but the elicitation of patients' goals and preferences is especially important in consideration of the use of palliative inotropic therapy, with a frank discussion of the quality of life versus longevity trade-off. As not all hospice agencies offer inotropic therapy, collaboration between cardiovascular and hospice and palliative care specialists is often crucial, especially in the transition to comfort care (35).

Treatment with implantable devices in heart failure

Implantable devices such as ICDs, left ventricular assist devices (LVADs), and CRT pacemakers have revolutionized the care of patients with HF. These devices prevent sudden cardiac death (ICDs) (37), improve functional status and quality of life (LVADs and CRT) (37, 38), and improve survival of HF (LVADs, ICDs, and CRT) (37–39). Informed consent for such devices must include the indications for the device and its potential risks and benefits, and any reasonable alternatives to device implantation. Importantly, patients and their families should understand the options for management at the end of life. Discussions regarding possible complications of device therapy and future deactivation should take place with patients and their caregivers prior to device implantation (40).

Implantable cardioverter-defibrillators and cardiac resynchronization therapy

By treating ventricular arrhythmias and preventing sudden cardiac death, ICDs can prolong survival. As older patients more commonly die of pump failure or progressive metabolic decline, the original intent of ICDs may not apply at the end of life (41). However, patients and their caregivers frequently do not understand the purpose of ICDs or lack awareness of the ability to deactivate tachytherapies (42). Furthermore, though discussions addressing the possibility of future deactivation are recommended prior to ICD implantation, they often do not happen (43–46). ICD deactivation may also raise ethical issues not only for patients but also for providers, as some clinicians may equate deactivation with physician-assisted suicide/physician aid in dying or euthanasia. Patients may suffer ICD shocks at the end of their lives that increase pain and anxiety, decrease quality of life, and disturb family members (47). Decisions about deactivation are especially important when initiating palliative inotropic therapy, as inotropes can increase tachyarrhythmias.

Many of the aforementioned issues with ICDs also pertain to the implantation of CRT devices, with the exception that for about two thirds of recipients, CRT devices improve symptoms by promoting atrioventricular and biventricular synchrony. As a result, deactivation of CRT may result in worsening of symptoms. It is important to ensure patient and family understanding about the potential effect of worsening symptoms with CRT deactivation. As combination defibrillator and CRT devices (CRT-D) are often implanted in the United States, providers should discuss the possibility of deactivating the defibrillator component at the end of life with all patients. Scientific statements that discuss these issues in greater detail have been published (45, 48).

LEFT VENTRICULAR ASSIST DEVICES

Few devices have carried both the promise and the ethical complexity associated with LVADs. The Centers for Medicare and Medicaid Services has mandated palliative care involvement in the multidisciplinary team as a condition for payment for patients under consideration for an LVAD as destination therapy (DT-LVAD: LVAD for the rest of the patient's life, with no intent to perform cardiac transplant). Originally developed as bridging devices for patients with cardiac injury expected to recover, and then for those awaiting cardiac transplant, destination therapy has become the most frequent indication for LVAD implantation. Many patients with end-stage HF do not qualify for heart transplantation due to factors such as age and obesity. For selected patients, these devices have demonstrated the ability to both prolong life and dramatically improve quality of life. There are, however, significant risks related to neurologic complications (both hemorrhagic and thrombotic stroke), gastrointestinal bleeding, infections, and repeated and prolonged hospitalizations (39). With potentially significant complications and burdens, it is recommended that patients and their families engage in preparedness planning as delineated in Table 29.4, including informed consent for LVAD implantation, designation of surrogate decision-makers, and elucidation of preferences and goals in the event of complications (e.g., stroke), device failure, development of debilitating comorbidities (e.g., dementia, cancer), and inadequate improvements or worsening of quality of life following implant (49). There is evidence of high caregiver burden with reports of high anxiety and negative impact on caregivers' health (50). The importance of a multidisciplinary team, including palliative care and sometimes ethics, is crucial in facilitating decision-making, preparedness planning, and caregiver support (51).

Table 29.4 Preparedness planning

Key components
Designation of surrogate decision-makers
Preferences and goals in the event of the following circumstances: • Inadequate quality of life • Debilitative comorbid conditions • Catastrophic complications due to LVAD-associated factors • Device failure

Source: Swetz KM et al., *Mayo Clin Proc*, 86, 493–500, 2011.

Palliative and end-of-life care in heart failure

With the aging of the population and increasing incidence and prevalence of HF, more clinicians will be involved in end-of-life care for patients with advanced, progressive HF. The systems of end-of-life and hospice care in both the United States and Europe were largely developed to manage oncologic patients. Studies in the United States suggest that some hospice organizations lack competence in management of HF at the end of life (52), in particular for managing cardiac medications and devices. Furthermore, CVD specialists may lack confidence in providing end-of-life care for their patients with HF (53). A solution to this dilemma is collaboration between cardiovascular specialists, hospice and palliative medicine specialists, and primary care providers in end-of-life care. The variable trajectory of HF makes identification of patients who may be eligible for hospice care difficult. Comorbid conditions such as pulmonary disease, dementia, and severe renal dysfunction decrease 6-month prognosis (54). Frequent hospitalizations, loss of functional status, and development of other comorbidities may signal overall decline and can also serve as triggers for discussions about goals and consideration of transitioning to comfort care (7).

Integration of palliative care throughout the course of HF care focuses on relief of patient symptoms, improving quality of life, and caregiver support. Involvement of palliative care earlier in the disease course results in improved symptom burden and timely and appropriate referrals to hospice (52).

Symptom management and life prolongation

Patients with HF have a symptom burden severity similar to that of patients with advanced malignancy (55). Prevalent symptoms include dyspnea, pain, fatigue, and depression (56). High symptom burden negatively impacts quality of life and functional status (57). Depression, pain, and spiritual suffering are underrecognized and undertreated in HF (58, 59). Symptom assessment instruments such as the Edmonton Symptom Assessment Scale (ESAS) and the Memorial Symptom Assessment Scale Modified for HF (MSAS-HF) are appropriate for a more comprehensive evaluation in patients with HF (60, 61). However, unlike management in many other diseases, including most end-stage cancers, life-prolonging cardiovascular therapies often have symptom benefit and improve quality of life (62). Thus, pursuing guideline-directed medical management with an angiotensin receptor neprilysin inhibitor, angiotensin receptor blockers, angiotensin-converting enzyme inhibitors, beta-adrenergic antagonists, aldosterone antagonists, and sodium-glucose cotransporter-2 inhibitors (62) can often be part of symptom management, as can interventions like CRT devices, transcatheter valve replacements, and LVADs. Inotropes can be considered for refractory symptoms in cases of cardiogenic shock and inability to escalate guideline-directed medications.

As HF progresses, patients may experience increased symptom burden and, consequently, poor quality of life. As goals evolve, there may be a shift from an emphasis on quantity to quality of life. This shift in focus should not automatically result in discontinuation of HF-directed medications. Adequate symptom management requires collaborative teamwork among providers from palliative care, primary care, and cardiovascular medicine. Social workers and clinical resource coordinators are crucial in mobilizing necessary services. This teamwork is also crucial in determining the benefit and burden of each therapy when considering discontinuation.

Care at the end-of-life in heart failure

As patient and family goals focus solely on comfort at the end of life, optimal care of HF patients requires nuanced utilization of cardiac medications and therapies, appropriate withdrawal of therapies, and application of palliative measures including inotropes. These complex decisions are governed by patients' goals, values, and preferences, as well as medical appropriateness. Hospice and palliative care specialists help providers, patients, and families transition to comfort care. Continued multidisciplinary teamwork in the end-of-life setting ensures expertise in cardiovascular and palliative measures. For example, hospice agencies may require guidance from electrophysiology and HF specialists in the management and deactivation of ICDs, CRT, and LVADs. In particular, consideration of LVAD deactivation may cause ethical distress on the part of providers who may believe that LVAD deactivation is similar to physician-assisted suicide and/or euthanasia, especially since death often ensues within minutes to hours after disabling the device. However, similar to the withdrawal of life support measures like mechanical ventilation and dialysis where there is progression of existing disease, LVAD deactivation results in the natural progression of end-stage cardiomyopathy and is ethically acceptable (62). Chaplains play important roles in addressing spiritual distress (63).

ETHICAL DECISIONS IN STROKE/ CEREBROVASCULAR ACCIDENTS

Cerebrovascular accidents (CVAs) affect those older than 65 three times as frequently as those younger than 65, and older patients have a substantially higher risk of dying after a stroke (64). In the acute stages of stroke, patients and families must make time-sensitive decisions such as proceeding with mechanical thrombectomy and decompressive craniectomy (64). As in HF, stroke patients have uncertain prognosis with possible outcomes ranging from full recovery to severe disability. As many as 15%–20% of patients die in the acute post-CVA period with another 10% dying in the 6–12 months following the acute CVA. Mortality is highest for hemorrhagic stroke and lowest for lacunar infarct, and it increases with age across all stroke types (65). However, even among those initially requiring mechanical ventilation, up to 25% may recover all or nearly all of their pre-CVA functional capacity (66). After CVA, patients and families must adapt to cognitive and functional deficits, as well as symptoms such as pain syndromes and incontinence specific to post-stroke patients. As a result, patients and their caregivers may experience significant distress. However, despite the need for palliative care, there is a lack of knowledge guiding symptom management, palliative care, and end-of-life care for stroke patients. This section discusses the ethical issues relating to artificial nutrition in the post-CVA period as well as palliative and end-of-life care after CVA.

Artificial nutrition in the post-stroke period

Nearly 80% of patients may have difficulty safely swallowing food and fluids after an acute CVA (67). For those who are expected to survive long term, or for those who wish to pursue aggressive interventions, artificial nutrition by feeding tube (FT) may be necessary. Though tube feeding in general does not prevent aspiration or prolong life in most patients with dysphagia, it may have a limited role in the acute post-CVA recovery period. Some patients and/or family members/surrogates may choose not to have a FT. The reasons for such a decision are varied and may include cognitive impairment or mood disorder caused by the stroke, misunderstanding of the role of artificial nutrition in recovery, or a well-informed desire not to prolong a life that is seen as unacceptable to the patient (68). Careful evaluation of the patient's understanding of the situation, cognitive ability, and motivations for refusing a FT are important to act with beneficence while avoiding harm and preserving autonomy. A formal capacity evaluation may be necessary in such a situation. If it is determined that patients have decision-making capacity, understand the risks and benefits of tube feeding, and wish to forgo this intervention to avoid life prolongation, clinicians should respect patients' autonomy and honor their wishes. Furthermore, many patients may wish to continue oral nutrition despite the risk of aspiration, pneumonia, and death. This decision should be supported in the competent patient who is able to give informed consent. In the unfortunate case of an incompetent patient with no available surrogate, health care professionals face a difficult dilemma. If a patient's previously expressed wishes are known, this should guide treatment—this may be true even if such preferences are not legally binding. In the absence of such expressed wishes, the health care professionals themselves (often with the assistance of ethics consultation) must be responsible for acting in the patient's best interest. If there is conflict or uncertainty among the health care team, legal counsel should be sought (69).

Symptom prevalence after a stroke

There is high symptom burden, disability, and caregiving burden among post-stroke patients and their caregivers. Families of patients dying after stroke frequently report inadequate symptom control, poor communication, and failure to address psychological morbidity (70). Pain syndromes specific to CVA patients include central post-stroke pain, hemiplegic shoulder pain, tension-type headache, and painful spasticity (71). As opioids may not be beneficial for these pain syndromes, physical therapy, consideration of antiepileptics, botulinum injections, and electrical stimulation should be considered (72). Other common symptoms include depression, anxiety, and emotional lability. Depression after CVA has been associated with dependency, poor functional outcome, and increased mortality (73). Fatigue also affects more than half of patients after a CVA. Incontinence, due to multiple factors including the effects of the stroke, immobility, and lack of communication (74), is a particularly distressing symptom for which there is a lack of guidance in treatment (75). A multidisciplinary approach, including neurology, palliative care, psychiatry, and physical, occupational, and speech therapy may be necessary for effective treatment and support of these symptoms.

Caregiving for stroke survivors

At least one quarter of stroke survivors will be dependent on others for activities of daily living (ADLs) 6 months after their CVA requiring assistance and caregiving. While many post-stroke patients reside in nursing homes or other care facilities, many receive care from family members or other caregivers. In contrast to conditions such as dementia or chronic heart disease, caregivers for stroke patients often have an abrupt transition from their previous routine to their new role in caring for their loved one. Stress and burnout are common in these caregivers and many report lack of support and poor quality of life (76). The degree of functional impairment of the stroke survivor is associated with decreasing quality of life in caregivers. Caregiver training has been shown to reduce depression and anxiety as well as improve quality of life in both caregivers and stroke survivors. Trained caregivers also experience less caregiver burden. Referral to a social worker familiar with resources in the community as well as connection with patient or caregiver advocacy groups may be beneficial (77).

Palliative care for stroke survivors

Patients and families have great palliative care needs throughout the stages of stroke. In the acute stages, patients and families can benefit from decision-making support and symptom management in times of crisis and uncertain prognosis. During post-stroke recovery, palliative care needs include support during adjustment to new functional and cognitive impairments, symptoms such as pain, and psychosocial distress (78). Patients and families often face decisions regarding CPR, mechanical ventilation, artificial nutrition, and dialysis. Palliative care involvement could help facilitate advance care planning and provide decision-making support, especially in consideration of withdrawal of life-sustaining support (79). As with other terminal illness, the use of hospice services can be of great benefit to patients dying of stroke and to their families. A 2010 study of US Medicare beneficiaries found that among patients dying within 30 days of an acute stroke, 23% utilized hospice services, which is on par with both malignant and other nonmalignant diseases (80).

ETHICAL ISSUES IN CARDIAC SURGERY

As the population ages, the prevalence of age-related illnesses such as aortic stenosis and coronary artery disease for which surgery is considered a therapeutic option has risen markedly. Advances in cardiopulmonary bypass pumps, minimally invasive options, anesthesia, hemostasis, and procedural time have improved the success and tolerability of surgical options (81). Since it was first performed in 1960, CABG has become a standard treatment for severe coronary artery disease (82). As techniques and outcomes have improved, CABG has been offered to increasingly complicated, medically ill, and older patients. It is now routine for centers in the United States, Canada, and Europe to perform CABG on patients in their 70s and

80s. Though the rate of perioperative complications and mortality is higher than for younger individuals, patients over age 80 have good long-term survival, improved quality of life, and an acceptable operative risk for CABG (83–86). These results come, however, with higher resource utilization in the postoperative period (87). As with CABG, similar results have been demonstrated for older patients undergoing valve replacement surgery, particularly with aortic valve replacement (88). Referring cardiology providers and surgeons must ensure a fully informed consent process, guiding patients and families through understanding of the indications, risks, benefits, and possible consequences of surgery and viable alternative options.

ETHICAL ISSUES IN INTERVENTIONS FOR AORTIC STENOSIS

Advanced age, end organ dysfunction, and multiple comorbid conditions are associated with higher mortality in patients with valvular heart disease, including aortic stenosis (87, 89). As the 1-year mortality increases to 40%–50% once patients develop severe symptoms, the decision to intervene in valvular disease in older patients can be complex (90, 91). Options include surgical aortic valve replacement (AVR), transcatheter aortic valve replacement (TAVR), or medical management. Since the first TAVR was performed in 2002 (92), advancing TAVR technologies and experience have resulted in increasingly improved symptoms and reduced all-cause mortality in comparison to medical therapy (93). For an expanding number of scenarios, TAVR is noninferior compared to surgical AVR with respect to major clinical outcomes and is associated with shorter length of stay and faster recovery (94). Many patients who are not candidates for surgical AVR experience improved longevity and quality of life after TAVR. Appropriate patient selection and procedural planning by a multidisciplinary heart team is mandated and is paramount for success. However, important factors such as frailty and liver dysfunction play significant roles but are not accounted for in common risk assessment tools such as the Society of Thoracic Surgeons Predicted Risk of Mortality (STS PROM) score (87, 89). Frailty and cognitive dysfunction have been shown to be associated with poorer outcomes, increased complications, and mortality (95, 96). In addition, cardiac disease may not be the primary driver of symptoms, disability, and mortality. As a result, not all patients benefit equally from TAVR (97).

Risks play a key part in any informed consent discussion, but especially in the case of TAVR and other nonsurgical interventions in older patients. Though there are declining rates of periprocedural risks with advancing TAVR technology and experience, risks include stroke and need for pacemaker placement (93). Post-procedurally, patients may experience delirium. Though cognition may improve, some patients could suffer cognitive decline following TAVR (98). Decreased mobility may complicate rehabilitation and put patients at risk for other disorders such as deep vein thrombosis.

The field of transcatheter interventions is expanding rapidly, with percutaneous devices for repair and replacement of the mitral and tricuspid valves joining the well-established percutaneous aortic and pulmonic valve replacements. The same decision-making, advance care planning, and preparedness planning principles that should direct the care of HF patients should also be applied to older patients under consideration for transcatheter procedures. As these devices have no impact on many of the comorbidities or frailty that preclude surgical options, palliative care should be a key component in the management of older patients undergoing transcatheter procedures. Although not mandated for payment, multidisciplinary teams caring for these patients should involve palliative care to help determine goals of care, support decision-making, and treat symptoms from multimorbid conditions (97).

CONCLUSION

As the burden of CVD and complexities of CVD management burgeon, patients and providers will be challenged by the ethical issues that arise throughout the disease course. Navigating complex ethical issues and communicating with patients and families can prove difficult, especially when providers have received little training in these areas. Key skills for providers include assessment of capacity, advance care planning, and basic symptom management. Shared decision-making requires these skills, and cardiovascular training programs should seek to provide venues for trainee education. Increasingly, cardiovascular providers will need to partner with ethics consultants and palliative care and hospice providers in a multidisciplinary format to improve the care of older patients. Efforts to address timely access, disparities, and cost, and to ensure goal-concordant care must be in parallel to optimize outcomes of older patients with CVD.

ACKNOWLEDGMENT

The author gratefully acknowledges and thanks Dr. Craig Tanner, Dr. Sarah J. Goodlin, and the late Dr. James N. Kirkpatrick for their contributions to this chapter in the previous edition of this text.

REFERENCES

1. Murad K, Goff DC Jr, Morgan TM et al. Burden of comorbidities and functional and cognitive impairment in elderly patients at initial diagnosis of heart failure and their impact on total mortality: The cardiovascular health study. *JACC Heart Fail* 2015; 3(7): 542–550.

2. Moye J, Marson DC. Assessment of decision-making capacity in older adults: An emerging area of practice and research. *J Gerontol B Psychol Sci Soc Sci* 2007; *62*: P3–P11.
3. Krumholz HM. Informed consent to promote patient centered care. *JAMA* 2010; *303*: 1190–1191.
4. Appelbaum PS. Clinical practice. Assessment of patients' competence to consent to treatment. *N Engl J Med* 2007; *357*: 1834–1840.
5. Dunn LB, Nowrangi MA, Palmer BW et al. Assessing decisional capacity for clinical research or treatment: A review of instruments. *Am J Psychiatry* 2006; *163*: 1323–1334.
6. Spilker B, ed. *Quality of Life and Pharmacoeconomics in Clinical Trials*, 2nd ed. Philadelphia, PA: Lippincott Williams & Wilkins, 1996.
7. Allen LA, Stevenson LW, Grady KL et al. Decision making in advanced heart failure: A scientific statement from the American Heart Association. *Circulation* 2012; *125*(15): 1928–1952.
8. Lautrette A, Peigne V, Watts J et al. Surrogate decision makers for incompetent ICU patients: A European perspective. *Curr Opin Crit Care* 2008; *14*: 714–719.
9. Sinuff T, Dodek P, You JJ et al. Improving end-of-life communication and decision making: The development of a conceptual framework and quality indications. *J Pain Symptom Manage* 2015; *49*(6): 1070–1080.
10. Fagerlin A, Schneider CE. Enough: The failure of the living will. *Hastings Cent Rep* 2004; *34*: 30–42.
11. Hickman SE, Hammes BJ, Moss AH, Tolle SW. Hope for the future: Achieving the original intent of advance directives. *Hastings Cent Rep* 2005; Spec No: S26–S30.
12. Hammes BJ, Rooney BL. Death and end-of-life planning in one midwestern community. *Arch Intern Med* 1998; *158*: 383–390.
13. Hickman SE, Nelson CA, Moss AH et al. The consistency between treatments provided to nursing facility residents and orders on the physician orders for life-sustaining treatment form. *J Am Geriatr Soc* 2011; *59*: 2091–2099.
14. Tolle SW, Tilden VP, Nelson CA, Dunn PM. A prospective study of the efficacy of the physician order form for life-sustaining treatment. *J Am Geriatr Soc* 1998; *46*: 1097–1102.
15. Hammes BJ, Rooney BL, Gundrum JD et al. The POLST program: A retrospective review of the demographics of use and outcomes in one community where advance directives are prevalent. *J Palliat Med* 2012; *15*: 77–85.
16. Loertscher L, Reed DA, Bannon MP, Mueller PS. Cardiopulmonary resuscitation and do-not-resuscitate orders: A guide for clinicians. *Am J Med* 2010; *123*: 4–9.
17. Ehlenbach WJ, Barnato AE, Curtis JR et al. Epidemiologic study of in-hospital cardiopulmonary resuscitation in the elderly. *N Engl J Med* 2009; *361*: 22–31.
18. Lannon R, O'Keeffe ST. Cardiopulmonary resuscitation in older people—A review. *Rev Clin Gerontol* 2010; *20*: 20.
19. De Vos R, Koster RW, De Haan RJ et al. In-hospital cardiopulmonary resuscitation: Prearrest morbidity and outcome. *Arch Intern Med* 1999; *159*: 845–850.
20. Burns JP, Edwards J, Johnson J et al. Do-not-resuscitate order after 25 years. *Crit Care Med* 2003; *31*: 1543–1550.
21. Anderson WG, Chase R, Pantilat SZ et al. Code status discussions between attending hospitalist physicians and medical patients at hospital admission. *J Gen Intern Med* 2010; *26*: 359–366.
22. Gorton AJ, Jayanthi NVG, Lepping P, Scriven MW. Patients' attitudes towards "do not attempt resuscitation" status. *J Med Ethics* 2008; *34*: 624–626.
23. Fried TR, O'Leary J, Van Ness P, Fraenkel L. Inconsistency over time in the preferences of older persons with advanced illness for life-sustaining treatment. *J Am Geriatr Soc* 2007; *55*: 1007–1014.
24. Puchalski CM, Zhong Z, Jacobs MM et al. Patients who want their family and physician to make resuscitation decisions for them: Observations from SUPPORT and HELP. Study to understand prognoses and preferences for outcomes and risks of treatment. Hospitalized elderly longitudinal project. *J Am Geriatr Soc* 2000; *48*: S84–S90.
25. Ardagh M. Futility has no utility in resuscitation medicine. *J Med Ethics* 2000; *26*: 396–399
26. Hilberman M, Kutner J, Parsons D, Murphy DJ. Marginally effective medical care: Ethical analysis of issues in cardiopulmonary resuscitation (CPR). *J Med Ethics* 1997; *23*: 361–367.
27. Beach MC, Morrison RS. The effect of do-not-resuscitate orders on physician decision-making. *J Am Geriatr Soc* 2002; *50*: 2057–2061.
28. Bosslet GT, Pope TM, Rubenfeld GD et al. An official ATS/AACN/ACCP/ESICM/SCCM policy statement: Responding to requests for potentially inappropriate treatments in intensive care units. *Am J Respir Crit Care Med* 2015; *191*(11): 1318–1330.
29. Chen JLT, Sosnov J, Lessard D, Goldberg RJ. Impact of do-not-resuscitation orders on quality of care performance measures in patients hospitalized with acute heart failure. *Am Heart J* 2008; *156*: 78–84.
30. Tanner CE, Fromme EK, Goodlin SJ. Ethics in the treatment of advanced heart failure: Palliative care and end-of-life issues. *Congest Heart Fail* 2011; *17*: 235–240.
31. Harding R, Selman L, Beynon T et al. Meeting the communication and information needs of chronic heart failure patients. *J Pain Symptom Manage* 2008; *36*: 149–156.

32. The AM, Hak T, Koeter G, van Der Wal G. Collusion in doctor-patient communication about imminent death: An ethnographic study. *BMJ* 2000; *321*: 1376–1381.
33. Levy WC, Mozaffarian D, Linker DT et al. The Seattle heart failure model: Prediction of survival in heart failure. *Circulation* 2006; *113*: 1424–1433.
34. Goodlin SJ, Quill TE, Arnold RM. Communication and decision-making about prognosis in heart failure care. *J Card Fail* 2008; *14*: 106–113.
35. Hauptman PJ, Mikolajczak P, George A et al. Chronic inotropic therapy in end-stage heart failure. *Am Heart J* 2006; *152*: 1096–1098.
36. Cox ZL, Calcutt MW, Morrison TB et al. Elevation of plasma milrinone concentrations in stage D heart failure associated with renal dysfunction. *J Cardiovasc Pharmacol Ther* 2013; *18*(5): 433–438.
37. Moss AJ, Zareba W, Hall WJ et al. Prophylactic implantation of a defibrillator in patients with myocardial infarction and reduced ejection fraction. *N Engl J Med* 2002; *346*: 877–883.
38. Cleland JG, Daubert JC, Erdmann E et al. The effect of cardiac resynchronization on morbidity and mortality in heart failure. *N Engl J Med* 2005; *352*: 1539–1549.
39. Long JW, Kfoury AG, Slaughter MS et al. Long-term destination therapy with the HeartMate XVE left ventricular assist device: Improved outcomes since the REMATCH study. *Congest Heart Fail* 2005; *11*: 133–138.
40. Berger JT, Gorski M, Cohen T. Advance health planning and treatment preferences among recipients of implantable cardioverter defibrillators: An exploratory study. *J Clin Ethics* 2006; *17*: 72–78.
41. MacIver J, Rao V, Delgado DH et al. Choices: A study of preferences for end-of-life treatments in patients with advanced heart failure. *J Heart Lung Transplant* 2008; *27*: 1002–1007.
42. Goldstein NE, Mehta D, Siddiqui S et al. "That's like an act of suicide" patients' attitudes toward deactivation of implantable defibrillators. *J Gen Intern Med* 2008; *23*: 7–12.
43. Goldstein NE, Lampert R, Bradley E et al. Management of implantable cardioverter defibrillators in end-of-life care. *Ann Intern Med* 2004; *141*: 835–838.
44. Goldstein NE, Mehta D, Teitelbaum E et al. "It's like crossing a bridge" complexities preventing physicians from discussing deactivation of implantable defibrillators at the end of life. *J Gen Intern Med* 2008; *23*: 2–6.
45. Lampert R, Hayes DL, Annas GJ et al. HRS expert consensus statement on the management of cardiovascular implantable electronic devices (CIEDs) in patients nearing end of life or requesting withdrawal of therapy. *Heart Rhythm* 2010; *7*(7): 1008–1026.
46. Kramer DB, Matlock DD, Buxton AE et al. Implantable cardioverter-defibrillator use in older adults: Proceedings of a Hartford change agents symposium. *Circ Cardiovasc Qual Outcomes* 2015; *8*(4): 437–446.
47. Kirkpatrick JN, Gottlieb M, Sehgal P et al. Deactivation of implantable cardioverter defibrillators in end of life care. *Am J Cardiol* 2012; *109*: 91–94.
48. Epstein AE, DiMarco JP, Ellenbogen KA et al. ACC/AHA/HRS 2008 Guidelines for device-based therapy of cardiac rhythm abnormalities: A report of the American College of Cardiology/American Heart Association Task Force on Practice Guidelines (Writing Committee to Revise the ACC/AHA/NASPE 2002 Guideline Update for Implantation of Cardiac Pacemakers and Antiarrhythmia Devices): Developed in collaboration with the American association for thoracic surgery and society of thoracic surgeons. *Circulation* 2008; *117*: e350–e408.
49. Brush S, Budge D, Alharethi R et al. End-of-life decision making and implementation in recipients of a destination left ventricular assist device. *J Heart Lung Transplant* 2010; *29*: 1337–1341.
50. Swetz KM, Freeman MR, Abou Ezzeddine OF et al. Palliative medicine consultation for preparedness planning in patients receiving left ventricular assist devices as destination therapy. *Mayo Clin Proc* 2011; *86*: 493–500.
51. Swetz KM, Ottenberg AL, Freeman MR, Mueller PS. Palliative care and end-of-life issues in patients treated with left ventricular assist devices as destination therapy. *Curr Heart Fail Rep* 2011; *8*: 212–218.
52. Goodlin SJ, Kutner JS, Connor SR et al. Hospice care for heart failure patients. *J Pain Symptom Manage* 2005; *29*: 525–528.
53. Bunzel B, Laederach-Hofmann K, Wieselthaler G et al. Mechanical circulatory support as a bridge to heart transplantation: What remains? Long-term emotional sequelae in patients and spouses. *J Heart Lung Transplant* 2007; *26*: 384–389.
54. Ahluwalia SC, Gross CP, Chaudhry SI et al. Change in comorbidity prevalence with advancing age among persons with heart failure. *JGIM* 2011; *26*(10): 1145–1151
55. Bekelman DB, Rumsfeld JS, Havranek EP et al. Symptom burden, depression, and spiritual wellbeing: A comparison of heart failure and advanced cancer patients. *J Gen Intern Med* 2009; *24*: 592–598.
56. Goodlin SJ, Trupp R, Bernhardt P et al. Development and evaluation of the "Advanced heart failure clinical competence survey": A tool to assess knowledge of heart failure care and self-assessed competence. *Patient Educ Couns* 2007; *67*: 3–10.
57. Zambroski CH, Moser DK, Bhat G, Ziegler C. Impact of symptom prevalence and symptom

burden on quality of life in patients with heart failure. *Eur J Cardiovasc Nurs* 2005; *4*: 198–206.
58. Goebel JR, Doering LV, Shugarman LR et al. Heart failure: The hidden problem of pain. *J Pain Symptom Manage* 2009; *38*: 698–707.
59. Cully JA, Johnson M, Moffett ML et al. Depression and anxiety in ambulatory patients with heart failure. *Psychosomatics* 2009; *50*: 592–598.
60. Chang VT, Hwang SS, Feuerman M. Validation of the Edmonton symptom assessment scale. *Cancer* 2000; *88*: 2164–2171.
61. Pak, E.S., Jones, C.A. & Mather, P.J. Ethical Challenges in care of patients on mechanical circulatory support at end-of-life. *Curr Heart Fail Rep* 2020. https://doi.org/10.1007/s11897-020-00460-4.
62. Blinderman CD, Homel P, Billings JA et al. Symptom distress and quality of life in patients with advanced congestive heart failure. *J Pain Symptom Manage* 2008; *35*: 594–603.
63. Goodlin SJ. Palliative care in congestive heart failure. *J Am Coll Cardiol* 2009; *54*: 386–396.
64. Roger VL, Go AS, Lloyd-Jones DM et al. Heart disease and stroke statistics–2012 update: A report from the American Heart Association. *Circulation* 2012; *125*: e2–e220.
65. Steiner T, Mendoza G, De Georgia M et al. Prognosis of stroke patients requiring mechanical ventilation in a neurological critical care unit. *Stroke* 1997; *28*: 711–715.
66. Creutzfeldt CJ, Holloway RG, Curtis R. Palliative care: A core competency for stroke neurologists. *Stroke* 2015; *46*: 2714–2719.
67. Martino R, Foley N, Bhogal S et al. Dysphagia after stroke: Incidence, diagnosis, and pulmonary complications. *Stroke* 2005; *36*: 2756–2763.
68. Sandman L, Agren Bolmsjo I, Westergren A. Ethical considerations of refusing nutrition after stroke. *Nurs Ethics* 2008; *15*: 147–159.
69. Blackmer J. Tube feeding in stroke patients: A medical and ethical perspective. *Can J Neurol Sci* 2001; *28*: 101–106.
70. Stevens T, Payne S, Burton C et al. Palliative care in stroke: A critical review of the literature. *Palliat Med* 2007; *21*: 323–331.
71. Kelly-Hayes M, Beiser A, Kase CS et al. The influence of gender and age on disability following ischemic stroke: The Framingham study. *J Stroke Cerebrovasc Dis* 2003; *12*: 119–126.
72. Creutzfeldt CJ, Holloway RG, Walker M. Symptomatic and palliative care for stroke survivors. *J Gen Intern Med* 2012; *27*: 853–860.
73. Hackett ML, Anderson CS, House A, Xia J. Interventions for treating depression after stroke. *Cochrane Database Syst Rev* 2008; (4): CD003437.
74. Thomas LH, Cross S, Barrett J et al. Treatment of urinary incontinence after stroke in adults. *Cochrane Database Syst Rev* 2008; *2008*: CD004462.
75. Nakayama H, Jorgensen HS, Pedersen PM et al. Prevalence and risk factors of incontinence after stroke: The Copenhagen Stroke Study. *Stroke* 1997; *28*(1): 58–62.
76. Han B, Haley WE. Family caregiving for patients with stroke: Review and analysis. *Stroke* 1999; *30*: 1478–1485.
77. Kalra L, Evans A, Perez I et al. Training carers of stroke patients: Randomised controlled trial. *BMJ* 2004; *328*(7448): 1099.
78. Braun LT, Grady KL, Kutner JS et al. Palliative care and cardiovascular disease and stroke: A policy statement from the American Heart Association/American Stroke Association. *Circulation* 2016; *134*: e198–e225.
79. Holloway RG, Arnold RM, Creutzfeldt CJ et al. Palliative and end of life care in stroke. *Stroke* 2014; *45*: 1887–1916.
80. DuPreez AE, Smith MA, Liou J-I et al. Predictors of hospice utilization among acute stroke patients who died within thirty days. *J Palliat Med* 2008; *11*: 1249–1257.
81. Cooley DA, Frazier OH. The past 50 years of cardiovascular surgery. *Circulation* 2000; *102*(20): IV87–IV93.
82. Weisse AB. Cardiac surgery: A century of progress. *Tex Heart Inst J* 2011; *38*: 486–490.
83. Baskett R, Buth K, Ghali W et al. Outcomes in octogenarians undergoing coronary artery bypass grafting. *CMAJ* 2005; *172*: 1183–1186.
84. Conaway DG, House J, Bandt K et al. The elderly: Health status benefits and recovery of function one year after coronary artery bypass surgery. *J Am Coll Cardiol* 2003; *42*: 1421–1426.
85. Stoica SC, Cafferty F, Kitcat J et al. Octogenarians undergoing cardiac surgery outlive their peers: A case for early referral. *Heart* 2006; *92*: 503–506.
86. Scott BH, Seifert FC, Grimson R, Glass PSA. Octogenarians undergoing coronary artery bypass graft surgery: Resource utilization, postoperative mortality, and morbidity. *J Cardiothorac Vasc Anesth* 2005; *19*: 583–588.
87. O'Brien SM, Shahian DM, Filardo G et al. The Society of Thoracic Surgeons 2008 cardiac surgery risk models: Part 2—Isolated valve surgery. *Ann Thorac Surg* 2009; *88*: S23–S42.
88. Ashikhmina EA, Schaff HV, Dearani JA et al. Aortic valve replacement in the elderly: Determinants of late outcome. *Circulation* 2011; *124*: 1070–1078.
89. Nashef SA, Roques F, Sharples LD et al. EuroSCORE II. *Eur J Cardiothorac Surg* 2012; *41*: 734–744.
90. Clark MA, Arnold SV, Duhay FG et al. Five-year clinical and economic outcomes among patients with medically managed severe aortic stenosis: Results from a Medicare claims analysis. *Circ Cardiovasc Qual Outcomes* 2012; *5*: 697–704.

91. Varadarajan P, Kapoor N, Bansal RC et al. Clinical profile and natural history of 453 nonsurgically managed patients with severe aortic stenosis. *Ann Thorac Surg* 2006; *82*: 2111–2115.
92. Cribier A, Eltchaninoff H, Bash A et al. Percutaneous transcatheter implantation of an aortic valve prosthesis for calcific aortic stenosis: First human case description. *Circulation* 2002; *106*: 3006–3008.
93. Leon MB, Smith CR, Mack M et al. Transcatheter aortic-valve implantation for aortic stenosis in patients who cannot undergo surgery. *N Engl J Med* 2010; *363*: 1597–1607.
94. Smith CR, Leon MB, Mack MJ et al. Transcatheter versus surgical aortic-valve replacement in high-risk patients. *N Engl J Med* 2011; *364*: 2187–2198.
95. Klein BE, Klein R, Knudtson MD et al. Frailty, morbidity, and survival. *Arch Gerontol Geriatr* 2005; *41*(2): 141–149.
96. Robinson, TN, Wu DS, Pointer LF et al. Preoperative cognitive dysfunction is related to adverse postoperative outcomes in the elderly. *J Am Coll Surg* 2012; *215*(1): 12–17.
97. Steiner JM, Cooper S, Kirkpatrick JN. Palliative care in end-stage valvular heart disease. *Heart* 2017; *103*: 1233–1237.
98. Auffret V, Campelo-Parada F, Regueiro A et al. Serial changes in cognitive function following transcatheter aortic valve replacement. *J Am Coll Cardiol* 2016; *68*(20): 2129–2141.

Index

For Product Safety Concerns and Information please contact our EU
representative GPSR@taylorandfrancis.com Taylor & Francis Verlag GmbH,
Kaufingerstraße 24, 80331 München, Germany

Printed and bound by CPI Group (UK) Ltd, Croydon, CR0 4YY
14/09/2026
02216253-0001